# Current Rhinology

Samy Elwany
Editor

# Current Rhinology

Springer

*Editor*
Samy Elwany
Department of Otolaryngology
Alexandria Faculty of Medicine
Alexandria, Egypt

ISBN 978-3-031-70076-7 ISBN 978-3-031-70077-4 (eBook)
https://doi.org/10.1007/978-3-031-70077-4



This Springer imprint is published by the registered company Springer Nature Switzerland AG
The registered company address is: Gewerbestrasse 11, 6330 Cham, Switzerland

*I dedicate this book to my small, lovely family: my wife, Maggie, my son Dino, and my daughter Nelly. I am deeply thankful to each of them for giving my life wonderful value and meaning. They are really the love of my life. I would also like to dedicate this book to all my students throughout my long career.*

*Samy Elwany*

# Preface

The field of rhinology has gained much scientific acclaim over the past few decades. A complete understanding of the diseases of the nose, paranasal sinuses, and related areas is best regarded as a work in progress and a field that is constantly developing. Medical technology has continued to rapidly improve, enabling high-quality imaging and visualization of previously obscured structures with exceptional clarity. In parallel with this, our understanding of the basic science of rhinology has greatly improved, facilitating better understanding of treatment strategies and protocols that improved patient outcomes.

The heightened use of the new 2D and 3D endoscopes has led to dramatic expansion in the scale and scope of various endoscopic techniques. Surgical procedures that were once considered challenging and dangerous are now rendered as routine operations. Image guidance has been added to enhance the precision and safety of advanced endoscopic procedures, ultimately leading to improved patient outcomes.

The book presents a comprehensive approach to the current science and practice of rhinology. It covers both the scientific and practical aspects of rhinology and provides clear practical advice on clinical and surgical management in both adults and children. This book included six chapters on basic and advanced rhinoplasty procedures. Therefore, it can be useful to a broad range of readers and practitioners, including ENT trainees, general otolaryngologists, and tertiary care rhinologists.

Several rhinologic conditions require multidisciplinary teams that provide the widest range of proficiency and greatest care to the patients. These conditions include, but not limited to, recalcitrant sinusitis, allergic rhinitis, vasculitis, as well as neoplasia involving the anterior skull base and sino-orbital interface. All of these topics are covered in this book, making it a valuable resource for specialists, such as allergists, immunologists, pulmonologists, oncologists, ophthalmologists, neurosurgeons, and rheumatologists.

The book has been written by an array of rhinology experts from several countries and with diverse subspecialty interests. As a result, this book is a collection of up-to-date global information on the current practice of rhinology.

I am extremely grateful to all the contributing authors who shared their fine expertise and knowledge in this book. Each author has made a state-of-the-art, valuable contribution, requiring countless hours of planning and writing. I extend my sincerest gratitude to each and every one of the authors for their commitment and support.

I hope that readers of this book will drive the utmost benefit from it, gaining a deeper understanding of the complexity of the nose and paranasal sinuses. I also hope that this will inspire an enduring passion for studying and continuing relentless research in this fascinating field. Finally I hope that this book will make a valuable contribution to the art and science of rhinology.

Alexandria, Egypt Samy Elwany

# About this Book

*Current Rhinology* presents a comprehensive approach to the current science and practice of rhinology and includes up-to-date knowledge for a broad range of topics, including applied radiology, olfactory disorders, epistaxis, as well as inflammatory and neoplastic sinonasal disorders. Sinonasal embryology, anatomy, and physiology were discussed wherever appropriate. This book's balance of applied science and clinical practicality makes it an ideal resource for anyone from trainee surgeons to established specialists in rhinology.

The book addresses the orbital and anterior skull base approaches and includes six basic and advanced rhinoplasty chapters. The book expands its scope beyond conventional boundaries by including dedicated chapters on nasal valves, biologics, odontogenic sinusitis, biomaterials in rhinology, and image guidance in endoscopic sinus surgery.

Throughout this book, the reader will find clear, state-of the-art practical advice on the clinical and surgical management of a wide range of rhinology disorders. The balance of applied science and clinical practicality makes this book an ideal resource for a broad range of readers and practitioners, including ENT trainee, general otolaryngologists, and tertiary care rhinologists.

This book has been written by a distinguished array of rhinology experts from various countries, each with diverse subspecialty interests. As a result, this book presents an all-inclusive collection of up-to-date global information on the current practice of rhinology. The controversies within the specialty are covered in a comprehensive and balanced manner.

The information in this book is supported by explanatory pictures, illustrations, and video clips. All chapters included key points to enhance understanding and retention. This book serves as both a book on fundamental aspects of rhinology and a reference guide for the recent advancements in the field.

## Contents

# Editors and Contributors

## About the Editor

**Samy Elwany** is a Professor of Otolaryngology at the Department of Otolaryngology, Alexandria University, Alexandria, Egypt. He earned his PhD degree from Alexandria University and held fellowship at Iowa University and research fellowship at Chicago University.

Dr. Elwany is the current President of the Egyptian Society of Otolaryngology and President of the Alexandria Society of Rhinology (RhinoAlex). He served as the Chairman of the Department of Otolaryngology, Alexandria University from 2007 to 2010. He is a member of the CORLAS (Collegium Oto-Rhino-Laryngologicum Amicitiae Sacrum) and of the American Academy of Otolaryngology.

Dr. Elwany has published several papers in national and international journals. Additionally, he has authored and co-authored four books. His last book *Rhinology Review* was published by Springer. He was the recipient of the Alexandria University and the Egyptian State awards. He serves on the editorial board of the Springer journal, *European Archives of Oto-Rhino-Laryngology and Head and Neck.*

## Contributors

**Khaled Gamal Dahy Ahmed** Department of Otolaryngology, Sohag University, Sohag, Egypt

**Ra'ed Al-Ashqar** Peninsula Medical School, University of Plymouth, Plymouth, UK
University Hospitals Plymouth NHS Trust, Plymouth, UK

**Rayan AlFallaj** Department of Otolaryngology–Head and Neck Surgery, King Saud University, Riyadh, Kingdom of Saudi Arabia

**Abdulmalik Alkhodair** Department of Otolaryngology-Head & Neck Surgery, King Saud Medical City, First Health Cluster, Riyadh, Saudi Arabia

**Abdulaziz AlQahtani** Department of Otolaryngology-Head & Neck Surgery, King Fahad Medical City, Second Health Cluster, Riyadh, Saudi Arabia

Faculty of Medicine, Alfaisal University, Riyadh, Saudi Arabia

**Ahmad Alroqi** Department of Otolaryngology-Head and Neck Surgery, College of Medicine, King Saud University, Riyadh, Saudi Arabia

**Saad Alsaleh** Department of Otolaryngology–Head and Neck Surgery, King Saud University, Riyadh, Kingdom of Saudi Arabia

**Sundus A. Alsedra** Al Yarmouk Teaching Hospital, Baghdad, Iraq

**Ahmed M. Arman, M.D** Department of Otolaryngology, Mansoura University, Mansoura, Egypt

**Nicolas Baldini, MD** University of Bordeaux College of Health Sciences, Bordeaux, France

Anatomy Laboratory, University of Bordeaux College of Health Sciences, Bordeaux, France

**Hussam Elbosraty** Department of Otolaryngology, Cairo University, Cairo, Egypt

**Paolo Castelnuovo** Division of Otorhinolaryngology, Department of Surgical Specialties, ASST Sette Laghi, Ospedale di Circolo, University of Insubria, Varese, Italy

Department of Otorhinolaryngology and Skull Base Surgery, University of Insubria, Varese, Italy

**Giuseppe Cottone** Milan, Italy

**Gianluca Dalfino** Division of Otorhinolaryngology, Department of Surgical Specialties, ASST Sette Laghi, Ospedale di Circolo, University of Insubria, Varese, Italy

**Kamal Ebeid** Otorhinolaryngology Department, Tanta University, Tanta, Egypt

**Mohamed El-Banhawy** Department of Otolaryngology, Delta University, Cairo, Egypt

**Omar El-Banhawy** Department of Otolaryngology, Menofyia University, Sheben El-Kom, Egypt

**Alaa Eldin Elfeky** Faculty of Medicine, Zagazig University, Zagazig, Egypt

**Noha Ahmed El-Kholy** Department of Otolaryngology, Mansoura University, Mansoura, Egypt

**Nelly Elwany** College of Dentistry, University of Kentucky, Lexington, KY, USA

**Samy Elwany** Department of Otolaryngology, Alexandria Faculty of Medicine, Alexandria, Egypt

Department of Otolaryngology, Alexandria University, Alexandria, Egypt

**Miguel Gonçalves Ferreira** Centro Hospitalar Universitário do Porto, Instituto Ciências Biomédicas Abel Salazar, Porto University, Porto, Portugal

Hospital Luz Arrábida, Vila Nova de Gaia, Portugal

Clínica Nariz e Face, Porto, Portugal

**Palmyra J. Geissler, MD** Rio de Janeiro, Brazil

Plastic Surgery Department, The University of Texas Southwestern Medical Center, Dallas, TX, USA

**Amr Gouda** Department of Otolaryngology, Ain Shams University, Cairo, Egypt

**Giacomo Gravante** Division of Otorhinolaryngology, Department of Surgical Specialties, ASST Sette Laghi, Ospedale di Circolo, University of Insubria, Varese, Italy

Department of Otorhinolaryngology and Skull Base Surgery, University of Insubria, Varese, Italy

**Nadine El Hadi** Department of Otolaryngology Head and Neck Surgery, American University of Beirut, Beirut, Lebanon

**Usamah El Hadi** Department of Otolaryngology Head and Neck Surgery, American University of Beirut, Beirut, Lebanon

**Hossam Abdel Hai** Department of Otolaryngology, Benha University, Banha, Egypt

**Mohamed Zaki Helal** Department of Otolaryngology, Aon Shams University, Cairo, Egypt

**Wael Khamis Hussien, MD, PhD** Department of Otolaryngology, Alexandria University, Alexandria, Egypt

**Ahmed A. Ibrahim** Alexandria University, Alexandria, Egypt

**Shimaa Ibrahim** ORL Department, Assiut University, Asyut, Egypt

**Mostafa Ismail** Otolaryngology Department, Minia University, Minia, Egypt

**Febin James** IQRAA Hospital, Elittil Hospital, Calicut, India

**Yazan Kanaan** University Hospitals Plymouth NHS Trust, Plymouth, UK

**Apostolos Karligkiotis** Division of Otorhinolaryngology, Department of Surgical Specialties, ASST Sette Laghi, Ospedale di Circolo, University of Insubria, Varese, Italy

**Ahmed Y. Khafagy, M.D** Faculty of Medicine, Mansoura University, Mansoura, Egypt

**Yasser W. Khafagy, M.D, PhD** Department of Otolaryngology, Mansoura University, Mansoura, Egypt

**Hisham Khalil** University Hospitals Plymouth NHS Trust, Plymouth, UK

Peninsula Medical School, University of Plymouth, Plymouth, UK

**Ali Abd Alameer Khazaal** Baghdad, Iraq

**Amr Kholief** Department of Otolaryngology, Alexandria University, Alexandria, Egypt

**Zeina Kurban** Department of Otolaryngology Head and Neck Surgery, American University of Beirut, Beirut, Lebanon

Louis Luke ENT Department, University Hospitals, Northamptonshire NHS Trust, Cliftonville, Northampton, UK

**Nasser Marran** Department of Otolaryngology Head and Neck Surgery, King Faisal Specialist Hospital and Research Center, Riyadh, Saudi Arabia

**Mostafa Mehana** University Hospitals Plymouth NHS Trust, Plymouth, UK

Ajit Mishra HCG Hospital, Borivali/Coloba, Mumbai, UK

**Ibrahim Rezk Mohamed** Department of Otolaryngology, Sohag University, Sohag, Egypt

**Haitham Morsi** Alexandria University Hospital/Canadian Hospital, Dubai, UAE

**Samiul Muquit** Department of Neurosurgery, Southwest Neurosurgery Centre, University Hospitals Plymouth NHS Trust, Plymouth, UK

Peninsula Medical School, University of Plymouth, Plymouth, UK

**Paresh Pramod Naik** University of Northamptonshire, Cliftonville, UK

**Veerasigamani Narendrakumar** Pragathi ENT & Endocrine Clinic, Chennai, India

**Usama Abdel Naseer** Department of Otolaryngology, Cairo University, Cairo, Egypt

**Yasser Nour** Department of Otolaryngology, Alexandria University, Alexandria, Egypt

**Enrico Robotti** Bergamo, Italy

**Matthew W. Ryan** Department of Otolaryngology, UT Southwestern Medical Center, Dallas, TX, USA

**Magdy Eisa Saafan** Department of Otolaryngology, Tanta University, Tanta, Egypt

**Mariline Santos** Centro Hospitalar Universitário do Porto, Instituto Ciências Biomédicas Abel Salazar, Porto University, Porto, Portugal

**Muhammad Shahzad** Department of Neurosurgery, Southwest Neurosurgery Centre, University Hospitals Plymouth NHS Trust, Plymouth, UK

**Ahmed G. Sholkamy** ORL Department, Assiut University, Asyut, Egypt

**Aarthi Sundararajan** Chennai, India

**Andrew C. Swift** Liverpool Head and Neck Centre, Liverpool University Hospitals NHS Foundation Trust, Liverpool, UK

**Mohamed K. Taha** Alexandria University Hospital, Alexandria, Egypt

**Mohamed Shehata Taha** Consultant ORL-HNS, Faculty of Medicine, Ain Shams University Hospitals, Ain Shams University, Cairo, Egypt

**Mohamed Ossama Tomoum** Department of Otolaryngology, Tanta University, Tanta, Egypt

**Ahmed Thabet** Department of Otolaryngology, Alexandria University, Alexandria, Egypt

**Mario Turri-Zanoni** Department of Otorhinolaryngology and Skull Base Surgery, University of Insubria, Varese, Italy

**Mustafa Wagdy** Alexandria University Hospital, Alexandria, Egypt

**Stephen P. Williams** Liverpool Head and Neck Centre, Liverpool University Hospitals NHS Foundation Trust, Liverpool, UK

# Applied Radiology of the Nose and Sinuses

1

Mohamed Zaki Helal

**Key Points**

- This chapter aims to refine imaging diagnosis and to emphasize the anatomical basis for surgery. Prior knowledge of basic anatomy is mandatory.
- Personal computer (PC) offers post-study manipulations of the thin series (0.5–1 mm dicom files) in the CD generated by the CT or MR machines. These modern post-processing techniques include Multiplanar Reconstruction (MPR), 3D Rendering (MIP, Volume Rendering and Surface Rendering) and Virtual Endoscopy. This is achieved with PC software like *OsiriX*™ and *Horos*™ on MAC computers. In the present time, IBM system does not yet have comparable advanced software [1].
- **3D MPR** images are used for proper understanding of anatomy, especially in dangerous areas and highlight the imaging anatomical basis for surgical procedures. MPR correlates coronal, axial, and sagittal planes together with the intersection of the two axes at the same point in the three planes.
- **3D Surface Rendering** is a 3D representation of different layers like skin and bones. It offers better delineation of deformities and fractures.
- **3D Volume Rendering** is a type of data visualization technique which creates a three-dimensional representation of data. It can delineate airways in nose and tracheobronchial tree.
- **Virtual Endoscopy** is PC software production of hundreds of cross-sectional images of the airway giving endoscopic-like view of intraluminal masses.

---

**Supplementary Information** The online version contains supplementary material available at https://doi.org/10.1007/978-3-031-70077-4_1.

M. Z. Helal (✉)
Department of Otorhinolaryngology, Ain Shams University, Cairo, Egypt
e-mail: mohamedzaki@med.asu.edu.eg


S. Elwany (ed.), *Current Rhinology*,
https://doi.org/10.1007/978-3-031-70077-4_1

## 1.1 Maxillary Ostium, Uncinate Process, Infundibulum, and Nasolacrimal Duct Relations (Fig. 1.1)

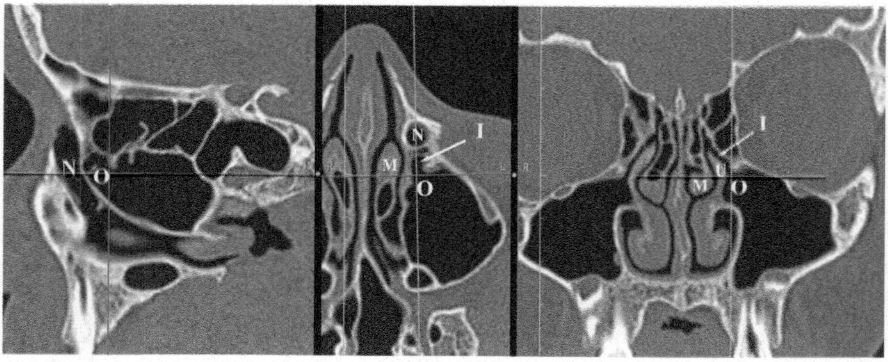


**Fig. 1.1** CT MPR with the intersection of X and Y points at the maxillary ostium (O). Note the position of the ostium is high and anterior in the medial wall of the sinus. The ostium is intimately related to the infromedial orbital wall and just posterior to the nasolacrimal duct (N). The ostium opens into the ethmoidal infundibulum (I)

## 1.2 Maxillary Ostium, Haller Cells [2], and Prelacrimal Recess (Fig. 1.2)

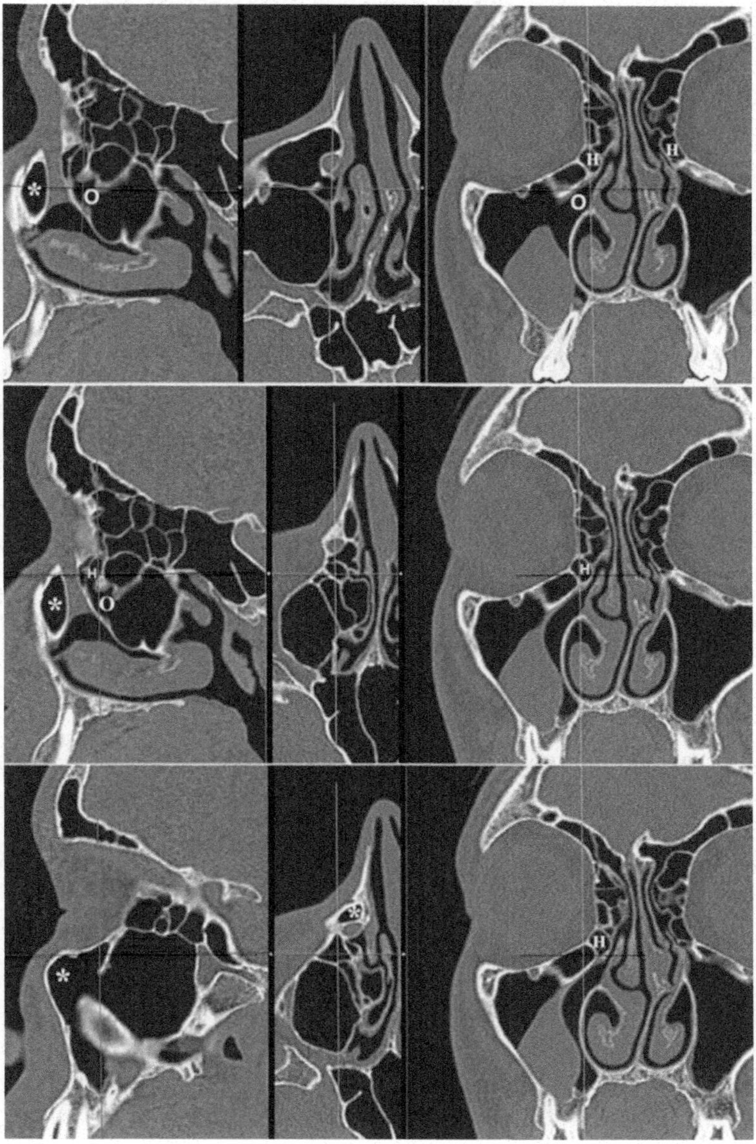


**Fig. 1.2** **CT MPR**: *In upper row*, the intersection of X and Y points at the maxillary ostium (O) while Haller cells (H) are extramural ethmoidal cells pneumatizing the inferomedial orbital wall narrowing the ostium. The asterisk (*) points to the prelacrimal recess of the anteromedial part of the antrum which is usually difficult to be mandibulated through middle meatal antrostomy. *In middle row*, the intersection of X and Y points at Haller cell (H) and its relation to maxillary ostium. *In lower row*, the intersections point at incomplete pneumatization of the inferior orbital wall lateral to Haller cell (H). Note the prelacrimal recess (*)

## 1.3 Uncinate Process and its Relation to Agger Nasi Cell and Frontal Sinus (Figs. 1.3 and 1.4)

The uncinate process has an anterior attachment to the ethmoidal crest of the ascending process of maxilla and posterior border of the lacrimal bone. Agger nasi cell [4] is the extramural ethmoidal pneumatization of these structures, therefore, the uncinate process forms most of its medial, superior, and posterior walls. The superior

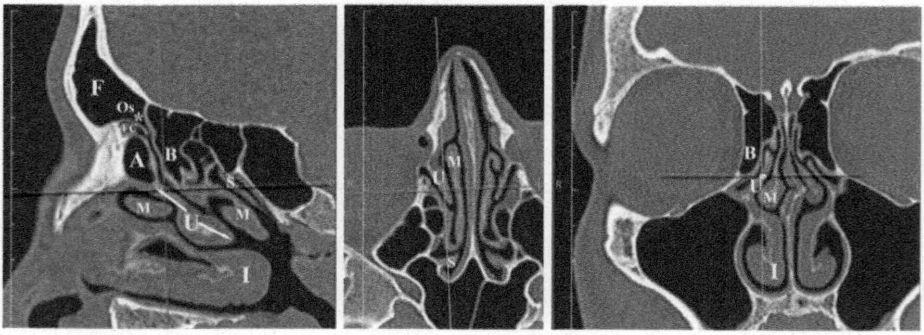


**Fig. 1.3** CT MPR with the intersection of X and Y points at the uncinate process (U). The white arrows show the uncinate in the sagittal plane, and the upper arrow points to the uncinate reaching the agger nasi cell (A). The frontal sinus (F) outlets into the superior end of the frontal recess (*) at the frontal ostium (Os). The ethmoidal bulla (B) reaches superiorly the skull base, and its anterior wall forms the posterior wall of the frontal recess. A small supra-agger cell (FC) [3] is seen anterior to the frontal ostium. Note the middle turbinate (M), inferior turbinate (I), and superior turbinate (S)

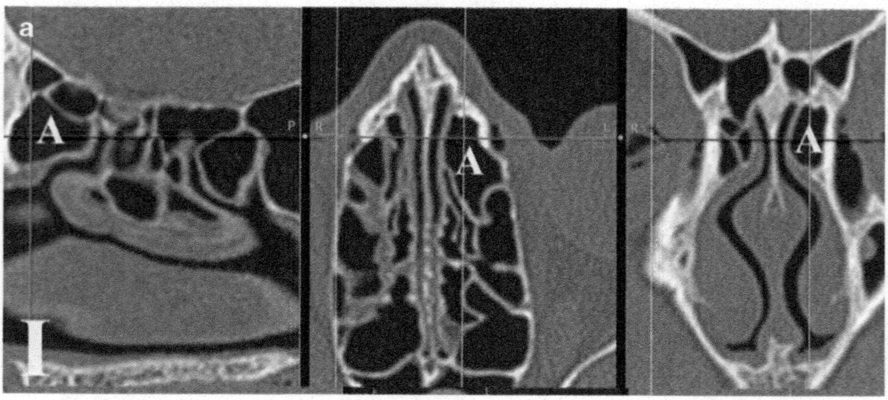


**Fig. 1.4** (**a**) *In row I*, the intersection of X and Y points at a left agger nasi cell (A) projected in coronal, axial, and sagittal planes. (**b**) *In row II*, the intersection of points at the uncinate process (U) in different planes and reaching the agger nasi cell (A) as shown in sagittal plane. *In row III*, the intersection of points at the uncinate process (U) reaching the posterior wall of the agger nasi cell (A) in sagittal and axial planes. *In row IV*, the intersection of points at a supra-agger frontal cell (FC) and the uncinate process reaching its posterior wall. *In row V*, the intersection of points at the frontal sinus (F) lateral to the supra-agger frontal cell (*)

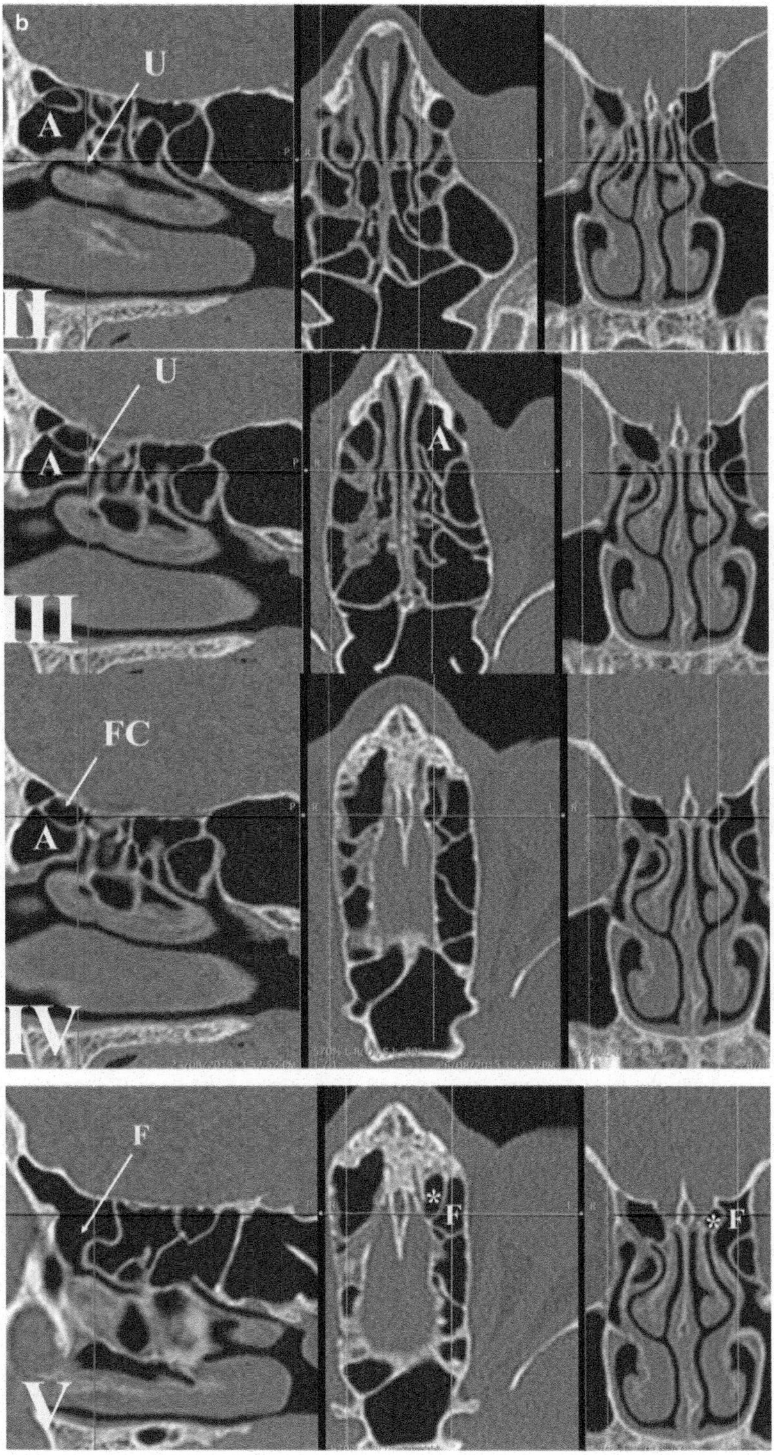


**Fig. 1.4** (continued)

insertion of the uncinate process will determine the outlet of the frontal sinus. In about 70% of individuals, it is attached to the medial wall of the orbit through the agger nasi cell, and subsequently, the frontal sinus drains into the middle meatus. In about 30% of individuals, it is attached to the fovea ethmoidalis or the middle turbinate insertion in a cribriform plate, and the frontal sinus drains into the ethmoidal infundibulum. This is the rational for *reaching the frontal sinus ostium during frontal sinusotomy through following the uncinate process superiorly.*

## 1.4 Frontal Sinus Ostium and Frontal Recess (Figs. 1.5 and 1.6)

The frontal sinus drains in an hourglass segment. The middle narrow part is considered as the frontal sinus ostium and the lower dilated segment is the frontal recess.

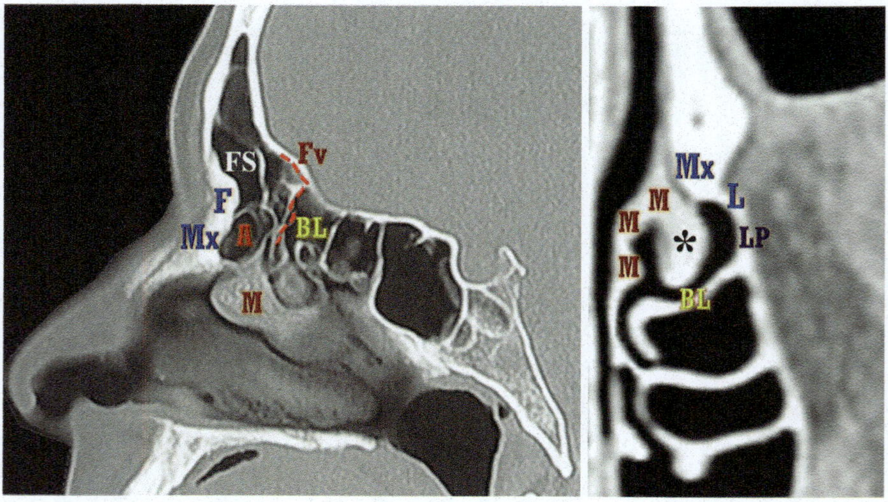


**Fig. 1.5** Frontal recess contents and walls. The frontal recess is six-walled cube with the upper wall tapered into the frontal ostium anteriorly and the first ethmoidal fovea (Fv) posteriorly. The lower end drains into the middle meatus. The anterior wall is the ascending process of maxilla (Mx) with its frontal beak (F) superiorly and the small lacrimal bone (L) medially. The medial wall is the lamina papyracea (LP). The posterior wall is the bullar lamella (BL) which is a thin structure connecting the ethmoid bulla anterior wall to the skull base. If the ethmoid bulla reaches the skull base, the upper part of its anterior wall will replace the bullar lamella. The frontal recess contains the agger nasi cell (A) and different frontal recess cells in addition to the uncinate process (*) in walls of the agger nasi cell

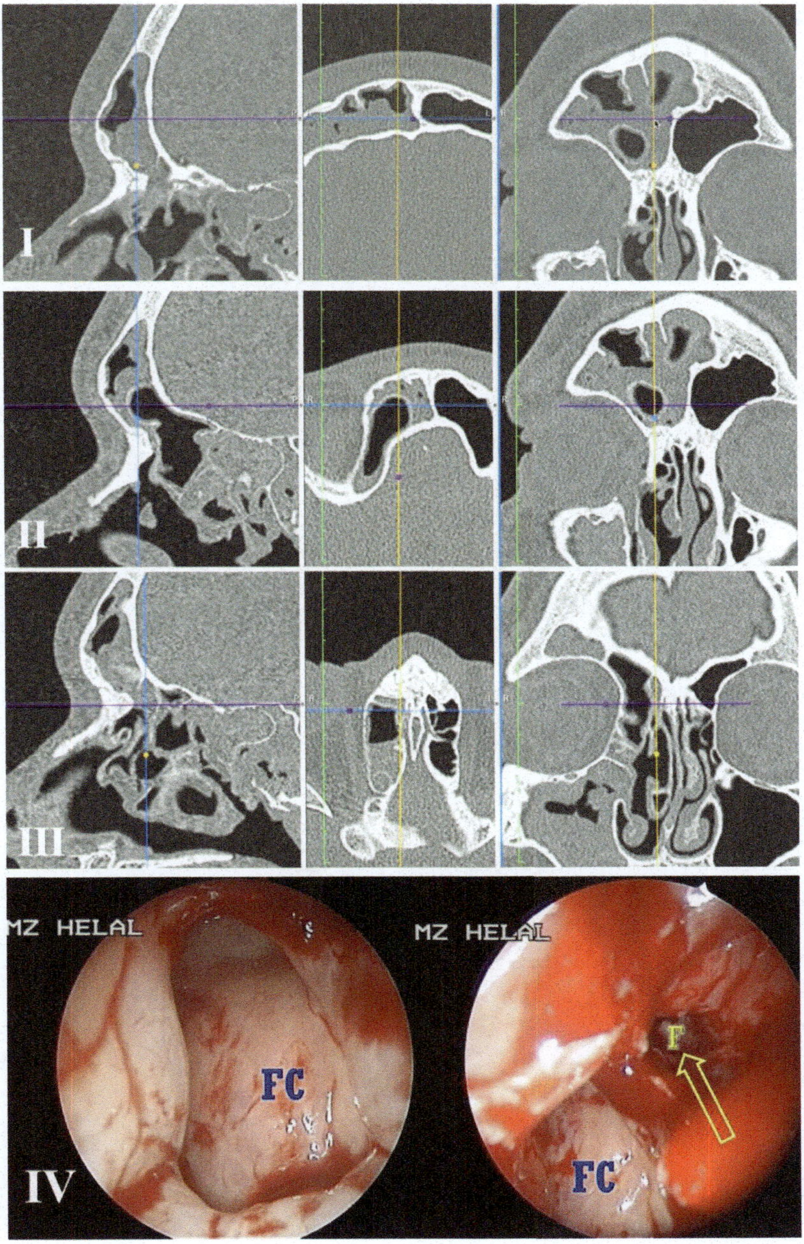


**Fig. 1.6** CT MPR of recurrent chronic rhinosinusitis (CRS). *In row I*, the intersection of X and Y points at the opaque frontal sinus. *In row II*, the intersections point at a huge suprabullar frontal cell intimately related to the posterior wall of the frontal sinus and having its same bulge pattern. *In row III*, the intersections point at frontal sinus ostium. *In row IV*, Operative snapshoot showing the huge suprabullar frontal cell (FC) intimately related to the posterior wall of the frontal sinus mimicking the endoscopic view of the frontal sinus having its same bulge pattern of its posterior wall. According to the forementioned MPR data, the real frontal sinus (F) was opened superomedial to FC (arrow)

## 1.5 Anterior Ethmoidal Artery (AEA) (Figs. 1.7, 1.8, 1.9, 1.10, 1.11, 1.12 and 1.13)

The ethmoidal artery emerges from lamina papyracea traversing the suprabullar ethmoid cell (SBC) to enter the cranial cavity at the thinnest point in skull base at the cribriform plate lateral lamella. The SBC anterior wall is known as bullar lamella and

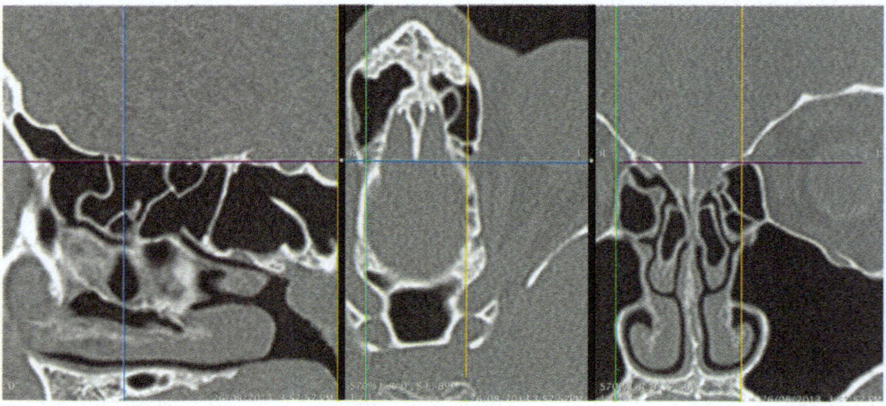

**Fig. 1.7** CT MPR: the intersections point at the AEA in coronal, axial, and sagittal planes. In the absence of frontal supraorbital pneumatization or supraorbital ethmoidal cell (SOC) the artery passes in the bony roof of the ethmoid or fovea ethmoidalis

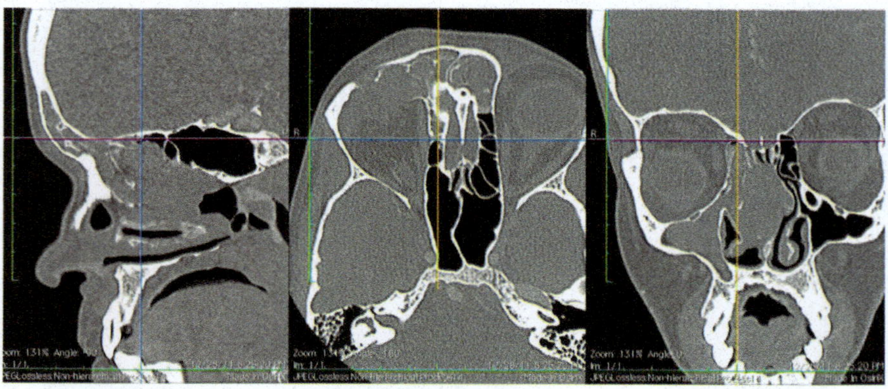

**Fig. 1.8** CT MPR: the intersections point at the AEA in coronal, axial, and sagittal planes. The AEA passes in fovea ethmoidalis above and behind a recurrent frontal lesion extending to the nasal cavity and obstructing the right maxillary outflow, which proved to be a mucocele. Preoperative visualization of the AEA avoided injury during surgery, and the sagittal plane projection was the most beneficial plane for the surgeon

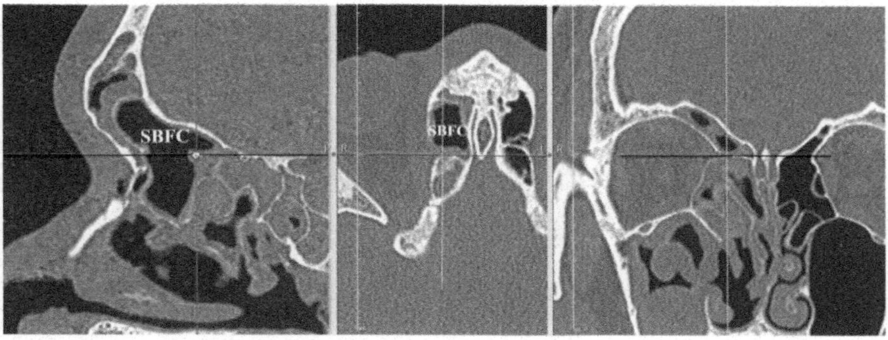


**Fig. 1.9** **CT MPR**: the intersections point at the AEA in coronal, axial, and sagittal planes. In presence of frontal supraorbital pneumatization and suprabullar frontal cell (SBFC) the artery passes in mesentery below the bony roof of the ethmoid or fovea ethmoidalis exposing it to possible injury during surgery. It passes in the floor of the supraorbital pneumatization, whether frontal or ethmoidal in origin, away from the elevated fovea. The skull base type here is type III according to Keros classification of skull base

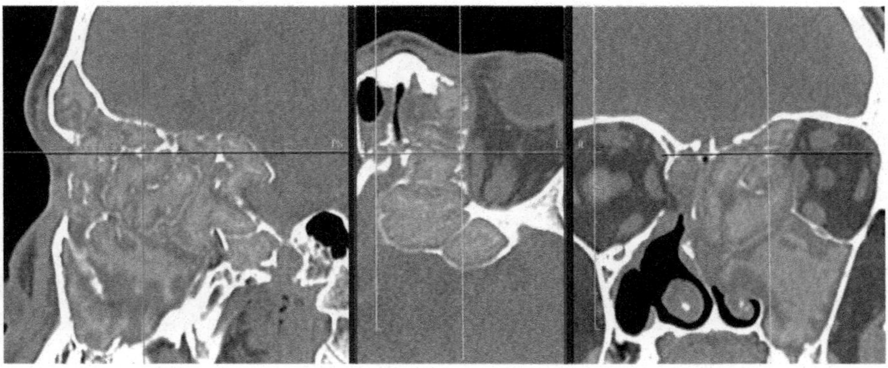

**Fig. 1.10** **CT MPR**: the intersections point at the AEA in coronal, axial, and sagittal planes in recurrent non-invasive fungal sinusitis with supraorbital pneumatization. To locate the AEA in huge recurrent non-invasive fungal sinusitis with its ground glass density is challenging. The artery here is running in mesentery inside the lesion and liable to surgical insult. Video 1.1. shows how the artery is searched for in a dynamic way where one moves the intersection point in one plane and the same point is simultaneously updated in the other two planes

separate the anterior ethmoidal artery from the frontal recess. If the ethmoidal bulla reaches the skull base, there will be no SBC and the artery will be inside the bulla itself, running in its superior wall or fovea. In the presence of a supraorbital ethmoidal cell (SOC); an extramural ethmoidal cell pneumatizing the fovea; the artery leaves the orbit at the floor of the SOC and runs in mesentery away from the fovea in SBC or ethmoidal bulla when reaching the skull base. Because of the presence of supraorbital pneumatization, the skull base type, according to Keros [5] will be type III.

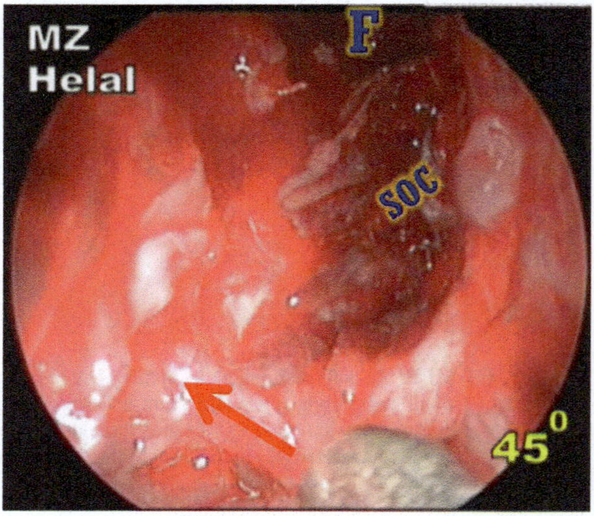


**Fig. 1.11** Operative snapshoot of the previous patient showing the left frontal sinus (F), SOC, and AEA (red arrow). Using the forementioned data, the artery was successfully identified and secured during surgery

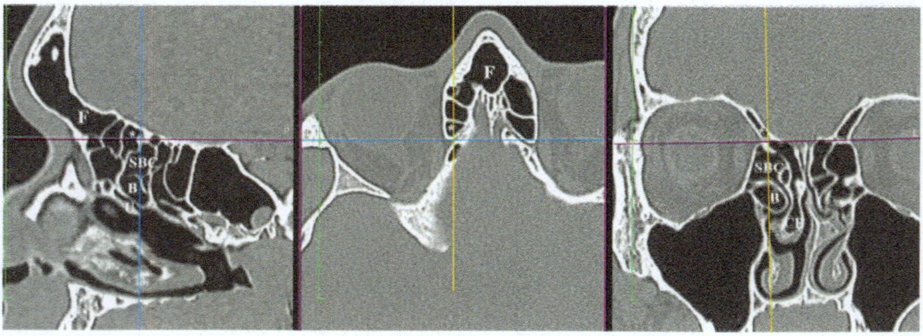


**Fig. 1.12** **CT MPR**: the intersections point at the AEA in coronal, axial, and sagittal planes. Usually, the AEA is located in suprabullar cell (SBC) or suprabullar space known as sinus lateralis (SL) which is the superior extension of the retrobullar space if present. Note the ethmoidal bulla (B), frontal sinus (F), uncinate process (U), supraorbital pneumatization (*) & middle turbinate anterior end pneumatization (concha bullosa, CB)

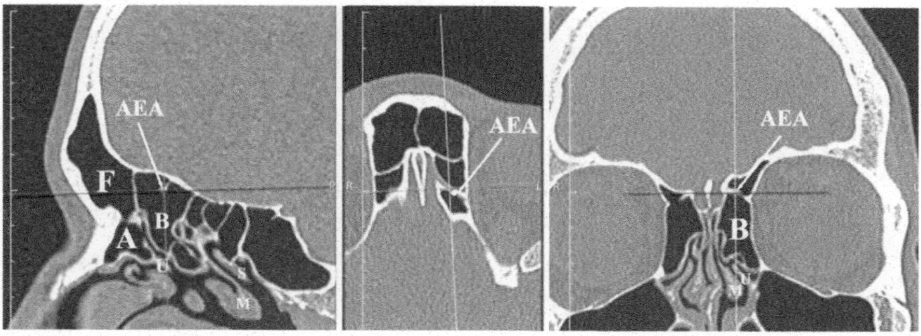


**Fig. 1.13** **CT MPR**: the intersections point at the AEA in coronal, axial, and sagittal planes. If the ethmoidal bulla reaches the skull base, there will be no suprabullar cell or space and subsequently the AEA will be inside the ethmoidal bulla. Note the ethmoidal bulla (B), frontal sinus (F), uncinate process (U), agger nasi cell (A), middle turbinate (M) & superior Turbinate (S)

## 1.6 Nasal Turbinates (Fig. 1.14)

The middle turbinate is turbinate of the anterior ethmoid sinus and its basal lamella (BL) is the partition between the anterior ethmoid sinus and the posterior ethmoid sinus. The superior turbinate is the turbinate of the posterior ethmoid sinus and it usually hides the sphenoid ostium.

Note the ethmoidal bulla (B), frontal sinus (F), uncinate process (U), agger nasi cell (A), middle turbinate (M), inferior turbinate (I), posterior ethmoid sinus (PE), sella turcica (SL), and AEA (arrow head).

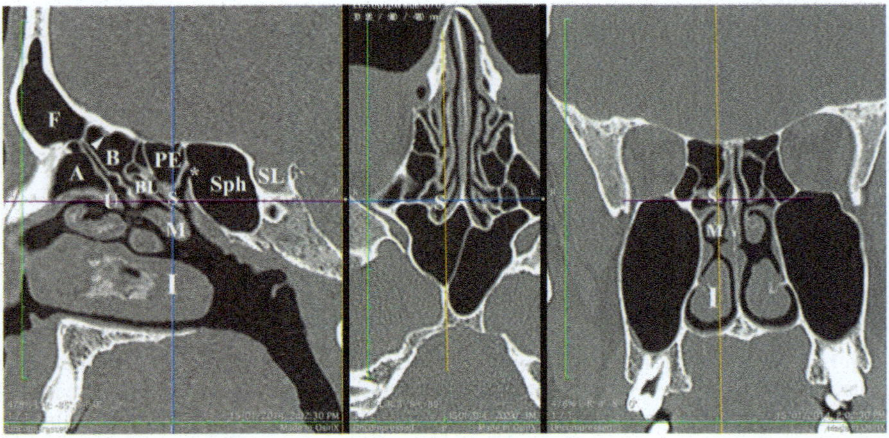


**Fig. 1.14** CT MPR: the intersections point at the superior turbinate (S) in coronal, axial, and sagittal planes. The basal lamella of middle turbinate (BL) is usually not a clean line but with much irregularity because of irregular pneumatization from both ethmoid sinuses. The sphenoid ostium (*) is usually hidden behind the superior turbinate (S) and its basal lamella (posterior wall of the posterior ethmoid sinus)

## 1.7 The Sphenoid Ostium (Fig. 1.15)

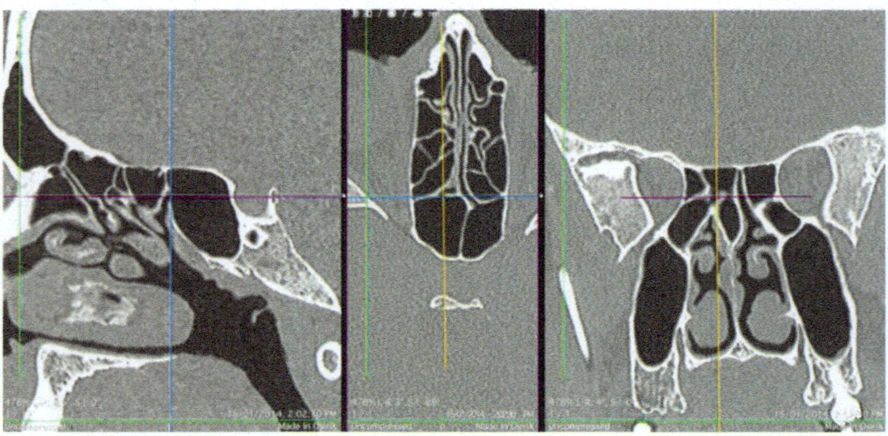

**Fig. 1.15** CT MPR: the intersections point at the sphenoid ostium in coronal, axial, and sagittal planes. It is located high in the anterior wall about 1 cm below the skull base

## 1.8 The Ethmosphenoid Junction (Figs. 1.16, 1.17 and 1.18)

Onodi cell [6] is an extramural ethmoidal cell pneumatizing the sphenoid bone. It is best delineated in CT MPR images.

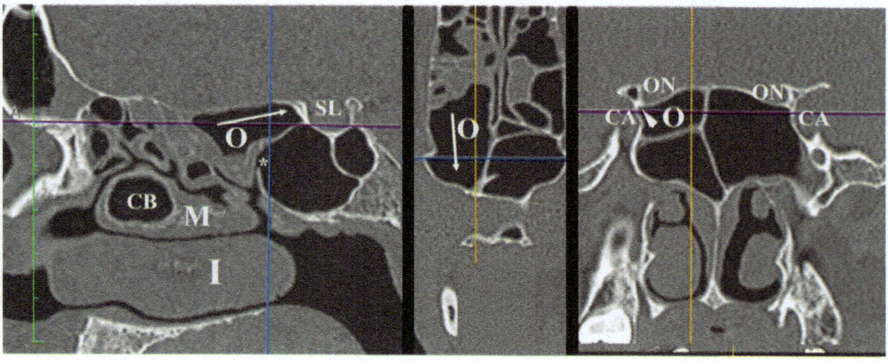


**Fig. 1.16** CT MPR: the intersections point at right Onodi cell (O) in coronal, axial, and sagittal planes. The cell starts in the posterior ethmoid and extends to the superior compartment of the sphenoid bone with the optic nerve (ON) in its upper lateral wall, the carotid artery (CA) in lower lateral wall and the opticocarotid recess (OCR) in between (arrowhead). Part of the sella turcica (SL) is also included in its posterior wall. The middle turbinate (M) has a concha bullosa (CB). The inferior turbinate (I) is hypertrophic with opacification in frontal and ethmoid sinuses

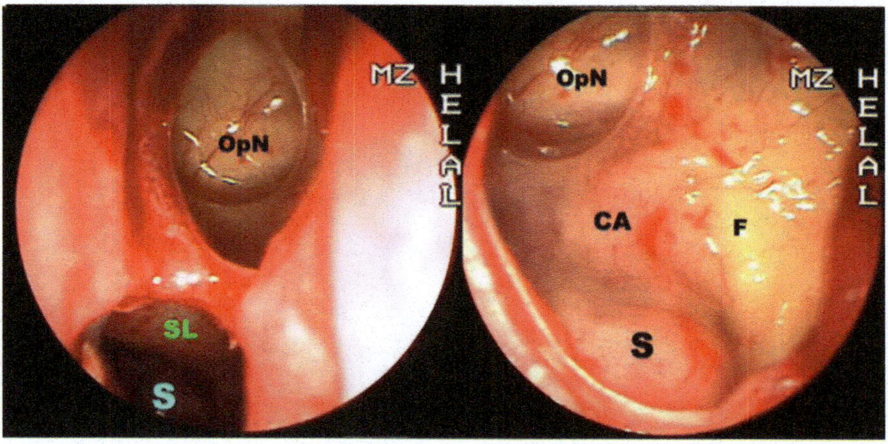


**Fig. 1.17** Operative snapshoots showing left Onodi cell with the optic nerve (OpN), carotid artery (CA), sphenoid sinus (S), sella turcica (SL), and the orbital apex with its shining fat (F). Note the relation of the sphenoid sinus to the posterior ethmoid (here to Onodi cell) is not posterior or posteromedial but strictly inferior

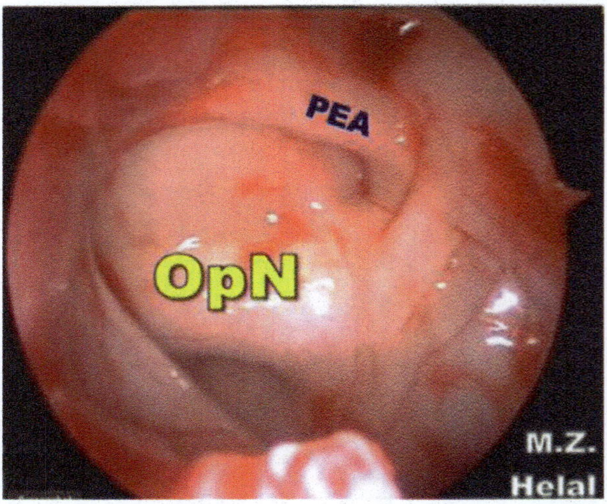


**Fig. 1.18** Operative snapshoot showing left Onodi cell with the optic nerve (OpN) and the posterior ethmoidal artery (PEA). The distance between them is about 6 mm. Onodi cell might be associated with a supreme turbinate; a small turbinate posterior to the superior turbinate

## 1.9 Complexity of Ethmoid Bone Pneumatization (Fig. 1.19)

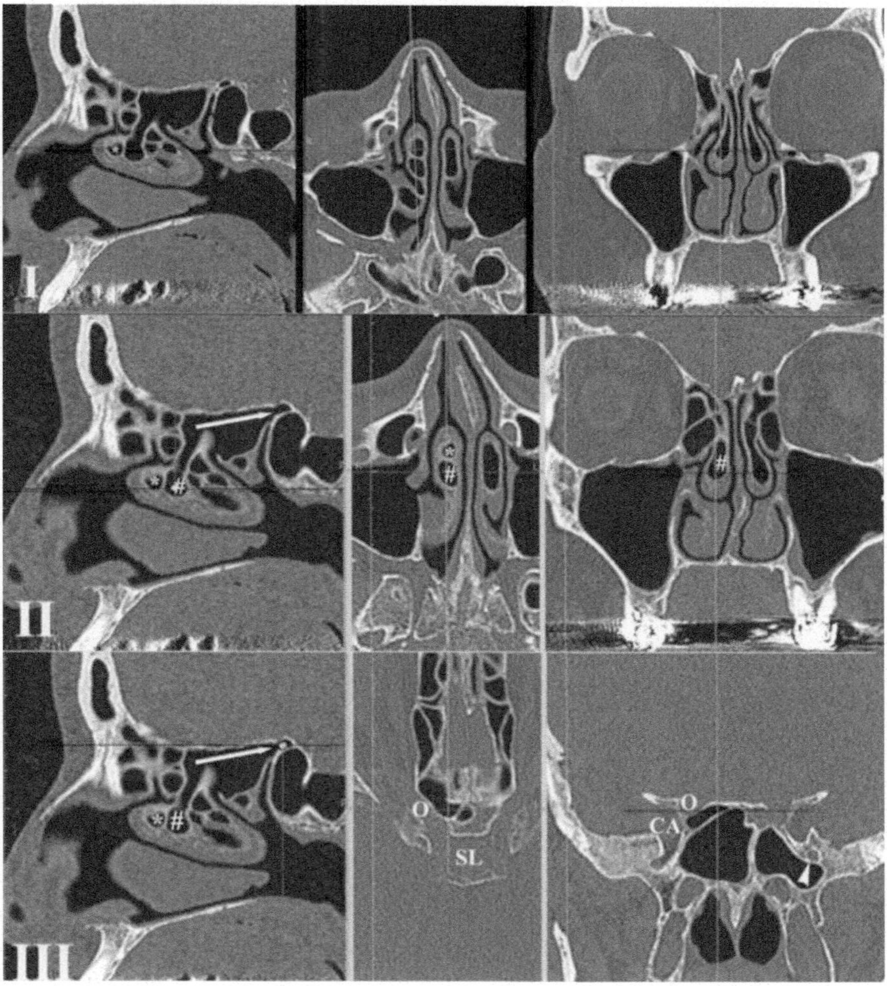


**Fig. 1.19** **CT MPR**: Middle turbinate anterior end pneumatization (concha bullosa; CB) is commonly from anterior ethmoid like here the left CB. The right one has dual pneumatization; the anterior one (*) from anterior ethmoid and the posterior one (#) from posterior ethmoid which is continued posteriorly as Onodi cell (arrow). *In row I*, the intersection points at right CB anterior cell (*). *In row II*, the intersection points at the CB posterior cell (#) with the arrow in Onodi cell. *In row III*, the intersection points at Onodi cell. Note the optic nerve (O), carotid artery (CA), foreman rotundum (arrow head), and sella turcica (SL)

## 1.10 The Maxillary Sinus and the Teeth (Fig. 1.20)

CT MPR discloses dental problems causing odontogenic maxillary sinusitis.

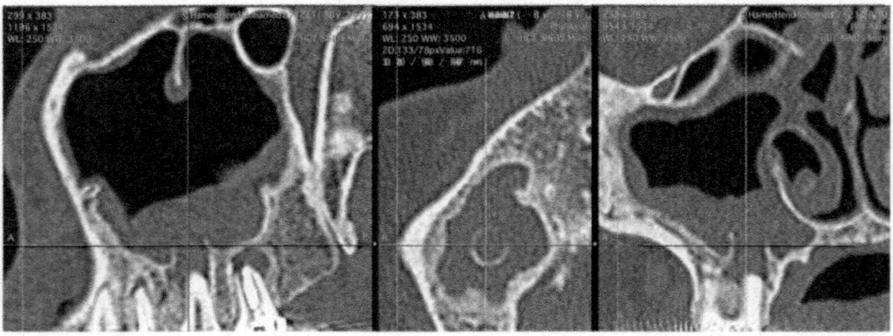

**Fig. 1.20** **CT MPR**: The intersections point at dental periapical cavity with disruption of the compact bone layer of the maxillary floor. Other teeth show periapical smaller cavities

## 1.11 CT MPR Offers Safety of Surgical Procedures (Fig. 1.21)

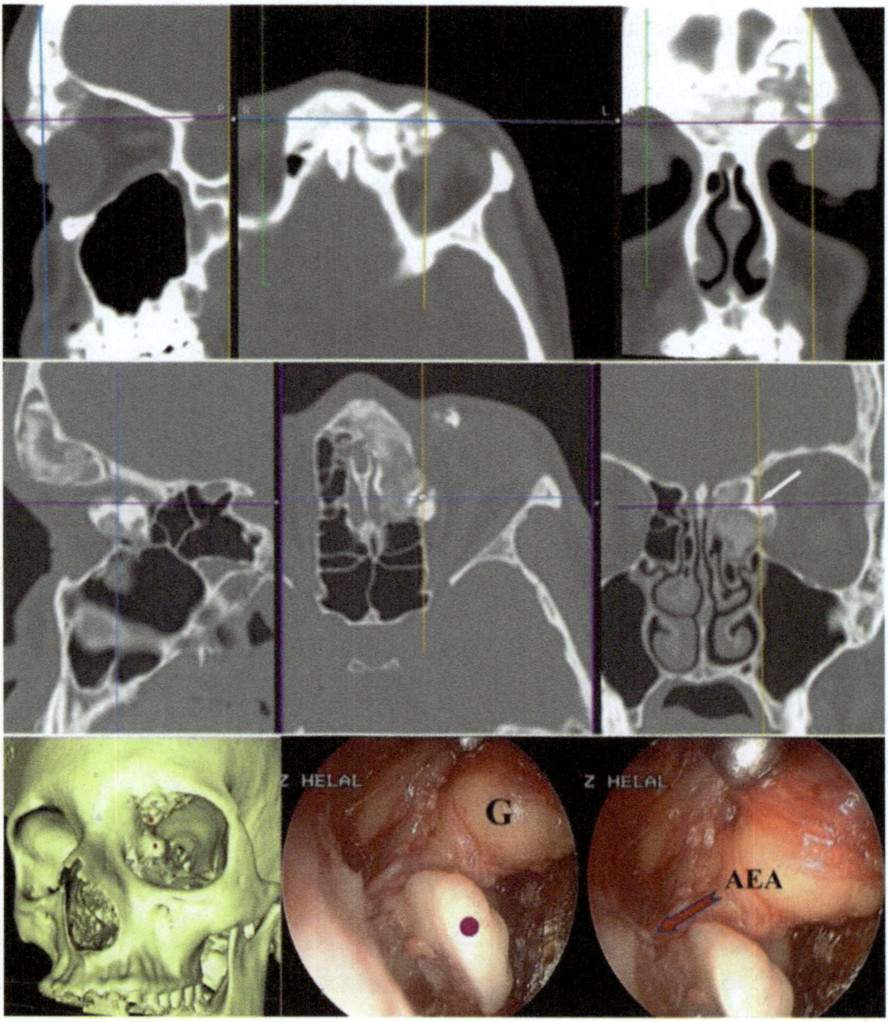


**Fig. 1.21** CT MPR of Frontoethmoid osteofibrosis with it mixed bony and soft tissue densities. The patient suffered from left eye pain due to bone overgrowths. *In upper row,* the overgrowth projecting downward from left frontal bone. *In middle row,* the overgrowth projects medially from the left ethmoid at the site of the AEA (arrow). The intersections point to AEA. *In lower row,* left is surface rendering showing the two projections (red *). Right and middle show operative snapshots with the lesion in medial orbital wall partially drilled (pink dot), the globe (G) retracted laterally with AEA (red arrow) secured based on the forementioned data

## 1.12 CT MPR Offers Safety in Revision Surgical Procedures (Figs. 1.22, 1.23, 1.24 and 1.25)

Revision endoscopic sinonasal surgery in absence of anatomical landmarks carries major risks for the orbit, cranial cavity, and neurovascular structures. Absence of the middle turbinate is an example that may call for navigation surgery (image-guided surgery, IGS) especially if MPR in OsiriX is insufficient to ensure safety without IGS. The following patient underwent multiple prior surgeries for non-invasive fungal rhinosinusitis, the middle turbinates were previously amputated. She developed bilateral fungal mucoceles in frontal lateral recesses and supraorbital pneumatization with wide dehiscence of orbital roof and marked proptosis and hypoglobia.

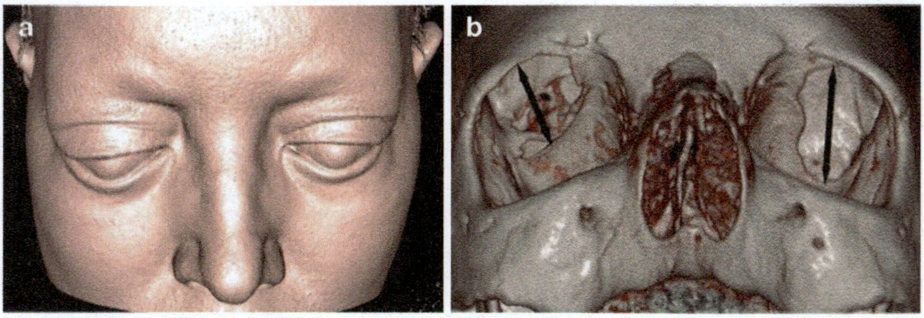


**Fig. 1.22** (**a**) Surface rendering showing bilateral proptosis and hypoglobia. (**b**) Volume rendering showing the large bone defects in orbital roofs (black arrows)

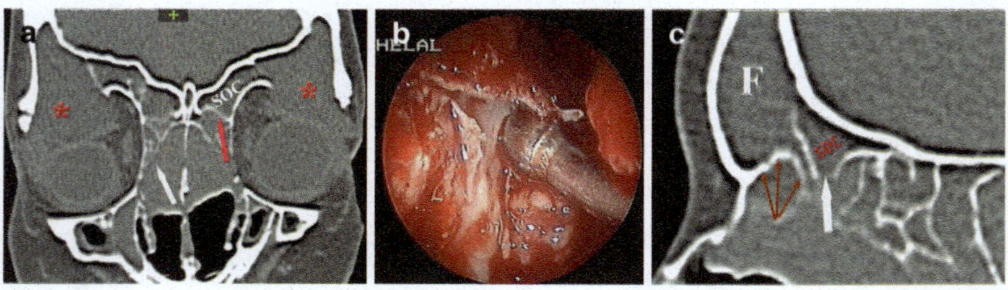


**Fig. 1.23** CT MPR data on the right side offers the middle turbinate axilla as a route to the right frontal sinus and left lamina papyracea and supraorbital cell (SOC) as a route for the left frontal sinus. The patient underwent successful surgery without navigation. In **a**, red asterisks (*) are huge mucoceles with big defects in orbital roof causing downward displacement of eye globes more on the right side. White arrow points to the expected middle turbinate axilla on the right side while the red arrow points to the pass along the left lamina papyracea to supraorbital cell (SOC). In **b**, operative snapshot showing the right axilla elevated by the suction tip and used as a safe route to right frontal sinus. In **c**, the white arrow points to the left supraorbital cell (SOC) and red arrows point to the cap in front to SOC which was removed to reach the left frontal sinus (F)

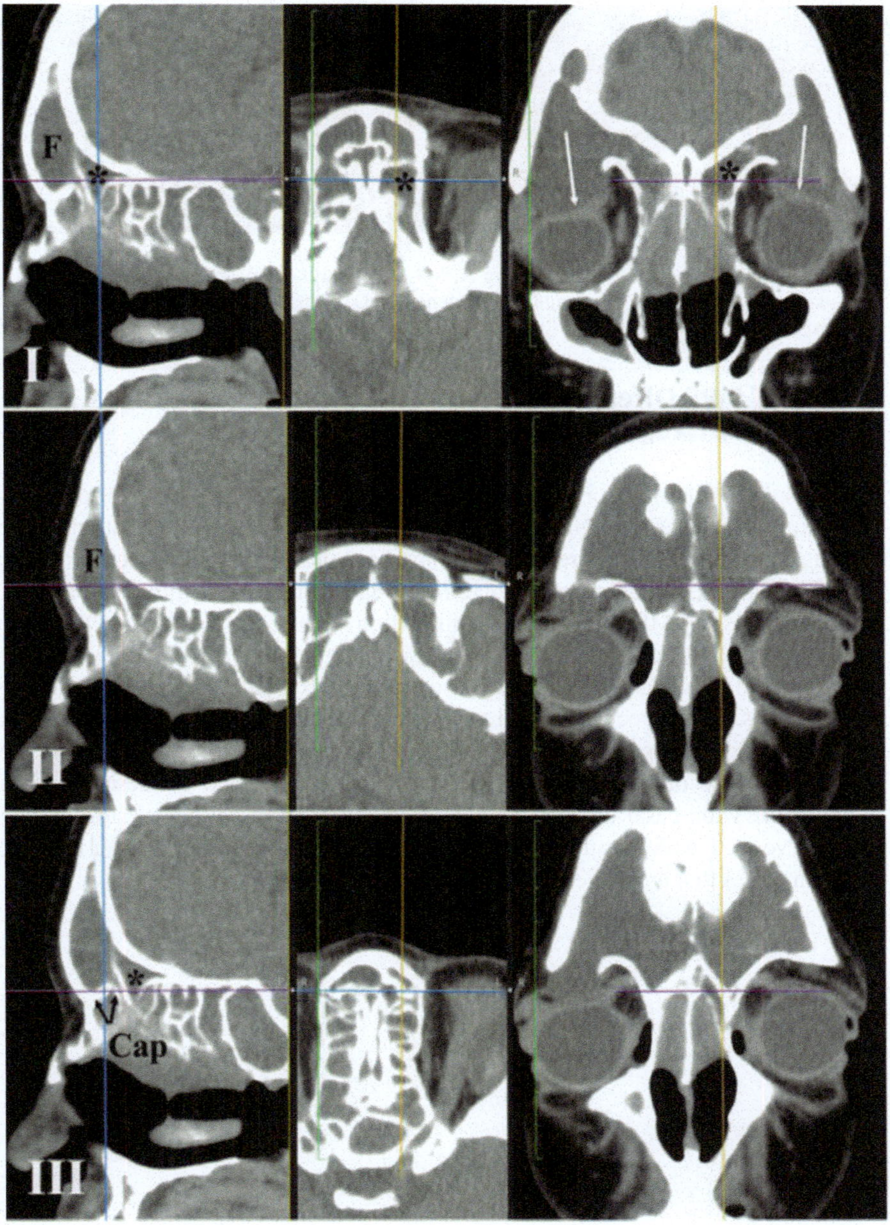


**Fig. 1.24** **CT MPR**: *In row I*, the intersections point to left supraorbital cell (*) used as a route to frontal sinus (F). The arrows demonstrate the extension of bilateral mucoceles pushing the globes downward. *In row II*, the intersections point to left frontal sinus (F). *In row III*, the intersections point to remnants of roof of agger nasi cell (Cap) which formed a cap anterior to SOC (*). Removal of such cap led to the frontal sinus

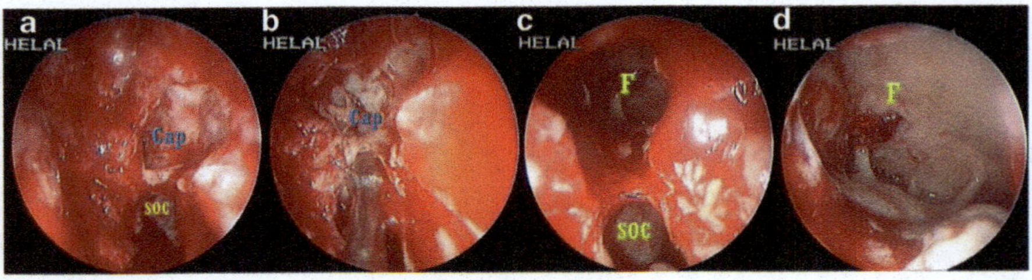


**Fig. 1.25** Operative snapshots showing in A, left SOC and the cap. In B, cap removal with a curved suction tip. In C, the left frontal sinus opened. In D, a closeup view of the left frontal sinus

## 1.13 CT MPR Offers Precision in Skull Base Defects (Fig. 1.26, 1.27, 1.28, 1.29 and 1.30)

Cerebrospinal rhinorrhea or CSF leaks might be traumatic, iatrogenic or spontaneous. Skull base defects might be tiny or wide enough to permit herniation of the meninges and brain tissues resulting in meningoceles or meningoencephaloceles. High-resolution CT is the primary imaging modality utilizing its thin series and PC software as OsiriX MPR to visualize obliteration of the olfactory fossa (OF) if the leak from the cribriform plate (CP). MRI Cisternography is a protocol to enhance CSF signal in T2 weighted cuts and is used as the secondary imaging modality for small lesions. It is especially useful with meningoencephaloceles and to highlight the possibility of idiopathic intracranial hypertension (IIH) which is commonly the etiological cause of spontaneous CSF leaks. IIH is suspected in presence of an empty sella, wide basal cisterns, deep cortical sulci, and CSF signal surrounding optic nerves. CT with intrathecal dye is an invasive technique which better to avoid except in cases that are difficult to diagnose.

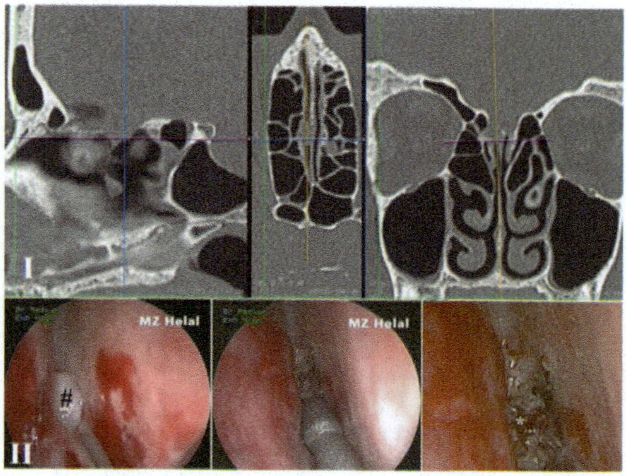


**Fig. 1.26** CT MPR: *In row I*, the intersections point to skull base defect in CP with localized opacity in right olfactory fossa. *In row II* from left to right, operative snapshots showing the lesion (#), CP after bipolar diathermy and the tiny bone defect (*)

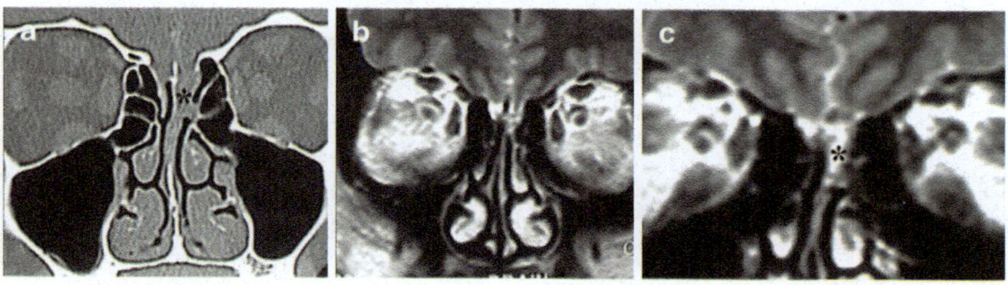


**Fig. 1.27** In A, left OF localized opacity (*) in CT. In B and C, same patient with MRI T2 showing the meningocele (*)

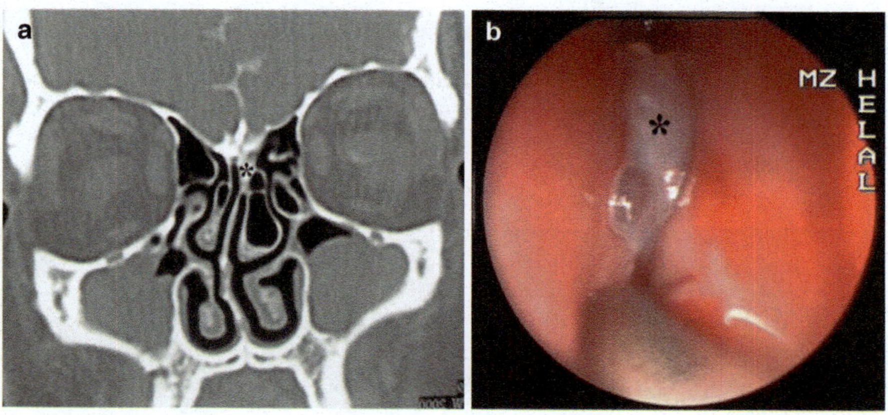


**Fig. 1.28** In A, CT with intrathecal metrizamide showing left CP meningocele (*).In B, operative snapshot of the lesion (*)

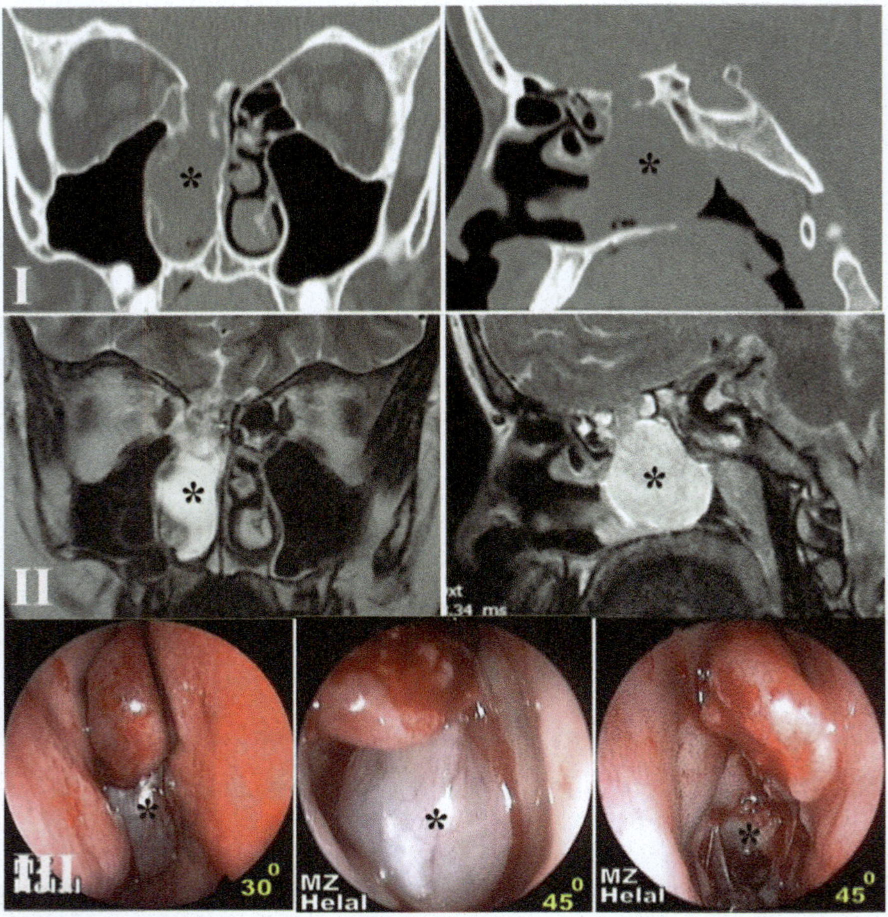


**Fig. 1.29** 11 years old female child presented with a nasal polyp-like swelling. *In row I*, CT study showed the lesion (*) and bone defect in fovea of posterior ethmoid roof. *In row II*, MRI T2 confirmed its nature as meningoencephalocele (*). *I row III*, operative snapshots of the lesion (*) before and during its removal

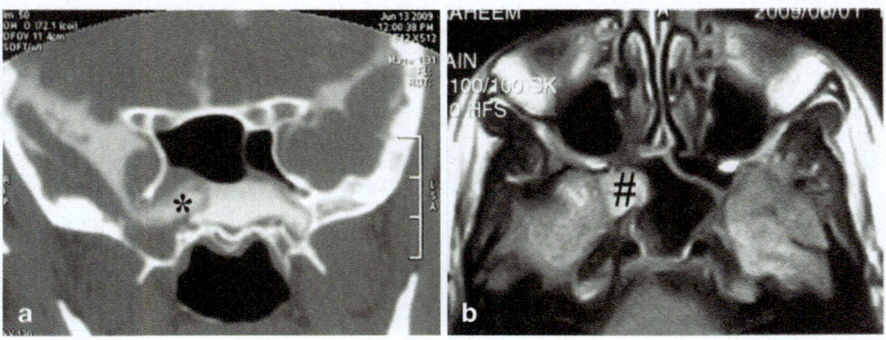


**Fig. 1.30** Leaks from right sphenoid lateral wall. In A, CT metrizamide showing meningocele (*). In B, MRI T1 showing meningoencephalocele (#)

## 1.14 CT MPR and MRI Data Offer Precision in Sinonasal Fungal Disorders

While CT is superior in delineating bones, MRI is superior in soft tissues, e.g., the orbit and intracranial cavity. Fungal sinusitis is classified into non-invasive and invasive types. Invasion means penetration of the fungi into mucus membrane while in non-invasive form the fungi are on top of the mucosal surface causing immunological reaction.

*In non-invasive fungal sinusitis,* the sinus lumen is filled with fungal colonies in allergic mucin with excess calcium and magnesium salts resulting in ground glass hyperdensity (higher attenuation than muscle) in CT and hypointensity in MRI T2 due to higher protein content and low water content of mucin. In MRI T2, the sinus mucous membrane preserves its hyperintense signal due to higher water content. (Fig. 1.31).

*In acute invasive fungal sinusitis,* CT findings may mimic non-fungal sinusitis except for early extra-sinus extension of infection. MRI is more specific with loss of the hyperintensity of the mucosa in T2 and variable degree of mucosal death (gangrene) due to vascular ischemia with hypointensity and non-enhancement in T1 (Fig. 1.32).

*In chronic granulomatous invasive fungal sinusitis,* CT finding is enhancible soft tissue granuloma, while in MRI T2 the hyperintense mucosal signal is lost and replaced by hypointense granuloma. In MRI T1, it is isointense and enhancible (Figs. 1.33, 1.34 and 1.35).

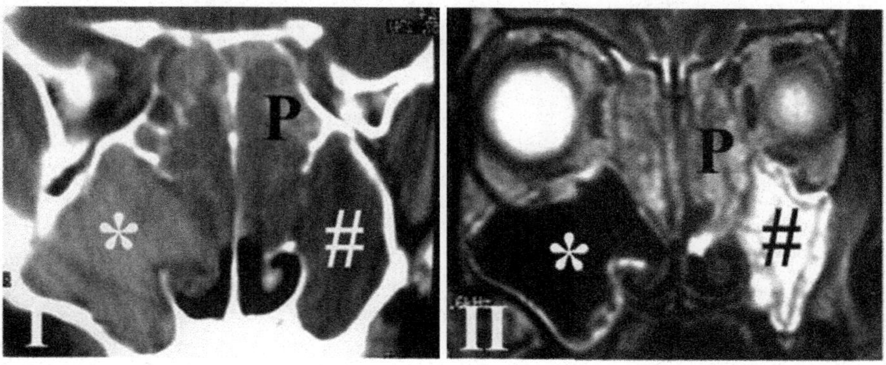


**Fig. 1.31** Non-invasive Fungal sinusitis. *In I,* CT showing hyperdense fungal mucin (*), isodense bacterial content (#) and polyps (P). *In II,* same patient MRI T2 showing hypointense mucin (*), hyperintense bacterial content (#) and polyps (P) with intermediate signal

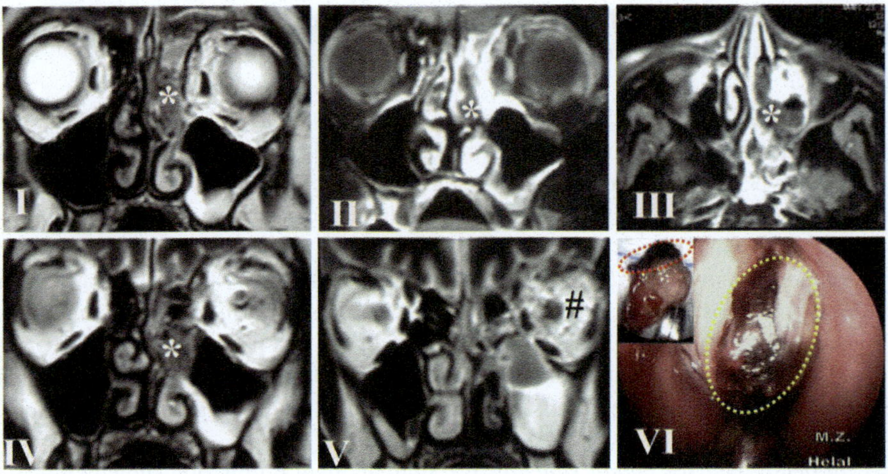


**Fig. 1.32** *Acute invasive fungal sinusitis with middle turbinate (MT) gangrene.* In I, coronal T2 with hypointense MT (*). In II and III coronal and axial T1 with contrast showing absent contrast uptake (*). In IV, T2 showing gangrene in left middle meatus and posterior fontanelle. In V, left orbital fat with an altered signal. In VI, operative snapshots of the gangrenous middle turbinate

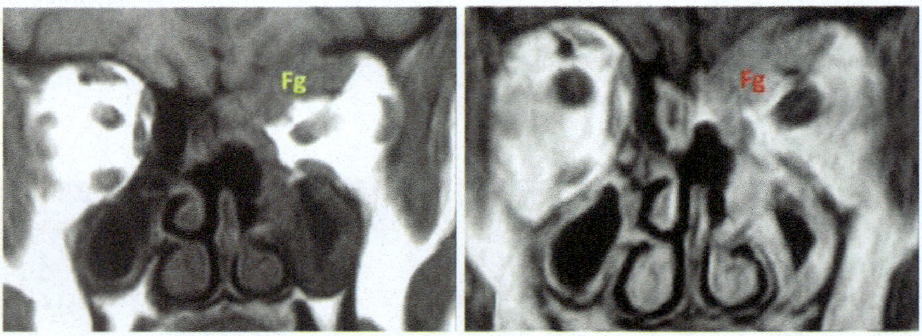


**Fig. 1.33** *Chronic granulomatous invasive fungal sinusitis.* The granuloma (Fg) in left ethmoid and maxillary sinuses extending to left orbital roof is isointense in T1 before contrast in (I) and enhancible after contrast in (II)

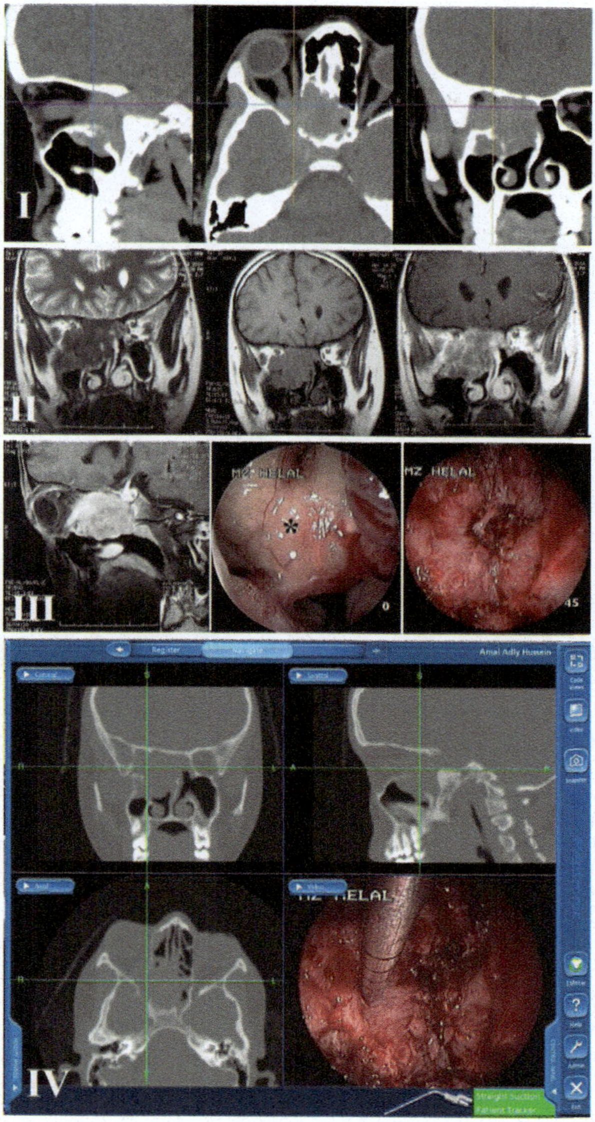


**Fig. 1.34** *Chronic granulomatous invasive fungal sinusitis.* A young female with recurrent lesion on the right side involving the maxillary sinus posterior wall, the posterior ethmoid and the sphenoid with extension to orbital apex causing total right oculomotor nerve paralysis. *In row I*, CT MPR showing the isodense soft tissue lesion. *In row II*, MRI T2 (hypointense), T1 before contrast (isointense) and T1 after contrast (hyperintense) respectively from left to right. *In row III* left, sagittal T1 with contrast showing the large lesion reaching the pituitary gland. *In row III* middle, the lesion covered with glistening mucosa. *In row III* right, operative snapshot after debulking the lesion. *In row IV*, image guided surgery (IGS) was mandatory to safeguard optic nerve and medial rectus muscle. Oculomotor palsy cured in two weeks' time. Histopathology demonstrated giant cells engulfing the septate fungal hyphae of Aspergillus and Voriconazole cured the patent in fifteen months treatment.

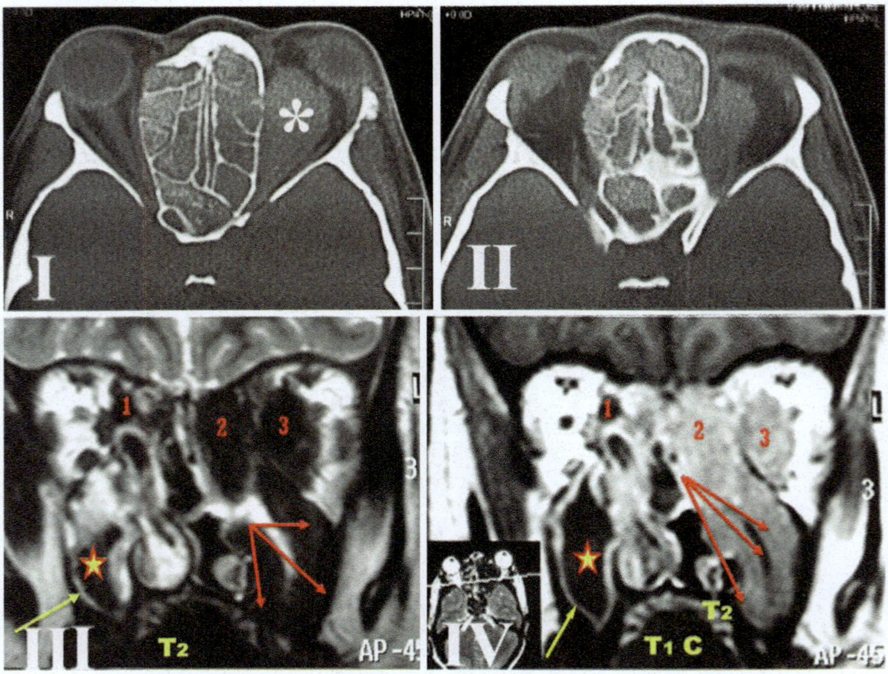


**Fig. 1.35** *Concomitant non-invasive and Chronic granulomatous invasive fungal sinusitis.* This association is rare but proper diagnosis is essential as the invasive form dictates the use of systemic antifungal treatment for months. *In I and II,* CT scan with pansinus hyperdense opacity of non-invasive fungal sinusitis and bilateral orbital granulomatous lesions right (*) more than left. *In III*, coronal T2 with multiple hypointense areas (1,2,3, star and red arrows). *In IV*, postcontrast coronal T1 with 1 (non-invasive, hypointense), 2, 3 and red arrows (Invasive with contrast uptake), star (non-invasive, hypointense) with hyperintense mucosa (yellow arrow)

## 1.15 Covid-Associated Mucormycosis (Figs. 1.36, 1.37, 1.38 and 1.39)

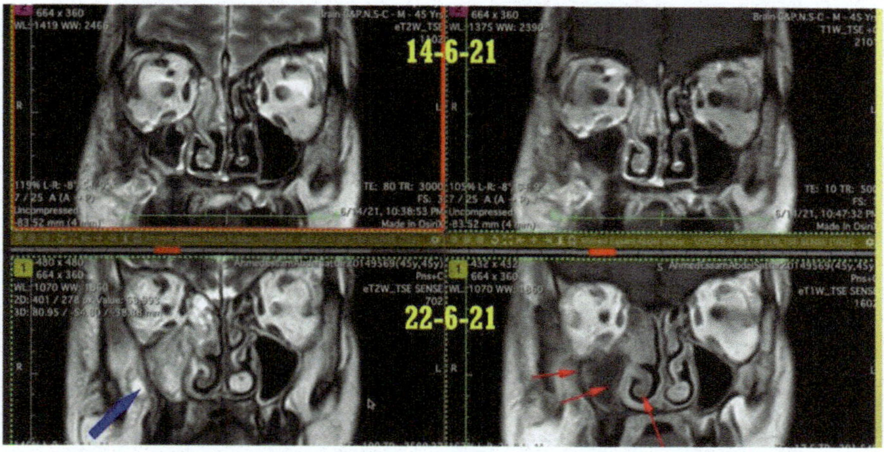


**Fig. 1.36** *Covid-19 associated Mucormycosis (CAM), Early findings. In upper row,* MRI with right acute ethmo-maxillary sinusitis with severe right facial pain. *In lower row*, 8 days later with extra-sinus extension of disease (blue arrow) and ischemia of right maxillary mucosa and right inferior turbinate (red arrows)

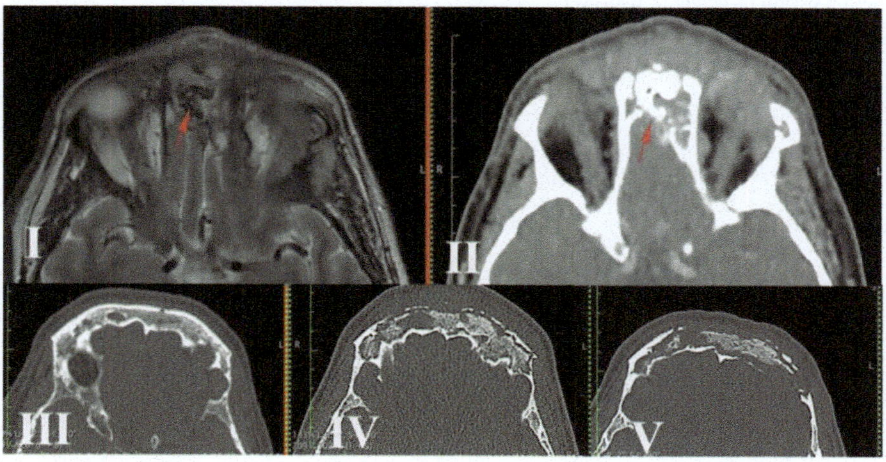


**Fig. 1.37** *Covid-19 associated Mucormycosis (CAM), Late findings.* CAM osteomyelitis of frontal bone with sequestrum (red arrow), *I:* MRI T2, *II:* CT with contrast, *III to V:* CT showing progress of the lesion every 2 months while being under Posaconazole treatment

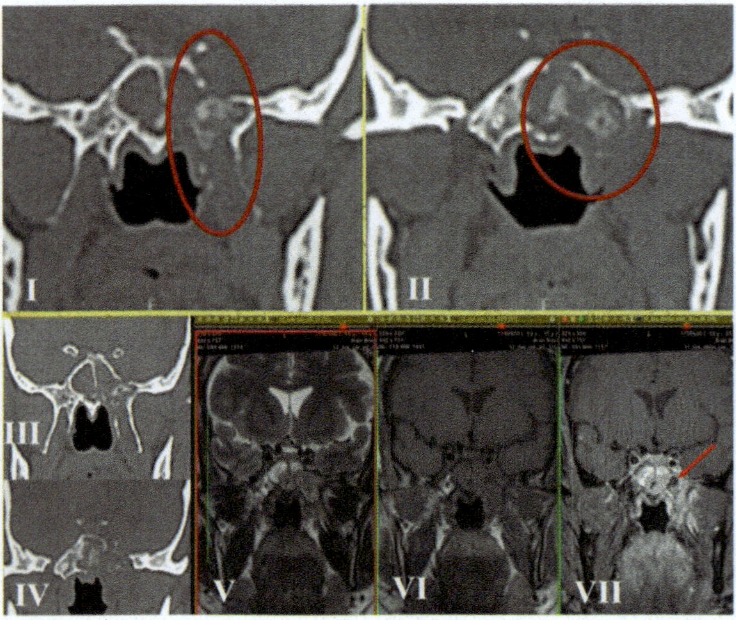


**Fig. 1.38** *Covid-19 associated Mucormycosis (CAM), Late findings. I to IV:* CAM osteomyelitis of left sphenoid bone with sequestrum (red circle) in CT coronal cuts. *V:* MRI T2 showing isointense lesion with hypointense center (sequestrum). *VI:* MRI T1 before contrast showing isointense lesion with hypointense center (sequestrum). *VII:* MRI T1 postcontrast with enhancement of the lesion except its center (red arrow)

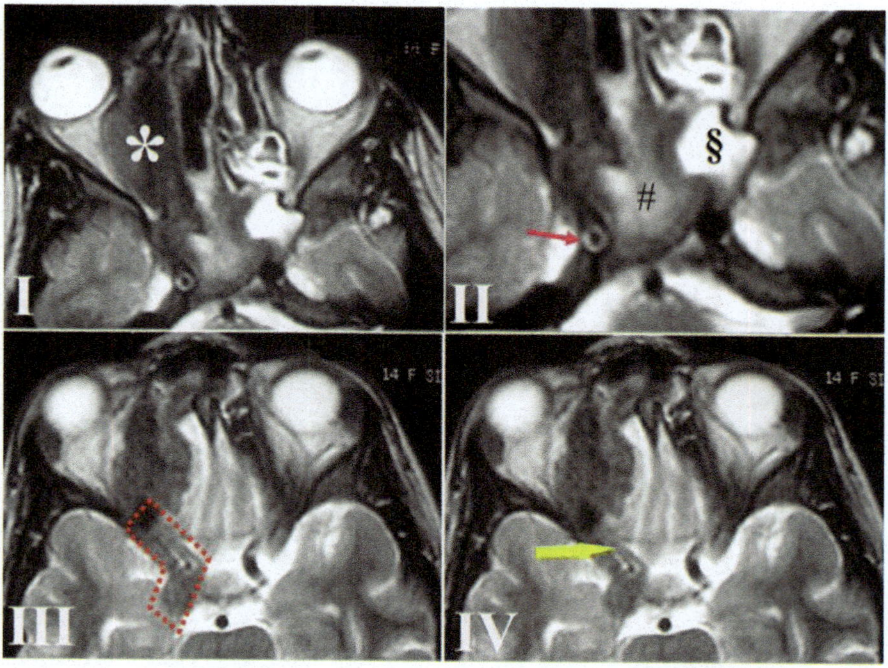


**Fig. 1.39** *Mucormycosis, Late findings. In I:* MRI T2 axial cuts showing intraorbital granuloma (*) with hypointensity. *In II:* close up view of *I* with mixed fungal/bacterial isointense signal (#) in right sphenoid sinus and hyperintense signal of bacterial content (§) in left sphenoid and posterior ethmoid sinus. Intra-cavernous carotid artery is constricted with hyperintense intimal signal denoting involvement in terminal stage of disease (red arrow in *II* and yellow arrow in *IV*). Extension was through superior orbital fissure (red shape in *III*)

## 1.16 CT MPR and MRI Data Offer Precision in Sinonasal Space-Occupying Lesions (Figs. 1.40, 1.41, 1.42, 1.43, 1.44, 1.45, 1.46, 1.47, 1.48, 1.49, 1.50, 1.51, 1.52 and 1.53)

Sinonasal benign space-occupying lesions like mucoceles and benign tumors cause sinus expansion with regular bone thinning leading to bone erosions, while malignant tumors cause little expansion but with irregular patchy bone erosions.

OsiriX™ is a trademark of Pixmeo.
Horos™ is a trademark of the Horos Project.

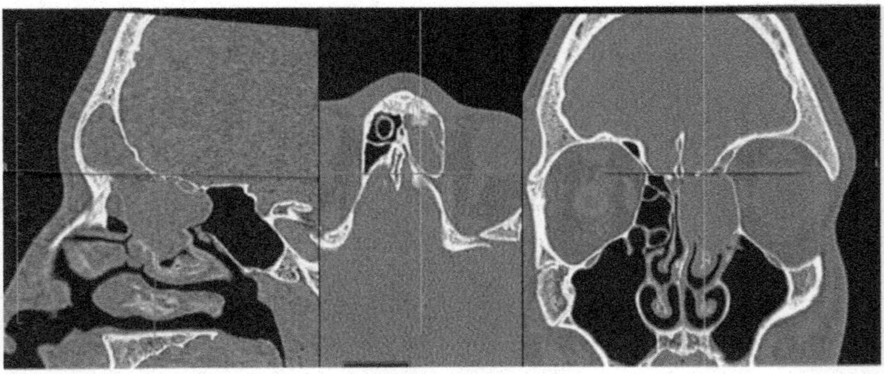

**Fig. 1.40** CT MPR: Left ethmoidal mucocele with left frontal opacity. The lesion caused regular expansion with lost ethmoid cellularity. The intersections point to AEA

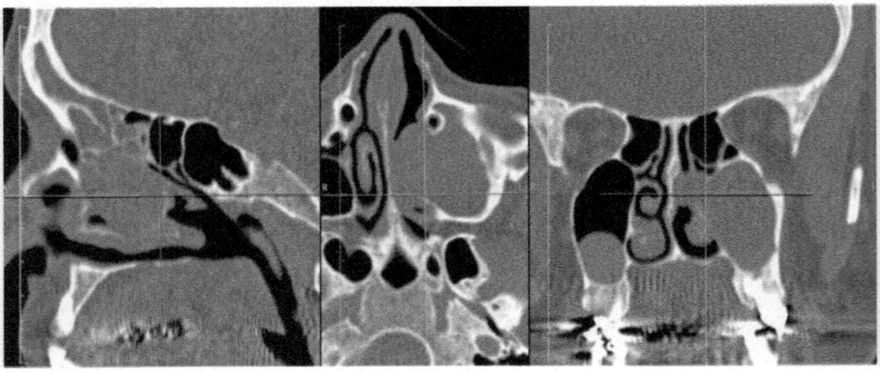

**Fig. 1.41** CT MPR: Left maxillary cystic lesion displacing posterior fontanelle medially with middle meatal polyp (? early antrochoanal polyp). The sclerosed maxillary walls denote chronicity. Right maxillary sinus shows floor cyst

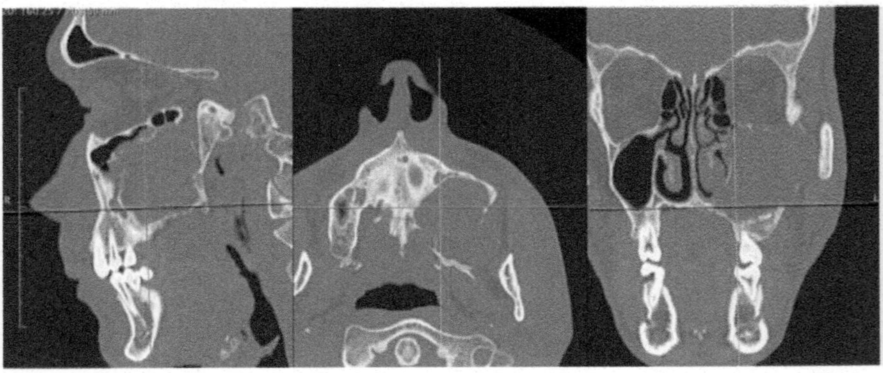

**Fig. 1.42** CT MPR: Left maxillary mucocele causing regular expansion with wide spread even bone erosions and lateral extension

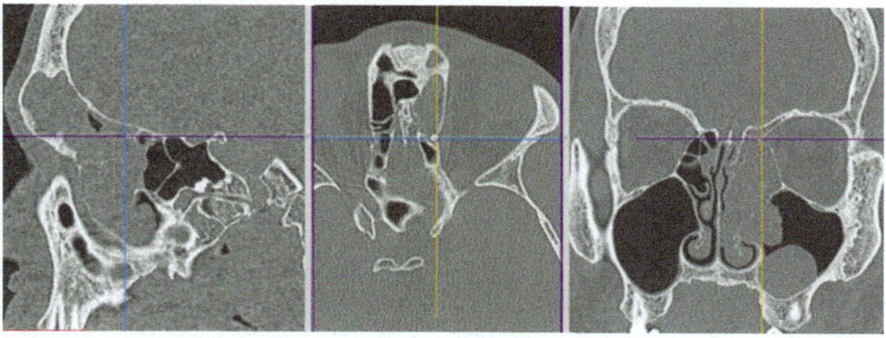

**Fig. 1.43** **CT MPR**: Left fronto-ethmoid inverted papilloma. The intersections point to AEA. The left maxillary sinus has a floor cyst

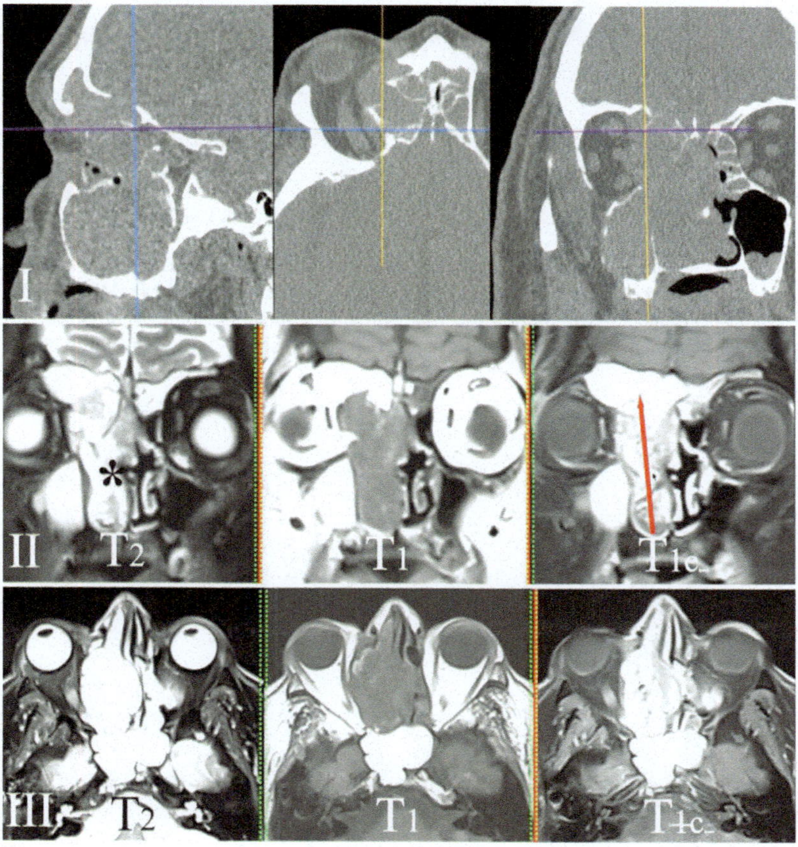


**Fig. 1.44** Right nasal inverted papilloma. *Row I,* CT MPR with extensive bone erosions and right orbital extension. The intersections point to AEA amidst the lesion. *Row II,* MRI T2, T1 and T1 with contrast from left to right. The tumor (*) size was well defined in MRI being best in T1c (arrow). IN MRT T2, the right frontal and maxillary sinuses had secretions with higher protein content than the left frontal sinus. *Row III,* shows the same findings in axial cuts. MRI differentiates well the tumor and retained secretions in sphenoid sinus

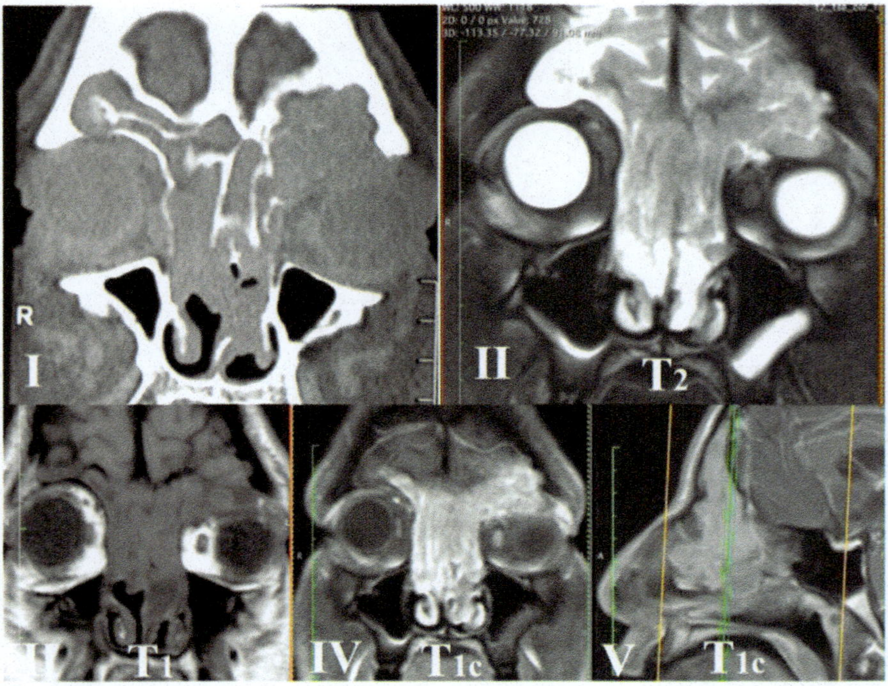


**Fig. 1.45** Recurrent Fronto-ethmoid inverted papilloma. *In upper row,* CT coronal cut (I) showing bilateral fronto-ethmoid tumor with mixed soft tissue and hyperdense shadows. MRI T2 (II) showing isointense striated soft tumor. *In lower row*, coronal T1 showing isointense tumor before contrast (III), T1 post contrast (IV) and sagittal post contrast (V) showing the enhancible tumor

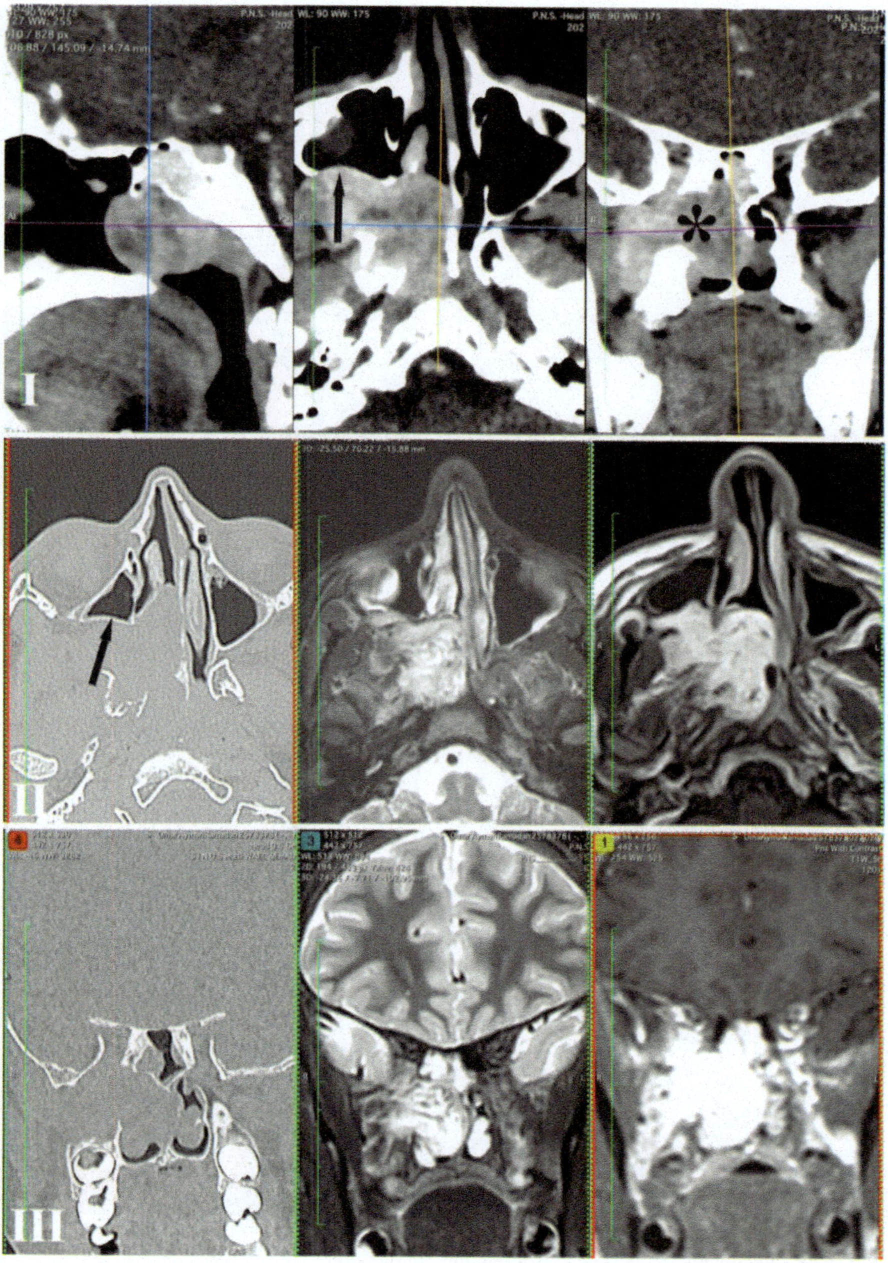


**Fig. 1.46** Juvenile angiofibroma. *In row I*, CT MPR of the tumor (*) in its typical location on the sphenoid face around the vidian foramen widening the pterygopalatine fossa (PPF), pushing the maxillary sinus posterior wall anteriorly (arrow) and extending laterally to the infratemporal fossa. *In row II*, PPF same findings (arrow) in axial CT, axial MRI T2 and axial MRI T1 with high contrast uptake (from left to right). *In row III*, PPF same findings in coronal CT, coronal MRI T2 and coronal MRI T1 with high contrast uptake (from left to right)

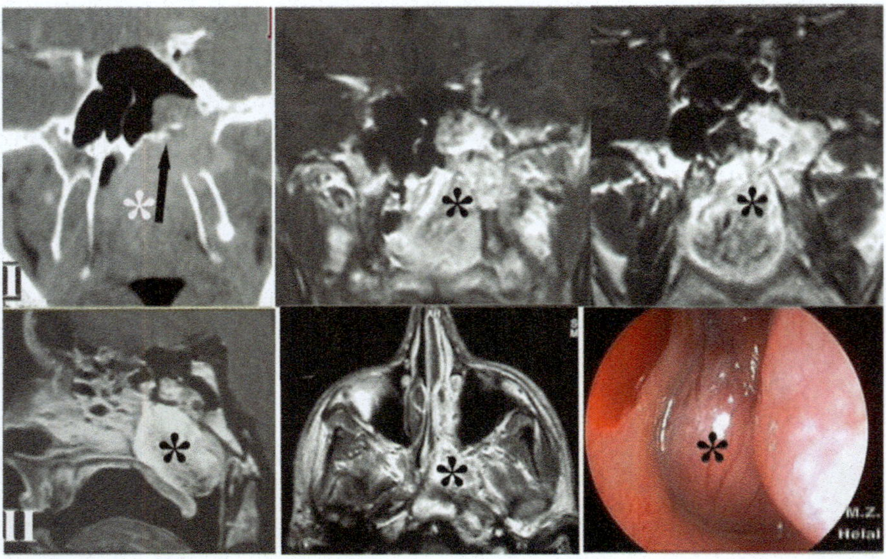


**Fig. 1.47** Juvenile angiofibroma (*). *In row I*, CT coronal cut, T1 with contrast and T2 from left to right, showing the typical origin from the vidian canal on the left side (arrow). *In row II*, MRI sagittal and axial T1 with contrast of the tumor (*) and operative snapshot of the tumor

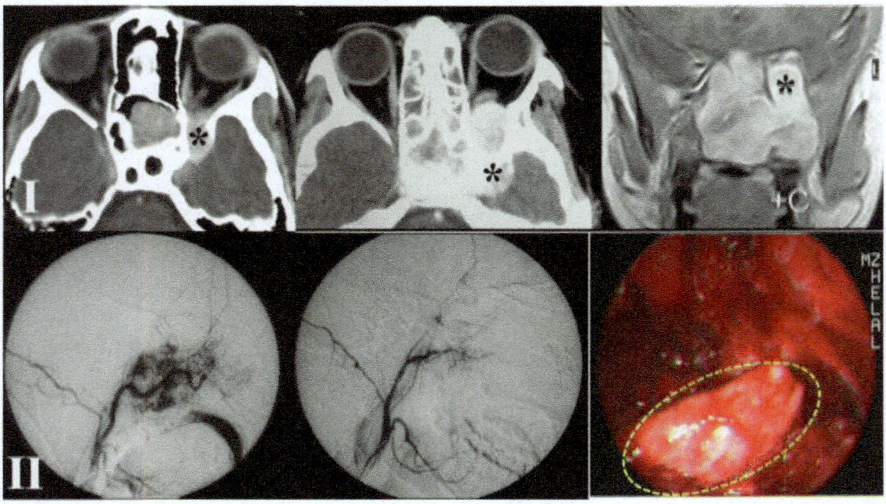


**Fig. 1.48** Juvenile angiofibroma extending intracranially through left superior orbital fissure (*). *In row I*, CT axial cuts with contrast and coronal MRI T1 with contrast.*In row II*, pre- and post-angiographic embolization of the feeding branches from maxillary artery, and operative snapshot of the part of the tumor delivered from superior orbital fissure

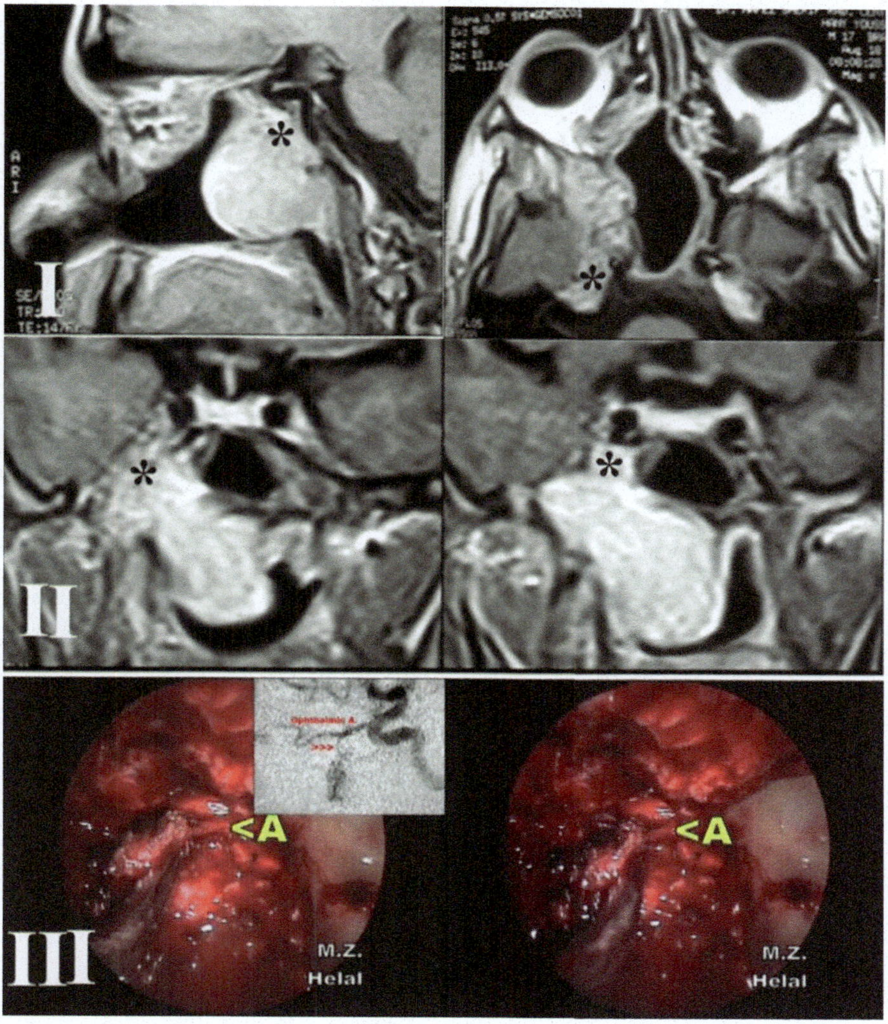


**Fig. 1.49** Recurrent Juvenile angiofibroma extending intracranially to right cavernous sinus (*). *In row I*, MRI post contrast sagittal and axial T1 cuts showing the tumor in lateral wall of the right posterior ethmoid and sphenoid and together with the right cavernous sinus. *In row II*, MRI coronal postcontrast T1 cuts showing the tumor in nasopharynx with its base in right cavernous sinus. *In row III*, prior angiography demonstrated unusual feeding blood supply from the right ophthalmic artery of the internal carotid artery. Operative snapshots showing the artery identified and cauterized in cavernous sinus

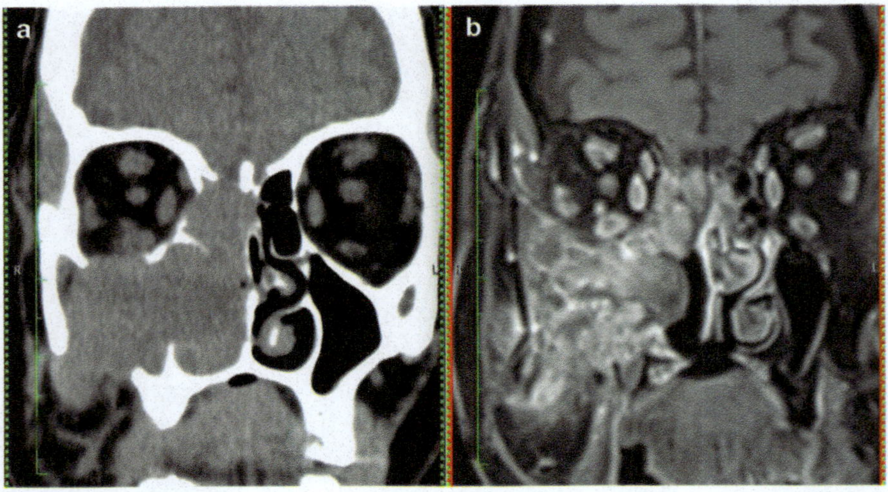


**Fig. 1.50** Right nasal Squamous cell carcinoma in recurrent inverted papilloma. (**a**) Coronal CT showing soft tissue lesion with bone erosions and extension to infratemporal fossa. (**b**) MRI T1 coronal cut with contrast showing heterogenous enhancement

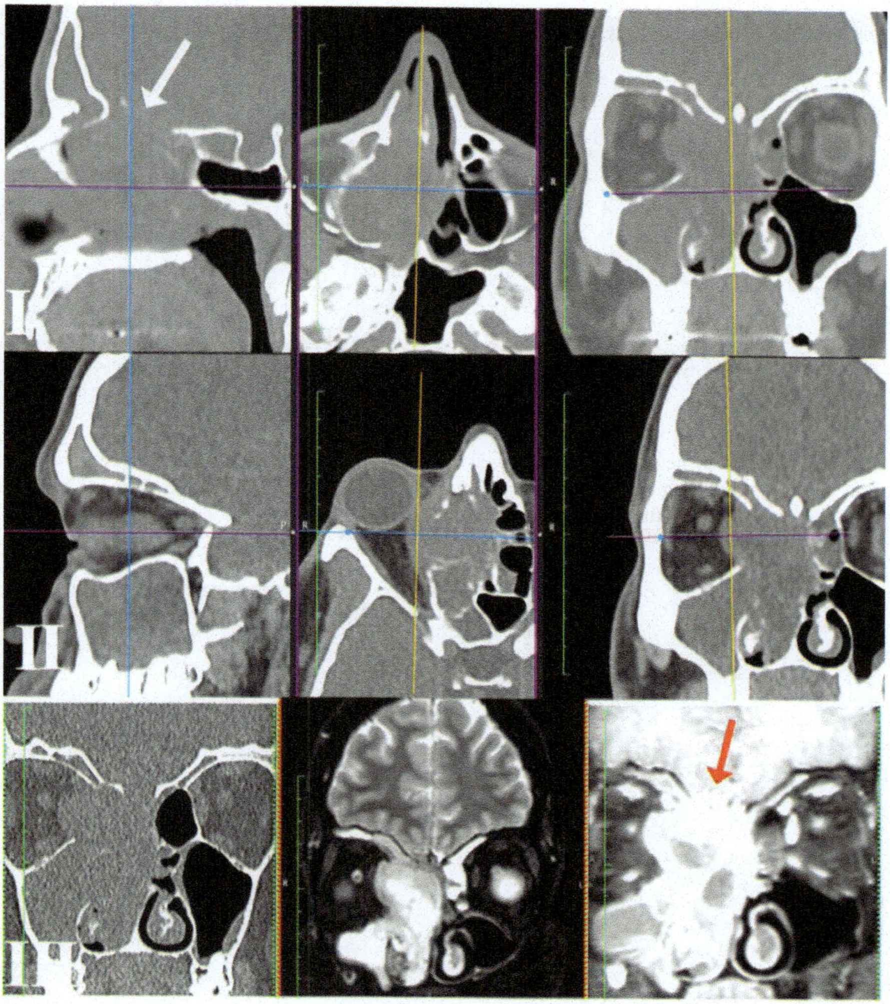


**Fig. 1.51** Rhabdomyosarcoma of right nasal fossa. *I row I*, CT MPR showing soft tissue mass causing wide spread bone loss (white arrow). *In row II*, CT MPR showing the tumor invading the right orbit. *In row III*, CT coronal cut (left) showing bone defects in nasal roof and right lamina papyracea. MRI T2 with fat suppression (middle) with slightly hyperintense tumor with central cystic degeneration. Adjacent sinuses were filled with secretions. MRI T1 with contrast (right) demonstrates contrast uptake and attachment to brain tissues (red arrow)

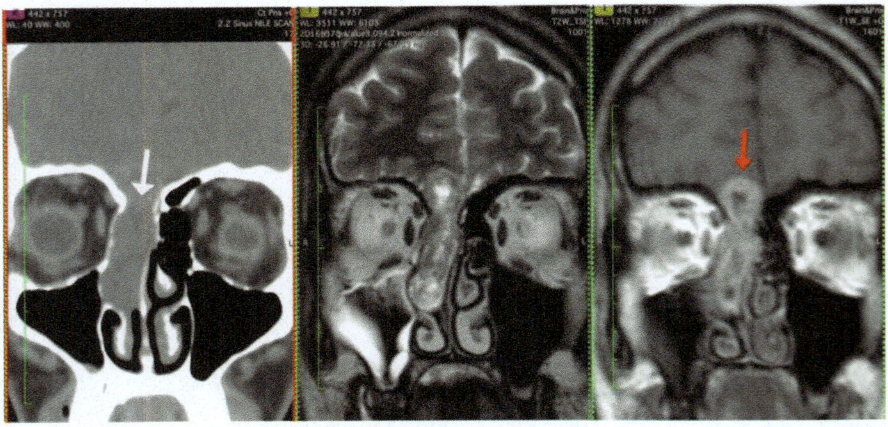

**Fig. 1.52** Olfactory neuroblastoma. Coronal CT (left) and MRI T2 (middle) showing right nasal roof defect with oblong soft tissue opacity mimicking meningoencephalocele. Coronal MRI T1 post-contrast (right) confirmed the enhancible nature of the tumor

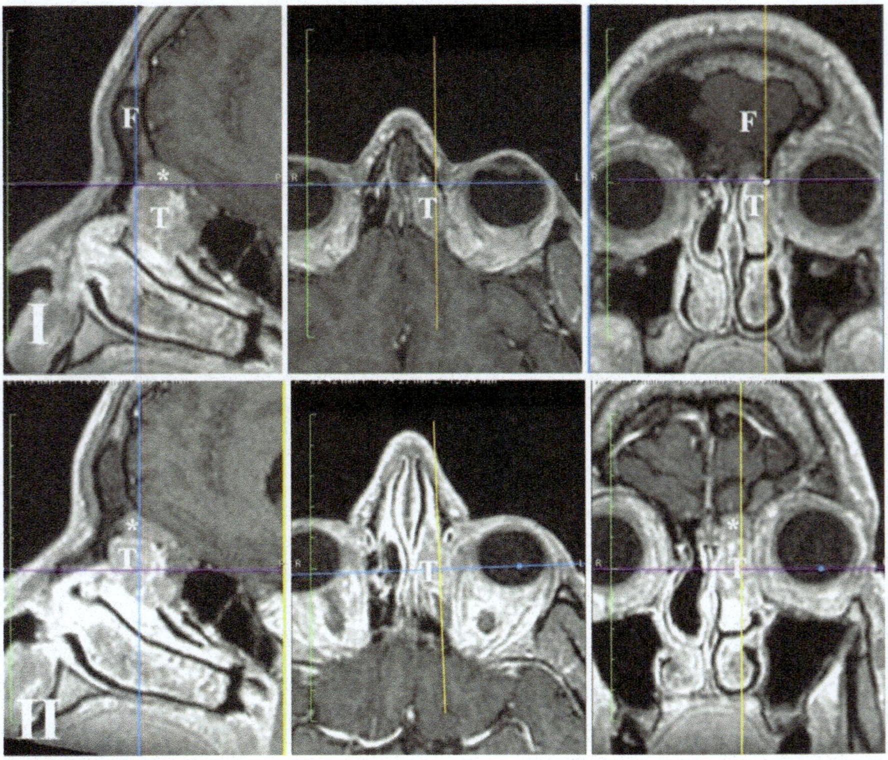


**Fig. 1.53** Ethmoid adenocarcinoma. MRI MPR can be achieved with clarity with cuts of around 1 mm thickness. *In row I*, the intersections point to the relation between the tumor (T) and the frontal sinus (F). In sagittal cut, secretions (*) intervene between the tumor and meninges. *In row II*, the intersections point to the relation between the tumor (T) and the orbit

## References

1. Rosset A, Spadola L, Ratib O. OsiriX: an open-source software for navigating in multidimensional DICOM images. J Digit Imaging. 2004;17:205–16.
2. Caversaccio M, Boschung U, Mudry A. Historical review of Haller's cells. Ann Anat. 2011;193:185–90.
3. Wormald PJ, Hoseman W, Callejas C, Weber RK, Kennedy DW, Citardi MJ, Senior BA, Smith TL, Hwang PH, Orlandi RR, Kaschke O, Siow JK, Szczygielski K, Goessler U, Khan M, Bernal-Sprekelsen M, Kuehnel T, Psaltis A. The international frontal sinus anatomy classification (IFAC) and classification of the extent of endoscopic frontal sinus surgery (EFSS). International Forum of Allergy & Rhinology. 2016;6(7):677–96.
4. Yousem DM. Imaging of sinonasal inflammatory disease. Radiology. 1993;188:303–14.
5. Keros P. On the practical value of differences in the level of the lamina cribrosa of the ethmoid. Z Laryngol Rhinol Otol. 1962;41:809–13.
6. Tomovic S, Esmaeili A, Chan NJ, Choudhry OJ, Shukla PA, Liu JK, Eloy JA. High-resolution computed tomography analysis of the prevalence of Onodi cells. Laryngoscope. 2012;122:1470–3.

# 2 Olfactory Disorders

Mohamed Shehata Taha

**Key Points**

- Olfactory disorders are universal; 5% of people are anosmic, and their frequency increases with age. Above 50, 25% of the population has an impaired sense of smell (presbyosmia).
- Olfactory dysfunction (OD) is divided into quantitative and qualitative impairments.
- The principal causes of OD include rhinosinusitis, nasal polyposis, trauma, viral infections and neurodegenerative illnesses such as Alzheimer's dementia or Parkinson's disease. The loss of smell is considered a clinical sign of early-stage disease and a marker of the disease's progression.
- The prognosis of OD depends on the cause and time of intervention.
- Treatment of the cause of OD is possible only when nasal diseases are responsible for the dysfunction. The primary options are surgery or the administration of corticosteroids.
- A new approach to the treatment of non-sinonasal OD is a course of olfactory training, artificial intelligence, platelets reach plasma, stem cell therapy, electrical stimulation and olfactory mucosa transplant.

M. S. Taha (✉)
Consultant ORL-HNS, Faculty of Medicine, Ain Shams University Hospitals, Ain Shams University, Cairo, Egypt


S. Elwany (ed.), *Current Rhinology*,
https://doi.org/10.1007/978-3-031-70077-4_2

## 2.1 Introduction

### 2.1.1 Definition

Olfactory dysfunction [OD] is defined as the reduced or distorted ability to smell during sniffing [orthonasal olfaction] or eating [retronasal olfaction] [1].

### 2.1.2 Olfaction and Smell Fundamental Importance

Although olfaction is critically important for a good quality of life, personal safety, and nutritional status, the sense of smell is underestimated by both patients and clinicians [2]. Not only does olfaction help us detect fragrances in the air around us, but it's also important in helping us enjoy the flavours of foods. You may have heard that "taste" primarily smells [3]. Correct assessment of the cause of olfactory impairment is important to determine which patients may benefit from therapy [4].

## 2.2 Anatomy and Physiology of Olfaction

The main role of the olfactory system is to detect and process odour signals. This function is essential for food selection by cognizance gustatory and olfactory gesture. The processing of odours by sensory signals obtained from different chemical stimuli has a fundamental role in physiological and emotional homeostasis, playing a critical role in reproductive and neuroendocrine regulation and is relevant for emotion, aggression memory, and recognition of predators and social organization [5].

The olfactory pathway starts with an olfactory epithelium that sits on the superior conchae deep in the nasal cavity. This pseudostratified ciliated columnar epithelium houses olfactory sensory neurons, basal stem cells and supporting cells. In addition, Bowman's glands located in the lamina propria under the epithelium send ducts to the surface of the epithelium and secrete a serous fluid that immerses the cilia of olfactory receptor neurons in a mucous layer to trap odorant molecules. Odorant molecules bind to olfactory receptor proteins in the cilia of olfactory sensory neuron dendrites.

Air-borne odorant molecules in the air that we breathe activate the olfactory receptor proteins in the olfactory cilia. It can find its way to the olfactory sensory neurons either through the nose [orthonasal stimulation] or from the mouth to the nose [retro nasal stimulation] [1]. The membrane of olfactory sensory neuron cilia houses odorant receptor proteins and thereby activates these neurons in the nasal epithelium. Each olfactory sensory neuron sends an axon through the cribriform plate of the ethmoid bone to the ipsilateral main olfactory bulb in the brain. The axons of olfactory sensory neurons coalesce to form the olfactory nerve [cranial nerve I] and olfactory nerve layer of the main olfactory bulb [6]. The olfactory epithelium displays a strong expression of angiotensin-converting enzyme 2 [ACE2] receptors. So it can be described as COVI-Philic epithelium [has high affinity to COVID-19 virus]. Inflammation in this area could be a cause of smell loss; although the olfactory receptor neurons lack the ACE2 receptor, the spread of inflammation to stem cells or olfactory receptor neurons may occur through the supporting cells, causing harm to the olfactory bulb and the central nervous system, leading to anosmia [7].

### 2.2.1 Kinship of Olfactory Cues with Health Maintenance

Olfactory stimuli by food impact energy balance, fortifying the body for digestion when food is eaten. Social chemosensory signals stimulate subsequent energetic overhaul needed for social interplay [8].

## 2.3 Quality of Life

All OD affect global quality of life, but each in different ways. Smell-impaired individuals are concerned with failing to detect hazards such as spoiled food, fire and gas. Phantasmic and anosmic/hyposmic individuals showed a higher concern for failing to detect fire and gas than parosmic individuals. There was a higher anxiety for cleanliness among those with phantosmia, whereas those with parosmia had a lower motivation to eat, cook, and socialize. Parosmic individuals also found it difficult to adjust to their disorder, which might be a result of its acute nature during recovery. Phantosmics reported changes in their weight, with some gaining and others losing weight since the onset of the disorder [9].

## 2.4 Classification of Olfactory Dysfunction

### 2.4.1 Qualitative Dysfunction

(i) Dysosmia: Distortion in the sense of smell.
(ii) Parosmia: Distortion in the perception of an odour. Euosmia is used to describe pleasant qualitative olfactory distortion in the presence of a stimulus and can therefore be considered a subtype of parosmia [10]. Troposmia is generally considered to be synonymous with parosmia [11].
(iii) Phantosmia: Distortion in the absence of an odour, "hallucinated smell".
(iv) Agnosia: Inability to classify or contrast odours, although able to detect odours.
(v) In special form of dysosmia, some patients interpret the smell of all odours as unpleasant [cacosmia].

### 2.4.2 Quantitative Dysfunction

(i) Normosmia: Normal sensitivity.
(ii) Hyposmia: A decreased ability to sense smells.

(iii) Anosmia [Functional and specific]: A total inability to sense smells.
- Complete anosmia: absolute loss of olfactory function; no sense of smell detectable.
- Functional anosmia: severe limitation of olfactory function; includes complete loss as well as residual odour perception.
- Partial anosmia: greatly reduced sensitivity to a particular odoriferous substance/group of substances compared with the general population, usually not viewed as pathological.

(iv) Hyperosmia is an overwhelming sensitivity to smells caused by a lower threshold for odour. This may be due to increased signals at any point between the olfactory receptors and the olfactory cortex. The causes of hyperosmia are genetics, hormone changes, migraines, environmental or the result of benzodiazepine withdrawal syndrome.

(v) Presbyosmia: the natural decline in the sense of smell in old age.

(vi) Heterosmia: inability to distinguish odours [12]. Olfactory reference syndrome—psychological disorder that causes the patient to imagine he or she has a strong body odour.

(vii) Osmophobia: aversion or psychological hypersensitivity to odours.

(viii) Multiple chemical sensitivity [MCS; also known as 'Idiopathic Environmental Intolerance'] is a condition in which patients describe a range of subjective symptoms following low-level exposure to various chemicals. Due to the range of organ systems affected, and the disparity of offending substances, it has been suggested that MCS is not an organic clinical entity, but rather a predominantly psychological condition. This view has been supported by studies demonstrating no significant difference in patient response to 'active' substances versus placebo [13].

## 2.5 Prevalence and Aetiology of OD

### 2.5.1 Prevalence

There is no widely accepted method to assess olfactory function in the general population, given the variability in measures used to determine OD [14]. Some investigations have reported prevalence rates ranging from 1.4% to 62.4% [15].

### 2.5.2 Aetiology

Factors and conditions that can cause dysosmia:

A. Congenital.
B. Ageing.
C. Trigeminal and olfactory Dysfunction.
D. Post-viral.

E. Sinonasal diseases.
F. Exposure to toxins or medications.
G. Head trauma.
H. Neurodegenerative disorders.
I. Other neurodegenerative diseases.
J. Epilepsy.
K. Psychiatric disorders.
L. Brain tumours.
M. Autoimmune and endocrine disease.
N. Smoking.
O. Idiopathic OD.
P. Medications.
Q. Head and neck radiation for cancer.
R. Diabetes: damage to the nerves involved in olfaction may likewise occur, similar to the nerve damage that can lead to peripheral neuropathy and retinopathy.
S. Vitamin deficiencies: A lack of thiamine or a lack of zinc are associated with a loss of the sense of olfaction.

**A. Congenital**

Certain genetic conditions are known to be associated with congenital dysfunction, most notably the developmental endocrine disorder Kallmann syndrome [hypogonadotropic hypogonadism]. The diagnosis is usually between 12 and 16 years. It is confederate with aplastic/hypoplastic olfactory sulci, olfactory bulb and olfactory sensory neurons OSN of varying number and maturity [16]. Patients mostly have severe hyposmia or functional anosmia, dating since birth. Also, olfactory dysfunction was diagnosed in Turner's syndrome [17].

Nowadays non-syndromic aplasia/hypoplasia of the olfactory bulb is recognized due to the advantage of magnetic resonance imaging (MRI). So non-syndromic, idiopathic congenital anosmia without genetic cause can be easily diagnosed [18]. Prerequisites for diagnosis are the olfactory sulcus should be shortened and the normal olfactory bulb structure should be absent hypoplastic [19].

**B. Age**

Olfactory function peaks around the third or fourth decade of life and then decreases with increasing age and is significantly reduced above the age of 55 years [20]. A decline in olfaction may be sharp in the sixth and seventh decades of life. The surface area of the olfactory mucosa decreases as a result of a loss of primary olfactory receptor neurons with replacement by respiratory epithelium [19]. Other pathological processes involved in the loss of olfactory function in ageing may include a reduced rate of basal cell proliferation, decreases in cilia and supporting cell microvilli, reduced metabolism, occlusion of the cribriform plate, changes of epithelial blood flow, or increased mucus viscosity [21].

**C. Trigeminal Nerve and OD**

The nasal cavity is innervated by two cranial nerves: the olfactory system and the trigeminal. Most odours stimulate both nervous systems and interaction between the two systems has a powerful influence on odour and touch perception. Many studies have shown that olfactory loss will lead to decreased responsiveness to trigeminal stimulation [22]. Atrophic rhinitis is a unique clinical setting which can result in the loss of both olfactory and trigeminal functions [23].

**D. Post-viral OD**

Post-viral anosmia is responsible for more than 40% of cases of anosmia, particularly in adults. The causative viruses known to be neurotropic for peripheral olfactory structures and capable of damaging the olfactory neuroepithelium are flu-like infections, the common cold, herpes simplex encephalitis, hepatitis, herpes simplex types 1 and 2, rabies [24] polio, the Indiana strain of wild-type vesicular stomatitis, mouse hepatitis, herpes simplex, Borna disease, and canine distemper viruses [25]. Human rhinovirus, picornavirus, parainfluenza virus type 2, and Epstein-Barr virus all were proven in post-viral OD.

Among them are the coronaviruses, which are first characterized in the 1960s and are accounting for 10–15% of cases [26]. A huge peer-reviewed report from UK and US indicates that two-thirds of positive COVID-19 self-reported cases state loss of smell or taste. Another systematic review states that 30% to 80% of confirmed COVID-19 patients complain of loss of smell or taste [27]. Olfactory/gustatory dysfunctions should be recognized for early detection of COVID-19 infection. Most recovery of olfactory/gustatory dysfunction in COVID-19 infection starts within 3 days and reaches the best recovery within 19 to 24 days [28].

A recent study examined 60 patients with anosmia and or ageusia using RT-PCR for COVID-19. Forty-six (76.7%) were positive and 14 (23.3%) were negative. Negative samples were tested by real-time multiplex PCR. Rhinovirus was the commonest isolated pathogen (5/14), followed by human parainfluenza (1/14), human adenovirus (1/14), and enterovirus (1/14). 2 bacterial pathogens were detected, while no pathogens could be detected in three patients [15].

Anosmia is less frequent than hyposmia in post-viral OD. Moreover, phantosmia and parosmia are related to post-viral OD. Increased susceptibility to viral damage can occur from the reduction or inhibition of mucociliary transport by disease, drugs, diet, or genetic factors, as well as from age-related changes in nasal function and normal defence mechanisms [29]. On rare occasions, OD has been seen with influenza vaccines likely as vaccine-related cases of Guillain–Barre syndrome and Bell's palsy [30].

**E. Sinonasal Diseases**

Loss of smell related to sinonasal diseases is almost always of gradual decrease over many years or a fluctuating course. The most common diseases causing olfactory dysfunction are chronic rhinosinusitis with and without nasal polyposis [CRSwNP and CRSsNP]. Olfactory loss is more frequent with CRSwNP than CRSsNP [31]. Due to inflammatory changes in the olfactory mucosa, olfactory loss in CRSwNP is conductive loss mixed with sensory-neural type. Moreover, altered olfactory receptor cells and olfactory mucus [Bowman's gland] may explain olfactory loss associated with CRSwNP. The olfactory epithelium of CRSwNP showed squamous metaplasia, a significant change in the normal cell-cycle dynamics and increased apoptosis [32]. 21.4% of allergic rhinitis patients are suffering from OD and nasal obstruction. Their olfactory threshold showed a correlation with radiographic changes number of sensitized allergens and blood eosinophilia [33]. However, the olfactory threshold was not related to nasal resistance measured by rhinomanometry [34].

**F. Toxins and Medications**

Local exposure to chemicals [formaldehyde, cadmium, benzene, gasoline, ammonia, hairdressing chemicals, herbicides, and zincs] can cause smell loss. Degrees of OD are correlated with the concentration of the toxins and the length of exposure. Toxin-induced olfactory dysfunction is usually permanent. Often, systemic drugs [chemotherapy, anticonvulsants, antidepressants, ant rheumatics, immunosuppressants, antimicrobials, antithyroid, and antihypertensive] appear to cause taste and OD [35]. The explanation of OD may be due to either central or peripheral neuroepithelial damage. In many cases, removing or changing the violating drugs will repudiate the effects on the olfactory functions [36].

**G. Head Trauma**

It was estimated that 15–30% of anosmia is related to head trauma, with an increased incidence of anosmia than hyposmia [37]. Recovery is unlikely in cases of loss of consciousness, post-traumatic amnesia, severe trauma, and the presence of radiological insults. Anosmia can occur despite minor blows, and more severe olfactory loss is produced by occipital blows and side impact rather than frontal blows. Causes of olfactory disorders following head trauma are secondary to oedema of the olfactory tract and bulb, stretching or shearing of the olfactory nerves at the site of the cribriform plate, haemorrhage [or contusion] in the olfactory brain area, olfactory mucosal damage and fibrosis and scar formation in the olfactory bulb, decreased volume of olfactory bulb injury of the connections between axons and the olfactory bulb [38]. Post-traumatic OD are always recognized soon after the injury; however, it can be delayed due to late-onset cell death. Recovery can occur due to regeneration of the olfactory nerve, but aberrant connections may lead to dysosmia. There are no specific treatments available for post-traumatic anosmia. The olfactory function returned in just 10–30% of cases while 20% of patients worsened. Poor prognosis is observed if the improvement is not obeyed within 6 months to 1 year of the insult [39].

**H. Neurodegenerative Disorders**

OD can be the earliest sign of degenerative processes of the central nervous system as [Alzheimer's disease AD and Parkinson's disease PD]. Those with AD or PD disease elicit changes in the identification of odour discrimination detection when compared with age-matched controls. The prognosis and severity of the disorder are correlated to disease progression. In most cases, olfactory loss is a complaint years before cognitive or motor symptoms. The risk of developing dementia is increased when OD occurs at the time of PD diagnosis [40]. Serious or unpleasant olfactory impairment was witnessed in patients with Down syndrome [41]. Impairments were found in patients with motor neuron diseases, spinocerebellar ataxia types 2 and 3 and Friedreich ataxia [42]. An association has also been recognized between smell loss and increased risk of mortality [43].

**I. Epilepsy**
Early threshold studies of patients with epilepsy reported heightened, not lessened, and overall bilateral sensitivity, particularly before an ictal event [44]. More recent work found normal thresholds, although this may reflect the influence of antiseizure medications [45].

**J. Psychiatric Disorders**
Various neuropsychiatric disorders such as bipolar disorder seasonal affective disorder and depression were linked to smell disorders due to involvement of the amygdala and cortex in these psychiatric diseases [46]. It has also been shown that patients with acute major depressive disorder or schizophrenia have not only decreased olfactory sensitivity but also reduced olfactory bulb volumes [47].

**K. Brain Tumours**
OD may be due to frontal and temporal lobe tumours, it was estimated that one-quarter of temporal lobe tumours cause olfactory loss. Anterior fossa tumours such as Foster-Kennedy syndrome and esthesioneuroblastoma show progressive hyposmia leading to anosmia [48].

**L. Autoimmune and Endocrine Disease**
OD can be caused by autoantibody [anti-ribosomal P] in patients with systemic lupus erythematosus [SLE]. Other endocrine diseases such as diabetes mellitus, hypothyroidism, and hypogonadism may be associated with OD [49].

**M. Smoking**
OD can be explained in smokers by changes in the morphology of the olfactory receptor neurons, increased apoptosis of these neurons, reduced volume of the olfactory bulb and nasal inflammation [50].

**N. Idiopathic OD**
OD may be considered idiopathic when a thorough evaluation showed no definite aetiology. Nearly 16% of cases are within this category [51].

## 2.6 Clinical Assessment

- History.
- Examination.
- Olfactory testing.

- Subjective assessment.
- Psychophysical testing.
- Electrophysiology and functional imaging.

## 2.6.1 History

Thorough history-taking should include:

- Is the patient had a problem with their smell or taste concerning flavour or taste concerning gustatory attributes [sour/bitter/salty/umami/sweet]?
- Is their dysfunction quantitative, qualitative or both?
- Are these affecting only specific odours or all odours and severity of dysfunction in terms of frequency [i.e. daily or less] and intensity [i.e. functional hyposmia or anosmia]?
- What treatment had been described to them, and what degree of success had it achieved in improving their condition?

### 2.6.1.1 Onset

Rapid OD is common in post-traumatic OD and post-infectious cases, although a gap of days and weeks between the trauma and recognition of the deficit may occur in the post-traumatic loss.

In neurodegenerative causes, such as ageing and sinonasal disease, smell loss is usually gradual.

### 2.6.1.2 Duration

Early childhood dysfunction indicates congenital anosmia. Dysfunction with long duration is a poor prognostic sign, as in post-traumatic and post-infectious smell loss.

### 2.6.1.3 Course

Chronic rhinosinusitis and nasal allergy are associated with fluctuating olfactory function. Progressive loss is a result of continuous exposure to toxins or drug side effects.

### 2.6.1.4 Other Nasal Symptoms

Symptoms of sinonasal disease must be assessed, including postnasal drip, rhinorrhoea, facial pain, nasal obstruction, itching and sneezing.

### 2.6.1.5 Effect on Quality of Life

- Does the patient describe anxiety or depression as a result of their dysfunction?
- Is their dysfunction causing problems with interpersonal communication or nutrition [including quantified weight change]?
- Does the patient rely on their sense of smell professionally [e.g. chef, sommelier, if the patient is suffering from significant psychological effects? Does the patient live alone?

- Did he experience any home accidents [gas leaks fires etc.]? These patients should be counselled regarding gas and smoke alarms.

#### 2.6.1.6 Past Medical History

Direct questioning about upper respiratory tract infections, nasal or neurosurgical procedures, previous head injuries, and any other chronic diseases that might affect olfaction [52].

#### 2.6.1.7 Medications

Previous and current medication history is important. When a patient has been treated with corticosteroids with improvement in smell, they are likely suffering from a sinonasal disease.

#### 2.6.1.8 History of Smoking, Toxins and Occupational Exposure

##### Family History

Congenital dysfunction may run in family. In older patients. Also, history of neurodegenerative diseases should be assessed.

### 2.6.2 Clinical Examination

A full ENT examination must be done. Nasal endoscopy, to visualize the olfactory cleft, [34]. Whilst nasal decongestant may be used [53]. The topical anaesthetic should be avoided until olfactory testing is performed because it may cause temporary OD [54]. Cranial nerve and peripheral nervous system examination should be done when a neurological aetiology is suspected [55].

### 2.6.3 Olfactory Testing

Three different types of olfactory testing can be undertaken:

1. Subjective, the patient reported an olfactory assessment.
2. Psychophysical olfactory assessment.
3. Olfactory assessment using electrophysiological studies or magnetic resonance imaging.

#### 2.6.3.1 Subjective Assessment

The commonly used Sino-Nasal Outcome Test [SNOT-22] assesses the overall disease burden. But it contains only one question regarding smell disorder [56]. A questionnaire of Olfactory Disorders [QOD], has a greater ability to differentiate between patients with normosmia versus hyposmia [57].

#### 2.6.3.2 Orthonasal Psychophysical Tools

Different features of olfaction can be quantitatively assessed. These features can be divided into suprathreshold and threshold olfactory function. The odour threshold is an odorant concentration where 50% of the stimuli are detected and 50% undetectable.

The suprathreshold olfactory test is the ability to detect odour stimuli of sufficient concentration [i.e. above the threshold level] in an unimpaired person. By varying the odour presented, such tools allow for the testing of odour discrimination and identification abilities. The **odour detection threshold** is not to be confused with the **odour recognition threshold**, which is the concentration of an odour required for recognition or identification. As this test involves the identification of the odorant, it combines elements of both suprathreshold and threshold tasks.

Other tests rely on changes in breathing behaviour with olfactory stimulation, e.g., the **Sniff Magnitude Test** or the recording of respiratory patterns with olfactometric stimulation [58]. The **Alcohol Sniff Test** uses the distance of the odour source from the nostrils as a measure of olfactory function. Subjects close their eyes and an opened alcohol pad is placed 30 cm below the nose. With each exhalation, the odour source is moved 1 cm closer until the patient reports smelling alcohol [59].

Olfactory threshold preferentially tests peripheral causes of olfactory loss, for example due to sinonasal disease, whereas the suprathreshold tests of discrimination and identification preferentially assess central or cognitive causes of olfactory dysfunction.

Some psychophysical olfactory tests were elaborated for research and clinical use. A number of these tests assess one aspect of olfaction, while others assess multiple components, [60] of which the 'University of Pennsylvania Smell Identification Test' [**UPSIT**] is a reliable test [61] UPSIT; known commercially as the Smell Identification Test TM can be self-administered in 10 to 15 minutes by most patients in the waiting room and scored in less than a minute by nonmedical personnel [62].

The "**Sniffin' Sticks**" are another popular psychophysical test battery, the classical version of which tests identification [I], discrimination [D], and odour threshold [T] [TDI] [63]. This tool utilizes reusable odorant 'pens' which are presented to the subject by an examiner. A three-alternate forced choice paradigm is employed for odour threshold and discrimination, whilst odour identification is tested using four-alternate forced choice written/visual cues. Composite 'TDI scores' from the individual subtests are used in diagnosis, and higher scores indicate better olfactory function. Also, the **Connecticut Chemosensory Clinical Research Centre Test** is used to assess odour identification and threshold [64].

### 2.6.4 Olfactory Testing in Children

Olfactory tests have been used in children as young as 5 years. For very young, as young as 4 years, and/or noncompliant children, the 'Smell Wheel' has been used [65]. It contains an 11-odour game-like test where odours are identified using pictures and words.

## 2.7 Diagnosis

Precise olfactory assessment is essential to

- Authorize the credibility of a patient's accusation.
- Delineate the exact fundamentals of the mystery.
- Faithful detector changes in function over time, for both medical treatments and interventions.
- Distinguish who pretends illness.
- Inaugurate reparation for everlasting impairment.

### 2.7.1 Electrophysiological Studies and Imaging

#### 2.7.1.1 Electrophysiological Studies

- Electroencephalography [EEG].
- Electro-olfactography [EOG—the recording of generator potential via an electrode in contact with the olfactory neuroepithelium] [66]. Instead, EEG is useful in medico-legal assessment as well as in patients who might not be able to comply with psychophysical testing.

#### 2.7.1.2 Imaging

- **Conventional imaging:**
- Traditional CT staging of the paranasal sinuses equate substantially with OD; however, it appears that volumetric techniques to assess opacification of the olfactory cleft may provide additional information regarding olfactory function in certain subsets of patients. CT scan is preserved for the detection of post-traumatic olfactory loss or detection of infectious sinonasal diseases, especially fungal sinusitis and to assess bone invasion in tumours [67].
- When the OD is established, but no definite cause is identified, conventional **MRI scanning** may be helpful, the olfactory apparatus [olfactory neuroepithelium, the olfactory bulb and higher pathways] can be assessed, intracranial neoplasms [benign or malignant] excluded, undetected neoplasms in the nasal cavity or paranasal sinuses and asymptomatic chronic inflammation of the paranasal sinuses excluded, and traumatic brain injury characterized [68]. MRI scanning additionally allows for the calculation of olfactory bulb volume, as well as olfactory sulcus depth [67].
- **Biological imaging.**
- It is the visualization, characterization, and measurement of biological processes at the molecular and cellular levels. Diffusion-weighted imaging [DWI] provides microscopic information from water protons which are not possible using conventional magnetic resonance imaging [MRI]. DWI measures the random [Brownian] motion of water protons that indirectly microstructures and cell density. This can be quantified in terms of apparent diffusion coefficients [ADC] [69].
- **Functional Imaging:**

- Functional magnetic resonance imaging [fMRI] and positron emission tomography [PET] allow for the recognition of brain activity in response to odorous stimuli [70]. Both of them exploit diversification in cerebral blood flow to map brain diversity in response to smell stimuli [71]. Diffusion tensor imaging [DTI] enables the delineation of white matter tracts as well as their connectivity in different brain areas [72]. DTI parameters can reveal brain tissue damage in the early clinical stages of neurodegenerative diseases [73].

## 2.8 Treatment of Olfactory Dysfunction

Effective and long-term treatments for OD are still elusive despite considerable efforts within both the clinical and research communities.

### 2.8.1 Medications

Straightaway, medical treatment is the maintainer of treatment in OD. Most clinicians in a previous European survey preferring topical steroids irrespective of aetiology [74].

- **Corticosteroids.**
- Current evidence conjectures the use of both systemic and topical steroids to olfactory loss secondary to chronic rhinosinusitis ± nasal polyposis [75]. Also, extensive guidelines exist for the management of CRS, where corticosteroids are recommended [76] concerning non-CRS-related causes of OD. The literature base is less robustious, and it is hard to draw firm conclusions about the utility of steroids in OD.
- Other studies advocate a possible benefit when systemic steroids are combined with other agents, such as Ginkgo Biloba, vitamin B and Zinc [77]. In addition to anti-inflammatory effects, corticosteroids may lead to the modification of olfactory gene expression [78]. Nowadays, the evidence supporting the use and frequency of systemic steroids, noteworthy in cases of non-CRS-related olfactory loss is penurious [79].
- **Phosphodiesterase inhibitors.**
- Phosphodiesterase inhibitors [pentoxifylline/theophylline] are proposed to ameliorate OD by averting debasement of intracellular cAMP [80].
- **Intranasal calcium buffers.**
- Free calcium within the nasal mucus layer plays a role in negative feedback inhibition of the intracellular olfactory signalling cascade [81]. It is therefore theorized that sequestration of such free calcium, using buffer solutions such as sodium citrate, may lead to amplification of the olfactory signal and consequent improvement in olfactory.
- **Miscellaneous:**

- Coffee: Hosseini A et al. have shown the astonishing result of caffeine in the recovery of smell [82].
- Insulin: Intranasal insulin films were used to manage anosmia in SARS-CoV-2 patients. They surpassed on tests of odour detection and discrimination [83].
- Melatonin: Melatonin is a well-known immune-stimulating, antioxidant, and anti-inflammatory, agent with exceptional safety. Melatonin has a good high permeability and cell diffusion capacity into the blood-brain barrier [BBB], because of its amphiphilic characteristics and tiny size. It restores BBB homeostasis by preventing microvascular hyperpermeability and counteracting SARS-CoV-2-induced neuroinvasion. Moreover, it has a protective effect on olfactory sensory neurons as demonstrated in rat models [84].

### 2.8.2 Platelets Rich Plasma [PRP]

PRP is an autologous biologic extract from fresh whole blood enclosing a high engrossment of platelets. It is reported to have pro-regenerative properties, including upregulation of neuro-regeneration and growth factors, plus an anti-inflammatory effect [85].

### 2.8.3 Olfactory Training

Olfactory training OT entangled inveterate daily exposure to a range of odorants. A group of patients with OD due to post-traumatic, post-infectious, and idiopathic aetiologies underwent OT by Humbell et al. [86]. Forty of their patient endured twice-daily smell training using four odorants: citronellal [lemon], eugenol [cloves], eucalyptol [eucalyptus] and phenyl ethyl alcohol [rose]. At 12 weeks statistically significant improvement in trained patients was noticed; in contrast, the non-training group did not [86]. These results indicated that OT was not related to sniffing but to olfactory stimulation. However, few studies have addressed the effect of training on patients with the sinonasal disease [87]. Despite the exact pathophysiological mechanism for recovery following smell training being hidden, it is hypothesized to involve the increased regenerative capacity of olfactory neurons as a result of repeated odourant exposure. Due to the low cost and high safety of olfactory training, it is an attractive treatment modality, which can be employed with relative indemnity [88].

### 2.8.4 Surgery

Surgery is considered the mainstay of treatment for patients with CRS ± polyps who failed extensive appropriate medical treatment. Many studies showed that olfaction generally improves after functional endoscopic sinus surgery [89]. The utility of surgery in addressing OD due to causes other than CRS is less well established. In a follow-up study, Schriever and colleagues demonstrated that nasal septoplasty had no beneficial effects on olfaction as measured at 1 year [90], though other studies have demonstrated benefit. The effect of septorhinoplasty on olfaction has not yet been sufficiently demonstrated, though some reports suggest that it may lead to improved function [91]. Surgical removal of the olfactory epithelium has been tried in a few patients. This procedure has not been validated and is high risk and should therefore be attempted only as a very last resort and only at an experienced, major medical centre [92].

### 2.8.5 Artificial Intelligence [AI]

Recently, an artificially intelligent olfactory [AIO] system for the diagnosis of OD was developed by a team from Zhejiang University in China. They built an "e-nose" that could "smell" sebum samples from PD patients. It was able to precisely diagnose OD in 70.8% of cases with a sensitivity of 91.7%. They concluded that AIO could distinguish OD, at a late or early stage, from healthy controls [93].

### 2.8.6 Olfactory Bulb Stimulation Using Olfactory Implant

Many studies clearly showed the possibility of placing intranasal stimulating electrodes, above or beneath the cribriform plate, intra- or extracranially. These procedures carry the risk of local or ascending infections like meningitis and CSF leaks. The integral technology of an olfactory implant consists of sensors which determine and distinguish odours [94].

### 2.8.7 Olfactory Mucosa Transplant

Olfactory mucosa can be transplanted into the cortex and the olfactory bulb (OB). Its survival rate is estimated to be 83%. The transplanted olfactory mucosa revealed vesicles in the vicinity of olfactory mucosal cells. Histological studies also showed that the multilayered structure of the olfactory mucosa was preserved, and ciliary-bearing cells were seen on the epithelial surface. Olfactory mucosa can be transplanted into different sites of the cortex, the fourth ventricle and the OB [95].

### 2.8.8 Stem Cell Transplantation

The bone marrow houses progenitor cells, differentiated cells, and a heterogeneous cell population with multipotent stem cells. The plasticity of bone marrow cells permits them to colonize different tissues and differentiate into diverse cell lineages. So bone marrow cells considered a good candidate for cell therapies [96].

An old study manifest that transplanted bone marrow cells can relocate into the olfactory mucosa of the recipient, grow there, and also differentiate into olfactory neuron. Stem cells can be introduced easily by nasal injection. However it is still in the stage of experimental study in animal models. Kurtenbach et al. showed very promising findings with regard to a possible functional restoration of the olfactory mucosa [96].

**Acknowledgements** The authors thank Prof. Essam Kerwash, leading senior clinical pharmacology assessor Medicines Regularity Agency Department of Health, London, United Kingdom, Dr. EH Abdel Goad, Head of the Urology Department, InkoziAlbert Lthuli Hospital South Africa, Prof. Anas M Askora, Prof. Mohamed Salah Mahmoud, and Dr. Ahmed Teaima [Ain Sham School of Medicine] and Dr. Azza Omran, Al-Mataria Teaching Hospital, for their help and support.

## References

1. Ennis M, Hamilton KA, Hayar A. Neurochemistry of the main olfactory system. In: Johnson DA, Lajtha A, editors. Handbook of neurochemistry and molecular neurobiology: sensory neurochemistry. New York, NY: Springer; 2007. p. 137–204.
2. Wilson RS, Schneider JA, Arnold SE, Tang Y, Boyle PA, Bennett DA. Olfactory identification and incidence of mild cognitive impairment in older age. Arch Gen Psychiatry. 2007;64:802–8.
3. Brämerson A, Johansson L, Ek L, et al. Prevalence of olfactory dysfunction: the Skövde population-based study. Laryngoscope. 2004;114(4):733–7.
4. Holbrook E. Clinical assessment and Management of Olfactory Disorders. In: Stucker F, de Souza C, Kenyon G, Lian T, Draf W, Schick B, editors. Rhinology and facial plastic surgery. Berlin, Heidelberg: Springer; 2009. https://doi.org/10.1007/978-3-540-74380-4_10.
5. Wrobel BB, Leopold DA. Clinical assessment of patients with smell and taste disorders. Otolaryngol Clin N Am. 2004;37(6):1127–42.
6. Mueller C, Temmel AF, Toth J, et al. Computed tomography scans in the evaluation of patients with olfactory dysfunction. Am J Rhinol. 2006;20(1):109–12.
7. Garratt M, Neyt C, Ladyman SR, Pyrski M, Zufall F, Leinders-Zufall T. Sensory detection of female olfactory cues as a central regulator of energy metabolism and body weight in male mice. iScience. 2023;26(4):106455.
8. Garratt M, Erturk I, Alonzo R, Zufall F, Leinders-Zufall T, Pletcher SD, Miller RA. Lifespan extension in female mice by early, transient exposure to adult female olfactory cues. elife. 2022;11:e84060. https://doi.org/10.7554/eLife.84060. PMID: 36525360; PMCID: PMC9904757
9. Pellegrino R, Mainland JD, Kelly CE, Parker JK, Hummel T. Prevalence and correlates of parosmia and phantosmia among smell disorders. Chem Senses. 2021;46:bjab046.
10. Landis BN, Frasnelli J, Hummel T. Euosmia: a rare form of parosmia. Acta Otolaryngol. 2006;126(1):101–3. https://doi.org/10.1080/00016480510043954.
11. Leopold D. Distortion of olfactory perception: diagnosis and treatment. Chem Senses. 2002;27(7):611–5. https://doi.org/10.1093/chemse/27.7.611.
12. Hawkes CH. Smell and taste complaints. Boston, MA: Butterworth-Heinemann; 2002. p. 49–50. isbn:978-0-7506-7287-0.
13. Das-Munshi J, Rubin GJ, Wessely S. Multiple chemical sensitivities: a systematic review of provocation studies. J Allergy Clin Immunol. 2006;118(6):1257–64. https://doi.org/10.1016/j.jaci.2006.07.046.
14. Desiato VM, Levy DA, Byun YJ, Nguyen SA, Soler ZM, Schlosser RJ. The prevalence of olfactory dysfunction in the general population: a systematic review and meta-analysis. Am J Rhinol Allergy. 2021;35(2):195–205.

15. Mansour OI, Taha MS, Mahmoud MS, et al. SARS COV-2 and other viral aetiology as a possible clue for the olfactory dilemma. Egypt J Otolaryngol. 2022;38:65. https://doi.org/10.1186/s43163-022-00251-9.
16. Hoffman HJ, Ishii EK, MacTurk RH. Age-related changes in the prevalence of smell/taste problems among the United States adult population. Results of the 1994 disability supplement to the national health interview survey [NHIS]. Ann N Y Acad Sci. 1998;855:716–22.
17. Ros C, Alobid I, Centellas S, Balasch J, Mullol J, Castelo-Branco C. Loss of smell but not taste in adult women with Turner's syndrome and other congenital hypogonadisms. Maturitas. 2012;73(3):244–50. https://doi.org/10.1016/j.maturitas.2012.07.012.
18. Iannaccone A, Mykytyn K, Persico AM, et al. Clinical evidence of decreased olfaction in Bardet-Biedl syndrome caused by a deletion in the BBS4 gene. Am J Med Genet. 2005;132 A(4):343–6.
19. Karstensen HG, Mang Y, Fark T, Hummel T, Tommerup N. The first mutation in CNGA2 in two brothers with anosmia. Clin Genet. 2014;2(607123):293–6. https://doi.org/10.1111/cge.12491.
20. Seiberling KA, Conley DB. Aging and olfactory and taste function. Otolaryngol Clin N Am. 2004;37(1209–28):vii.
21. Hummel T, Smitka M, Puschmann S, Gerber JC, Schaal B. Buschhüter D [2011] correlation between olfactory bulb volume and olfactory function in children and adolescents. Exp Brain Res. 2011 Oct;214(2):285–91.
22. Hummel T, Barz S, Lotsch J, Roscher S, Kettenmann B, Kobal G. Loss of olfactory function leads to a decrease of trigeminal sensitivity. Chem Senses. 1996;21:75–9.
23. Huart C, Eloy P, Collet S, Rombaux P. Chemosensory function assessed with psychophysical testing and event-related potentials in patients with atrophic rhinitis. Eur Arch Otorrinolaringol. 2012;269:135–41.
24. Suzuki M, Saito K, Min W-P, et al. Identification of viruses in patientswith postviral olfactory dysfunction. Laryngoscope. 2007;117(2):272–7.
25. Baker H, Genter MB. The olfactory system and the nasal mucosa as portals of entry of viruses, drugs, and other exogenous agents into the brain. In: Doty RL, editor. Handbook of olfaction and gustation. New York, NY: Marcel Dekker; 2003. p. 549–73.
26. Teaima AA, Salem OM, Teama MAEM, et al. Patterns and clinical outcomes of olfactory and gustatory disorders in six months: prospective study of 1031 COVID-19 patients. Am J Otolaryngol. 2022;43(1):103259.
27. Tong JY, Wong A, Zhu D, Fastenberg JH, Tham T. The prevalence of olfactory and gustatory dysfunction in COVID-19 patients: a systematic review and meta-analysis. Otolaryngol - Head Neck Surg [United States]. 2020;163(1):3–11. https://doi.org/10.1177/0194599820926473.
28. Mahmoud MS, Taha MS, Mansour OI, et al. Prevalence and outcomes of olfactory and gustatory dysfunctions in hospitalized SARS-CoV-2-infected patients. Egypt J Otolaryngol. 2022;38:19. https://doi.org/10.1186/s43163-022-00207-z.
29. Brownstein DG. Resistance/susceptibility to lethal Sendai virus infection genetically linked to a mucociliary transport polymorphism. J Virol. 1987;61(5):1670–1.
30. Fiser DJ, Borotski L. Anosmia after administration of influenza vaccine. Med Pregl. 1979;32:455–7.
31. Delank KW, Stoll W. Olfactory function after functional endoscopic sinus surgery for chronic sinusitis. Rhinology. 1998;36:15–9.
32. Kern RC, Conley DB, Haines GK 3rd, Robinson AM. Pathology of the olfactory mucosa: implications for the treatment of olfactory dysfunction. Laryngoscope. 2004;114:279–85.
33. Rydzewski B, Pruszewicz A, Sulkowski WJ. Assessment of smell and taste in patients with allergic rhinitis. Acta Otolaryngol. 2000;120:323–6.
34. Cowart BJ, Flynn-Rodden K, McGeady SJ, Lowry LD. Hyposmia in allergic rhinitis. J Allergy ClinImmunol. 1993;91:747–51.
35. Gaines AD. Anosmia and hyposmia. Allergy Asthma Proc. 2010;31:185–9.
36. Murphy C, Doty RL, Duncan HJ. Clinical disorders of olfaction. In: Doty RL, editor. Handbook of olfaction and gustation. 3rd ed. New York, NY: Marcel Dekker; 2003. p. 461–78.

37. Doty RL, Yousem DM, Pham LT, Kreshak AA, Geckle R, Lee WW. Olfactory dysfunction in patients with head trauma. Arch Neurol. 1997;54(9):1131–14.
38. Jiang RS, Chai JW, Chen WH, Fuh WB, Chiang CM, Chen CC. Olfactory bulb volume in Taiwanese patients with posttraumatic anosmia. Am J Rhinol Allergy. 2009;23:582–4.
39. Schechter PJ, Henkin RI. Abnormalities of taste and smell after head trauma. J NeurolNeurosurg Psychiatry. 1974;37:802–10.
40. Domellof ME, Lundin KF, Edström M, Forsgren L. Olfactory dysfunction and dementia in newly diagnosed patients with Parkinson's disease. Parkinsonism Relat Disord. 2017;38:41–7.
41. Cecchini MP, Viviani D, Sandri M, Hahner A, Hummel T, Zancanaro C. Olfaction in people with down syndrome: a comprehensive assessment across four decades of age. PLoS One. 2016;11(1):e0146486.
42. Hüttenbrink KB, Hummel T, Berg D, Gasser T, Hähner A. Olfactory dysfunction: common in later life and early warning of neurodegenerative disease. Dtsch Arztebl Int. 2013;110(1–2):1–7, e1. https://doi.org/10.3238/arztebl.2013.0001.
43. Pinto JM, Wroblewski KE, Kern DW, Schumm LP, McClintock MK. Olfactory dysfunction predicts 5-year mortality in older adults. PLoS One. 2014;9(10):e107541.
44. Santorelli G, Marotta A. Olfactometric threshold of the epileptic in basal conditions and after crises: experimental confirmation of data registered in the clinic. Osp Psichiatr. 1964;32:185–90.
45. Martinez BA, Cain WS, de Wijk RA, Spencer DD, Novelly RA, Sass KJ. Olfactory functioning before and after temporal lobe resection for intractable seizures. Neuropsychology. 1993;7(3):351–63.
46. Temmel AF, Quint C, Schickinger-Fischer B, Klimek L, Stoller E, Hummel T. Characteristics of olfactory disorders in relation to major causes of olfactory loss. Arch Otolaryngol Head Neck Surg. 2002;128:635–41.
47. Rochet M, El-Hage W, Richa S, Kazour F, Atanasova B. Depression, olfaction, and quality of life: a mutual relationship. Brain Sci. 2014;8(5):80.
48. Cho SH. Clinical diagnosis and treatment of olfactory dysfunction. Hanyang Med Rev. 2014;34(3):107–15. https://doi.org/10.7599/hmr.2014.34.3.107.
49. Shoenfeld N, Agmon-Levin N, Flitman-Katzevman I, Paran D, Katz BS, Kivity S, et al. The sense of smell in systemic lupus erythematosus. Arthritis Rheum. 2009;60:1484–7.
50. Schriever VA, Reither N, Gerber J, Iannilli E, Hummel T. Olfactory bulb volume in smokers. Exp Brain Res. 2013;225(2):153–7.
51. Fonteyn S, Huart C, Deggouj N, Collet S, Eloy P, Rombaux P. Non-sinonasal-related olfactory dysfunction: a cohort of 496 patients. Eur Ann Otorhinolaryngol Head Neck Dis. 2014;131(2):87–91. https://doi.org/10.1016/j.anorl.2013.03.006.
52. Ottaviano G, Frasson G, Nardello E, Martini A. Olfaction deterioration in cognitive disorders in the elderly. Aging ClinExp Res. 2016;28(1):37–45. https://doi.org/10.1007/s40520-015-0380-x.
53. Hummel T, Rothbauer C, Pauli E, Kobal G. Effects of the nasal decongestant oxymetazoline on human olfactory and intranasal trigeminal function in acute rhinitis. Eur J ClinPharmacol. 1998;54(7):521–8. https://doi.org/10.1007/s002280050507.
54. Welge-Lüssen A, Wille C, Renner B, Kobal G. Anesthesia affects olfaction and chemosensory event-related potentials. Clin Neurophysiol. 2004;115(6):1384–91. https://doi.org/10.1016/j.clinph.2003.12.028.5.
55. Soler G. Evaluación clínica del sentido del olfato: conceptos clínicos básicos y explicación del CCCRC o Test de Connecticut. In: Soler G, Gusto OY, editors. Enfoque Multidisciplinario. Buenos Aires: Acadia Editorial; 2013. p. 65–76.
56. Hopkins C, Gillett S, Slack R, Lund VJ, Browne JP. Psychometric validity of the 22-item Sinonasal outcome test. Clin Otolaryngol. 2009;34(5):447–54. https://doi.org/10.1111/j.1749-4486.2009.01995.x.
57. Soler ZM, Smith TL, Alt JA, Ramakrishnan VR, Mace JC, Schlosser RJ. Olfactory-specific quality of life outcomes after endoscopic sinus surgery. Int Forum Allergy Rhinol. 2016;6(4):407–13. https://doi.org/10.1002/alr.21679.

58. Frank RA, Gesteland RC, Bailie J, et al. Characterization of the sniff magnitude test. Arch Otolaryngol Neck Surg. 2006;132(5):532. https://doi.org/10.1001/archotol.132.5.532.
59. Davidson TM, Murphy C. Rapid clinical evaluation of anosmia. The alcohol sniff test. Arch Otolaryngol Head Neck Surg. 1997;123(6):591–4. https://doi.org/10.1001/archotol.1997.01900060033005.
60. Eibenstein A, Fioretti AB, Lena C, Rosati N, Amabile G, Fusetti M. Modern psychophysical tests to assess olfactory function. Neurol Sci. 2005;26(3):147–55. https://doi.org/10.1007/s10072-005-0452-3.
61. Picillo M, Iavarone A, Pellecchia MT, et al. Validation of an Italian version of the 40-item University of Pennsylvania Smell Identification Test that is physician-administered: our experience on one hundred and thirty-eight healthy subjects. Clin Otolaryngol. 2014;39(1):53–7. https://doi.org/10.1111/coa.12212.
62. Voznessenskaya VV, Klyuchnikova MA, Rodionova EI, et al. A standardized test for evaluation of olfactory function for the Russian population. Biol Bull Russ Acad Sci. 2018;45:485–9. https://doi.org/10.1134/S1062359018050175.
63. Hummel T, Sekinger B, Wolf SR, Pauli E, Kobal G, Hummel T. "Sniffin" Sticks': olfactory performance assessed by the combined testing of odor identification, odor discrimination and olfactory threshold. Chem Senses. 1997;22(1):39–52.
64. Cain WS, Gent JF, Goodspeed RB, Leonard G. Evaluation of olfactory dysfunction in the Connecticut chemosensory clinical research center. Laryngoscope. 1988;98(1):83–8. https://doi.org/10.1288/00005537-198801000-00017.
65. Cameron EL, Doty RL. Odor identification testing in children and young adults using the smell wheel. Int J Pediatr Otorhinolaryngol. 2013;77(3):346–50. https://doi.org/10.1016/j.ijporl.2012.11.022.
66. Gottschlich M, Hummel T. Effects of handedness on olfactory event-related potentials in a simple olfactory task. Rhinology. 2015;53:149–53. https://doi.org/10.4193/Rhino14.204.
67. Herzallah IR, Askar SM, Amer HS, Ahmed AF, El-Anwar MW, Eesa MH. Olfactory bulb volume changes in patients with sinonasal polyposis: a magnetic resonance imaging study. Otolaryngol Head Neck Surg. 2013;148(4):689–93.
68. Lotsch J, Reither N, Bogdanov V, et al. A brain-lesion pattern based algorithm for the diagnosis of posttraumatic olfactory loss. Rhinology. 2015;53(4):365–70. https://doi.org/10.4193/Rhino15.010.
69. Savic I. Imaging of brain activation by odorants in humans. Curr Opin Neurobiol. 2002;12(4):455–61. https://doi.org/10.1016/S0959-4388[02]00346-X.
70. Taha T, Megahed AA, Taha MS, et al. Diffusion tensor imaging: a smart move to olfactory pathway imaging; comparative study of chronic sinonasal polyposis patients and normal control. Egypt J RadiolNucl Med. 2020;51:34.
71. Lundstrom JN, Boesveldt S, Albrecht J. Central processing of the chemical senses: an overview. ACS Chem Neurosci. 2011;2(1):5–16. https://doi.org/10.1021/cn1000843.
72. Torresa CV, Manzanaresb R, Solac RG. Integrating diffusion tensor imaging-based tractography into deep brain stimulation surgery: a review of the literature. Stereotact Funct Neurosurg. 2014;92:282–90. https://doi.org/10.1159/000362937.
73. Le Bihan D. Looking into the functional architecture of the brain with diffusion MRI. Nature Rev Neurosc. 2003;4(6):469–80.
74. Damm M, Temmel A, Welge-Lussen A, et al. Riechstorungen: Epidemiologie und Therapie in Deutschland, Österreich und der Schweiz. HNO. 2004;52(2):112–20.
75. Federspil P, Wilhelm-Schwenk RCJ. Kinetics of olfactory function following endonasal sinus surgery for nasal polyposis. Rhinology. 2008;46:184–7.
76. Orlandi RR, Kingdom TT, Hwang PH, et al. International consensus statement on allergy and rhinology: rhinosinusitis. Int Forum Allergy Rhinol. 2016;6(Suppl 1):S22–209. https://doi.org/10.1002/alr.21695.
77. Jiang RS, Twu CW, Liang KL. Medical treatment of traumatic anosmia. Otolaryngol Head Neck Surg. 2015;152(5):954–8. https://doi.org/10.1177/0194599815571272.

78. Tian J, Pinto JM, Xin Y, et al. Dexamethasone affects mouse olfactory mucosa gene expression and attenuates genes related to neurite outgrowth. Int Forum Allergy Rhinol. 2015;5(10):907–18. https://doi.org/10.1002/alr.21586.276.
79. Guo KJ, Zhao FC, Guo Y, Li FL, Zhu L, Zheng W. The influence of age, gender and treatment with steroids on the incidence of osteonecrosis of the femoral head during the management of severe acute respiratory syndrome: a retrospective study. Bone Joint J. 2014;96-B(2):259–62. https://doi.org/10.1302/0301-620X.96B2.31935.
80. Gudziol V, Hummel T. Effects of pentoxifylline on olfactory sensitivity. Arch Otolaryngol Head Neck Surg. 2009;135(3):291–5. https://doi.org/10.1097/00006534-198006000-00008.
81. Kurahashi T, Shibuya T. $Ca^{2+}$-dependent adaptive properties in the solitary olfactory receptor cell of the newt. Brain Res. 1990;515(1–2):261–8. https://doi.org/10.1016/0006-8993[90]90605-B.
82. Hosseini A, Mirmahdi E, Moghadam MA. Treatment of anosmia and Ageusia in COVID-19 patients by using coffee. Res Square. 2020; https://doi.org/10.21203/rs.3.rs-76002/v2.
83. Mohamad SA, Badawi AM, Mansour HF. Insulin fast-dissolving film for intranasal delivery via olfactory region, a promising approach for the treatment of anosmia in COVID-19 patients: design, in-vitro characterization and clinical evaluation. Int J Pharm. 2021;601:120600. https://doi.org/10.1016/j.ijpharm.2021.120600.
84. Koc S, Cayli S, Aksakal C, Ocakli S, Soyalic H, Somuk BT, Yüce S. Protective effects of melatonin and selenium against apoptosis of olfactory sensory neurons: a rat model study. Am J Rhinol Allergy. 2016;30:62–6. https://doi.org/10.2500/ajra.2016.30.4313.
85. Everts P, Onishi K, Jayaram P, Lana JF, Mautner K. Platelet-rich plasma: new performance understandings and therapeutic considerations in 2020. Int J Mol Sci. 2020;21(20):7794. https://doi.org/10.3390/ijms21207794.
86. Hummel T, Reden KRJ, Hähner A, Weidenbecher M, Hüttenbrink KB. Effects of olfactory training in patients with olfactory loss. Laryngoscope. 2009;119(3):496–9. https://doi.org/10.1002/lary.20101.
87. Fleiner F, Lau L, Goktas O. Active olfactory training for the treatment of smell disorders. Ear Nose Throat J. 2012;91(5):198–203.
88. Bérubé S, Demers C, Bussière N, et al. Olfactory training impacts olfactory dysfunction induced by COVID-19: a pilot study. ORL J Otorhinolaryngol Relat. 2022;85(2):1–10. https://doi.org/10.1159/000528188.
89. Heian IT, Helvik AS, Hummel T, et al. Measured and self-reported olfactory function in voluntary Norwegian adults. Eur Arch Otorrinolaringol. 2022;279:4925–33.
90. Schriever VA, Gupta N, Pade J, Szewczynska M, Hummel T. Olfactory function following nasal surgery: a 1-year follow-up. Eur Arch Otorrinolaringol. 2013;270(1):107–11.
91. Leopold DA, Hornung DE. Olfactory cocainization is not an effective long-term treatment for phantosmia. Chem Senses. 2013;38(9):803–6.
92. Wei F, Linxin X, Qiwen Y, Fang J, Zhao G, Li Y, Pan C, Dong H, Wang D, Ren H, Guo Y, Liu Q, Liu J, Chen X. Artificial intelligent olfactory system for the diagnosis of Parkinson's disease. ACS Omega. 2022;7(5):4001–10.
93. Chiu SW, Tang KT. Towards a chemiresistive sensor-integrated electronic nose: a review. Sensors. 2013;13(10):14214–47.
94. Yagi S, Costanzo RM. Grafting the olfactory epithelium to the olfactory bulb. Am J Rhinol Allergy. 2009;23:239–43.
95. Landis BN, Konnerth CG, Hummel T. A study on the frequency of olfactory dysfunction. Laryngoscope. 2004;114:1764–9.
96. Kurtenbach S, Goss GM, Goncalves S, et al. Cell-based therapy restores olfactory function in an inducible model of hyposmia. Stem Cell Rep. 2019;12:1354–65.

# Epistaxis

3

## An Update on Current Management

Nadine El Hadi, Zeina Kurban, and Usamah El Hadi

**Key Points**

- Epistaxis is a frequent emergency condition in Otorhinolaryngology as well as other specialties in medicine. It spans all age groups and across all genders.
- Hypertension, local nasal trauma, and systemic hematologic diseases as well as coagulopathy were among the most common etiological/risk factors that affects these patients.
- A certain percent who presents with epistaxis remain without an explainable cause for their condition.
- Conservative or nonsurgical methods, ranging from cautery to packing, can be helpful to control epistaxis in many patients.
- More invasive surgical or intervention treatment were reserved for those patients that fail conservative and nonsurgical methods.

## 3.1 Introduction

The accepted definition of epistaxis is that of bleeding occurring from within the inner surfaces and structures of the internal nose. Epistaxis is a common issue that confronts many physicians across different specialties and subspecialties in medicine, many times requiring hospital admissions [1].

**Supplementary Information** The online version contains supplementary material available at https://doi.org/10.1007/978-3-031-70077-4_3.

N. El Hadi · Z. Kurban · U. El Hadi (✉)
Department of Otolaryngology Head and Neck Surgery, American University of Beirut, Beirut, Lebanon


S. Elwany (ed.), *Current Rhinology*,
https://doi.org/10.1007/978-3-031-70077-4_3

It is thought that approximately 60% of the population will be affected by epistaxis during their lifetime, with 6% requiring medical attention [2]. Epistaxis can be either minor, arising from the anterior region of the nose, or more major, arising from the posterior part of the nose [3].

Anterior epistaxis is more common than posterior epistaxis [4]. Kiesselbach plexus, which is a rich vascular anastomotic area formed by end arteries in the nose over the anterior aspect of the nasal septum is the commonest site of anterior epistaxis (80%–90%) [5].

Epistaxis may occur secondary to both local and systemic factors:

- Local causes may be due to different anatomical, inflammatory, infective, traumatic, and neoplastic causes.
- The systemic reasons for epistaxis are diseases that result in coagulopathy, hypertension, liver disease, renal disease, and anticoagulant drugs.

However, in majority of patients (80–90%), the reason remains unknown and is termed as "idiopathic" [6].

Other risk factors associated with nosebleed include prior nasal or sinus surgery, catheters inserted into the nose, CPAP usage, Intranasal application of drugs that lead to nasal mucosa abrasions or septal perforation, and intake of medications that interfere with coagulation or platelet function.

Aggravating factors for the epistaxis can range from nose blowing habit, nose picking that can cause injury to the Kiesselbach plexus that results in anterior epistaxis, excessive coughing, straining in constipation, and benign prostatic hyperplasia (BPH), and upon lifting heavy objects. Diabetes mellitus results in degenerative changes in blood vessels, making them more brittle with secondary bleeding during sudden changes in blood pressure.

Pallin et al. [6] found that epistaxis is more frequent in children younger than 10 years and elderly people above 60 years of age. Males were affected more often than females, with a ratio of 1.6 [7, 8].

Evaluation of patients presenting with epistaxis requires the performance of CBC as well as bleeding and coagulation profile.

Computed tomography (CT) might be ordered in patients for whom the suspicion for a vascular tumor of the sinonasal tract exists.

Varshney and Saxena [9] consider hypertension as the second most common cause of epistaxis. Hypertension is thought to extend the bleeding when it starts due to arterial muscle degeneration that leads to defective contracture of smooth muscles of the blood vessel leading to persistent bleeding. The fact that patients with epistaxis are usually anxious and apprehensive might lead in it is self to transient hypertension due to anxiety.

A study by Min looking at the association between hypertension and epistaxis arrived at the conclusion that hypertension was associated with the risk of epistaxis, yet the association does not provide a contributory relationship between hypertension and epistaxis. Other studies also fail to support any direct relationship [10]. Recently, it was reported that atherosclerosis is one of the potential risk factors in hypertensive patients with epistaxis, and this may have an impact on treatment choices [11].

Nosebleeds are also known to occur in inherited bleeding disorders, such as von Willebrand disease or hemophilia, or in hereditary hemorrhagic telangiectasia [12] it can also be a complication in patients taking anticoagulants and pills or herbal supplements that impair platelet function [13–16].

Hereditary hemorrhagic telangiectasia (HHT) is a hereditary disorder that results in vascular dysplasia and the formation of arteriovenous malformations. Frequent epistaxis is a common presenting symptom of the disease.

The Curacao Criteria published in 2000 traditional diagnostic criteria required for the diagnosis of HHT include (1) recurrent epistaxis; (2) multiple telangiectasias of the face, lips, oral cavity, nasal cavity, and/or fingers; (3) visceral AVMs, typically found in the lungs, liver, gastrointestinal tract, or brain; and (4) a first-degree relative with HHT [16]. The presence of three or more criteria is considered a "definite" diagnosis, whereas two criteria equate to a "possible or suspected" diagnosis. One or zero criterion makes a diagnosis of HHT unlikely [17].

## 3.2 Management

Management of any patient with epistaxis begins with supporting the patient hemodynamically, determining the magnitude of the bleeding and the amount of blood loss and to try to identify the offending bleeder, controlling the bleeding vessel, and trying to treat the underlying disease.

A systematic review on medical treatment is provided by Halderman [18]. There is no definite protocol for the control of bleeding, and methods range from the application of local pressure, topical vasoconstrictor, nasal packing, cauterization (chemical/electric) to embolization or ligation of vessels [19].

The American Academy of Otolaryngology–Head and Neck Surgery (AAO-HNS) created guideline for recommended management of epistaxis:

- Clinicians should treat active nasal bleeding with firm compression to the lower third of the nose (grade C/medium).
- Clinicians should perform anterior rhinoscopy and/or nasal endoscopy to identify a source of bleeding (grade C/medium).
- Clinicians should treat ongoing active bleeding with nasal packing (nonresorbable or resorbable) when source of bleeding is not identified (grade C/medium).
- Resorbable packing should be used for patients with suspected bleeding disorders and those using anticoagulation or antiplatelet medications (grade C/medium).
- Patients with an identified source of bleeding should be treated with topical vasoconstrictors, nasal cautery (anesthetized, directed cautery [grade C]), and/or moisturizing agents (grade B/medium).

- Clinicians should evaluate patients with persistent or recurrent bleeding for candidacy for surgical arterial ligation or endovascular embolization (grade C/high) [20, 21].

The scheme for the treatment of epistaxis depends on site, severity, and etiology of bleeding. Broadly, they are divided into nonsurgical and surgical methods.

A. Nonsurgical/noninterventional treatment:
    1. Observation with topical vasoconstrictor only
    2. Chemical cauterization
    3. Electrocauterization
    4. Anterior nasal packing
    5. Posterior nasal packing
B. Surgical/interventional treatment
    1. Endoscopic sphenopalatine artery (SPA) clipping or coagulation
    2. Endoscopic anterior ethmoid artery coagulation
    3. Embolization
    4. Excision of bleeding mass
    5. Septoplasty

Approximately 80% to 90% of nosebleeds arise from the anterior segment of the nasal septum and can be controlled with constant finger pressure to the lower third of the nose to squeeze the offending blood vessels. Occasionally, applying local vasoconstrictors, such as oxymetazoline, helps to aid in the final control [5].

Anterior nasal packing might be needed to control larger bleeders, whereas posterior epistaxis often requires posterior nasal packing or arterial ligation. Anterior nasal pack was usually held in place for 48 h, whereas posterior nasal pack was removed after 48–72 h. Antibiotic was prescribed to reduce infectious complications.

Chemical cauterization consists of using silver nitrate or trichloroacetic acid or using bipolar diathermy and or suction electrocautery. Monopolar diathermy was associated with a risk of optic or oculomotor nerve damage when used in or close to the orbit [22, 23].

When children present with recurrent epistaxis, it was found that combining cautery with antiseptic cream was not more beneficial than using the antiseptic cream alone. The cream consisted of an antiseptic as well as antibiotic substance, such as Naseptin, that is made up of two active ingredients: chlorhexidine-dihydrochloride, an antiseptic, and neomycin sulfate antibiotic. The antiseptic cream acts as a lubricant to reduce the crusting, thus decreasing recurrent epistaxis whereas the antibiotic further reduces infection [24, 25]. However, there are reports that states that the incidence and seriousness of the nose bleed may be lessened by blending together the antiseptic cream with the nasal cautery versus using the cream alone [26].

Recently, innovative approaches, such as the use of fibrin glue, have been introduced to control bleeding. Fibrin glue is a cryoprecipitate that binds to the injured vessels, thus sealing them and preventing further bleeding. Complications due to fibrin glue were [lesser than those of electrocautery, chemical cautery, and nasal packing. Rebleeding following the application of glue was found to be in the range of 15%, similar to that of electrocautery [27].

Laser was found to be suitable for the treatment of hereditary hemorrhagic telangiectasia [28].

Another medical option for the treatment of epistaxis was the use of tranexamic acid. Both topical and intravenous forms were found to be helpful in controlling epistaxis, and IV tranexamic acid reduced the need for transfusion in emergency or urgent surgery [29].

However, there is some controversy in evaluating the usefulness and safety of tranexamic acid in epistaxis. The study of Janapala et al. [30] showed that patients who were treated with TXA were 3.5 times more likely to attain control of bleeding compared to other standardized methods for the management of epistaxis. Their conclusion is that Topical TXA is helpful in reducing epistaxis compared to the standard practice. Zahed et al. studied 32 patients with anterior epistaxis in the emergency department and found that topical tranexamic acid resulted in rapid control of epistaxis and early discharge from the unit [31, 32].

No trials for the usage of intravenous TXA are available for the control of epistaxis. On the other hand, oral tranexamic acid had no significant benefit, probably due to its inadequate absorption). Two studies assessing oral tranexamic acid in hereditary hemorrhagic telangiectasia showed some benefit [33].

Recently, bipolar cautery devices with integrated suction tips are available, allowing the surgeon to suction and remove blood clots, thus facilitating the identification of the bleeder with prompt cauterization and cessation of the epistaxis. Ahmed and Woolford reported an 89% success rate with endoscopic electrocautery in patients with epistaxis [34].

Anterior nasal packing are usually done with either non-resorbable material such as Merocel, bismuth iodoform paraffin paste impregnated pack (BIPP), Vaseline impregnated gauze, Inflatable 2-balloon catheter [35] and Foley urinary catheters.

Absorbable nasal packing materials that can be used for epistaxis include Surgicel (oxidized regenerated cellulose), Surgiflo (hemostatic gelatin thrombin matrices), Floseal (hemostatic gelatin thrombin matrices), Posisep (chitosan-based polymers), Gelfoam (Purified porcine skin), and Merogel (hyaluronic acid) [36].

In a study done by Corbridge et al., Merocel nasal packing was found to be effective in 85% of cases, with no major benefit compared to regular conservative gauze Strips [37]. The meta-analysis favored absorbable hemostatic agents versus packing [38].

The role of resorbable nasal packing is vital when it is used to control bleeding from patient who are anticoagulated or suffer from HHT whereby removal of non-absorbable packs will pose the risk of abrasion of the nasal mucosa and recurrence of bleeding. It is also of great value in children where removing packs can be both traumatic and predispose to recurrent bleeding.

Absorbable hemostats act as a mesh that stimulate clotting and denote a possible treatment alternative. The three main types of hemostatically active agents are:

1. Adhesive hemostats, which contain fibrinogen or thrombin (e.g., bovine thrombin and fibrin sealants).
2. Mechanical hemostats, which provide platelet activation and aggregation (e.g., oxidized cellulose polymers such as Surgicel®).
3. Antifibrinolytic drugs (e.g., tranexamic acid).

Insertion of nasal packs can cause nasal mucosal disruption, which, in combination with antiplatelet or anticoagulation agents, may in fact contribute to further bleeding during the management episode and/or lead to longer-term sequalae, such as adhesions [39].

Occasionally the nasal packs fail to control the bleeders as it is located in a position where the nasal pack cannot reach and will only be identified by using the endoscope.

Posterior nasal packing becomes an option when anterior packing or other methods fail to control profuse bleeding. It also a vital option when the source of bleeding is not identified and the availability of an experienced endoscopists is unavailable. It can be done either by using conventional pack made from gauze piece or Foley's catheter, or by using a commercially available Inflatable balloon catheter or a combination of packs (Figs. 3.1, 3.2 and 3.3).

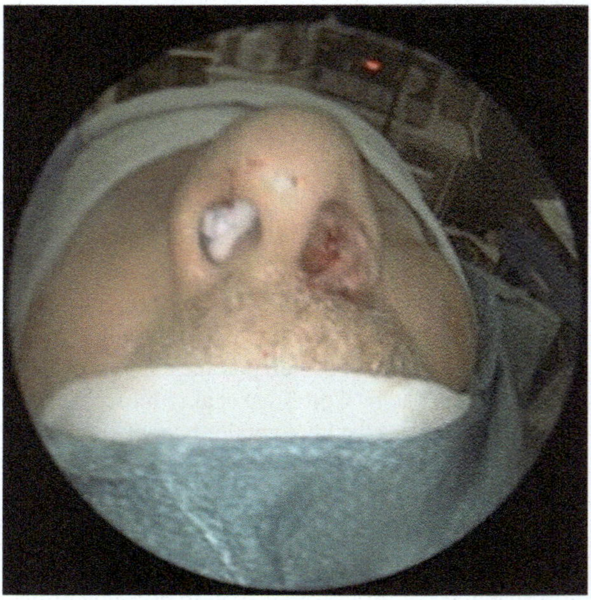

**Fig. 3.1** Nasal packing

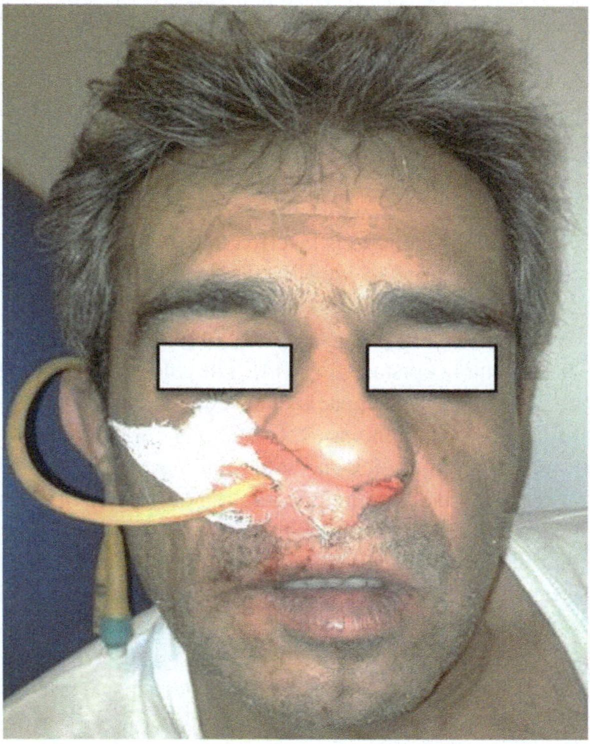

**Fig. 3.2** Foley's catheters

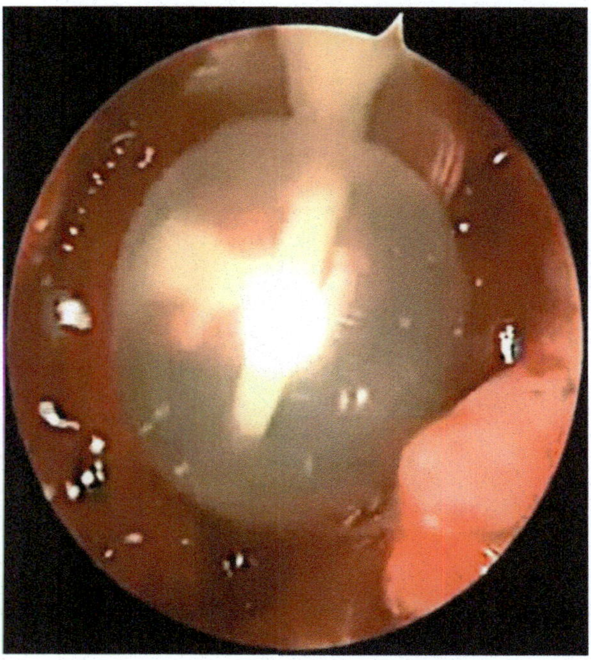

**Fig. 3.3** Pneumatic balloon in place

### 3.2.1 Complications of Nasal Packing

Insertion of nasal packing is not a comfortable process, nor is tolerating it for 48 h. a pleasant experience. Posterior packing is a hazardous procedure and can result in airway compromise or can get dislodged or mispositioned. Synechiae can occur following nasal packing, resulting in nasal obstruction. Nasal septal perforation is another occurrence with bilateral nasal packs (Fig. 3.4). It is prudent to be careful when a Foley catheter is inserted to avoid necrosis of the ala secondary to umbilical clam that is used to hold the Foley in position or from the catheter trunk that is secured to the face [40].

Almost 6% of patients will need more aggressive treatment to control recurrent or intractable epistaxis [41–44]. The role of the endoscope to detect posterior bleeders and control the epistaxis has reduced the need for prolonged nasal packing [45]. In fact, the location and isolation of the SPA has become easy with the endoscope thus facilitating quick and safe route for control (Fig. 3.5).

Endoscopic clipping/coagulation of SPA or endovascular embolization has drastically reduced the need for posterior nasal packing and significantly reduced the morbidity and complication rate with a reported success rate of up to 98% [46]. The procedure is associated with a low rate of postoperative hemorrhage (3.4%) as well as morbidity rate that is comparable to embolization.

The sphenopalatine artery divides posteriorly into two branches, the PLNB and the PSB. The SPA divides into the lateral nasal artery and the posterior septal nasal artery, which supply the lateral nasal wall and posterior septum, respectively. The SPA has 2+ branches immediately medial to the crista ethmoidalis in 97%, 3+ branches in 67%, and 4+ branches in 35% of individuals [47].

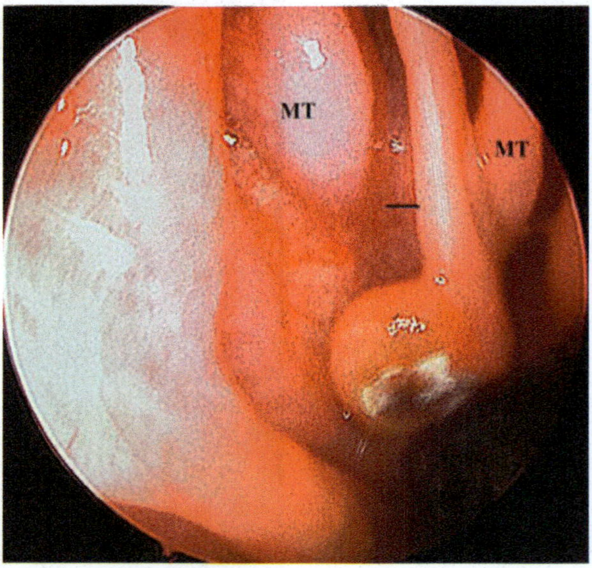


**Fig. 3.4** Septal perforation: The posterior edge of the perforation (arrow) and both middle turbinates (MT) are seen

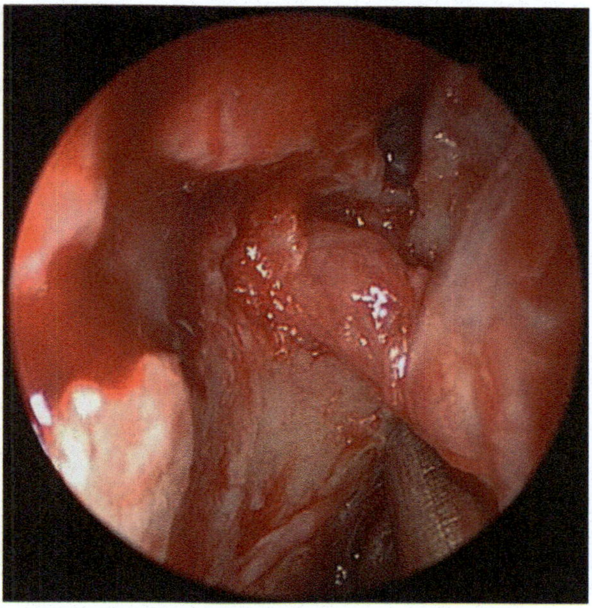

**Fig. 3.5** Sphenopalatine artery

Lee et al. [48] studied the sphenopalatine artery in cadaver heads and found that the SPA has two major branches in 76, three branches in 22%, and four branches in 2% of the explored.

Due to this variation in anatomy of the SPA, failure to recognize and identify all the potential branches can lead to failure to adequately control the offending vessels. Figure 3.6 shows two clipped branches, and Fig. 3.7 shows three clipped branches. Clipping of all branches is necessary for achieving hemostasis. This technique is highly valuable for elderly sick patients with a lot of comorbidities and cannot tolerate nasal packing.

Several surgical techniques exist for ligation of the anterior/posterior ethmoidal artery, the internal maxillary artery, or external carotid artery. These approaches are resorted to when the bleeding vessel is suspected to arise from the roof of the nose or when SPA ligation has failed to control the bleeding (Fig. 3.8). Transnasal endoscopic anterior ethmoid artery ligation requires a preoperative CT scan to check the location of the artery and its proximity to the skull base in order to avoid inadvertently injuring the skull base and resulting in CSF leak or inadvertent penetration of the orbit [49]. Intraoperative bleeding emanating from the anterior ethmoid artery suspended by a pedicle can safely be controlled by bipolar electrocautery unless it is close to the fovea or the orbit.

Ligation of the external carotid artery is a nonspecific method of decreasing blood flow to the nose, with a high failure rate due to the presence of collateral circulation from the opposite external carotid artery [50].

Embolization procedures control nosebleeds in up to 87%, with minor complications in 20% and major complications in up to 2.1%–3.8%. Blindness and stroke are the most feared complications of embolization. These complications are rare but are

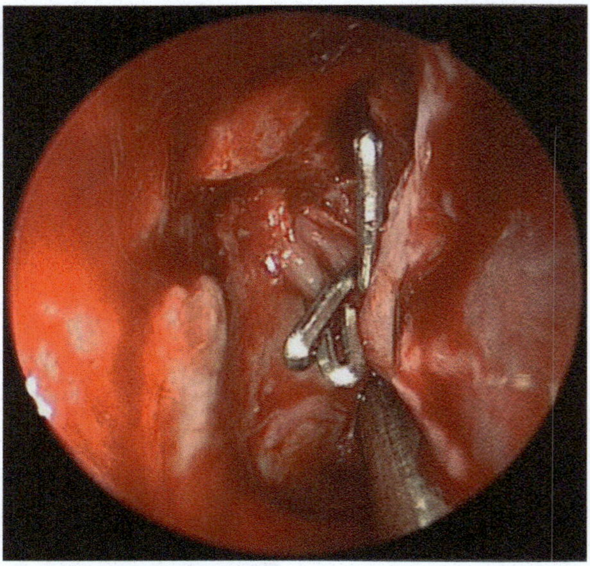

**Fig. 3.6** Two clipped branches of SPA

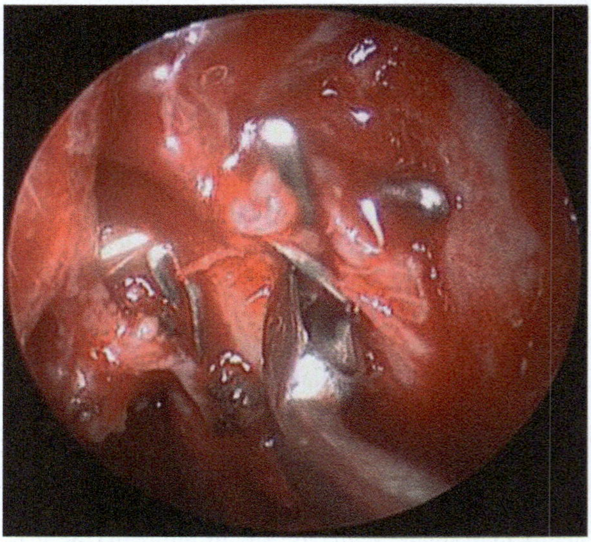

**Fig. 3.7** Three clipped branches of SPA

more frequent than in patients undergoing surgical arterial clipping or coagulation [51, 52].

Angiographic embolization uses coils, gel foam, or polyvinyl alcohol to embolize the bleeding vessel. However, this procedure might be associated with stroke, hemiplegia, ophthalmoplegia, facial nerve palsy, and soft tissue necrosis [53].

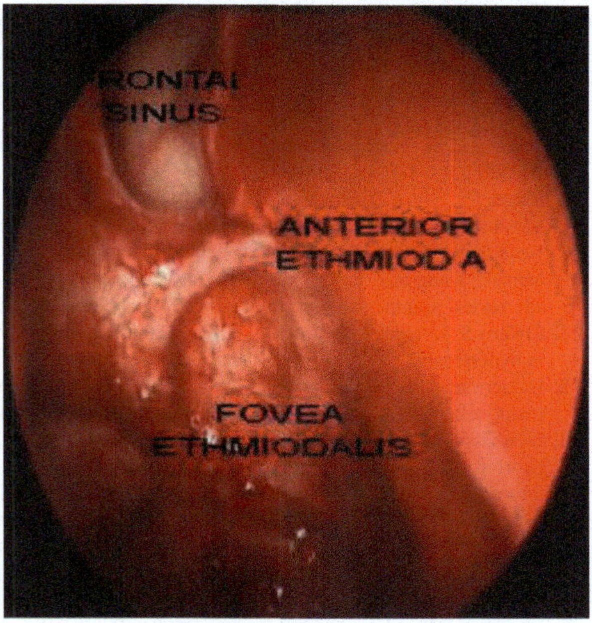


**Fig. 3.8** Anterior ethmoid hanging from the roof close to the fovea ethmoidalis

## 3.3 Conclusion

Epistaxis is a frequent emergency condition in otorhinolaryngology and other specialties in medicine. It spans all age groups and across all genders. Hypertension, local nasal trauma, and systemic hematologic diseases as well as coagulopathy were among the most common etiological/risk factors that affect these patients. A certain percentage of those who present with epistaxis do not have an explainable cause for their condition.

Conservative or nonsurgical methods, ranging from cautery to packing, can be helpful to control epistaxis in many patients.

More invasive surgical or intervention treatments were reserved for those patients that fail conservative and nonsurgical methods.

## References

1. Tunkel DE, Anne S, Payne SC, et al. Clinical practice guideline: nosebleed (epistaxis). Otolaryngol Head Neck Surg. 2020;162(1_suppl):S1–S38.
2. Small M, Murray JA, Maran AG. A study of patients with epistaxis requiring admission to hospital. Health Bull. 1982;40(1):20–9.
3. Walker TWM, MacFarlane TV, McGarry GW. The epidemiology and chronobiology of epistaxis: an investigation of Scottish hospital admissions 1995–2004. Clin Otolaryngol. 2007;32(5):361–5.

4. Ciaran SH, Owain H. Update on management of epistaxis. West Lond Med J. 2009;1:33–41.
5. Seikaly H. Epistaxis. N Engl J Med. 2021;384(10):944–51.
6. Pallin DJ, Chng YM, McKay MP, Emond JA, Pelletier AJ, Camargo CA Jr. Epidemiology of epistaxis in US emergency departments, 1992 to 2001. Ann Emerg Med. 2005;46(1):77–81.
7. Payne SC, Feldstein D, Anne S, Tunkel DE. Hypertension and epistaxis: why is there limited guidance in the nosebleed clinical practice guidelines? Otolaryngol Head Neck Surg. 2020;162:33–4.
8. Huang CL, Shu CH. Epistaxis: a review of hospitalized patients. Chin Med J. 2002;65(2):74–8.
9. Varshney S, Saxena RK. Epistaxis: a retrospective clinical study. Indian J Otolaryngol Head Neck Surg. 2005;57(2):125–9.
10. Min HJ, Kang H, Choi GJ, Kim KS. Association between hypertension and epistaxis: systematic review and metanalysis. Otolaryngol Head Neck Surg. 2017;157:921–7.
11. Elwany S, Ibrahim AA, Soliman AI, Bazak R, Ibrahim HA. The significance of atherosclerosis in hypertensive patients with epistaxis. J Laryngol Otol. 2018;132(4):323–6.
12. Halderman AA, Ryan MW, Clark C, et al. Medical treatment of epistaxis in hereditary hemorrhagic telangiectasia: an evidence based review. Int Forum Allergy Rhinol. 2018;8:713–28.
13. Escabasse V, Bequignon E, Verillaud B, et al. Guidelines of the French Society of Otorhinolaryngology (SFORL): managing epistaxisunder coagulation disorder due to antithrombotic therapy. Eur Ann Otorhinolaryngol Head Neck Dis. 2017;134:195–9.
14. Biggs TC, Baruah P, Mainwaring J, Harries PG, Salib RJ. Treatment algorithm for oral anticoagulant and antiplatelet therapy in epistaxis patients. J Laryngol Otol. 2013;127:483–8.
15. Williams A, Biffen A, Pilkington N, et al. Haematological factors in the management of adult epistaxis: systematic review. J Laryngol Otol. 2017;131:1093–107.
16. Faughnan ME, et al. Second international guidelines for the diagnosis and management of hereditary hemorrhagic telangiectasia. Ann Intern Med. 2020;173(12):989–1001.
17. Shovlin CL, Guttmacher AE, Buscarini E, et al. Diagnostic criteria for hereditary hemorrhagic telangiectasia (Rendu-Osler-weber syndrome). Am J Med Genet. 2000;91:66–7.
18. Halderman AA, Ryan MW, Clark C, Sindwani R, Reh DD, Poetker DM, Invernizzi R, Marple BF. Medical treatment of epistaxis in hereditary hemorrhagic telangiectasia: an evidence-based review. Int Forum Allergy Rhinol. 2018;8(6):713–28. https://doi.org/10.1002/alr.22094.
19. Klotz DA, Winkle MR, Richmon J, Hengerer AS. Surgical management of posterior epistaxis: a changing paradigm. Laryngoscope. 2002;112(9):1577–82.
20. Kasle DA, Fujita K, Manes RP. Review of clinical practice guideline: nosebleed (epistaxis). JAMA Surg. 2021;156(10):974–5. https://doi.org/10.1001/jamasurg.2021.2873.
21. Tunkel DE, Anne S, Payne SC, Ishman SL, Rosenfeld RM, Abramson PJ, Alikhaani JD, Benoit MM, Bercovitz RS, Brown MD, Chernobilsky B, Feldstein DA, Hackell JM, Holbrook EH, Holdsworth SM, Lin KW, Lind MM, Poetker DM, Riley CA, Schneider JS, Seidman MD, Vadlamudi V, Valdez TA, Nnacheta LC, Monjur TM. Clinical practice guideline: nosebleed (epistaxis). Otolaryngol Head Neck Surg. 2020;162(1_suppl):S1–S38. https://doi.org/10.1177/0194599819890327.
22. Schietroma JJ, Tenzel RR. The effects of cautery on the optic nerve. Ophthalmic Plast Reconstr Surg. 1990;6(2):102–7. https://doi.org/10.1097/00002341-199006000-00004.
23. Green KMJ, Board T, O'Keeffe LJ. Oculomotor nerve palsy following submucosal diathermy to the inferior turbinates. J Laryngol Otol. 2000;114(4):285–6.
24. Alsaif A, Karam M, Alhaider A, Almazeedi A, Aldubaikhi A, Alfayez A. The addition of silver nitrate cautery to antiseptic nasal cream for patients with epistaxis: a systematic review and meta-analysis. Int J Pediatr Otorhinolaryngol. 2020;138:110365.
25. Meccariello G, Georgalas C, Montevecchi F, Cammaroto G, Gobbi R, Firinu E, De Vito A, Vicini C. Management of idiopathic epistaxis in adults: what's new? Acta Otorhinolaryngol Ital. 2019 Aug;39(4):211–9. https://doi.org/10.14639/0392-100X-2155.
26. McGarry MG. Recurrent epistaxis in children. BMJ Clin Evid. 2013;2013:0311.
27. Vaiman M, Segal S, Eviatar E. Fibrin glue treatment for epistaxis. Rhinology. 2002;40(2):88–91.

28. Stankiewicz JA. Nasal endoscopy and control of epistaxis. Curr Opin Otolaryngol Head Neck Surg. 2004;12(1):43–5.
29. Perel P, Ker K, Morales UCH, et al. Tranexamic acid for reducing mortality in emergency and urgent surgery. Cochrane Database Syst Rev. 2013;1:CD010245. https://doi.org/10.1002/14651858.CD010245.pub2.
30. Janapala RN, Tran QK, Patel J, Mehta E, Pourmand A. Efficacy of topical tranexamic acid in epistaxis: a systematic review and meta-analysis. Am J Emerg Med. 2022;51:169–75. https://doi.org/10.1016/j.ajem.2021.10.043.
31. Zahed R, Moharamzadeh P, Alizadeharasi S, Ghasemi A, Saeedi M. A new and rapid method for epistaxis treatment using injectable form of tranexamic acid topically: a randomized controlled trial. Am J Emerg Med. 2013;31:1389–92.
32. Zahed R, Mousavi Jazayeri MH, Naderi A, Naderpour Z, Saeedi M. Topical tranexamic acid compared with anterior nasal packing for treatment of epistaxis in patients taking antiplatelet drugs: randomized controlled trial. Acad Emerg Med. 2018;25:261–6.
33. Kamhieh Y, Fox H. ENT department, Royal Glamorgan Hospital, Llantrisant, Wales, UK tranexamic acid in epistaxis: a systematic review. Clin Otolaryngol. 2016;41:771–6.
34. Ahmed A, Woolford TJ. Endoscopic bipolar diathermy in the management of epistaxis: an effective and cost-efficient treatment. Clin Otolaryngol Allied Sci. 2003;28(3):273–5.
35. Elwany S, Kamel T, Mekhamer A. Pneumatic nasal catheters: advantages and drawbacks. J Laryngol Otol. 1986;100(6):641–7.
36. Miller RS, Steward DL, Tami TA, et al. The clinical effects of hyaluronic acid ester nasal dressing (Merogel) on intranasal wound healing after functional endoscopic sinus surgery. Otolaryngol Head Neck Surg. 2003;128(6):862–9.
37. Corbridge RJ, Djazaeri B, Hellier WP, Hadley J. A prospective randomized controlled trial comparing the use of merocel nasal tampons and BIPP in the control of acute epistaxis. Clin Otolaryngol Allied Sci. 1995;20(4):305–7.
38. Milinis K, Swords C, Hardman JC, Slovick A, Hutson K, Kuhn I, Smith ME. INTEGRATE (the UK ENT trainee research network). Dissolvable intranasal haemostatic agents for acute epistaxis: a systematic review and meta-analysis. Clin Otolaryngol. 2021;46(3):485–93.
39. Schlosser RJ. Clinical practice. Epistaxis. N Engl J Med. 2009;360:784–9.
40. Civelek B, Kargi AE, Sensoz O, Erdogan B. Rare complication of nasal packing: alar region necrosis. Otolaryngol Head Neck Surg. 2000;123:656–7.
41. Brinjikji W, Kallmes DF, Cloft HJ. Trends in epistaxis embolization in the United States: a study of the Nationwide inpatient sample 2003-2010. J Vasc Interv Radiol. 2013;24:969–73.
42. Goddard JC, Reiter ER. Inpatient management of epistaxis: outcomes and cost. Otolaryngol Head Neck Surg. 2005;132:707–12.
43. Rudmik L, Leung R. Cost-effectiveness analysis of endoscopic sphenopalatine artery ligation vs arterial embolization for intractable epistaxis. JAMA Otolaryngol Head Neck Surg. 2014;140:802–8.
44. Villwock JA, Jones K. Recent trends in epistaxis management in the United States: 2008-2010. JAMA Otolaryngol Head Neck Surg. 2013;139:1279–84.
45. Limura J, Hatano A, Ando Y, et al. Study of hemostasis procedures for posterior epistaxis. Auris Nasus Larynx. 2016;43:298–303.
46. Kumar S, Shetty A, Rockey J, Nilssen E. Contemporary surgical treatment of epistaxis: what is the evidence for sphenopalatine artery ligation? Clin Otolaryngol Allied Sci. 2003;28:360–3.
47. Man L-X, Fakhri S, Luong AU, Citardi MJ. Chapter 3—Sphenopalatine/internal maxillary artery ligation. In: Chiu AG, Palmer JN, Adappa ND, editors. Atlas of endoscopic sinus and skull base surgery. 2nd ed; 2019. p. 19–24.e1. https://doi.org/10.1016/C2015-0-01193-5.
48. Lee HY, Kim HU, Kim SS, et al. Surgical anatomy of the sphenopalatine artery in lateral nasal wall. Laryngoscope. 2002;112(10):1813–8.
49. Rudmik L, Smith TL. Management of intractable spontaneous epistaxis. Am J Rhinol Allergy. 2012;26:55–60.

50. Spafford P, Durham JS. Epistaxis: efficacy of arterial ligation and long-termoutcome. J Otolaryngol. 1992;21(4):252–6.
51. Dubel GJ, Ahn SH, Soares GM. Transcatheter embolization in the management of epistaxis. Semin Intervent Radiol. 2013;30:249–62.
52. Strach K, Schrock A, Wilhelm K, et al. Endovascular treatment of epistaxis: indications, management, and outcome. Cardiovasc Intervent Radiol. 2011;34:1190–8.
53. Bent JP III, Wood BP. Complications resulting from treatment of severe posterior epistaxis. J Laryngol Otol. 1999;113(3):252–4.

# 4 Biomaterials in Rhinology

Samy Elwany

**Key Points**

- Numerous commercially available sinonasal biomaterials are available. Although several studies compared the utility of these material regarding postoperative hemostasis, several confounding factors existed in most studies. It is interesting to note that PVA appears to be the most popular "standard" to which other biomaterials are compared.
- Collagen-based biomaterials seem to be generally effective in achieving hemostasis, especially when mixed with a coagulation cascade participant, such as thrombin. However, the evidence supporting the wound healing capabilities of these compounds is weak.
- Hyaluronic acid (HA) biomaterials seem to promote wound healing as a class, yet their hemostatic abilities have not been well demonstrated.
- Fibrin glue shows promising results in early trials, although drawbacks unique to this product (e.g., risk for viral transmission) have limited its popularity.
- Among the natural and synthetic biopolymers, chitosan gel appears to stand out as a material that exhibits both hemostatic and wound healing properties.
- A number of studies that found no statistical difference in hemostasis or wound healing between packing (removable or absorbable biomaterials) and no packing after ESS. This may be due to the unnecessity of routine packing post-ESS in many patients.
- Steroid-releasing implants have shown promising results so far in decreasing the inflammatory load and redeciding the rates of adhesion formation. However, it is still too early to predict the long-term benefits that these stents may have on disease course.

S. Elwany (✉)
Department of Otolaryngology, Alexandria University, Alexandria, Egypt
e-mail: samy.elwany@alexmed.edu.eg


S. Elwany (ed.), *Current Rhinology*,
https://doi.org/10.1007/978-3-031-70077-4_4

## 4.1 Introduction

The National Institutes of Health defines a biomaterial as "any substance (other than a drug) or combination of substances synthetic or natural in origin, which can be used for any period of time, as a whole or part of a system which treats, augments, or replaces tissue, organ, or function of the body" [1].

Different types of biomaterials, both nonabsorbable and absorbable, have been developed over the years and used in rhinologic practice to achieve hemostas, and allow better drug, prevent adhesions formation, and allow better topical drug delivery.

The initial reason that nasal packing was developed was to prevent postoperative hemorrhage, a common complication after nasal surgery. Nasal packing and hemostatic gels and foams diminish bleeding via either direct physical pressure on the mucosa or enzymatic activation of the clotting cascade [2].

Another potential complication after ESS is the development of synechiae, which can occur in up to 36% of patients. Adhesions can be particularly problematic when they occur between the middle turbinate and lateral nasal wall, which can prevent access for postoperative debridement, impair adequate mucociliary clearance, and reduce the delivery of topical therapies into the sinus cavities [3, 4].

Third, there has been considerable research to develop implantable spacers capable of delivering continuous, high potency anti-inflammatory medications directly to the sinus mucosa after ESS in the hopes of preventing disease relapse and reducing the need for systemic therapy.

## 4.2 Nonabsorbable Nasal Biomaterials

Nonabsorbable nasal biomaterials are used to prevent postoperative hemorrhage via pressure tamponade. They can also serve as a physical barrier to adhesion formation.

The more commonly used materials used today, including expandable polyvinyl acetate (PVA) foam tampons (Merocel; Medtronic Xomed, Jacksonville, Florida) and related products, polyethylene terephthalate–coated cotton fleece (Telfa; The Kendall Company, Boston, Massachusetts), and carboxymethylcellulose-coated fabric sponges (Rapid Rhino Riemann; Applied Therapeutics, Obernberg, Germany).

There have been numerous trials comparing the efficacy of various nonabsorbable biomaterials in ESS [5]. Investigators have studied various sleeves and coatings on PVA foam. Kim and colleagues found that when PVA was inserted into a latex glove finger, the sheath caused significantly less pain and bleeding on pack removal and improved endoscopic scores during follow-up when compared with plain PVA [6]. Similar findings were produced by Akbari et al. [7]. A recent study compared the efficacy of various PVA coatingsand found that the polyethylene film coating (Merocel 2000) provided best comfort during removal,, followed by oxidized cellulose (Merocel Hemox) and then plain PVA. For hemostasis following removal, the oxidized cellulose coating was most effective, followed by polyethylene film and then standard PVA. All differences reported were statistically significant [8].

Cruise et al. showed that polyethylene terephthalate–coated cotton fleece effectively reduces bleeding, crusting, and adhesion formation after ESS but causes significantly more pain on removal when compared with a carboxymethylcellulose-coated fabric sponge [9].

A major drawback of nonabsorbable packs, which is that they must be removed following their insertion, an event that can cause significant pain and can also induce mucosal tearing and bleeding. Other potential include complications patient's discomfort and toxic shock syndrome [10]. Extensive damage to the nasal has also been reported in animal models [11].

## 4.3 Absorbable Biomaterials

Absorbable biomaterials were first described in the otolaryngologic literature in 1969 with a report on oxidized regenerated plant cellulose for control of hemorrhage [12]. Since then, an increasing number of different classes of absorbable substances have been developed.

### 4.3.1 Classes of Absorbable Biomaterials

- Extracellular matrix-based materials: gelatin film, gelatin foam, flowable gelatin matrix with thrombin, hyaluronic acid (HA) gels, and foams
- Coagulation cascade precipitants: fibrin glue
- Natural and synthetic biopolymers: oxidized cellulose, carboxymethylcellulose, microporous polysaccharide hemospheres (MPH), chitosan, polyurethane foam (PUF), thermosensitive polyethylene glycol poloxamer
- Steroid delivery compounds: PVA, carboxymethylcellulose, PUF, polylactide-co-glycolide stent

### 4.3.2 Extracellular Matrix-Based Biomaterials

Biomaterials belonging to this category are derived from either collagen or HA and are usually formulated as a porous sponge, foam, or gel.

The expansile qualities of **collagen-based substances** are exploited when exposed to blood, which results in tamponade of hemorrhage. These materials also achieve hemostasis through activation of the coagulation cascade through the intrinsic pathway. Some products that incorporate thrombin into the collagen matrix to augment this effect. They may also serve as a temporary spacer, which prevents adhesion formation. The collagen in these materials usually takes the form of gelatin and is often derived from purified porcine or bovine tissue. Complete liquefaction is generally seen in 3–5 days after being placed in the nasal cavity.

Tom et al. examined the utility of middle metal stenting with gelatin film The authors found no significant difference in adhesion formation after the insertion of gelatin films in the middle meatus, arguing against the wound healing efficacy of this product [13].

Multiple proprietary porous, water-insoluble hemostatic gelatin sponge or foam formulations are commercially available (Gelfoam, Cutanplast, and Spongostan). In comparison with PVA, gelatin foam caused significantly less discomfort while in situ and less bleeding on pack removal, although there was no difference in Lund-Mackay scores [14]. Two proprietary formulations of gelatin foam have also been compared and were found to provide equivalent wound healing and hemostatic benefits, although differences were noted in patient comfort [15]. Wee et al. evaluated gelatin foam against an unpacked control and found no differences in subjective symptoms, endoscopic findings, or bleeding events between the two groups [16].

Bovine-derived, granulated gelatin matrix admixed with thrombin has been developed as a flowable compound (FloSeal) for injection into sinus cavities. This admixture was initially has been repeatedly shown to be an effective hemostatic agent in ESS. When compared with unpacked control, the flowable gelatin-thrombin admixture significantly reduced the postoperative bleeding time and the amount of pain while in situ [17]. No difference in crusting or adhesions was noted at 1–3 months. Flowable gelatin-thrombin admixture has also exhibited comparable hemostatic capabilities to a plant-based polysaccharide (HemoStase) [18].

Gelatin sponges can be infused with a solution containing thrombin immediately prior to their insertion for enhanced hemostatic effect but this may result in more granulation tissue and adhesions [19].

As a class, collagen-based biomaterials appear to be effective hemostatic agents in the setting of ESS. While collagen and thrombin are coagulation cascade precipitants and are theoretically proinflammatory, the studies presented here do not demonstrate an increased propensity for adverse wound healing outcomes with the use of these materials [1].

Several **HA-based products** are available for use in ESS and are formulated as a gel, mesh, or foam. Hybrid foams composed of HA and collagen also exist. HA compounds are postulated to increase the rate of re-epithelialization and prevent adhesion formation.

A nasal pack composed of esterified HA (MeroGel) has been on the market for several years. There are conflicting reports about its hemostatic properties and ability to synechiae formation [20–24].

Few studies have evaluated the efficacy of water-insoluble HA polymer gel (Sepragel Sinus) after ESS and reported less edema and granulation tissue after HA gel treatment arm [25].

The hemostatic properties of HA gel were investigated by Frenkiel et al., who found no significant difference in total blood loss between HA gel and unpacked control [26].

Cross-linked HA gel and hyaluronan hydrogel appear to confer good benefit in terms of wound healing, although the evidence consists of a single study for each product. More studies are needed to evaluate the hemostatic abilities of these compounds [27].

### 4.3.3 Coagulation Cascade Precipitants

This class includes agents that primarily promote the coagulation cascade. Fibrin sealants are the sole member of this category in wide use today.

Fibrin glue (Evicel) is a surgical sealant composed of purified human-origin cryoproteins and thrombin that induces clot formation at the site of bleeding. Because this product is composed of pooled human blood products, there is a very small risk of virus transmission. Fibrin glue has been shown to be an effective hemostatic agent when used post-ESS [28]. Although concerns about the proinflammatory properties of this biomaterial have been raised [29]. Unfortunately, this product has not been trialed against negative control.

#### 4.3.3.1 Natural and Synthetic Absorbable Biopolymers

This class of biomaterials includes plant-sourced products, such as oxidized cellulose and carboxymethylcellulose (CMC), MPH, crustacean-derived polymers (e.g., chitosan), and purely synthetic materials (e.g., polyurethane and polyethylene glycol).

Oxidized cellulose, a vegetable-derived product, promotes hemostasis by precipitating platelet aggregation. Despite their widespread use, there is a paucity of literature documenting their effectiveness in rhinology. A powdered formulation of oxidized cellulose (Bloodcare) was reported to be more effective than PVA in preventing postoperative hemorrhage and leads to roughly the same incidence of crusting and adhesion formation [30].

Carboxymethylcellulose is a plant-sourced polysaccharide biomaterial that is a potent activator of the coagulation cascade and is available as a mesh, foam, or gel. Randomized controlled trials have failed to demonstrate the efficacy of the gel or mesh formulations with respect to hemostasis [31] or wound healing [32] when compared with unpacked control.

MPH is a hemostatic nasal packing material produced from potato starch. MPH has been shown to significantly reduce bleeding on postoperative day 1 when compared with negative control [33]. However, the incidence of adhesion formation was equivalent to that of the unpacked control [34].

Chitosan is a biopolymer synthesized via deacetylation of chitin, a major component of crustacean exoskeletons. In addition to its bacteriostatic properties, it is believed to potentiate the coagulation cascade and is commercially available in gel and aerosolized formulations. When [35] compared with a negative control, chitosan gel significantly sinus ostial stenosis [36, 37].

There are currently two purely synthetic absorbable biomaterials on the market: PUF (Nasopore) and polyethylene glycol thermosensitive poloxamer (TPX). Nasopore is a freeze-dried PUF with hydrophilic properties that allow it to function as a metal spacer while permitting fragmentation. It has performed inconsistently with respect to postoperative hemostasis and synechia prevention [38]. Verim et al. showed no difference between PUF and PVA with regard to mucosal healing and re-epithelialization, although PUF caused significantly less pain and nasal obstruction [39]. PUF has not been trialed against negative control.

A TPX composed of polyethylene glycol has been studied as an antiadhesion agent, given its hydrophilic, biodegradable properties. The authors found no significant difference between TPX and HA with respect to adhesion formation [35].

### 4.3.4 Steroid Delivery Compounds

While the above biomaterials may function to prevent postoperative hemorrhage and synechiae formation after endoscopic sinus surgery, they do not ameliorate underlying mucosal inflammation. While oral and topical steroids remain critical components of the medical management of CRS, each has its limitations. Oral steroids are poorly suited for long-term therapy due to their systemic side effects. Topical steroid sprays and irrigations are difficult to reach anatomic regions such as the frontal or sphenoid sinuses. In addition, patients who have issues with compliance are not ideally suited for long-term daily medication treatment. The theoretical advantages of drug-eluting biomaterials include controlled, sustained release of medication to the affected mucosa, as well as adhesion prevention and maintenance of ostial patency.

A variety of different biomaterials, such as budesonide-soaked Merocel and CMC foam impregnated with dexamethasone, have been investigated as possible drug delivery systems with very limited beneficial effect on epithelial healing and adhesion formations [40, 41].

Côté and Wright compared triamcinolone-soaked PUF with saline control inserted after ESS. As determined via endoscopic scores, nasal cavities receiving triamcinolone-soaked PUF had significantly improved wound healing when compared with the saline control, suggesting that steroid-soaked PUF may be effective at reducing local inflammation after ESS [42].

An expandable polylactide-co-glycolide polymer impregnated with mometasone furoate (Propel) has been studied as a steroid-releasing implant. Each implant contains 370 μg of steroid medication, 90% of which is released by day 13; 85% of the implant is reabsorbed by day 30. Two prospective trials investigated the efficacy of this steroid-releasing implant, the first of which was conducted by Murr et al. [43]. The cavities that received the steroid implant had significant reductions in inflammation, frequency of polyp formation, and incidence of adhesions when compared with nasal cavities that received the untreated implant. The authors reported no detectable systemic steroid exposure [43]

In a similar study design, Marple et al. focused on how the steroid-releasing implant affected postoperative interventions [44] Compared with the negative control cavity, the authors showed a significant relative reduction in overall postoperative interventions, as well as a significant decrease in incidence of frank polyposis [44].

Preliminary evidence suggests improved wound healing and reduced inflammation when steroid-releasing implants are used post-ESS. Other steroid-soaked biodegradable foam applications appear less efficacious in reducing inflammation but might represent a less expensive alternative. Further investigations need to be performed before this new technology can be considered for widespread use, taking into consideration its long-term results and cost-effectiveness regimens.

## 4.4 Conclusions

Biomaterials continue to play a vital role in rhinology, as they have for the past 60 years. Ideally, a rhinologic biomaterial would decrease postoperative bleeding, improve healing, and decrease inflammation after ESS. A large number of biomaterials with differing properties have been studied to varying degrees. Certain products do seem to be more effective than others in reducing postoperative complications and producing better outcomes, although the heterogeneity among studies does not allow for the selection of a superior biomaterial for ESS.

While nonabsorbable biomaterials are still effective in providing certain important functions, newer, absorbable substances may be just as effective in avoiding the morbidity associated with packing removal.

Given that CRS is a disease characterized primarily by inflammation, drug-eluting systems may play an increasingly important role in preventing disease recurrence and improving outcomes. However, more studies are needed on this newer technology before it can be considered for widespread use. As evidenced by the growing number of products released over the past decade, there will likely be many more exciting developments to come in this continually expanding field.

## References


1. Massey CJ, Suh JD, Tessema B, Gray ST, Singh A. Biomaterials in rhinology. Otolaryngol Head Neck Surg. 2016;154:606–17.
2. Stankiewicz JA, Lal D, Connor M, Welch K. Complications in endoscopic sinus surgery for chronic rhinosinusitis: a 25-year experience. Laryngoscope. 2011;121:2684–701.
3. Ramadan HH. Surgical causes of failure in endoscopic sinus surgery. Laryngoscope. 1999;109:27–9.
4. Thornton RS. Middle turbinate stabilization technique in endoscopic sinus surgery. Arch Otolaryngol Head Neck Surg. 1996;122:869–72.
5. Budu V, Panfiloiu A, Guliga A, Decuseara T, Costache A-N, Mistra D, Sava L, Bulescu IA, Tusaliu M. Compatible biomaterials used in rhinology surgery—our expertise. Sci Bull Electr Eng Faculty. 2017;17:35–7.
6. Kim DW, Lee E-J, Kim S-W, Jeon S-Y. Advantages of glove finger-coated polyvinyl acetate pack in endoscopic sinus surgery. Am J Rhinol Allergy. 2012;26:e147–9.
7. Akbari E, Philpott CM, Ostry AJ, Clark A, Javer AR. A double-blind randomised controlled trial of gloved versus ungloved merocel middle meatal spacers for endoscopic sinus surgery. Rhinology. 2012;50:306–10.
8. Melis A, Karligkiotis A, Bozzo C, Machouchas N, Volpi L, Castiglia P, Castelnuovo P, Meloni F. Comparison of three different polyvinyl alcohol packs following functional endoscopic nasal surgery. Laryngoscope. 2015;125:1067–71.
9. Cruise AS, Amonoo-Kuofi K, Srouji I, Kanagalingam J, Georgalas C, Patel NN, Badia L, Lund VJ. A randomized trial of rapid rhino Riemann and Telfa nasal packs following endoscopic sinus surgery. Clin Otolaryngol. 2006;31:25–32.

10. Weber RK. Nasal packing and stenting. GMS Curr Top Otorhinolaryngol Head Neck Surg. 2009;8:Doc02.
11. Shaw CL, Dymock RB, Cowin A, Wormald PJ. Effect of packing on nasal mucosa of sheep. J Laryngol Otol. 2000;114:506–9.
12. Huggins S. Control of hemorrhage in otorhinolaryngologic surgery with oxidized regenerated cellulose. Eye Ear Nose Throat Mon. 1969;48:420–3.
13. Tom LW, Palasti S, Potsic WP, Handler SD, Wetmore RF. The effects of gelatin film stents in the middle meatus. Am J Rhinol. 1997;11:229–32.
14. Cho K-S, Shin S-K, Lee J-H, Kim J-Y, Koo S-K, Kim Y-W, Kim M-J, Roh H-J. The efficacy of Cutanplast nasal packing after endoscopic sinus surgery: a prospective, randomized, controlled trial. Laryngoscope. 2013;123:564–8.
15. Cho K-S, Park C-H, Hong S-L, Kim M-J, Kim J-Y, Kim Y-W, Koo S-K, Roh H-J. Comparative analysis of Cutanplast and Spongostan nasal packing after endoscopic sinus surgery: a prospective, randomized, multicenter study. Eur Arch Otorrinolaringol. 2015;272:1699–705.
16. Wee JH, Lee CH, Rhee CS, Kim J-W. Comparison between Gelfoam packing and no packing after endoscopic sinus surgery in the same patients. Eur Arch Otorrinolaringol. 2012;269:897–903.
17. Gall RM, Witterick IJ, Shargill NS, Hawke M. Control of bleeding in endoscopic sinus surgery: use of a novel gelatin-based hemostatic agent. J Otolaryngol. 2002;31:271–4.
18. Jameson M, Gross CW, Kountakis SE. FloSeal use in endoscopic sinus surgery: effect on postoperative bleeding and synechiae formation. Am J Otolaryngol. 2006;27:86–90.
19. Chandra RK, Conley DB, Kern RC. The effect of FloSeal on mucosal healing after endoscopic sinus surgery: a comparison with thrombin-soaked gelatin foam. Am J Rhinol. 2003;17:51–5.
20. Franklin JH, Wright ED. Randomized, controlled, study of absorbable nasal packing on outcomes of surgical treatment of rhinosinusitis with polyposis. Am J Rhinol. 2007;21:214–7.
21. Wormald PJ, Boustred RN, Le T, Hawke L, Sacks R. A prospective single-blind randomized controlled study of use of hyaluronic acid nasal packs in patients after endoscopic sinus surgery. Am J Rhinol. 2006;20:7–10.
22. Miller RS, Steward DL, Tami TA, Sillars MJ, Seiden AM, Shete M, Paskowski C, Welge J. The clinical effects of hyaluronic acid ester nasal dressing (Merogel) on intranasal wound healing after functional endoscopic sinus surgery. Otolaryngol Head Neck Surg. 2003;128:862–9.
23. Berlucchi M, Castelnuovo P, Vincenzi A, Morra B, Pasquini E. Endoscopic outcomes of resorbable nasal packing after functional endoscopic sinus surgery: a multicenter prospective randomized controlled study. Eur Arch Otorrinolaringol. 2009;266:839–45.
24. Hu K-H, Lin K-N, Li W-T, Huang H-M. Effects of Meropack in the middle meatus after functional endoscopic sinus surgery in children with chronic sinusitis. Int J Pediatr Otorhinolaryngol. 2008;72:1535–40.
25. Kimmelman CP, Edelstein DR, Cheng HJ. Sepragel sinus (hylan B) as a postsurgical dressing for endoscopic sinus surgery. Otolaryngol Head Neck Surg. 2001;125:603–8.
26. Frenkiel S, Desrosiers MY, Nachtigal D. Use of hylan B gel as a wound dressing after endoscopic sinus surgery. J Otolaryngol. 2002;31(Suppl 1):S41–4.
27. Shi R, Zhou J, Wang B, Wu Q, Shen Y, Wang P, Wang J, Wang Y, Chen Y, Shu XZ. The clinical outcomes of new hyaluronan nasal dressing: a prospective, randomized, controlled study. Am J Rhinol Allergy. 2013;27:71–6.
28. Vaiman M, Eviatar E, Shlamkovich N, Segal S. Use of fibrin glue as a hemostatic in endoscopic sinus surgery. Ann Otol Rhinol Laryngol. 2005;114:237–41.
29. Erkan AN, Cakmak O, Kocer NE, Yilmaz I. Effects of fibrin glue on nasal septal tissues. Laryngoscope. 2007;117:491–6.
30. Al-Shaikh S, Muddaiah A, Lee RJ, Bhutta MF. Oxidised cellulose powder for haemostasis following sinus surgery: a pilot randomised trial. J Laryngol Otol. 2014;128:709–13.
31. Kastl KG, Betz CS, Siedek V, Leunig A. Control of bleeding following functional endoscopic sinus surgery using carboxy-methylated cellulose packing. Eur Arch Otorrinolaringol. 2009;266:1239–43.

32. Kastl KG, Betz CS, Siedek V, Leunig A. Effect of carboxymethylcellulose nasal packing on wound healing after functional endoscopic sinus surgery. Am J Rhinol Allergy. 2009;23:80–4.
33. Akiyama K, Karaki M, Yonezaki M, Goto R, Inamoto R, Hoshikawa H, Mori N. Usefulness of nasal packing with silver-containing carboxy methylated cellulose in endonasal sinus surgery. Auris Nasus Larynx. 2014;41:264–8.
34. Antisdel JL, West-Denning JL, Sindwani R. Effect of microporous polysaccharide hemospheres (MPH) on bleeding after endoscopic sinus surgery: randomized controlled study. Otolaryngol Head Neck Surg. 2009;141:353–7.
35. Song KJ, Lee HM, Lee EJ, Kwon JH, Jo KH, Kim K-S. Anti-adhesive effect of a thermosensitive poloxamer applied after the removal of nasal packing in endoscopic sinus surgery: a randomised multicentre clinical trial. Clin Otolaryngol. 2013;38:225–30.
36. Ngoc Ha T, Valentine R, Moratti S, Robinson S, Hanton L, Wormald P-J. A blinded randomized controlled trial evaluating the efficacy of chitosan gel on ostial stenosis following endoscopic sinus surgery. Int Forum Allergy Rhinol. 2013;3:573–80.
37. Valentine R, Athanasiadis T, Moratti S, Hanton L, Robinson S, Wormald P-J. The efficacy of a novel chitosan gel on hemostasis and wound healing after endoscopic sinus surgery. Am J Rhinol Allergy. 2010;24:70–5.
38. Shoman N, Gheriani H, Flamer D, Javer A. Prospective, double-blind, randomized trial evaluating patient satisfaction, bleeding, and wound healing using biodegradable synthetic polyurethane foam (NasoPore) as a middle meatal spacer in functional endoscopic sinus surgery. J Otolaryngol Head Neck Surg. 2009;38:112–8.
39. Verim A, Seneldir L, Naiboğlu B, Karaca ÇT, Külekçi S, Toros SZ, Oysu Ç. Role of nasal packing in surgical outcome for chronic rhinosinusitis with polyposis. Laryngoscope. 2014;124:1529–35.
40. Rudmik L, Mace J, Mechor B. Effect of a dexamethasone Sinu-foam™ middle meatal spacer on endoscopic sinus surgery outcomes: a randomized, double-blind, placebo-controlled trial. Int Forum Allergy Rhinol. 2012;2:248–51.
41. Chang EH, Alandejani T, Akbari E, Ostry A, Javer A. Double-blinded, randomized, controlled trial of medicated versus nonmedicated merocel sponges for functional endoscopic sinus surgery. J Otolaryngol Head Neck Surg. 2011;40(Suppl 1):S14–9.
42. Côté DWJ, Wright ED. Triamcinolone-impregnated nasal dressing following endoscopic sinus surgery: a randomized, double-blind, placebo-controlled study. Laryngoscope. 2010;120:1269–73.
43. Murr AH, Smith TL, Hwang PH, Bhattacharyya N, Lanier BJ, Stambaugh JW, Mugglin AS. Safety and efficacy of a novel bioabsorbable, steroid-eluting sinus stent. Int Forum Allergy Rhinol. 2011;1:23–32.
44. Marple BF, Smith TL, Han JK, Gould AR, Jampel HD, Stambaugh JW, Mugglin AS. Advance II: a prospective, randomized study assessing safety and efficacy of bioabsorbable steroid-releasing sinus implants. Otolaryngol Head Neck Surg. 2012;146:1004–11.

# Headache and Facial Pain

5

Usama Abdel Naseer

**Key Points**

- Rhinologists frequently encounter patients with headache and/or facial pain.
- Many of these cases are part of a primary headache disorder or less frequently related to secondary head and neck diseases, making the diagnostic process more difficult.
- Rhinologists have a responsibility to be familiar with both primary and secondary headaches to reach the correct diagnosis and provide appropriate, timely treatment.
- The key to finding the correct diagnosis in each individual presenting with headache is to perform a stepwise, comprehensive evaluation of the patient, appropriate medical examination, and imaging if indicated.

## 5.1 Classification

Headache is probably the most common complaint that leads people to seek medical advice [1]. It is estimated that approximately one-half of the adult population is affected by a headache disorder every year [2]. In addition to primary care doctors and emergency room physicians, otolaryngologists, neurologists, and internists see most of these patients.

Headaches are classified as primary or secondary headaches. Primary headaches are idiopathic and have no underlying cause, with the most common being tension-type headaches, migraines, and cluster headaches, which affect approximately 40%, 10%, and 1% of the adult population, respectively [3].

U. A. Naseer (✉)
Department of Otolaryngology, Cairo University, Cairo, Egypt


S. Elwany (ed.), *Current Rhinology*,
https://doi.org/10.1007/978-3-031-70077-4_5

**Table 5.1** International classification of headache disorders, 3rd ed. (ICHD-3) [4]

| |
|---|
| **Primary headaches** |
| • Migraine |
| • Tension-type |
| • Trigeminal autonomic cephalalgias (e.g., cluster headache) |
| • Other primary headache disorders (e.g., cold-stimulus headache and primary cough headache) |
| **Secondary headaches** |
| • Headache attributed to any of the following: Head or neck trauma, cranial or cervical vascular disorder, nonvascular intracranial disorder, substance use or withdrawal, infection, disturbance of homeostasis, psychiatric disorder |
| • Headache or facial pain attributed to a disorder of the cranium, neck, eyes, ears, nose, sinuses, teeth, mouth, or other facial or cranial structures (e.g., acute, chronic, or recurring rhinosinusitis, temporomandibular disorder). |
| **Painful lesions of the cranial nerves and other facial pain** |
| • Pain attributed to a lesion or disease of the trigeminal nerve, glossopharyngeal nerve, nervus intermedius, and central idiopathic pain. |

Secondary headache disorders occur when a definitive cause or relevant underlying pathology is present. Therefore, secondary headaches include headaches attributed to infection, trauma, hypertension, and so forth.

The International Headache Society (IHS) has published a system of classification and operational diagnostic criteria for headaches based on clinical consensus, including primary headaches, secondary headaches, painful lesions of the cranial nerves, and other facial pain disorders. The classification thus established criteria based on the characteristics of the headache and describes 14 different categories (Table 5.1) [4].

## 5.2 Evaluation and Diagnostic Approach

Despite being a common symptom, it is difficult to evaluate, given its wide range of clinical presentations and etiologies. The diagnostic and therapeutic approach to these patients, therefore, requires a working knowledge of common headache diagnostic criteria and a straightforward algorithm for clinical decision-making that facilitates the initial evaluation and appropriate treatment of the patients [5].

Headache is defined in terms of frequency, duration, and severity and in terms of quality, size, and accompanying factors such as photophobia, nausea, or vomiting. The most critical question in evaluating headache history is to establish whether the headache is of primary or secondary type. The new-onset headache should undergo assessment for the secondary causes.

Many of patients with headache / facial pain often present to the rhinologist with "sinus headache," which is a widely used terminology in the medical field. Patients with pain or pressure in or around the maxillary, ethmoid, or frontal regions as well as mandibular or temporal pain, often blame the sinuses for this pain based on the rationale that if a structure is in direct proximity where the pain or pressure is located, it is likely the cause of the problem [3]. These cases frequently represent a diagnostic challenge because of the associated systemic complaints and overlapping symptomatology common to many headache etiologies.

Primary headaches are essentially recurrent headaches. When headache is recurrent, the next important question is if the current episode is like prior headaches. If this headache is like the previous headaches, a primary headache disorder is the most likely diagnosis. If the present headache is different from the previous headache episodes or it is a new-onset headache, an evaluation for the secondary causes is necessary [3].

Asking about the intensity and pain distribution is helpful because higher pain levels and unilaterality are associated with migraines or cluster headache. Daily and constant pain is unlikely to be of sinonasal origin. Pressing symmetric pain in the face and temples is indicative of tension-type pain, which is rarely severe and may be associated with "trigger points" located in the neck, shoulders, and head muscles. Palpation of the temporomandibular joints for tenderness on jaw opening and percussion of the teeth may be helpful, as is the examination of cranial nerves, particularly the trigeminal nerve [6].

The key to finding the correct diagnosis in each individual presenting with headache to the otolaryngology clinic is to perform a stepwise, comprehensive evaluation of the patient, including an extensive history, nasal endoscopy, thorough head and neck examination, and imaging, if indicated. The main goal is to diagnose the true cause of the symptoms and confirm or rule out any potential otolaryngologic causes. It is also important to consider that headache can be multifactorial, and the combination of different diagnostic modalities can provide more of the information necessary to elucidate each case [7].

## 5.3 Primary Headaches

A general understanding of primary headaches will assist in timely diagnosis and treatment. According to the ICHD, there are four broad categories of primary headaches including migraine, tension-type, trigeminal-autonomic cephalgia, and other primary headache disorders. There are more than 20 subclassifications within these categories.

In general, it is important to differentiate the duration of episodes as less than or greater than 4 h per day, and the frequency as less than or greater than 15 days per month [8].

### 5.3.1 Tension-type Headaches

Tension-type headaches are the most prevalent headache globally, with a lifetime prevalence of 78%. This type of headache is most prevalent between the ages of 30–39 and is higher in females. Tension-type headaches are usually described as mild to moderate, bilateral or band-like pressure and tightness.

Episodes last from a few minutes to several days can be waxing and waning. Usually, they are not exacerbated by routine physical activity. With more severe cases, patients may also experience throbbing or pulsatile pain and photophobia, which can make it difficult to differentiate from migraine [9, 10]. In frequent episodic tension-type headaches here are at least 10 episodes occurring on less than 15 days/month for more than 3 months.

## 5.3.2 Migraines

Migraines are the second most prevalent primary headache and are the third-highest cause of disability globally in people younger than 50 years old.

Episodes can start as early as childhood or teenage years. They are categorized into two major types: migraine with or without aura. An aura is described as a focal neurologic symptom that occurs before or at the onset of a migraine and fully resolves spontaneously. These auras can range from visual disturbances, sensory abnormalities, aphasia, hemiplegia, or vertigo.

Migraine is usually described as unilateral pulsating pain in the temple but can also be bitemporal or involve the whole head. It has a gradual onset with a crescendo of pain rated moderate to severe. Associated symptoms include nausea, emesis, photophobia, and phonophobia. The episodes last 4–72 h and are worse with activity, resulting in patients seeking a dark and quiet room for relief. Also, there is a known association between migraines and vestibular symptoms.

Episodic vertigo can occur in up to 25% of migraine patients, and these vertiginous episodes can have an abrupt onset, last days, and often occur during headache-free times [9, 11–13].

### 5.3.2.1 Migraine Without Aura

The patient should have at least five attacks fulfilling the following criteria and not attributed to another disorder:

- Headache attacks lasting 4–72 h (untreated or unsuccessfully treated).
- Headache has at least two of the following characteristics:
  - Moderate or severe pain intensity.
  - Pulsating quality.
  - Unilateral location.
  - Aggravation by routine physical activity (e.g., walking or climbing stairs).
- During headache at least 1 of the following:
  - Photophobia and phonophobia.
  - Nausea and/or vomiting.

### 5.3.2.2 Migraine With Aura

- At least two attacks of typical aura with migraine headache.
- Aura lasts <1 h and immediately precedes headache and may be precipitated by certain foods, or bright lights.

- Aura consists of at least one of the following:
  - Fully reversible visual symptoms including positive features (e.g., flickering lights, spots, or lines) and/or negative features (i.e., loss of vision).
  - Fully reversible sensory symptoms including positive features (i.e., pins and needles) and/or negative features (i.e., numbness).
  - No motor weakness.
  - At least one aura symptom develops gradually over 5 or more minutes and/or different aura symptoms occur in succession over 5 or more minutes. Each symptom lasts more than 5 and less than 60 min.
- Headache fulfilling the same criteria as migraine without aura begins during the aura or follows aura within 60 min.

Other types of migraine include typical aura with non-migraine headache, typical aura without headache, familial hemiplegic migraine, sporadic hemiplegic migraine, and Basilar-type migraine.

### 5.3.3 Cluster Headaches

Cluster headaches are a subcategory of trigeminal-autonomic cephalgia and are separated into episodic and chronic and are considered as one of the most severe primary headache disorders.

Cluster headaches are more common in middle-aged patients. They affect around 1 in 1000 people worldwide. Cluster headache has historically been considered a male disorder as it's reported to be two to five times more common among men. The headaches are more common in autumn and spring.

Cluster headaches are usually described as quick onset, unilateral, deep, and constant pain near the temple or eye. It reaches maximum intensity within minutes, and episodes last 15 min to 3 h. Associated symptoms include ipsilateral lacrimation, ocular erythema, nasal congestion, rhinorrhea, pallor, diaphoresis, or Horner syndrome. The attacks have a frequency from 1 every other day to 8/day. They may also tend to happen at night. The headaches occur several times per day for several weeks and then have symptom-free periods (Episodic cluster headaches) [9, 11]. In chronic cluster headache. The attacks recur over more than 1 year without remission periods or with remission periods lasting less than 1 month.

Diagnosis of cluster headaches requires at least five attacks fulfilling the following criteria:

- Severe or very severe unilateral orbital, supraorbital, and/or temporal pain lasting 15–180 min if untreated.
- Headache is accompanied by at least 1 of the following:
  - Ipsilateral conjunctival injection and/or lacrimation
  - Ipsilateral nasal congestion and/or rhinorrhea
  - Ipsilateral eyelid oedema
  - Ipsilateral forehead and facial sweating

- Ipsilateral miosis and/or ptosis
- A sense of restlessness or agitation

## 5.4 Secondary Headaches

Secondary headache or facial pain attributed to disorders of the sinuses, cranium, eyes, ears, teeth, or other facial structures is a distinct category. Table 5.2 lists the causes of secondary headaches organized by anatomic location [5].

Secondary headaches with red flag symptoms, such as fever, neurologic signs, papilledema, or postural changes, should also be considered with high degree of suspicion [14]. Other warning signs include sudden onset (thunderclap headache), age of onset less than 5 years or more than 65 years, and changes in the pattern of headaches.

Systemic signs such as fever, chills, weight loss, myalgia, or diaphoresis can point toward infection, malignancy, vasculitis, or inflammatory disease. If a patient has a history of malignancy, then metastasis should always be kept in mind.

**Table 5.2** Causes of secondary headache [5]

| |
|---|
| **Nose/paranasal sinuses** |
| Sinonasal and nasopharyngeal tumors |
| Acute rhinosinusitis |
| **Ears** |
| Otitis externa |
| Acute otitis media |
| Vestibular migraine |
| **Eyes** |
| Glaucoma |
| Ocular inflammatory diseases |
| **Teeth/ temporomandibular joint** |
| Dental impaction or infection |
| Temporomandibular joint disorders |
| Myofascial pain |
| **Arterial hypertension** |
| **Intracranial** |
| Infectious and noninfectious inflammatory diseases |
| Tumors and cysts |
| Hemorrhage |
| High CSF pressure syndromes |
| Trauma |
| Pituitary apoplexy |
| **Neurovascular** |
| Arteriovenous malformation |
| Trigeminal neuralgia |
| **Other causes** |
| As an adverse effect of some drugs |
| Narcotics use or its withdrawal |

### 5.4.1 Rhinogenic Headache

Sinus headache is controversial. For centuries, conceptual understanding of headache causation has been attributed to anatomic abnormalities of the nose and paranasal sinuses. In fact headache has historically been a catch-all term for head and facial pain, leading to overdiagnosis of sinusitis in patients meeting criteria for migraine [15].

Sinusitis must be confirmed by its own diagnostic criteria before attributing a headache to the sinuses Tables 5.3, 5.4 and 5.5 [4]. In 1988, Stammberger and Wolf hypothesized that headaches of sinus origin were caused by (1) referred pain due to intense and constant mucous contact, (2) hypoxia of the paranasal sinuses due to poor or absent ventilation, and (3) pressure caused by secretions and polyps.

The location of the headache or facial pain should match sites of disease on imaging, and there should be a temporal relationship between the headache and the sinonasal symptoms. The headache resolves with appropriate sinusitis treatment.

A newer controversial cause of rhinogenic headache has been attributed to intranasal mucosal contact points from anatomic variations such as septal deviation and concha bullosa. This correlation between rhinogenic headache and mucosal contact points is not novel and was first described by John Roe in 1888. However, the relationship between headache and anatomic abnormalities in the nose is questionable since many subjects with nasal anatomic variants are totally asymptomatic.

Some authors differentiated between rhinogenic headache and sinus headache. Rhinogenic headache is classified when the pain has no relation to inflammatory sinus diseases. On the other hand, sinus headache is associated with inflammatory sinus conditions, such as acute bacterial rhinosinusitis.

**Table 5.3** Headache attributed to acute rhinosinusitis [4]

| |
|---|
| *Description:* |
| Headache caused by acute rhinosinusitis and associated with other symptoms or clinical signs of this disorder. |
| *Diagnostic criteria:* |
| A. Any headache fulfilling criterion C. |
| B. Clinical, nasal endoscopic, or imaging evidence of acute rhinosinusitis. |
| C. Evidence of causation shown by at least 2 of the following: |
| 1. Headache has developed in temporal relation to the onset of the rhinosinusitis. |
| 2. Either or both of the following: |
| a. Headache has significantly worsened in parallel with the worsening of the rhinosinusitis. |
| a. Headache has significantly improved or resolved in parallel with the improvement in or resolution of the rhinosinusitis. |
| 3. Headache is exacerbated by pressure applied over the paranasal sinuses |
| 4. In the case of a unilateral rhinosinusitis, headache is localized ipsilateral to it |
| D. Not better accounted for by another international classification of headache disorders, third edition diagnosis |

**Table 5.4** Headache attributed to chronic or recurring rhinosinusitis [4]

| |
|---|
| *Description:* |
| Headache caused by a chronic infectious or inflammatory disorder of the paranasal sinuses and associated with other symptoms or clinical signs of the disorder. |
| *Diagnostic criteria:* |
| A. Any headache fulfilling criterion C. |
| B. Clinical, nasal endoscopic, or imaging evidence of current or past infection or other inflammatory process within the paranasal sinuses. |
| C. Evidence of causation shown by at least 2 of the following: |
| 1. Headache has developed in temporal relation to the onset of sinusitis |
| 2. Headache waxes and wanes in parallel with the degree of sinus congestion, drainage, and other symptoms of CRS |
| 3. Headache is exacerbated by pressure applied over the paranasal sinuses |
| 4. In the case of unilateral rhinosinusitis, headache is localized ipsilateral to it |
| D. Not better accounted for by another international classification of headache disorders, third edition diagnosis |

**Table 5.5** Headache attributed to disorder of the nasal mucosa, turbinates, or septum [4]

| |
|---|
| *Diagnostic criteria:* |
| A. Any headache fulfilling criterion C |
| B. Clinical, nasal endoscopic, or imaging evidence of a hypertrophic or inflammatory process within the nasal cavity (a) |
| C. Evidence of causation shown by at least 2 of the following: |
| 1. Headache has developed in temporal relation to the onset of the intranasal lesion |
| 2. Headache has significantly improved or significantly worsened in parallel with improvement in (with or without treatment) or worsening of the nasal lesion |
| 3. Headache has significantly improved after local anesthesia of the mucosa in the region of the lesion |
| 4. Headache is ipsilateral to the site of the lesion |
| D. Not better accounted for by another international classification of headache disorders, third edition diagnosis |
| (a) Examples are concha bullosa and nasal septal spur. |

A potential mechanism for mucosal contact point headaches postulates that axonal reflex arcs are generated upon stimulation between the two mucosal surfaces within the nose. This reflex triggers the release of substance P, a vasodilating neuropeptide found in unmyelinated group C nerve fibers. Substance P causes vasodilation, plasma leak (neurogenic edema), and histamine release, among other inflammatory events. This vascular phenomenon may be responsible for migraine-like headache secondary to referred pain, as the dura mater, nasal cavity, and paranasal sinuses are innervated by the trigeminal branches. Additionally, constant mucosal contact would lead to localized or referred pain following the distribution of the first and second trigeminal branch dermatomes. The peripheral stimulus responsible for triggering the axonal reflex may be chemical, caloric, or mechanical.

Some controversy exists on this topic because surgical correction has been found to help a subset of patients with refractory headaches [16]. However, there are similar rates of contact points in patients with and without headaches. The causality of the headache and the mucosal contact being a trigger for primary headaches are not well understood.

### 5.4.2 Post-Traumatic Headache

Post-traumatic headache is attributed to moderate or severe head injury and has no typical characteristics.

Physical trauma leads to cellular injury, resulting in an unregulated ion-exchange neurotransmitter release. The increased neuronal activity results in metabolic stress (lactate and free radicals), leading to axonal damage [16].

Symptoms of post-traumatic headache can include nausea, vomiting, dizziness, sensitivity to light and noise, insomnia, poor concentration, fatigue and personality changes like depression or nervousness. The headache might also have a pulsating quality that worsens with activity and may progress to chronic and possibly debilitating conditions [17].

The headache usually develops within 7 days after head trauma or after regaining consciousness following head trauma. It may persist for few months after head trauma. Head trauma should have at least one of the following criteria:

- Loss of consciousness for >30 min.
- Glasgow Coma Scale <13.
- Posttraumatic amnesia for >48 h.
- Imaging demonstration of a traumatic brain lesion (skull fracture, cerebral hematoma.

### 5.4.3 Atypical Facial Pain/Persistent Idiopathic Facial Pain

Atypical facial pain is a collective term used for otherwise unclassifiable pain syndromes of the face. It describes mostly unilateral lancinating and burning pain, which is constantly present but fluctuating in intensity and may be accompanied by paraesthesias over a period of several years. The pain is usually confined at onset to a limited area on one side of the face. It is attributed to deficient tyramine metabolism, which causes centrally disinhibition of pain neuroregulation. The disease is more common in females and often confused with dental disease [18].

Both the International Headache Society (IHS) and the International Association for the Study of Pain (IASP) have adopted the term persistent idiopathic facial pain to replace atypical facial pain.

It is a diagnosis of exclusion. There is no sensory loss or other physical signs, and investigations are normal. Patients have other non-specific complaints such as irritable bowel syndrome, chronic fatigue. Depression common. Among those patients and antidepressants and psychotropic agents are worth considering.

### 5.4.4 Trigeminal Neuralgia

Trigeminal neuralgia is described as Paroxysmal attacks of pain lasting from a fraction of a second to 2 min, affecting one or more divisions of the trigeminal n (usually V2 and/or 3). Ipsilateral twitching may occur it is more common in females above 50 years. Neuralgic attacks are stereotyped in the individual patient, and there is no clinically evident neurological deficit.

Pain has at least one of the following characteristics:

- Intense, sharp, superficial, or stabbing.
- Precipitated from trigger areas or by trigger factors.

## References


1. Patel ZM, Setzen M, Poetker DM, DelGaudio JM. Evaluation and management of "sinus headache" in the otolaryngology practice. Otolaryngol Clin N Am. 2014;47(2):269–87. https://doi.org/10.1016/j.otc.2013.10.008.
2. Hainer BL, Matheson EM. Approach to acute headache in adults. Am Fam Physician. 2013;87(10):682–7.
3. Velasquez N, DelGaudio JM. The role of the otolaryngologist in the evaluation and management of "sinus headache". Otolaryngol Clin N Am. 2022;55(3):501–18. https://doi.org/10.1016/j.otc.2022.02.009.
4. Headache classification committee of the international headache society (IHS) the international classification of headache disorders, 3rd edition. Cephalalgia. 2018;38(1):1–211. https://doi.org/10.1177/0333102417738202.
5. Cady RK, Dodick DW, Levine HL, et al. Sinus headache: a neurology, otolaryngology, allergy, and primary care consensus on diagnosis and treatment. Mayo Clin Proc. 2005;80(7):908–16.
6. Bigal ME, Lipton RB. The differential diagnosis of chronic daily headaches: an algorithm-based approach. J Headache Pain. 2007;8(5):263–72.
7. Baraness L, Baker, AM. Acute headache. In: StatPearls [internet]. StatPearls Publishing. doi:32119397. Available at: https://www.ncbi.nlm.nih.gov/books/NBK554510/. Accessed September 28, 2021.
8. Crystal SC, Robbins MS. Epidemiology of tension-type headache. Curr Pain Headache Rep. 2010;14(6):449–54.
9. Feoktistov A, Diamond M. Diagnosing and understanding adult headache. Otolaryngol Clin N Am. 2014;47(2):175–85.
10. Baloh RW. Neurotology of migraine. Headache. 1997;37(10):615–21.
11. Murthy HD, Mowry SE. The role of the otolaryngologist in the evaluation and Management of Headache. Otolaryngol Clin N Am. 2022;55(3):493–9. https://doi.org/10.1016/j.otc.2022.02.001. Epub 2022 Apr 27
12. Chiang BC, Vanderpluym J. Diagnosing secondary headaches. Pract Neurol. 2020:31–5.
13. Al-Hashel JY, Ahmed SF, Alroughani R, et al. Migraine misdiagnosis as a sinusitis, a delay that can last for many years. J Headache Pain. 2013;14(1):97.
14. Welge-Luessen A, Hauser R, Schmid N, et al. Endonasal surgery for contact point headaches: a 10-year longitudinal study. Laryngoscope. 2003;113(12):2151–6.
15. Abu-Bakra M, Jones NS. Prevalence of nasal mucosal contact points in patients with facial pain compared with patients without facial pain. J Laryngol Otol. 2001;115(8):629–32.

16. Ashina H, Porreca F, Anderson T, Amin FM, Ashina M, Schytz HW, Dodick DW. Post-traumatic headache: epidemiology and pathophysiological insights. Nat Rev Neurol. 2019;15(10):607–17.
17. Tessler J, Horn LJ. Posttraumatic headache. In: StatPearls treasure. Islands, FL: StatPearls Publishing; 2024.
18. Paulson GW. Atypical facial pain. Oral Surg Oral Med Oral Pathol. 1977;43(3):338–41.

# Paediatric Rhinology

# 6

Paresh Pramod Naik

**Key Points**

- An understanding of complete developmental process of paranasal sinus is necessary for surgical planning and management.
- Child presenting with CRS should be screened for cystic fibrosis.
- Unilateral nasal discharge should raise a suspicion of retained foreign body.
- Encourage role of multidisciplinary management in pediatric rhinology.
- Image guidance surgery in skull base pediatric cases should be encouraged.

## 6.1 Introduction

While diseases may share the same name between children and adults, it's crucial to recognize that they are not identical conditions. This is primarily due to the distinct symptomatology and clinical manifestations observed in children. Certain diseases and anomalies are exclusive to or predominantly affect the pediatric population. Therefore, managing these conditions necessitates specialized knowledge and skills tailored to pediatric care.

Moreover, the growth of the skull base is characterized by an asynchronous pattern, wherein the anterior portions exhibit delayed growth compared to other areas.

**Supplementary Information** The online version contains supplementary material available at https://doi.org/10.1007/978-3-031-70077-4_6.

P. P. Naik (✉)
University of Northamptonshire, Cliftonville, UK
e-mail: pareshnaikp@gmail.com


S. Elwany (ed.), *Current Rhinology*,
https://doi.org/10.1007/978-3-031-70077-4_6

## 6.2 Embryology

The nose and paranasal sinus development is not finished until puberty.

Due to the constant change, sinus diseases in pediatric face surgical challenges. The nasal apparatus formation starts as early as 3–4 weeks of fetal life [1].

### 6.2.1 Ethmoturbinals and Lamella

*Ethmoturbinals derivatives.*

- First: Ascending portion forms agger nasi, while descending portion forms uncinate process.
- Second: Middle turbinate.
- Third: Superior turbinate.
- Fourth fuses with fifth to form supreme turbinate.
- Supreme turbinate usually gets reabsorbed during puberty.

*Furrows are structures formed between ethmoturbinals.*

- First furrow is between the first and second ethmoturbinal. Derivates of first furrow are the ascending portion, which forms the frontal recess, descending portion, which forms the ethmoidal infundibulum, hiatus semilunaris, middle meatus.
- Second furrow forms the superior meatus.
- Third furrow forms the supreme meatus.

The attachments of ethmoturbinals are called as *lamella.*

| Lamella | Future derivative |
|---|---|
| First lamella | Lateral extension of uncinate process |
| Second lamella | Lateral extension of ethmoid bulla |
| Third lamella | Attachment of middle turbinate |
| Fourth lamella | Attachment of the superior turbinate |
| Fifth lamella | Attachment of the supreme turbinate (if present) |

*Most constant* lamella is the *basal lamella* of the middle turbinate. It represents the boundary between anterior and posterior ethmoids.

## 6.3 Congenital Nose Block

### 6.3.1 Congenital Pyriform Aperture Stenosis: [2, 3]

**Clinical Features**

- Nasal obstruction.
- Apnoeic episodes.
- Respiratory distress.

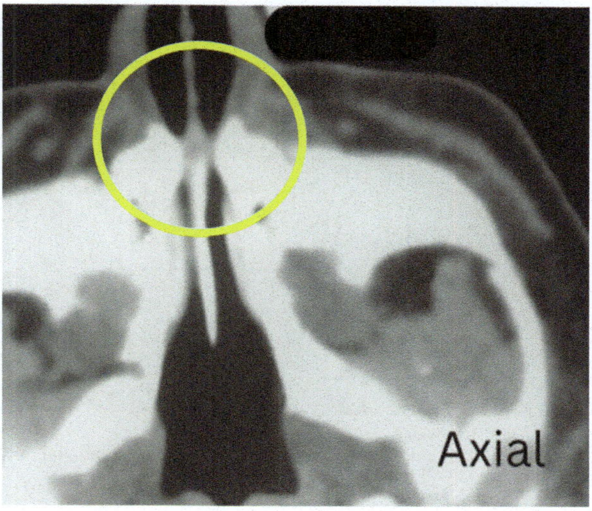


**Fig. 6.1** Congenital pyriform aperture stenosis encircled in yellow

- Feeding difficulty.
- Often central single mega-incisor.
- Axial CT scan shows the stenosis (Fig. 6.1).
- Differential diagnosis, bilateral choanal atresia.

**Surgery**
- Trans nasal approach.
- Sublabial approach.
- The excess pyriform rim is drilled out.
- Stenting nasopharyngeal airway post procedure for 2–4 weeks.

### 6.3.2 Choanal Atresia: [4, 5]

- Can be unilateral or bilateral.
- Unilateral more common, often late diagnosis.
- Most common presentation is persistent unilateral nasal discharge.
- Bony atresia more common than membranous.
- Bilateral choanal atresia often presents with respiratory distress.
- Cyanosis disappears as soon as child starts crying.
- McGroven Nipple can be used to temporary relief.
- Size 6 Fr Catheter can be passed to see if it comes in the oropharynx.
- Associated with CHARGE syndrome, Apert Syndrome, DiGeorge, trisomy 18, trisomy 21.
- Gold standard diagnosis: CT scan (Fig. 6.2).

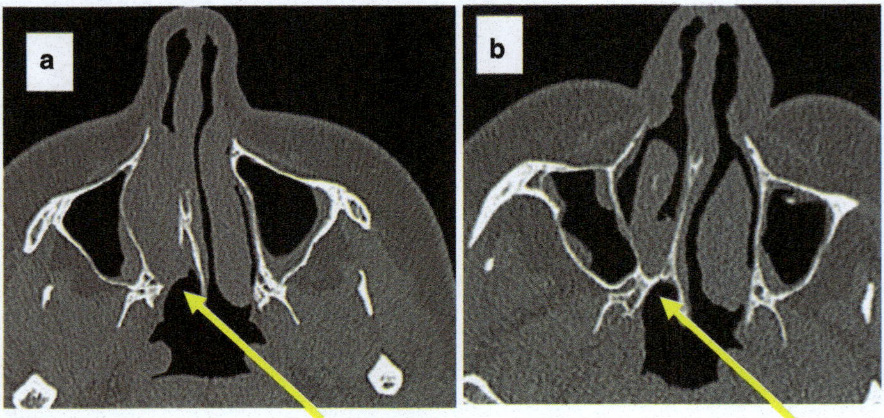


**Fig. 6.2** Axial cut CT scan, showing unilateral choanal atresia. (**a**) Membranous type, (**b**) Bony type

**Surgical Management**

- Endoscopic transnasal approach is by far most popular for opening the posterior choana.
- By excising a segment of the posterior nasal septum, a passage is created between the two nasal cavities.
- Extending the repair towards the posterior region ensures the formation of a single central choana instead of separate nasal ports, which may be prone to stenosis.
- The removal of the bony septum is typically carried out using bone forceps or a drill.
- The bony area is covered by superior and inferior-based mucosal flap.

**Syndromes Associated with Nasal Block**

- Treacher Collin, Cruzons syndrome.

## 6.4 Epistaxis

- **Causes of epistaxis** (Table 6.1).
- **Management of epistaxis** (Fig. 6.3).

**Table 6.1** Causes of epistaxis

| |
|---|
| **Hematological conditions** |
| Platelet abnormalities |
| HHT |
| Bleeding disorders |
| Leukaemia |
| von Willebrand disease |
| Haemophilia |
| Liver diseases |
| **Neoplasms** |
| Juvenile nasopharyngeal angiofibroma |
| Papilloma |
| Hemangioma |
| Rhabdomyosarcoma |
| Lymphoma |
| **Inflammation** |
| Upper respiratory tract infection |
| Allergic rhinitis |
| Vestibulitis |
| Non allergic rhinitis with eosinophilia |
| Foreign body |
| **Trauma** |
| Nose picking |
| Facial fracture |
| Dry air |
| Post-surgery |
| Nasogastric tube insertion |

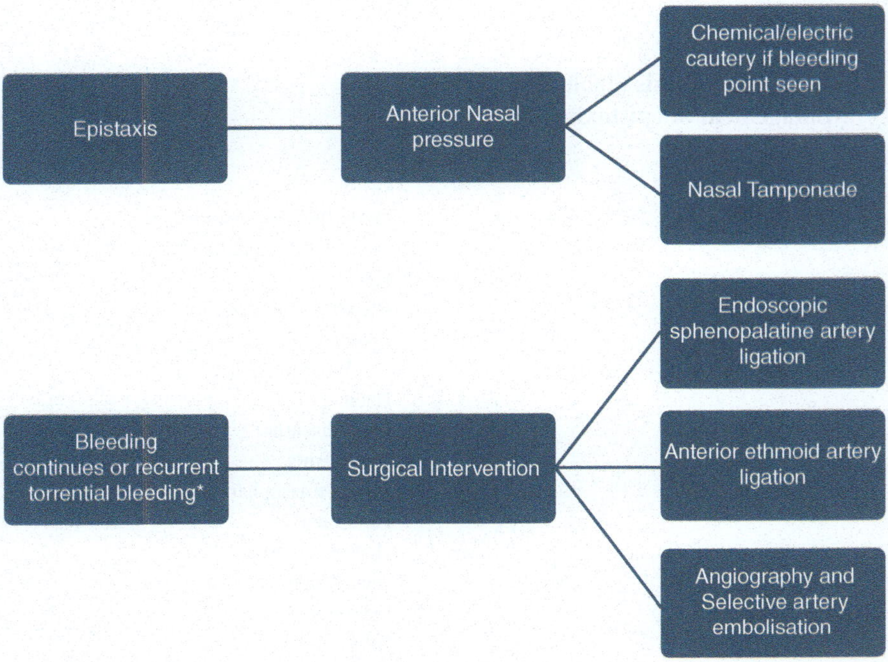


**Fig. 6.3** Management of epistaxis. * at this stage one must try to evaluate underlying cause by conducting investigations like screening for coagulopathy, radiological imaging CT or MRI scan

## 6.5 Chronic Rhinosinusitis

Chronic rhinosinusitis (CRS) is characterized by inflammation of the sinonasal tract lasting for a minimum of 12 weeks. The key indicators of CRS encompass mucopurulent drainage, nasal obstruction, facial pain/pressure, and hyposmia.

details on this topic are provided in the previous chapter.

When encountering sinonasal polyposis or persistent chronic rhinosinusitis (CRS) in a child, it is essential to consider conditions such as cystic fibrosis (CF), ciliary dyskinesia, and immunodeficiency.

## 6.6 Cystic Fibrosis

Cystic fibrosis (CF), is an autosomal recessive condition, characterised by mutations in the cystic fibrosis transmembrane conductance regulator (CFTR). Mutations in the CFTR gene disrupt the proper transport of chloride and bicarbonate across epithelial surfaces, representing a key pathogenic mechanism in CF. This aberrant ion transport leads to the dehydration of the airway surface liquid volume, ultimately impairing mucociliary clearance (MCC) & hence affecting sinuses. CRS

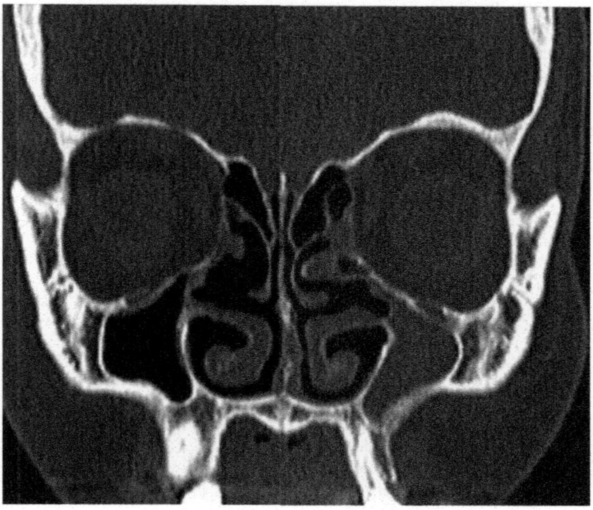

**Fig. 6.4** CT scan coronal section of child with CF. Left maxillary sinus showing mucosal disease with maxillary sinus hypoplasia

with or without nasal polyps is the most common ENT. Cystic fibrosis is known to affect ciliary movement. Patients with cystic fibrosis have more changes of chronic rhinosinusitis than the general population [6].

### 6.6.1 Investigations

CT sinus: presence of mucosal thickening, retention cysts, isolated maxillary sinus opacification, maxillary sinus hypoplasia [7]. (Fig. 6.4).

### 6.6.2 Treatments

- Saline inhalation [8].
- Betamethasone nasal drops [9].
- Sinonasal inhalation of tobramycin has be proven (level I evidence) to reduce Pseudomonas aureginosa colonisation [10].
- *Dornase alfa*: A genetically engineered version of naturally occurring human enzyme which cleaves extracellular DNA, has been shown to reduce CRS symptoms.
  - **Dosage:** 2500 units once daily, administered by jet nebuliser, >5 years. Management of cystic fibrosis. It has also proven for significant increase in FEV1 [11]..

## 6.7 Allergic Rhinitis

- **Pathophysiology of allergic rhinitis** (Fig. 6.5).
- **Clinical picture:**

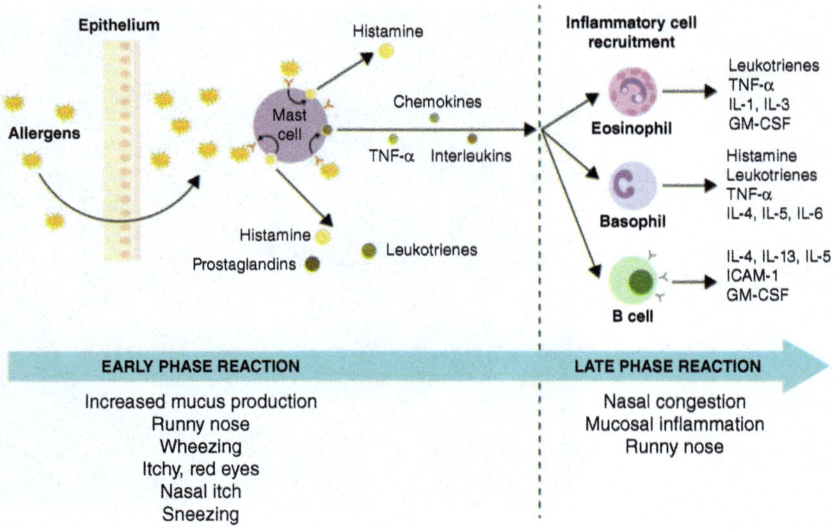


**Fig. 6.5** Pathophysiology of allergic rhinitis [12] with permission

| **Symptoms** [13] |
|---|
| Rhinorrhoea |
| Pruritis |
| Sneezing |
| Nasal congestion |
| Hyposmia |

| **Associated features** [13] |
|---|
| Redness of eyes |
| Allergic salute/allergic crease |
| Family history of allergic rhinitis |
| Co-morbidities: Asthma, atopic dermatitis, behavioral changes |
| Hyposmia |

- **Management of Allergic Rhinitis** (Fig. 6.6):

As per ARIA (Allergic Rhinitis and its Impact of Asthma) Guidelines [14].

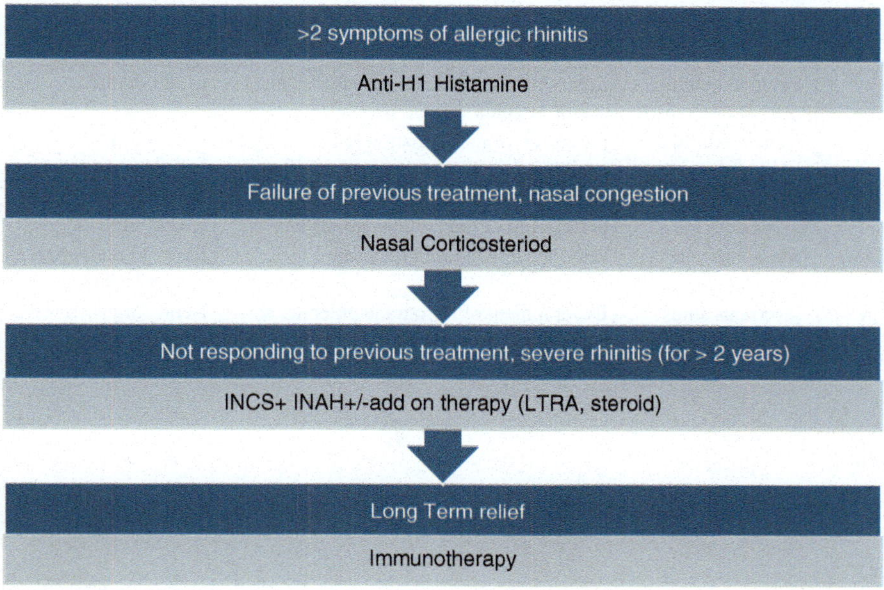


**Fig. 6.6** Treatment flowchart for allergic rhinitis. INCS—intranasal corticosteroid, INAH—intranasal antihistamine, LTRA—Leukotriene Receptor Antagonists

## 6.8 Complications of Chronic and Acute Rhinosinusitis

### 6.8.1 Orbital Complications

#### 6.8.1.1 Chandler's Classification of Orbital Complications [15] (Table 6.2)

All cases should be under joint Ophthalmology and ENT care.

#### 6.8.1.2 Orbital Cellulitis

A child with orbital swelling represents diagnostic challenge that demands multidisciplinary input for diagnosis and management. (Figs. 6.7,6.8, 6.9).

**Table 6.2** Chandler's classification

| Stage | Name | Classification | Management |
|---|---|---|---|
| I | Preseptal cellulitis | Inflammation & edema anterior to the orbital septum | i.v. antibiotics |
| II | Orbital cellulitis | Extension of inflammation to include the orbital contents posterior to the septum | i.v. antibiotics |
| III | Subperiosteal abscess | Collection of purulent exudate beneath periosteum of the lamina papyracea | External drainage + i.v. antibiotics |
| IV | Orbital abscess | Purulent collection in the orbit | External drainage + i.v. antibiotics |
| V | Cavernous sinus thrombosis | Development of retrograde phlebitis & coagulation. B/L eye findings, proptosis. | Neurosurgery review<br>i.v. heparin<br>i.v. antibiotics |

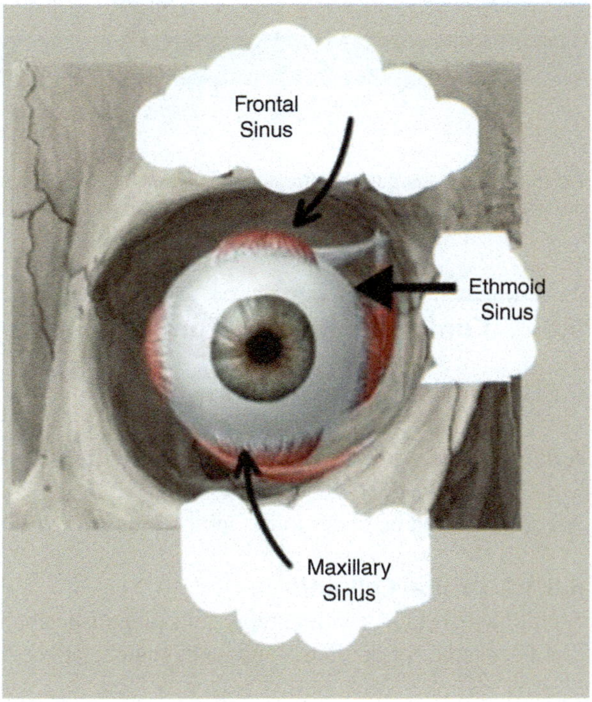


**Fig. 6.7** —Spread of infection from sinus to orbit

## 6.8.2 Potts Puffy Tumour

### 6.8.2.1 Definition

Potts puffy tumor is defined as osteomyelitis of the frontal bone with associated subperiosteal secondary to frontal sinusitis.

Timely diagnosis and prompt intervention are paramount to prevent intracranial complications. Treatment usually entails surgical intervention alongside extended courses of intravenous antibiotics, aiming for a favorable recovery outcome.

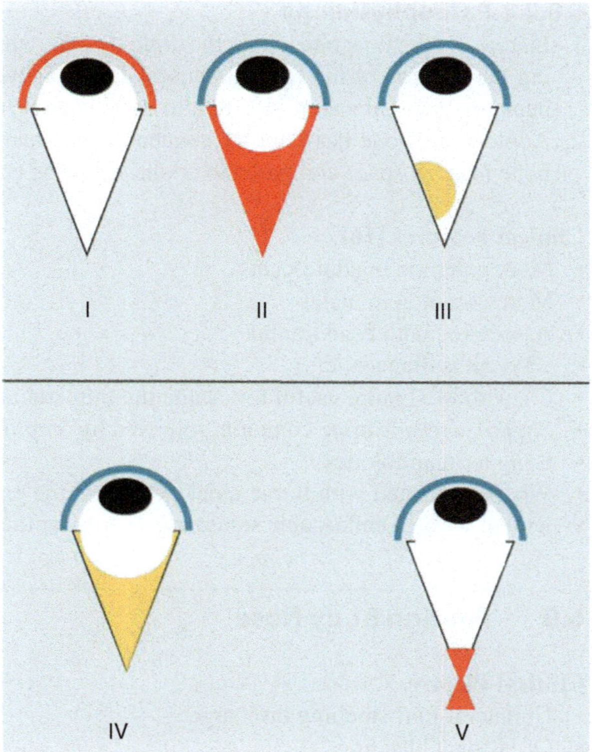


**Fig. 6.8** Graphic representation of orbital cellulitis. Red color—cellulitis, yellow color—abscess, blue—normal septum

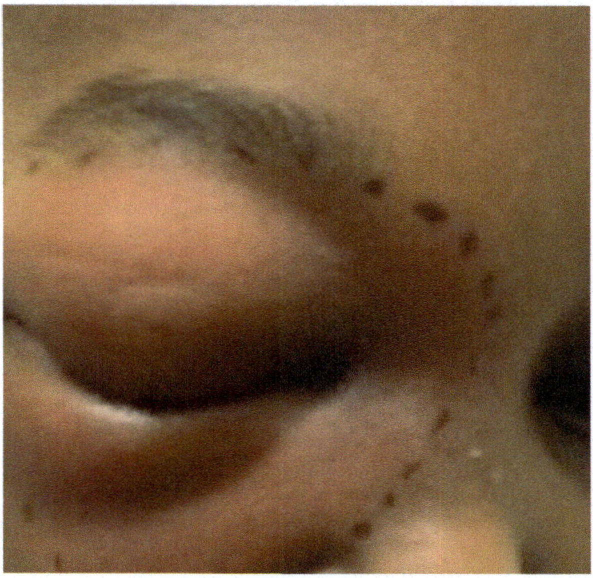

**Fig. 6.9** Orbital cellulitis

#### 6.8.2.2 Pathophysiology

1. Increase in the flow rate within the diploic veins, which are responsible for draining the mucosa of the frontal sinuses. This heightened flow rate facilitates the hematogenous spread of infection to both the bone and the brain.
2. Adolescents bone has a looser connection between the frontal sinuses and the bone marrow space compared to adults, allowing easy spread.

**Clinical Features [16]**

- More common in adolescents
- More common in males
- Associated with head trauma
- CT scan is diagnostic.
- CT with MRI more useful for evaluating intracranial involvement
- *Streptococcus* is more common, followed by *Staphylococcus*.
- Long term antibiotics
- When associated with intracranial extension, the external approach is favorable with or without endoscopic sinus surgery to clear the primary source of infection.

## 6.9 Foreign Body Nose

**Clinical Picture**

- Unilateral foul-smelling discharge.
- Occasional bleeding.
- Use of nasal decongestants may improve visualization.
- Topical anaesthetic spray/drops will increase the compliance of the patient.

**Management**

- Outpatient nasal endoscopy, with the use of nasal decongestant and topical anesthetic spray.
- CT scan can be used as primary radiological investigation. However, CT scan in young pediatric age group may need sedation.
- Batteries require urgent attention and need removal under emergency.
- While removing outpatients, for young children, make sure the child is in an upright position on parents' lap.
- For children with intellectual disability and special needs, retrieval should be done under short GA.
- Examination under GA with retrieval of the foreign body and wash out.

## 6.10 Congenital Midline Nasal Malformation [17, 18]

### 6.10.1 Classification: (Fig. 6.10)

### 6.10.2 Encephaloceles, Glioma, Dermoid (Table 6.3)

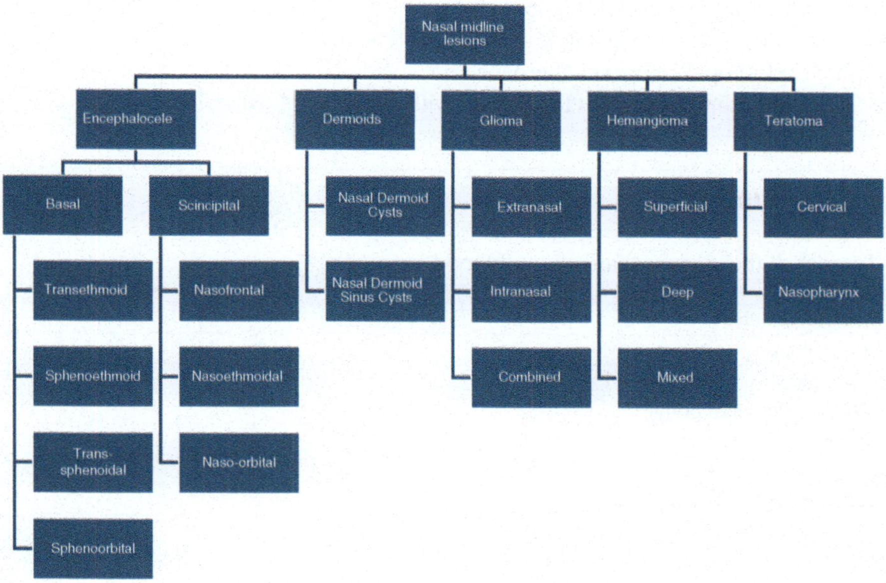


**Fig. 6.10** Nasal midline lesions

**Table 6.3** Encephaloceles, glioma, dermoid

| | Encephaloceles | Glioma | Dermoid |
|---|---|---|---|
| Age | Infants, adolescents | Infants and adolescents | Children and adolescents |
| Clinical features | Bluish, soft, compressible | Reddish blue, firm, non-compressible | Solid groove with hair follicle |
| Pulsation | + | – | – |
| Transillumination | + | – | – |
| CSF leak | Yes | Rarely | Rarely |
| Furstenberg sign | + | – | – |

### 6.10.3 Management

**Investigation**
- CT scan paranasal sinus with brain
- MRI scan with contrast of paranasal sinus with Brain

**Surgery**
- Depending on the size of the lesion, following approaches can be used:
  1. Open septorhinoplasty approach.
  2. Direct median incision.
  3. Endoscopic sinonasal approach.
  4. Craniotomy approach for lesions with intracranial extension.

## 6.11 Tumors

Tumors of the sinonasal area in childhood are rare.

| Clinical features |
| --- |
| Nose block |
| Nose bleed |
| Widening of nasal bridge |
| Epiphora |
| Proptosis |
| Swelling of the nose and cheek/face |
| Neck nodes/distant nodes (lymphoma) |

### 6.11.1 Hemangioma

- Most common benign tumor in infancy
- Can be superficial (superficial dermis) or deep (lower dermis)
- Nasal obstruction
- Epistaxis
- Blue-red mass on rhinoscopy
- MRI: Isodense on T1; hyperintense on T2
- Differential diagnosis: hemangiopericytoma, pyogenic granuloma
- Most lesions resolve as the age progresses.
- *Management* [19].
- Medical management: Oral propranolol 2 mg/kg/day
- High dose oral prednisolone
- Intralesional steroid for small lesions.

- Sclerosing agent injection.
- Superficial lesions: Nd:YAG laser excision
- In case of surgical excision, preoperative selective embolization is warranted.

**Juvenile Nasopharyngeal Angiofibroma** and other tumors are described in dedicated chapters.

## References


1. Lee S, Fernandez J, Mirjalili SA, Kirkpatrick J. Pediatric paranasal sinuses-development, growth, pathology, & functional endoscopic sinus surgery. Clin Anat. 2022;35(6):745–61. https://doi.org/10.1002/ca.23888. Epub 2022 Apr 26. PMID: 35437820; PMCID: PMC9544638
2. Marrugo Pardo GE, Parra Charris JS, Parra Charris AE, Villa Zuluaga DF. Congenital nasal pyriform aperture stenosis: diagnosis, management and technical considerations. Acta Otorrinolaringol Esp (Engl Ed). 2020;71(3):154–9. https://doi.org/10.1016/j.otorri.2019.05.001. Epub 2019 Sep 5. PMID: 31495444
3. Bazak R, Ibrahim AA, Hussein WKA, Abdelnaby MM, Elwany S. Extramucosal pyriplasty without stenting for management of pyriform aperture stenosis. Eur Arch Otorrinolaringol. 2018;275(6):1469–75. https://doi.org/10.1007/s00405-018-4969-5. Epub 2018 Apr 16. PMID: 29663112
4. Ramsden JD, Campisi P, Forte V. Choanal atresia and choanal stenosis. Otolaryngol Clin N Am. 2009;42(2):339–52. https://doi.org/10.1016/j.otc.2009.01.001. PMID: 19328897
5. Attya H, Callaby M, Thevasagayam R. Choanal atresia surgery: outcomes in 42 patients over 20 years and a review of the literature. Eur Arch Otorrinolaringol. 2021;278(7):2347–56. https://doi.org/10.1007/s00405-020-06506-6. Epub 2021 Jan 2. PMID: 33386964
6. Krajewska J, Zub K, Słowikowski A, Zatoński T. Chronic rhinosinusitis in cystic fibrosis: a review of therapeutic options. Eur Arch Otorrinolaringol. 2022;279(1):1–24. https://doi.org/10.1007/s00405-021-06875-6. Epub 2021 Jul 22. PMID: 34296343; PMCID: PMC8739462
7. Eggesbø HB, Søvik S, Dølvik S, Eiklid K, Kolmannskog F. CT characterization of developmental variations of the paranasal sinuses in cystic fibrosis. Acta Radiol. 2001;42(5):482–93. https://doi.org/10.1080/028418501127347214. PMID: 11552886
8. Mainz JG, Schumacher U, Schädlich K, Hentschel J, Koitschev C, Koitschev A, et al. Sino nasal inhalation of isotonic versus hypertonic saline (6.0%) in CF patients with chronic rhinosinusitis—results of a multicenter, prospective, randomized, double-blind, controlled trial. J Cyst Fibros. 2016;15(6):e57–66.
9. Hadfield PJ, Rowe-Jones JM, Mackay IS. A prospective treatment trial of nasal polyps in adults with cystic fibrosis. Rhinology. 2000;38(2):63–5.
10. Mainz JG, Schaedlich K, Schien C, Michl R, Schelhorn-Neise P, Koitschev A, et al. Sinonasal inhalation of tobramycin vibrating aerosol in cystic fibrosis patients with upper airway *Pseudomonas aeruginosa* colonization: results of a randomized, double-blind, placebo-controlled pilot study. Drug Des Dev Ther. 2014;8:209. https://doi.org/10.2147/DDDT.S54064.
11. Cimmino M, Nardone M, Cavaliere M, Plantulli A, Sepe A, Esposito V, et al. Dornase alfa as postoperative therapy in cystic fibrosis sinonasal disease. Arch Otolaryngol Neck Surg. 2005;131(12):1097. https://doi.org/10.1001/archotol.131.12.1097.
12. Meltzer EO, Rosario NA, Van Bever H, et al. Fexofenadine: review of safety, efficacy and unmet needs in children with allergic rhinitis. Allergy Asthma Clin Immunol. 2021;17:113. https://doi.org/10.1186/s13223-021-00614-6.

13. Scadding GK, Smith PK, Blaiss M, Roberts G, Hellings PW, Gevaert P, Mc Donald M, Sih T, Halken S, Zieglmayer PU, Schmid-Grendelmeier P, Valovirta E, Pawankar R, Wahn U. Allergic rhinitis in childhood and the new EUFOREA algorithm. Front Allergy. 2021;2:706589. https://doi.org/10.3389/falgy.2021.706589. PMID: 35387065; PMCID: PMC8974858
14. Brożek JL, Bousquet J, Agache I, Agarwal A, Bachert C, Bosnic-Anticevich S, Brignardello-Petersen R, Canonica GW, Casale T, Chavannes NH, Correia de Sousa J, Cruz AA, Cuello-Garcia CA, Demoly P, Dykewicz M, Etxeandia-Ikobaltzeta I, Florez ID, Fokkens W, Fonseca J, Hellings PW, Klimek L, Kowalski S, Kuna P, Laisaar KT, Larenas-Linnemann DE, Lødrup Carlsen KC, Manning PJ, Meltzer E, Mullol J, Muraro A, O'Hehir R, Ohta K, Panzner P, Papadopoulos N, Park HS, Passalacqua G, Pawankar R, Price D, Riva JJ, Roldán Y, Ryan D, Sadeghirad B, Samolinski B, Schmid-Grendelmeier P, Sheikh A, Togias A, Valero A, Valiulis A, Valovirta E, Ventresca M, Wallace D, Waserman S, Wickman M, Wiercioch W, Yepes-Nuñez JJ, Zhang L, Zhang Y, Zidarn M, Zuberbier T, Schünemann HJ. Allergic rhinitis and its impact on asthma (ARIA) guidelines-2016 revision. J Allergy Clin Immunol. 2017;140(4):950–8. https://doi.org/10.1016/j.jaci.2017.03.050. Epub 2017 Jun 8. PMID: 28602936
15. Chandler JR, Langenbrunner DJ, Stevens ER. The pathogenesis of orbital complications in acute sinusitis. Laryngoscope. 1970;80(9):1414–28. https://doi.org/10.1288/00005537-197009000-00007. PMID: 5470225
16. Koltsidopoulos P, Papageorgiou E, Skoulakis C. Pott's puffy tumor in children: a review of the literature. Laryngoscope. 2020;130(1):225–31. https://doi.org/10.1002/lary.27757.
17. Saettele M, Alexander A, Markovich B, Morelli J, Lowe LH. Congenital midline nasofrontal masses. Pediatr Radiol. 2012;42(9):1119–25. https://doi.org/10.1007/s00247-012-2409-z. Epub 2012 May 22. PMID: 22648391
18. Fitzpatrick E, Miller RH. Congenital midline nasal masses: dermoids, gliomas, and encephaloceles. J La State Med Soc. 1996;148(3):93–6. PMID: 8984139
19. Holland KE, Drolet BA. Infantile hemangioma. Pediatr Clin N Am. 2010;57(5):1069–83.

# Congenital Nasal Anomalies

# 7

Yasser W. Khafagy, Noha Ahmed Elkholy, and Ahmed Y. Khafagy

**Key Points**

- Congenital nasal anomalies have a relatively low incidence, but highlighting its basic features is critical for appropriate management of these anomalies.
- Losee et al., classified congenital nasal anomalies into the following categories; Aplasia, hypoplasia, clefts, neoplasms and associated syndromes.
- Choanal atresia is one of the most common anomalies and the mixed bony and membranous type enjoys the highest incidence among cases.
- Bilateral choanal atresia is an airway emergency at birth while repair of unilateral choanal atresia is usually delayed to the pre-school age.
- Endoscopic transnasal repair is the primary procedure to treat choanal atresia.
- Endoscopic repair should be done within a "Working Zone" to avoid injury of the important surrounding structures.
- Nasal clefts are usually associated with cleft lip and palate and the worse the cleft lip, the worse the cleft nose.
- Nasal dermoid is the most common midline nasal cyst and usually associated with midline pit.
- In midline nasal lesions, a magnetic resonance imaging is mandatory to detect any associated intracranial connection.

**Supplementary Information** The online version contains supplementary material available at https://doi.org/10.1007/978-3-031-70077-4_7.

Y. W. Khafagy (✉) · N. A. Elkholy
Department of Otolaryngology, Mansoura University, Mansoura, Egypt
e-mail: ykhafagy@mans.edu.eg

A. Y. Khafagy
Department of Otolaryngology, Mansoura University, Mansoura, Egypt

Faculty of Medicine, Mansoura University, Mansoura, Egypt


S. Elwany (ed.), *Current Rhinology*,
https://doi.org/10.1007/978-3-031-70077-4_7

Congenital nasal anomalies are considered relatively rare, being detected in 1: 40,000 live births [1]. This is a relative estimate as the exact prevalence is difficult to determine as minor anomalies may pass overlooked or remain confined to certain specialized medical centers. Basic knowledge of the nasal embryology, classification systems, and clinical considerations is critical for appropriate management of these anomalies.

## 7.1 Nasal Embryology

Nasal development begins around the fourth or fifth weeks of gestation and is usually completed by the eighth week. Embryonic stomodeum is surrounded by the five facial processes involved in nasal development. These processes are two maxillary, two mandibular, and nasofrontal prominences [2]. Of these five primordia, the frontonasal prominence is the main structure responsible for nasal development. Neural crest cells proliferate on the lateral aspects of the frontal prominence, forming the nasal placodes. Then, the nasal placodes invaginate to form the olfactory pit and then the lateral and medial nasal processes [3].

Nasal septum develops as a fusion between the nasal laminae and the nasofrontal process in an anterior to posterior direction. These nasal laminae are the posterior continuation of the lateral rounded edges of the medial nasal prominences [4]. At the ninth week of gestation, the nasal septum fuses posteriorly with the palatine processes. Chondrification and ossification begin around the twelfth week, but complete ossification occurs at puberty [3]. The philtrum and the columella are formed by fusion between the maxillary processes and the medial nasal processes. Also, the maxillary processes give rise to the lower part of the lateral nasal walls and the posterior borders of the nares. The nares are occluded with epithelium initially, which then breaks down by the 24th week, leaving permanent choana [2].

The contact between the ectoderms of both the nasal sac and the roof of the mouth results in the formation of the oronasal septum. Attenuation of the oronasal septum leads to the creation of the oronasal membrane separating the nasal cavity from the pharynx, and then this membrane degenerates, forming the choanae. Ectodermal folds appear in the ethmoid region as the nasal cavity heightens, giving rise to superior, middle, and inferior conchae [2].

## 7.2 Classification System

Losee and colleagues developed the most recent classification for congenital nasal anomalies in 2004 [1, 4].

This system divides the nasal anomalies into six types:

- Type I: Atrophy and hypoplasia
- Type II: Hyperplasia and duplications
- Type III: Clefts

- Type IV: Neoplasms and vascular anomalies
- Type V: Congenital syndromes with nasal malformation

## 7.3 Type I: Atrophy and Hypoplasia

These are the most common class of congenital nasal anomalies in which there is underdevelopment of nasal structures. They range from complete aplasia (arrhinia) to a hypoplasia of a part of the nose.

### 7.3.1 Total Arrhinia (Complete Nasal Agenesis)

It is a condition in which the external nose, nasal cavities, and olfactory apparatus are completely absent. It is an extremely rare condition with unknown etiology. Associated abnormalities in chromosomes 9, 13, and 21 have been reported. The underlying embryological background is the failure of the invagination of the nasal placode [1, 5]. There are possible coexistent other midline anomalies such as holoprosencephaly, hypotelorism, meningoencephalocele, and orofacial clefting. Therefore, these associated conditions should be evaluated before any surgical intervention [5].

Unilateral agenesis is also reported and defined as heminasal aplasia. It can also be associated with other anomalies on the ipsilateral side of the face. The most common associated problem is the absence of the cribriform plate, due to developmental loss of the ipsilateral nasal placode [6]. Also, hypoplasia is often associated with orofacial clefting, such as columellar agenesis and partial nasal bone agenesis [7, 8]. In fact, isolated hypoplastic nasal anomalies may represent a carrier state of orofacial clefting [9].

### 7.3.2 Nasal Hypoplasia

Nasal hypoplasia can be a part of the craniofacial syndrome as Binder syndrome, Fraser syndrome, Apert and Crouzon syndromes. Binder syndrome, nasomaxillary hypoplasia, is a combined hypoplasia of the anterior nasal spine, columella, and midface. In Fraser syndrome, there is hypoplastic nares, underdeveloped nasal dorsum, and cryptopthalmos [1]. Apert and Crouzon syndromes have common features in the form of midface hypoplasia, nasal cavity stenosis, and maxillary sinus hypoplasia [10].

Atresia of the nasal cavity can occur in its anterior, middle, or posterior parts. Atresia of the anterior nasal cavity, pyriform aperture stenosis, and posterior nasal cavity obstruction (choanal atresia) will be discussed here. However, stenosis of the nasal cavity itself, although rare, should also be considered in any newborn presenting with nasal obstruction.

### 7.3.3 Pyriform Aperture Stenosis

Pyriform aperture stenosis (PAS) results as a bony overgrowth of the nasal process of maxilla. This condition is rare and subtle, thus it has been overlooked as a cause of respiratory distress in neonates. PAS is characterized by narrowing the anterior bony opening of the nose with subsequent increase in nasal resistance and occurrence of cyclic cyanosis [3, 11]. The condition often presents in the early few months of life, either alone or combined with holoprosencephaly. A clue for its diagnosis is the presence of a solitary maxillary central incisor [11, 12]. This condition can be easily differentiated from choanal atresia by an axial CT [11].

Treatment of this condition is variable according to the degree of stenosis. Mild cases can improve with growth and may not require surgical intervention [12]. Severe cases with persistent respiratory distress, cyanosis, apnea, or poor feeding are candidates for surgical correction [12]. Surgery entails reaching the premaxilla through a sublabial approach, and then the narrowed nasal aperture is enlarged by submucosal drilling of the nasal process of the maxilla (Extramucosal Pyriplasty) [13].

### 7.3.4 Choanal Atresia and Stenosis

#### 7.3.4.1 Introduction, Embryology, and Historical Background

Choanal atresia (CA) is one of the most common causes of congenital nasal airway abnormalities. It was first described by Roederer in 1755 as the most common major congenital nasal anomaly. The incidence is twice more common in girls [11]. In 1910, the deformity was found to be 90% bony and 10% membranous [14]. In a recent study, it is discovered to be pure bony in 29%, mixed membranous and bony in 71% with no pure membranous atresia reported [15].

The disease results from failure of degeneration of the bucconasal membrane during the fifth or sixth week of gestation with subsequent anatomical closure of the posterior nasal choanae. The anatomic boundaries of the posterior choanae are the following: under surface of the sphenoid body superiorly, medial pterygoid plate laterally, vomer medially, and horizontal plate of the palatine bone inferiorly. The atresia can be caused by any of those anatomical components [3].

Notably, CA follows a "2–1" rule, having a ratio of 2:1 for unilateral to bilateral, female to male and right side to left side [16]. In a previous study of 129 patients with choanal atresia and stenosis (CA/S), about 51% of case were found to be a part of (CHARGE) syndrome [17]. Also, cases with choanal atresia have a possible coexistence with Treacher Collins syndrome [3]. Bilateral cases were more common in patients having other associated congenital anomalies while unilateral CA was found in isolated cases more frequently [17].

Although the theory of persistence of buccopharyngeal membrane is the most accepted one, other theories have also been described. Those include abnormal persistence of the mesoderm forming adhesions in the naso-choanal region, abnormal persistence of the nasobuccal membrane of Hochstetter, and misdirection during migration of the neural crest cells [16].

To obtain further insights in the pathogenesis of CA, various molecular and genetic models have been studied. Those include the role of retinoic acid deficiency during gestation in development of many malformations [18]. Retinoic acid (RA) is produced from vitamin A by an enzyme called retinaldehyde dehydrogenase (Raldh). It is important for ontogenesis and homeostasis of various tissues [19]. Its role in development of CA was described by Dupe et al. who linked impaired RA synthesis to over-expression of fibroblast growth factor 8 (FGF-8), which in turned led to CA [19]. This link was also supported by the presence of high levels of FGF-8 in patients with craniosynostosis syndromes [20].

Moreover, there is a potential association between CA and prenatal use of thioamides. Thioamides, such as methimazole, carbimazole, and propylthiouracil, are used as a medical treatment for hyperthyroidism [21]. Barbero et al., in their series, found an association between prenatal maternal hyperthyroidism treated with methimazole and CA development [22]. However, the possibility of a causal association between maternal hyperthyroidism itself and CA has been described [22]. Further studies are still required to delineate this link.

#### 7.3.4.2 Clinical Presentation and Diagnosis

Clinical presentation of CA is variable. This variability depends on many factors including side of obstruction whether unilateral or bilateral and associated other congenital anomalies. It can range from acute airway obstruction to chronic recurrent sinusitis. In bilateral choanal atresia, infants usually present with a respiratory distress and intermittent cyanosis characteristically relieved by crying. This can be attributed to the elevated laryngeal position in neonates and being obligate nasal breathers. Due to inability to breathe and feed simultaneously, feeding difficulty may be the initial presenting feature. Also, a history of multiple failed extubation attempts in a neonate, should raise the possibility of bilateral CA.

Infants with unilateral CA often present later in life and rarely have respiratory distress. A persistent unilateral mucoid rhinorrhea with obstruction in childhood can be the first presentation for unilateral cases. Occasionally, it may not be diagnosed until late in adulthood due to the non-specific symptoms of unilateral nasal obstruction. Due to the low morbidity of unilateral CA, its surgical treatment is usually delayed as the chances of successful repair increase with age owing to the more favorable anatomy [23].

Diagnosis of choanal atresia at birth can be done through various tests. It can be suspected if a French catheter of size 5 or 6 cannot be passed through the nose to the nasopharynx. Other methods include methylene blue dye test, cotton wisp test, and laryngeal mirror test. However, the preferred method of diagnosis is through endoscopic visualization of the atretic plate closing the choana.

Although plain radiographs have been used widely to determine the patency of the choana by using a contrast material, the procedure of choice nowadays is CT with or without contrast. CT is used not only to confirm the diagnosis, but also to determine exactly the extent of atresia [3]. A careful review of the CT scan can give an idea about the thickness of obliteration of the posterior choana and, also the width and height of the nasopharynx (Figs. 7.1, 7.2, 7.3). This is crucial for an

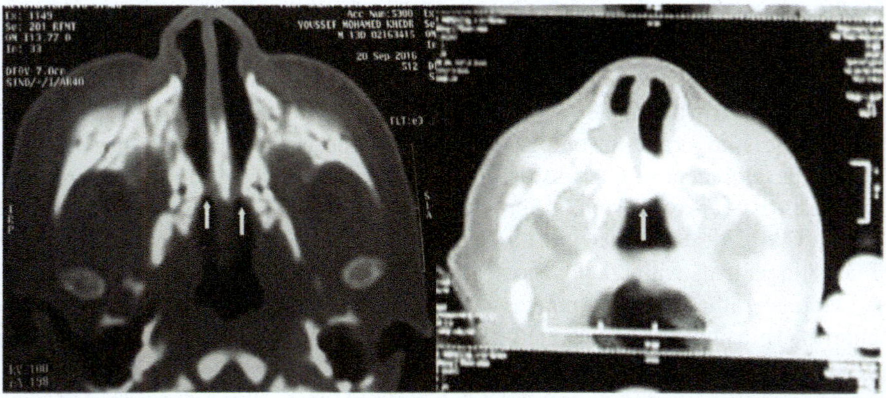

**Fig. 7.1** Computed tomography scans demonstrating bilateral bony choanal atresia, arrow points to a very thick atretic plate

**Fig. 7.2** Computed tomography scan showing passage of dye through the right side of the nose and arrest of passage through the left side of the nose confirming the diagnosis of left side choanal atresia

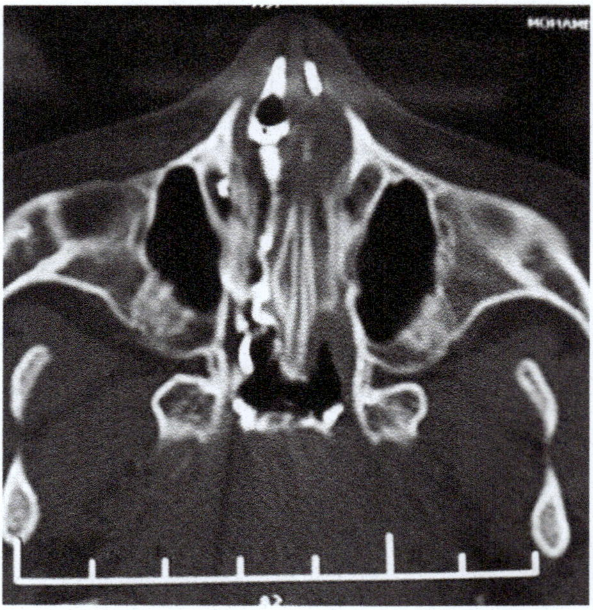

accurate surgical plan. If difficult surgery is suspected like in cases of partially atretic nose or very thick atretic plate, certain precautions can be implemented to facilitate surgery and reduce complications as the use of laser, powered instrumentation, shortening the duration of the procedure and avoiding working laterally [24].

Slovis et al. reviewed the CT findings in 11 CA patients and 66 control patients to compare the choanal space between CA and normal infants [25]. According to his findings, the normal mean choanal air space of a newborn was about 0.67 mm and increases by 0.27 mm per year up to 20 years old. In comparison to CA, the choanal space was absent in bony atresia while in membranous atresia, it was reduced to 1/3

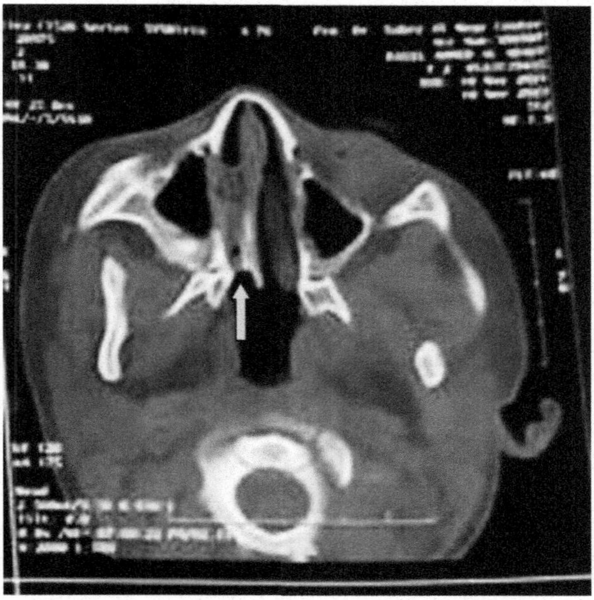

**Fig. 7.3** Computed tomography scan showing right side bony and membranous choanal atresia

of the normal size. The mean normal vomer thickness was 2.3 mm in children less than 8 years of age and reached 2.8 mm at the age of 8 years. In CA, the vomer thickness was found to be around 6.0 mm in bony atresia and 3.0 mm in membranous type. The thickness of the bony atretic plate is always variable, between 1 and 12 mm, depending on the medial pterygoid plate and vomer [25].

#### 7.3.4.3 Treatment

##### Initial Airway Management

The primary presentation of bilateral CA is an airway emergency at birth. Therefore, the goal of initial treatment here is to ensure an adequate oral airway through a McGovern nipple. It is an artificial intraoral nipple with a large opening secured in the mouth and can pass a small feeding tube to provide simultaneous feeding. If this method fails, the second option will be an endotracheal intubation to secure the airway.

Tracheostomy is usually restricted to cases with other comorbidities where the definitive surgical correction will be delayed. These conditions include cardiopulmonary instability and multi-level airway obstruction. It has been noted that cases of bilateral CA and CHARGE syndrome are more likely to fail surgical repair due to the severely contracted nasopharynx in a lateral or vertical dimension with poor pharyngeal muscle control [26].

#### 7.3.4.4 Surgical Management

Various surgical approaches had been proposed starting from the mid-nineteenth century with different outcomes and success rates. Not only the surgical technique itself is variable, but also the use of postoperative stenting and adjunct therapy is variable among authors [27].

- **Transnasal Puncture**

  This method was first described by Emmertin in 1851 in neonates with bilateral CA [28, 29]. Instruments used included the urethral sounds and Fearson dilators. At first puncturing the atretic plate was done blindly, then the laryngeal mirror and the 120° endoscope were used to visualize the nasopharyngeal side of the atretic plate. This method had a high restenosis rate, so a combination with post-operative stenting was recommended. This approach had become restricted to cases with a thin membranous CA with a very narrow nose making the endoscopic visualization very difficult [16]. This is attributed to the potential complications linked to the blind nature of the procedure, such as septal and turbinate injury, intranasal adhesion, clival injury causing Gradenigo syndrome, CSF rhinorrhea with possible meningitis [28].
- **Transpalatal Repair**

  Transpalatal CA repair was first described by Owens in 1965. Its main aim was to optimize exposure of the atretic plate. It starts with elevation of a U-shaped posteriorly based mucosal flap behind the hard-soft palatal junction. After that, bone drilling is commenced involving the atretic plates, the posterior part of the vomer and the medial pterygoid plates.

  This approach enjoys a high primary success rate, up to 84% [30], but has significant associated complications such as maxillary growth affection with subsequent cross-bite and high palatal arch deformity [16]. Other reported complications include palatal flap breakdown and fistula, palatal muscle dysfunction resulting in velopharyngeal incompetence [31]. Owing to these mentioned complications, the transpalatal approach is not recommended now before the age of 6 years [32–34].
- **Transnasal Endoscopic Repair**

  The transnasal endoscopic repair has become the primary procedure for CA repair, as stated by Park et al. [30]. The endoscopic technique was first demonstrated by Stankiewicz [35]. Since then, several modifications have been described. First it is very important to identify the working zone which includes the superior limit of the obliterated choana which should be below the attachment of the middle turbinate. Working above this limit will cause bleeding and may cause injury to the skull base. Medially, the superior limit should be parallel to the level of the choana. Higher dissection of the septum is not helpful. Anteriorly, the dissection should be few millimeters, and it ends where the lateral and medial walls are parallel (where the posterior narrowing start). Inferiorly, incision is made at the junction of the floor of the nose and the septum extending horizontally over its junction with the atretic plate (Figs. 7.4 and 7.5). Variable flaps have been described, as superiorly based, or laterally based. The flaps aim to preserve mucosa as far as possible. It is important to avoid cartilage exposure. The procedure is usually done using a 2.9- or 4.0-mm rigid endoscope, 4.0 mm rigid endoscope is much better as it gives more panoramic view of the working

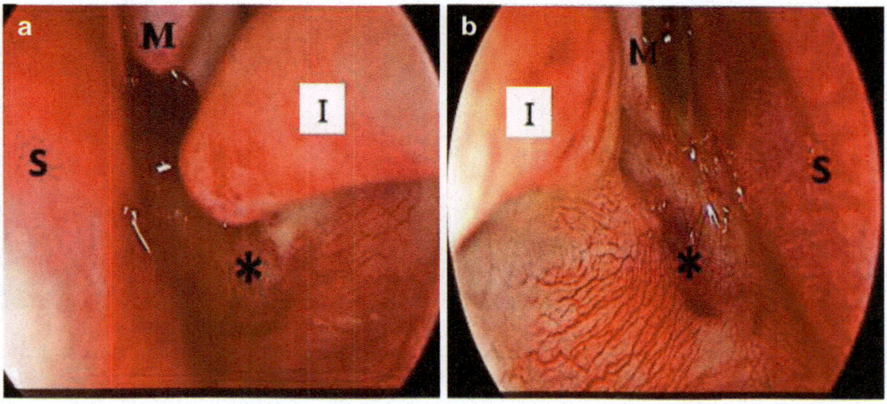


**Fig. 7.4** Endoscopic view of bilateral choanal atresia (**a**): Left side and (**b**): Right side. S: Septum, M: Middle turbinate, I: Inferior turbinate, asterisk: Atretic plate

**Fig. 7.5** Illustration of the direction of flap elevation during endoscopic repair of choanal atresia (right side). S: Septum, it: inferior turbinate, mt: middle turbinate

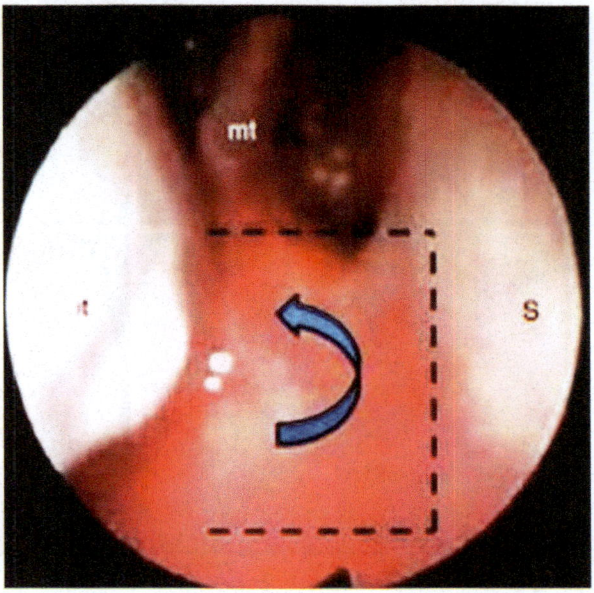


zone. The ideal point of entry into the nasopharynx is the junction between the hard palate and the vomer inferiorly and medially, as this is the thinnest part of the atresia (Figs. 7.6, 7.7, and 7.8).

After mucosal elevation, the vomer is removed to create the neo-choana [36]. To prevent affection of the nasal growth canters, no more than 1/3 of the bony septum can be removed. CT scan of these infants after few years showed significant loss of the posterior septum. Sometimes, the lateral boundary of the atresia needs widening by ear curettes or by drilling. Any exposed bone should be covered with mucosa to prevent post-operative restenosis [37]. It is very important

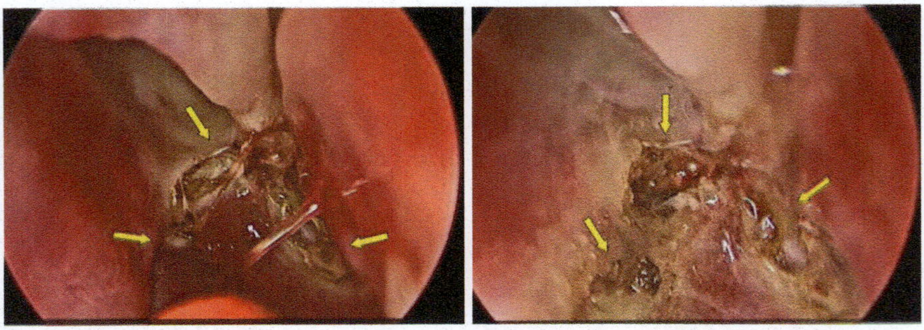

**Fig. 7.6** Endoscopic view of left choanal atresia showing the marks done by diathermy to define the limits of the working zone at the beginning of endoscopic repair

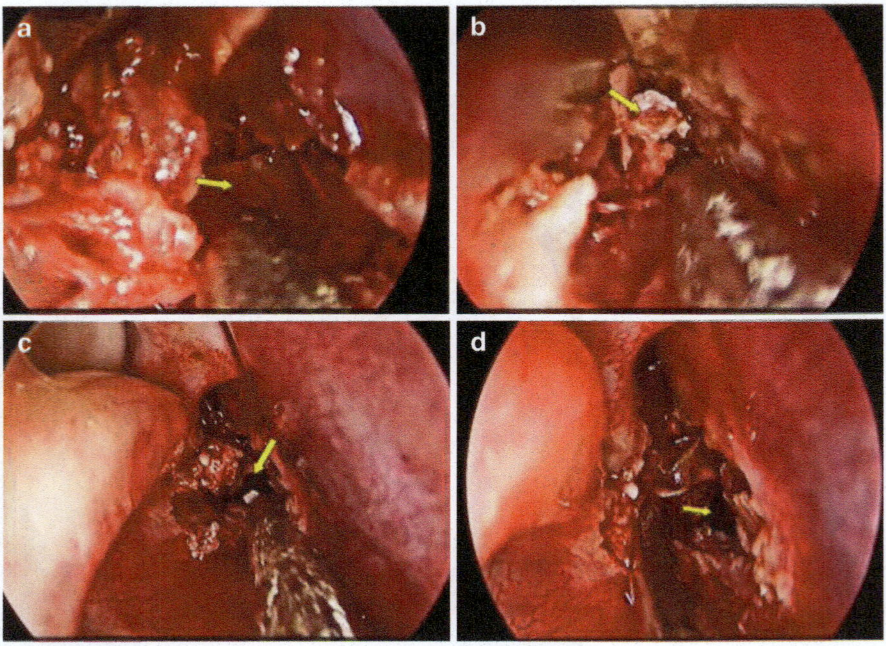


**Fig. 7.7** Endoscopic repair of a left choanal atresia. (**a**) the yellow arrow refers to the atretic bony plate, (**b**) the yellow arrow refers to the bone removed to open the atretic plate, (**c**) the picture after opening the atresia with the arrow refers to the nasopharynx starting to be visible through the new choana, (**d**) the picture after widening of the new choanal opening

to avoid any inadvertent injury to the nasal vestibule or the columella from heat during drilling. A posterior septal window may be added if the nostril is too small to accommodate the endoscope and the instruments [38].

Surgical steps are demonstrated in Videos 7.1 and 7.2.

In a previous meta-analysis of 20 studies, the mean success rate with the transnasal endoscopic repair was 85.3% [39]. As there is no strict definition of

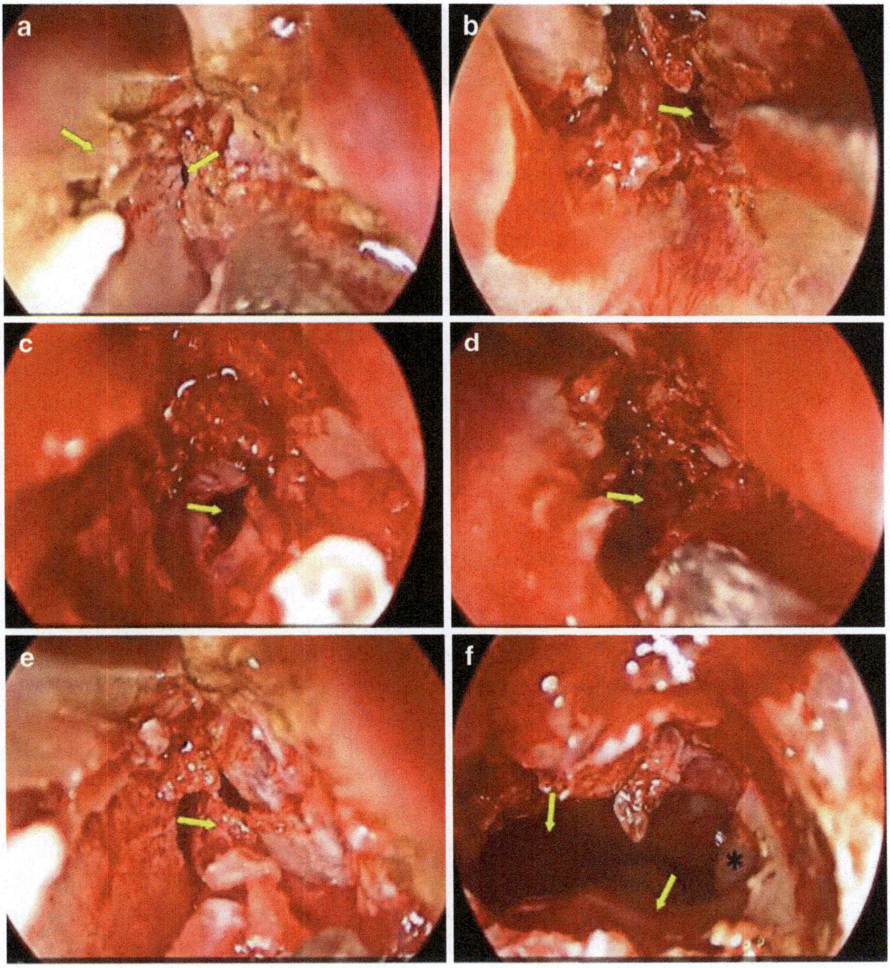


**Fig. 7.8** Endoscopic repair of bilateral choanal atresia. (**a**) Endoscopic demonstration of the right side of the nose showing the atretic plate and the beginning of opening of the new choana, (**b**) Endoscopic picture of the right side of the nose after opening of the atretic plate, (**c**) Endoscopic visualization of the left side of the choanal atresia while starting to open it, (**d**) Endoscopic picture showing the new left choana, (**e**) The arrow refers to the vomer in between the two new choanal openings, (**f**) Final endoscopic picture after removal of the vomer and connecting the two new choanal openings, asterisk refers to the left tubal elevation, the upper arrow refers to the nasopharynx, the lower arrow refers to the upper surface of the soft palate

the surgical failure, the success rate is difficult to interpret and compare across various studies. Revision is defined, by some authors, as the need for removal of excess granulation tissue, while others consider any need for general anesthesia as for stent removal is a revision procedure. A common complication of this approach is the post-operative restenosis. Its risk factors include; nasopharyngeal and gastroesophageal reflux, cases younger than 10 days of age, pure bony atretic plate and presence of associated malformations. It is highly recommended to use saline irrigation frequently postoperatively with scheduled second look evaluations to reduce the chance of restenosis.

- **Post-operative Stenting**

  Stent use after CA repair is a controversial topic with different opinions throughout literature. Traditionally, it was used as an adjunctive measure to reduce the incidence of restenosis. Commercial or custom-made stents, from endotracheal tube, are available [40]. In early author's experience, empirical stent use was done in all cases for a duration of 5–8 weeks as a prophylactic for restenosis [41]. Recently, stenting is only reserved for some selected cases with persistent narrow choana even after drilling, difficult follow-up situations and patients with associated congenital anomalies. On evaluation of the difference in overall success rate in cases with and without stenting, there was no superior results in either group. However, the incidence of postoperative granulation tissue and subsequently, restenosis was found to be higher when the stents were used making non-stent surgery more favorable [42].

  Many researches had discussed this topic with no clear-cut evidence on the effectiveness of stents use. There is still disagreement in the recommended stent duration, its type and the way it is fixed to the nostril leaving this point with many inconsistencies. The most adopted concept until now is that a combined close post-operative follow-up, early removal of nasal crusting and regular saline irrigation are the key points for successful repair of CA without stenting [43].

- **Mitomycin C**

  Mitomycin C is an aminoglycoside that inhibits DNA synthesis by generating oxygen radicals that alkylate and crosslink DNA. Due to this mechanism of action, it has been used to inhibit fibroblast proliferation and thus reducing post-surgical restenosis. In early 2000s, studies revealed better surgical outcome in CA repair when mitomycin C was used [44]. However, when subsequent comparative studies were conducted between mitomycin group and a control group, there was no significant difference in the incidence of postoperative stenosis [45].

  Carter et al., in their study, had concluded that there is no change in the restenosis rate with topical mitomycin C, but the postoperative granulation tissue and subsequent surgical debridement are markedly decreased [45]. There is no supporting evidence till now for the use of mitomycin in children with remaining concerns regarding its potential carcinogenic effect in this young age [46].

#### 7.3.4.5 Surgery with Navigators

Most of operative procedures for surgical correction of choanal atresia are usually done without using navigators provided that there available pre-operative high-quality CT scans and appropriately sized instrumentations and endoscopes. There are few reports discussing the use of navigators in endoscopic transnasal CA repair [47].

#### 7.3.4.6 Laser-Assisted Surgery

Laser-assisted $CO_2$ CA repair was first described in 1978 by Healy et al. [48]. However, it was found ineffective when bone thickness exceeds 1 mm. Other types of laser have been described with limited experience, such as Nd-YAG, potassium titanyl phosphate (KTP), and diode laser (CDL).

The lack of significant advantage of laser use over the conventional cold methods, associated reported fire risks and some reported deaths from air embolism with Nd-YAG laser limited the widespread acceptance of laser-assisted repair in CA [49].

## 7.4 Type II: Hyperplastic and Duplication Anomalies

These anomalies include a wide range from supernumerary nostrils to duplicate columella up to polyrhinia. The underlying embryological explanation is the presence of an accessory olfactory pit or duplicated olfactory placode [1]. Polyrhinia results from duplication of the medial nasal process only while the lateral nasal process develops normally [50]. These duplicate structures may be the presentation of a midline craniofacial cleft [1]. A pre-operative radiological evaluation is very important in these cases as they are always associated with other underlying bony anomalies. The classically described duplicate nasal anomaly is the proboscis lateralis. By definition, it is typically a tubular tract arising from the lateral nose or medial canthus. It is usually lined by squamous and ciliated respiratory epithelium and is associated with sinonasal hypoplasia or aplasia on the ipsilateral side [51, 52]. As proboscis is often associated with ipsilateral absence of olfactory nerve, olfactory lobe, and cribriform plate, it is thought to be caused by lesion or absence of the olfactory placode early in development. The condition also has an effect on the eye and eyelid development with resulting hypertelorism and/or coloboma of the eyelid, iris or retina [1, 51].

## 7.5 Type III: Nasal Clefts

Nasal clefts anomalies often occur in association with cleft lip and palate. The worse the cleft lip, the worse the nasal deformity [3]. These clefts can be unilateral or bilateral. In unilateral cases, the premaxilla and maxilla tether the nose, causing the septum to deviate. As development continues, maxillary growth is also affected by the tethered septum, leading to maxillary hypoplasia. Complete clefting of the nose results from the failure of development of the frontal processes, either medial or lateral clefts [53, 54].

Tessier, in 1976, developed the well-known classification system for craniofacial clefts using the orbit as the primary structure of reference [55]. The craniofacial clefts that involve the nose are Tessier No. 0, 1, 2, and 3 clefts, and their cranial extensions: Tessier No. 11, 12, 13, and 14 [1].

Frontonasal dysplasia, Tessier No. 0/14 cleft or median facial cleft, is the most severe form being presented by frontonasal encephalocele, hypertelorism, broad nasal dorsum, failure of closure of the anterior neuropore and a V-shaped forehead [1]. The intermediate presentation of this condition is called Frontorhiny. It is characterized by hypertelorism, wide nasal dorsum, bifid nasal tip, broad columella and widely separated narrow nostrils [56]. There is association between the midline clefts and midline nasal masses, so a concurrent presence of a nasal dermoid or encephalocele should be ruled out in cases of midline clefts [5].

In Tessier No. 1/13, the bony cleft includes the alveolus, pyriform aperture, nasal bone, and frontal process of maxilla while the soft tissue involvement includes the cupid's bow and nasal ala, causing lateral displacement of the medial canthus [1].

Cleft lip and nasal deformity are considered a part of Tessier No. 2/12 clefts. The complete form of this anomaly is rare and involves a soft-tissue defect of the lip up to the alar rim, with involvement of the upper lateral cartilage and the frontal process of the maxilla [1]. The embryological explanation of this cleft is failure of the fusion of the medial and lateral nasal processes with the maxillary process [57]. Also, heminasal aplasia, supernumerary nostrils, and proboscis lateralis may be considered a variation of type 2 cleft [55] (Fig. 7.9).

In unilateral cleft lip, there is associated medial and inferior rotation of the medial nasal crus and retrodisplacement of the nasal ala with flat flared nostril. The nasal tip and base are usually wide with nasal septal deviation to the normal side of the nose. In bilateral clefts, there are other defects in addition to those mentioned with unilateral cleft as shortened columella and prognathism due to hypoplastic maxilla [3].

The most appropriate timing for surgical correction of these clefts are still controversial. Delayed correction is sometimes favored by some surgeons to wait until

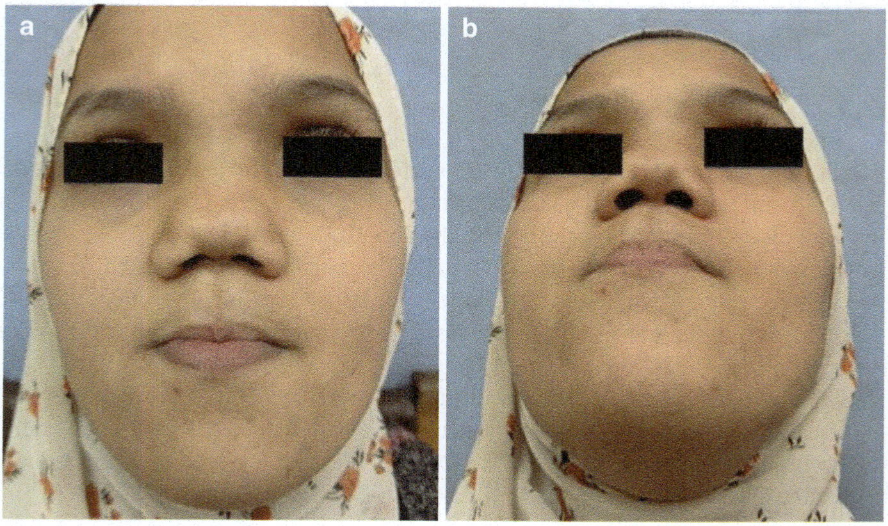


**Fig. 7.9** Cleft lip and nose, (**a**) frontal view, (**b**) basal view

the facial growth is complete and nasal structures are matured to give the best results. In contrary, other surgeons prefer early intervention in these cases especially those associated with inadequate breathing and respiratory distress [3, 11, 54, 58, 59].

## 7.6 Type IV: Congenital Masses, Neoplasms, and Vascular Anomalies

Congenital nasal masses are rare lesions that can present anywhere in the nose; external nose, the nasal cavity, paranasal sinuses, nasopharynx, oral cavity, and orbit [60]. The reported common congenital nasal masses include meningo-encephalocele, glioma, dermoid cyst, vascular malformations, and, rarely, malignant and benign neoplasms [61].

The three most frequently described anomalies include; dermoid cysts, encephaloceles, and gliomas. The underlying mechanism of occurrence of these anomalies is faulty closure of the anterior neuropore with subsequent persistence of an anterior cranial defect [62, 63].

### 7.6.1 Nasal Dermoid Cysts

Nasal dermoid cysts are the most common of congenital midline nasal lesions. They usually present as non-compressible cystic mass, sinus, or a combination of both over the nasal dorsum with a midline pit [64]. Dermoid cysts may occur anywhere from the glabella to nasal tip, but the most common site, 60%, is in the lower third [65]. Less commonly, they can be present intranasally and in 10% can be combined. The nasal dermoid usually terminate in a subcutaneous tract with hair at its opening. Intracranial extension can be found in 20–45% of these cases, but they don't enlarge with crying or straining (Fig. 7.10). They can be presented as a recurrent septal abscess or osteomyelitis and with intracranial extension, they can be the cause of meningitis or brain abscess [40].

Grunwald [66] in 1910, stated the mechanism behind development of this anomaly. It starts as a protrusion of a dural diverticulum in the space between the nasal bones and nasal capsule and as the nasal processes of the frontal bones grow, they surround the diverticulum to form the foramen cecum, separating the dura from the skin. Normally, this diverticulum is involved. Incomplete closure of its pathway results in a persistent attachment of the dura to the dermis. When the dura recedes, it pulls nasal ectoderm upward trapping epithelium in the diverticulum path. When this epithelium proliferates, it produces the dermoid with associated glands and hair [67].

Nasal dermoids are not part of certain named clinical syndromes. However, there other associated anomalies reported in up to 41% of these cases including cleft defects, aural atresias, and hydrocephalus [64]. According to Wardinksi, In those

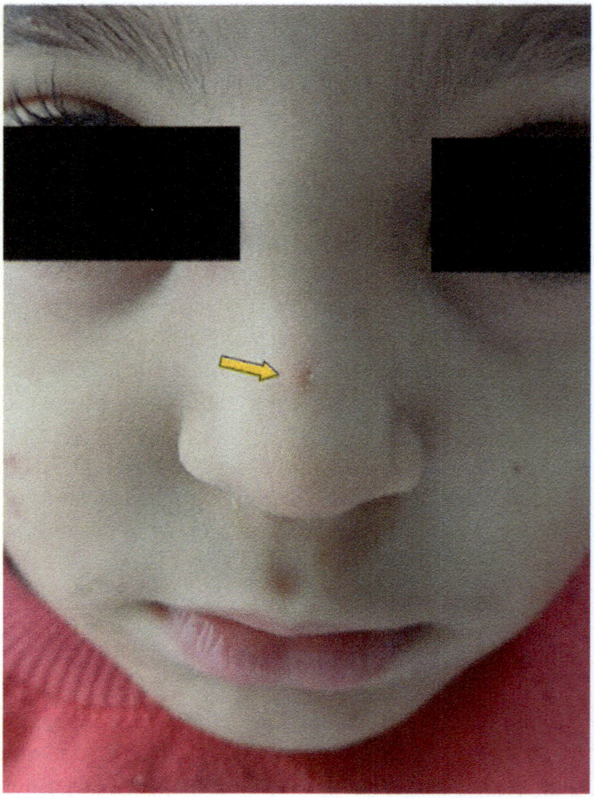

**Fig. 7.10** Photographic view of a nasal dermoid cyst with pit in the middle part of the nasal dorsum slightly to the left side

cases presenting with other congenital anomalies, the frequency of intracranial extension increases from 31% to 65% [68].

Thorough CT and MRI are considered the preoperative gold standard radiographic evaluations to detect any intracranial extension and to prepare the surgical plan. The CT findings suspecting intracranial involvement are enlarged foramen cecum and bifid crista galli [40, 69]. High-resolution MRI with contrast helps in differentiation between avascular dermoids and hemangiomas or vascular teratomas [70]. Notably, the crista galli in infants is unossified and does not contain marrow fat. Subsequently, any high-intensity enhancement in MRI T1 images in the area of the crista galli in an infant is strongly suggestive of an intracranial dermoid [70] (Fig. 7.11).

The standard treatment for nasal dermoids is surgical excision of the lesion and its tract. Early intervention with complete excision prevents its recurrence and avoids distortion of the nose [67]. There is a reported recurrence rate of 5.5% by Denoyelle and colleagues [64] in their series. The recommended criteria for successful surgical excision of the nasal dermoid, as stated by Pollock [71], are all related to the approach used. These include that the approach should permit access to all midline cysts, allows for medial and lateral osteotomies, facilitates repair of any associated cerebrospinal fluid rhinorrhea, permit reconstruction of a distorted

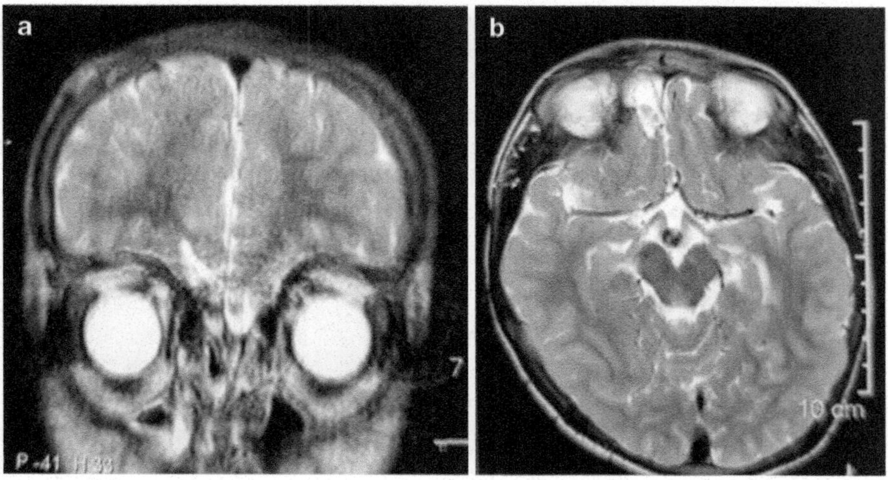


**Fig. 7.11** Magnetic resonance imaging, (**a**) Coronal and (**b**) Axial, demonstrating intranasal dermoid with an intracranial connection

nasal dorsum with an acceptable facial scar [40.67]. Endoscopic approach in nasal dermoid is limited to totally intranasal dermoids with little or no cutaneous extension. Sometimes, it can be combined with a small external midline excision of the cutaneous punctum in cases extending to the skin [72].

### 7.6.2 Nasal Encephaloceles

Nasal encephaloceles are an extracranial herniation of meninges and brain tissue. They are usually classified by their site of herniation, with nasofrontal, nasoethmoidal, and naso-orbital encephaloceles present at the forehead, nasal dorsum, and orbit, respectively. With all these different locations, the internal defect is always located in the midline. Encephaloceles, like demoids, are soft, compressible masses, but they characteristically transilluminate and may be mistaken for polyps. Also, encephaloceles have a positive Furstenberg test, as crying or straining cause enlargement of the mass. They can be identified easily in MRI imaging as a continued signal with the intracranial space. The risk of CSF leak, meningitis, or even intracranial abscess can occur with infected encephaloceles [60].

### 7.6.3 Nasal Gliomas

Nasal gliomas represent a persistent brain tissue through a cranial defect, but with lost meningeal connection, unlike encephaloceles. The term glioma is a misnomer as it is not a true neoplasm. Other terms as encephaloma, nasal cerebral heterotopia, or neuroglial heterotopia can describe the lesion more accurately reflecting its nature [73]. They are typically firm, non-compressible, and can be anywhere from the glabella to the nasal tip. 60% of the cases are extranasal, 30% intranasal, and 10% are combined [60]. Although they are less translucent, gliomas can be mistaken for nasal polyps. In about 15 to 20% of cases, there may be a dural connection with a pedicle of glial tissue. However, absence of extracranial continuity of CSF flow should be present on MRI [63]. Gliomas have a lower risk of intracranial complications due to lack of meningeal continuity, but they can become infected with subsequent deformed septum or nasal bones [73].

### 7.6.4 Vascular Anomalies of the Nose

The most described nasal vascular anomaly haemangioma. They are benign vascular tumors that usually appear during the first weeks of birth. During the first year of life, they are characterized by rapid proliferation followed by a quiescent stage and then involution stage that can last for several years.

Treatment of nasal hemangioma was restricted to those cases with functional problems as nasal obstruction or visual affection, or lesions with ulceration and bleeding. With discovery of propranolol, it is considered an effective and common treatment for accelerating involution stage with rare side effects [74]. Some authors suggested use of topical β-blockers with lower risk of associated side effects than the systemic treatment. Other treatment possibilities include intralesional steroid injections, pulse dye laser therapy, and surgical removal [75].

### 7.6.5 Neoplasms

The previously reported nasal neoplastic lesions include pilomatrixoma, lipoma, neurofibroma, neuroblastoma, rhabdomyosarcoma, and teratoma [76]. The most common lesion of those is teratoma, as it has the greatest potential for causing life-threatening airway complications. Given the incidence of 1:20,000 live births, head and neck teratomas represent only 5% of neonatal teratomas. They are formed of the three germ layers and can often be diagnosed on prenatal ultrasound. Cervical teratomas are the most common while those present in the nasopharynx are the second common. Resection of these teratomas are usually done in early newborn period provided that the airway is wide enough [77].

## 7.7 Type V: Congenital Syndromes with Malformed Nasal Structures

The coexistence of more than one craniofacial anomaly usually characterizes a certain syndrome. Maxillary hypoplasia is a common finding in craniofacial syndromes as it usually produces a contracted nasal cavity with other respiratory problems [11].

### 7.7.1 Crouzon Syndrome

This syndrome was first described in 1912. The main characteristics of this autosomal dominant condition include craniosynostosis, midface retrusion, and proptosis [78]. It accounts for 5% of cases of craniosynostosis, with a prevalence of 1 in 25,000 births. The underlying genetic mutation is related to the FGFR2 gene on chromosome 10q26. Multiple sutures can be involved in this syndrome; however, the coronal suture is the most common being involved in nearly 95% of cases. Other features include maxillary hypoplasia with a small nasopharynx, narrowed or obliterated anterior nares, hypertelorism, nasal septum deviation, and a "parrot-beak" nose. These cases can have a normal intelligence level if they are managed properly as associated brain malformations are uncommon [79].

### 7.7.2 Apert Syndrome

It is similar to Crouzon syndrome in many aspects. It is also autosomal dominant and results from a mutation in the FGFR2 gene, but its prevalence is only 1:160,000 births [79]. As it is associated with high mortality, its prevalence is closer to 1 in 2 million [80]. The syndrome is characterized by fused coronal sutures, mental retardation, brain malformations, craniosynostosis, midface hypoplasia, and choanal stenosis [81]. Other nasal abnormalities may involve a saddle nose with a bulbous tip and a high-arched palate (Fig. 7.12). Unlike Crouzon syndrome, cases with

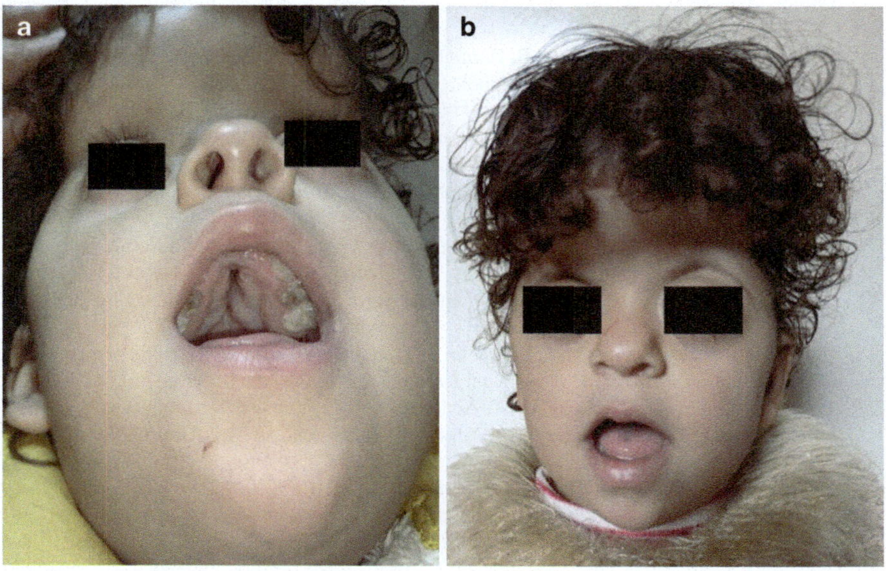


**Fig. 7.12** Very high arched palate in a case of Apert syndrome

Apert syndrome usually have symmetric syndactyly of the extremities with possible other axial skeletal problems.

### 7.7.3 Stickler Syndrome

Stickler syndrome is also an autosomal dominant syndrome and affects approximately 1 in 10,000 people [3]. The underlying genetic defect is related to the COL2A1 gene on chromosome 12, which codes for type II procollagen. This protein is found in vitreous gel and cartilage. Therefore, the disease is primarily characterized by ophthalmic abnormalities, but various orofacial anomalies may also develop [82]. This includes a flattened midface, depressed nasal bridge, long philtrum, and hypoplastic maxilla [83]. Other problems may involve high-frequency sensorineural hearing loss, bifid uvula, mandibular hypoplasia, and cleft palate. This syndrome is the most common association with the Robin sequence [82].

## References


1. Losee JE, Kirschner RE, Whitaker LA, Bartlett SP. Congenital nasal anomalies: a classification scheme. Plast Reconstr Surg. 2004;113(2):676–89.
2. Szeremeta W, Parikh TD, Widelitz JS. Congenital nasal malformations. Otolaryngol Clin N Am. 2007;40(1):97–112.
3. Cummings C. Otolaryngology head and neck surgery. 4th ed. Philadelphia, PA: Elsevier Mosby; 2005.
4. Netter F. Atlas of human anatomy. Teterboro, NJ: Icon Learning Systems; 2003.
5. Otteson TD. Congenital malformations of the nose and paranasal sinuses. In: Bluestone CD, Simons JP, Healy GB, editors. Bluestone and stool's pediatric otolaryngology, vol. 1. Shelton, CT: PMPH; 2014. p. 1017–35.
6. Van Kempen A, Nabben F, Hamel B. Heminasal aplasia: a case report and review of the literature of the last 25 years. Clin Dysmorphol. 1997;6(2):147–52.
7. Guerrissi JO. Congenital absence of nasal bones. Ann Plast Surg. 1993;30(3):260–3.
8. Manning K, Singh S. Hypoplasia of the nasal bones. J Laryngol Otol. 1977;91(12):1085–91.
9. Tollefson TT, Humphrey CD, Larrabee WF, Adelson RT, Karimi K, Kriet JD. The spectrum of isolated congenital nasal deformities resembling the cleft lip nasal morphology. Arch Facial Plast Surg. 2011;13(3):152–60.
10. Ginat DT, Robson CD. CT and MRI of congenital nasal lesions in syndromic conditions. Pediatr Radiol. 2015;45:1056–65.
11. Lee WT, Koltai PJ. Nasal deformity in neonates and young children. Pediatr Clin. 2003;50(2):459–67.
12. Vercruysse J-P, Wojciechowski M, Koninckx M, Kurotova A, Claes J. Congenital nasal pyriform aperture stenosis: a rare cause of neonatal nasal obstruction. J Pediatr Surg. 2006;41(4):e5–7.
13. Bazak R, Ibrahim AA, Hussein WKA, Abdelnaby MM, Elwany S. Extramucosal pyriplasty without stenting for management of pyriform aperture stenosis. Eur Arch Otorrinolaringol. 2018;275(6):1469–75.
14. Frasee J. Congenital atresia of the choanae. Br Med J. 1910;2(2604):1698–701.
15. Brown OE, Pownell P, Manning SC. Choanal atresia: a new anatomic classification and clinical management applications. Laryngoscope. 1996;106(1):97–101.
16. Hengerer AS, Brickman TM, Jeyakumar A. Choanal atresia: embryologic analysis and evolution of treatment, a 30-year experience. Laryngoscope. 2008;118(5):862–6.

17. Burrow TA, Saal HM, de Alarcon A, Martin LJ, Cotton RT, Hopkin RJ. Characterization of congenital anomalies in individuals with choanal atresia. Arch Otolaryngol Head Neck Surg. 2009;135(6):543–7.
18. Wilson JG, Roth CB, Warkany J. An analysis of the syndrome of malformations induced by maternal vitamin a deficiency. Effects of restoration of vitamin a at various times during gestation. Am J Anat. 1953;92:189–217.
19. Dupé V, Matt N, Garnier J-M, Chambon P, Mark M, Ghyselinck NB. A newborn lethal defect due to inactivation of retinaldehyde dehydrogenase type 3 is prevented by maternal retinoic acid treatment. Proc Natl Acad Sci. 2003;100(24):14036–41.
20. Hehr U, Muenke M. Craniosynostosis syndromes: from genes to premature fusion of skull bones. Mol Genet Metab. 1999;68(2):139–51.
21. Chabrolle J, Bruel H, El Khoury E, et al. Methimazole and choanal atresia. Archives de pediatrie: organe officiel de la Societe francaise de pediatrie. 2003;10(5):463–4.
22. Barbero P, Valdez R, Rodríguez H, et al. Choanal atresia associated with maternal hyperthyroidism treated with methimazole: a case–control study. Am J Med Genet A. 2008;146(18):2390–5.
23. Newman JR, Harmon P, Shirley WP, Hill JS, Woolley AL, Wiatrak BJ. Operative management of choanal atresia: a 15-year experience. JAMA Otolaryngol Head Neck Surg. 2013;139(1):71–5.
24. Khafagy YW. Endoscopic repair of bilateral congenital choanal atresia. Laryngoscope. 2002;112(2):316–9.
25. Slovis T, Renfro B, Watts F, Kuhns L, Belenky W, Spoylar J. Choanal atresia: precise CT evaluation. Radiology. 1985;155(2):345–8.
26. Coniglio JU, Manzione JV, Hengerer AS. Anatomic findings and management of choanal atresia and the CHARGE association. Ann Otol Rhinol Laryngol. 1988;97(5):448–53.
27. Cedin AC, Atallah AN, Andriolo RB, Cruz OL, Pignatari SN. Surgery for congenital choanal atresia. Cochrane Database Syst Rev. 2012;2:CD008993. https://doi.org/10.1002/14651858.CD008993.
28. Gujrathi C, Daniel S, James A, Forte V. Management of bilateral choanal atresia in the neonate: an institutional review. Int J Pediatr Otorhinolaryngol. 2004;68(4):399–407.
29. Emmert C. Stenochorie und Atresie der Choannen, Lehrbach der Speciellen Chirurgie, vol. 2. Stuttgart: Dann; 1854. p. 535–8.
30. Park AH, Brockenbrough J, Stankiewicz J. Endoscopic versus traditional approaches to choanal atresia. Otolaryngol Clin N Am. 2000;33(1):77–90.
31. Stieve M, Kempf H, Lenarz T. Management of choanal atresia in cases of craniofacial malformation. J Maxillofacial Oral Surg. 2009;8:52–4.
32. Freng A. Growth in width of the dental arches after partial extirpation of the mid-palatal suture in man. Scand J Plast Reconstr Surg. 1978;12(3):267–72.
33. Hengerer AS, Strome M. Choanal atresia: a new embryologic theory and its influence on surgical management. Laryngoscope. 1982;92(8):913–21.
34. Pirsig W. Surgery of choanal atresia in infants and children: historical notes and updated review. Int J Pediatr Otorhinolaryngol. 1986;11(2):153–70.
35. Stankiewicz JA. The endoscopic repair of choanal atresia. Otolaryngol Head Neck Surg. 1990;103(6):931–7.
36. Ibrahim AA, Magdy EA, Hassab MH. Endoscopic choanoplasty without stenting for congenital choanal atresia repair. Int J Pediatr Otorhinolaryngol. 2010;74(2):144–50.
37. Rodríguez H, Cuestas G, Passali D. A 20-year experience in microsurgical treatment of choanal atresia. Acta Otorrinolaringol (English Edition). 2014;65(2):85–92.
38. Peixoto MC, Spratley J, Oliveira G, Martins J, Bastos J, Ribeiro C. Effectiveness of cochlear implants in children: long term results. Int J Pediatr Otorhinolaryngol. 2013;77(4):462–8.
39. Durmaz A, Tosun F, Yldrm N, Sahan M, Kvrakdal C, Gerek M. Transnasal endoscopic repair of choanal atresia: results of 13 cases and meta-analysis. J Craniofac Surg. 2008;19(5):1270–4.
40. Manning SC, Bloom DC, Perkins JA, Gruss JS, Inglis A. Diagnostic and surgical challenges in the pediatric skull base. Otolaryngol Clin N Am. 2005;38(4):773–94.

41. Khafagy Y, Mokbel K, El Morsy S. Endoscopic management of congenital choanal atresia: second look procedure is mandatory. Mansoura Med J. 2004;33(1):259–65.
42. Eladl HM, Khafagy YW. Endoscopic bilateral congenital choanal atresia repair of 112 cases, evolving concept and technical experience. Int J Pediatr Otorhinolaryngol. 2016;85:40–5.
43. Teissier N, Kaguelidou F, Couloigner V, François M, Van Den Abbeele T. Predictive factors for success after transnasal endoscopic treatment of choanal atresia. Arch Otolaryngol Head Neck Surg. 2008;134(1):57–61.
44. Holland BW, McGuirt WF Jr. Surgical management of choanal atresia: improved outcome using mitomycin. Arch Otolaryngol Head Neck Surg. 2001;127(11):1375–80.
45. Carter JM, Lawlor C, Guarisco JL. The efficacy of mitomycin and stenting in choanal atresia repair: a 20 year experience. Int J Pediatr Otorhinolaryngol. 2014;78(2):307–11.
46. Agrawal N, Morrison G. Laryngeal cancer after topical mitomycin C application. J Laryngol Otol. 2006;120(12):1075–6.
47. Ramsden JD, Campisi P, Forte V. Choanal atresia and choanal stenosis. Otolaryngol Clin N Am. 2009;42(2):339–52.
48. Healy GB, McGill T, Jako GJ, Strong MS, Vaughan CW. Management of choanal atresia with the carbon dioxide laser. Ann Otol Rhinol Laryngol. 1978;87(5):658–62.
49. Yuan H-B, Poon K-S, Chan K-H, Lee T-Y, Lin C-Y. Fatal gas embolism as a complication of Nd-YAG laser surgery during treatment of bilateral choanal stenosis. Int J Pediatr Otorhinolaryngol. 1993;27(2):193–9.
50. Williams A, Pizzuto M, Brodsky L, Perry R. Supernumerary nostril: a rare congenital deformity. Int J Pediatr Otorhinolaryngol. 1998;44(2):161–7.
51. Abou-Elhamd K-EA. Proboscis lateralis: a report of two cases. Int J Pediatr Otorhinolaryngol. 2004;68(4):503–5.
52. Leung M, Krakovitz P, Koltai P. Congenital sinonasal disorders. In: Rhinology: diseases of the nose, sinuses, and skull base. New York: Thieme; 2012. p. 381–93.
53. Cutting CB. Secondary cleft lip nasal reconstruction: state of the art. Cleft Palate Craniofac J. 2000;37(6):538–41.
54. Moore CC, MacDonald I, Latham R, Brandt MG. Septopalatal protraction for correction of nasal septal deformity in cleft palate infants. Otolaryngol Head Neck Surg. 2005;133(6):949–53.
55. Tessier P. Anatomical classification of facial, cranio-facial and latero-facial clefts. J Maxillofac Surg. 1976;4:69–92.
56. Pham NS, Rafii A, Liu J, Boyadjiev SA, Tollefson TT. Clinical and genetic characterization of frontorhiny: report of 3 novel cases and discussion of the surgical management. Arch Facial Plast Surg. 2011;13(6):415–20.
57. Rontal M, Duritz G. Proboscis lateralis: case report and embryologic analysis. Laryngoscope. 1977;87(6):996–1006.
58. Wong K-S, Lin J-L. An underrecognized cause of respiratory distress in a neonate. CMAJ. 2006;174(11):1558–9.
59. Murali H, Hurt H. Nasal molding: a cultural practice causing respiratory distress in a term infant. J Pediatr. 2004;144(3):403–4.
60. Rahbar R, Resto VA, Robson CD, et al. Nasal glioma and encephalocele: diagnosis and management. Laryngoscope. 2003;113(12):2069–77.
61. Bradley P, Singh S. Congenital nasal masses: diagnosis and management. Clin Otolaryngol Allied Sci. 1982;7(2):87–97.
62. Hughes GB, Sharpino G, Hunt W, Tucker HM. Management of the congenital midline nasal mass: a review. Head Neck Surg. 1980;2(3):222–33.
63. Hedlund G. Congenital frontonasal masses: developmental anatomy, malformations, and MR imaging. Pediatr Radiol. 2006;36:647–62.
64. Denoyelle F, Ducroz V, Roger G. Nasal dermoid sinus cysts in children. Laryngoscope. 1997;107(6):795–800.
65. Pratt LW. Midline cysts of the nasal dorsum: embryologic origin and treatment. Laryngoscope. 1965;75(6):968–80.

66. Grunwald L. Beitrage zur Kenntinis Kongenitoter Geschwulste unt Missbildungen an Ohrunt Nase. Zeitschr f Ohrenheilk. 1910;60:270–317.
67. Hanikeri M, Waterhouse N, Kirkpatrick N, Peterson D, Macleod I. The management of midline transcranial nasal dermoid sinus cysts. Br J Plast Surg. 2005;58(8):1043–50.
68. Wardinsky TD, Pagon RA, Kropp RJ, Hayden PW, Clarren SK. Nasal dermoid sinus cysts: association with intracranial extension and multiple malformations. Cleft Palate Craniofac J. 1991;28(1):87–95.
69. Posnick JC, Bortoluzzi P, Armstrong DC, Drake JM. Intracanial nasal dermoid sinus cysts: computed tomographic scan findings and surgical results. Plast Reconstr Surg. 1994;93(4):745–54.
70. Fornadley JA, Tami TA. The use of magnetic resonance imaging in the diagnosis of the nasal dermal sinus-cyst. Otolaryngol Head Neck Surg. 1989;101(3):397–8.
71. Pollock RA. Surgical approaches to the nasal dermoid cyst. Ann Plast Surg. 1983;10(6):498–501.
72. Weiss DD, Robson CD, Mulliken JB. Transnasal endoscopic excision of midline nasal dermoid from the anterior cranial base. Plast Reconstr Surg. 1998;102(6):2119–23.
73. Adil E, Robson C, Perez-Atayde A, et al. Congenital nasal neuroglial heterotopia and encephaloceles: an update on current evaluation and management. Laryngoscope. 2016;126(9):2161–7.
74. Hogeling M, Adams S, Wargon O. A randomized controlled trial of propranolol for infantile hemangiomas. Pediatrics. 2011;128(2):e259–66.
75. Hochman M, Mascareno A. Management of nasal hemangiomas. Arch Facial Plast Surg. 2005;7(5):295–300. https://doi.org/10.1001/archfaci.7.5.295.
76. Zeitouni AG, Shapiro RS. Congenital anomalies of the nose and anterior skull base. In: Tewfik TL, Der Kaloustian VM, editors. Congenital anomalies of the ear, nose, and throat. New York: Oxford University Press; 1997. p. 189–200.
77. April MM, Ward RF, Garelick JM. Diagnosis, management, and follow-up of congenital head and neck teratomas. Laryngoscope. 1998;108(9):1398–401.
78. Crouzon O. Dysostose cranio-faciale hereditaire. Bull Mem Soc Med Paris. 1912;33:545–55.
79. Am PCN. Capitolo 592 Anomalie congenite del sistema nervoso centrale Stephen L. Kinsman e Michael V. Johnston. Pediatr Clin N Am. 2004;51:237–70.
80. Blank C. Apert's syndrome (a type of acrocephalosyndactyly)–observations on a British series of thirty-nine cases. Ann Hum Genet. 1959;24(2):151–64.
81. Kabbani H, Raghuveer TS. Craniosynostosis. Am Fam Physician. 2004;69(12):2863–70.
82. Rose PS, Levy HP, Liberfarb RM, et al. Stickler syndrome: clinical characteristics and diagnostic criteria. Am J Med Genet A. 2005;138(3):199–207.
83. Herrmann J, France TD, Spranger JW, Opitz JM, Wiffler C. The Stickler syndrome (hereditary arthroophthalmopathy). Birth Defects Orig Artic Ser. 1975;11(2):76–103.

# Nasal Trauma

8

Kamal Ebeid

**Key Points**

- Nasal fractures rank third in the incidence of all human fractures.
- The hallmarks of nasal fracture are mobility, crepitus, and bony angulation.
- Photographic documentation is highly recommended.
- Most nasal and septal fractures can be managed with closed reduction.
- It is important to have a plan for open reduction in certain instances.

## 8.1 Pathophysiology

The protruding and delicate skeleton of the nose makes it prone to soft tissue injuries and fractures. Nasal fractures rank third in the incidence of all human fractures, behind clavicle and wrist fractures. Many fractures of the nasal bone and septal skeleton go undiagnosed and untreated at the time of initial injury but account for a high percentage of subsequent septoplasty procedures for nasal obstruction or deviation [1].

Nasal fractures can be open, closed, or both. Nose fractures that occur in urban areas usually occur during fights, car accidents, or playing sports. In rural areas, nose fractures occur as a result of accidents on the farm, at work, during sports or during leisure time. The injuries sustained in traffic accidents are usually the most serious. While lap belts save lives, they often set the stage for serious nasal fractures (extreme fragmentation or damage to the nasoethmoidal complex).

K. Ebeid (✉)
Otorhinolaryngology Department, Tanta, Egypt
e-mail: kamal.ebeid@med.tanta.edu.eg


S. Elwany (ed.), *Current Rhinology*,
https://doi.org/10.1007/978-3-031-70077-4_8

The injury caused by a blow to the nose varies with the following factors: (a) age of the patient (tissue flexibility), (b) the amount of force applied, (c) the direction of the force, and (d) the nature of the striking object.

Common soft-tissue injuries include lacerations, ecchymosis, and hematoma of the external or internal nose. Skeletal injuries comprise fractures (comminution is more common among older patients), dislocations (more common among children), Dislocation injuries can involve any articulation of the external nasal skeleton or the septum.

The pattern of nasal fractures varies with the direction of applied forces; a distinct difference is found between frontal and lateral forces. Colton and Beekhuis [2] described a third class of fractures, those produced by force applied from below. A force of 25–75 pounds per square inch is needed to produce a nasal fracture. If the force is applied from a frontal direction, the injury varies from minor (lower margin of nasal bones) to marked (flattening of the external skeleton). Lateral forces can cause only a depressed fracture of the ipsilateral nasal bone or can be strong enough to outfracture the contralateral nasal bone as well. The injuries from below can cause telescoping of fragments and shortening of the nose or blockage of one side of the nasal airway due to septal fractures and dislocations, particularly dislocation of the quadrangular cartilage from the crest of the maxilla.

Septal fracture lines usually are vertical when they are located anteriorly and horizontal when located posteriorly. Septal fractures are said to activate interlocked stresses, and during the process of healing by fibrosis, they can produce septal twisting of various configurations (C-shaped, S-shaped, or spurs) [2].

## 8.2 Clinical Evaluation and Diagnosis

### 8.2.1 Clinical Examination

The history includes questions about the force, direction, and nature of the injury. When epistaxis has occurred, the probability of open fracture is high. When the patient also reports a change in nasal appearance or the onset of nasal airway obstruction, nasal fracture is almost certainly present.

The nose should be examined externally and internally to rule out deformities, deviations or abnormal contours. Lacerations, mucosal tears, petechiae, and hematomas are strong indications of a fracture. Other symptoms of a fractured nose include swollen eyelids, scleral edema, periorbital petechiae, and subconjunctival hemorrhage. Subcutaneous emphysema can be caused by the patient's attempts to push blood clots out through the nose. The intranasal examination is preceded by cleaning of the mucosa and careful suction of clotted blood.

The hallmarks of fracture are mobility, crepitus, and bony angulation. It can be helpful to place a nasal fracture elevator inside the nose and a fingertip on the outside to check for nasal bone mobility. Palpation of the external nose for tenderness, mobility, and stability is the most reliable step for diagnosing pyramid fracture [1].

You should exclude common associated injuries such as dental fractures, ocular trauma, involvement of the lacrimal system, and cerebrospinal fluid (CSF) fistula which may appear after several days of injury, but suspicion runs quite high if the patient has anosmia [1].

### 8.2.2 Radiological Evaluation

Plain radiological studies may be helpful in assessing nasal fractures, but they are reliable only when correlated with physical examination findings (Fig. 8.1). The bony septum, dorsal pyramid, and lateral nasal walls can be evaluated on the Waters view. For some patients, the nasal bones can be seen with an occlusal view or with the use of a soft-technique lateral radiograph. Many experts believe that these studies are not necessary [3].

CT scan evaluation is valuable in certain patients especially those of severe facial trauma (Fig. 8.2).

### 8.2.3 Photographic Documentation

Photographic documentation is recommended and can serve as an important part of the record, along with the radiographs. Clinicians must obtain preinjury photographs for their records, when possible, because 30% of patients have previous nasal deformities.

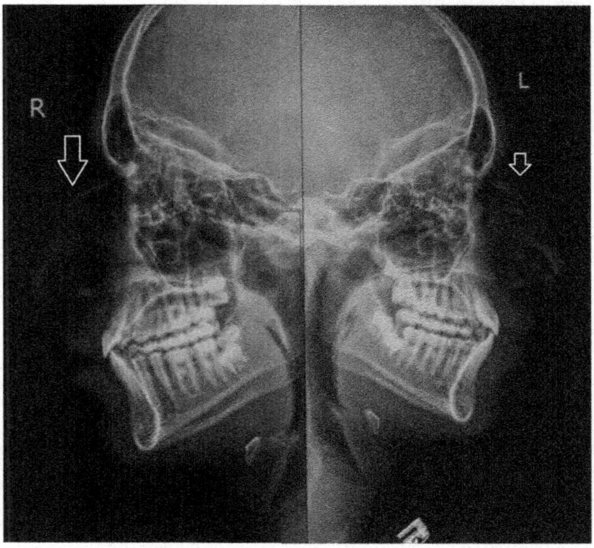


**Fig. 8.1** Plain radiograph showing fractured nasal bones (arrows)

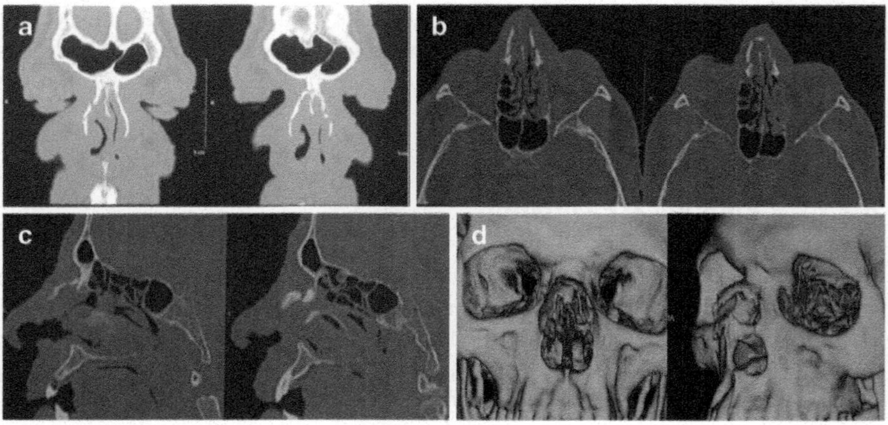


**Fig. 8.2** A CT scan of nose and paranasal sinuses of a patient presented with nasal fracture with an evident comminution of the nasal skeleton; corona cuts (**a**), axial cuts (**b**), sagittal cuts (**c**), and 3D reconstruction images (**d**)

## 8.3 Treatment

The best opportunity for successful management is during the first 3 h after trauma. If this is impossible, most authors agree that reduction is performed within 3–7 days. Colton and Beekhuis stated that no harm is found in waiting until swelling has diminished, and surgery is convenient for the patient and surgeon [2].

The treatment options are closed or open reduction of the fractured external pyramid or septum.

### 8.3.1 Closed Reduction

The indications for closed reduction are (a) unilateral or bilateral fracture of the nasal bones and (b) fracture of the nasal septal complex with nasal deviation less than one-half the width of the nasal bridge (Figs. 8.3 and 8.4).

Some surgeons prefer to use general anesthesia in the treatment of most patients, but other authors have observed that nasal fractures can be managed as well with local anesthesia as they can with general anesthesia, if the injuries are similar. One evaluation of results 3 months after reduction showed the rates of postreduction nasal obstruction or external deformity were equivalent whether general or local anesthesia had been used.

Using 0.25% phenylephrine and Cetacaine as the first application and adding five drops of 1:10,000 epinephrine to the 4% cocaine used on the four cotton pledgets. The pledgets are applied at (a) Roof of nose, (b) lateral nasal wall, (c) floor of nose and (d) septal mucosa. Topical anesthesia is supplemented with injection of 2% lidocaine with 1:100,000 epinephrine along the dorsum of the nose lateral to the nasal pyramid and at the base of the anterior septum. These injections block the pain

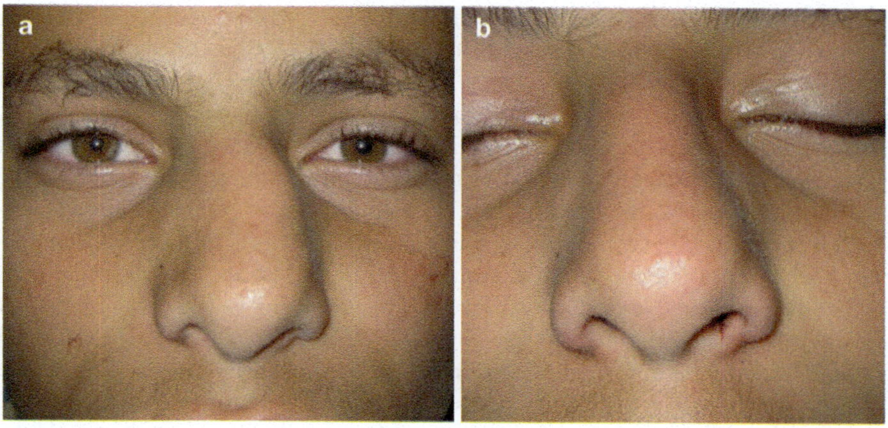


**Fig. 8.3** A 14-year-old male patient presented with nasal fracture with an evident deviation to the left side (**a**). Evident adequate immediate reduction with closed technique (**b**)

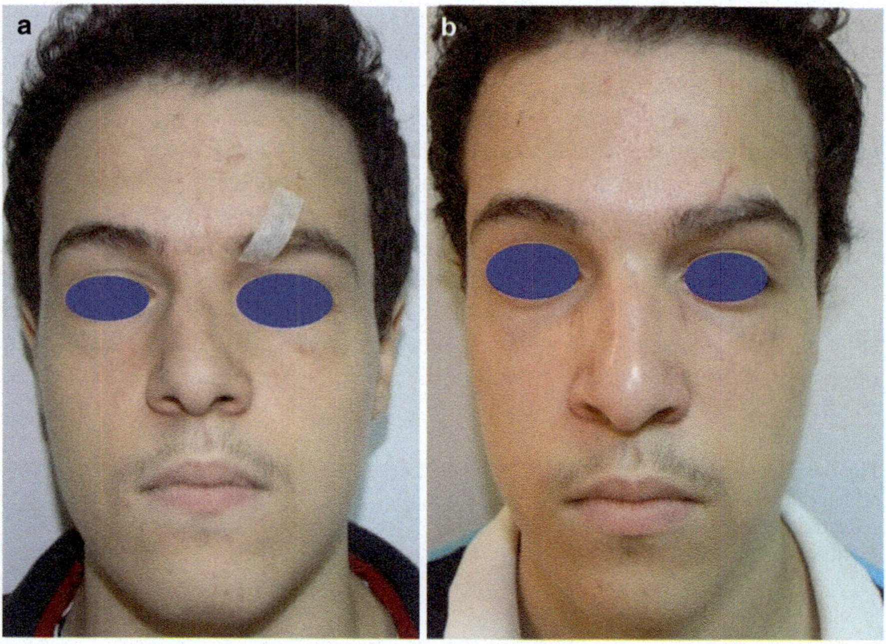


**Fig. 8.4** A 17-year-old male patient presented with nasal fracture with an evident deviation to the right side (**a**). Evident adequate immediate reduction with closed technique (**b**)

fibers in the infratrochlear, infraorbital, greater palatine, and superior alveolar nerves. The physician allows 15–20 min for anesthesia to become effective. Giving 5–10 mg of diazepam about 30 min before surgery helps with sedation. For more extensive procedures, intravenous sedation provides adequate anesthesia in most instances [4].

Even simple depressed fractures of the nasal bones are best managed in the operating room. Preferred instruments for closed reduction are Boies or Ballenger elevators, Asch or Walsham forceps, or large Kelly forceps with rubber tubing on each of the blades. The distance from the nostril rim to the nasofrontal angle is measured, and the instrument is inserted to a point about 1 cm less than the measured distance. The depressed fragment is elevated by means of force in the direction opposite the fracturing force, usually anterolaterally. If the opposite nasal bone is displaced laterally, that bone is moved medially to its normal position. The Asch or Walsham forceps can be inserted one blade in each nostril, or one blade inserted in the nose under the nasal bone and the other placed on the overlying skin. Pressure must not be exerted too high in the nose (under the thick nasal bone near the nasofrontal suture) because this area rarely is fractured, and mucosal tears and bleeding can be produced. Reduction usually can be accomplished with the fragments in position, but digital molding may be necessary for some patients. Inadequate reduction of the nasal septum prevents satisfactory repositioning of the external nose in the case of bilateral pyramidal fracture dislocation.

Reducing the fragments of nasal bone first often reduces the septum simultaneously; if not, the nasal pyramid can usually be gently elevated with an Asch or a Walsham forceps while pressure is applied over the displaced septal region.

A few difficult cases of septal fracture dislocation do not respond to closed reduction. In these instances, elevating the mucoperichondrium on one side often exposes an overriding or interlocked cartilage fracture that necessitates segmental resection. Any loose or devitalized fragments of bone or cartilage are removed. Early stabilization via septoplasty or open techniques has become increasingly popular by some authors. These authors have found improved outcomes in certain patients who are treated early with an aggressive protocol [5–8].

The septum can be stabilized with polymeric silicone splints sutured in place (Fig. 8.5), and gauze packing is placed in each nasal passage. An external dressing of paper tape, 2-inch-wide (5 cm) orthopedic plaster (Fig. 8.6), and an external layer

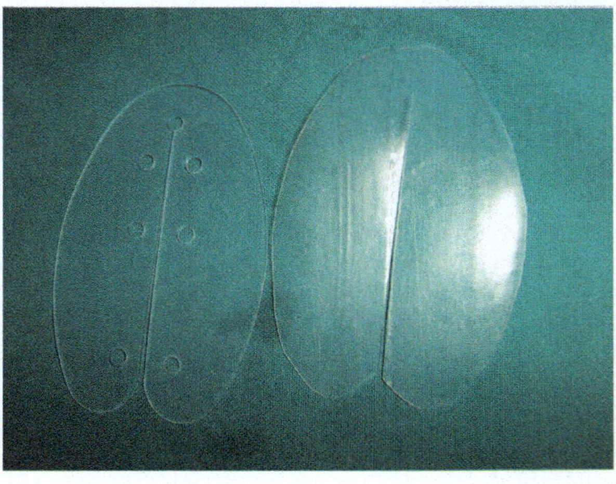

**Fig. 8.5** Septal splint which can be inserted after reduction of septal fractures

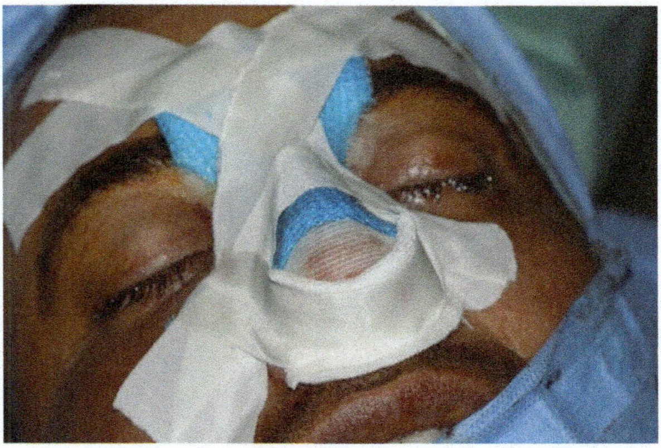

**Fig. 8.6** Orthopedic plaster is fixed with tape after the first layer of dressing

of tape is applied. The use of intranasal dressing is controversial. Some authors advise routine use of antibiotic-impregnated gauze for 2–3 days, whereas others caution against this practice because of the danger of toxic shock syndrome. The splints are removed 10 days after the operation. Various nasal splints are available, including several made of heat-sensitive, thermoplastic materials. After closed reduction and application of paper-tape strips, a thermoplastic splint is placed in hot water and applied over the paper tape. It hardens in a few seconds and adheres tightly to the underlying tape.

The first opportunity for reduction provides the best chance for a good result. Although most nasal and septal fractures can be managed with closed reduction, some remain suboptimally reduced despite the surgeon's best efforts. It is important to have a plan for progressing to open reduction in these instances.

### 8.3.2 Open Reduction

Open reduction is generally recommended for (a) extensive fracture dislocation of the nasal bones and septum (Fig. 8.7), (b) nasal pyramid deviation exceeding one-half the width of the bridge of the nose, (c) fracture dislocation of the caudal septum, (d) open septal fractures, and (e) persistent deformity after closed reduction. Other indications for open reduction include septal hematoma, inadequate bony reduction due to septal deformity, combined deformities of septal and alar cartilages, displaced fractures of the anterior nasal spine, and a history of recent intranasal surgery.

The septum can be approached through a hemitransfixion incision on the side of dislocation. Further access to the fracture lines is gained through bilateral intercartilaginous incisions. The dorsal skin is elevated off the upper lateral cartilages, and the periosteum is elevated from the nasal bones. Incisions in the piriform aperture provide access to the lateral fracture lines (Fig. 8.8). The cartilaginous segments are exposed and reduced. Sometimes, a segment of cartilage must be resected adjacent to the fracture. A Cottle elevator or Ballenger swivel knife is used to excise small

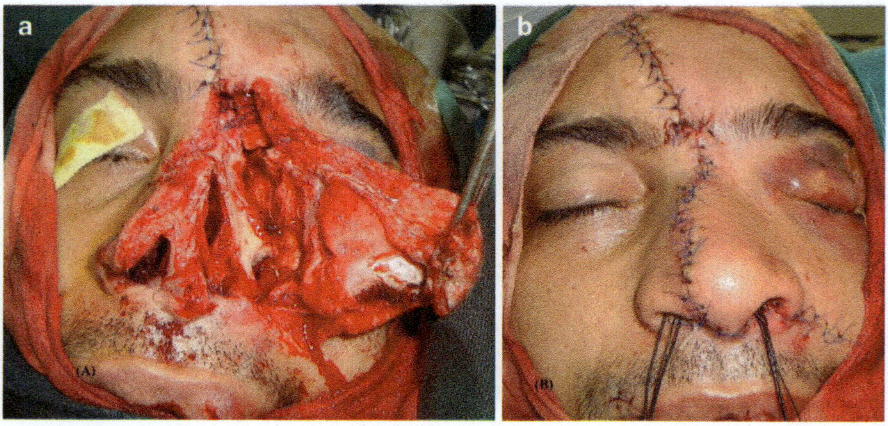


**Fig. 8.7** A 28-year-old male patient presented with open nasal fracture with extensive soft tissues and skeletal injuries (**a**), result after adequate reconstruction of the skeleton and soft tissues repair (**b**)

strips of cartilage. Radical resection of cartilage or bone is avoided to preserve support and limit fibrosis and contracture.

After septal surgery of this type, satisfactory reduction almost always can be accomplished. In view of the trend toward open procedures, a note of caution is added regarding periosteal elevation over nasal bone fragments, lest they be displaced, devitalized, or lost. Rasping is not attempted near fracture fragments, and efforts to improve preinjury appearance are minimized [9].

Packing and splinting are for closed reduction. Antibiotic coverage is routine. Cold compresses are recommended for 24–48 h to reduce existing edema and prevent additional edema.

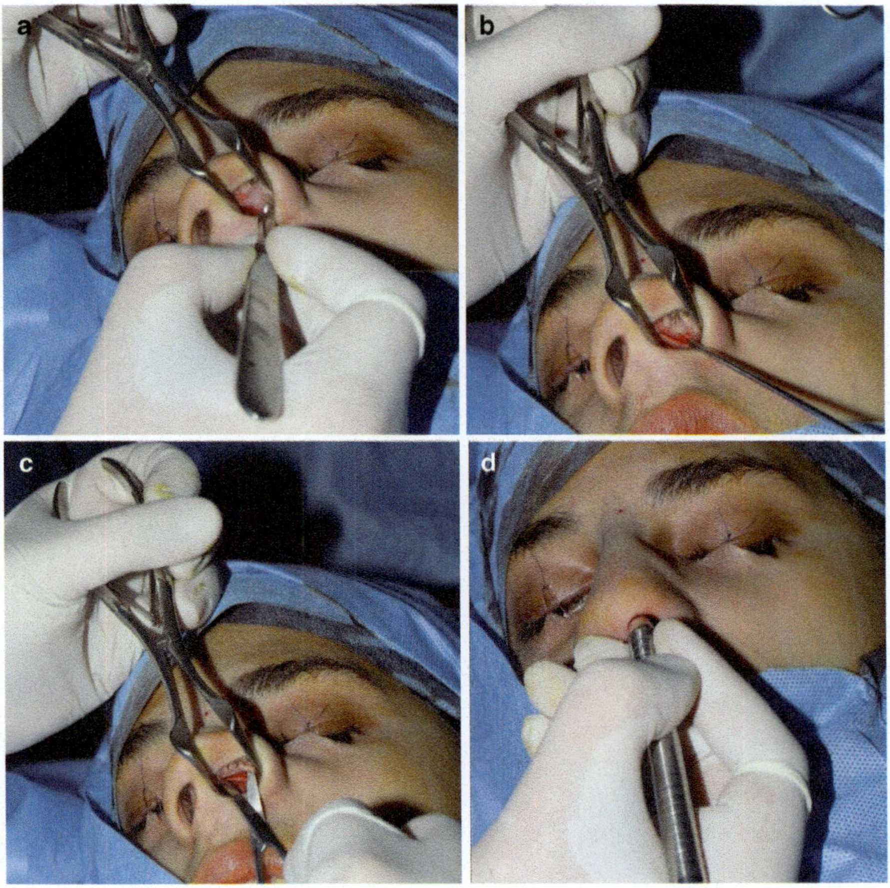


**Fig. 8.8** An open technique for reduction of nasal fractures through intercartilagenous incision (**a**–**c**), then mucoperiosteal elevation and subsequent bony reduction (**d**)

## References


1. Holt GR. Biomechanics of nasal septal trauma. Otolaryngol Clin N Am. 1999;32:615–9.
2. Colton JJ, Beekhuis GJ. Management of nasal fractures. Otolaryngol Clin N Am. 1986;19:73.
3. JF, Denholm S. Routine x-rays in nasal trauma: the influence of audit on clinical practice. J R Soc Med. 1994;87:153.
4. Newton CR, White PSA. Nasal manipulation with intravenous sedation: is it an acceptable and effective treatment? Rhinology. 1998;38:114–6.
5. Davis RE, Chu E. Complex nasal fractures in the adult—a changing management philosophy. Facial Plast Surg. 2015;31:201–15.
6. Staffel JG. Optimizing treatment of nasal fractures. Laryngoscope. 2002;112:1709–19.
7. Defatta RJ, Ducic Y, Adelson RT, Sabatini PR. Comparison of closed reduction alone versus primary open repair of acute nasoseptal fractures. J Otolaryngol Head Neck Surg. 2008;37:502–6.
8. Arnold MA, Yanik SC, Suryadevara AC. Septal fractures predict poor outcomes after closed nasal reduction: retrospective review and survey. Laryngoscope. 2019;129(8):1784–90.
9. Bailey BJ. Nasal fractures in head & neck surgery—otolaryngology. Philadelphia, PA: Lippincott Williams & Wilkins; 2006.

# Maxillofacial Trauma

# 9

Kamal Ebeid

**Key Points**
- Traumatic injury has been identified as the leading cause of reduced productivity, accounting for the loss of more working years than heart disease and cancer combined.
- Multislice CT is an imaging modality of choice for most facial skeletal fractures, while MRI remains for evaluation of brain and adjacent soft tissue injuries.
- Classification of mandibular fractures is of relevance with respect to treatment and therefore should assign the location of the fracture to the anatomic region involved.
- Maxillofacial trauma is classified into fractures affecting the central midface and those affecting the lateral midface, Central midface fractures are classified into LeFort I and LeFort II types, fractures of the nose and nasoethmoid complex. Lateral midface fractures consist of zygomatic bone and zygomatic arch fractures.

Cranio-maxillofacial injuries affect a significant proportion of trauma patients either in isolation or concurring with other serious injuries. It can be classified as mandibular, midfacial, and upper facial traumatic injuries.

K. Ebeid (✉)
Otorhinolaryngology Department, Tanta University, Tanta, Egypt
e-mail: kamal.ebeid@med.tanta.edu.eg


S. Elwany (ed.), *Current Rhinology*,
https://doi.org/10.1007/978-3-031-70077-4_9

## 9.1 Mandibular Trauma

Mandible fractures are among the most common skeletal injuries in humans due to blunt or penetrating trauma. They are often associated with other craniofacial, cervical, and systemic trauma. Mandibular fractures may destabilize the airway and may create malocclusion, joint dysfunction, pain, infection, and paresthesia. In facial trauma management, emergent consideration must be given to secure the airway and obtain hemostasis before initiating definitive treatment of any fracture [1].

### 9.1.1 Classification of Mandibular Fractures

Mandibular fractures are most referred to their anatomic location as symphyseal, parashymphaseal, body, angle, ramus, alveolar, condyle, or coronoid.

A. **Condyle Fractures**

   Condyle fractures are considered the most common fracture of the mandible. Ellis et al. classified condylar fractures as condylar head fracture (intracapsular fracture located at the border between the condylar head and neck), condylar neck fracture (located below the condylar head but on or above the lowest point of the sigmoid notch), and condylar base fracture (the fracture line isolated below the lowest point of the sigmoid notch) [2].

   Most condylar fractures are currently treated by closed techniques. Evidence supporting open reduction of condylar fractures is growing, specifically sub condyle fractures and endoscopic techniques (Fig. 9.1) [3, 4].

B. **Mandibular Coronoid Fractures**

   The coronoid process serves as the attachment of the temporalis muscle. Coronoid fractures are rare and usually do not require treatment, unless they are involved in an impingement from a zygomatic fracture.

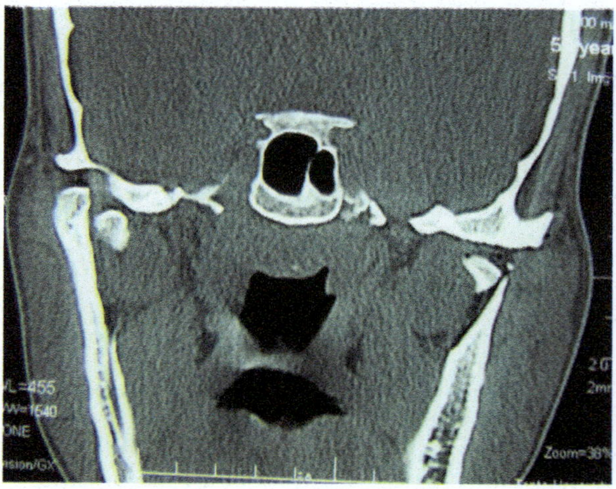

**Fig. 9.1** A coronal CT scan demonstrating medial displacement of condylar head fracture

C. **Mandibular Ramus Fractures**

The ramus is the vertical portion of the mandible above the horizontal plane of the alveolar ridge, ending at the sigmoid notch. Fractures in the ramus are rare. They can be vertical but are more often horizontal.

D. **Mandibular Angle Fractures.**

Fractures of this angle are common. They occur in 25 percent of adult fractures and result from the area weakened by the third molar tooth.

E. **Mandibular Body Fractures.**

The mandibular body is the horizontal mandible from distal symphysis to a vertical line distal to the third molar tooth (Fig. 9.2). Body fractures and angle fractures will be affected by muscle pull, which can produce a favorable fracture by reducing the fracture or an unfavorable fracture if the depressors and elevator muscles distract the fracture.

F. **Mandibular Symphyseal and Parasymphyseal Fractures**

Symphyseal and parasymphyseal fractures (Fig. 9.3) are usually caused by direct trauma to the chin. The symphysis is the area between vertical lines drawn distal to the mandibular canine teeth. A symphyseal fracture is a midline mandibular fracture between the central incisors. A parasymphyseal fracture is a non-midline fracture occurring within the symphysis. Bilateral fractures may cause posterior displacement of the tongue and airway compromise. They may also involve contralateral condyle fractures in up to 37% of the cases.

G. **Dentoalveolar Fractures.**

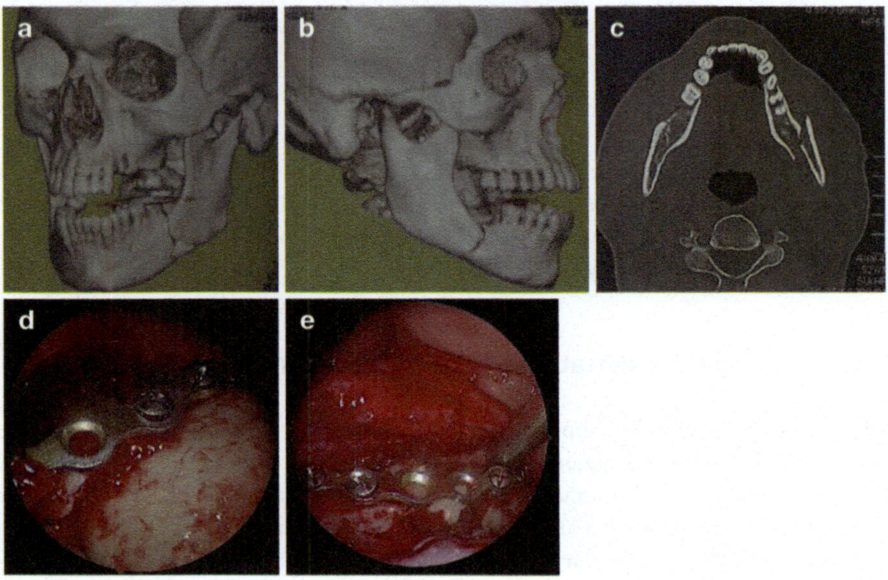


**Fig. 9.2** A 3D, axial CT scan demonstrating bilateral mandibular body fractures with unfavorable left one (**a**–**c**), surgical reduction and fixation was done using miniplates and screws on both sides (**d**, **e**)

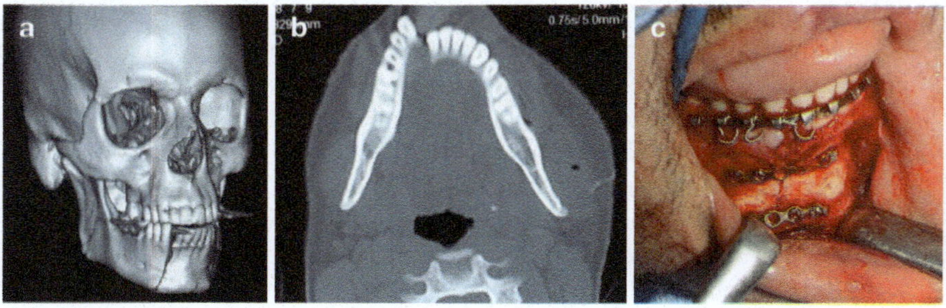


**Fig. 9.3** A 3D, axial CT scan demonstrating right parasymphyseal mandibular fractures (**a**, **b**), surgical reduction and fixation was done using miniplates and screws with occlusion restoration using MMF by arch bar (**c**)

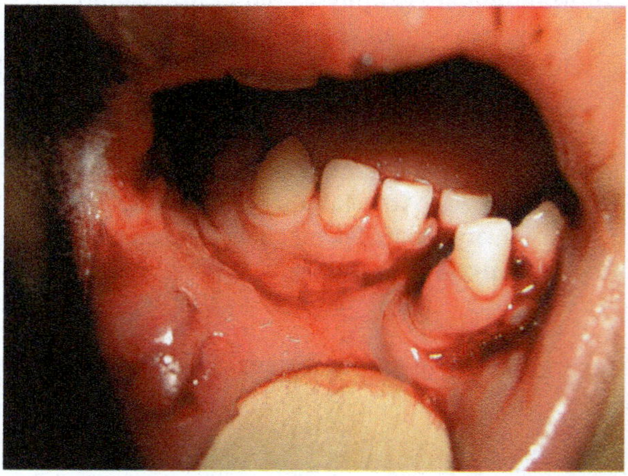

**Fig. 9.4** Intraoral view of fractured mandible showing displaced fracture and discrepancy of occlusion

The alveolar bone houses the dentition. This bone atrophies in the absence of teeth. Dentoalveolar fractures are common, but isolated alveolar fractures are rare. Dental luxation and alveolar segments may be fixated in the MMF, by separate ligatures, or by wire composite splinting. (Fig. 9.4) [5].

### 9.1.2 Clinical Presentation of Mandibular Fractures

A- Advanced trauma life-support protocols

The traumatized patient is best evaluated from a trauma team approach. Once the advanced trauma life-support protocols have been instituted, the airway has been stabilized, and breathing, circulation, and neurological status have been addressed, secondary surveys can be initiated. The intact mandible supports the airway by anterior tongue attachment.

B- Trauma History

The site (chin, body), direction and size, and source (fist, pipe) of the traumatic force are very helpful in identifying direct and indirect fractures of the mandible.

Medical history should include identification of the following prior to surgery: previous mandibular trauma, occlusal abnormalities, TMJ disease, and bleeding, endocrine, neurological, bone, and collagen disorders.

C- Head and neck examination

Evaluate the entire head and neck for facial lacerations, swellings, and hematomas. Bimanually palpates the inferior border of the mandible from the symphysis to the angle on each side. Note areas of swelling, step deformity, or tenderness. Palpate the movement of the condyle through the external auditory meatus. Pain elicited through palpation of the preauricular region should alert the clinician to a possible condylar fracture.

D- Oral examination

A change in occlusion may be due either to a displaced fracture (Fig. 9.4), fractured teeth, and alveolus or to injury to the TMJ. Tears in the unattached mucosa or attached gingiva and ecchymosis in the floor of the mouth usually indicate a mandibular symphyseal or body fracture, also test of mobility by gentle manipulation of bone around the suspected site of fracture.

### 9.1.3 Radiological Evaluation

1- Panorex: Panorex offers low radiation, low cost, and excellent detail, and is excellent for follow-up evaluation.
2- CT Scan: CT is generally the preferred method of imaging for multiple mandibular fractures and is especially helpful in the multiply traumatized patient requiring images of the cervical spine, cranium, and carotid arteries. Also, 3-D CT scanning capabilities add immeasurably to the diagnosis and treatment planning of complex facial fractures.
3- Periapical Radiographs: Periapical radiographs show dental root fractures next to mandible and alveolar fractures.
4- Magnetic resonance imaging (MRI): is better for evaluating associated soft-tissue trauma [6].

### 9.1.4 Management of Mandibular Trauma

Traditional 6-week treatment of closed reduction with MMF or open reduction has given way to early mobilization and restoration of jaw function, improved airway control, improved nutrition, improved patient comfort and hygiene, and an earlier return to work [7].

A- Closed reduction is indicated in the following conditions:
   (a) Nondisplaced favorable fractures.

(b) Pediatric Fractures involving the developing dentition, open reduction can injure developing tooth buds or partially erupted teeth [8]. Pediatric condyle fractures are best managed by closed reduction and early mobilization after 2–3 weeks of MMF.
(c) Grossly Comminuted Fractures can be treated by closed reduction to minimize periosteal stripping of bone fragments.
(d) Coronoid Fractures Coronoid fractures are rarely treated unless there is an impingement on the zygomatic arch.
(e) Adult Condyle Fractures Adult condyle fractures are controversial topics in maxillofacial trauma. Closed treatment is generally the appropriate choice, unless the patient meets Valiati et al.'s criteria for open treatment [8]. If condylar fractures do not fall within these criteria, the patient can be treated with closed reduction for 2–3 weeks. When a condylar fracture is in association with other fractures of the mandible, the other fractures should be treated with ORIF, and the condylar fracture should be treated with closed reduction.

Contraindications to closed reduction MMF include patients with compromised pulmonary function with severe asthma or severe chronic obstructive pulmonary disease, poorly controlled seizures, psychiatric or neurologic disorders, and severe nausea or eating disorders.

Closed reduction can be accomplished with a variety of techniques with and without the dentition. When teeth are present, circumdental wire, arch bars, IMF screws, acid etch brackets are used [9].

B- Open Reduction:
A- Displaced unfavorable fractures through the angle of the mandible.
B- Atrophic edentulous mandibles, minimal cancellous bone, and poor osteogenesis and healing potential.
C- Complex facial fractures requiring a stable mandibular base.
D- Specific groups of condylar fractures benefit from surgical intervention.

Surgical approaches must be tailored to meet the demand of soft tissue and bony fracture repair. The ideal osteosynthesis system of mandibular fractures must meet hardness and durability criteria to handle functional charges and allow bone healing.

Intraoral Approaches have many advantages include expediency, no facial scar, low risk to facial nerve, and performed under local anesthesia. Symphysis and parasymphysis fractures are easily accessed through a labial sulcus incision. Body, angle, and ramus fractures can be accessed through a vestibular incision.

External approaches can be used to manage certain types of mandibular fractures, The submental approach is used to treat fractures of the anterior mandibular body and symphysis. The retromandibular approach may be used to access the ramus and subcondylar region of the mandible.

The preauricular approach is excellent for exposure to the TMJ. the facelift approach provides the same exposure as the retromandibular and preauricular approaches combined. However, the skin incision is placed in a more esthetic location [10, 11].

**Osteosynthesis** is the reduction and fixation of a bone fracture with implantable devices. Wire osteosynthesis is used for limited definitive fixation and is helpful in alignment of fractures prior to rigid fixation. Though wire osteosynthesis is now rarely used for definitive fixation since the advent of rigid fixation. Plate fixation can be a "load-bearing" or "load-sharing" osteosynthesis [12–14]. Load-bearing osteosynthesis requires a rigid plate to bear the entire force of movement at the fracture during function. Load-bearing plates are indicated for comminuted fractures and fractures of atrophic mandible. Load-sharing osteosynthesis creates fracture stability with shared buttressing by significant bone contact and the plate used for fixation. This requires adequate bone stock at the fracture site to create resistance to movement. Examples of load-sharing osteosynthesis include lag-screw fixation, compression plating, and a miniplate fixation technique popularized by Champy [15].

## 9.2 Midfacial Trauma

### 9.2.1 Maxillary and Orbital (and Zygomatic) Fractures

A- **Le Fort Series of Fractures:** Around the end of the nineteenth century, René Le Fort, a French military surgeon, created a series of fractures by traumatizing cadaver faces. He noticed several patterns that seemed to occur that tended to separate the tooth-bearing bone from the solid cranium above. These patterns tended to occur at three general anatomic levels that have come to be known as Le Fort I, II, and III fractures (Fig. 9.5). While few fractures precisely match the Le Fort definitions, these approximations are extremely useful in communicating the nature of an injury among physicians, and they are also useful in planning treatment planning. Le Fort I, II, and III basically define the level at which the bones holding the teeth are separated from the remaining bone above [16].

(a) **Le Fort I:** The Le Fort I classification describes a fracture that extends across both maxillae above the dentition. It crosses each inferior maxilla from lateral to medial through the pyriform apertures and across the nasal septum. Posteriorly, it generally severs the pterygoid plates inferiorly. This frees the tooth-holding maxillary alveoli from the remaining facial bones above.

(b) **Le Fort II:** The Le Fort II classification starts in the maxilla laterally but extends more superiorly into the orbital floor. It crosses the anterior inferior and medial orbits and crosses the nasal bones superiorly or separates the nasal bones from the frontal bones at the frontonasal suture. It continues posteriorly across the nasal septum and pterygoid plates. It is commonly called the pyramidal fracture due to the pyramidal shape of the inferior facial fragment.

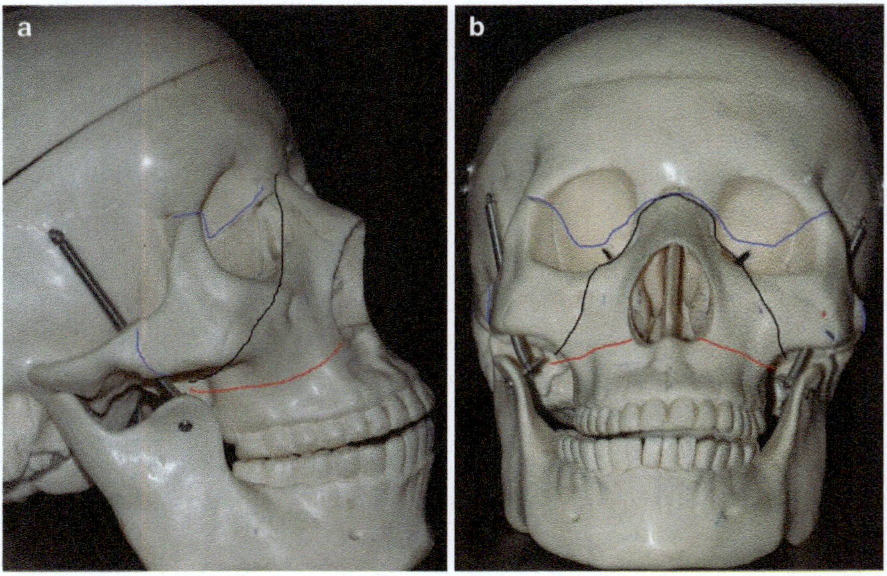


**Fig. 9.5** Demonstration of Le Fort Series of Fractures, lateral view (**a**) and frontal view (**b**). Le Fort I (Red line), II (Black line), and III fractures (Blue Line)

(c) **Le Fort III:** Finally, the Le Fort III classification completely separates the facial bones from the skull, resulting in what is known as a complete craniofacial separation. It traverses the zygomatic arches laterally and the lateral orbital rims and walls, crosses the orbital floors more posteriorly, crosses the medial orbits (lamina papyracea), and is completed at the frontonasal junction. Posteriorly, like the Le Fort II, it traverses the nasal septum and the pterygoid plates, thus completely separating the facial structure from the skull.

### 9.2.2 Zygomatic Fractures

Zygomatic fractures have sometimes been called "tripod" or "quadrapod" fractures, due to the perceived three or four attachments of the zygoma to the surrounding bones—mainly, the frontal bone at the lateral orbital rim, the temporal bone along the zygomatic arch, and the maxillary bone along its broad attachment. The zygoma's broad lateral expanse near the pterygoid plates leads to confusing nomenclature since it can be considered a single attachment (tripod) or double attachment at the inferior orbital rim and zygomaticomaxillary suture (quadrapod). Either way, when these attachments are fractured, the malar eminence is generally displaced posteriorly, laterally, or medially. When the inferior orbital rim rotates medially, it is considered medially displaced; when it rotates laterally, it is considered laterally displaced; and when it is impacted posteriorly, it is considered posteriorly displaced.

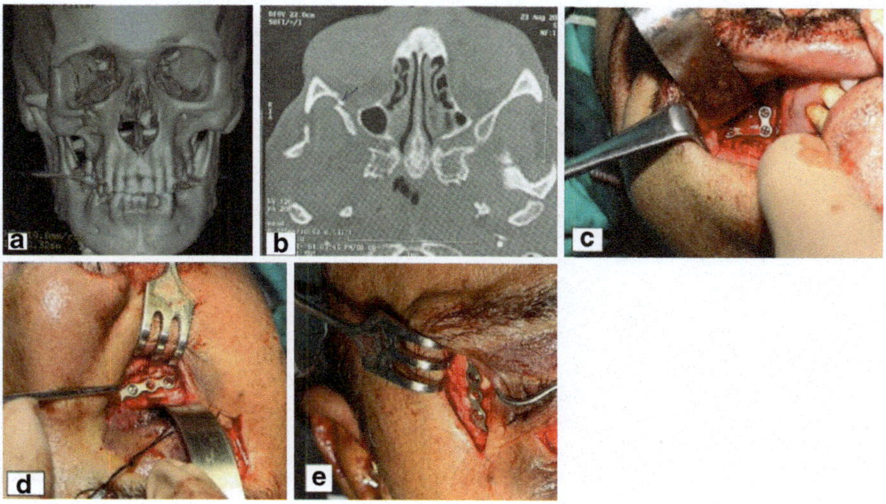

**Fig. 9.6** A 3D and axial CT scan showing right zygomaticomaxillary fracture (**a**, **b**). Fixation of zygomaticomaxillary buttress through transoral incision (**c**). Fixation of the orbital rim through transcutaneous subciliary incision (**d**). Fixation of the right frontozygomatic area through lateral incision just below eyebrow (**e**)

Obviously, the direction of displacement determines the approach to repair (Fig. 9.6) [16].

### 9.2.3 Orbital Fractures

Orbital fractures are usually described by the status of the walls and rims. A pure blowout fracture occurs when a wall is "blown out" without an identifiable fracture of the rim. Floor fractures are both the most common and most severe, presumably since there is ample space for significant displacement. Medial fractures are common but are typically less severe. Lateral wall displacement is generally associated with displacement of the zygoma, and roof fractures are uncommon (Fig. 9.7).

#### 9.2.3.1 Clinical Assessment of Midfacial Trauma

Assessing movement of the tooth-bearing maxillary bones relative to the cranium, making sure that the teeth themselves are not moving separately from the bone. The anterior maxillary arch is held and rocked relative to a second hand on the forehead. If there is movement of the maxillary arch and maxillae relative to the frontal bones, then a Le Fort fracture can be presumed. The level of movement may be difficult to detect, but the CT scan will sort that out.

Eye assessment including vision, evidence of extraocular muscle entrapment.an ophthalmological evaluation to rule out ocular and/or retinal injury is mandatory.

CT scan is the key to the diagnosis of midfacial fractures. In general, axial CTs are best for visualizing vertical bone structures, and coronal CTs are best for

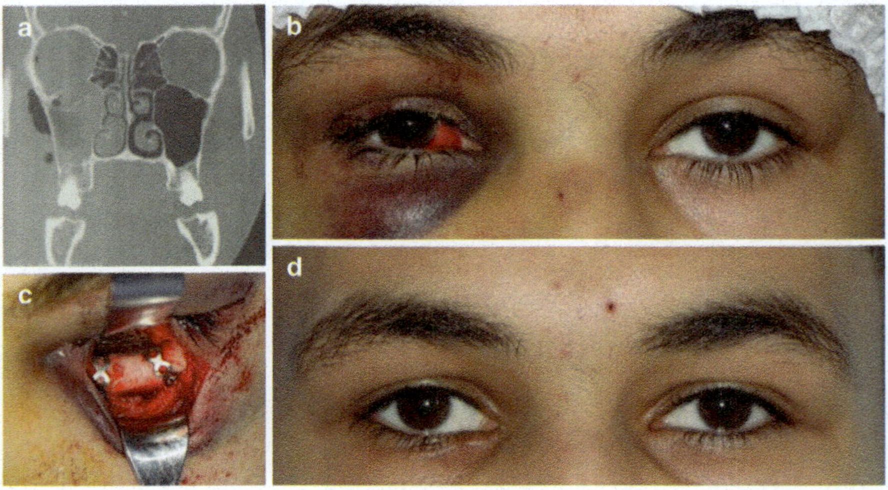


**Fig. 9.7** A coronal CT scan showing right orbital floor fracture (**a**). An evident enophthalmos of the right eye (**b**). A subciliary incision was done and orbital floor is reconstructed with a titanium mesh (**c**). 3 months post-operative photograph showing improvement of enophthalmos without evident scar (**d**)

visualizing horizontal structures, though with modern CT algorithms and high-resolution scanning, both can be easily produced and should be utilized. The three-dimensional (3D) CT is helpful for creating a gestalt for the surgeon, but it is less accurate than the axial and coronal CTs from which it is created.

#### 9.2.3.2 Reconstruction of Midfacial Trauma

Midfacial bones are repaired for two main reasons: to restore normal function and to restore normal facial contour (cosmesis). Le Fort fractures can affect the position of the dentition and result in significant malocclusion. Because this will interfere with chewing, repair is very important. Zygomatic fractures may be another cause of globe dysfunction/malposition, because of the contribution of the zygoma to the orbital structure. More commonly, however, a displaced zygoma, particularly a depressed arch, may lead to impingement on the temporalis muscle, causing trismus and/or painful mouth opening and difficulty with mastication. More commonly, however, zygomatic fractures are reduced for cosmetic reasons. It is also common for patients to refuse repair when the problem is only cosmetic. The main dysfunction for which orbital repair is performed is diplopia, which is usually due to muscle entrapment of one of the extraocular muscles, though it can occur because of significant globe malposition as well. Globe malposition can also cause significant cosmetic deformity [16].

#### 9.2.3.3 Approaches for Reconstruction of Midfacial Trauma

1- **Le Fort Fractures**

Most Le Fort fractures will require fixation at the lower maxillary level, to build a proper foundation for the remainder of the fracture stabilization. A sublabial transmucosal exposure provides excellent exposure of the front face of the maxillae bilaterally, allowing repair at the Le Fort I level. Arch bars are generally applied first to assist with reduction of the occlusion. Fractures at the nasofrontal junction are exposed via a coronal incision when necessary. Otherwise, a direct horizontal incision can sometimes be used when only limited exposure is needed for repair. The main goal of repair is to reestablish the correct bony architecture by repositioning the bones into their correct anatomical positions and fixating them in those correct positions. Fixation is most performed using rigid fixation devices typically plates and screws.

Le Fort I fractures must be repaired along the strong medial and lateral vertical buttresses.

If a complex Le Fort III (i.e., craniofacial separation along with zygomatic and lower maxillary fractures) is repaired from the top down, fixation of the zygomas to the skull will change these complex fractures from a Le Fort III to a Le Fort I fracture, and repair of the nasofrontal junction and inferior orbital rims will convert the remainder to Le Fort I fractures.

2- **Zygomatic Fractures**

The rotated fractures need to be corrected by rotation contrary to the rotation created by the injury. If the zygoma was impacted, then reduction requires direct pull counter to the direction of the impaction. This disimpaction technique involves placing a sturdy instrument, such as a Dingman elevator, beneath the malar eminence and applying a firm, but not excessive, distractive force. The instrument can be placed through an incision in the temporalis fascia from above or the mucoperiosteum from below. Reduction is often monitored along the zygomaticomaxillary buttress intraorally. When the bone is adequate to ensure reduction, fixation along the zygomaticomaxillary buttress using an appropriate plate and screw will often suffice. However, if there is comminution in this area, not only will reduction be more difficult to determine, but fixation will be more difficult as well. Additional reduction and fixation may be applied along the inferior orbital rim and along the lateral orbital wall at the zygomaticosphenoid junction. The frontozygomatic area provides strong bone for fixation when necessary. If the zygomatic arch needs to be explored and repaired (which is less common, typically occurs only in severely displaced and comminuted fractures), fixation should be performed using either wires or the thinnest plates available, since plates in this area can be visible and can alter the facial width (Fig. 9.6) [16].

3- **Orbital Fractures**

(a) **Orbital Floor Approaches**

1. Subciliary Incision

The orbital floor fractures can be accessed by a lower eyelid subciliary incision (Fig. 9.1). Nam and colleagues performed 405 subciliary incisions with Frost suture removal on postoperative day 3 and subsequent vigorous lower lid massage and reported no cases of lid retraction or ectropion [17].

This transcutaneous approach is generally placed 1–2 mm below and parallel to the lash line (Fig. 9.7). The incision can be made through skin and muscle, and dissection can be carried out under the muscle to the inferior orbital rim. Alternatively, the incision can be made through skin, carried inferiorly for several mm, whereupon the orbicularis muscle is dissected away from the orbital septum, exposing the inferior orbital rim. Care must be taken to avoid damaging the thin skin. It is also important to avoid injury to the orbital septum, to minimize the risk of ectropion developing because of scarring.

2. Infraorbital Incision

   This incision is performed more inferiorly than the subciliary incision, usually at the junction of the lower lid and cheek skin. It is a very direct approach to the bone. However, the scar tends to be more visible, and if the dissection is continued laterally, there is a tendency for prolonged lower lid edema.

3. Transconjunctival Approaches

   The transconjunctival incision provides the obvious advantage of a lack of an external scar. Appling and colleagues found 12% transient ectropion and 28% permanent increased scleral show in subciliary incisions compared with no ectropion and 3% increased scleral show with transconjunctival incisions. Patel and colleagues also report highly favorable results using a transconjunctival incision [18, 19].

4. Endoscopic Transmaxillary Approach

   This approach involves making a window in the anterior wall of the maxillary sinus. Generally, a small plate may be placed and removed prior to making the bone cuts, so that the bony window can be replaced after fracture reduction has been achieved. The orbital floor is then visualized through the maxillary sinus.

5. Endoscopic Transnasal Approach

   Access is more difficult with this approach since visualization is limited by the pyriform aperture and nasal septum. However, the orbital floor can be visualized via a large middle meatal antrostomy.

6. Combined approaches.

   Kakibuchi and colleagues reported 12 cases of fresh blowout fractures were treated with combination of transconjunctival approach and transantral endoscopic approach, ocular movement recovered, and symptomatic diplopia disappeared after surgery in all eight cases which were symptomatic preoperatively. And improvement of enophthalmos of more than 2 mm in all five cases which were symptomatic preoperatively. One early case showed temporary entropion. Transient numbness of the cheek appeared in five cases and temporary maxillary sinusitis recovered in one case. Postoperative infection was not observed [20].

(b) **Approaches for Medial Orbital Wall**

1- External Skin Incision

   A vertical skin incision halfway between the nasal dorsum and the medial canthus can be made and taken down through periosteum to bone. Elevation can then proceed posteriorly under the periosteum. Note that the medial canthal ligaments are detached but will reattach when the periosteum is allowed to reposition itself). The Lynch incision provides good access but carries the risk of scarring or webbing, and injury to the lacrimal system or canthal tendon.

2- Coronal Incision

The coronal incision offers the greatest exposure and access, and this approach is optimal in cases of massive facial trauma. However, concerns such as scarring in male pattern baldness, alopecia, frontalis palsy, scalp numbness, and increased surgical time make other more direct approaches desirable in most cases [21].

3- Transconjunctival Incisions

The transcaruncular and precaruncular incisions have been described with satisfactory results. These incisions reportedly provide sufficient exposure without notable scarring [22–24].

4- Endoscopic Transnasal

This approach is performed endoscopically through the ethmoid sinus. Care must be taken when opening the ethmoid bulla, since the orbital contents are in the sinus, and when the bulla is opened, the orbital fat is generally right there. Bae and colleagues reported 14 patients with fractured medial orbital wall underwent surgery using the endoscopic transnasal approach. Preoperative computed tomography was used to calculate the size of the bone defect, and the titanium mesh was designed to be shorter than the anteroposterior length of the defect and longer than its height (Figs. 9.3 and 9.4). The titanium mesh was inserted into the orbit under an endoscopic view. The authors then confirmed that the titanium mesh supported the orbital contents by pressing the eyeball and finished the operation. Immediately after surgery, CT results were evaluated. Results Postoperative CT scans confirmed that the titanium mesh was well-inserted and in the correct position. All patients were discharged without any complications [25].

The standard endoscopic techniques involve partial ethmoidectomy and exposure of the lamina papyracea. With reduction of the herniated orbital contents, and application of intranasal splint or packing is placed between the lamina and the middle turbinate for a period (approximately 2 months) until healing is completed. Alternatively, an intranasal endoscopic approach to assist in placement of an orbital implant by means of a periorbital incision has been described [26, 27].

(c) **Combined Medial Orbital Wall and Floor Fractures**

Jeon and colleagues described repair of medial and orbital floor fractures with an endonasal endoscopic approach, using a feeding tube inflated balloon for floor support, and a silastic sheet with Merocel packing retained for 4 weeks for medial wall support. These investigators reported 2 cases of resultant diplopia in 11 isolated floor fractures, 1 case of enophthalmos in 17 medial wall fractures, and 4 cases of diplopia in the 12 combined floor and medial wall fractures. They conclude that this technique should be considered a safe alternative for isolated floor or medial wall fractures but should perhaps not be considered for combined fractures or if there is an orbital rim fracture [28].

(d) **Approaches for the Lateral Orbital Wall**

1- Infrabrow Incision

Incisions through the brow are not recommended since scars separate the hair follicles and become quite visible. An incision can be made either above or below the brow.

2- Upper Blepharoplasty incisionupper lid blepharoplasty incision is preferred since it hides nicely once it heals The incision goes through the skin and orbicularis muscle, and then extends superiorly to the bone.

3- Extended Lower Lid Transconjunctival (with or without Lateral Canthotomy).

The lower lid transconjunctival incision described above can be extended laterally, either (1) within the orbit (posterior to the lateral canthus), though this limits access anteriorly, or (2) preferably, by incising the lateral canthus, separating the upper and lower lid attachments, and performing an inferior cantholysis. This can be extended laterally through the skin as needed for exposure of the lateral orbital rim. It is important to reattach the ligament to the lateral orbit inside and behind the rim at the end of the procedure.

4- Extended Subciliary Incision

The lower lid subciliary incision can be extended laterally for exposure of the lateral orbital rim.

(e) Orbital Roof

1- Upper Blepharoplasty incision.
2- External Ethmoidectomy incision.
3- Coronal incision.
4- The coronal incision can be elevated to a level below the superior orbital rims for access to the orbital roof.

#### 9.2.3.4 Aim of the Reconstruction of Orbital Fractures

The purpose of the reconstruction of the internal orbital walls is the faithful anatomical reconstruction in 3D considering shape and volume. The reduction of thin bone fragments is often not possible or insufficient. There is often an indication to cover or bridge the defect to prevent further displacement of the soft tissue. Therefore, it is often indicated to use alloplastic material to support the soft tissue and reshape the cavity. Depending on the size and location of the defect, materials of different stiffness were recommended for the repair of orbital lesions [29–32].

#### 9.2.3.5 Reconstruction Materials for Orbital Fractures

Reconstruction using autologous bones such as iliac crest, calvarium or microvascular bone offer a possibility for rebuilding and augmenting orbital contours especially after tumor resection. However, to reconstruct the traumatic defects the morbidity is too high, the bone parts cannot have a truly anatomical shape and bone Volume lost by resorption. But alloplastic materials such as titanium and porous polyethylene are used, however, these materials, except titanium, were have by some complications and a faithful reconstruction that requires 3D anatomy of the orbital walls rarely reached.

The accurate 3D reconstruction of the complex anatomy of the bony orbit is time-consuming and technique dependent. To solve this problem, some surgeons use sterilized skull models for precise execution. CT scan data can be analyzed to make this possible stereolithography models or alloplastic implants for reconstruction. When these techniques are combined with intraoperative navigation, can improve the accuracy of surgical repair. But these are of high cost and time consuming and not available for all institutions.

As regard the anatomical S-shaped of the orbital floor has an initial shallow convex section behind the rim, inclines upward to meet the medial wall, creating these convex curves of the medial wall and floor create a "post bulbar constriction" of the orbital cavity, this anatomical information was included into the design of the orbital implants for accurate reconstruction [33–43].

## 9.3 Upper Facial Trauma

### 9.3.1 Frontal Sinus and Anterior Skull Base Trauma

The thick bone of the anterior wall of the sinus as well as its curved convexity, acts as a first barrier to the effects of cranial trauma resists fracture. Considerable force—up to 1600-foot pounds of impact is required to fracture the anterior wall [44].

The sinus has a mid-line septum that divides it into two halves. The drainage connection to the anterior aspect of the middle meatus of the lateral nasal wall begins as a funnel-shaped structure at the anterior medial extremity of the insertion of the mid-line septum in the frontal sinus floor. The space into which the frontal sinus drains is called the frontal recess. It is the space posterior to the frontal beak (nasal process of the frontal bone), between the lamina papyracea and the vertical lamella of the middle turbinate continuing to the lateral wall of the olfactory fossa and is anterior to the basal lamella of the middle turbinate [45].

The frontal sinus floor has an area of common wall with the orbital roof, superiormedially, and the posterior wall forms the anterior wall of the anterior cranial fossa. The posterior wall has a central spine that projects intracranially, upon which lies the superior sagittal sinus [46].

Very often the patients presenting with a fracture of the frontal sinus are victims of violent crime, gunshot wounds, or industrial accidents. They commonly have multiple other, more immediately life-threatening injuries, so the sinus injury is often overlooked. Appropriate treatment of these fractures is essential, because of the potential for the formation of a frontal sinus mucocele or pyocele. With the proximity of the posterior sinus wall to the anterior cranial fossa, these pathological entities can lead to life-threatening complications of meningitis and brain abscess [46, 47].

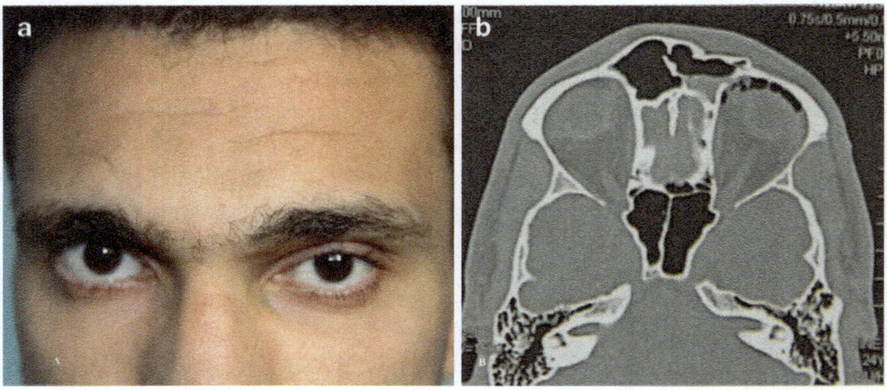


**Fig. 9.8** A 24-year-old male patient presented with frontal blunt trauma (**a**), an axial CT scan of the paranasal sinuses demonstrating minimal displacement of the anterior table (**b**) the patient was managed conservatively

#### 9.3.1.1 Anterior Wall Fractures

*Linear fractures:* linear fractures of the anterior wall are often overlooked, but even if detected, there would be no mandate to treat them (Fig. 9.8). They may present with a subgaleal hematoma.

*Depressed fractures:* If the fracture is depressed, it will appear as a distinct depression in fracture. However, if the patient is seen sometime after the occurrence of the injury, the depression may fill with blood, and the displaced area will be effaced. Displaced fractures should be reduced for two principal reasons. The most important is that if there is any entrapped mucosa between the edges of the fracture, there is the potential to develop a mucocele. The second reason is to prevent the inevitable deformity of a dent in the forehead that will result if the displaced fragment is not properly reduced (Fig.9.9).

*Compound fractures* are by definition in continuity with forehead laceration. These fractures are often comminuted. and depressed bone fragments are seen in the depths of the cutaneous wound. Blood, CSF, and even brain may be seen coming through the laceration. If the fracture is compounded, it can sometimes be reduced through an overlying laceration. If the laceration is too small to effectively reduce the fracture, then additional exposure can be gained by extending the laceration horizontally along a natural crease line in the forehead skin (Fig. 9.10). The two other incisions that can be used are the "gull-wing" or "butterfly" incision in a glabellar crease connected to the upper medial aspects of the eyebrows. This incision is best applied in patients with short sinuses or in bald men. The coronal scalp flap provides the best surgical exposure and is the most used. The fracture fragments are disimpacted with a stout bone hook and, as much as possible, the bone fragments are left with periosteum as a vascular pedicle. A mucosal strip adjacent to the fracture is incised and removed, and a thin layer of the underlying bone is resected with a diamond bur. The fracture fragments are fixed in place with a series of miniplates and square plates.

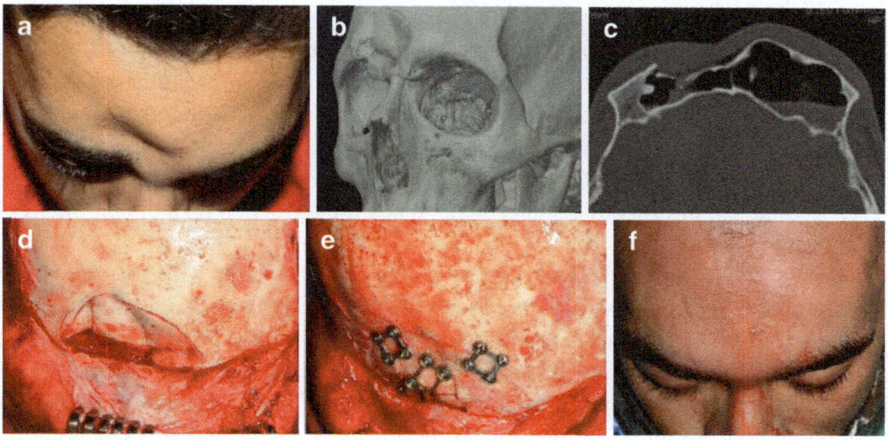


**Fig. 9.9** A 22-year-old male patient presented with frontal blunt trauma (**a**), a 3 D and axial CT scan of the paranasal sinuses demonstrating considerable displacement of the anterior table (**b**, **c**) surgical exposure was done through coronal approach showing displaced anterior table, which was reduced and fixed with miniplates and screws (**d**, **e**). Restoration of anterior table contour was achieved (**f**)

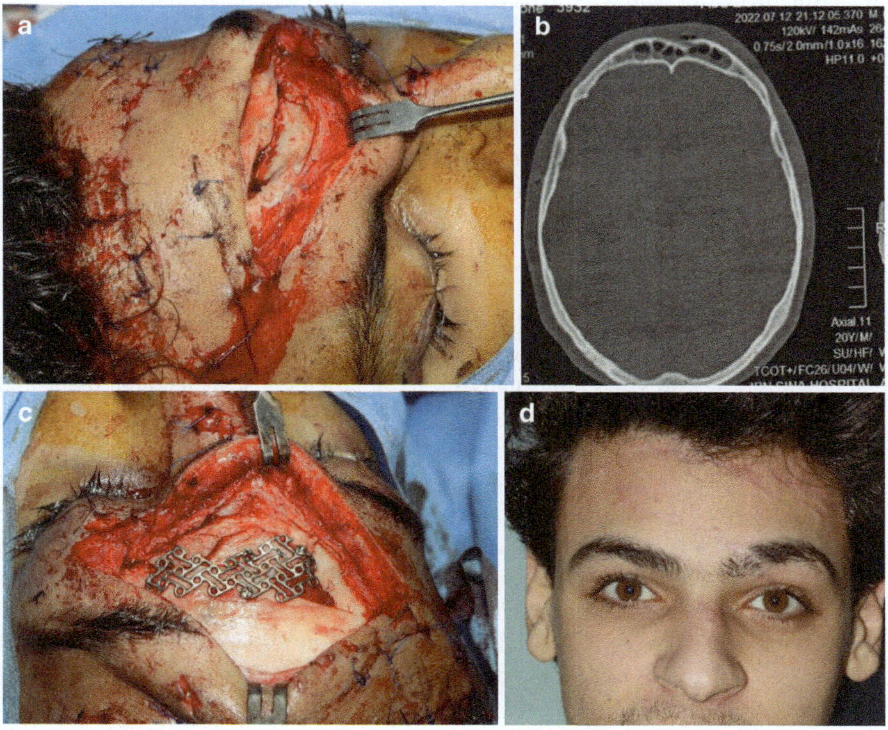


**Fig. 9.10** A 22-year-old male patient presented with compound frontal trauma, demonstrating laceration with exposed anterior table fractures (**a**), an axial CT scan of the skull demonstrated considerable displacement of the anterior table (**b**) surgical exposure was done through the laceration showing displaced anterior table which was reduced and fixed with titanium mesh and screws (**c**). Restoration of anterior table contour was achieved (**d**)

#### 9.3.1.2 Posterior Wall Fractures

*Linear fractures:* Isolated posterior wall fractures are very uncommon. If present, they are often part of a calvarial vault fracture. There are no presenting differentiating symptoms. The dilemma regarding treatment centers on distinguishing between a linear-only fracture versus a displaced fracture. Only a fine-cut computed tomography (CT) scan taken in the axial and sagittal planes will give enough definition to clearly establish or rule out displacement. When the physician is in doubt, the fracture should be treated.

*Displaced fractures:* A clear sign of a displaced posterior wall fracture is the presence of CSF rhinorrhea. If mixed with blood, the CSF leak can be identified by looking for the "halo sign." A drop of nasal drainage is allowed to fall on a surgical towel. If the halo spreading from the central blood clot is more than double the width of the clot, then this is a sign of a CSF leak and thus an anterior dural tear. If any doubt concerning posterior wall displacement exists, frontal sinus exploration is indicated. This is usually done through a coronal scalp incision, then creating an osteoplastic bone flap of the anterior wall of the frontal sinus. A clear view of the interior of the sinus is obtained, and any disruption of the posterior wall is identified. If a CSF leak is seen, the limits of the anterior fossa dural rent are exposed by removing posterior wall bone. The dural tear is closed with interrupted sutures, and the area is reinforced with a patch of fascia Lata or temporalis fascia.

If an area of bone greater than 2 cm in diameter is removed, the anticipated sinus drillout and obliteration with fat are abandoned, and a frontal sinus cranialization procedure is performed. If fat grafting and obliteration of the sinus are performed, then careful attention to complete removal of all mucosae is mandatory. The drilling of the bone of the interior of the sinus is essential to remove all remnants of mucosal lining prior to obliteration of the sinus cavity with a carefully harvested abdominal wall fat graft [47].

#### 9.3.1.3 Frontal Sinus Outflow Tract Fractures

Fractures of the frontal sinus outflow tract have no particularly distinguishing clinical diagnostic features and are usually picked up on a CT scan. Though the actual fracture may not be seen, an opacified frontal sinus that does not clear in 2 weeks raises a strong suspicion of disruption of the outflow tract. The duct is often fractured as part of a Le Fort III maxillary fracture. If in 2 weeks the sinus does not clear, a test can be done to establish patency of the duct. A small trephine hole in the floor of the sinus is made through a small incision in or just below the brow. The sinus is irrigated through the trephine with a saline solution containing cocaine or epinephrine. A solution containing methylene blue is instilled in the sinus, and the appearance of the dye in the middle meatus of the nose is observed with a sinus endoscope. The appearance of the dye indicates duct patency; the dye's absence is an indication for surgery [47].

All methods of opening the frontal sinus floor to the nasal cavity have been attempted with varying degrees of success. Currently, the use of the Draf III endoscopic version of the Lothrop operation has become very popular. The two classic open techniques are the Lynch operation using the Sewell-Boyden flap to line the widely open tract, and the osteoplastic flap procedure with fat obliteration [48].

#### 9.3.1.4 Through-and-Through Fractures

The through-and-through fracture is the most serious of all frontal sinus fractures. It is a compound comminuted fracture involving the anterior and posterior walls, entering the anterior cranial fossa (Fig. 9.11). The skin is torn often extensively, the dura is ripped, and the frontal lobes are lacerated and contused.

This devastating injury was formerly managed by the neurosurgeon by craniectomy, often discarding the skull fragments because of their contamination at the scene of the accident, and not cleansing them and restoration of the cranial vault because of the concern of brain swelling. The otolaryngologist classically did a Riedel ablation, with the two procedures leaving the patient with unprotected brain as well as a significant cosmetic defect. In 1975, Donald and Bernstein and Derome and Merville described the cranialization procedure for these through-and-through fractures [49, 50].

The neurosurgeon controls intracranial problems by stopping intracranial bleeding, debriding necrotic brain, and providing a water-tight dural repair. The otolaryngologist initially ensures all the bony fragments from the anterior wall of the frontal sinus have been saved. The posterior wall of the sinus is completely removed, so that the cavity of the frontal sinus is now in continuity with the anterior cranial fossa. The frontal sinus mucosa is now completely stripped out with an elevator from the floor and the remaining anterior wall, such that the remaining sinus cavity

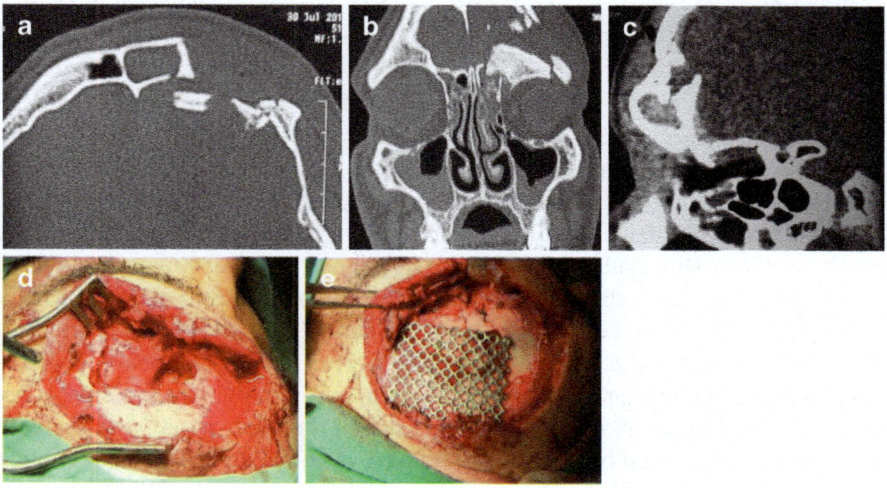


**Fig. 9.11** A 45-year-old male patient presented with extensive frontal trauma with comminution and displacement of anterior and posterior tables, which is evident in CT scan, axial, coronal, and sagittal sections (**a**–**c**), surgical exposure was done through forehead laceration showing displaced anterior and posterior table with dural laceration, dural repair was done using artificial dural material, cranialization was done (**d**). Restoration of anterior table contour was achieved using titanium mesh and screws (**e**)

is completely divested of mucosa. Total removal of all mucosal remnants of the sinus is ensured by removing 1–2 mm of bone with a cutting burr. The outflow tract is eliminated with sinus mucosal inversion inside it, together with plugging by temporalis muscle. The cleansed anterior wall fragments are similarly divested of all their mucosa with a cutting bur, and then fixed in place with square plates and miniplates.so the frontal sinus is thus eliminated as a potential source of infection, and the esthetic contour of the forehead is preserved.

### 9.3.2 Naso-orbital-ethmoid Fractures

Fractures of the naso-orbital-ethmoid (NOE) region are typically due to blunt trauma injuries. Etiologies may range from motor vehicle accidents to falls and sports, but the force and focus of the blow determine the extent of the injuries to the structures located in this region of the face, including the orbital contents and the anterior skull base structures.

NOE fractures can involve damage to multiple important osseous, vascular, cranial nerve, and supporting structures located within the NOE complex, including: nasal bones, perpendicular plate of the ethmoid/septum, nasal process of the frontal bone, cribriform plate and olfactory nerve, lamina papyracea, medial orbit, ethmoid sinus, orbital fat, medial rectus muscle, superior oblique muscle with trochlea, ethmoid arteries, ethmoid nerves, medial canthal attachments, lacrimal fossa, lacrimal sac, superior and inferior canaliculi, superior portion of the nasal-lacrimal duct and nasal process of the maxilla and lateral-superior nasal wall.

The subjective symptoms of injuries to the NOE complex include the following: diplopia. Nasal stuffiness. Epistaxis, visual disturbances, pain, dizziness, vertigo, and anosmia.

Traumatic telecanthus is one of the most common objective signs, The average intercanthal distance of approximately 30–31 mm. The diagnosis of traumatic telecanthus requires a measurement more than those normative value. The pathology can be either unilateral or bilateral, with the former more difficult to measure. Diplopia can be due to injuries to the medial rectus muscle, superior oblique muscle and/or trochlear slip, oculomotor nerve, trochlear nerve, and entrapment of medial orbital structures into a fracture of the lamina papyracea. Nerve injury is usually neuropraxia, so if forced duction tests are normal, observation is warranted. Retrobulbar hematoma is a very serious condition, in which periglobal blood vessels have been ruptured and blood accumulates around or within the muscular cone.

Nasal obstruction can be due to compression of the upper nasal passages, with infracturing of the nasal bones; and generalized mucosal edema. Epistaxis is quite common with NOE fractures. It usually represents the disruption of the nasal mucoperiosteum caused by blunt trauma or shearing forces and displaced bony fractures. Severe epistaxis may indicate disruption of the ethmoid arteries and/or the sphenopalatine arteries.

Imbalance may be present in patients with NOE injuries, primarily in patients with serious trauma to the face that can cause a concussion, anterior skull base contusion, cerebral edema, or injury to the medial longitudinal fasciculus. Contrecoup injuries to the brainstem and vestibular/cerebellar pathways may have occurred; these signs are ominous for more serious intracranial pathology. Nystagmus may be a feature of contrecoup trauma.

Anosmia is another worrisome sign that can be due to accumulation of blood, mucus, and swollen nasal membranes, but could also be due to a disruption of the olfactory nerve at the level of the cribriform plate. If this injury is suspected, the patient should be tested for CSF rhinorrhea, using filter paper in the front-leaning-head position, or collected and tested for beta-2 transferrin.

Epiphora is usually due to tissue edema surrounding the medial eyelids. However, fractures and soft tissue injuries involving the lacrimal drainage system will produce epiphora, which requires further evaluation with lacrimal probing at the time of the surgical repair.

The preferred imaging modality for naso-orbital ethmoid injuries is axial and coronal computed tomography (CT) scans. Images between 1.5 and 2.0 mm in thickness provide adequate detail to determine the extent and the nature of injuries. The CT scan also provides information as to the integrity of the nasal bones and nasal septum. In addition, associated injuries to the frontal sinuses, nasofrontal ducts, and orbits must not be overlooked. By combining the valuable imaging data obtained from the CT scans with the physical examination findings, one can then formulate a management plan [6].

### 9.3.3 Classification of NOE Injuries

Two major classification systems for naso-orbital ethmoid complex fractures currently exist.

A. **Gruss** in 1985 characterized fractures of the naso-orbital ethmoid complex as either isolated or in combination with adjacent maxillofacial injuries [51].
   - Type 1 Isolated bony NOE injury.
   - Type 2 Bony NOE and central maxilla 2A Central maxilla only, 2B Central and one lateral maxilla, 2C Central and bilateral lateral maxillae.
   - Type 3 Extended NOE injury, 3A With craniofacial injuries, 3B With LeFort II and III fractures.
   - Type 4 NOE with orbital displacement, 4A With oculo-orbital displacement 4B With orbital dystopia.
   - Type 5 NOE with bone loss.

B. ***Markowitz* et al.** in 1991 focused their classification to various fracture patterns of the nasoorbital ethmoid complex itself [52].
   - Type I: Single-fragment bone segment with intact canthal tendon insertions.
   - Type II: Comminuted central bone segment with fractures remaining external to the medial canthal tendon insertion.
   - Type III: Comminuted single fragment with fractures extending into bone bearing the canthal insertion.

### 9.3.4 Surgical Management of NOE Fractures

Surgical intervention is indicated in compressed NOE complex, Traumatic telecanthus, Persistent epistaxis, despite local hemostatic measures, medial orbital fracture with entrapment demonstrated on forced duction testing, fracture(s) seen on imaging studies of the floor of the frontal sinus, which could block outflow, fractures of the NOE involving the medial canthal tendons, disruption of the lacrimal fossa and superior nasolacrimal duct, obvious injury to the region of the lacrimal canaliculi, evidence of a developing retrobulbar hematoma, which requires urgent ophthalmologic intervention, CSF rhinorrhea due to a fracture of the cribriform plate or posterior wall of the inferior frontal sinus seen in imaging studies.

### 9.3.5 Primary Objectives of the Surgical Repair/Reconstruction of the NOE Complex [47].

1- Stop nasal bleeding through compression and/or clipping/cautery of vessels as needed.
2- Reduce the compressed and widened NOE bones and splint or fixate them into proper position. Reduce any fracture edges that may be involving the cribriform plate.
3- Re-establish normal intercanthal distance and maintain it in proper position for healing, usually by internal fixation.
4- Re-establish continuity to the nasolacrimal drainage system through closure of lacerations and internal stenting.
5- Reduce medial orbital entrapped tissues, if present, while protecting the globe.
6- Explore and repair frontal sinus floor and/or posterior sinus wall fractures as required.
7- Re-attach the trochlea of the superior oblique muscle if it has been disrupted from its normal osseous/periosteal attachment.
8- Re-establish a normal frontal and profile appearance to the NOE complex region.
9- Repair any lacerations with a fine plastic closure, especially those that may be used for exposure of the fractures.
10- Repair CSF leak at the anterior skull base if conservative measures and time have not led to closure.

### 9.3.6 Surgical Incisions for Repair of NOE Fractures

If one or more lacerations are in the NOE complex, it may be possible to expose the fractures and associated injured structures through these lacerations. It can be extended for adequate exposure. Fine-plastic closure of the lacerations, whether used for exposure or not, will be necessary.

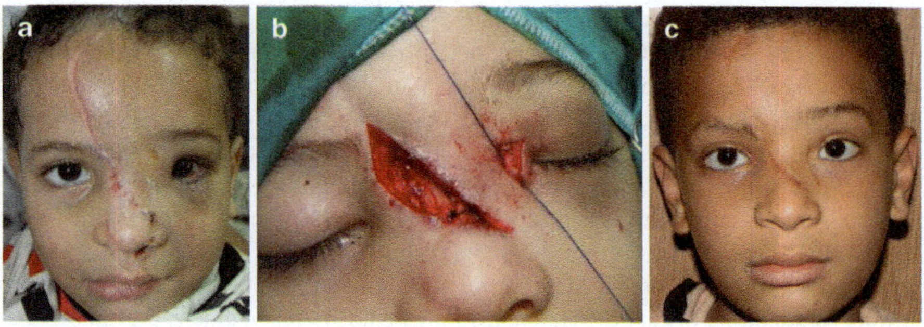


**Fig. 9.12** A 4-year-old male patient presented with NOE fracture with an evident left side telecanthus (**a**), Surgical exposure through laceration was done and medial canthal tendon was explored through left medial canthal incision then anchored with 4 zero prolene suture and fixed to the frontonasal area (**b**), 4 years post-operative with accepted cosmetic outcome (**c**)

Transconjunctival approaches can be utilized to approach the medial orbital wall injuries through either transcaruncular or retrocaruncular incisions.

An extended medial canthal/lateral nasal approach is often utilized to reduce and fixate the NOE complex fractures and to reconstruct the medial canthal tendons to their proper position. The incision is usually gull-wing shaped, placed approximately 8–10 mm from the inner palpebral angle, extending superiorly and inferiorly for approximately 15–20 mm. The periosteum can be elevated laterally, exposing the lacrimal fossa, medial orbit (lamina papyracea), and ethmoid arteries. The exposure is sufficient to reduce medial orbit entrapments and fixate the intercanthal distance to the proper width (Fig. 9.12). The incision can be extended superiorly (as with a Lynch incision) to expose the region of the trochlear slip, if that structure needs repair, or can be reattached to the superior-medial orbital wall. If the incision is extended much beyond 1 cm, it is wise to incorporate a small Z-plasty to reduce the risk of web formation in this concave anatomic area.

For severe NOE fractures that involve the anterior skull base, nasal process of the frontal bone, inferior/anterior/posterior frontal sinus or that extend into the cribriform plate, it is usually necessary to approach the reconstruction through a bifrontal (coronal) forehead flap, elevating in the subperiosteal plane. This exposure will also allow for repair of an avulsed trochlea, and obliteration of the frontal sinus, if indicated.

## 9.4 Reconstructive Options

The reconstruction of NOE injuries usually involves the reduction and fixation of the nasal bones, medial orbit, nasolacrimal system, and medial canthal tendons, with the goals of obtaining near-normal cosmetic appearance and function, as well as reducing immediate and late complications.

Reduction of the NOE fractures in the operating room are normally a simple maneuver of manually compressing the splayed fractures at the level of the medial canthi to obtain a more normal intercanthal distance, based on half of the patient's interpupillary distance. Often, this reduction sufficiently produces adequate NOE anterior/profile projection, and the bones maintain their position without internal fixation. Only an external nasal cast may be required in most patients. If the NOE fractures are unstable, requiring internal stabilization particularly to maintain the proper intercanthal distance then several fixation options are commonly used. Internal transnasal wiring can be applied after the medial canthal region has been exposed bilaterally. The preferred method of fixating the NOE fractures is to apply low-profile miniplates to the fracture sites after reducing the fractures and achieving proper intercanthal distances. The plates may be left in place unless they cause discomfort to the patient in the future.

Reconstruction of a damaged lacrimal drainage system will likely require the insertion of a polymer canalicular tube. If there is a medial orbital wall fracture (lamina papyracea and ethmoid sinus complex), this area must be explored and reconstructed.

Most CSF leaks at the level of the cribriform plate will self-seal after reduction of the fractures. Consideration may also be given to placing the patient in the semi-upright position and inserting an epidural drain. For persistent leaks, an endoscopic approach to repair is usually successful [53].

### 9.4.1 Complications After NOE Repair

The complications seen after NOE fracture management relate to the status of the medial canthal tendon and the nasolacrimal duct. The most annoying complication is persistent telecanthus (Fig. 9.13). This is almost impossible to adequately treat secondarily. If one does approach it, typically the area needs to be refractured and the medial canthal bone fragment reduced more medially. In these situations, the soft tissue overlying this area needs to be thinned to rid it of the fibrosis that typically adds to the poor appearance [54].

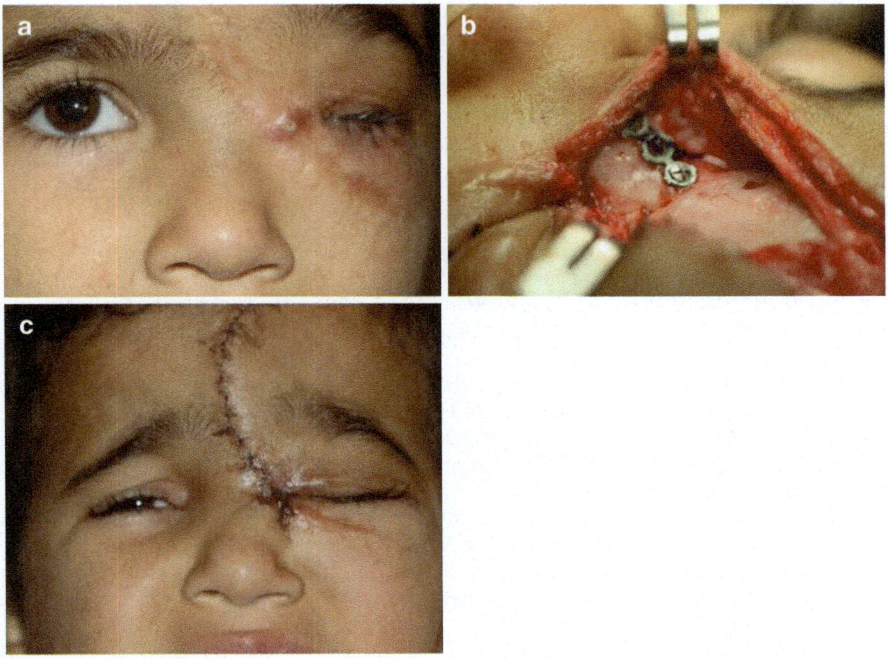

**Fig. 9.13** A 4-year-old female patient presented with neglected NOE fracture with an evident left side telecanthus (**a**), Surgical exposure through laceration was done and medial canthal tendon was anchored with 4 zero prolene suture and fixed with low profile miniplate to the frontonasal area (**b**), 1 week post-operative with accepted cosmetic outcome (**c**)

## References


1. Gilardino MS, Chen E, Bartlett SP. Choice of internal rigid fixation materials in the treatment of facial fractures. Craniomaxillofac Trauma Reconstr. 2009;2(1):49–60.
2. Ellis E 3rd, Moos KF. el-attar a. ten years of mandibular fractures: an analysis of 2,137 cases. Oral Surg Oral Med Oral Pathol. 1985;59(2):120–9.
3. Palmieri C, Ellis E 3rd, Throckmorton G. Mandibular motion after closed and open treatment of unilateral mandibular condylar process fractures. J Oral Maxillofac Surg. 1999;57(7):764–75. discussion 775-776
4. De Riu G, Gamba U, Anghinoni M, Sesenna E. A comparison of open and closed treatment of condylar fractures: a change in philosophy. Int J Oral Maxillofac Surg. 2001;30(5):384–9.
5. Olson RA, Fonseca RJ, Zeitler DL, Osbon DB. Fractures of the mandible: a review of 580 cases. J Oral Maxillofac Surg. 1982;40(1):23–8.
6. Schuknecht B, Graetz K. Radiologic assessment of maxillofacial, mandibular, and skull base trauma. Eur Radiol. 2005;15(3):560–8.
7. Schneider M, Erasmus F, Gerlach KL, Kuhlisch E, Loukota RA, Rasse M. Open reduction and internal fixation versus closed treatment and mandibulomaxillary fixation of fractures of the mandibular condylar process: a randomized, prospective, multicenter study with special evaluation of fracture level. J Oral Maxillofac Surg. 2008;66(12):2537–44.
8. Valiati R, Ibrahim D, Abreu ME, Heitz C, de Oliveira RB, Pagnoncelli RM. The treatment of condylar fractures: to open or not to open? A critical review of this controversy. Int J Med Sci. 2008;5(6):313–8.

9. Eusterman VD. Mandibular trauma in resident manual of trauma to the face, head, and neck. 1st ed. Alexandria, VA: American Academy of Otolaryngology—Head and Neck Surgery Foundation; 2012.
10. Baker S, Betts NJ. Mandibular angle fractures. Oral Maxillofac Surg Knowled Update. 1998;2:25.
11. Zide MF, Kent JN. Indications for open reduction of mandibular condyle fractures. J Oral Maxillofac Surg. 1983;41(2):89–98.
12. Hinds EC, Girotti WJ. Vertical subcondylar osteotomy: a reap appraisal. Oral Surg Oral Med Oral Pathol. 1967;24(2):164–70.
13. Kempers KG, Quinn PD, Silverstein K. Surgical approaches to mandibular condylar fractures: a review. J Craniomaxillofac Trauma. 1999;5(4):25–30.
14. Theriot BA, Van Sickels JE, Triplett RG, Nishioka GJ. Intraosseous wire fixation versus rigid osseous fixation of mandibular fractures: a preliminary report. J Oral Maxillofac Surg. 1987;45(7):577–82.
15. Champy M, Loddé JP, Schmitt R, Jaeger JH, Muster D. Mandibular osteosynthesis by miniature screwed plates via a buccal approach. J Maxillofac Surg. 1978;6(1):14–21.
16. Kellman RM, Morehead JM. Midfacial trauma in resident manual of trauma to the face, head, and neck. 1st ed. Alexandria VA: American Academy of Otolaryngology—Head and Neck Surgery Foundation; 2012.
17. Nam SB, Bae YC, Moon JS, et al. Analysis of the postoperative outcome in 405 cases of orbital fracture using 2 synthetic orbital implants. Ann Plast Surg. 2006;56(3):263–7.
18. Appling WD, Patrinely JR, Salzer TA. Transconjunctival approach vs subciliary skin-muscle flap approach for orbital fracture repair. Arch Otolaryngol Head Neck Surg. 1993;119(9):1000–7.
19. Patel PC, Sobota BT, Patel NM, et al. Comparison of transconjunctival versus subciliary approaches for orbital fractures: a review of 60 cases. J Craniomaxillofac Trauma. 1998;4(1):17–21.
20. Kakibuchi M, Fukazawa K, Fukuda K, Yamada N, Matsuda K, Kawai K, Tomofuji S, Sakagami M. Combination of transconjunctival and endonasal-transantral approach in the repair of blow-out fractures involving the orbital floor. Br J Plast Surg. 2004;57(1):37–44.
21. Liss J, Stefko ST, Chung WL. Orbital surgery: state of the art. Oral Maxillofac Surg Clin North Am. 2010;22(1):59–71.
22. Edgin WA, Morgan-Marshall A, Fitzsimmons TD. Transcaruncular approach to medial orbital wall fractures. J Oral Maxillofac Surg. 2007;65(11):2345–9.
23. Holck DEE, Ng JD. Evaluation and treatment of orbital fractures. Philadelphia, PA: WB Saunders; 2006. p. 290–3.
24. Moe KS. The precaruncular approach to the medial orbit. Arch Facial Plast Surg. 2003;5(6):483–7.
25. Bae SH, Jeong DK, Go JY, Park H, Kim JH, Lee JW, Kang T. A novel technique for placing titanium mesh with porous polyethylene via the endoscopic transnasal approach into the orbit for medial orbital wall fractures. Arch Plast Surg. 2019;46(5):421–5.
26. Rhee J, Lynch J, and. Loehrl T. Intranasal endoscopy-assisted repair of medial Orbital Wall fractures. Archives of. Facial Plast Surg. 2000;2(4):269–73.
27. Sanno T, Tahara S, Nomura T, et al. Endoscopic endonasal reduction for blowout fracture of the medial orbital wall. Plast Reconstr Surg. 2003;112:1228–37.
28. Jeon SY, Kwon JH, Kim JP, et al. Individual preformed titanium meshes for orbital fractures. Oral Surg Oral Med Oral Pathol Oral Radiol Endod. 2006;102(4):442–7.
29. Guo L, Tian W, Feng F, Long J, Li P, Tang W. Reconstruction of orbital floor fractures: comparison of individual prefabricated titanium implants and calvarial bone grafts. Ann Plast Surg. 2009;63(6):624–31.
30. Tang W, Guo L, Long J, et al. Individual design, and rapid prototyping in reconstruction of orbital wall defects. J Oral Maxillofac Surg. 2010;68(3):562–70.
31. Jank S, Emshoff R, Schuchter B, Strobl H, Brandlmaier I, Norer B. Orbital floor reconstruction with flexible Ethisorb patches: a retrospective long-term follow-up study. Oral Surg Oral Med Oral Pathol Oral Radiol Endod. 2003;95(1):16–22.

32. Gosau M, Schöneich M, Draenert FG, Ettl T, Driemel O, Reichert TE. Retrospective analysis of orbital floor fractures—complications, outcome, and review of literature. Clin Oral Invest. 2011;15(3):305–13.
33. Gierloff M, Seeck NG, Springer I, Becker S, Kandzia C, Wiltfang J. Orbital floor reconstruction with resorbable polydioxanone implants. J Craniofac Surg. 2012;23(1):161–4.
34. Schramm A, Gellrich N-C, Naumann S, Bühner U, Schön R, Schmelzeisen R. Non-invasive referencing in computer assisted surgery. Med Biol Eng Comp Suppl. 1999;37:644–5.
35. Schmelzeisen R, Gellrich NC, Schoen R, Gutwald R, Zizelmann C, Schramm A. Navigation-aided reconstruction of medial orbital wall and floor contour in cranio-maxillofacial reconstruction. Injury. 2004;35(10):955–62.
36. Ellis E III, Tan Y. Assessment of internal orbital reconstructions for pure blowout fractures: cranial bone grafts versus titanium mesh. J Oral Maxillofac Surg. 2003;61(4):442–53.
37. Scolozzi P, Momjian A, Heuberger J. Computer-aided volumetric comparison of reconstructed orbits for blow-out fractures with non-preformed versus 3-dimensionally preformed titanium mesh plates: a preliminary study. J Comput Assist Tomogr. 2010;34(1):98–104.
38. Gear AJ, Lokeh A, Aldridge JH, Migliori MR, Benjamin CI, Schubert W. Safety of titanium mesh for orbital reconstruction. Ann Plast Surg. 2002;48(1):1–7. discussion 7–9
39. Kuttenberger JJ, Hardt N. Long-term results following reconstruction of craniofacial defects with titanium micro-mesh systems. J Craniomaxillofac Surg. 2001;29(2):75–81.
40. Kermer C, Lindner A, Friede I, Wagner A, Millesi W. Preoperative stereolithographic model planning for primary reconstruction in craniomaxillofacial trauma surgery. J Craniomaxillofac Surg. 1998;26(3):136–9.
41. Metzger MC, Schön R, Tetzlaf R, et al. Topographical CT-data analysis of the human orbital floor. Int J Oral Maxillofac Surg. 2007;36(1):45–53.
42. Gellrich NC, Schramm A, Hammer B, et al. Computer-assisted secondary reconstruction of unilateral posttraumatic orbital deformity. Plast Reconstr Surg. 2002;110(6):1417–29.
43. Bittermann G, Metzger MC, Schlager S, Largesse WA, Gross N, Cornelius CP, Schmelzeisen R. Orbital reconstruction: prefabricated implants, data transfer, and revision surgery. Facial Plast Surg. 2014;30(5):554–60.
44. Nahum AM. The biomechanics of maxillofacial trauma. Clin Plastic Surg. 1975;2:59.
45. Wormald PJ, Hoseman W, Callejas C, Weber RK, Kennedy DW, Citardi MJ, Senior BA, Smith TL, Hwang PH, Orlandi RR, Kaschke O, Siow JK, Szczygielski K, Goessler U, Khan M, Bernal-Sprekelsen M, Kuehnel T, Psaltis A. The international frontal sinus anatomy classification (IFAC) and classification of the extent of endoscopic frontal sinus surgery (EFSS). Int Forum Allergy Rhinol. 2016;6(7):677–96.
46. Lang J. Paranasal sinuses. In: Lang J, editor. Clinical anatomy of the nose, nasal cavity and paranasal sinuses. New York: Thieme Medical Publishers, Inc.; 1989. p. 63.
47. Donald PJ, Holt GR. Upper facial trauma in in resident manual of trauma to the face, head, and neck. 1st ed. Alexandria VA: American Academy of Otolaryngology—Head and Neck Surgery Foundation; 2012.
48. Draf W. Endonasal micro-endoscopic frontal sinus surgery: the Fulda concept. Opera Tech Otolaryngol Head Neck Surg. 1991;2:234–40.
49. Donald PJ, Bernstein L. Compound frontal sinus injuries with intracranial penetration. Laryngoscope. 1978;88(225–232):7.
50. Merville LC, Derome PJ. Concomittant dislocations of the face and skull. J Maxillofac Surg. 1978;6(1):2–14.
51. Gruss J. Naso-ethmoid-orbital fractures: classification and role of primary bone grafting. Plast Reconstr Surg. 1985;75:303–15.
52. Markowitz B, Manson P, Sargent L, Vander Kolk C, Yaremchuk M, Glassman D, Crawley W. Management of the medial canthal tendon in nasoethmoid orbital fractures: the importance of the central fragment in classification and treatment. Plast Reconstr Surg. 1991;87:843–53.
53. Vora NM, Fedok FG. Management of the central nasal support complex in naso-orbital ethmoid fractures. Facial Plast Surg. 2000;16(2):181–91.
54. Nguyen M, Koshy JC, Hollier LH Jr. Pearls of nasoorbitoethmoid trauma management. Semin Plast Surg. 2010;24(4):383–8.

# Septal Surgery

# 10

Stephen P. Williams and Andrew C. Swift

**Key Points**

- Septoplasty is a long-established procedure in rhinological practice. It has been shown to be effective at alleviating nasal obstruction in patients with significant nasal septal deviation, though appropriate patient selection and pre-operative counseling are crucial to achieve optimal outcomes.
- A range of procedures have been developed and it is important for the surgeon to match the specific problems of each individual case with specific technical solutions to achieve the most optimal outcome. This remains challenging as there remains no clear consensus on the relative indications for endonasal, endoscopic, endoscope-assisted, combined, and open approaches to the nasal septum.
- Furthermore, it is important that future studies consider longer follow-up periods to allow a greater appreciation of the durability of symptom improvement as well as detailed information about post-operative nasal symptoms that should facilitate meaningful analysis.

## 10.1 Introduction

It is estimated that greater than 70% of the adult population have some form of appreciable deviation of their nasal septum [1]. Nasal obstruction is a non-specific symptom with a vast range of different etiologies and many of such nasal septal deviations will be incidental findings. However, septal deviation will be causative or contributory in many of those with symptoms of significant nasal blockage.

S. P. Williams · A. C. Swift (✉)
Liverpool Head and Neck Centre, Liverpool University Hospitals NHS Foundation Trust, Liverpool, UK


S. Elwany (ed.), *Current Rhinology*,
https://doi.org/10.1007/978-3-031-70077-4_10

Accordingly, septoplasty continues to represent a commonly performed procedure, with pre-COVID estimates suggesting more than 250,000 cases are performed per annum in the USA [2], with approximately 16,000 carried out each year in the UK [3].

Whilst septal surgery has been performed since the nineteenth century [4], and undergone sequential refinement since, the adoption of the endoscope into regular rhinological practice has facilitated additional approaches to the deviated septum. More recently, concerns over potential restriction of septoplasty in the publicly funded health care setting have sparked multiple studies seeking to establish an evidence base for what has been established clinical practice for more than a century [5, 6].

## 10.2 Applied Anatomy

The nasal septum forms the midline support of the nasal cavity, acting as a key determinant in both the external structure, and so appearance, of the nose and the establishment of laminar flow during nasal respiration.

There are three main component sections: the membranous, cartilaginous and bony septum. Beginning at the nasal tip, the membranous septum represents the fibrofatty tissue between and posterior to the medial crura of the lower lateral cartilages. The cartilaginous septum is referred to as the quadrangular cartilage due to its shape when viewed in the sagittal plane. The caudal edge of the quadrangular cartilage runs from the anterior nasal spine (the most anterior projection of the maxillary bone and representing a key attachment of the septum) to the anterior septal angle where it turns to form the dorsal edge and so the cartilaginous nasal dorsum until it meets the nasal bones at the keystone area. The bony septum forms its posterior component, consisting of the perpendicular plate of the ethmoid bone superiorly, forming the upper third of the nasal septum, and the vomer inferiorly. The vomer articulates inferiorly with the bony maxillary crest which emanates anteriorly from the maxillary bone and posteriorly from the palatine bone (Fig. 10.1).

Functionally, the septum forms a part of an external and an internal valve. Whilst the use of the word 'valve' is technically incorrect, due to the passage of air in both directions through the nasal passage, it reflects an area of an anatomical narrowing generating a significant amount of nasal resistance. The internal valve is formed by the union of the septum with the upper lateral cartilage and the angle between the two. The external valve is caudal to the internal valve and is bounded by the columella and septum medially, the nasal floor, and the caudal border of the lower lateral cartilage.

Nasal airway resistance is also generated by the nasal septal body, a thickened region of mucosa located superior to the inferior turbinate and anterior to the middle

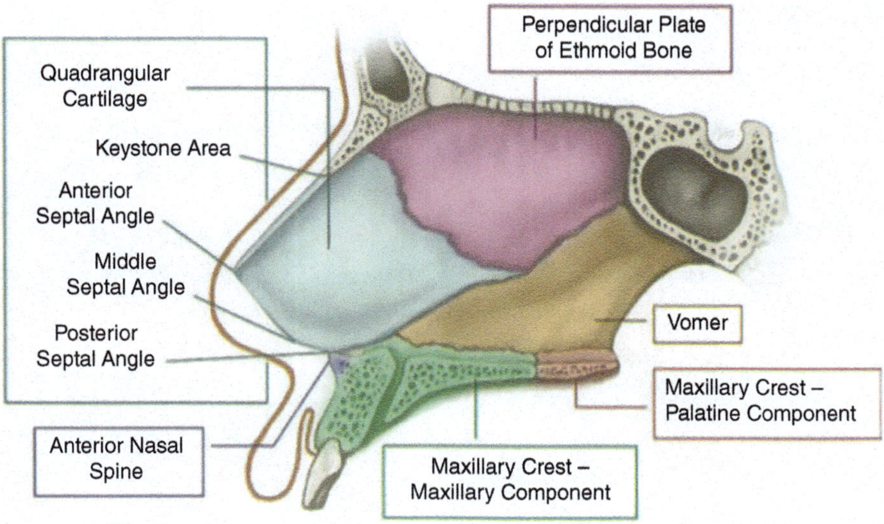


**Fig. 10.1** Cartilaginous and bony anatomy of the nasal septum (reproduced, with permission, from Ref. [15])

turbinate that is rich in both glandular and sinusoidal vascular tissue. It is thought to be involved in the regulation of nasal airflow during the nasal cycle.

The nasal septum has a rich blood supply drawn from the anastomosis of multiple vessels, particularly in its anterior aspect—classically referred to as Little's area or Kiesselbach's plexus. A reliable triangular plexus of vessels with contribution from the anterior ethmoidal artery, branches of the sphenopalatine artery, and superior labial artery is found, with variable contributions from the greater palatine and posterior ethmoidal arteries [7].

Whilst the basic anatomical layout of the nasal septum looks apparently simple, there are significant individual anatomical variations that affect the shape, angles, and thickness of the various component parts. Also, as surgeons, we generally only see these whilst operating in the coronal plain. Such variation is demonstrated in Fig. 10.2. Of particular interest is the thickness of the bone in the anterior section of the ethmoid plate, compared to the relatively thin bone posterior to this region. Appreciation of this area is important to understand whilst addressing deformity during surgery of the bony nasal septum.

Understanding the anatomy is important for also understanding the anatomical deformity and how to best correct this. Such deformities may be localized to a septal spur formed by the vomer and maxillary crest to complex deformities that will block both sides of the nose.

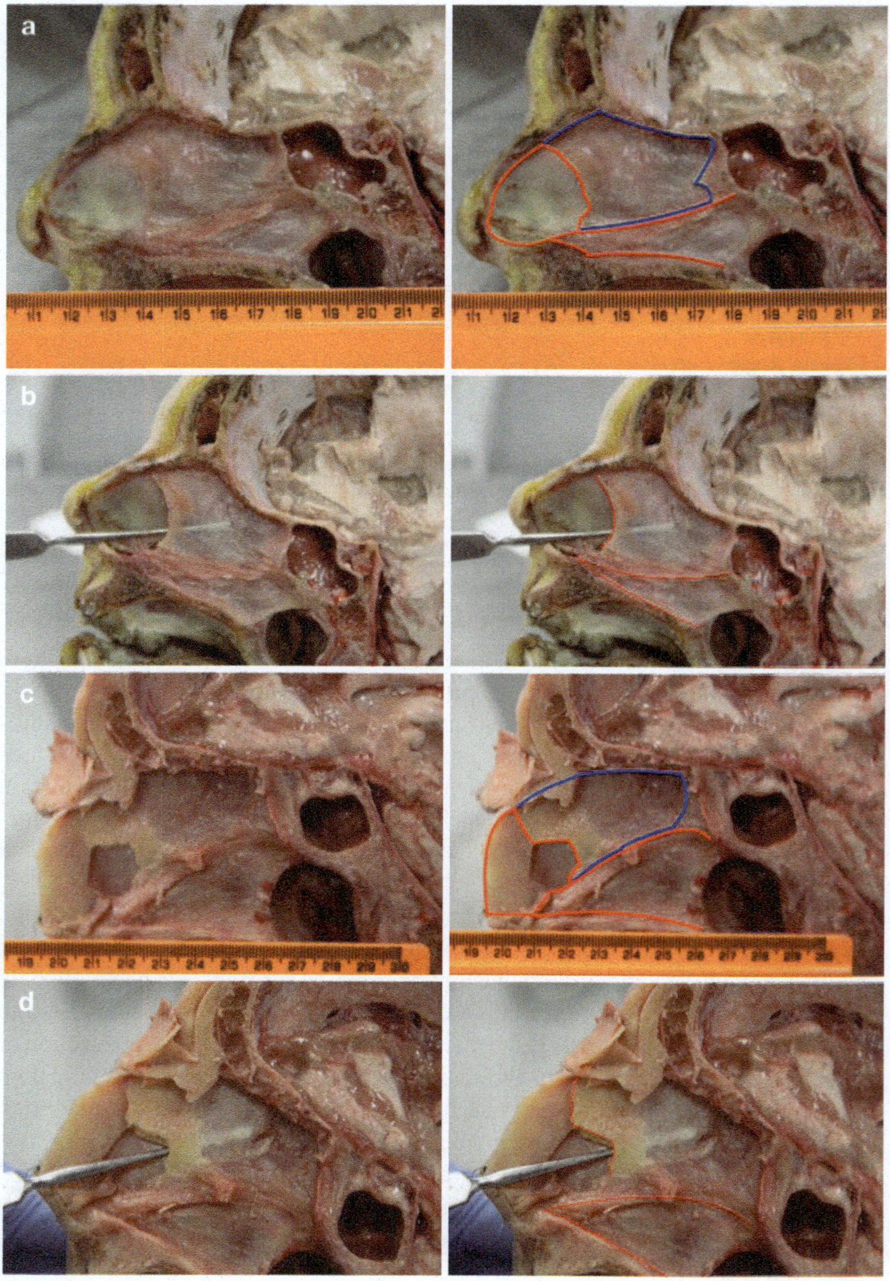


**Fig. 10.2** Anatomy of the nasal septum (**a**) Sagittal cadaveric dissection of the nasal septum. The perpendicular plate of the ethmoid (PPE) is shown within the blue line. The quadrangular cartilaginous septum is shown in red anterior to the PPE. The vomer is sited inferior to the PPE, outlined in red. (**b**) Cartilaginous septum separated from the PPE, demonstrating the junction between bone and cartilage and the thin, transparent area of the PPE. (**c** and **d**) Cartilaginous septum partially removed, demonstrating anatomical variation at the cartilaginousosseous junction and the thick anterior bar of the PPE anterior to the paper-thin area of the PPE

## 10.3 Assessment of the Nasal Septum

### 10.3.1 Clinical Assessment

A thorough history and examination are obviously of paramount importance in all patients with symptoms of nasal obstruction. Deviation of the nasal septum can be congenital or acquired, when it usually follows trauma, but, as alluded to above, care should be taken to exclude other coexistent inflammatory or neoplastic conditions, which, when present, can often be the key driver of sinonasal symptom burden. If ignored, such coexistent pathology can significantly confound the expected post-operative outcomes following septal surgery.

Within the UK, a national review has noted significant variance in rates of septal surgery between centers [8], which betrays the lack of standardization and consistency in terms of both patient assessment and, crucially, indication for surgical intervention.

### 10.3.2 External Examination

Examination of the nose in patients with nasal obstruction is often focused on the nasal cavities and septum. It is therefore very easy to miss external nasal deformity that may co-exist with septal deformity. Such deformity is important to document or record by photographic evidence before undertaking any form of septal surgery, should there be an unexpected change in nasal shape after septal surgery.

### 10.3.3 Internal Examination

Sequential examination of the nasal passages, both before and after topical mucosal decongestion remains the most appropriate form of examination and this is commonly performed with a headlight and nasal speculum. Endoscopic assessment is helpful to examine the posterior septum and nasopharynx, and also exclude sinonasal disease which may go unnoticed with anterior rhinoscopy alone. Ultimately, assessment of the nasal septum remains subjective, though the following grading system has been suggested to quantify severity of deviation more formally: [5].

**Mild deviation**—obstruction <50% of nasal passage

**Moderate deviation**—obstruction ≥50% nasal passage

**Severe deviation**—septum in contract with lateral nasal wall

### 10.3.4 Airway Metrics

Objective measurements of nasal airflow can also be used during assessment, such as rhinomanometry, to measure nasal airway resistance, or rhinospirometry, to determine relative airflow between the two nasal passages, though such investigations are rarely performed in routine clinical practice with most centers favoring more simple assessments of nasal misting [9].

Indeed, whilst such objective findings find a use in the research and medicolegal setting, they have been noted to add little to clinical examination in terms of diagnosis of nasal septal deviation [10].

Symptom burden can be quantified using patient-reported outcome measures, such as the Nasal Obstruction Symptom Evaluation (NOSE) scale. This is a five-item fixed-response survey designed and validated within the context of patients with nasal obstruction undergoing septal surgery. Scores can range from 0 to 100, and it has been reported to have a minimal clinically important difference of 19.4 (which represents the minimum sum score change required for detectable symptom improvement) [11].

The 22-item Sino-Nasal Outcome Test (SNOT-22) has also been utilized, to good effect, in the setting of septoplasty surgery [6, 12], though, as it is specifically designed for a somewhat different context (that of chronic rhinosinusitis), there are some concerns with its validity as a standalone measure in this setting [13].

## 10.4 Indications and Contraindications

Septoplasty is indicated in patients with nasal obstruction where the septum is deemed to be causing significant nasal obstruction or where surgical access to the ethmoid, nasolacrimal sac/duct, or skull base is required. The decision to operate may be straightforward, where there has been a history of unilateral obstruction after nasal trauma. However, the effect of mucosal congestion from rhinitis or rhinosinusitis must be fully appreciated and ideally treated prior to finally deciding on proceeding to septal surgery. Septal surgery may also be considered in patients with sleep-disordered breathing, especially in patients with obstructive sleep apnea where reliance is made on effective Continuous Positive Airways Pressure (CPAP).

The decision to operate on the septum can fall in an uncertain area where the degree of likely improvement and success must be balanced against surgical risk, possible outcomes, and treatment of associated sinonasal disease. However, with careful selection, the outcome of nasal septoplasty is very effective. Caution should be applied with surgery in patients with chronic granulomatous/vasculitic disease such as sarcoidosis, substance abuse such as cocaine, pre-existing cartilaginous perforation, or those in whom surgery would carry high risk.

## 10.5 Surgical Technique

Surgery of the nasal septum has been practiced for over a century and was originally performed under local anesthesia with the patient sitting upright. The operation performed in this way was the classic submucous resection (SMR) in which the deviated section of the septum was excised. This technique remained popular for decades, but in the 1930s, Cottle described his more conservative concept of septal reconstruction via a series of mucosal tunnels in contrast to resection. This led to the operation that became known as septoplasty, and a debate as to which procedure was best subsequently followed.

Whilst septoplasty was less destructive, submucous resection was fast, well-established, and frequently practiced. However, with the advent of operation health coding, septoplasty became the operation of choice, but this was in practice a merger of techniques, with a wide range of septal resection versus septal reconstruction of the cartilaginous septum. Preservation or reconstruction of the bony septum is of lesser importance, but preservation of the cartilaginous septum is advantageous for nasal support, resilience to future trauma, reducing the likelihood of septal perforation, and facilitating revision septal surgery should the need arise.

Currently, septal surgery is performed by three different techniques: the most recent being endoscopic septoplasty; the conventional endonasal route (via headlight or loupes); or external/open septoplasty. However, the divisions are, in practice, not so clear-cut and can be combined in endoscope-assisted septoplasty.

The choice of approach will be driven by a multitude of factors such as anatomy, septal deformity, symptoms of obstruction, equipment, and local facilities. However, it will also reflect a surgeon's training, expertise, experience, and philosophy, in a world where information transfer is rapid and pressure to conform is significant, even in surgery. The chosen or preferred technique should be which one that is best for the individual problem, and surgeons should acquire skills that allow then to perform all techniques with expertise, as required.

### 10.5.1 Preparation of the Nose

All techniques benefit from the use of pharmacological vasoconstrictors to limit bleeding and are recommended to reduce the vascularity of tissues d.

uring dissection. There is a widely held belief that injection of a combination local anesthetic/vasoconstrictor preparation (e.g., Lignospan® Special; Septodont, UK) will 'hydro-dissect' the mucoperichondrium from its underlying cartilage and so facilitate surgical dissection. However, the perichondrium in this region consists of multiple layers, and the chance of reliably infiltrating the vasoconstrictor solution beneath the lowest and most resilient of these layers is extremely unlikely [14].

The patient is placed supine with head elevation to further limit bleeding, also assisted by modern anesthetic techniques.

#### 10.5.1.1 Submucosal Resection

Now strictly considered a precursor of what is considered a septoplasty, submucosal resection begins with an incision placed around a centimeter from the causal end of the nasal septum, historically known as the Killian's incision. Mucoperichondrial flaps are elevated bilaterally, and the deviated portion of the septum is excised in its entirety, preserving a region known as the "L-strut", representing the portion of quadrangular cartilage providing crucial dorsal and caudal support (corresponding to a 1 cm strip of cartilage, Fig. 10.3). This thereby aims to remove the deviated

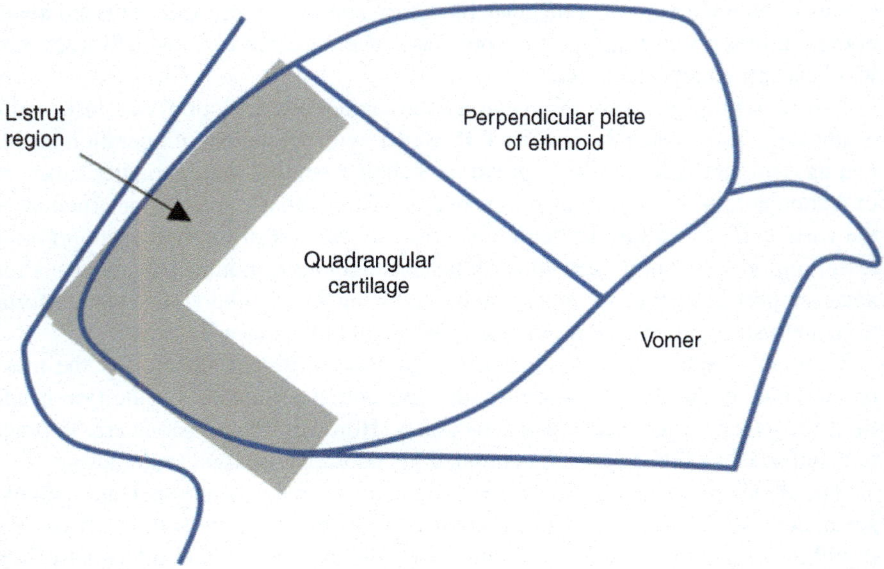


**Fig. 10.3** L-strut region, comprising a 1 cm strip of cartilage consisting of the dorsal and caudal borders of the quadrangular cartilaginous septum

segment of the septum *en bloc*, whilst preserving the structural support for the external nose.

### 10.5.2 Endonasal Septoplasty

Subsequent techniques popularised for septoplasty focus on the preservation of cartilage and bone whenever possible with an emphasis on more conservative resection, largely due to concerns over higher rates of complication (particularly septal perforation and nasal saddling) in patients undergoing classical submucosal resection.

#### 10.5.2.1 The Incision

Whilst endonasal septoplasty can be performed through a Killian's incision (as above), the use of a hemi-transfixion incision is recommended, especially for caudal deviations and dislocation of the columella septal cartilage. The hemi-transfixion incision is made at the most caudal point of the quadrangular cartilage as it adjoins the membranous septum and extends inferiorly to provide access to the anterior nasal spine.

Dissection down to the avascular subperichondrial plane is more challenging than via a Killian's incision due to a cap of fibrous attachments between the mucoperichondrium and cartilage at its caudal edge and can be technically difficult in the setting of surgery after trauma or previous septal surgery.

Such dissection will often benefit from the use of sharp dissection, with a scalpel (15 blades with long, thin handle) or Iris scissor, alongside the use of a sharp Cottle or Freer elevator. Precision blood-free surgery is facilitated using operating loupes and good soft tissue retraction by an assistant, in contrast to single-handed surgery utilizing a Cottles bivalve retractor. However, for single-handed surgery, a sharp elevator with inbuilt suction can facilitate raising of the mucoperichondrial flaps.

#### 10.5.2.2 Mucosal Elevation

Working through a hemi-transfixion incision, a mucosal flap is generally elevated in the concave side of the septum, although it is acknowledged that some surgeons may have a preference to always elevate on a particular side (usually a right-handed surgeon elevating the left-sided flap).

Some surgeons will routinely elevate bilateral flaps whilst others will restrict elevation to a single side if possible. The latter may maintain greater cartilage support, but in complex or S-shaped deformity (with deviation affecting both sides of the nose at different points), elevation of bilateral flaps will facilitate better correction of the deformity.

Deviations in the septum can be addressed through a variety of different strategies and specific situations and techniques below:

#### 10.5.2.3 Mobilization of the Quadrangular Cartilage

Mobilization of the quadrangular cartilage is achieved through its disarticulation at the level of the osteocartilaginous junction. This is generally described as performed through the application of medial pressure to the cartilage just ahead of where it meets the perpendicular plate of the ethmoid bone. Frequently, what is observed in practice is a chondrotomy fracture through the cartilage itself, just anterior to this junction, which is then referred to as a ‘vertical’ chondrotomy. A vertical chondrotomy such as this can also be placed at, or just ahead, of an existing fracture line to allow for mobilization, and either the subsequent reposition or limited resection, of fractured parts.

An inferior “chondrotomy” is now created just above the bony crest of the septum. Technically, the inferior edge of the septum is separated from the maxillary crest, and then an inferior strip of septum is excised to shorten the septum if too long. The established historical term for mobilizing the margins of the cartilaginous septum is a ‘swinging door’ (Fig. 10.4). Should an over-long cartilaginous septum overlap one side of the maxillary crest it is likely to form a cartilaginous/bony maxillary crest spur. This can be addressed by resecting a small strip of excess cartilage by sharp dissection and addressing the bony spur if necessary. Care should be taken to preserve the keystone area and L-strut superiorly, wherever possible, and to be conservative with any resection in this region to limit loss of tip support.

#### 10.5.2.4 Correction of the Cartilaginous Septum

Deformity of the caudal septum, which includes the columella region and cartilaginous dorsum, can be challenging and easily underestimated. Surgery to the L-strut region carries inherent risks of undermining the stability and support of the nasal tip

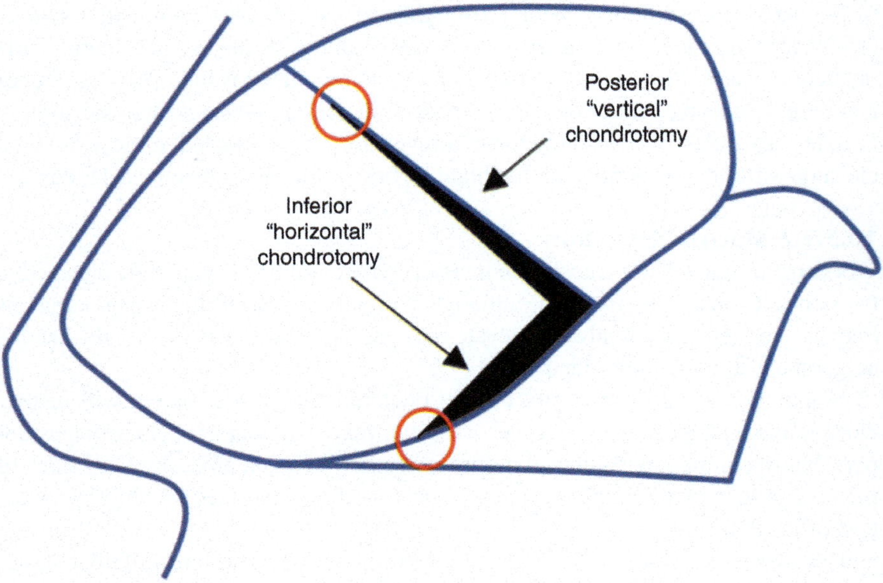


**Fig. 10.4** "Swinging door" mobilization of septal cartilage via posterior 'vertical chondrotomy' and inferior 'horizontal chondrotomy'. Note the limits of both incisions, marked in red circles, preserving the L-strut region

and dorsum. A range of techniques, often in combination, can be employed, determined by specific facets of individual cases and expertise of the operating surgeon.

Relieving tension within a deformed section of the caudal septum and body of the quadrangular cartilage has long been addressed by either dividing healed fracture lines or scoring the concave surface of the septal cartilage (Fig. 10.5b). Such methods will often benefit from extra support by splinting the septum against a fixed batten graft, harvested as a rectangular section of posterior cartilage. Batten grafts are secured in place with a transeptal quilted mattress suture (Fig. 10.5c).

It is not unusual for the caudal septal base to be positioned on one side of the anterior nasal spine rather than on the superior aspect of the spine (Fig. 10.5a). Favored options to correct for such findings include conservative excision of the 'excess' septal length (to allow the septum to again sit upon the spine in the midline; Fig. 10.5b)) or the 'door stop' method, in which the inferior caudal end of the septum is left intact but pushed across to the contralateral side. Both techniques are then secured with a septospinal suture (Fig. 10.5c), in which a slowly absorbable material (such as a 4–0 polydioxanone; PDS, Ethicon, Johnson & Johnson, New Brunswick, NJ, USA) is used to reattach the base of the septum to either the anterior nasal spine or the premaxilla. This is helped by first creating a hole within the bone of the nasal spine with either a 19-gauge needle or a fine drill. Such techniques are favored in preference to the removal of sections of septal cartilage as they reconstruct the septum, thus favoring a more robust septum with less risk of perforation.

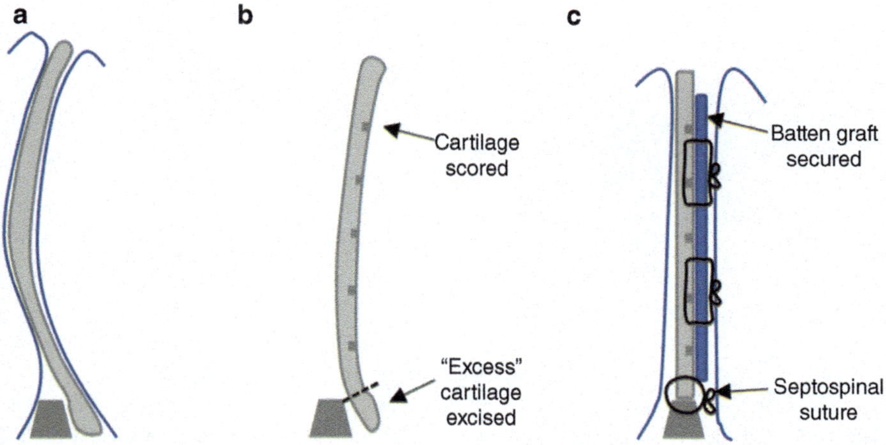


**Fig. 10.5** Management of the deviated caudal septum (**a**) Deviated caudal septum with septal base slippage from anterior nasal spine; (**b**) Scoring and straightening of the septum with conservative excision of "excess" cartilage to allow septum to sit in midline; (**c**) Supporting the septum with both a batten graft and septospinal suture

#### 10.5.2.5 The Posterior Bony Septum

The bony septum is exposed by elevation of mucosa on both sides. Deviations of the vomer and perpendicular ethmoid plate may splint the position of the cartilaginous septum or contribute to airway impairment. Torsional force on the perpendicular ethmoid plate should be avoided to prevent inducing a fracture running superiorly to the skull base. Sections of bone can be removed using various techniques such as sharp Jansen-Middleton punch forceps, placement of bony cuts by turbinectomy scissors or an osteotome, or the use of a drill. Which method is chosen will be determined to some extent by the thickness of the bone in the anterior section of the perpendicular ethmoidal plate.

##### Septal Spurs

Septal spurs can prove challenging, and mucosal elevation often risks iatrogenic tears from very thin mucosa that is least resilient at the apex of the spur.

Some spurs are accentuated from cartilage overlying one side of the maxillary crest, whereas those that are most posterior arise from the vomer or junction of the vomer with the ethmoid plate.

More subtle posterior spurs may not cause significant nasal obstruction or need correction. Surgical reduction/resection will entail mucosal elevation in a 'back to front' approach, with elevation in a sub-perichondrial plane both dorsally and posteriorly above the spur before mobilization of the spur [15].

Larger septal spurs warrant an approach in a 'front to back' manner, and this is best performed via development of septal tunnels—with one above and another below the spur itself (Fig. 10.6) [14]. When both tunnels are elevated beyond the spur, its apex can then be dissected (working from either the inferior or superior

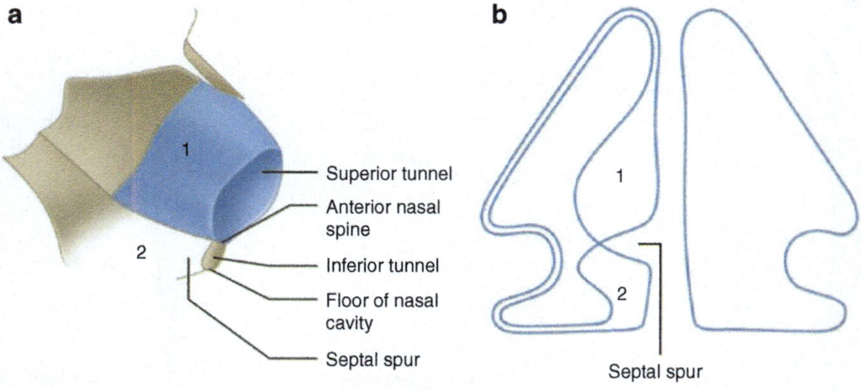


**Fig. 10.6** Elevation of superior [1] and inferior [2] mucosal tunnels viewed in sagittal (**a**) and coronal (**b**) section (reproduced, with permission, from Ref. [15])

tunnel), confident that the risk of an iatrogenic flap tear is reduced by decreased tension and tethering of the mucosa around the spur. Once the mucosa is dissected free, the spur can be resected with sharp dissection (as described above), whilst preserving mucosa and minimizing the risk or degree of mucosal tearing.

### 10.5.3 Open External Approach Septoplasty

Though often a reflection of the preferences of a particular surgeon, open external approaches have long been favored for more complex deviation, especially that involving the L-strut region of the septum. Enhanced visibility is also why an open approach is frequently employed when placing grafts. Indeed, significant dorsal deformity is often corrected by way of open septoplasty to facilitate the placement of spreader grafts, set between the upper lateral cartilage and dorsal septum, to straighten or conceal the deviation of dorsal L-strut.

Though discussed in greater detail within dedicated chapters on septorhinoplasty, an open approach to the septum is achieved through transcolumellar and marginal incisions, with the septum exposed through transdomal division of the lower lateral cartilages and subsequent dissection in a subperichondrial plane.

In the setting of severe deviation of the dorsal and/or caudal end of the quadrangular cartilage, an open approach can be utilized to perform extracorporeal septoplasty, in which the entirety of the cartilaginous septum is removed and then reconstructed. Though originally described in the 1950s [16], its contemporary description is found presented alongside a large series published by Gubisch in 1995 [17].

Its component steps involve the initial mobilization of the septal cartilage by way of posterior and inferior chondrotomy, and subsequent release from its attachments at the keystone area. The resected septal cartilage is then rebuilt upon a PDS plate (Ethicon, Johnson & Johnson, New Brunswick, NJ, USA) as scaffold. Reconstructive options include reorientating or reshaping existing pieces of septal cartilage or augmenting existing cartilage with sections of either septal bone or auricular cartilage. Cadaveric allograft material can also be utilized, if such autograft options are depleted, and the priority is to rebuild a straight L-strut. This neoseptum is then returned and secured within the nasal cavity by way of three-point fixation: at the keystone area to the upper lateral cartilages, at the anterior nasal spine with a septo-spinal suture, and with a quilted mattress suture through the neoseptum and both mucosal flaps.

Extracorporeal septoplasty remains an advanced procedure and though a recent systematic review has demonstrated that it is an effective technique with a low overall complication rate of 2%, irregularities in the nasal dorsum are reported in up to 83% of patients postoperatively [18]. The use of camouflage dorsal onlay grafts, placed over the reattachment point at the rhinion, has been recommended to attempt to reduce this [17].

### 10.5.4 Endoscopic Septoplasty

In general, the principles of endoscopic septoplasty are identical to those described above for endonasal surgery. Endoscopic septoplasty is generally performed with a 0 degree endoscope with an endoscopic lens cleaning sheath (e.g. Endo-Scrub®; Medtronic, Minneapolis, MN, USA) that facilitates continuous endoscopic surgery in a narrow, confined nasal cavity.

Access is typically through a Killian incision made with the scalpel tip just behind the leading edge of the upper lateral cartilage (Fig. 10.7a). The incision is extended down to the level of the floor of the nasal cavity (Fig. 10.7b) and dissection begins in a subperichondrial plane (Fig. 10.7c) as with a conventional endonasal approach. Bilateral mucosal flaps can be elevated once a vertical chondrotomy has been performed (Fig. 10.7d). For localized spurs, the incision can be localized either just anterior to the spur or along the length of the spur to preserve nasal mucosa as best as possible.

Endoscopic septoplasty has been shown to have clinical equipoise, in terms of both outcomes and operative time, to an endonasal approach [19], and utilizing an endoscope also allows for the adoption of a more tailored approach to focal septal spurs, with mucosal incisions placed either immediately anterior (or more simply placed along their length) allowing direct access for mobilization and precise excision whilst preserving nasal mucosa. The enhanced optics of an endoscope are of particular value in observing both the posterior septum and the dorsum of the nose, both of which can be challenging with an endonasal approach. However, limitations are the difficulty of correcting anterior septal deformities and accommodating the wide-angle distortion of the endoscope. Advantages include the magnified clear screen view for teaching and for theatre staff to appreciate and maintain attention during surgery.

Endoscopic septoplasty is not best suited to cases with significant caudal deviation or anterior cartilaginous deformity. However, a hybrid approach commencing

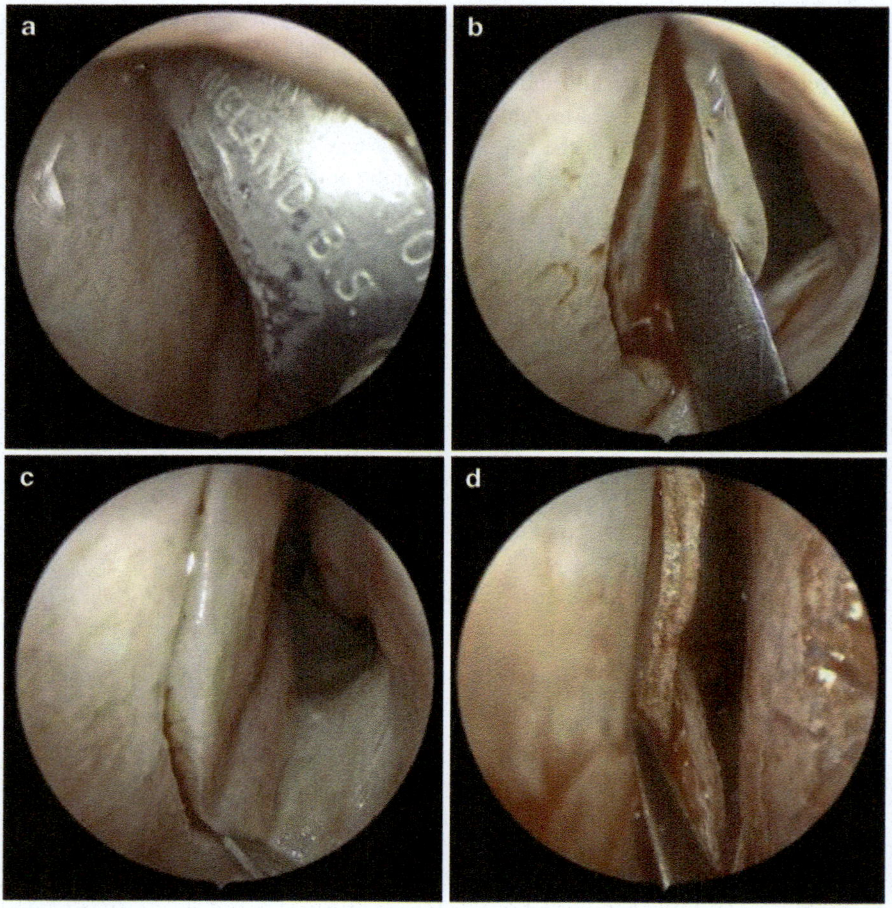


**Fig. 10.7** Endoscopic septoplasty—(**a**) Killian incision begun behind leading edge of upper lateral cartilage; (**b**) incision extended to floor of the nose; (**c**) dissection begins in the subperichondrial plane with a Freer dissector; (**d**) Vertical chondrotomy

with a hemi-transfixion incision, will facilitate conventional septal surgery anteriorly and superiorly, which progresses to an endoscope for the posterior bony component of the deformity.

### 10.5.5 Local Anesthetic Surgery

Partly driven by restrictions created by the COVID pandemic, local anesthetic rhinological procedures, including septoplasty, continue to gain in popularity. This is especially true within the USA, with an increased adoption of office-based procedures. This trend is likely to increase in the UK given the difficulty accessing conventional theatre time that will result in 'office-based' surgery becoming much more predominant to secure patient care. Many of the more advanced procedures discussed above will not be possible in the setting of an awake patient, but more limited surgery will be feasible in many. Ultimately, patient selection is key though there exist a series of extensive published recommendations covering pre-operative patient education, operative set-up, and peri-operative procedure [20, 21].

### 10.5.6 Paediatric Septal Surgery

Septoplasty in children is best avoided, especially in young children, unless deemed essential. Often, if surgery is performed, it is termed a limited septoplasty, which may provide sufficient relief. Ideally, there should be minimal resection of cartilage to facilitate revision surgery in later years should this be required. More extensive septal surgery, and particularly extracorporeal septal surgery, carries a small but significant risk of interfering with septal growth, risking nasal deformity and obstruction in later years.

### 10.5.7 Post-Operative Management

For many years post-operative management following surgery on the nasal septum was insertion of a Vaseline gauze pack that was removed the next day. Such packs were replaced by the more convenient and better tolerated polyvinyl acetate non-absorbable sponge packs (Merocel®) and later by fragmentable dressings (Nasopore®). However, this practice has, in many cases, been replaced by suturing the mucosal flaps together with absorbable polyglactin 910 (Vicryl®) sutures, thus obviating the need to pack the nose.

Post-operative infection is uncommon and prophylactic antibiotics are generally unnecessary.

The nasal cavities can be kept clear of crusts by the regular use of saline sprays or sometimes saline rinses.

## 10.6 Complications

The overall complication rate after septoplasty is relatively low, though a large series reports that 12% are treated with antibiotics for an infection in the post-operative period, 11% report transient altered sensation of their upper teeth, 10% note changes in the external appearance of their noise and 4% represent post-operatively with secondary hemorrhage that may require intervention and re-admission. Risk factors for infection include obesity, smoking and diabetes [6].

### 10.6.1 Uncommon Complications (1 in 20)

Infection: Infection after septoplasty is unusual but would present with increasing nasal pain, tenderness, redness, feeling unwell, and pyrexia.

Septal hematoma: Post-operative septal hematoma from a collection of blood beneath the raised mucosal septal flaps is a potential complication after septal surgery. A hematoma needs formal surgical drainage to prevent infection, abscess formation, cartilage necrosis, perforation, and saddle deformity. Techniques to prevent a hematoma include the insertion of nasal packs or dressings, quilting sutures, septal splints, and inferior mucosal incisions to facilitate drainage.

### 10.6.2 Rare Complications (<1 in 100)

Cerebrospinal fluid (CSF) leaks: CSF leaks after septal surgery are rare. However, they may arise from intraoperative cribriform plate damage from forceful twisting of the perpendicular plate of the ethmoid bone, that is firmly attached to the skull base as a single bony unit.

Alteration in nasal shape to correct cartilaginous deviation or improve tip support is usually done intentionally, but unintentional deformity such as saddle formation is fortunately rare.

Smell and taste may be impaired temporarily, but loss of smell (anosmia) is extremely rare.

### 10.6.3 Long-Term Risks

Difficulties with healing during the post-operative period may lead to nasal septal perforation between 2 and 3% of patients and nasal synechiae/adhesions in at least 3–4% [5, 6].

Revision surgery rates vary in reported series, and systematic review of longer-term follow up data suggests patient satisfaction may wane with time [5]. Whilst dissatisfaction rates have been reported to be as high as 24–29% [22, 23], recent data suggests revision surgery is only performed in 1.1% of adult cases overall.

## 10.7 Outcomes

The last 5 years have seen publication of the first two randomized controlled trials (RCTs) comparing the effectiveness of septoplasty to medical treatment alone.

In 2018, van Egmond et al. reported a multi-center RCT of 203 patients undergoing septoplasty (with or without concurrent turbinate surgery). Outcomes included subjective survey measures including the NOSE scale, SNOT-22, a battery of generic quality of life scales, and objective measures of peak nasal inspiratory flow (PNIF). Results demonstrated surgical intervention, via septoplasty, to be more effective than medical treatment alone, both at 6–12 months post-operatively. Indeed, there was also a 30% crossover from the medical to the surgical treatment arm during the study window [5].

Such results were echoed in a more recent RCT, by Carrie et al., considering 378 patients randomized to either septoplasty (again with or without concurrent turbinate surgery) versus 6 months of medical treatment with both a topical steroid spray and nasal saline. Septoplasty was again shown to be more effective than medical treatment when measured using the NOSE scale, SNOT-22, and PNIF. Rhinospirometry results also demonstrated a consistent treatment-related shift, in those undergoing surgery, from a predominantly uninarial pattern to one of equal binarial airflow. Indeed, results suggest that patients with nasal obstruction, septal deviation (without coexistent sinonasal disease), and a baseline NOSE score > 30 can be reliably recommended septoplasty and that patients with higher baseline NOSE scores are more likely to demonstrate measurable post-operative benefit [6].

A range of septal surgical procedures have been developed and it is important for the surgeon to match the specific problems of each individual case with specific technical solutions to achieve the most optimal outcome. This remains challenging as there remains no clear consensus on the relative indications for endonasal, endoscopic, endoscope-assisted, combined, and open approaches to the nasal septum. Future outcome studies should include details of the individual surgical techniques and consider longer follow-up periods to allow a greater appreciation of the durability of symptom improvement as well as detailed information about post-operative nasal symptoms that should facilitate meaningful analysis.

## References

1. Stallman JS, Lobo JN, Som PM. The incidence of concha bullosa and its relationship to nasal septal deviation and paranasal sinus disease. AJNR Am J Neuroradiol. 2004;25(9):1613–8.
2. Bhattacharyya N. Ambulatory sinus and nasal surgery in the United States: demographics and perioperative outcomes. Laryngoscope. 2010;120:635–8.
3. NHS Digital Hospital Episode Statistics. Admitted Patient Care—England, 2019–2020. https://digital.nhs.uk/data-and-information/publications/statistical/hospital-admitted-patient-care-activity/2019-20 [Last accessed Mar 2024].
4. Adams W. On the treatment of broken-nose by forcible straightening and mechanical retentive apparatus. Br Med J. 1875;2(770):421–2.
5. van Egmond MMHT, Rovers MM, Hannink G, Hendriks CTM, van Heerbeek N. Septoplasty with or without concurrent turbinate surgery versus non-surgical management for nasal obstruction in adults with a deviated septum: a pragmatic, randomised controlled trial. Lancet. 2019;394:314–21.
6. Carrie S, O'Hara J, Fouweather T, Homer T, Rousseau N, Rooshenas L, Bray A, Stocken DD, Ternent L, Rennie K, Clark E, Waugh N, Steel AJ, Dooley J, Drinnan M, Hamilton D, Lloyd K, Oluboyede Y, Wilson C, Gardiner Q, Kara N, Khwaja S, Leong SC, Maini S, Morrison J, Nix P, Wilson JA, Teare MD. Clinical effectiveness of septoplasty versus medical management for nasal airways obstruction: multicentre, open label, randomised controlled trial. Br Med J. 2023;383:e075445.

7. Chiu T, Dunn JS. An anatomical study of the arteries of the anterior nasal septum. Otolaryngol Head Neck Surg. 2006;134(1):33–6.
8. Balai E, Jolly K, Bhamra N, Osborne MS, Barraclough J. The changing face of rhinology in the NHS: a study of septoplasty, septorhinoplasty and rhinoplasty hospital episode statistics. Ann R Coll Surg Engl. 2021;103(4):291–5.
9. Andrews P, Joseph J, Li CH, Nip L, Jacques T, Leung T. A UK survey of current ENT practice in the assessment of nasal patency. J Laryngol Otol. 2017;131(8):702–6.
10. Aziz T, Biron VL, Ansari K, Flores-Mir C. Measurement tools for the diagnosis of nasal septal deviation: a systematic review. J Otolaryngol Head Neck Surg. 2014;43(1):11.
11. Stewart MG, Witsell DL, Smith TL, Weaver EM, Yueh B, Hannley MT. Development and validation of the nasal obstruction symptom evaluation (NOSE) scale. Otolaryngol Head Neck Surg. 2004;130(2):157–63.
12. Buckland JR, Thomas S, Harries PG. Can the Sino-nasal outcome test (SNOT-22) be used as a reliable outcome measure for successful septal surgery? Clin Otolaryngol. 2003;28(1):43–7.
13. Williams SP, Hughes DM, Leong SC. An examination of the internal validity of the Sino-nasal outcome Test-22 in patients with septal deviation. Eur J Rhinol Allergy. 2023;6(2):49–54.
14. Huizing EH, de Groot JAM. Septal surgery. In: Functional reconstructive nasal surgery. 2nd ed. Stuttgart: Thieme; 2015. p. 158–91.
15. Green R, Carrie S. Septoplasty. In: Swift AC, Carrie S, de Souza C, editors. Contemporary rhinology: science and practice. Cham: Springer Nature; 2023. p. 555–67.
16. King ED, Ashley FL. The correction of the internally and externally deviated nose. Plast Reconstr Surg. 1952;10:116–20.
17. Gubisch W. The extracorporeal septum plasty: a technique to correct difficult nasal deformities. Plast Reconstr Surg. 1995;95(4):672–82.
18. Spataro EA, Saltychev M, Kandathil CK, Most SP. Outcomes of extracorporeal septoplasty and its modifications in treatment of severe L-strut septal deviation: a systematic review and meta-analysis. JAMA Facial Plast Surg. 2019;21(6):542–50.
19. Hwang PH, McLaughlin RB, Lanza DC, Kennedy DW. Endoscopic septoplasty: indications, technique, and results. Otolaryngol Head Neck Surg. 1999;120(5):678–82.
20. Kao R, Rabbani CC, Ting JY, Shipchandler TZ. In-office functional nasal surgery. Otolaryngol Clin N Am. 2019;52(3):485–95.
21. Local Anaesthetic Rhinological Surgery Guideline. ENT-UK / British Rhinological Society; 2022. https://www.entuk.org/_userfiles/pages/files/guidelines/local_anaesthetic_rhinological_surgery_lars_guideline.pdf [Last accessed Mar 2024].
22. Illum P. Septoplasty and compensatory inferior turbinate hypertrophy: long-term results after randomized turbinoplasty. Eur Arch Otorrinolaringol. 1997;254(Suppl 1):S89–92.
23. Siegel NS, Gliklich RE, Taghizadeh F, Chang Y. Outcomes of septoplasty. Otolaryngol Head Neck Surg. 2000;122(2):228–32.

# The Nasal Valves

# 11

Samy Elwany

**Key Points**

- Each nasal cavity has two valves, external and internal. The external nasal valve (ENV) is defined by the alar rim at the nasal vestibule. The internal nasal valve (INV) is the angle (10–15°) between the upper lateral cartilage and nasal septum.
- The nasal valve area includes the internal nasal valve, the inferior turbinate, and the area between them.
- Nasal valve dysfunction is an important cause of persistent nasal obstruction and can be static, dynamic, or a combination of the two.
- Nasal valve dysfunction may be iatrogenic, post-traumatic, or developmental.
- There are a variety of surgical interventions and a number of medical devices that are available for the treatment of nasal valve obstruction.
- Correct anatomical diagnosis is key to planning nasal valve surgery.

The primary function of the nose is to allow for proper airflow into the human body. We rely on the nose not only to permit adequate volumes of air to reach the lungs but also to humidify, warm, and filter the inspired air to optimize pulmonary gas exchange. The nose is also the organ of olfaction. When functional, it allows us to experience the joys of pleasurable scents and tastes and to beware potentially harmful environmental pathogens. Finally, being a central facial feature, the nose is a major determinant of facial aesthetics.

Nasal valves (Fig. 11.1) compromise results in significant disturbance of nasal air flow. Nasal valves dysfunction is frequently overlooked by rhinologist as well as

S. Elwany (✉)
Department of Otolaryngology, Alexandria University, Alexandria, Egypt
e-mail: samy.elwany@alexmed.edu.eg


S. Elwany (ed.), *Current Rhinology*,
https://doi.org/10.1007/978-3-031-70077-4_11

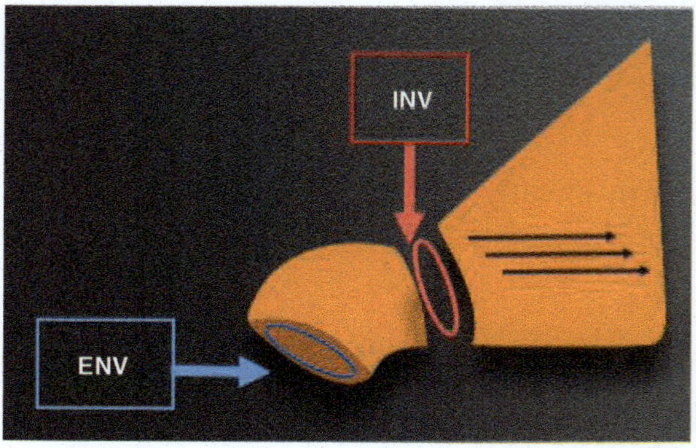


**Fig. 11.1** Internal (INV) and external (ENV) nasal valves

facial plastic surgeons. Understanding the anatomy, physiology, and pathophysiology of the nasal valve and nasal valve area is essential for restoration of the primary function of the nose and avoidance of iatrogenic dysfunction of the nasal valves [1, 2].

## 11.1 Applied Anatomy

The nasal valves are the narrowest portion of the nasal airway, accounting for over half of the total nasal airway resistance. The internal nasal valve is the primary regulator of nasal airflow [1].

**The external nasal valve (ENV)** is located in the nasal vestibule and is bounded by the alar rim laterally and columella medially and also includes the anterior naslspine and the soft tissues covering the nasal sill and floor of the vestibule of the nose (Fig. 11.2).

**The internal nasal valve (INV)** is the acute angle between by the nasal septum medially and the caudal edge of the upper lateral cartilage laterally. The **nasal valve area (NVA)** Also includes the head of the inferior turbinate infero-laterally and the floor of the nose inferiorly (Fig. 11.3).

The normal angle between the upper lateral cartilage and nasal septum is 10–15°, and the cross-sectional area of this region is approximately 55–64 mm squared (Fig. 11.4). A smaller cross-sectional area or a narrowed internal nasal valve angle (Fig. 11.5) will cause increased airway resistance and the sensation of nasal airway obstruction [3].

The external skin covering, the internal mucosal covering, the intrinsic cartilage, and the subcutaneous muscles all contribute to the strength and stability of both the internal and external nasal valves [4, 5].

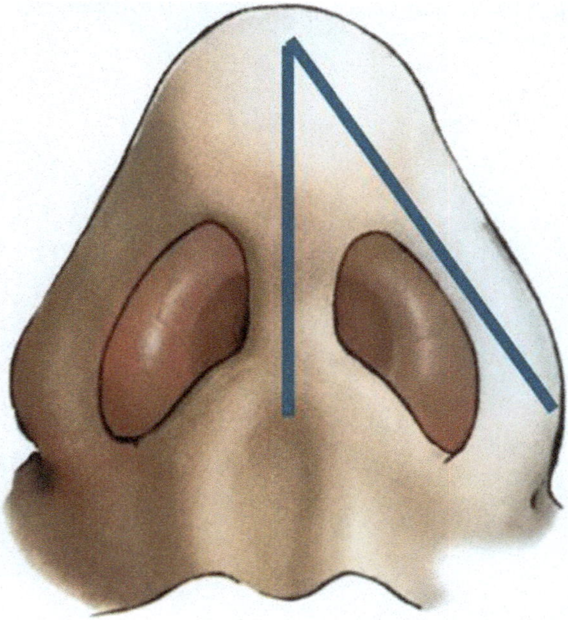

**Fig. 11.2** External nasal valve between the ala of the nose and the columella

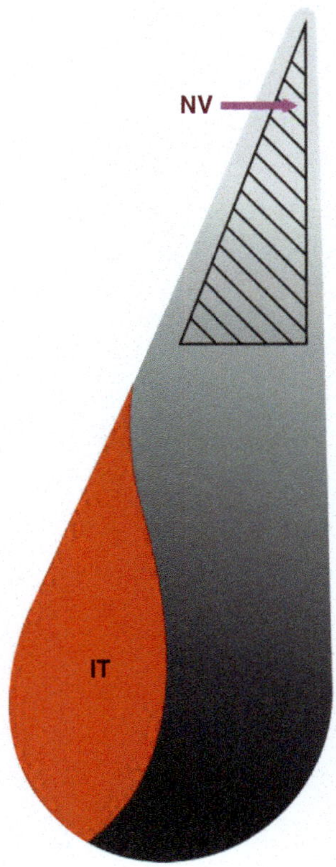


**Fig. 11.3** The internal nasal valve between the upper lateral cartilage and the septum. The nasal valve area includes also the anterior end of the inferior turbinate (IT) and opposing septum. NV: nasal valve

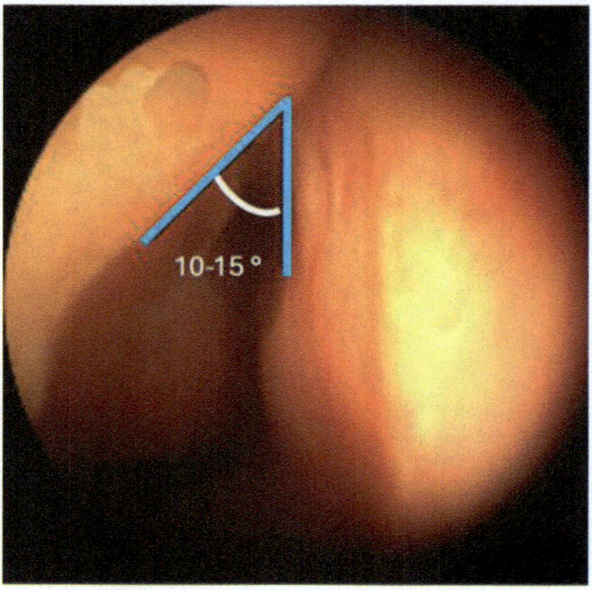


**Fig. 11.4** Normal internal nasal valve angle

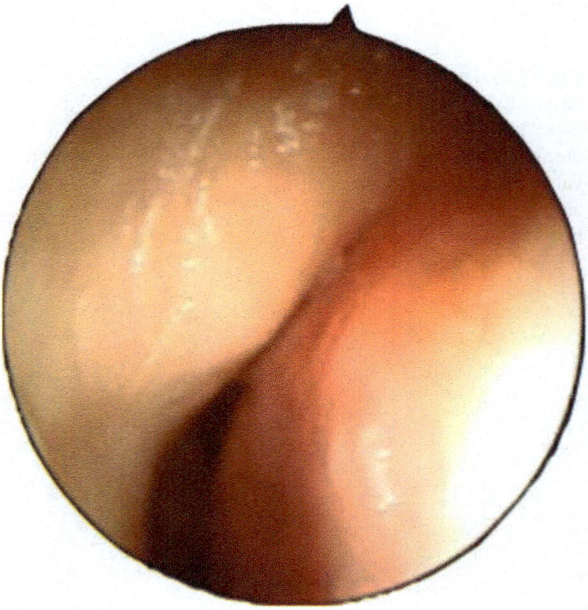

**Fig. 11.5** Narrowed or occluded internal nasal valve angle

## 11.2 Nasal Valve Assessment

When examining a patient with external nasal valve collapse, it is important to observe the behavior of the nasal valves during normal inspiration. The collapse of the nasal valve with forced inspiration is common and should be considered to avoid unnecessary surgery.

The traditional Cottle's maneuver (Fig. 11.6) is of little use in the assessment of the nasal valve dysfunction since almost all patients experience an improved airway when the test is performed.

The internal tenting test (Fig. 11.7) with a probe to hold open the nasal valve is a valuable tool in assessing the nasal valves and correcting the degree of collapse.

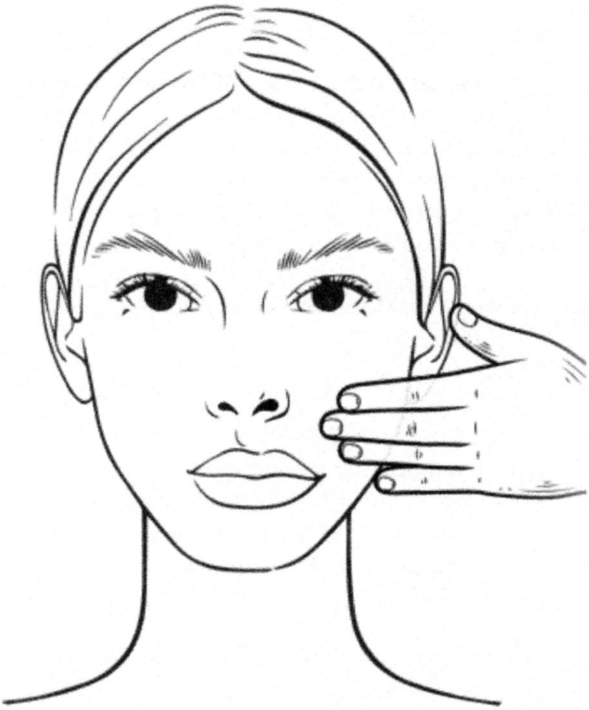

**Fig. 11.6** Cottle's Test

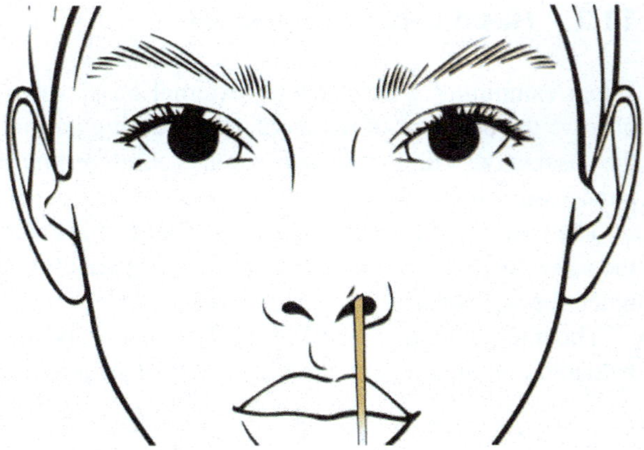

**Fig. 11.7** Internal tenting test

## 11.3 Types and Causes of Nasal Valve Dysfunction

Narrowing of the nasal valve causing nasal obstruction is either static due to anatomical narrowing, dynamic caused by inspiration, or a combination of the two. The dysfunction may be post-surgical, post-traumatic, or developmental. Iatrogenic dysfunction is the most frequent type.

A. **External nasal valve:**
   (a) **Static:**
      1. Dislocated caudal edge of the septal cartilage (Fig. 11.8).
      2. Alar scars.
      3. Over/under projected tip.
   (b) **Dynamic:** Alar rim collapse.

   Dynamic external nasal valve collapse occurs when the valve appears normal at rest, but upon inspiration through the nose, there is collapse of the alar rims (Fig. 11.9). It occurs due to weakness of the lower lateral cartilage and malposition of the lower lateral cartilage (as with vertically oriented lower lateral cartilages)

   In examining a patient with external valve collapse, it is best to simply observe the nose during quiet breathing and watch the nasal vestibule for narrowing of the alar rim on gentle nasal inspiration. The internal tenting test will help to identify the precise area of weakness and may further help demonstrate to the patient what may be achieved with surgical correction of the external nasal valve weakness.

B. **Internal nasal valve:**
   (a) **Static:**
      1. Septal deviation involving the dorsal part of the nasal septum.
      2. Scars and adhesions. Static internal valve dysfunction results from scarring of the medial seg, the upper lateral cartilage to the nasal following

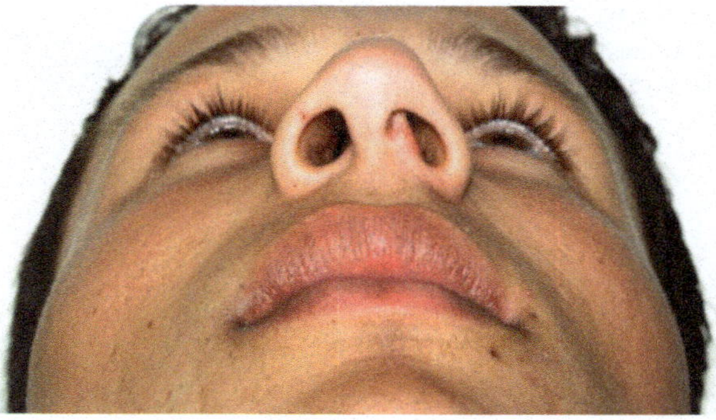

**Fig. 11.8** Caudal dislocation of the septum

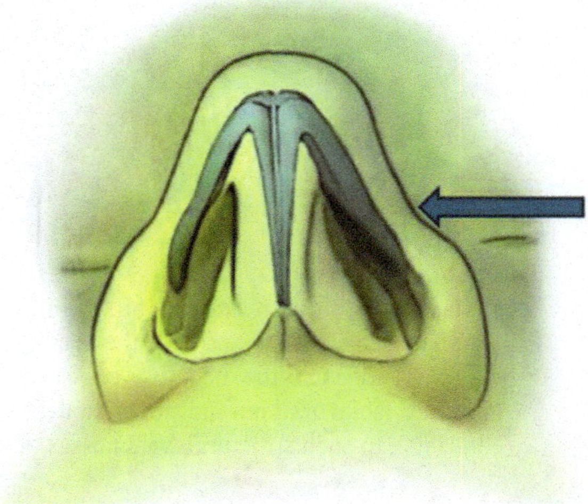

**Fig. 11.9** Alar collapse

the separation of those structures along with their intervening mucosa (Fig. 11.10).

3. Weakening of the lateral wall of the internal valve. Elevation of the skin-soft tissue envelope, damage to the nasal dilator muscles, and weakening of the mucosal support of the middle third cartilages contribute to a weakening of nasal valve support.
4. Iatrogenic narrowing (Inverted V). Classically, the inverted V deformity has been linked to the separation of the upper lateral cartilage from the overlying nasal bones during rhinoplasty. However, it may also be seen either in patients with internal nasal valve collapse who have never undergone previous rhinoplasty or in patients who have had a standard dorsal reduction rhinoplasty without disarticulation of the upper lateral cartilages from the nasal bones.

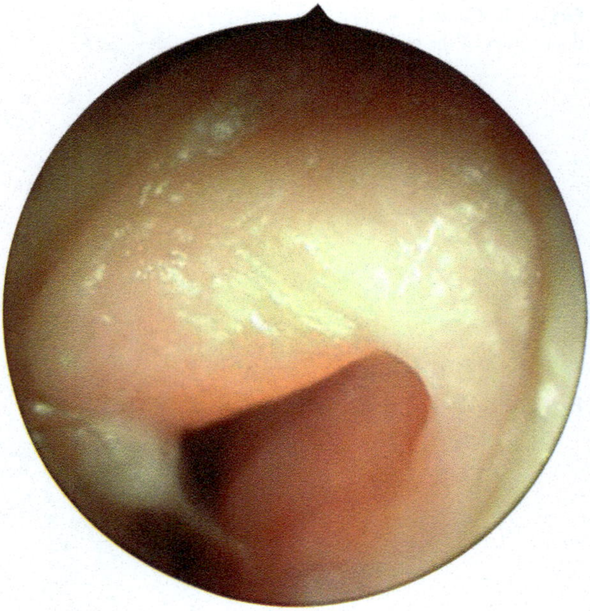

**Fig. 11.10** Scarring and adhesions of the internal nasal valve

(b) **Dynamic:**

Collapse/weakness of lateral wall. Thin, weak, detached, or absent upper lateral cartilages cannot provide the necessary strength along the nasal sidewall to withstand the negative pressures created by inspiratory nasal. Previous facial trauma and congenital or developmental factors may all contribute to such structural weaknesses of the nasal sidewall.

## 11.4 Management of Nasal Valve Dysfunction

Over the past 10–15 years, there has been an increased awareness of the nasal valve as a contributor to nasal airway obstruction, resulting in several innovations and scientific publications on the matter [6–10]. No single technique stands out as the "gold standard," as being able to solve all causes and types of nasal valve collapse. The overall goal of nasal valve surgery is to widen the existing nasal valve area and to strengthen the structural support elements that maintain a patent valve area at rest and which minimize dynamic collapse of the nose that results from the negative inspiratory forces of nasal breathing.

If the collapse is simply occurring at night, the use of some form of nasal dilator can suffice and is often all that is required for patients and are a safe alternative to potentially complex nasal surgery.

Correct anatomical localization of the site and cause of valve dysfunction is key if surgery is planned taking in consideration the possible poor correlation between clinical findings and the patient symptoms.

## 11.4.1 Surgical Treatment of the External Nasal Valve

### 11.4.1.1 The Lateral Crural J-Flap

Minor degrees of fibro-fatty collapse can be addressed using a lateral crural J-flap. This is essentially a procedure where a 'boomerang' area of internal nasal skin is excised and then the posterior part of the flap is dissected free from the fibrofatty tissue then advanced into the defect. This leads to tensioning the lateral part of the external valve [11].

### 11.4.1.2 Repositioning of the Lower Lateral Cartilages (LLCs)

Cephalic orientation of lower lateral cartilage causes weakening of the corresponding lateral wall of the external nasal valve. Mobilization and repositioning of the cartilages caudally can add support to the valve and reduce collapse [12].

### 11.4.1.3 Lateral Crural Strut Grafts

Lateral crural strut graft may be used to strengthen the lateral wall of the external valve. In many cases, this problem is caused by over resection if the LLC during rhinoplasty. These grafts are harvested from septal cartilage and are placed between the lateral crus and the underlying vestibular skin. The graft can be extended to rest on the bony pyriform aperture to increase support [13].

### 11.4.1.4 Alar Batten/Rim Grafts

Batten grafts are versatile grafts that may be used for both internal and external nasal valve collapse, depending on where they are positioned [14].

A marginal incision is made along the inferior margin of the lower lateral cartilage and a sharp scissor is used to dissect a pocket along the nasal rim to the alar-facial groove. A cartilage graft is harvested from either the septum or the conchal bowl and inserted into the pocket. The graft should extend from the alar-facial groove either to the dome or to the area just lateral to the soft tissue triangle in order to avoid a sharp edge being seen through the skin of the soft tissue triangle. If less support is needed, a smaller graft may be used which has been referred to as an alar rim graft.

Alar rim grafts are thin strips of cartilage placed in a subcutaneous pocke close to the alar margin. The main benefit of these grafts is usually aesthetic and if used alone they are usually insufficient to correct the collapse.

## 11.4.2 Surgical Treatment of the Internal Nasal Valve

### 11.4.2.1 Batten Grafts

These grafts are used in cases where an area of weakness is identified on the nasal sidewall in the region of the alar crease. The grafts are positioned over the point of maximum weakness, often opposite the scroll region [14].

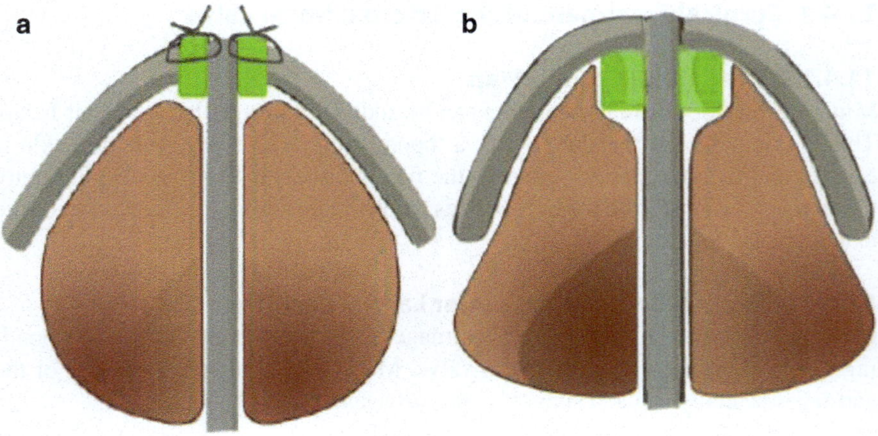


**Fig. 11.11** Spreader grafts. a: Correct placement. b: Incorrect placement

#### 11.4.2.2 Spreader Grafts

Spreader grafts are thin strips of cartilage positioned between the septum and the upper lateral cartilages ULCs to correct the narrowing of the mid-third of the nose and the internal nasal valve [15].

The grafts are usually harvested from the septum, with pinna used in cartilage-depleted patients. Spreader grafts are better inserted through an open approach to facilitate precise placement and fixation [16]. Occasionally, wider grafts may be required in which case a layering of multiple pieces of septal cartilage may be stacked together to provide adequate thickness. The grafts may be combined with suture suspension for greater, more stable widening of the internal valve angle (Figs. 11.11 and 11.12).

#### 11.4.2.3 Auto-Spreader Flaps

Auto-spreader flaps are a technique where the ULCs are folded medially to reconstruct the mid-third. This technique may be used to improve aesthetic mid-third width and improve internal valve function [17]. (Figs. 11.13).

#### 11.4.2.4 Other Surgical Procedures

Other techniques include correction of septal deformities (Fig. 11.14), columellar struts (Figs. 11.15 and 11.16), flaring sutures [18] to splay the ULC and open the internal nasal valve [8], Butterfly cartilage grafts [6], and generally from the pinna and bridging the ULC to widen the internal valve, and modified Z-plasty technique [19].

Flaring sutures may be used alone or in combination with various other techniques in order to maximize the widening of the valvular airway. A horizontal mattress stitch (is thrown from one upper lateral cartilage to the other and tied tightly over the nasal dorsum. As the suture is tied down, the upper lateral cartilages elevate outward, thereby widening the nasal valve angle and area [20].

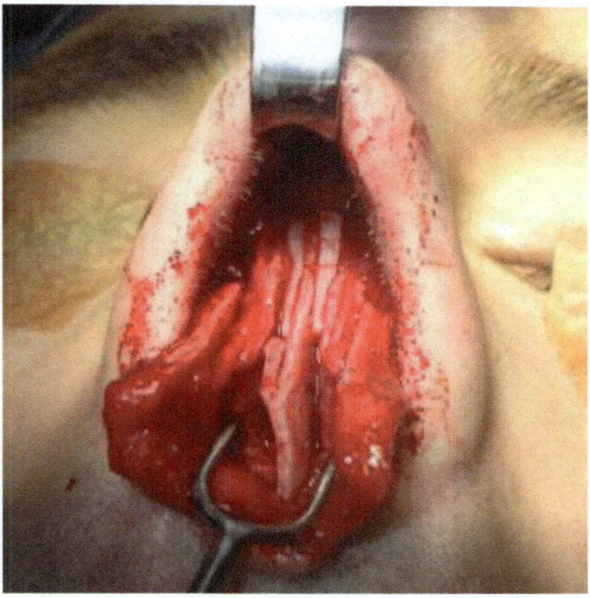

**Fig. 11.12** Spreader grafts in place between the septal cartilage and upper lateral cartilages

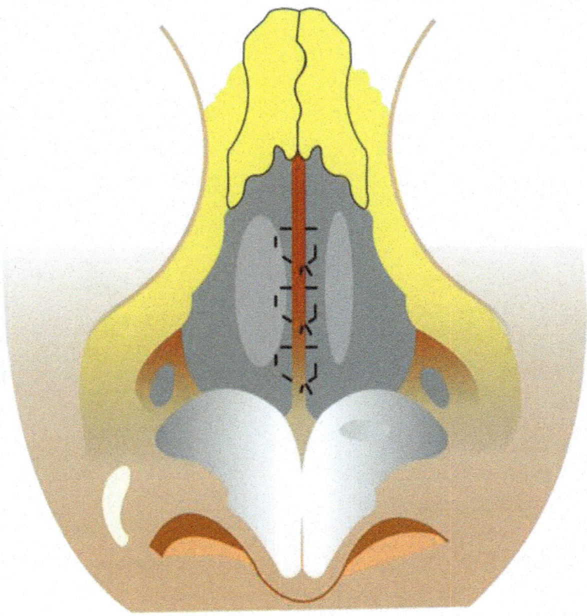

**Fig. 11.13** Autospreader flaps

The "butterfly graft" relies on the elastic nature of conchal cartilage to spring open the internal nasal valve. The graft may cause irregularities, especially in patients with thin skin. In this case, crushed cartilage grafts are used to camouflage the edges of the graft and create a smooth dorsal contour.

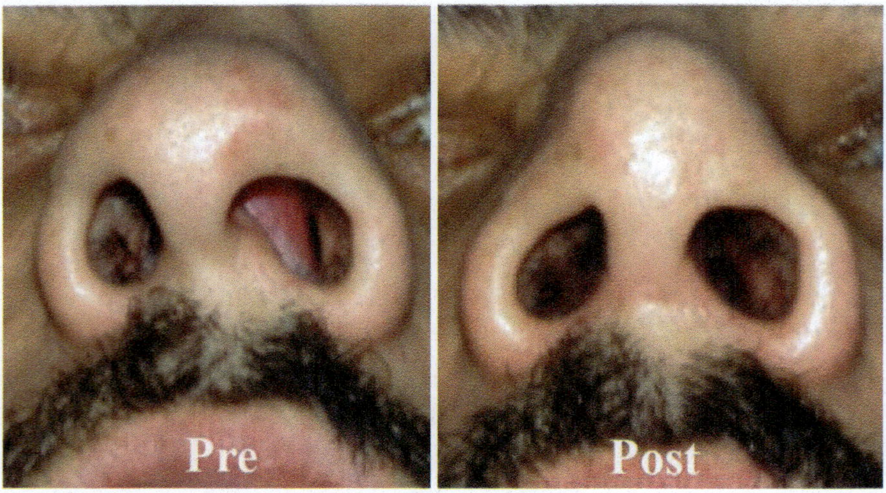


**Fig. 11.14** Correction of caudal dislocation of the nasal septum

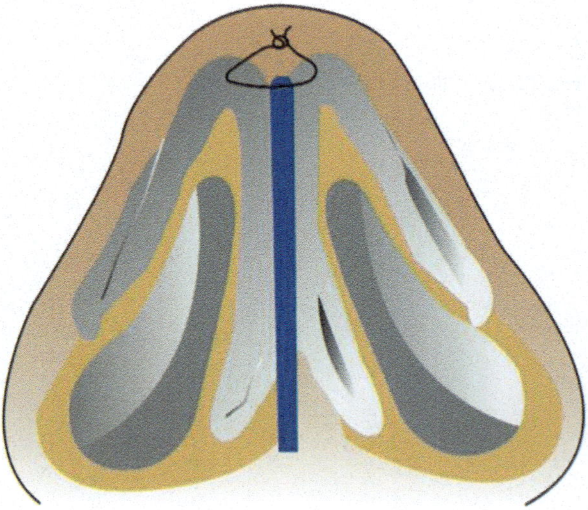

**Fig. 11.15** Columellar strut inserted medial the medial crura of the lower lateral cartilages

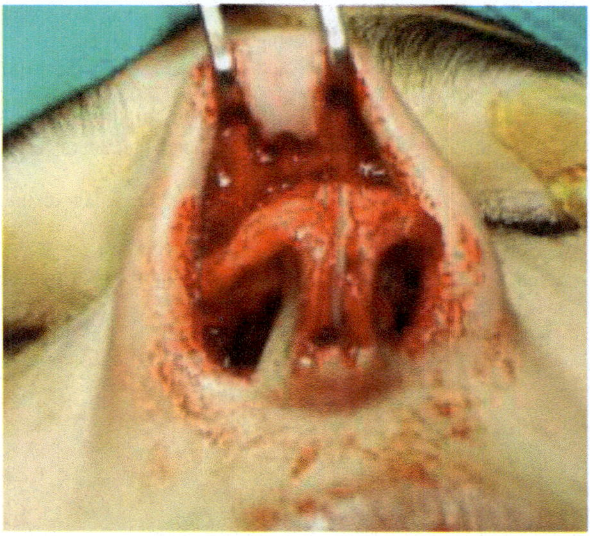

**Fig. 11.16** Columellar strut in place

## References


1. Elwany S, Thabet H. Obstruction of the nasal valve. J Laryngol Otol. 1996;110:221–4.
2. Constantian MB, Clardy RB. The relative importance of septal and nasal valvular surgery in correcting airway obstruction in primary and secondary rhinoplasty. Plast Reconstr Surg. 1996;98:38.
3. Bridger GP. Physiology of the nasal valve. Arch Otolaryngol. 1970;92:543–53.
4. Aksoy F, Veyseller B, Yildirim YS, Acar H, Demirhan H, Ozturan O. Role of nasal muscles in nasal valve collapse. Otolaryngol Head Neck Surg. 2010;142:365–9.
5. Vaiman M, Eviatar E, Segal S. Muscle-building therapy in treatment of nasal valve collapse. Rhinology. 2004;42:145–52.
6. Clark JM, Cook TA. The "butterfly" graft in functional secondary rhinoplasty. Laryngoscope. 2002;112:1917–25.
7. Akcam T, Friedman O, Cook TA. The effect on snoring of structural nasal valve dilatation with a butterfly graft. Arch Otolaryngol Head Neck Surg. 2004;130:1313–8.
8. Gassner HG, Friedman O, Sherris DA, Kern EB. An alternative method of middle vault reconstruction. Arch Facial Plast Surg. 2006;8:432–5.
9. Mendelsohn MS, Golchin K. Alar expansion and reinforcement: a new technique to manage nasal valve collapse. Arch Facial Plast Surg. 2006;8:293–9.
10. Byrd HS, Meade RA, Gonyon DLJ. Using the autospreader flap in primary rhinoplasty. Plast Reconstr Surg. 2007;119:1897–902.
11. O'Halloran LR. The lateral crural J-flap repair of nasal valve collapse. Otolaryngol Head Neck Surg. 2003;128:640–9.
12. Hamra ST. Repositioning the lateral alar crus. Plast Reconstr Surg. 1993;92:1244–53.
13. Gunter JP, Friedman RM. Lateral crural strut graft: technique and clinical applications in rhinoplasty. Plast Reconstr Surg. 1997;99:943–5.
14. Toriumi DM, Josen J, Weinberger M, Tardy MEJ. Use of alar batten grafts for correction of nasal valve collapse. Arch Otolaryngol Head Neck Surg. 1997;123:802–8.

15. Teymoortash A, Fasunla JA, Sazgar AA. The value of spreader grafts in rhinoplasty: a critical review. Eur Arch Otorrinolaringol. 2012;269:1411–6.
16. Sheen JH. Spreader graft: a method of reconstructing the roof of the middle nasal vault following rhinoplasty. Plast Reconstr Surg. 1984;73:230–9.
17. Hussein WK, Elwany S, Montaser M. Modified autospreader flap for nasal valve support: utilizing the spring effect of the upper lateral cartilage. Eur Arch Otorrinolaringol. 2015;272:497–504.
18. Park SS. The flaring suture to augment the repair of the dysfunctional nasal valve. Plast Reconstr Surg. 1998;101:1120–2.
19. Varadharajan K, Choudhury N, Saleh HA. Modified Z-plasty of the internal nasal valve-to treat mechanical nasal obstruction: how we do it. Clin Otolaryngol. 2019;44:1203–4.
20. Ismail A, Hussein W, Elwany S. Combining spreader grafts with suture suspension for management of narrow internal nasal valve angles. Turk Arch Otorhinolaryngol. 2018;56:25–9.

# Nasal Septal Perforation 12

Abdulmalik Alkhodair, Nasser Marran, Ahmad Alroqi, and Abdulaziz AlQahtani

**Key Points**

- Nasal septal perforation (NSP) results from the necrosis of nasal septum layers, impairs nasal airflow, and may produce symptoms.
- For a successful repair, it is essential to comprehend the anatomy of the septum and its arterial supply.
- The etiology of NSPs is varied and includes trauma, inflammatory, infectious, drug-induced, and neoplastic causes.
- Nasal endoscopy, imaging, and laboratory testing can help identifying the underlying cause.
- Medical treatment, which is frequently adequate in asymptomatic cases, depends on nasal emollients and could involve silicone septal buttons.
- Surgical success rates vary depending on the location and size of the perforation, patient's condition as well as the surgical technique.
- Prior to surgery, patient selection is an important procedure that needs to be thought through. Various surgical procedures, such as endonasal approaches, endoscopic techniques, and external rhinoplasty, provide a range of surgical techniques.

A. Alkhodair
Department of Otolaryngology-Head & Neck Surgery, King Saud Medical City, First Health Cluster, Riyadh, Saudi Arabia

N. Marran
Department of Otolaryngology Head and Neck Surgery, King Faisal Specialist Hospital and Research Center, Riyadh, Saudi Arabia

A. Alroqi
Department of Otolaryngology-Head and Neck Surgery, College of Medicine, King Saud University, Riyadh, Saudi Arabia

A. AlQahtani (✉)
Department of Otolaryngology-Head & Neck Surgery, King Fahad Medical City, Second Health Cluster, Riyadh, Saudi Arabia

Faculty of Medicine, Alfaisal University, Riyadh, Saudi Arabia


S. Elwany (ed.), *Current Rhinology*,
https://doi.org/10.1007/978-3-031-70077-4_12

## 12.1 Introduction

Nasal septal perforations (NSPs) are essentially full-thickness defects in the nasal septum that arise from necrosis affecting various layers like mucoperichondrium, mucoperiosteum, cartilage, and/or bone. (Fig. 12.1) These perforations result in a communication between the two nasal cavities, disrupting the normal laminar airflow inside the nose. This disruption leads to turbulent air patterns which can cause damage to the septal respiratory epithelium and impair overall nasal function [1–3].

The presentation of peripherally located septal perforation differs significantly from central septal perforation. An example of peripheral perforation includes septectomy associated with Draf III frontal sinus surgery and posterior septectomy in transsellar and expanded endoscopic transnasal skull base surgeries. Unlike anterior septal perforations, peripherally located perforations are typically asymptomatic.

NSPs can manifest a range of symptoms based on their location. Superior and posterior NSPs often present asymptomatically, differing in presentation and etiology from anterior perforations. In contrast, anterior NSPs are more likely to cause noticeable symptoms. These include nosebleeds (reported in 58% of cases), crusting (43%), nasal blockage (39%), facial pain (17%), and whistling sounds (15%). The severity of symptoms varies, ranging from being completely asymptomatic to causing significant issues such as severe epistaxis, nasal cosmetic deformities, crust formation, and nasal obstruction [2, 4].

The influence of nasal septal perforation (NSP) on sleep parameters remains under-explored in medical literature. However, a study suggests that NSP might be a contributing factor to sleep apnea, especially when sleeping in the supine position. Furthermore, treatment for NSP shows a potential positive impact on sleep-disordered breathing, though this effect has not reached statistical significance [5].

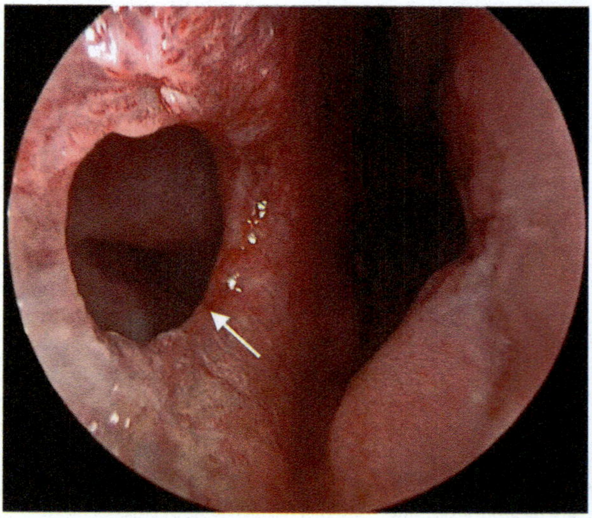

**Fig. 12.1** Endoscopic view of the left nasal cavity demonstrates the nasal septal perforation (white arrow)

## 12.2 Brief Overview of Relevant Nasal Anatomy

### 12.2.1 Nasal Septum

The nasal septum, a key structural component of the nose, consists of a small anterior membranous section, cartilage, and several bones, including the vomer, the bony crests of the maxilla and palatine bones, and the ethmoid's perpendicular plate (Fig. 12.2). Its cartilaginous part is made up of the quadrilateral cartilage, which thickens from 3–4 mm at its midpoint to 4–8 mm anteroinferiorly. The anterior septal angle, a crucial structural element, is created where the upper margin of the cartilage expands at its junction with the upper lateral cartilages, above the domes of the lower lateral cartilages. This cartilage is firmly connected to the nasal bones, ethmoid's perpendicular plate, and the vomer through collagenous fibers [6–8].

The perpendicular plate, forming the superior and anterior bony portion of the septum, extends above to the cribriform plate and crista galli and is closely associated with parts of the nasal bones. The vomer, constituting the posterior and inferior part of the septum, connects with the sphenoid's rostrum through its alae, creating the vomerovaginal canals for the pharyngeal branches of the maxillary artery. It is

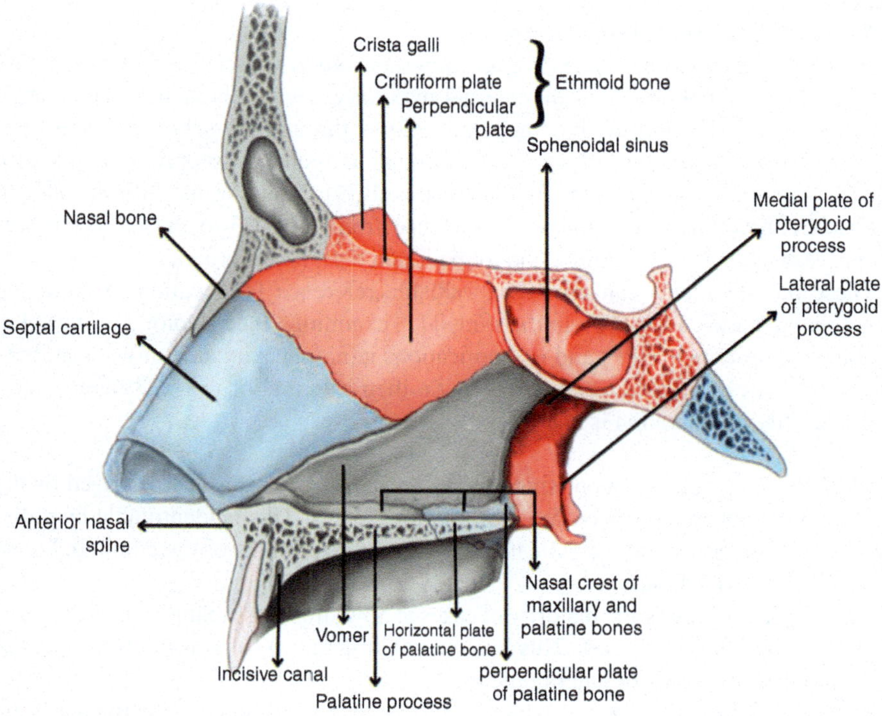


**Fig. 12.2** Schematic drawing of a sagittal view of the nasal septum with cartilaginous/bony structures

not uncommon for the sphenoid sinus to extend into the vomer and pneumatize it [6, 7].

The vomer's inferior border connects with the nasal crest made by the maxillae and palatine bones, while its anterior border articulates with the perpendicular plate and quadrilateral cartilage. Its posterior edge forms the septum's posterior free edge. Serving as the primary support structure for the external nose, the nasal septum not only facilitates nasal cavity ventilation but also contributes to the nose's structural integrity and esthetic appearance [7, 8].

### 12.2.2 Blood Supply

The blood supply to the nasal septum is a complex network provided by both the external and internal carotid arteries. The external carotid artery branches into the maxillary and facial arteries, which play a crucial role in supplying blood to the nose. Additionally, the internal carotid artery, through its ophthalmic artery branch, contributes significantly to the nasal septum's blood supply. This intricate vascular system ensures adequate and consistent blood flow to various parts of the nasal septum (Figs. 12.3 and 12.4). Below is a list of important arteries that supply the nasal septum:

#### 12.2.2.1 Sphenopalatine Artery

The sphenopalatine artery (SPA), an important blood vessel for the nasal cavity mucosa, is the end-artery of the internal maxillary artery, a branch of the external carotid artery. Exiting the pterygopalatine fossa through the sphenopalatine foramen to enter the nasal cavity, the SPA, through its branches, supplies the posterior nasal septum and most of the lateral nasal wall [9]. Studying the SPF distance to nose's anterior part. The measured distance from the SPF to the nasal sill was approximately 59.4 ± 4.2 mm, and to the limen nasi, it was around 49.1 ± 3.7 mm. These measurements can provide a valuable reference for locating the foramen within the nasal cavity [10]. In the study [11] examining the osteology of the sphenopalatine foramen (SPF) and its implications in nasal cavity anatomy, the authors proposed a classification system based on their observations of 238 lateral nasal walls. This classification is as follows:

Class I: This category, comprising 35% of the studied cases, is characterized by the SPF opening exclusively into the superior meatus. This is identifiable by a distinctive notch or foramen situated in the middle turbinate or the ethmoidal crest of the palatine bone.

Class II: Representing the majority of cases at 56%, this class features the SPF spanning the ethmoidal crest. This anatomical structure results in the SPF opening into both the superior and middle meati.

Class III: The least common, observed in 9% of cases, this class is distinguished by the presence of two separate SPF openings, one each into the superior and middle meati.

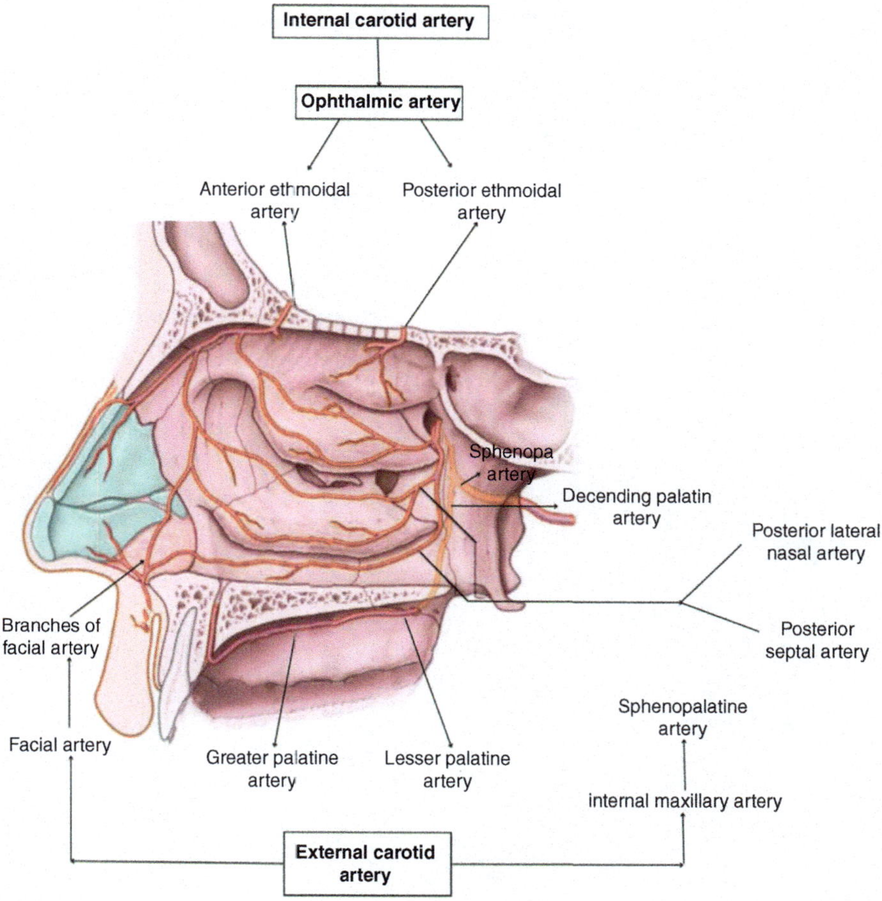


**Fig. 12.3** Schematic drawing of a sagittal view of the lateral nasal wall showing the blood supply derived from both internal and external carotid arteries

In surgical procedures, the crista ethmoidalis, a small crest originating from the palatine bone located anterior to the sphenopalatine artery (SPA), serves as a critical anatomical landmark [12]. In a study conducted by Bolger et al. [13]., which involved dissections of 22 cadavers, the proximity of the crista ethmoidalis to the SPA was consistently observed. In all 22 dissections, the artery was found to be closely associated with the crista ethmoidalis. Specifically, in 21 of these cases, the SPA was situated posteriorly, and in one case, it was positioned 3 mm inferior to the crista ethmoidalis.

It primarily bifurcates into the posterior septal artery (PSA) and the posterior-lateral nasal artery (PLNA), which supply the septum and lateral wall, respectively. The posterior septal artery (PSA) is detailed as traversing the sphenoid rostrum to the posterior septum and is divided into three segments: pterygopalatine, sphenoidal, and septal. The PSA, after emerging from the sphenopalatine foramen (SPF),

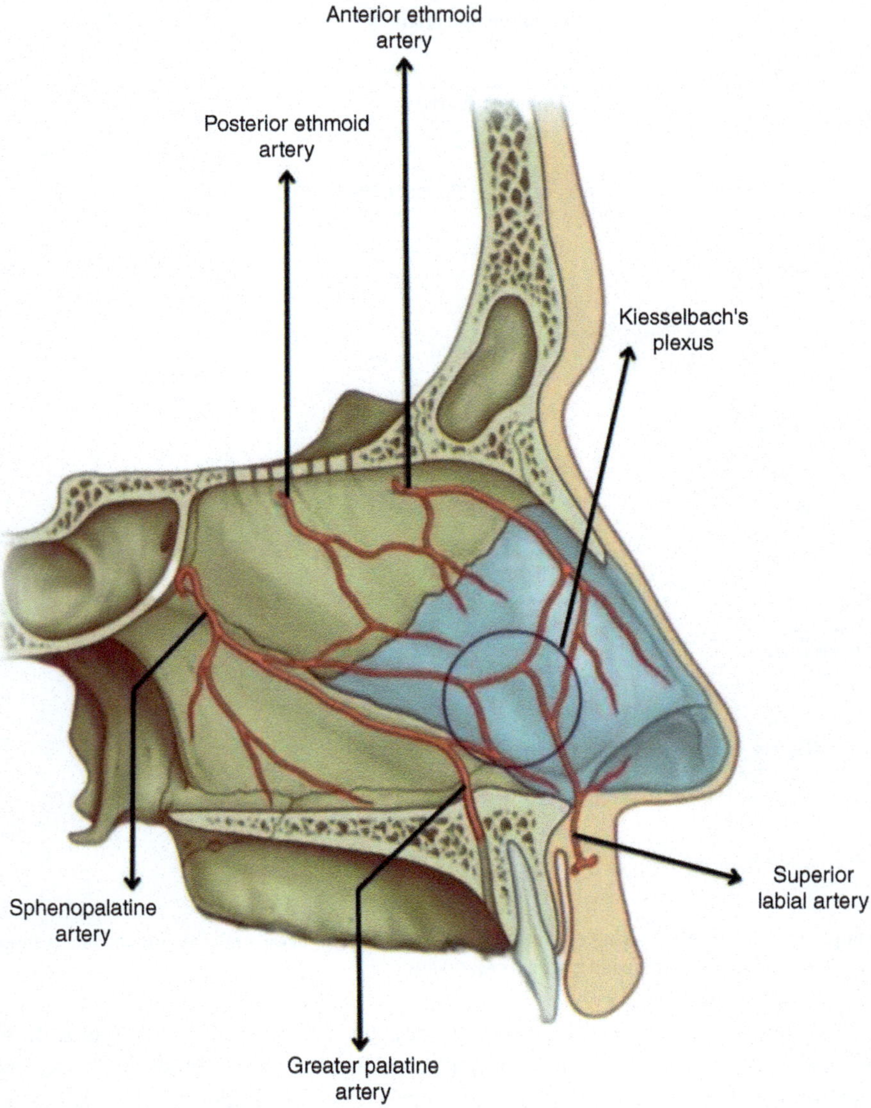


**Fig. 12.4** Schematic drawing of a sagittal view of the nasal septum showing the blood supply

bifurcates near the sphenoid rostrum into two branches that extend onto the septum. These branches can anastomose or split, with connections to the anterior ethmoidal artery, superior labial artery at Kiesselbach's plexus, posterior ethmoidal artery, and the greater palatine artery at the incisive canal. The posterior-lateral nasal artery (PLNA) originates separately from the sphenopalatine foramen (SPF), branching into the inferior turbinate artery (ITA) and the middle turbinate artery (MTA) to supply the turbinates. Occasionally, the MTA is observed as a third distinct artery emerging from the SPF. Additionally, the anterior lateral nasal wall receives blood supply from the lateral branch of the anterior ethmoidal artery (AEA) and the anterior lateral nasal artery (ALNA), a branch of the facial artery. These two arteries form an anastomosis near the axilla of the inferior turbinate [14].

#### 12.2.2.2 Greater Palatine Artery

The descending palatine artery (DPA), branching from the internal maxillary artery, divides into the lesser and greater palatine arteries. The greater palatine artery exits the greater palatine foramen to supply the hard palate and related structures, while also connecting with the sphenopalatine artery's terminal branch. The DPA presents three variations: type I as a singular artery, type II consisting of the greater and lesser palatine arteries (most common), and the less common type III with more than two arteries, occasionally extending through the lateral wing of the pterygoid process [15].

#### 12.2.2.3 Anterior and Posterior Ethmoid Arteries

The anterior ethmoid artery (AEA), deriving from the ophthalmic artery connected to the internal carotid artery, supplies blood to the ethmoid and frontal sinuses, anterior nasal septum, and meninges. It follows a course from posterior-lateral to anterior-medial along the skull base. The AEA may sometimes be located slightly below the skull base. A key surgical reference point for the AEA is the anterior lacrimal crest, with the artery positioned about 22–25 mm behind it. The posterior ethmoid artery (PEA), another ophthalmic artery branch, provides blood to the posterior ethmoids and septum. It runs in a bony canal near the ethmoid roof, just anterior to the sphenoid sinus [16, 17].

A study on the biomechanical strength of the nasal septal lining involved dissecting and testing different layers from human cadaver specimens. It compared the tensile strength of mucosa-only, perichondrium-only, and composite specimens. Findings indicated that the perichondrium layer possessed the greatest biomechanical strength, emphasizing its importance in septal surgeries. Flaps containing both mucosa and perichondrium were shown to be stronger than those with individual layers. This highlights the benefit of preserving the perichondrial layer to strengthen the septal flap and prevent nasal septal perforation. The measured tensile strengths were 662 g for mucosa, 1370 g for perichondrium, and 2340 g for the composite layer. The mechanical testing system measured the highest tensile force in grams for each specimen, indicating the force required to cause failure. Once the specimen failed and tension was lost, the force value immediately dropped to zero. This measurement was crucial in determining the strength of each nasal septal lining sample [18].

Comprehending the anatomy of the anterior ethmoidal artery is crucial for flap harvesting in septal perforation repair, and factors like active smoking, a history of intranasal drug use, and diabetes mellitus are significantly linked to surgical failure, underscoring their importance in preoperative planning and patient counseling [19].

## 12.3 Epidemiology

The incidence of nasal septal perforation is variable according to the underlying etiology. Post-septoplasty, the incidence of nasal septal perforation is observed to be between 1.6% and 6.7%. Higher rates of nasal septal perforation are observed in septoplasty cases when combined with inferior turbinate reduction. These perforations may result from various factors, such as the devascularization of septal mucosa, excessive use of electrocautery during surgery causing mucosal damage, and the alignment of bilateral mucosal tears post-cartilage resection. Tight sutures leading to ischemia and local trauma from intranasal steroid or saline sprays can also contribute to septal perforations [20].

An animal study has determined that prolonged nasal splint placement in rabbits is associated with increased inflammation. The study found that extended use of nasal splints led to histopathological changes in the nasal mucosa, consequently increasing the risk of septal perforation. Notably, splint placement for a duration of 15 days was linked to a greater likelihood of septal perforation compared to shorter usage periods [21].

Another common cause of NSP is drug abuse. A study conducted in an urban hospital in New York, USA, focused on determining the prevalence of NSP in this setting. The study found that 2.05% of CT imaging cases showed evidence of NSP, with the most common risk factor being a history of drug abuse, particularly cocaine use [22].

Other than septoplasty as a cause of NSP, pituitary surgeries are rising and accessed trans nasally with the advances in instruments, visualization, and understanding of skull base anatomy. In a study comparing endoscopic and microscopic approaches for transsphenoidal hypophyseal surgery, Group 1 (microscopic) experienced a higher incidence of nasal septal perforations (41.9%) compared to Group 2 (endoscopic), predominantly in the middle septum. While one patient in Group 1 developed a pan-septal perforation leading to saddle nose deformity, Group 2 had perforations in the posterior septum as part of the surgical technique, with no complications in the anterior and middle septum. The difference in septal perforation rates between the two groups was statistically significant, particularly for middle septal perforations [23].

Nasal complications, including nasal septum perforation (0.8%), were observed following endonasal transsphenoidal resection of pituitary neoplasms, indicating that nasal septum perforation is a potential postoperative complication. To minimize this risk, it is essential to conduct surgeries with precision and care, focusing on minimizing mucosal injury, protecting the nasal cavity, and supporting tissue regeneration to prevent nasal adhesion and facilitate swift healing [24].

In a five-year retrospective case-control study, 145 patients undergoing endoscopic resection of pituitary tumors or Rathke's cleft cysts were assessed to compare the Hemi-T approach with traditional skull base reconstruction methods. Of these, the Hemi-T technique was applied in 105 cases, and the traditional method, similar to Rivera-Serrano's "rescue flap" with superior and posterior incisions in the nasoseptal flap, was used in the remaining cases. The study noted a significant difference in septal perforation rates: 4.9% (5 out of 102 cases) in the Hemi-T group versus 16.2% (6 out of 37 cases) in the traditional group ($p = 0.029$) [25, 26].

The Hemi-T approach typically involves a Killian incision on the left side for submucoperichondrial/mucoperiosteal dissection up to the sphenoid rostrum. This method includes removing the bony septum for a binasal approach and creating a mucoperiosteal flap for reconstruction, allowing for bimanual surgery with minimal dissection. Postoperatively, the right posterior septum mucosal flap covers the surgical area. For larger defects, a full-length nasoseptal flap is harvested from the left side, repositioned, and sutured back after removing the sphenoid floor's mucosa [27].

While the transseptal transsphenoidal approach is another described method for accessing pituitary tumors, the associated risk of nasal septal perforation (NSP) with this technique remains unclear.

In a study examining 111 cases of nasoseptal flaps used for skull base reconstruction, it was found that anterior septal perforations were the most common complication, accounting for 14.4% of cases and typically manifesting within 3 months following the surgery. Most of these perforations occurred in primary procedures where patients had not undergone previous septoplasty. The suspected cause of these perforations is a decreased vascular supply to the contralateral septal mucosa, potentially leading to ischemic conditions and resulting in mucosal and cartilaginous necrosis. To reduce the risk of perforations, employing free mucosal grafts or biomaterials to cover the septal donor site has been proposed as an effective preventive measure. This method could further lower the rate of septal perforations by promoting better protection and healing at the donor site [28].

Pediatric nasal septal perforations, while less common and less reported than in adults, are often associated with complications from nasal foreign bodies like batteries. Surgical considerations for these perforations in children include the severity of symptoms, the cause of the perforation, existing comorbidities, and the potential impact on nasal growth. The challenges in pediatric septal repair involve determining the optimal age for surgery and selecting the most effective surgical technique [29–32].

Cullen et al. successfully developed and validated the NOSE-Perf scale, a reliable and efficient instrument for evaluating symptoms in nasal septal perforation (NSP) patients, adept at differentiating between NSP, nasal obstruction, and absence of rhinologic complaints; however, further validation in various languages is necessary for its broader applicability [33].

A study used two main tools to measure the success of nasal septum perforation repair. Subjective outcomes were assessed using the Nasal Obstruction Symptom Evaluation (NOSE) instrument, which evaluated patients' perceptions of nasal obstruction before and after surgery. Objective outcomes were measured using active anterior rhinomanometry, a technique that quantitatively assesses nasal airway resistance. The findings indicated complete closure of nasal septal perforations in all patients, significant improvement in NOSE scores, and changes in nasal airway resistance, demonstrating both anatomical and physiological restoration postoperatively [34].

## 12.4 Pathophysiology

Numerical simulations reveal that while anterior caudal septal perforations disrupt the temperature and humidity of inhaled air, anterior cranial and posterior caudal perforations have minor effects on air conditioning, and septal perforations can lead to reduced humidity and heating of the air [35]. Nasal bleeding and pain may be related to high pressure and shear at the perforation site [36].

Patients with symptoms exhibited significantly elevated wall shear stress (WSS) and heat flux, particularly around the posterior margin of the perforation, with WSS being the shear force per unit surface area of nasal mucosa, indicative of airflow-mucosa interactions. A WSS threshold of 0.72 Pa effectively distinguishes between asymptomatic and symptomatic NSP with 87% sensitivity and 100% specificity. High WSS can cause nasal crusting, dryness, or pain, while heat flux, representing the heat transfer per unit mucosal surface area during restful breathing, along with WSS, serves as indicators of the extent of airflow-mucosa interactions [37].

The strategy of enlarging the nasal septum, especially beyond the middle turbinate, is based on Bernoulli's principle, aiming to reduce the high-velocity airflow and resultant turbulence through large symptomatic perforations. This technique, effective for patients with limited reconstructive options, lowers airflow velocity, thereby diminishing symptoms like whistling, mucosal drying, crusting, and bleeding at the perforation edges [38].

Bing et al.'s study [39] concluded that airflow communication in the upper nasal cavity minimally impacts ventilation, while disruptions in airflow distribution occur in the lower part, necessitating repair procedures, especially for nasal septal perforation which not only causes symptoms but also increases wall shear stress around the communication site, in contrast to the Draf III procedure where this stress is lower. Complementarily, Daniel et al.'s research [40] highlighted the significant role of perforation size and position, demonstrating that anterior and posterior perforations more substantially affect nasal airflow compared to superior ones. Moreover, the alterations in wall shear stress and airflow velocity at the perforation site are intensified with increased size of anterior perforations or decreased size of posterior ones, underscoring the direct correlation between the perforation's size and location and its impact on nasal airflow dynamics.

Following the repair of septal perforation, crossflows disappeared and stream lines appeared in the olfactory cleft area and high-shear stress areas decreased [41]. Even if complete closure was not achieved, the modification of size and position of the septal perforation (SP) through surgical intervention can effectively mitigate symptoms. In daily clinical practice, it is commonly observed that patient symptoms improve postoperatively, even if the perforation is not fully closed, as long as it is reduced in size and relocated to a more cranial and posterior position [42].

In a study involving 10 patients with nasal septal perforation (NSP), five underwent posterior septectomy and five received conventional flap or button repair. Computational fluid dynamics (CFD), based on CT scans, was used to simulate nasal aerodynamics and compare surgical outcomes and airflow features between the two treatments. Patients treated with posterior septectomy had larger perforations and higher airflow rates across the perforation site. This procedure significantly reduced wall shear stress along the posterior margin. The study concluded that NSP causes flow disturbance and increased wall shear stress, contributing to symptoms. The effectiveness of posterior septectomy as a treatment option may be due to the removal of high-stress points along the posterior margin [43].

Post-septoplasty, these perforations frequently occur due to direct trauma during the elevation of mucosal flaps, resulting in tears on opposing sides. Moreover, overly tight suturing that causes ischemia and necrosis in nearby tissues, as well as infections, are also known to be contributing factors to such perforations [44]. Another important factor is the development of septal hematoma that leads to the detachment of the mucoperichondrium from the underlying quadrangular cartilage. This separation disrupts the blood supply, causing ischemia and eventually the necrosis of the cartilage tissue, which in turn can lead to the formation of a perforation. A frequent surgical pitfall during nasal septal procedures involves mistakenly dissecting in a supraperichondrial and submucosal plane. This action often results in removing the perichondrium or periosteum along with the cartilage and bone, leaving only mucosal flaps in contact with each other. Flaps composed solely of mucosa, lacking the reinforcement and strength provided by the perichondrial layer, may increase the risk of immediate or delayed septal perforation [18].

Epistaxis, a common emergency, is often treated with silver nitrate; a study on nasal septum tissue showed that the depth and intensity of coagulative necrosis from silver nitrate application depend more on contact time than concentration, recommending a maximum of 20 s for adults and 10 s for children using a 75% solution [45].

Nasal septal perforation (NSP) progresses through four stages: initial local inflammation with mucosal damage and swelling, followed by reduced blood flow and inflammation causing ischemia and loss of mucosal layers, then irregular healing leading to cartilage necrosis, and finally, the development of fragile atrophic epithelium around the perforation, susceptible to bleeding and crusting. Poor hygiene can exacerbate NSP, causing further enlargement, infections, and continuous low-grade perichondritis [1, 2].

Squamous cell carcinoma arising from nasal septal perforations (NSP) is an uncommon occurrence, indicating that NSPs do not significantly increase the risk of developing such malignancies. This rarity underscores the importance of considering other potential causes in the diagnosis and treatment of NSPs [46].

Certain systemic medications can put patients at risk of NSP. The use of bevacizumab, a humanized monoclonal antibody targeting vascular endothelial growth factor (VEGF) that inhibits angiogenesis, has been linked to nasal septum perforation. A case report highlighted a 34-year-old woman with metastatic breast cancer who developed nasal septum perforation during treatment with paclitaxel and bevacizumab. Bevacizumab's mechanism, which prevents VEGF from binding to its receptors and thereby inhibits new blood vessel formation, has also been associated with increased wound healing complications, particularly in patients undergoing major surgery. In this patient's case, the impaired angiogenesis-dependent wound healing due to anti-VEGF therapy likely caused a cycle of mucosal irritation, itching, and nonhealing erosions in the nasal septum, ultimately leading to its perforation. This vulnerability of the nasal septum to perforation is exacerbated when mucosal irritation or mechanical trauma exposes the underlying avascular cartilage [47, 48].

In a study on bevacizumab's intranasal use for hereditary hemorrhagic telangiectasia-associated epistaxis, it was administered to 58 patients either as a submucosal injection or as a spray. Additional KTP laser treatment was used in some cases. Notably, 8.6% of patients developed septal perforations, particularly when both bevacizumab and laser were applied to the cartilaginous septum. After modifying treatment protocols to avoid the cartilaginous septum, no new perforations were reported, suggesting bevacizumab is a safe treatment when applied with caution [49].

The pathogenesis of cocaine-induced midline destructive lesions (CIMDL) involves inflammatory, infective, proapoptotic, and autoimmune mechanisms. Nasal septal perforation, a common manifestation of CIMDL, highlights its rarity among cocaine users. Treatment for CIMDL is challenging, as immunosuppressive therapy is ineffective. The only effective intervention is complete abstinence from cocaine use, which is necessary to halt disease progression and enable successful surgical reconstruction [50].

A study focused on 25 patients with untreated symptomatic nasal septal perforations to investigate microbial flora. Swabs were collected around the perforations for culture analysis and compared with a healthy control group. Major findings included a significantly higher prevalence of *S. aureus* (88%) in patients with septal perforations, compared to the control group (13%). Corynebacterium spp. and Propionibacterium spp. were more commonly found in the control group. The study also noted high genetic heterogeneity in *S. aureus* strains, as no specific genotypes were linked to septal perforation [51].

## 12.5 Differential Diagnosis

NSP can arise from various causes, including piercings, exposure to industrial chemicals, illicit drug and intranasal steroid use, surgical trauma, and bilateral cautery, though the precise mechanisms behind substance induced NSP formation remain unclear [1, 2].

Vasculitic diseases are among the systemic causes of NSP. They often present with nasal symptoms like rhinitis, sinusitis, and epistaxis, with septal perforation being a notable feature. Among these, granulomatosis with polyangiitis (GPA, formerly Wegener's granulomatosis) and eosinophilic granulomatosis with polyangiitis (EGPA, formerly Churg-Strauss syndrome) are relatively common in the sinonasal tract. Specifically, in GPA, patients frequently experience persistent bleeding, crusting, and nasal obstruction, with septal perforation being a potential complication. This highlights the importance of considering vasculitic diseases in the differential diagnosis of nasal septal perforations [52].

Cocaine-induced midline destructive lesions (CIMDL) mimic systemic diseases and are prevalent in about 4.8% of cocaine users, presenting clinically with symptoms like hyposmia, facial pain, ulcers, and nasal septal perforation. Differentiating between them can be challenging, especially when there is no history of cocaine use. Anti-neutrophil cytoplasmic antibodies (ANCA) are a notable distinguishing feature [50].

Cocaine-induced midline destructive lesion (CIMDL) is a destructive process resulting from chronic cocaine use, primarily through sniffing, leading to repeated vasoconstrictions, ischemia, and necrosis of nasal mucosal and cartilaginous structures, often mimicking diseases like granulomatosis with polyangiitis. A diagnosis of CIMDL is typically suspected with the presence of nasal septal perforation, palatal perforation, or lateral nasal wall destruction, alongside a complete workup that includes ruling out other differential diagnoses and toxicological screening to confirm cocaine abuse [53].

The intranasal abuse of combined opioid-acetaminophen medications (COAMs) has been identified as a cause of septal perforation, with talc, a commonly used binder in these medications, likely contributing to septal necrosis. The incidence of septal perforation is notably higher in cases of COAM abuse compared to cocaine abuse. For effective treatment, it is crucial for patients to cease intranasal use of COAMs and seek early intervention from an addiction specialist. Talc, a hydrated magnesium silicate crystal, is utilized in various industries, including medicine and drug production. In medical applications, talc pleurodesis is used to induce local inflammation and create adhesion between the parietal and visceral pleura to prevent recurrent pleural effusion or pneumothorax. This same substance serves as a binder in COAMs and acetaminophen-only tablets. Pathologically, nasal biopsies from individuals abusing drugs intranasally often reveal a polarizable birefringent substance, identified in 57% of cases, which is likely talc from COAM tablets. This finding underscores the potential harm caused by the intranasal abuse of medications containing talc, leading to tissue necrosis and septal perforation due to a localized inflammatory response [54].

In a study assessing abnormal rhinological findings in Sjögren's syndrome patients, hyposmia was significantly more prevalent compared to controls, and nasal septal perforation was observed in 10% of the Sjögren's syndrome group, along with nasal mucosal dryness, suggesting that Sjögren's syndrome should be considered in patients with smell deprivation and/or nasal septal perforation [55].

Other immunological disorders in which NSP reported is the IgG4-related disease. In IgG4-related disease (IgG4-RD), the involvement of midline structures often manifests as nasal septum perforation or bone erosion [56].

Button batteries (BBs) in the nasal cavity, a common issue in children under 6 years, can lead to serious complications such as ulceration and septal perforation. Lou [57] reported septal perforation in 7 of 9 cases involving BBs, suggesting that neutralizing the BB's alkaline effect with weak acidic seawater spray may prevent such outcomes. Huang et al. [58] found preoperative perforation in 21 out of 97 nasal BB cases and one postoperative case, highlighting that prolonged exposure increases the risk of septal damage. However, Jatana et al. [59] and others demonstrated that neutralizing alkali injury without causing thermal injury is feasible through serial irrigation with weak acidic liquids like lemon or orange juice, or using honey and Carafate (Allergan, Dublin, Ireland), which are more effective than saline in reducing BB discharge and neutralizing tissue pH, thereby preventing septal perforation [60, 61].

It is important to consider neoplasms in the differential diagnosis of NSP. T-cell lymphomas are associated with septal perforation in sinonasal lymphoma [62].

Clinicians should keep a high index of suspicion for infections as a cause of NSP. Mucosal leishmaniasis (ML) can lead to septal perforation and facial deformities due to the erosion of nasal bone and cartilage, with nasal septum perforation commonly linked to Leishmania braziliensis. Diagnosing ML usually involves biopsy, culture, or PCR of the affected region. Detection is often challenging as ML has fewer parasites than cutaneous leishmaniasis (CL), leading to lower smear and culture positivity rates. Culture and PCR sensitivities for Leishmania are reported to be between 42–46% and 80–98%, respectively. However, smear positivity in ML cases is only about 17%, while PCR positivity is higher at 71% [63].

In patients with ex-lepromatous leprosy who also suffer from atrophic rhinitis, there is a notable incidence of septal perforation, with approximately 46.2% of these patients experiencing this condition [64]. (Table 12.1).

## 12.6 Workup

Diagnosing septal perforations is complex due to the variety of potential causes, making a comprehensive medical history essential. Incorporating the visual analog scale (VAS) into the workup of nasal septal perforation (NSP) is highly recommended. VAS, a tool that measures symptom severity on a scale from 0 (no symptoms) to 10 (maximum symptoms), is crucial for evaluating pre- and postoperative symptoms such as epistaxis, crusting, whistling, nasal obstruction, and pain. Studies utilizing VAS have demonstrated significant post-surgical improvements in these symptoms, including complete resolution of epistaxis, crusting, and whistling, along with a 92% improvement in nasal blockage. This approach offers a quantitative method to assess the effectiveness of treatments and track patient outcomes over time [3].

In evaluating nasal septal perforations, measuring their size is critical. This measurement, usually done via CT scans or during surgery, is key to predicting repair success. Smaller perforations typically have higher chances of complete closure, whereas larger perforations, particularly those over 2 cm, tend to have a higher rate of surgical failure. This information is crucial for guiding treatment strategies [65]. The size of the perforation can be also gauged using barium paste along its edges, followed by a lateral head X-ray, as detailed by Rettinger and Hosemann [66].

Intranasal corticosteroids (INCSs) are generally safe to use, though they can have some adverse effects like nasal irritation, epistaxis, septal perforation, suppression of the hypothalamic-pituitary-adrenal (HPA) axis, and growth suppression. However, septal perforation is extremely rare, and HPA axis suppression is

**Table 12.1** Causes of septal perforation

| Class | Causes |
|---|---|
| Traumatic/iatrogenic | • Post-septal surgery.<br>• Chemical cautery.<br>• Nasal packing.<br>• Nasal fracture.<br>• Septal hematoma.<br>• Foreign body.<br>• Nasogastric tube.<br>• Prolonged nasal intubation.<br>• Nasal pricking. |
| Inflammatory | • Granulomatosis with polyangiitis GPA.<br>• Eosinophilic granulomatosis with polyangiitis EGPA.<br>• Systemic lupus erythematosus SLE.<br>• Rheumatoid arthritis RA.<br>• Crohn's disease.<br>• Dermatomyositis.<br>• Sarcoidosis. |
| Infectious | • Syphilis.<br>• HIV.<br>• Invasive fungal infections.<br>• Septal abscess.<br>• Leprosy.<br>• Tuberculosis. |
| Drug-induced | • Vasoconstrictive nasal spray.<br>• Intranasal steroids.<br>• Cocaine abuse. |
| Neoplasm | • Non-Hodgkin lymphoma.<br>• Squamous cell carcinoma.<br>• Adenoid cystic carcinoma.<br>• Basal cell carcinoma.<br>• Esthesioneuroblastoma.<br>• Rhabdomyosarcoma. |

inconsistent and not considered clinically significant. Long-term studies have not found evidence of nasal atrophy associated with INCSs. For instance, a study of 315 patients using intranasal beclomethasone propionate for over 5 years showed no mucosal damage, and another study with 87 patients treated for 1–6 years also found no mucosal atrophy. Isolated cases of septal perforation have been reported, often linked to devascularization due to trauma, septal surgery, decongestant abuse, or cocaine use. Therefore, in patients with septal perforation who are on INCS, it is advised to conduct a thorough workup and search for more common etiologies before attributing the perforation to INCS use [67].

For patients presenting with septal perforation or necrosis of midline nasal and palatal structures, routine drug testing should be considered. This recommendation is based on the fact that many illicit drugs are consumed transnasally, and repeated exposure to stimulants or narcotics via this route can lead to local tissue destruction. This often manifests as chronic rhinosinusitis or nasoseptal perforation. Sinusitis and septal perforation associated with illicit drug use were initially identified in cocaine abuse cases. Cocaine use is relatively widespread, particularly among 15- to 34-year-olds, ranking as the fourth most commonly used illegal drug following marijuana, heroin, and ecstasy [68].

Diagnosing NSP typically involves straightforward methods like using a nasal speculum or endoscopy. These tools effectively reveal the presence of a perforation. It is important to include examining the external nose for deformities such as a saddle nose as it can be indicative of conditions like GPA. Additionally, imaging techniques, such as CT scans, can not only confirm the diagnosis but also assist in mapping the extent and location of the NSP. In cases where the patient's history suggests specific causes, imaging can also provide clues about the underlying reasons for the NSP, aiding in forming a more comprehensive understanding of the condition [4].

In the workup of nasal septal perforation, a notable advancement includes the use of three-dimensional (3-D) printing for sizing prostheses. This method, originating from the Mayo Clinic since 1972 for patients unsuitable for surgical intervention, has significantly improved prosthesis retention rates. Earlier approaches saw about 27% of patients opting not to retain their prosthesis. However, the introduction of 3D printing, utilizing CT scans to create precise templates of the patient's septal perforation, has led to better-fitted, medical-grade silastic prostheses and enhanced patient comfort and compliance. In a study of 21 patients who received these custom-sized prostheses, 20 reported symptom relief, and the retention rate of the prosthesis improved to 90%. This marked increase from previous rates highlights the effectiveness of 3D printing in the management of challenging nasal septal perforations, making it a valuable addition to the workup and treatment process [69].

The relationship between olfaction and nasal septal perforation (NSP) is not extensively documented in existing literature. However, a study has objectively demonstrated improvements in smell for NSP patients after repair, as assessed by an olfactory performance test using an olfaction test kit. This finding underscores the significance of conducting olfaction tests in individuals with NSP to evaluate and monitor changes in their sense of smell [70].

If the cause of nasal septal perforation is unclear, a series of laboratory tests can be conducted to aid in the diagnosis of potential systemic diseases. These tests include the erythrocyte sedimentation rate, rheumatoid factor, C-ANCA, and angiotensin-converting enzyme levels. Biopsy is to be considered in suspected malignancy. (Table 12.2).

## 12.7 Treatment

### 12.7.1 Medical Management

Generally, when a patient with NSP is asymptomatic, conservative management focusing on regular application of nasal emollients is usually satisfactory. However, for patients who continue to experience symptoms despite nasal emollients, nonsurgical interventions are commonly employed. These interventions often include the

**Table 12.2** Causes of septal perforation and related diagnostic tests

| Class | Disease | Manifestations | Diagnostic test |
|---|---|---|---|
| Vasculitis and autoimmune disease | Granulomatosis with polyangiitis GPA | Conjunctivitis, chronic sinusitis, saddle nasal deformity, stridor, dyspnea, cough, arthralgias, glomerulonephritis. | • C-ANCA.<br>• Biopsy (small to medium vessel vasculitis). |
| | Eosinophilic granulomatosis with polyangiitis EGPA | Fatigue, fever, asthma, chronic sinusitis, hemoptysis, skin rash, peripheral neuropathy | • P-ANCA.<br>• Eosinophilia.<br>• Biopsy (granulomas and vasculitis with extravascular eosinophilia). |
| | Systemic lupus erythematosus SLE | Malar rash, fever, kidney involvement, seizure, anemia | • Ana.<br>• Anti-dsDNA.<br>• Anti-RO/SSA. |
| | Rheumatoid arthritis RA | Joint swelling deformity and pain, rheumatoid nodules, cardiovascular involvement, interstitial lung fibrosis | • RF.<br>• Anti-CCP. |
| | Sarcoidosis | Dyspnea on exertion, cough, chest pain, fever, violaceous rash on the cheeks, anterior or posterior granulomatous uveitis | • Hypercalcemia/ hypercalciuria.<br>• Pulmonary biopsy.<br>• High ACE. |
| Neoplastic | Benign vs. malignant | – | • Biopsy. |

(continued)

**Table 12.2** (continued)

| Class | Disease | Manifestations | Diagnostic test |
|---|---|---|---|
| Infections | Invasive fungal sinusitis | Fever, headache, decrease vision, diplopia, nasal discharge | • Biopsy (vascular invasion with fungal hyphae). |
| | Tuberculosis | Cough, weight loss, fever, hemoptysis | • Culture.<br>• AFB.<br>• Biopsy (granuloma with central caseous necrosis). |
| | Leprosy | Hypopigmented skin lesions, peripheral neuropathy, erythema nodosum leprosum | • AFB.<br>• Skin biopsy (epithelioid granuloma with giant cells). |
| | Syphilis | Painless genital ulcers, skin rash, fever, fatigue | • RPR.<br>• VDRL.<br>• FTA-ABS treponemal tests.<br>• PCR.<br>• Biopsy (*Treponema pallidum).* |
| | Rhinoscleroma | Chronic sinusitis, external nasal deformity, dysphagia, stridor | • Biopsy (Mikulicz cells). |

Abbreviations: C-ANCA (cytoplasmic anti-neutrophil cytoplasmic antibody), P-ANCA (perinuclear anti-neutrophil cytoplasmic antibody), ANA (anti-nuclear antibody), anti-dsDNA (anti-double-stranded DNA)
anti-RO/SSA (autoantibodies directed against the Ro/SSA antigens), RF (rheumatoid factor), anti-CCP (anti-cyclic citrullinated peptide), ACE (angiotensin-converting enzyme), AFB (acid fast bacilli), PRP (rapid plasma reagin), VDRL (Venereal Disease Research Laboratory), FTA-ABS (fluorescent treponemal antibody absorption), PCR (polymerase chain reaction)

use of silicone septal buttons. These devices mechanically close the defect without the need for tissue manipulation. The placement of a septal button can be easily conducted in a clinic setting using topical anesthesia. In the past, buttons were predominantly made from acrylic and plastic, but nowadays, they are primarily composed of soft silicone [71]. As mentioned earlier, new 3D printing technology has produced a more precise silastic prosthesis to fit the septal perforation. It improves the patient's comfort and reduces the retention rate. Long-term studies have verified the effectiveness of this treatment approach in managing epistaxis, nasal airway obstruction, and whistling [69].

On the other hand, there are potential negative effects associated with it, including an increase in nosebleeds, pain and discomfort, erosion of the perforation's edges, and the possibility of crust formation at the site [72, 73]. Patients often experience intolerance due to local irritation, nasal blockage, or the buildup of thick secretions. Those who wish to have them removed typically do so within 6 months [74].

### 12.7.2 Surgical Management

Surgical interventions are typically considered for symptomatic patients who have not achieved satisfactory results with conservative therapy. Various surgical approaches and techniques have been developed to repair nasal septal perforations (NSP) [74].

The objective of surgical repair is to restore normal nasal physiology by reconstructing laminar airflow, promoting the warming and humidification of inspired air, facilitating mucus production, and enhancing mucociliary transport. As NSP involves a defect across three layers, a three-layered repair is pursued whenever feasible, involving both right and left septal mucoperichondrial flaps and the intervening cartilage [75].

The reported success rates in the literature for closing septal perforations of all sizes range from 30% to 100% [71–73, 75–80]. In a systematic literature review, Kim and Rhee [65] reported an aggregate successful closure rate of 93% for perforations smaller than 2 cm and 78% for perforations larger than 2 cm. A recent community survey self-reported success rates for closing perforations smaller than 1 cm, 1–2 cm, and larger than 2 cm were 84%, 64%, and 31%, respectively [75]. The figures in the survey are notably lower than those documented in the literature, possibly because proficient surgeons are more inclined to share favorable experiences, influencing the perception of achievable results. Despite these modest outcomes, it is plausible that the actual success rate may be even lower than reported in this survey.

#### 12.7.2.1 Patient's Selection

The wide range of success rates indicates that the procedure can be influenced by various factors, including the size and location of the perforation, the underlying etiology, surgical technique, tissue quality, the quantity of remaining cartilage, the presence of scar tissue on the mucosa, postoperative care, individual patient characteristics, and, most importantly, the expertise and proficiency of the surgeon [75]. Therefore, patient selection becomes a crucial aspect in achieving successful results. Large perforation size is associated with low success rate. In a review conducted by Kridel and Delaney involving 139 patients who underwent NSP repair, it was found that the closure rate is only 71.4% of patients with perforations exceeding 1.5 cm [75]. The presence of active autoimmune disease and diabetes millets can affect the healing process and immune response, potentially impacting the outcomes of surgical interventions [19]. Autoimmune diseases or chronic inflammatory conditions are typically deferred until the patient achieves a stable remission state for a minimum of 6 months, during which they continue their maintenance medical therapy, and lab markers indicating the underlying chronic inflammatory condition remain consistently stable [81]. Therefore, patients with systemic diseases like GPA should be in a remission state before considering the repair. Literature reports have documented successful repair outcomes for patients in a remission state [82]. However, it should be noted that a higher rate of revision may be expected in these patients [83]. It is important to highlight that the risk of failure in these conditions is amplified by factors such as prominent crust formation, colonization of *Staphylococcus aureus*, and the risk of relapse [76]. Smoking can compromise the healing process of the repair, with reported odds of surgical failure for smokers being three times higher than for non-smokers [19, 75]. Cocaine abuse causes nasal defects ranging from minor septal perforation to loss of dorsal support. Patients with NSP resulting from cocaine use should undergo a psychiatric assessment to evaluate their mental status prior to undergoing any surgical intervention. However, consumption of cocaine is an absolute contraindication for surgery, as the repair is likely to fail [76].

#### 12.7.2.2 Surgical Approaches

The repair procedure is mostly performed by rhinologists, general otolaryngologists, or facial plastic surgeons. Hence, a wide range of surgical treatment methods for nasal septal perforation have been reported [74]. Nevertheless, there is a lack of standardization in surgical approaches and techniques [84]. The most reported surgical approaches include open external rhinoplasty, closed endonasal, and endoscopic approaches [74].

As previously stated, the surgical approach is determined by many factors but mainly by the surgeon's experience and training background.

1. The **external rhinoplasty approach** provides the surgeon with excellent binocular vision and facilitates the use of both hands simultaneously. Performing a concomitant rhinoplasty and nasal septal perforation repair is often advantageous, as both procedures can be surgically approached using the open method. Moreover, certain routine rhinoplasty techniques, such as medial osteotomies and dorsal lowering, create additional mucosal redundancy [85]. In contrast, the open rhinoplasty approach is associated with specific cosmetic drawbacks, primarily affecting the appearance of the nose. These techniques demonstrate modest success rates and may result in complications associated with open procedures, such as scarring and donor site morbidity [74, 75]. The reported closure rates for the open rhinoplasty approach are 90%, 75%, and 42% for small, moderate, and large perforation sizes, respectively [86].
2. The **endonasal approach**, using a standard Killian or hemi-transfixion incision, is primarily employed by general otolaryngologists [74]. This approach is deemed effective for addressing small defects measuring less than 5 mm. However, it can be notably challenging, especially when dealing with large perforations or patients with small nostrils. In some instances, a lateral alotomy may be necessary to enhance access and visualization; nevertheless, this carries the risk of creating an external nasal scar for the patient [85]. This technique demonstrates a modest success rate, particularly for large perforations [86].
3. Recently, purely **endoscopic approach** has gained popularity among rhinologists. This approach offers excellent visualization and exposure without the need for extensive dissection, providing effective control of the margins of the perforation. Since the advent of the endoscopic approach, several innovative intranasal repair methods have been developed. However, it is essential to highlight that

these techniques demand proficient endoscopic skills, presenting a challenge for less experienced surgeons. Moreover, endoscopic techniques may lead to longer operating times and the potential drawback of limited surgical visibility during flap suturing [75]. The overall success rate of endoscopic techniques has reached up to 90% [84]. Further details of the endoscopic approach will be discussed in the subsequent section.

4. The external open approaches, such as midfacial degloving, bicoronal flap, and lateral rhinotomy, have been documented as surgical methods for addressing large septal perforations exceeding 2 cm [87]. Nevertheless, it seems that this approach is seldom necessary due to its notable drawbacks. These disadvantages include extensive exposure, significant intraoperative blood loss, prolonged surgical duration, potential risk of neurovascular injury, vestibular stenosis, and the possibility of asymmetry [77].

#### 12.7.2.3 Surgical Techniques

A diverse array of surgical techniques is employed for NSP repair. In this section, our focus will be on endoscopic approaches and techniques. Various local and regional flaps, as well as autologous and synthetic grafts, have been utilized for defect repair. Local flaps can be categorized into two types: random pattern flaps, which lack a significant named blood supply, and axial flaps, which have a specific pedicled arterio-venous system along their long axis. Both types are considered rotational advancement flaps that can be employed unilaterally or bilaterally, with or without interposition grafts. The random pattern flap can be harvested from the nasal septum, lateral nasal wall, middle turbinate, inferior turbinate, or nasal floor, while axial flaps should be pedicled to a specific blood supply such as the anterior ethmoidal artery (AEA), sphenopalatine artery (SPA), or greater palatine artery (GPA) [88].

The axial flap is considered more robust and reliable; however, its successful utilization requires meticulous harvesting to encompass the pedicled artery, prevent pedicle rotation, and ensure minimal tension during closure. Consequently, a unilateral axial flap has been reported to be less successful than a unilateral random flap (87.5% vs. 93.4%). However, when combined with an additional layer, such as an interposition graft or flap, the success rate was higher in the axial flap group (79.1 vs. 92.3%). Adding a third layer of free mucosal graft elevated the success rate of the axial flap to 100% compared to 95% for the random flap [89].

Multilayered reconstruction has demonstrated a higher success rate compared to a single layer. This is primarily attributed to the bilateral coverage of the perforation, increased vascularity, and reduced tension closure for each flap [85, 86]. This can be accomplished through a combination of unipedicled vs. bipedicled axial/random flaps with or without interposition grafts or free mucosal grafts. However, the unipedicled advancement flap alone has been reported as effective in achieving complete closure of NSP. It is associated with favorable closure rates, shorter operative times, and the preservation of a greater amount of nasal respiratory mucosa [79, 90–93]. The critical limitation of the unipedicled nasal mucosal flap is its insufficient size in the case of a large perforation [94]. Nevertheless, a high success rate has been reported with the use of a single-layer axial flap, particularly for large perforations up to 3 cm [95]. A precise surgical technique, combined with the achievement of tension-free closure, could be the critical factor in successfully repairing a sizable defect using a unipedicled flap alone.

The AEA flap stands out as an example of an axial pedicled flap known for its versatility, robust blood supply, and expansive surface area. In the initial description by Castelnuovo et al., a remarkable 100% success rate was reported. Nevertheless, a subsequent longitudinal follow-up study uncovered a success rate of 81% [96, 97]. Following this, the AEA flap has been employed as a single layer using various techniques. Rusetsky et al. implemented the cross-septal technique, wherein the AEA flap is advanced anteriorly to cover the perforation, then passed through an anterior septal incision to the contralateral nasal cavity and turned backward to cover the perforation on the opposite side. This technique demonstrated success rates of 83% and 89% in pediatric and adult age groups, respectively [30, 97, 98]. Another approach was adopted by Santamaría et al., who utilized an extended version of the AEA flap, incorporating the mucosa of the choana to cover large septal perforations [98]. Notably, all patients in this study achieved complete closure of the perforation. Studies detailing the multilayer closure of septal perforations by the AEA flap in combination with other flaps or grafts have consistently reported a 100% success rate [29, 30, 99].

The greater palatine artery (GPA) flap serves as an alternative axial flap due to its proximity to the NSP. This flap utilizes the nasal floor and nasal septal mucoperiosteum to effectively cover the perforation. Notably, it has been employed in both single and multilayered repair techniques, consistently demonstrating a high closure rate [100].

The inferior turbinate flap demonstrates potential advantages, including abundant vascular supply and a wide rotation range. However, despite these merits, authors have documented unexpectedly high failure rates, rendering it an unfavorable choice as a primary treatment option [101]. The major disadvantages include the need for a second-stage procedure to release the pedicle, and the flap may lead to nasal obstruction due to its bulky nature [92].

The application of a buccal mucosal flap, rotated from beneath the upper lip and introduced through an incision into the nasal floor, has been examined for the repair of NSP. Nonetheless, the procedure has not gained widespread adoption primarily because the buccal mucosa does not undergo a transformation into ciliated, mucus-producing, self-cleansing mucosa [101].

The pericranial flap is considered appropriate for addressing large or total NSP. It is introduced into the nasal cavity through a small horizontal opening in the frontal bone leading to the frontal sinus [102]. Despite its effectiveness in closing perforations, the procedure is associated with persistent postoperative crusting, a dry nose, and the potential for flap necrosis. Given the procedural risks and accompanying morbidity, the utilization of these regional flaps has not been widely embraced [74]. It is typically reserved for challenging cases where septal mucosa is unavailable for reconstruction.

#### Interposition Grafts

Interposition graft plays a vital role as a template to facilitate the migration of mucosa during the healing phase. It helps in minimizing the shrinkage of mucosal flaps after rotation [89]. Furthermore, the graft acts as a protective barrier between the repaired flaps during the healing process, thereby reducing the risk of incisional breakdown [103]. Surgeons have documented utilization of a diverse range of graft materials such as autologous septal or conchal cartilage, pericranium, periosteum, temporalis fascia, ethmoid bone, mastoid cortex, polydioxanone plate, porcine intestinal submucosa, collagen matrix, and acellular human dermal allograft [77, 85, 93, 103]. Septal cartilage remnants are widely regarded as the optimal choice for intervention due to their ease of procurement and minimal donor site morbidity [94, 104]. Connective tissue allografts and xenografts have demonstrated clinical efficacy equal to that of autologous connective tissue when interposed between repaired septal flaps [86, 87, 105]. Considerations for the selection of interposition graft material should weigh the operative time and potential morbidity related to harvesting autografts against the costs of non-autografts.

#### Tunnel Technique

This technique has been described by the authors of this chapter. It is a modified technique to the original flap described by Castelnuovo et al. which is based on the AEA axial flap [95, 106]. A local anesthetic agent is infiltrated in the mucosa around the septal perforation and at the incision lines over the nasal septum, nasal floor, and inferior meatus. The anterior flap incision is started at 0.5 cm posterior to the septal perforation and extend over the nasal septum down to the inferior meatus. The posterior incision is located 1 cm to the free edge of the middle turbinate and extended vertically the same way as the anterior incision. The third incision is made laterally at the inferior meatus to communicate the previous two incisions. Mucoperichondrium/mucoperiosteum is elevated carefully (Fig. 12.5). The second part of the procedure is to elevate the flap around the perforation. It is started with a hemi-transfixion incision that is made as in the septoplasty procedure. The mucoperichondrial flap is elevated 360 degree all around the perforation. This flap is called a "peri-perforation flap." The main flap is then advanced beneath the "peri-perforation flap" that works as a tunnel and advanced anteriorly until it reaches the hemi-transfixion incision. The flap is secured with 2 absorbable sutures, one superiorly and one anteriorly with the hemi-transfixion incision. Silastic sheets are applied and kept for 1 week.

The advantage of the tunnel technique is that it provides extra support to the AEA flap and holds it against the exposed cartilage. Applying the flap over the bare cartilage enhance the healing process. This also helps in minimizing the need for multiple sutures and shorten the duration of silastic sheet application. This technique showed a success rate of 94% (17/18 patients). The only one failure case was a revision surgery. There were no significant postoperative complications.

### 12.7.2.4 Postoperative Care

Silastic sheets are typically applied bilaterally to the nasal septum at the conclusion of the procedure and secured with nonabsorbable sutures. The use of silastic sheets

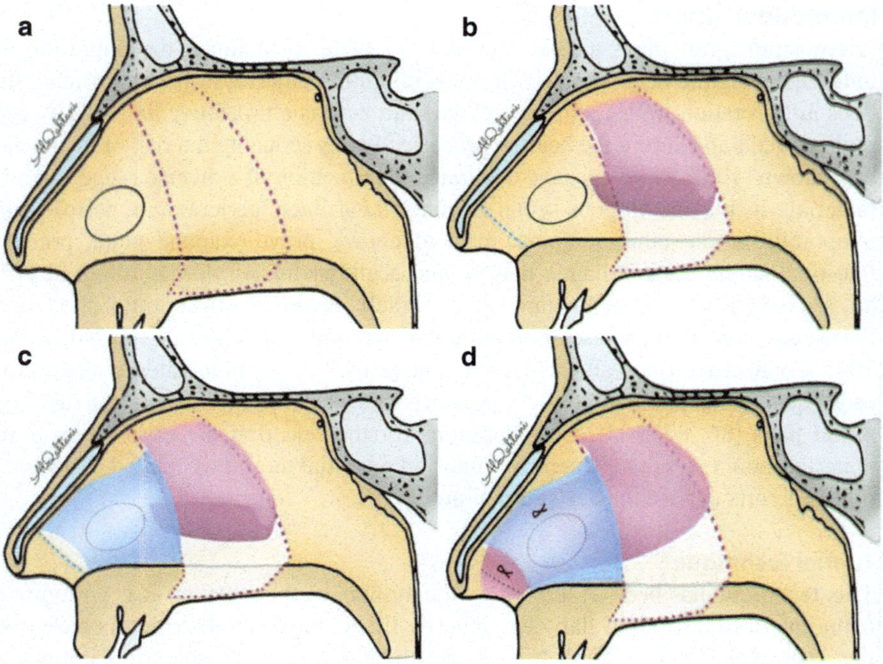

**Fig. 12.5** Schematic drawing of the tunnel technique. (**a**) The purple dots represent the incision lines of the AEA flap. (**b**) The AEA flap is harvested (the purple color). (**c**) The light blue color represents the peri-perforation flap. (**d**) The AEA flap is advanced beneath the peri-perforation flap, and two sutures are applied to hold the flaps together with the septum. AEA: anterior ethmoid artery

is essential for reducing swelling and aiding in mucosal healing, as reported by 89% of respondents in a recent community survey. However, the duration of sheet placement varies, with removal typically occurring within 1–3 weeks.

In instances of bleeding or when it is necessary to stabilize the mucosa, lubricated packing is applied for a period ranging from 24 to 48 h. Additionally, all patients are advised to maintain nasal moisture by frequently using nasal douches with saline. Some authors recommend the application of both antibiotic ointment and topical vitamin A ointment on both sides of the reconstruction until the healing process is complete. These ointments play a role in hydrating and promoting the regeneration of nasal mucosa post-surgery. Furthermore, patients are instructed to refrain from using vasoconstrictive sprays, smoking, digital manipulation, and exposure to noxious fumes during the postoperative period.

## 12.8 Pediatric Consideration

Septal perforations are relatively rare in the pediatric population. The predominant symptom observed in children with nasal perforations is nasal crusting, occurring in approximately 73% of cases [32].

The management of septal perforations in children generally follows the same protocols as in adults. However, repairing a perforation can pose greater challenges in this age group. These challenges arise from limitations in accessing the affected area, ensuring an adequate supply of mucosal flaps, and ensuring compliance with postoperative instructions.

There is a notable scarcity of literature exploring the impact of repairing pediatric septal perforations on future nasal growth. Nevertheless, existing literature on pediatric septoplasty suggests that raising unilateral or bilateral mucoperichondrial flaps does not adversely affect facial growth [91]. A case series conducted by D.T. Chang et al. involved 27 patients with an average age of 10 years. Among these patients, six underwent surgical treatment using a combination of free graft and mucosal flap repairs. The study reported a success rate of 66% [32]. However, reperforation occurred in two patients, attributed to active granulomatous disease and septal hematomas. It is crucial to thoroughly assess the cause of the perforation and the level of patient cooperation before considering definitive repair of pediatric septal perforations.

## 12.9 Conclusion

In conclusion, nasal septal perforations, caused by necrosis of various nasal septum layers, disrupt the nasal airflow, potentially leading to symptoms like nosebleeds and nasal blockage. Understanding the anatomy of the nasal septum's arterial supply is vital for successful repair, especially considering risk factors such as smoking, drug use, and diabetes. NSPs have diverse etiologies, ranging from chemical exposure to surgical trauma. Their size influences the severity of symptoms. Diagnosis typically involves endoscopy or imaging like CT scans, with additional lab tests aiding in identifying specific conditions like Churg-Strauss syndrome or Wegener's granulomatosis, although these tests have limited specificity.

NSP management involves both medical and surgical approaches. Medical management, often sufficient for asymptomatic cases, relies on nasal emollients and may include silicone septal buttons. Surgical interventions, employed for symptomatic patients, exhibit varying success rates influenced by factors such as perforation size, location, patient health, and surgical technique. Patient selection is a critical process that should be considered before surgery. Different surgical approaches, including external rhinoplasty, endonasal approaches, and endoscopic techniques, offer diverse options with associated benefits and drawbacks. Axial flaps like the anterior ethmoidal artery (AEA) flap, along with multilayered repairs and interposition grafts, enhance closure success. Postoperative care, including silastic sheets, nasal douching, and careful avoidance of exacerbating factors, contributes to optimal outcomes.

## References


1. Lanier B, Kai G, Marple B, Wall GM. Pathophysiology and progression of nasal septal perforation. Ann Allergy Asthma Immunol. 2007;99:473–9. quiz 480-471, 521
2. Pereira C, Santamaria A, Langdon C, Lopez-Chacon M, Hernandez-Rodriguez J, Alobid I. Nasoseptal perforation: from etiology to treatment. Curr Allergy Asthma Rep. 2018;18:5.
3. Wong S, Raghavan U. Outcome of surgical closure of nasal septal perforation. J Laryngol Otol. 2010;124:868–74.
4. Martinez Neto EE, Dolci JE. Nasal septal perforation closure with bacterial cellulose in rabbits. Braz J Otorhinolaryngol. 2010;76:442–9.
5. Boynuegri S, Cayonu M, Tuna EU, et al. The effect of nasal septal perforation and its treatment on objective sleep and breathing parameters. Med Sci Monit. 2016;22:501–7.
6. Henson B, Drake TM, Edens MA. Anatomy, Head and Neck, Nose Sinuses *StatPearls*. Treasure Island (FL) ineligible companies. Disclosure: Taylor Drake declares no relevant financial relationships with ineligible companies. Disclosure: Mary Ann Edens declares no relevant financial relationships with ineligible companies.: StatPearls Publishing Copyright © 2023, StatPearls Publishing LLC., 2023.
7. Oneal RM, Beil RJ Jr, Schlesinger J. Surgical anatomy of the nose. Clin Plast Surg. 1996;23:195–222.
8. Sobiesk JL, Munakomi S. Anatomy, Head and Neck, Nasal Cavity *StatPearls*. Treasure Island (FL) ineligible companies. Disclosure: Sunil Munakomi declares no relevant financial relationships with ineligible companies.: StatPearls Publishing Copyright © 2023, StatPearls Publishing LLC., 2023.
9. Padgham N, Vaughan-Jones R. Cadaver studies of the anatomy of arterial supply to the inferior turbinates. J R Soc Med. 1991;84:728–30.
10. Lee HY, Kim HU, Kim SS, et al. Surgical anatomy of the sphenopalatine artery in lateral nasal wall. Laryngoscope. 2002;112:1813–8.
11. Wareing MJ, Padgham ND. Osteologic classification of the sphenopalatine foramen. Laryngoscope. 1998;108:125–7.
12. Pothier DD, Mackeith S, Youngs R. Sphenopalatine artery ligation: technical note. J Laryngol Otol. 2005;119:810–2.
13. Bolger WE, Borgie RC, Melder P. The role of the crista ethmoidalis in endoscopic sphenopalatine artery ligation. Am J Rhinol. 1999;13:81–6.
14. MacArthur FJ, McGarry GW. The arterial supply of the nasal cavity. Eur Arch Otorrinolaringol. 2017;274:809–15.
15. Toure G. Distribution of the maxillary artery in the deep regions of the face and the maxilla: clinical applications. J Plast Reconstr Aesthet Surg. 2019;72:1020–4.
16. Ogle OE, Weinstock RJ, Friedman E. Surgical anatomy of the nasal cavity and paranasal sinuses. Oral Maxillofac Surg Clin North Am. 2012;24:155–166, vii.
17. Manjila S, Cox EM, Smith GA, et al. Extracranial ligation of ethmoidal arteries before resection of giant olfactory groove or planum sphenoidale meningiomas: 3 illustrative cases with a review of the literature on surgical techniques. Neurosurg Focus. 2013;35:E13.
18. Kim DW, Egan KK, O'Grady K, Toriumi DM. Biomechanical strength of human nasal septal lining: comparison of the constituent layers. Laryngoscope. 2005;115:1451–3.
19. Tumlin P, Assi S, Armeni M, Ramadan HH, Reyes C, Makary CA. Outcome of endoscopic repair of nasal septal perforation. Ann Otol Rhinol Laryngol. 2023;132:1617–20.
20. Ketcham AS, Han JK. Complications and management of septoplasty. Otolaryngol Clin N Am. 2010;43:897–904.

21. Tan M, Kalcioglu MT, Sahin N, Bayindir T, Samdanci E, Filiz A. Assessment of mucosal changes associated with nasal splint in a rabbit model. Braz J Otorhinolaryngol. 2015;81:184–9.
22. Gold M, Boyack I, Caputo N, Pearlman A. Imaging prevalence of nasal septal perforation in an urban population. Clin Imaging. 2017;43:80–2.
23. Kiraz M, Gunaldi O, Tanriverdi O, et al. Comparison of sinonasal complications of microscopic and endoscopic approaches for transsphenoidal hypophyseal surgery: prospective study. Turk Neurosurg. 2018;28:915–22.
24. Cheng Y, Xue F, Wang TY, et al. Analyses and treatments of postoperative nasal complications after endonasal transsphenoidal resection of pituitary neoplasms. Medicine (Baltimore). 2017;96:e6614.
25. Fnais N, Maio SD, Edionwe S, et al. Hemi-transseptal approach for pituitary surgery: a follow-up study. J Neurol Surg B Skull Base. 2017;78:145–51.
26. Rivera-Serrano CM, Snyderman CH, Gardner P, et al. Nasoseptal "rescue" flap: a novel modification of the nasoseptal flap technique for pituitary surgery. Laryngoscope. 2011;121:990–3.
27. Tewfik MA, Valdes CJ, Zeitouni A, Sirhan D, Di Maio S. The endoscopic hemi-transseptal approach to the Sella turcica: operative technique and case-control study. J Neurol Surg B Skull Base. 2014;75:415–20.
28. Soudry E, Psaltis AJ, Lee KH, Vaezafshar R, Nayak JV, Hwang PH. Complications associated with the pedicled nasoseptal flap for skull base reconstruction. Laryngoscope. 2015;125:80–5.
29. Nassif SJ, Scott AR. Pediatric septal perforation repair with the endoscopic anterior ethmoid artery flap. Otolaryngol Head Neck Surg. 2021;164:448–50.
30. Rusetsky Y, Mokoyan Z, Meytel I, Spiranskaya O, Malyavina U. Endoscopic repair of septal perforation in children. Int J Pediatr Otorhinolaryngol. 2020;130:109817.
31. Jennings JJ, Shaffer AD, Stapleton AL. Pediatric nasal septal perforation. Int J Pediatr Otorhinolaryngol. 2019;118:15–20.
32. Chang DT, Irace AL, Kawai K, Rogers-Vizena CR, Nuss R, Adil EA. Nasal septal perforation in children: presentation, etiology, and management. Int J Pediatr Otorhinolaryngol. 2017;92:176–80.
33. Taylor CM, Bansberg SF, Marino MJ. Assessing patient symptoms due to nasal septal perforation: development and validation of the NOSE-perf scale. Otolaryngol Head Neck Surg. 2021;165:739–44.
34. Ozturk S, Zor F, Ozturk S, Kartal O, Alhan D, Isik S. A new approach to objective evaluation of the success of nasal septum perforation. Arch Plast Surg. 2014;41:403–6.
35. Lindemann J, Reichert M, Kroger R, Schuler P, Hoffmann T, Sommer F. Numerical simulation of humidification and heating during inspiration in nose models with three different located septal perforations. Eur Arch Otorrinolaringol. 2016;273:1795–800.
36. Nomura T, Ushio M, Kondo K, Kikuchi S. Effects of nasal septum perforation repair on nasal airflow: an analysis using computational fluid dynamics on preoperative and postoperative three-dimensional models. Auris Nasus Larynx. 2018;45:1020–6.
37. Li C, Maza G, Farag AA, et al. Asymptomatic vs symptomatic septal perforations: a computational fluid dynamics examination. Int Forum Allergy Rhinol. 2019;9:883–90.
38. Chen PG, Floreani S, Wormald PJ. The utility of enlarging symptomatic nasal septal perforations. Ear Nose Throat J. 2018;97:E41–3.
39. Zhou B, Huang Q, Cui S, Liu Y, Han D. Impact of airflow communication between nasal cavities on nasal ventilation. ORL J Otorhinolaryngol Relat Spec. 2013;75:301–8.
40. Cannon DE, Frank DO, Kimbell JS, Poetker DM, Rhee JS. Modeling nasal physiology changes due to septal perforations. Otolaryngol Head Neck Surg. 2013;148:513–8.
41. Nomura T, Ushio M, Kondo K, Yamasoba T. Effects of nasal septum perforation repair surgery on three-dimensional airflow: an evaluation using computational fluid dynamics. Eur Arch Otorrinolaringol. 2015;272:3327–33.
42. Lindemann J, Rettinger G, Kroger R, Sommer F. Numerical simulation of airflow patterns in nose models with differently localized septal perforations. Laryngoscope. 2013;123:2085–9.

43. Otto BA, Li C, Farag AA, et al. Computational fluid dynamics evaluation of posterior septectomy as a viable treatment option for large septal perforations. Int Forum Allergy Rhinol. 2017;7:718–25.
44. Dabrowska-Bien J, Skarzynski PH, Gwizdalska I, Lazecka K, Skarzynski H. Complications in septoplasty based on a large group of 5639 patients. Eur Arch Otorrinolaringol. 2018;275:1789–94.
45. Rana AK, Sharma R, Sharma VK, Mehrotra A, Upadhyay D, Pandey S. Is chemical cauterization safe on septal cartilage in treatment of recurrent epistaxis? Indian J Otolaryngol Head Neck Surg. 2022;74:1322–7.
46. Cukurova I, Gumussoy M, Kaptaner S, et al. Squamous cell carcinoma originating from the nasal septal perforation: a rare nasal tumor. Kulak Burun Bogaz Ihtis Derg. 2014;24:177–80.
47. Rodriguez CA, Martin T, Lozano R, Gomez A, Cruz JJ. Spontaneous nasal perforation in a bevacizumab-treated patient with metastatic breast cancer. Breast J. 2017;23:745–6.
48. Geltzeiler M, Steele TO. Nasal septal perforation secondary to systemic bevacizumab. Am J Otolaryngol. 2017;38:354–5.
49. St C, Karnezis T, Davidson TM. Safety of intranasal bevacizumab (Avastin) treatment in patients with hereditary hemorrhagic telangiectasia-associated epistaxis. Laryngoscope. 2011;121:644–6.
50. Trimarchi M, Bertazzoni G, Bussi M. Cocaine induced midline destructive lesions. Rhinology. 2014;52:104–11.
51. Hulterstrom AK, Sellin M, Monsen T, Widerstrom M, Gurram BK, Berggren D. Bacterial flora and the epidemiology of staphylococcus aureus in the nose among patients with symptomatic nasal septal perforations. Acta Otolaryngol. 2016;136:620–5.
52. Fokkens WJ, Lund VJ, Hopkins C, et al. European position paper on rhinosinusitis and nasal polyps 2020. Rhinology. 2020;58:1–464.
53. Nitro L, Pipolo C, Fadda GL, et al. Distribution of cocaine-induced midline destructive lesions: systematic review and classification. Eur Arch Otorrinolaringol. 2022;279:3257–67.
54. Vosler PS, Ferguson BJ, Contreras JI, Wang EW, Schaitkin BM, Lee S. Clinical and pathologic characteristics of intranasal abuse of combined opioid-acetaminophen medications. Int Forum Allergy Rhinol. 2014;4:839–44.
55. Kamel UF, Maddison PJ. Rhinological manifestations of Sjogren's syndrome: a cohort-matched, prospective, cross-sectional, observational study. J Laryngol Otol. 2021;135:932–6.
56. Lanzillotta M, Campochiaro C, Trimarchi M, et al. Deconstructing IgG4-related disease involvement of midline structures: comparison to common mimickers. Mod Rheumatol. 2017;27:638–45.
57. Lou ZC. Analysis of nasal foreign bodies in 341 children. J Laryngol Otol. 2019;133:908–12.
58. Huang T, Li WQ, Xia ZF, Li J, Rao KC, Xu EM. Characteristics and outcome of impacted button batteries among young children less than 7 years of age in China: a retrospective analysis of 116 cases. World J Pediatr. 2018;14:570–5.
59. Jatana KR, Rhoades K, Milkovich S, Jacobs IN. Basic mechanism of button battery ingestion injuries and novel mitigation strategies after diagnosis and removal. Laryngoscope. 2017;127:1276–82.
60. Anfang RR, Jatana KR, Linn RL, Rhoades K, Fry J, Jacobs IN. pH-neutralizing esophageal irrigations as a novel mitigation strategy for button battery injury. Laryngoscope. 2019;129:49–57.
61. Jatana KR, Barron CL, Jacobs IN. Initial clinical application of tissue pH neutralization after esophageal button battery removal in children. Laryngoscope. 2019;129:1772–6.
62. Shirazi N, Bist SS, Puri N, Harsh M, Ahmad S. Primary sinonasal lymphoma in immunocompetent patients: a 10 years retrospective clinicopathological study. J Oral Maxillofac Pathol. 2018;22:280–1.
63. Gul HC, Tosun F, Karakas A, et al. A case of mucosal leishmaniasis: mimicking intranasal tumor with perforation of septum. J Microbiol Immunol Infect. 2016;49:604–7.
64. Suzuki J, Oshima T, Watanabe K, Suzuki H, Kobayashi T, Hashimoto S. Chronic rhinosinusitis in ex-lepromatous leprosy patients with atrophic rhinitis. J Laryngol Otol. 2013;127:265–70.

65. Kim SW, Rhee CS. Nasal septal perforation repair: predictive factors and systematic review of the literature. Curr Opin Otolaryngol Head Neck Surg. 2012;20:58–65.
66. Rettinger G, Hosemann W. Measuring the size of nasal septal perforations. A simple radiological method. Rhinology. 1988;26:157–9.
67. Bensch GW. Safety of intranasal corticosteroids. Ann Allergy Asthma Immunol. 2016;117:601–5.
68. Gonik NJ, Bluth MH. Otolaryngology concerns for illicit and prescription drug use. Clin Lab Med. 2016;36:745–52.
69. Onerci Altunay Z, Bly JA, Edwards PK, et al. Three-dimensional printing of large nasal septal perforations for optimal prosthetic closure. Am J Rhinol Allergy. 2016;30:287–93.
70. Altun H, Hanci D. Olfaction improvement after nasal septal perforation repair with the "cross-stealing" technique. Am J Rhinol Allergy. 2015;29:e142–5.
71. Taylor RJ, Sherris DA. Prosthetics for nasal perforations: a systematic review and meta-analysis. Otolaryngol Head Neck Surg. 2015;152(5):803–10.
72. Brain DJ. Septo-rhinoplasty: the closure of septal perforations. J Laryngol Otol. 1980;94(5):495–505.
73. Pallanch JF, Facer GW, Kern EB, Westwood WB. Prosthetic closure of nasal septal perforations. Otolaryngol Head Neck Surg. 1982;90(4):448–52.
74. Watson D, Barkdull G. Surgical management of the septal perforation. Otolaryngol Clin N Am. 2009 Jun;42(3):483–93.
75. Delaney SW, Kridel RWH. Contemporary trends in the surgical Management of Nasal Septal Perforations: a community survey. Facial Plast Surg. 2019;35(1):78–84.
76. Pedroza F, Patrocinio LG, Arevalo O. A review of 25-year experience of nasal septal perforation repair. Arch Facial Plast Surg. 2007;9(1):12–8.
77. Romo T 3rd, Foster CA, Korovin GW, Sachs ME. Repair of nasal septal perforation utilizing the midface degloving technique. Arch Otolaryngol Head Neck Surg. 1988;114:739–42.
78. Romo T 3rd, Jablonski RD, Shapiro AL, McCormick SA. Long-term nasal mucosal tissue expansion use in repair of large nasoseptal perforations. Arch Otolaryngol Head Neck Surg. 1995;121:327–31.
79. Lee HR, Ahn DB, Park JH, et al. Endoscopic repairment of septal perforation with using a unilateral nasal mucosal flap. Clin Exp Otorhinolaryngol. 2008;1:154–7.
80. Kridel RWH, Appling WD, Wright WK. Septal perforation closure utilizing the external septorhinoplasty approach. Arch Otolaryngol Head Neck Surg. 1986;112:168–72.
81. Dedhia RD, Davis SJ, Stephan SJ. Optimizing septal perforation repair techniques. Curr Opin Otolaryngol Head Neck Surg. 2020;28(4):212–7.
82. Duffy FJ Jr, Rossi RM, Pribaz JJ. Reconstruction of Wegener's nasal deformity using bilateral facial artery musculomucosal flaps. Plast Reconstr Surg. 1998;101(5):1330–3.
83. Rasmussen N. Management of the ear, nose, and throat manifestations of Wegener granulomatosis: an otorhinolaryngologist's perspective. Curr Opin Rheumatol. 2001;13(1):3–11.
84. Goh AY, Hussain SSM. Different surgical treatments for nasal septal perforation and their outcomes. J Laryngol Otol. 2007;121:419–26.
85. Fairbanks DNF. Nasal septal perforation repair: 25-year experience with the flap and graft technique. Am J Cosmet Surg. 1994;11:189–94.
86. Giacomini PG, Ferraro S, Di Girolamo S, Ottaviani F. Large nasal septal & perforation repair by closed endoscopically assisted approach. Ann Plast Surg. 2011;66:633–6.
87. Stoor P, Gre'nman R. Bioactive glass and turbinate flaps in the repair of nasal septal perforations. Ann Otol Rhinol Laryngol. 2004;113:655–61.
88. Woolford TJ, Jones NS. Repair of nasal septal perforations using local mucosal flaps and a composite cartilage graft. J Laryngol Otol. 2001;115(1):22–5.
89. Gravina A, Pai KK, Shave S, Eloy JA, Fang CH. Endoscopic techniques for nasal septal perforation repair: a systematic review. Ann Otol Rhinol Laryngol. 2023;132(5):527–35. https://doi.org/10.1177/00034894221098704. Epub 2022 Jun 8. PMID: 35676865
90. Lee KC, Lee NH, Ban JH, Jin SM. Surgical treatment using an allograft dermal matrix for nasal septal perforation. Yonsei Med J. 2008;49:244–8.

91. Teymoortash A, Hoch S, Eivazi B, Werner JA. Experiences with a new && surgical technique for closure of large perforations of the nasal septum in 55 patients. Am J Rhinol Allergy. 2011;25:193–7.
92. Moon IJ, Kim SW, Han DH, et al. Predictive factors for the outcome of nasal septal perforation repair. Auris Nasus Larynx. 2011;38:52–7.
93. Mansour HA. Repair of nasal septal perforation using inferior turbinate graft. J Laryngol Otol. 2011;125:474–8.
94. Kridel RWH. Considerations in the etiology, treatment, and repair of septal perforations. Facial Plast Surg Clin North Am. 2004;12:435–50.
95. Castelnuovo P, Ferreli F, Khodaei I, Palma P. Anterior ethmoidal artery septal flap for the Management of Septal Perforation. Arch Facial Plast Surg. 2011;13(6):411–4. https://doi.org/10.1001/archfaci.2011.44.
96. Zocchi J, Russo F, Volpi L, Elhassan HA, Pietrobon G, Arosio A, Bignami M, Castelnuovo P. Long term outcomes of Nasoseptal perforation repair with an anterior ethmoidal artery flap. Am J Rhinol Allergy. 2022;36(1):18–24. https://doi.org/10.1177/19458924211012120. Epub 2021 Apr 20. PMID: 33878936
97. Rusetsky Y, Mokoyan Z, Spiranskaya O, Arutyunyan S. Cross-septal returned flap: modified endoscopic technique for bilateral closure of septal perforation. Int J Oral Maxillofac Surg. 2020;49(10):1260–3. https://doi.org/10.1016/j.ijom.2020.01.026. Epub 2020 Feb 20. PMID: 32088131
98. Santamaría-Gadea A, Langdon C, Alobid I. Extended anterior ethmoidal artery flap: novel endoscopic technique for large septal perforation. Laryngoscope. 2022;132(2):298–300. https://doi.org/10.1002/lary.29748. Epub 2021 Aug 6. PMID: 34357591
99. Cavada MN, Orgain CA, Alvarado R, Sacks R, Harvey RJ. Septal perforation repair utilizing an anterior ethmoidal artery flap and collagen matrix. Am J Rhinol Allergy. 2019;33(3):256–62. https://doi.org/10.1177/1945892418816959.
100. Santamaría-Gadea A, Vaca M, de Los SG, Alobid I, Mariño-Sánchez F. Greater palatine artery pedicled flap for nasal septal perforation repair: radiological study and case series. Eur Arch Otorrinolaringol. 2021;278(6):2115–21. https://doi.org/10.1007/s00405-020-06230-1.
101. Teichgraeber JF, Russo RC. The management of septal perforations. Plast Reconstr Surg. 1993;91:229–35.
102. Alobid I, Langdon C, Santamaria A. Technique to repair total septal perforation with a pericranial flap: the money box approach. JAMA Facial Plast Surg. 2018;20(4):324–5.
103. Friedman M, Ibrahim H, Ramakrishnan V. Inferior turbinate flap for repair of nasal septal perforation. Laryngoscope. 2003;113:1425–8.
104. Rokkjaer MS, Barrett TQ, Petersen CG. Good results after endonasal cartilage closure of nasal septal perforations. Dan Med Bull. 2010;57:A4196.
105. Schultz-Coulon HJ. Three-layer repair of nasoseptal defects. Otolaryngol Head Neck Surg. 2005;132:213–8.
106. Almahbub AJ, Alsabih MI, Solaim MN, Alwihaibi WM, Alsuliman YA, Alfawwaz FS, AlQahtani AA. Endoscopic repair of nasal septal perforation with anterior ethmoidal artery flap using tunnel technique. Eur Arch Otorhinolaryngol. 2024. https://doi.org/10.1007/s00405-024-08843-2. Epub ahead of print. PMID: 39044061.

# Surgery of the Inferior Turbinate

# 13

Omar El-Banhawy and Mohamed El-Banhawy

**Key Points**

- The nasal turbinates are important anatomical structures in the lateral wall of the nose. They arise from the cartilaginous nasal capsule. The inferior nasal turbinate is a separate bone formed from the maxilloturbinal structure at the tenth week of gestation. The function of the nasal turbinates is to warm and humidify air entering the nasal cavity, and their curvature increases the overall surface area to assist in this function. The inferior turbinates alter their size by contracting or enlarging to permit or obstruct airflow, which regulates the moisture levels.
- Nasal obstruction is one of the most frequently reported symptoms in clinical practice, with up to one-third of the population affected. Beside septal deviation, hypertrophied turbinates are the second most frequent cause of obstructions to nasal breathing. Inferior turbinate hypertrophy is defined as the enlargement of the turbinate that may involve the bone and the mucosa. The main causes of inferior turbinate hypertrophy include septal deviation, allergic rhinitis, vasomotor rhinitis, and chronic hypertrophic rhinitis.
- Initial treatment of inferior turbinate hypertrophy is conservative, and the first-line therapy is antihistamines, systemic or topical decongestants, and corticosteroids. However, when conservative therapy fails, the next step is surgery. Except for the compensatory turbinate hyperplasia, a surgical reduction of the turbinate should only be indicated if a three-month conservative therapy has not had any subjective and success.

O. El-Banhawy
Department of Otolaryngology, Menofyia University, Shebeen El-Kom, Egypt

M. El-Banhawy (✉)
Department of Otolaryngology, Delta University, Dakahlia, Egypt


S. Elwany (ed.), *Current Rhinology*,
https://doi.org/10.1007/978-3-031-70077-4_13

- The treatment for inferior turbinate hypertrophy is tissue volume reduction surgery, a procedure aimed at reducing the volume of the mucosa of the lower nasal turbinates. Depending on the method, the surgery targets both the bone and submucosal tissue. The fibrosis on the submucosal tissue minimizes engorgement of the turbinates, while the bone reductions increase the intranasal space, relieving the nasal obstruction.
- The fact that there are several methods for turbinate reduction are used clearly demonstrates that there is apparently no ideal technique which guarantees long-term therapy success.
- The objective of this chapter was to demonstrate the effectiveness of different surgical procedures for inferior turbinate hypertrophy on functional and symptomatic outcomes in patients with nasal obstruction due to inferior turbinate hypertrophy that have failed medical management. The primary aim is to improve patient quality of life.

## 13.1 Inferior Turbinate

Each nasal cavity contains three turbinates: the superior, middle, and inferior turbinates. The nasal turbinates are important anatomical structures that arise from the cartilaginous nasal capsule. The inferior turbinate is the largest of all turbinates and lowest of the three and is covered with a mucous membrane. It extends horizontally from the lateral wall of the nasal cavity. Its length, on average, is 48.7 mm in men and 47.3 mm in women [1].

The inferior nasal turbinate is a separate bone formed from the maxilloturbinal structure at the tenth week of gestation. The inferior nasal turbinate consists of turbinate bone, mucoperiosteum, soft erectile tissue, and mucosa. The inferior turbinates are lined with mucosa consisting of ciliated pseudostratified columnar epithelium. The submucosal lamina propria supports this epithelial layer and contains parasympathetic nerve fibers, mucous glands, Goblet cells, and abundant vasculature. The venous capacity vessels (sinusoids) are subepithelially localized in the lamina propria of the inferior and middle turbinates. They are significantly involved in the regulation of the thickness of the mucosa. In a swollen condition, the volume of the inferior turbinate can increase by three to four times compared with its subsided state, and can then almost completely block the lower nasal passage [2].

The inferior nasal turbinate is expansible due to the presence of the submucosal cavernous plexus, especially well developed at its anterior part. The vasculature within the inferior turbinate most commonly exhibits a nasal cycle of engorgement on one side, whereas the opposite side is decongested. The inferior turbinates alter their size by contracting or enlarging to permit or obstruct airflow, which regulates the moisture levels. This pattern switches every 2–6 h [3].

The function of the nasal turbinates is to warm and humidify air entering the nasal cavity, trap particles >4 μm, and direct airflow throughout the nasal cavity, and their curvature increases the overall surface area to assist in this function [1].

## 13.2 Inferior Turbinate Hypertrophy

The most common cause of nasal obstruction is nasal septum deviation, followed by inferior turbinate hypertrophy. Inferior turbinate hypertrophy is defined as the enlargement of the turbinate that may involve the bone and the mucosa. Although this enlargement is mostly reversible, it can persist, as in cases of vasomotor rhinitis, allergic rhinitis, or compensatory hypertrophy, because of septal deviation [4].

There are several classification systems for inferior turbinate hypertrophy. Three of them are based on clinical examination of the inferior turbinate size, while one is based on computed tomography scan imaging [4]. Friedman et al. [4] used the three-grading system; grade 1 is mild enlargement with no obvious obstruction, grade 2 is incomplete obstruction, and grade 3 complete occlusion of the nasal cavity (Fig. 13.1).

Many different medical therapies have been applied to treat hypertrophied inferior turbinate, including the use of antihistamines, systemic decongestants, or intranasal sprays which are commonly used to treat those conditions, principally to reduce nasal obstruction and restore comfortable nasal breathing. However, surgical reduction may be a good option in those cases in which medical treatment has failed [5]. The treatment for ITH is tissue volume reduction surgery, a procedure aimed at reducing the volume of the mucosa of the lower nasal turbinates which aimed to increase the cross-sectional area of the nasal valve to relieve nasal blockage. Depending on the method, the surgery targets both the bone and submucosal tissue. The fibrosis on the submucosal tissue minimizes engorgement of the turbinates, while the bone reductions increase the intranasal space, relieving the nasal

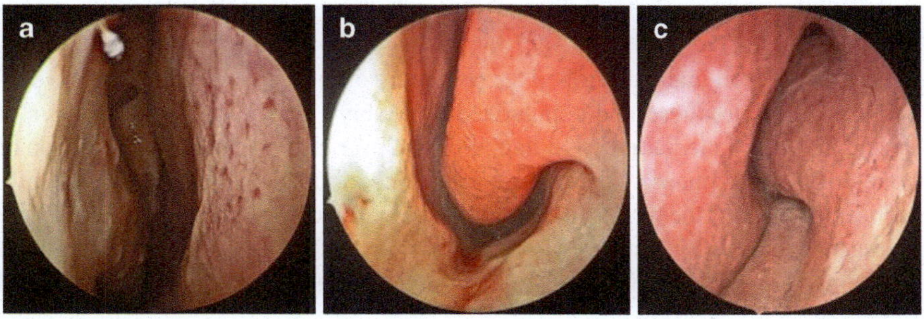


**Fig. 13.1** Endoscopic grading system of inferior turbinate hypertrophy according to Friedman et al. [4]. (A) Grade 1: is mild enlargement of right nasal cavity. (B) Grade 2 is incomplete obstruction left nasal cavity. (C) Grade 3 is complete obstruction of inferior turbinate left cavity

obstruction [5]. The main aim of turbinate surgery has to be the preservation of a well-functioning mucosa membrane while at the same time creating a sufficiently large air space to ensure the humidification and purification of air and the maintenance of a physiological airway resistance.

### 13.2.1 The Most Common Surgical Procedures Applied for Turbinate Hypertrophy

The goal of turbinate surgery is to reduce the erectile submucosal tissue volume and the bony turbinate.

Types of surgical technique for turbinate reduction.

| Nonmucosal preservation surgery | Mucosal preservation surgery |
|---|---|
| Conventional turbinectomy (partial or total) | Conventional turbinoplasty |
| Electrocautery turbinectomy | Microdebrider turbinoplasty |
| Laser turbinectomy | Coblation turbinoplasty |
| Cryoturbinectomy | Radiofrequency turbinoplasty |
| | Ultrasound turbinoplasty<br>Quantum molecular resonance |

## 13.3 Mucosal Preservation Surgery

### 13.3.1 Conventional Turbinoplasty

This surgery is designed to remove the nonfunctional obstructive part of the turbinate while preserving the functional medial mucosa, which plays the key role in the warming and humidification of air through the nasal passages. The term turbinoplasty covers various methods of intraturbinal surgical reduction of the inferior turbinate volume with preservation of the mucosa. The other term used for this technique is "submucosal resection," as a reference to its submucosal dissection procedure.

Freer [6] in originally described the procedure of inferior turbinoplasty. The procedure was reintroduced and popularized by Mabry [7]. The operation consists of development of a medial mucosal flap of the inferior turbinate and then resection of bone and lateral mucosa. The advantage of this procedure is that it significantly reduces the bulk of the turbinate, but preserves the functional medial mucosa. There is less bleedings and lower formation of crusts. According to the surgeon training, it can be performed in a satisfactory time without increasing for too long the surgical time [7].

In a study done by El Henawi et al. [8], they found that endoscopic turbinoplasty was associated with lesser intraoperative blood loss, and it was also associated with a longer operative duration in comparison with submucous resection of inferior turbinate. Also, the learning curve for endoscopic turbinoplasty may be steeper, and hence, the role of surgical experience must be borne in mind while interpreting these results, as an experienced endoscopic surgeon may take lesser duration for the procedure as compared to a novice.

### 13.3.2 Microdebrider Turbinoplasty

Microdebrider turbinoplasty, a surgical procedure, involves the use of a microdebrider, which is a powered rotary instrument with a cutting tip that rapidly oscillates back and forth with the capability of continuously suctioning blood from the operative site, allowing better surgical visual field and permitting precise tissue removal in a mucosal-sparing manner. It is selected to accomplish partial inferior turbinectomy, allowing for controlled and rapid removal of hypertrophic soft tissue while preserving the general turbinate form. Procedure disadvantages are obvious: The need of general anesthesia and the relative cost of equipment, in the other hand, the surgery is safe with low morbidity rate, well-tolerated, mucosal preservative, and easily can combine with other sinonasal procedures. In terms of complications, microdebrider may has a higher incidence of postoperative bleeding compared to radiofrequency but a smaller amount of intraoperative blood loss and shorter operative time compared to submucosal resection [9].

### 13.3.3 Coblation Turbinoplasty

Coblation is a unique method of delivering radiofrequency energy to the soft tissue for applications in otolaryngology. Coblation turbinoplasty is performed by inserting electrodes into tissues, which produces radiofrequency currents. These currents induce coagulative necrosis and fibrotic atrophy around tissues, and this necrosis induces healing which eventually decreases the volume of the inflammation caused edema [4]. Moreover, this procedure can conserve nasal mucosa and minimizes postoperative complication and discomfort with less pain and faster recovery for cases where tissue is excised [4]. Coblation turbinoplasty can be consider as an effective and safer procedure in inferior turbinate hypertrophy than other conventional turbinoplasty technique as it operates at relatively low temperatures compared to traditional electrocautery, allowing for controlled tissue removal with minimal damage to surrounding structures. The disadvantage of coblation turbinoplasty is that it may cause more postoperative crusting and bleeding [4].

### 13.3.4 Radiofrequency Turbinoplasty

Radiofrequency turbinoplasty is a minimally invasive technique that reduces the turbinate volume in a precise and targeted manner. It uses radiofrequency to reduce the tissue volume with minimal impact on surrounding tissues. Radiofrequency thermal ablation principle is to transfer low-frequency energy into the submucosa by a specially designed electrode. The transferred energy triggers an ionic agitation in the tissue and causes a temperature rise, thus forming a thermal lesion in the submucosa. Although there is a temperature of on average no more than 75 °C, this is nevertheless sufficient to induce thermonecrosis. During the healing period, contraction of tissues due to fibrosis leads to a decrease in the total volume of the turbinate. It is a reliable method that can be performed even in office settings under local anesthesia. However, relapses are likely to occur in the long-term follow-up, similar to other techniques of inferior turbinate surgery [10].

### 13.3.5 Ultrasound Turbinoplasty

In recent years, high-intensity focused ultrasound (HIFU) has been used for the treatment of benign lesions in obstetrics, gynecology, and urology. It is a noninvasive treatment that effectively coagulates and necrotizes target tissues (mainly solid tumors) that are located deep within the body without damaging the surrounding tissue. Ultrasound turbinoplasty, also known as sonoturboplasty or ultrasound-guided turbinoplasty, is a relatively novel approach for treating nasal obstruction caused by enlarged turbinates. The procedure is performed by inserting an activated ultrasonic nasal probe submucosally through the inferior turbinate and advancing it along its length. Then, the probe was moved in a forward–backward movement in a slow and gentle manner. At the end of this process, the nasal probe was withdrawn from the turbinate tissue [11].

Kim et al. [11], findings showed better mucosal preservation in HIFU-treated turbinates than in radiofrequency-treated turbinates. The volume of the nasal cavity calculated by CT scans was higher in the HIFU-treated turbinates than in the non-treated turbinates, and this effect was similar to the changes observed in radiofrequency-treated turbinates. Therefore, HIFU turbinoplasty is a useful technique to reduce inferior turbinate hypertrophy as it showed better results, with decreased nasal resistance, increased nasal flow, and significant increase in nasal patency with minimal complications. This technique is a relatively newer, and its widespread adoption and long-term outcomes may still be under evaluation [11].

### 13.3.6 Quantum Molecular Resonance

Quantum molecular resonance (QMR) devices have been applied as energy-based devices in many head and neck surgeries. QMR devices are powered using electron energy quanta, which is generated by alternate current and high-frequency electron

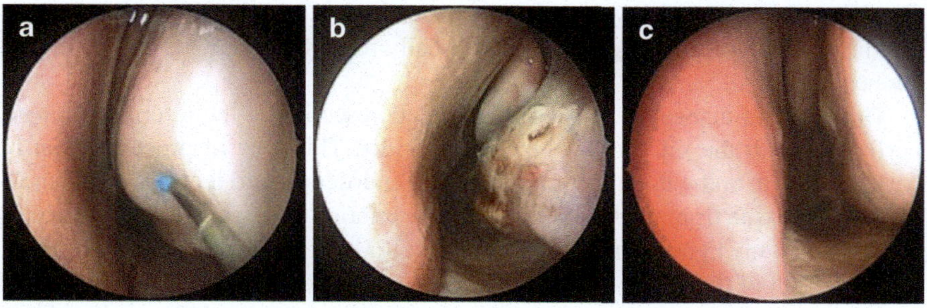


**Fig. 13.2** Endoscopic view of grade 3 inferior turbinate hypertrophy: (A) Grade 3 Left inferior turbinate hypertrophy. Intraoperative during application of quantum probe submucosal. (B) Immediate post-application of molecular quantum probe showing the shrinkage of the turbinate. (C) The size of the turbinate 6 months postoperative

waves, and it is characterized by a well-defined dominant wave at 4 MHz, followed by waves at 8, 12, and 16 MHz with reduced amplitude [5]. As the electron energy quanta is delivered, cell molecular bonds in human tissue resonate, followed by subsequent bond breakage and a minimal temperature increase. The process also activates the physiological coagulation cascade without the need for necrotic plugs, which is contrary to methods that use other cauterization methods [12]. The mechanism of action is based on molecular bound breaking: QMR generates frequencies that makes bounds resonate and break keeping the surrounding tissues at a low temperature (<45 °C) [12].

Quantic molecular resonance treatment is an outpatient procedure that can be performed under minimally invasive local anesthesia, and it is a rapid (about 10 min of treatment) and accurate technique (the wound is extremely localized with minimal effects on the surrounding tissues (Fig. 13.2). If necessary, this procedure can be repeated, and the rate of postoperative complications such as pain, early and late bleeding, synechiae, scabs, infections, and nasal dryness is substantially minimal.

## 13.4 Non Mucosal Preservation Surgery

### 13.4.1 Conventional Turbinectomy (Partial or Total)

There are two main types of turbinectomy:

**Partial Turbinectomy** where a portion of the inferior turbinate, usually the posterior is removed, typically the part that is causing the obstruction. This procedure aims to alleviate nasal congestion while preserving some of the turbinate tissue to maintain their important functions. The procedure may be performed by direct visualization or with the aid of an endoscope [4].

Friedman also use the shaver intraturbinally and suggest this variation as a technically safe alternative [4].

**Total Turbinectomy** It involves the complete removal of either the inferior or middle turbinates. This is less common and usually reserved for severe cases of turbinate enlargement.

This surgical maneuver consists in complete resection of the inferior turbinate, performed with the scissors or the microdebrider. This type of procedure can be performed with and without the use of a nasal endoscope, and it consists in removing the soft tissue from the lateral aspect of the inferior turbinate and the underlying bone, when bony hypertrophy is also involved [13].

As a result of the partial or total turbinectomy, an important improvement of the nasal breathing can be observed, the recurrence being exceptional. Some side effects can be observed after this procedure. The exposed raw mucosal edges and bone may lead to nasal crusting with need for postoperative debridement. Despite the electrocautery control, the mucosal edges may continue to bleed and nasal packing may be required for hemostasis. Sometimes, postoperative pain is very important. Atrophic rhinitis is also a threat to the patients submitted to these procedures [13].

Some evidence exists that turbinectomy may lead to a high incidence of empty nose syndrome, an iatrogenic syndrome of chronic nasal impairment due to extended. Unfortunately, this type of surgery, extremely aggressive, can later lead to dry nose syndrome or even the syndrome of the empty nose with a paradoxical obstruction. The obstructive event is due to the loss of normal nasal resistance and the formation of a laminar air column. This situation causes a poor contact between the air and the nasal walls, the mucosa, due to the absence of the sensory fibers of the inferior turbinate, and shows a reduction or even a loss of the respiratory flow. Some authors considered total turbinectomy is a nasal crime, and they do not consider it useful to perform the resection of more than a third or half of the inferior turbinate.

Elwany et al. [13] compared partial turbinectomy against three other techniques for inferior turbinate reduction to determine their subjective and objective outcomes. Their study found both partial turbinectomy and laser turbinectomy outperformed the other two techniques of inferior turbinoplasty and cryoturbinectomy in terms of relieving nasal obstruction and improving olfaction. In addition, all four techniques did not affect mucociliary clearance. However, the authors observed those patients who underwent partial turbinectomy developed nasal discomfort, headache, atrophic changes, and postoperative bleeding more than others.

### 13.4.2 Electrocautery Turbinectomy

Electrocautery (EC) is the oldest method of treating inferior turbinate hypertrophy. It was first applied by Heider in 1845; however, it was not quite preferred until Neres and Horn reinvented it by applying EC submucosally in the early nineteenth century [14]. It has become more popular after World War II, when it was found that submucosal coagulation has better results and fewer undesirable effects on the nasal mucosa. On a mucosal and submucosal level, atrophic and metaplastic changes up to and including the loss of cilia can be found, which has a negative effect on the mucociliary transport. The effect of submucosal cauterization is based on coagulation of venous sinusoids within the turbinate, leading to a submucosal fibrosis and reduction of inferior turbinate volume. Despite being the oldest surgical option, EC is still used as a first-choice treatment by many otorhinolaryngologists [14]. It is considered by some authors as the least effective in improving nasal airway resistance and reducing turbinate volume, with higher rates of postoperative crusting and nasal synechiae reported [15]. Therapeutic success is short-lived; the recurrence of turbinate hyperplasia cannot be prevented in the long-term [15].

### 13.4.3 Laser Turbinectomy

Tissue ablation procedures, using diode lasers, carbon dioxide lasers, argon lasers, neodymium-yttrium aluminum garnet lasers, holmium yttrium aluminum garnet lasers, and potassium-titanyl phosphate lasers, have been widely used in developed countries. These laser types differ on emitted laser wavelength, output power, wave emission, and mode of application. Different laser systems have been used increasingly and, to some extent successfully, to shrink turbinates and good outcome with minimum morbidity [16].

Various modes of laser are available for inferior turbinate reduction. Carbon dioxide laser is used when there is hyperplastic head of the turbinate, and if the entire length of turbinate is hypertrophied, the Nd:YAG laser has been preferred. Diode laser in addition to Hog:YAG laser is opted for outpatient procedure under local anesthesia with good long-term results [13]. Although the outcomes using conventional modalities are known since a long time, there are limited studies with the usage of diode lasers for turbinate reduction. Further as it is cost-effective, the present study was undertaken to compare outcomes to diode laser turbinate reduction (LTR) and conventional partial inferior turbinectomy (PIT) [16].

The advantages of the laser surgical procedure include lack of bleeding and limited tissue trauma as well as the ability to offer it as an outpatient treatment [16]. It has been widely used recently due to good outcome with minimum morbidity. The lasers commonly used for inferior turbinate reduction are diode and $CO_2$ lasers. Carbon dioxide laser is used when there is hyperplastic head of the turbinate, and if the entire length of turbinate is hypertrophied, the Nd:YAG laser has been preferred [16, 17].

Laser reduction of inferior turbinate may confer many advantages. Freedom from postoperative packing should be distinct advantage especially in children. Laser turbinectomy offers less intraoperative bleeding, postoperative pain, and discomfort and less use of analgesia and less stay in the hospital [16]. Laser reduction of inferior satisfies most of the criteria to fulfill to be an ideal treatment of choice in addition to preserving physiological functions. Although not as cost-effective as conventional methods, better quality of life with laser definitely makes it an important tool to replace the era of cold knife in turbinate surgeries in the modern-day world.

### 13.4.4 Cryoturbinectomy

Cryosurgery for chronic rhinitis was first introduced by Ozenberger [18]. Cryotherapy is a minimally invasive procedure that uses nitrous oxide or liquid nitrogen as a cooling agent and induces necrosis by freezing the turbinate. This method under local anesthesia with the help of cryoprobe cooling agent (nitrous oxide or liquid nitrogen) is applied on the surface of turbinates. There is intracellular ice crystal formation and protein denaturation and subsequent tissue destruction which lead to debulking of turbinates. The duration of application time varied from 5 s to 3 min. The overall short-term results are satisfactory, but the benefit is usually not sustainable and amount of volume reduction is hard to predict in comparison with other methods, and it has dismal long-term results [5]. Cryosurgery was later gradually abandoned due to the availability of new techniques enabling better procedures to be performed.

## 13.5 Turbinate Surgery in Children

The anatomical dimensions of a child's nose are tiny: The length of the inferior turbinate in a three-year old is about 30 mm, and an adult's is around 35–50 mm. The distance to the nasal floor in a one-year old is about 4 mm, in an adult 6.8 mm [19].

In their study, Siméon et al. [20], claimed very high prevalence of turbinate hypertrophy in children with allergic rhinitis: about 81%. Therefore, this sign may represent a relevant clinical characteristic of allergic rhinitis in childhood especially among children with asthma, bronchial and simultaneous cortisone resistance, pathologically enlarged turbinates can be found regularly. The turbinate hypertrophy can become problematic, leading to conditions such as chronic nasal congestion, difficulty breathing, and recurrent sinus infections. The surgery aims to alleviate these symptoms and improve the overall nasal function.

The children met criteria for surgery, with nasal obstruction resistant to antihistamines and local corticosteroids and, in some cases, to attempted specific desensitization. In such cases of failure, management guidelines recommend surgical inferior turbinate reduction.

When compared to adults, turbinate reduction surgery in children is contentious and debatable. Medical therapy should always be optimized before surgical therapy is contemplated. The surgical therapy of turbinates in childhood should be carried out as cautiously and as conservatively as possible in order to avoid growth disorders resulting from surgery. Hence, any surgery of turbinates in childhood should be limited to avoid unwarranted complication. For this reason, gentle methods for reduction of the turbinate mucosa which may be repeated are recommended [19].

Radiofrequency turbinoplasty seems to provide an optimal combination of turbinate volume and hence obstruction, reduction, and conserved nasal function. It has been shown to conserve mucociliary function, with lower associated morbidity [19]. Coblation turbinoplasty differs from the radiofrequency technologies based on a thermal process of molecular ionization: It achieves low-temperature molecular disintegration, with minimal necrosis of neighboring tissue. Coblation turbinoplasty is associated with less pain, improved healing, and no excessive crusts which are essential preconditions for treatment in pediatrics [20].

Due to limited data and uncertainty over the long-term adverse effects, the decision to perform surgical turbinate reduction in children depends on clinical judgment and the preference of patients or their guardians/parents. In terms of surgical steps, there are no differences between children and adults.

## 13.6 Adjunct Techniques

Out-fracture of the inferior turbinate may be performed with other turbinate reduction techniques. It involves lateral displacement of broken out inferior turbinate by an initial in-fracture, moving it medially from its attachment at the lateral nasal wall. The basis of doing this procedure is to create additional space when inferior turbinate is lateralized. Its efficacy is variable, resulting in much criticism over its role. As there is a tendency for the turbinate to return to its original position, it is not recommended as a single procedure, but it may be used to supplement the other techniques [5].

### 13.6.1 What Is the Ideal Surgical Technique for the Reduction of Inferior Turbinate Hypertrophy?

There is no gold standard procedure in treating turbinate hypertrophy either mucosal or osseous hypertrophy or both. Any procedure must improve or preserve the mucosal morphology. Both microdebrider turbinoplasty and radiofrequency technology have the advantage of most effective safe, widespread use, and familiarity. Ultrasound turbinoplasty is the next most promising technology.

In 2010, a review by plastic surgeons and otorhinolaryngologists by "American Society for Aesthetic Plastic Surgery" [21]:

61.9% of prefer conventional turbinoplasty.
35.2% prefer out-fracture of inferior turbinate (as a sole procedure).
8.6% give radiofrequency technology.

## 13.7 Empty Nose Syndrome

Empty nose syndrome (ENS) is a clinical entity without consensual definition. The descriptive term "empty nose syndrome" (ENS), or more exactly "empty nose syndrome of Stenkvist," was originally coined in 1994 by Kern and Stenkvist who, when investigating coronary CT images of paranasal sinuses, recognized a considerable loss of tissue in the region of the inferior and middle turbinates, and who described this condition as "empty nose" [22]. It is a rare complication of nose or

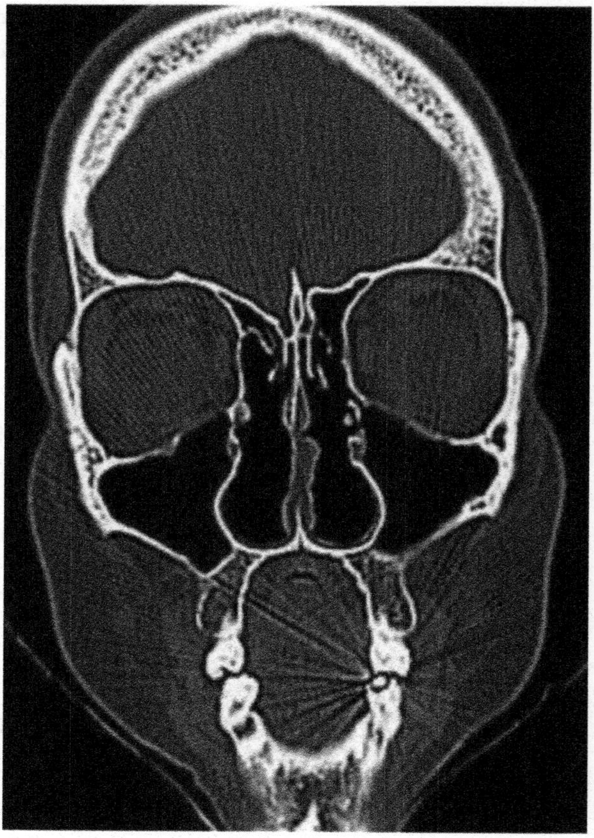

**Fig. 13.3** Coronal CT scan showing extensive resection of both the inferior and middle turbinates representing empty nose syndrome

sinus surgery, and of inferior turbinectomy in particular. Physiopathology remains unclear, but probably involves disorder caused by excessive nasal permeability affecting neurosensitive receptors and inhaled air humidification and conditioning functions [22].

In Anglo-American usage, ENS is divided up into three subtypes: The ENS inferior turbinate (ENS-IT) refers to the situation when the inferior turbinate has been removed. ENS middle turbinate (ENSMT) describes the condition after removal of the middle turbinate, and ENS-both refers to the resection of all turbinates (Fig. 13.3) [23].

Pathogenesis of ENS is multifactorial and includes changes in laminar physiological airflow, disruption of mucosa functions, and deficient neural sensation. This leads to the development of ENS symptomatology such as dyspnea, nasal dryness, nasal burning, nasal obstruction, feeling of suffocation, and even comorbid psychiatric disorders that significantly impairs life quality. ENS symptom development is usually delayed, from months to years postoperatively, and the symptom severity is not strictly dependent on the resected tissue volume [24].

The treatment strategy for ENS should be complex and overcome the three main challenges: (1) Reconstitute the nasal anatomical structure that will allow the nasal airway resistance increasing; (2) Recover damaged nasal mucosa that will result in edema decreasing, normalizing air heating and humidifying; and (3) Stimulate nerve recovery and renew tissue sensitivity [25, 26]. In recent years, stem cell-based therapies were extensively studied, and promising results were acquired for various stem cell types combined with different grafts and biomaterials. However, there remain some challenges to be solved, such as the low survival rate of transplanted cells and the difficulty of restoring the proper volume and normal architecture of the organ tissue [27].

## References

1. Georgakopoulos B, Hohman MH, Le PH. Anatomy, head and neck, nasal concha. In: StatPearls publishing, FL. Treasure Island, FL: StatPearls Publishing; 2022.
2. Berger G, Hammel I, Berger R, Avraham S, Ophir D. Histopathology of the inferior turbinate with compensatory hypertrophy in patients with deviated nasal septum. Laryngoscope. 2000;110:2100–5.
3. Ozcan KM, Selcuk A, Ozcan I, Akdogan O, Dere H. Anatomical variations of nasal turbinates. J Craniofac Surg. 2008;19:1678–82.
4. Friedman M, Tanyeri H, Lim J, Landsberg R, Caldarelli D. A safe, alternative technique for inferior turbinate reduction. Laryngoscope. 1999;109:1834–7. https://doi.org/10.1097/00005537-199911000-00021.
5. Passali D, Passali FM, Damiani V, Passali GC, Bellussi L. Treatment of inferior turbinate hypertrophy: a randomized clinical trial. Ann Otol Rhinol Laryngol. 2003;112:683–8.
6. Freer OT. The inferior turbinate: its longitudinal resection for chronic intumescence. Laryngoscope. 1911;21:1136–44.
7. Mabry RL. Inferior turbinoplasty. Arch Otolaryngol Head Neck Surg. 1988;114(10):1189.
8. El Henawi DEDM, Ahmed MR, Madian YT. Comparison between power-assisted turbinoplasty and submucosal resection in the treatment of inferior turbinate hypertrophy. ORL J Otorhinolaryngol Relat Spec. 2011;73(3):151–5.
9. Kanesan N, Norhayati MN, Hamid SSA, Abdullah B. Microdebrider-assisted inferior turbinoplasty versus other surgical techniques. Acta Otorhinolaryngol Ital. 2022;42(5):415–26.
10. Utley DS, Goode RL, Hakim I. Radiofrequency energy tissue ablation for the treatment of nasal obstruction secondary to turbinate hypertrophy. Laryngoscope. 1999;109:683–6.
11. Kim JK, Cho SW, Kim H, Jo SC, Kim HG, Won TB, Kim JW, Lim JH, Rhee CS. Development of high-intensity focused ultrasound therapy for inferior turbinate hypertrophy. Clin Exp Otorhinolaryngol. 2022;15(2):160–7.
12. Vescovi P, Manfredi M, Merigo E, Fornaini C, Rocca J-P, Nammour S, et al. Quantic molecular resonance scalpel and its potential applications in Oral surgery. Br J Oral Maxillofacial Surg. 2008;46(5):355–7.
13. Elwany S, Harrison R. Inferior turbinectomy: comparison of four techniques. J Laryngol Otol. 1990;104:206–9.
14. Hol MK, Huizing EH. Treatment of inferior turbinate pathology: a review and critical evaluation of the different techniques. Rhinology. 2000;38(157–166):2.
15. Zhang K, Pipaliya RM, Miglani A, Nguyen SA, Schlosser RJ. Systematic review of surgical interventions for inferior turbinate hypertrophy. Am J Rhinol Allergy. 2023;37(1):110–22.
16. Ohyama M, Yamashita K, Furuta S, Nobori T, DaikuzonoN. Applications of the Nd:YAG laser in otorhinolaryngology. In: Joffe SN, Oguro Y, editors. Advances in Nd:YAGLaser surgery. New York, NY: Springer; 1988. p. 156–65.

17. Sroka R, Janda P, Killian T, Vaz F, Betz CS, Leunig A. Comparison of long term results after Ho:YAG and diode laser treatment of hyperplastic inferior nasal turbinates. Lasers Surg Med. 2007;39:324–31.
18. Ozenberger JM. Cryosurgery in chronic rhinitis. Laryngoscope. 1970;80:723–34.
19. Komshian SR, Cohen MB, Brook C, Levi JR. Inferior turbinate hypertrophy: a review of the evolution of management in children. Am J Rhinol Allergy. 2019;33:212–9.
20. Siméon R, Soufflet B, Souchal Delacour I. Coblation turbinate reduction in childhood allergic rhinitis. Eur Ann Otorhinolaryngol Head Neck Dis. 2010;127(2):77–82.
21. Feldman EM, Koshy JC, Chike-Obi CJ, Hatef DA, Bullocks JM, Stal S. Contemporary techniques in inferior turbinate reduction: survey results of the American Society for Aesthetic Plastic Surgery. Aesthet Surg J. 2010;30(5):672–9.
22. Scheithauer MO. Surgery of the turbinates and "empty nose" syndrome. GMS Curr Top Otorhinolaryngol Head Neck Surg. 2010;9:Doc03.
23. Houser SM. Empty nose syndrome associated with middle turbinate resection. Otolaryngol Head Neck Surg. 2006;135:972–3. https://doi.org/10.1016/j.otohns.2005.04.017.
24. Payne SC. Empty nose syndrome: what are we really talking about? Otolaryngol Clin N Am. 2009;42:331–7 [ix-x].
25. Modrzynski M. Hyaluronic acid gel in the treatment of empty nose syndrome. Am J Rhinol Allergy. 2011;25:103–6.
26. Jang YJ, Kim JH, Song HY. Empty nose syndrome: radiologic findings and treatment outcomes of endonasal microplasty using cartilage implants. Laryngoscope. 2011;121:1308–12.
27. Gordiienko IM, Gubar OS, Sulik R, Kunakh T, Zlatskiy I, Zlatska A. Empty nose syndrome pathogenesis and cell-based biotechnology products as a new option for treatment. World J Stem Cells. 2021;13(9):1293–306.

# Rhinitis

# 14

Samy Elwany and Hossam Abdel Hai

**Key Points**

- Rhinitis is a widespread condition that causes significant morbidity worldwide and profoundly affects patients' quality of life.
- Rhinitis is still an ill-defined disease that includes controversial entities and few proven facts. The term "rhinopathy" is a more correct term than rhinitis since the common symptoms of rhinitis may exist in the absence of actual inflammation.
- The united airway concept is based upon the strong association between allergic rhinitis and asthma.
- Rhinitis is usually, and broadly, classified into infectious and non-infectious categories.
- The infectious category is the better-defined type. Non-infectious rhinitis may be allergic or non-allergic.
- Non-allergic rhinitis includes several categories: vasomotor, occupational, hormonal, drug-induced, and some other less common types.
- Allergic rhinitis may be over-diagnosed and/or under-treated, and it may considerably downgrade quality of life.
- Most types of rhinitis share several treatment options. However, some types require specific therapies.

S. Elwany (✉)
Department of Otolaryngology, Alexandria University, Alexandria, Egypt
e-mail: samy.elwany@alexmed.edu.eg

H. A. Hai
Department of Otolaryngology, Benha University, Benha, Egypt



S. Elwany (ed.), *Current Rhinology*,
https://doi.org/10.1007/978-3-031-70077-4_14

## 14.1 Introduction

Rhinitis is a prevalent condition that affects patients' quality of life [1], causes substantial morbidity worldwide, and has significant economic impact [2–4]. It has been reported that allergic rhinitis is a strong risk factor for asthma in adults and that 30% of patients with allergic rhinitis are predisposed to develop asthma along the course of the disease (The united airway concept) [5].

Despite the prevalence of rhinitis, it is still an ill-defined disease that includes many unclear entities and few proven facts. The term "rhinitis" is debatable as it denotes an inflammatory disease of the nasal mucosa. However, the usual symptoms of rhinitis such as itching, sneezing, rhinorrhea, and blockage may occur without actual inflammation. The term "rhinopathy" is a more correct term, but it is seldom used.

There is no universally established scheme for the definition, classification, or the terminology of different types of rhinitis. Use of the different terms for the same disease and of the same term for diverse diseases has, in part, made reports of rhinitis confusing and difficult to analyze and compare. The introduction of the term "rhinosinusitis" further complicated the issue since sinusitis may coexist with rhinitis many patients [6].

Both allergic and non-allergic rhinitis increase bronchial hyperreactivity and are risk factors for asthma. Allergic rhinitis may increase the risk of asthma about three-fold. It is estimated that about 70% of asthmatic patients have history of allergic rhinitis, and about 30% of patients with allergic rhinitis have tendency to develop asthma later. The close association between allergic rhinitis and bronchial asthma and the fact that upper respiratory tract infections trigger exacerbations of asthma led to the development of the "United Airway" concept [5, 7].

For all non-infectious rhinitis phenotypes, clinical presentation is similar with patients presenting withy nasal obstruction, rhinorrhea/postnasal drip, nasal itch, or sneezing. Symptoms should be present for two or more consecutive days and for more than 1 h on most days.

In practice, the clinical diagnosis can be complicated by the presence of two or more phenotypes. An overlap is also possible between mucosal and structural pathologies both contributing to the patients' symptom.

## 14.2 Classification of Rhinitis

Rhinitis is broadly classified into infectious and non-infectious groups, the infectious category being the better-defined type. Mixed forms of rhinitis do exist and can be confusing [6].

A. **Infectious:**
   a. Viral (e.g., common cold)
   b. Bacterial (e.g., rhinoscleroma)
   c. Fungal (e.g., Rhinosporidiosis)

B. **Non-infectious:**
  a. Allergic
  b. Non-allergic
    i. Non-allergic rhinitis mimicking allergic rhinitis
      1. Vasomotor rhinitis
      2. Non-allergic rhinitis with eosinophilia (NARES)
    ii. Occupational rhinitis
    iii. Gustatory rhinitis
    iv. Hormonal rhinitis
    v. Rhinopathy of pregnancy

## 14.3 Infectious Rhinitis

### 14.3.1 Acute Viral Rhinitis (Coryza—Common Cold)

Acute viral rhinitis is a common cause of bilateral nasal obstruction. The infection is caused by one of a multitude of rhinoviruses transmitted as droplets and mists from person to person. The disease is more common during winter, in children, in schools, and in crowded inadequately aerated areas.

Although the disease is self-limited, it may be complicated by secondary bacterial infection. The usual bacterial invaders include Streptococcus pneumoniae, Staphylococcus aureus, Hemophilus influenzae, and Moraxella catarrhalis. The distinction between viral and bacterial infections is usually based on clinical grounds including the duration of the disease and the presence of purulent discharge rather than recognition of the causative organisms.

#### 14.3.1.1 Clinical Picture

The disease has three stages following incubation period of 1–3 days:

a. Prodromal Stage (Stage of Invasion): This stage lasts for few hours and is characterized by sneezing, burning sensation in the nasopharynx, nasal obstruction, and headache.
b. Hyperemic Stage (Stage of Secretion): This stage lasts for 4–5 days and is characterized by low grade fever, arthralgia, malaise, nasal obstruction, and watery nasal discharge. The nasal mucosa appears congested, and a clear discharge may be seen in the nasal cavity (Fig. 14.1).
c. Resolution Stage: This is the natural course of an uncomplicated disease and is characterized by gradual resolution of symptoms within 5–7 days.

Symptoms lasting more than 7 days or worsening instead of improving indicate that secondary bacterial infection has occurred. Complications of the disease include acute bacterial rhinosinusitis, acute otitis media, and lower respiratory infections.

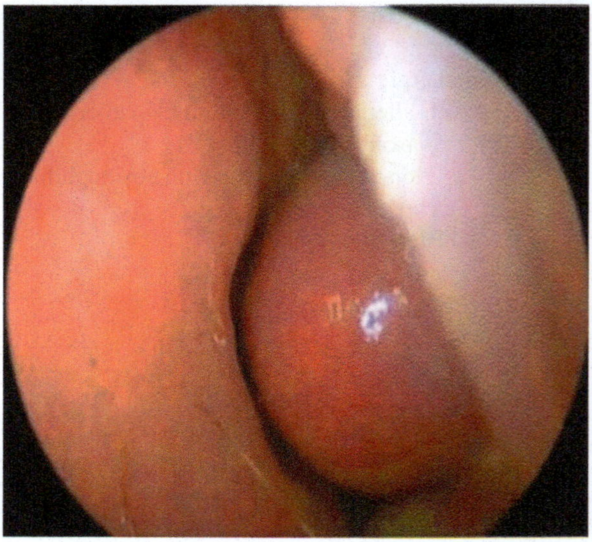

**Fig. 14.1** Acute vital rhinitis (common cold). The nasal mucosa appears red and congested

#### 14.3.1.2 Treatment

Only supportive treatment is required since the disease is self-limiting. Treatment may include bed rest, antipyretic-analgesics, nasal decongestants (local and/or systemic), and steam inhalations.

Antibiotics should be used only for cases complicated by secondary bacterial infections in order to avoid the development of resistant bacterial strains.

### 14.3.2 Scleroma

Scleroma is a one of the specific granulomata of the respiratory tract that is typically characterized by granulomatous lesions with characteristic hardness giving it the name scleroma (Fig. 14.2).

The disease was initially described by Von Hebra (in 1870) as a lesion involving the nose (rhinoscleroma). Now, it is known to also involve the larynx, trachea, and bronchi [8]. Atypical presentations are not uncommon in endemic areas (Fig. 14.3).

Scleroma is caused by gram-negative bacilli called Frisch bacillus or *Klebsiella rhinoscleromatis*. Special stains such as periodic acid–Schiff and Warthin-Starry silver stains can reveal the bacterial rods within histiocytes.

Scleroma is endemic in Egypt, Eastern Europe, Russia, and Central and South America (scleroma belt). It is more common in adults and has a higher incidence among low socio-economic classes. The mode of transmission of infection is not yet known.

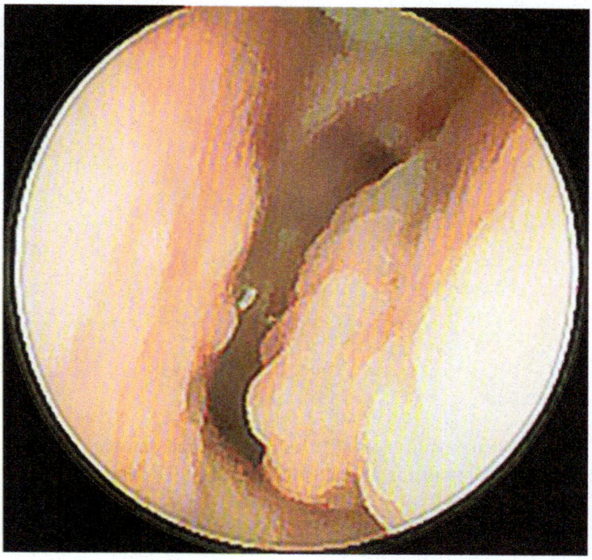

**Fig. 14.2** Granulomatous lesion at the early stage of scleroma

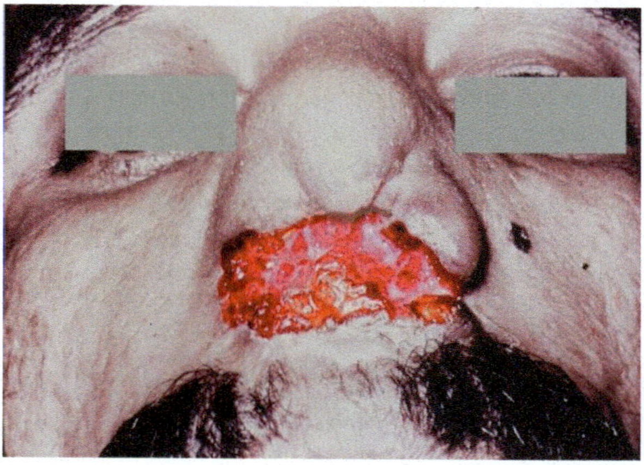

**Fig. 14.3** The granulomatous mass of scleroma extended outside the nasal cavities and destroyed the columella and anterior part of the nasal septum

## 14.3.2.1 Pathology

Scleroma exists in three forms: granulomatous, fibrotic, and atrophic. The granulomatous form is the most characteristic and common one. The three forms may overlap.

The granulomatous form is the active stage. In this stage, the submucosa is infiltrated by lymphocytes, plasma cells, and three characteristic components:

a. *Mikulicz cells* which are large vacuolated foam cells containing the scleroma bacilli. They are derived from histiocytes.
b. *Russell bodies* which are degenerated plasma cells staining red with eosin.

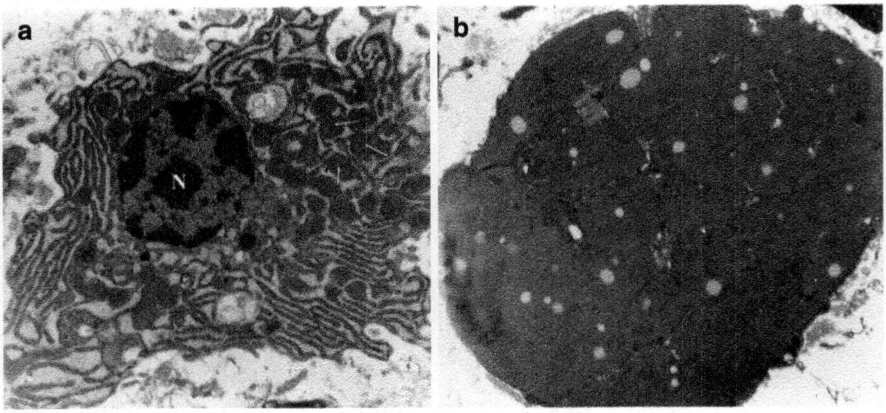


**Fig. 14.4** Transmission electron micrograph showing Mott call (**a**) and Russell body (**b**). The Mott call contains many inclusions (arrows). N = nucleus

c. *Mott* cells which are detected by transmission electron. Mott cells are plasma cells with numerous inclusion bodies and are thought to be the precursors of Russell bodies (Fig. 14.4).

In the fibrotic stage, the cellular infiltration is gradually replaced by fibroblasts and dense fibrous tissue giving the lesions its characteristic hardness and name. Contraction of the fibrous tissue may lead to partial or complete obliteration of the nasal cavity as well as external deformities.

In few cases, the nasal mucosa appears atrophic rather than granulomatous (secondary atrophic rhinitis). The epithelium shows squamous metaplasia with profound or total loss of cilia and goblet cells and scarce seromucinous glands [9, 10].

#### 14.3.2.2 Clinical Picture

Three clinical presentations have been described corresponding with the pathological features. These presentations are frequently intermingled together:

a. Granulomatous Presentation: This is the classical presentation where the nasal cavity shows firm pale pink granulomatous masses starting anteriorly near the mucocutaneous junction of the nose and extending posteriorly. The granulomatous masses may extend to the external nose and upper lip (Hebra nose).
b. Fibrotic Presentation: The nasal cavities are stenosed or obliterated by firm unyielding concentric fibrous tissue. External deformities are commonly present.
c. Atrophic Presentation: The mucosa appears thin, atrophic, and covered with crusts. The nasal cavity appears roomy with small turbinates.

#### 14.3.2.3 Involvement of Other Regions

Involvement of other regions is usually secondary to nasal involvement. Uncommonly, it is primary. The following sites may be involved:

a. The Pharynx (Pharyngoscleroma):

The nasopharynx may be stenosed and the soft plate may be fibrosed and tilted up (uvula sign). The tonsils also may be involved.

b. The Larynx (Laryngoscleroma):

Laryngeal involvement is more common in females, and it usually involves the subglottic region. In the granulomatous stage, the lesions usually appear as cushions in the subglottic region. In the fibrotic stage, contraction of the fibrous tissue produces concentric subglottic stenosis and stridor. The granulomata may extend to the trachea, and bronchi.

c. The lacrimal sac (dacryoscleroma).
d. The middle ear (tympanoscleroma).
e. The maxillary sinuses.

#### 14.3.2.4 Investigations

1. Biopsy. The characteristic pathological feature (Mikulicz cells and Russel bodies) usually confirms the diagnosis of scleroma.
2. Scrapings and culture for bacilli in difficult-to-treat cases-
3. Radiological Evaluation: CT scans show the granulomatous masses filing and expanding the nasal cavity and external nose. CT scans of the larynx and trachea, preferably with 3D reconstructions, will disclose the stenotic segments (Figs. 14.5 and 14.6).

#### 14.3.2.5 Differential Diagnosis

1. Sinonasal neoplasms.
2. Other granulomatous lesions.

#### 14.3.2.6 Treatment

1. Long course of antibiotics is the main treatment. The preferred antibiotic groups include the quinolones, aminoglycosides, and tetracyclines. Specific antibiotics may be also given after culture and sensitivity testing.

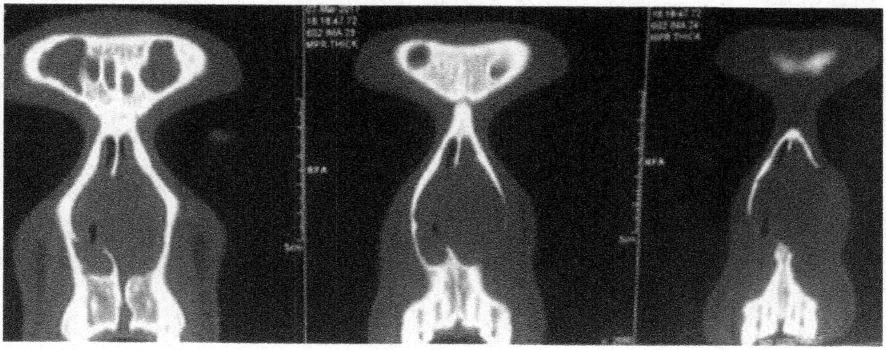

**Fig. 14.5** The granulomatous masses of scleroma filling both nasal cavities, destroying the nasal septum, and expanding the external nose

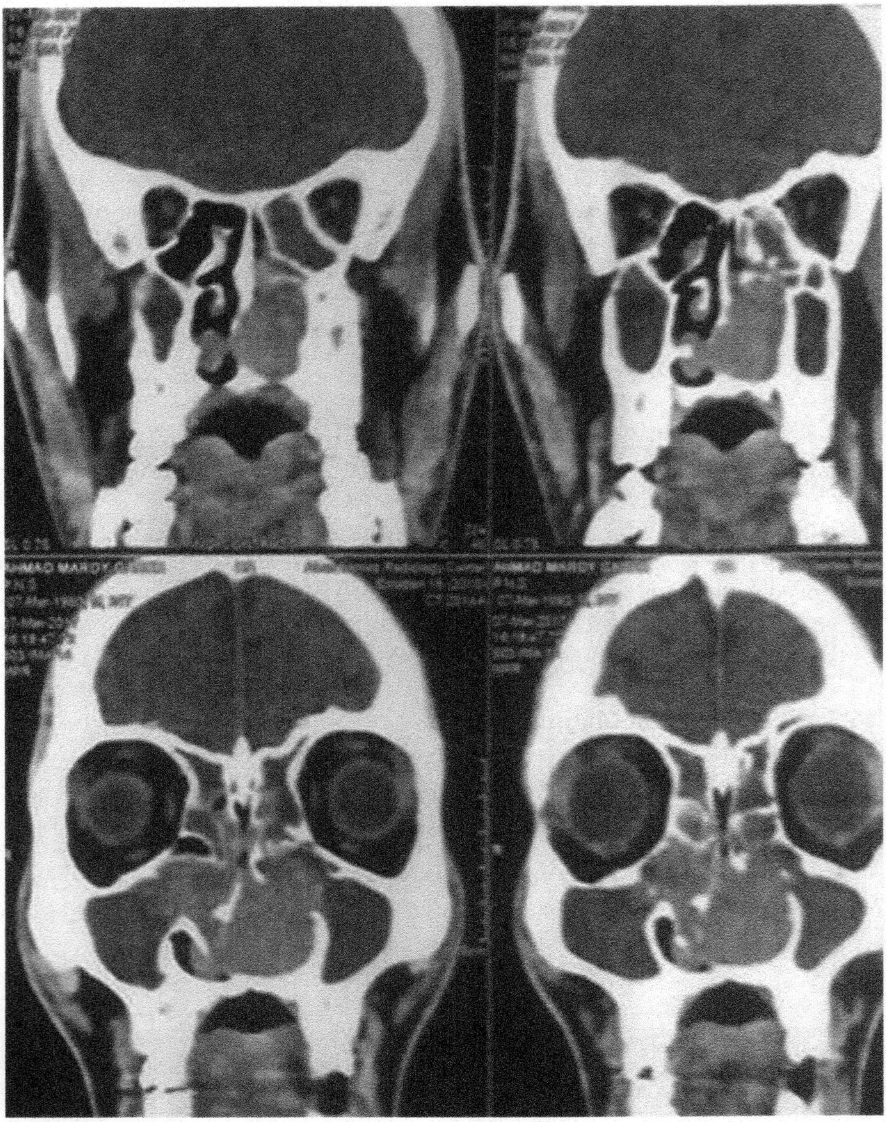

**Fig. 14.6** The granulomatous masses of scleroma fill both nasal cavities and destroy the nasal septum

2. Surgery may be needed to open the nasal airway and to correct external deformities. Patients with laryngotracheal stenosis may need dilatations, segmental resections, or tracheostomy.

### 14.3.3 Rhinosporidiosis

Rhinosporidiosis is a chronic granulomatous infection of the mucous membranes caused by Rhinosporidium seeberi. It is endemic in in India, Sri Lanka, South America, and Africa.

The disease usually presents with vascular friable strawberry-like polyps that arise from the nasal mucosa. Histologically, the polyps show pseudoepitheliomatous hyperplasia. The disease may also involve the conjunctiva and urethra.

The treatment of rhinosporidiosis is surgical excision of the polyp(s). Recurrences may infrequently occur [11, 12].

## 14.4 Allergic Rhinitis

### 14.4.1 Introduction

Allergic rhinitis is an immunoglobulin E (IgE)-mediated inflammatory nasal condition resulting from allergen introduction in a sensitized individual [13]. Presumptive diagnosis of allergic rhinitis is usually clinical and is made if someone experiences one or more of rhinorrhea, sneezing, itching of nose/palate/eyes, or nasal congestion in response to allergen exposure. Cough is also a common symptom. The diagnosis is confirmed with demonstration of specific IgE reactive to environmental allergens. Food allergy testing is not recommended in the routine evaluation of rhinitis. Treatment includes allergen avoidance (reducing exposure to relevant allergens such as dander, dust mite, and pollen), pharmacotherapy, and immunotherapy. Intranasal corticosteroids remain the single most effective class of medications for treating allergic rhinitis. Immunotherapy is often recommended for patients with persistent symptoms.

### 14.4.2 Definition

Allergic rhinitis (AR) is an immunoglobulin E (IgE)-mediated inflammatory nasal condition resulting from allergen exposure in a sensitized individual and resulting in the characteristic symptoms of nasal itching, sneezing, rhinorrhea, and nasal congestion. Frequently, there is itching in the palate and ocular symptoms such as itching, conjunctival redness, eyelid discoloration, and puffiness, and as well as increased lacrimation. Allergic rhinitis may cause depressed mode and decreased productivity [3, 14].

Atopy means genetic predisposition to develop allergic IgE-mediated response to allergens. Patients with a family history of allergies have a higher risk of developing allergic rhinitis. Patients who suffer from asthma or eczema are also more likely to develop allergic rhinitis [15].

The term the atopic (or allergic) march refers to the progressive development of allergic symptoms in childhood onwards. This starts with atopic dermatitis (allergic eczema) and may progress first to short-lasting food allergy and then to allergic asthma and allergic rhinitis.

### 14.4.3 Prevalence

Allergic rhinitis has been estimated to affect 20–25% of the population worldwide. It is more common in children and younger age groups. It is not uncommon for children to "grow out of their allergies" due to environmental or immunologic changes. There is usually a decrease in the number of allergic individuals in the geriatric population [2, 4].

### 14.4.4 Allergens

Inhalant allergens are the principal triggers of allergic rhinitis. Food allergens are less frequent. Allergic rhinitis may sometimes be triggered by exposures to proteins that do not commonly provoke IgE-mediated responses such as wood dusts and grain dusts.

### 14.4.5 Pathophysiology

Sensitization to an allergen occurs in genetically predisposed people. Allergens are captured by dendritic allergen-presenting cells and presented to T-helper (Th) cells. Activated Th cells are called Th2 cells. These activated Th2 cells trigger plasma cells to produce specific IgE antibodies that bind to a mast cell, therefore sensitizing it to degranulate when the same allergen crosslinks the bound IgE on subsequent exposure. This causes the release of histamine, tryptase, and other newly synthesized inflammatory mediators such as leukotrienes and prostaglandin.

The most significant cytokines are interleukin 4 (IL-4), interleukin 5 (IL-5), and interleukin 13 (IL-13). IL-4 stimulates B cells to produce allergen-specific IgE that binds through its high-affinity receptor, to effector cells especially mast cells and basophils.

On later exposure to the same allergen, the allergen binds with two molecules of allergen-specific IgE on the surface of a mast cell and triggers the release of inflammatory mediators such as histamine, leukotrienes, and prostaglandin. These mediators start the early-phase allergic reaction associated with sneezing and watery rhinorrhea.

The cytokines also stimulate migration of leucocytes, predominantly eosinophils and basophils to the sensitized mucosa. The leucocytes in turn release their mediators including the major basic protein leading to the late-phase allergic reaction usually occurring few hours later and are associated with increased nasal congestion.

The early-phase reaction is mainly driven by histamine causing nerve irritation (sneezing and itching), stimulation of submucosal glands and hyperpermeability of blood vessels (running), and vasodilatation (block). Other mediators involved in the late-phase reaction cause continued block and other systemic effects such as wheeze.

### 14.4.6 Classifications of Allergic Rhinitis

A. **Seasonal**: Limited to definite season, e.g., hay fever. Allergic symptoms appear when weeds and flowers bloom, and pollen counts are higher.
B. **Perennial**: Continuous or constant, sometimes with seasonal exacerbations. Indoor allergies, such as those from pets and dust mites, can induce allergy throughout the year.

### 14.4.7 ARIA Classification [16]

A. **Intermittent**: Symptoms are present fewer than 4 days a week or for fewer than 4 consecutive weeks.
B. **Persistent**: Symptoms present for 4 or more days a week or for 4 or more consecutive weeks.

Intermittent and persistent allergic rhinitis can each be subdivided into mild or severe:

A. **Mild**: Symptoms are not troublesome and do not affect quality of life (sleep, work, education…. etc.)
B. **Moderate to Severe**: Symptoms are troublesome and do affect quality of life.

If a patient has one or more of the symptoms that affect quality of life (disturbed sleep, impairment of daily life …etc.), then they are categorized as having moderate to severe disease.

A more accurate assessment of quality of life can be made with a variety of tools such as the 36-Item Short Form Health Survey (SF-36), Rhino conjunctivitis Quality of Life Questionnaire (RQLQ), or the 22-item Sinonasal Outcome Test (SNOT-22) [17, 18]. A visual analog scale (VAS) has been lately introduced follow up the patients and document their response to treatment [19].

**Local allergic rhinitis** is a subtype of allergic rhinitis that is defined as: rhinitis due to nasal production of specific immunoglobulins in the absence of atopy. This is termed "entopy." Skin prick test and RAST test are typically negative. This is sometimes termed "entopy." Local allergic rhinitis is frequently misdiagnosed as vasomotor rhinitis and may upgrade to classic allergic rhinitis [20].

The allergic mucosa is usually primed for non-allergic stimuli. The presence of both of allergic and non-allergic elements in the same patient is called "**Mixed allergic rhinitis.**"

### 14.4.8 Allergic Rhinitis and Asthma

The term "unified allergic airway" refers to the association of allergic rhinitis and asthma. It is estimated that 65–75% of patients with allergic asthma will have symptomatic AR. In patients with allergic rhinitis, approximately 25% will develop asthma. It appears that the inflammatory mediators released in the respiratory mucosa have systemic as well as local effects.

### 14.4.9 The Association between Allergic Rhinitis and COVID-19

Coronavirus disease 2019 (COVID-19) is a contagious disease whose symptoms and risk factors are newly described. It has been proposed that a patient's COVID-19 prognosis can be worsened by the underlying diseases that affect their immune system. The tissue alterations and inflammation inherent in allergic diseases can make allergy patients vulnerable to infections.

Some allergic diseases, including asthma, have been defined as risk factors for a poor outcome in COVID-19. Although the nose is the entry port and site of the early infection of viruses, including SARS-CoV-2, the situation for allergic rhinitis is still controversial [21].

A cohort survey conducted in South Korea reported that COVID-19 patients who had allergic rhinitis required longer periods of hospitalization [22]. Another study found that allergic rhinitis did not affect the severity of COVID-19 [23]. A recent metanalysis found that allergic rhinitis did not affect the severity of COVID-19 [24]. At the present time, it seems that allergic rhinitis, in the absence of associated asthma, does not have significant effect on the course of COVID-19.

### 14.4.10 Clinical Picture

Presumptive diagnosis of allergic rhinitis is usually clinical and is made if someone experiences one or more of the symptoms of allergic rhinitis in response to allergen exposure.

A. **Symptoms of Allergic Rhinitis.**
   1. Nasal congestion (stuffiness), sneezing, and runny nose. "The nasal block is often variable, cycling from side to side. Nasal discharge is typically bilateral, watery, and clear.
   2. Itchy nose, throat, and eyes.
   3. Red watery eyes.
   4. Headaches and sinus pressure.
   5. postnasal drip.
   6. Irritant coughing.

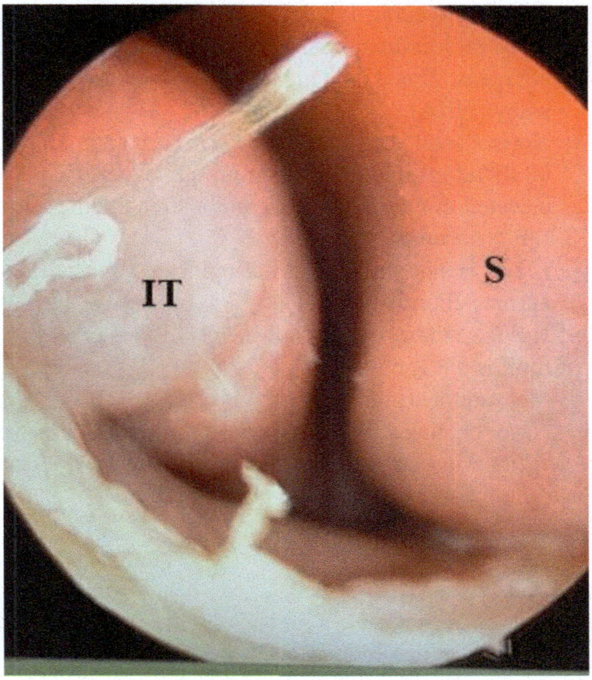


**Fig. 14.7** Allergic rhinitis. The inferior turbinate (IT) appears swollen and pale unlike that of acute viral rhinitis. S = nasal septum

B. **Signs:**
   a. Facial signs
      1. Shiners: bluish discoloration and mild edema around the eyes
      2. Allergic gap (open mouth—mouth breathing)
      3. Supratip crease (allergic salute)
   b. Nasal signs.
      1. Pale, moist nasal mucosa with occasional blue hue (Fig. 14.7)
      2. Swollen inferior turbinates
      3. Signs of chronic rhinosinusitis may be present with or without nasal polyps.

### 14.4.11 Investigations

- Skin prick test.
  - A battery of common allergens is placed on the skin of the flexor aspect of the forearm. If the patient has an allergy to any of the allergens, then a wheal and flare will appear within 15–20 min.
  - A negative control (carrier substance) and a positive control (histamine-containing solution) should be included to ensure accuracy of the results.
  - Positive SPT must be correlated with the patient's symptoms to be useful, and if several are positive, it may be that only one or two are clinically relevant."

- Allergen-specific IgE level (RAST test—radioallergosorbent test): RAST is a blood radioimmunoassay test that can detect specific IgE antibodies to suspected allergens. This is now more commonly performed as a fluoroenzymatic immunoassay (FEIA).
- Normal total serum IgE values are less than 100 IU/mL in adults and less than 60 IU/ml in children total serum IgE levels (PRIST test): Total serum IgE may be elevated in type I allergies, and also including helminthic infections and hyper-IgE syndrome.
- Blood eosinophilia may occur in an acute allergic reaction but is unusual in chronic allergic rhinitis.
- Nasal Smears: An increase in eosinophils in a nasal smear may occur in allergic rhinitis but is not specific.
- Measurements of local nasal IgE.
- Nasal challenge A drop of the suspected allergen squeezed into the nose may cause rhinitis symptoms. The obstructive effect can be measured objectively by rhinomanometry pre- and post-challenge.

### 14.4.12 Treatment

The treatment of allergic rhinitis includes lessening exposure to allergens and other triggers, reduction of the symptoms, by drug therapy, and modification of the disease process by immunotherapy. In most people, this combined approach can effectively control symptoms [25, 26].

A. **Avoidance**

   Avoiding precipitating antigens/triggers sounds like the ideal method of controlling symptoms. Sometimes people can get rid of their allergy by avoiding the allergens that trigger symptoms. However, many allergens are hard to avoid. Pet allergens are persistent and will be widespread within a house. House dust mites are found in high levels in pillows and mattresses, and an anti-allergen cover may help to reduce their allergenic effect. Cockroach and mold levels can be controlled by appropriate pesticides and attention to damp within the home.

B. **Pharmacotherapy**

   The vast majority of patients with allergic rhinitis will be treated symptomatically according to the ARIA guidelines. A visual analog score (VAS) may be used to follow up symptom control [16].

   1. Steroid nasal sprays

      Nasal glucocorticoid sprays are the first-line treatment for the symptoms of allergic rhinitis. They act on early and late phases of nasal allergy and are and effective for all symptoms of allergic rhinitis including nasal congestion because in most patients of their anti-inflammatory effects [27]. They work by inhibiting inflammatory gene transcription in the cell nucleus (among other actions) and therefore take some time to have an effect.

Steroid sprays differ regarding the frequency of doses, the spray device, and cost, but all have comparable efficacy. They work best when they are used properly, and the medication remains in the nose rather than draining down the back of the throat. If nasal blockage is severe, the patient may need to use a low concentration nasal decongestant before applying the steroid spray to reduce mucosal swelling. This allows the nasal spray to reach more areas within your nasal passages.

Nasal steroids are most effective when used regularly. However, some people can use lower doses when symptoms are less severe.

Systemic absorption or bioavailability of nasal steroids is generally less than 2%, and their main side effects are irritation, occasional crusting, and minimal bleeding. These side effects can be easily treated by using a moisturizing nasal gel or spray. Nasal steroids are generally safe when used for many years. However, it is always recommended to prescribe the lowest effective dose.

Steroid sprays may be prescribed to children older than 2 years. There is no clinical evidence that their use in children may slow down the growth rate.

Steroid sprays seem to have no adverse effects on HbA1c and serum glucose levels in diabetic patients. Their long-term use appears to be safe, provided that the patients are carefully monitored, especially those receiving triamcinolone acetonide.

There is no sufficient clinical trials on the use of steroid sprays in pregnancy. It is suggested that the use of fluticasone furoate, mometasone, and budesonide is safe if they are used at the recommended therapeutic dose after a proper medical evaluation. Risk-benefit ratio should always be considered in every patient [28].

2. Oral second-generation non-sedating oral antihistamines.

   These are fast-acting and effective for rhinorrhea and sneezing but less so for nasal congestion. They will also reduce throat itching and ocular symptoms.

   Using them along with nasal steroids may provide greater symptom relief than using one of these medications alone. This is not evidence-based so far.

   First-generation antihistamines are no longer used for treatment of allergic rhinitis because of their sedation and anticholinergic actions.

3. Nasal antihistamine spray.

   Nasal antihistamine sprays have similar actions to oral antihistamines with the benefit of absent systemic side effects and higher concentrations in the nasal mucosa. Antihistamine sprays start to work within minutes after use. They can be used daily or when needed to relieve the symptoms. Their most annoying side effect is bad aftertaste in the throat after use. This can be minimized by keeping the head tilted forward while spraying to prevent the medicine from draining down the throat.

4. Combination glucocorticoid/antihistamine sprays improve symptoms of allergic rhinitis better than either drug alone. The combination spray has the

benefits and side effects of both when used at the recommended dose (one spray in each side of the nose twice per day). The spray is approved for use in people over 6 years old [29].

5. Decongestants

   Oral decongestants are available in combination with antihistamines and may be used to relieve nasal stuffiness. The decongestant agent is usually pseudoephedrine. Oral decongestants may elevate blood pressure and are not appropriate for people with high blood pressure, certain cardiovascular conditions, benign hypertrophy of prostate, and glaucoma.

   Decongestant nasal sprays may be used occasionally but are generally not recommended for treating allergic rhinitis. The active agents include phenylephrine, oxymetazoline, and xylometazoline. They should not be used for more than 3–5 days at a time, because they may cause a type of rhinitis called "rhinitis medicamentosa," with shortening of the duration of the action of the drug and more constant nasal congestion [30–32] (Fig. 14.8).

6. Sodium cromoglycate (Cromolyn)

   Cromolyn stabilizes mast cell membranes and reduces the release of the mediators that are responsible for the allergic reaction. It is a safe drug but needs to be used 4–6 times per day. It is generally not as effective as other treatments, but it is especially useful in children. Cromoglicate eyedrops may relieve allergic conjunctivitis.

7. Topical anticholinergic drugs (e.g., ipratropium bromide).

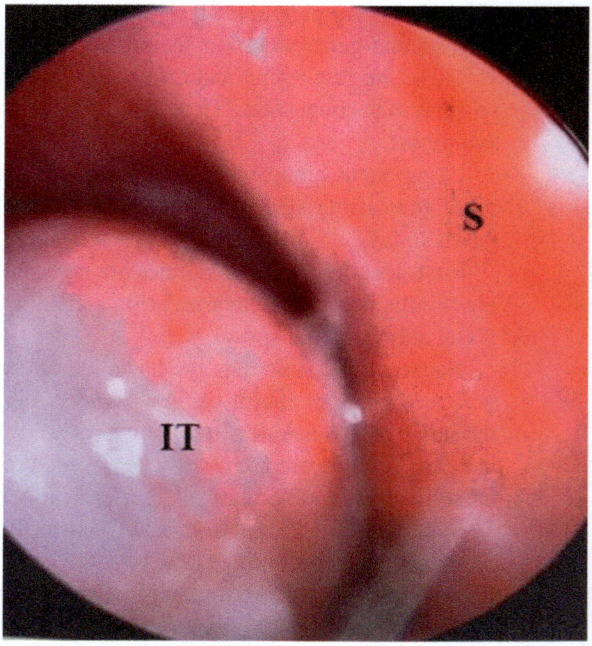


**Fig. 14.8** Rhinitis medicamentosa following long use of decongestant nasal drops. The nasal mucosa appears red and dry

Topical anticholinergics may be used if watery discharge is the predominant symptom. They are more frequently used for treatment of geriatric and gustatory rhinitis.

8. Leukotriene receptor antagonists/modifiers.

   Leukotriene receptor antagonists block the actions of leukotrienes released from mast cells and can be useful in some patients with both asthma and allergic rhinitis. However, they are less effective than nasal steroids.

9. Nasal irrigation and saline sprays.

   Nasal irrigation with saline, with or without additives, helps to remove out allergens and irritants from the nose. They can be used before applying a spray-containing medication to get a better effect from the medication. Nasal irrigation carries few risks when done correctly and with saline made with sterilized water. Saline is also available in a standard nasal spray, although this is not as effective as using larger amounts of water in an irrigation [33, 34].

10. Monoclonal Antibodies: A variety of humanized monoclonal antibodies are now becoming available for the treatment of allergic disease taking in consideration their costs. Omalizumab binds to circulating IgE, thus inhibiting it from binding to mast cells. This both prevents mast cell degranulation and reduces cellular expression of IgE-binding sites, therefore giving a longer mode of action. It is generally only used for patients with severe allergic rhinitis and asthma.

    Mepolizumab, reslizumab, and benralizumab block IL5 (or the IL5 receptor). Dupilumab targets the receptor for IL4 and IL13. These drugs are not widely used for the treatment of allergic rhinitis alone but can be useful in patients with combined allergic rhinitis and asthma.

11. Short courses of oral steroids for 7–10 days are very effective and may be used cautiously in poor responders and certain other situations.

C. **Immunotherapy (Desensitization)**

Immunotherapy (injection SCIT or sublingual SLIT) involves exposure to regular small but increasing doses of an allergen. This causes the production of regulatory T cells (Treg) that switch the immune response from the excess production of Th2 cells to a Th1 profile. There is also a production of IgG4 that acts as a blocking antibody preventing IgE-binding. After a few-year course of treatment, patients should experience a long-lasting reduction in symptoms and a halt in disease progression.

Immunotherapy is especially used for those with known allergens, and patients do not respond to pharmacotherapy. In children, immunotherapy can help prevent the development of allergic asthma later in life.

Immunotherapy is more often given by injections (SCIT). Treatment begins with several months of weekly injections of gradually increasing doses, followed by monthly maintenance injections. Immunotherapy is usually continued for a minimum of three (SLIT) years. Its main complication is anaphylaxis.

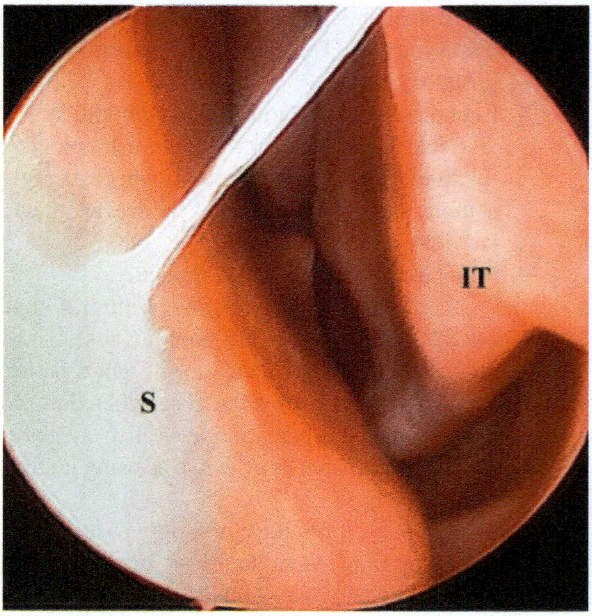


**Fig. 14.9** The inferior turbinate after radiofrequency submucosal turbinoplasty. The mucosa of the turbinate is well healed and the size of the turbinate is adequately reduced

Patients initially stay on medications when they start immunotherapy and then gradually reduce the medications as their symptoms improve.

Sublingual immunotherapy is a form of immunotherapy given as a daily pill that is given every day for several months of the year. The allergen given is taken up by antigen-presenting cells in the oral mucosa and then works in much the same way as SCIT.

This type of treatment does not involve getting shots, and it is very safe because it rarely causes severe allergic reactions. However, it is only available for a few types of allergies, and if the patient frequently forgets to take the pills daily, the treatment might not work [35–37].

D. Surgical treatment

a. Turbinate surgery to reduce the size of hypertrophied inferior turbinates in selected patients (Fig. 14.9) [38]. Surgical reduction of the size of the turbinate should be done wisely to avoid the irreversible complication of empty nose syndrome (Fig. 14.10).

b. Surgical procedures to interrupt the parasympathetic supply to the nasal mucosal: vidian neurectomy, posterior nasal neurectomy, and application of botulinum toxin to the sphenopalatine foramen area [39, 40].

Posterior nasal neurectomy is easier to perform than vidian neurectomy and avoids postoperative dryness of the eyes and palatal numbness that are common after vidian neurectomy. The procedures should be performed on both sides of the nose [41, 42].

Recurrence of symptoms is common after these procedures. These procedures have been also used for vasomotor rhinitis [43]

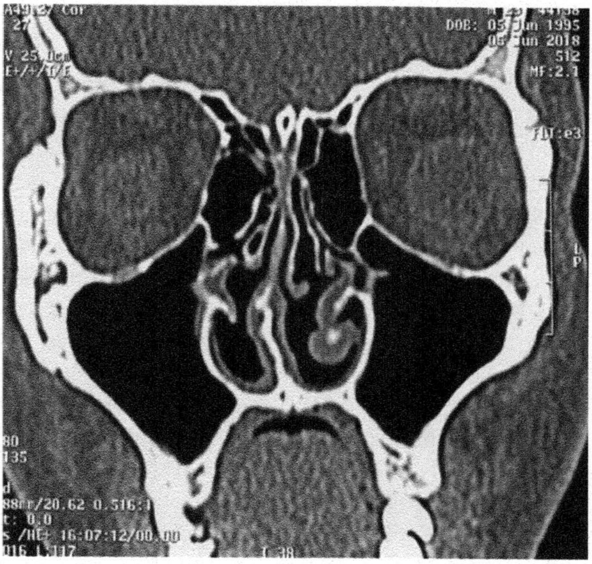

**Fig. 14.10** The right inferior turbinate is almost totally excised (Empty Nose Syndrome)

### 14.4.13 Aspirin-Exacerbated Respiratory Disease (AERD—Samter's Triad)

AERD is a hypersensitivity reaction induced by aspirin and other non-steroidal anti-inflammatory drugs (NSAIDs, N-NERD) that inhibit an enzyme called cyclooxygenase. Acetaminophen is usually safely tolerated at low doses (up to 500 mg at a time) [44, 45].

AERD affects about 10% of adults with asthma and 20–30% of patients with combined asthma and nasal polyps and starts usually between the ages of 20–50 due to intrinsic disorder of prostaglandin metabolism.

The clinical picture is a combination of asthma and chronic rhinosinusitis with nasal polyps.

#### 14.4.13.1 Investigations

1. Aspirin challenge test.
2. Examination of blood and nasal smears for eosinophils,

#### 14.4.13.2 Treatment

Steroids (oral, intranasal, and inhalers) are the main treatment. Aspirin desensitization as a steroid-sparing treatment in some patients.

Non-steroid medications include drugs that inhibit the production of leukotrienes (zileuton) or block the function of leukotrienes (montelukast) may be beneficial as an additive therapy.

Endoscopic sinus surgery is reserved for obstructing nasal polyps. The recurrence rate after surgery is high. Nasalization procedures or reboot surgery may be needed in recalcitrant cases [44].

## 14.5 Non-Allergic Rhinitis

Non-allergic rhinitis (NAR) includes broad group of diverse nasal diseases that are not allergic in origin and are elicited by a variety of environmental changes. Literally speaking, the term non-allergic rhinitis can include many types of rhinitis, e.g., infectious, hormonal, occupational, gustatory, and geriatric rhinitis [46, 47].

Non-allergic rhinitis is usually an under-estimated entity. However, it is reported that at least half of all patients presenting with rhinitis may have a non-allergic form. A national survey of allergists conducted by the National Rhinitis Classification Task Force (NRCTF) found that a total of 57% of patients presenting with chronic rhinitis had either pure or mixed NAR. Moreover, 44% of patients with allergic rhinitis were classified as also having some component of NAR.

Non-allergic rhinitis is a diagnosis of exclusion. Many clinicians empirically treat allergic rhinitis without paying enough attention to the differences between AR and NAR. This lowers the outcome of treatment since research has not shown oral antihistamines to be beneficial in relieving symptoms of non-allergic rhinitis. This, also, may be the reason why some patients with allergic rhinitis report that their symptoms are not completely controlled.

However, in clinical practice when we talk about non-allergic rhinitis, we usually mean the group that have similar symptoms to allergic rhinitis. It includes two main types: idiopathic rhinitis (previously called vasomotor) and non-allergic rhinitis with eosinophilia (NARES). Itching and sneezing are less common with non-allergic rhinitis than with allergic rhinitis, but nasal congestion/obstruction and anterior and posterior rhinorrhea are usually prominent. The pathophysiology of these two types is caused by dysregulation of the neurogenic pathway and can originate from either afferent or efferent neuronal abnormalities. By definition, the patients should have neither clinical sign of infection nor signs of allergic inflammation such as allergen-specific IgE in serum or positive skin prick tests.

Several provocation tests have been developed to diagnose patients with NAR. A cold, dry air provocation test has a high sensitivity and specificity in diagnosing nasal hyperreactivity, a common feature in idiopathic rhinitis patients. Patients are exposed to air of <−10 °C and a relative humidity of <10% for 15 min, delivered via a common anesthesia mask at a flow of 25 L/min. Before and after the provocation, peak nasal inspiratory flow (PNIF). A reduction of 20% or more is taken as a threshold for diagnosis [48].

Other provocation tests using chemical compounds have been used, such as mannitol, capsaicin, methacholine, and histamine. However, these tests have several limitations such as low sensitivity and specificity and possible adverse reactions.

### 14.5.1 Etiology

Non-allergic rhinitis typically occurs in reaction to environmental triggers, which may include:

1. Changes in relative humidity and temperature.
2. Odors (such as bleach, solvents, or fragrances),
3. Active and passive smoking [49, 50].
4. Occupational irritants and pollutants such as automotive fumes.
5. Bright lights and spicy foods.
6. Nasal mucosal hyperreactivity following viral rhinitis.
7. Emotional factors, including stress and sexual arousal, may also affect nasal symptoms probably due to stimulation of the autonomic nervous system.
8. Endocrine factors: menstruation and pregnancy.
9. Drugs: ACE inhibitors, β-blockers, and oral contraceptives.

### 14.5.2 Idiopathic Rhinitis (Vasomotor Rhinitis—VMR)

Vasomotor rhinitis is the most common entity of non-allergic rhinitis especially in older patients. Settipane and Klein found that VMR affects about 50–60% of NAR patients. It is sometimes called perennial non-allergic rhinitis. Unfortunately, the term is erroneously used to describe entities without vasomotor pathogenesis. Allergy tests are characteristically absent, and immunotherapy is not indicated [51, 52].

#### 14.5.2.1 Pathogenesis

Vasomotor rhinitis results from fluctuations in vascular tone and permeability of the mucosal blood vessels due to activation of transient receptor potential channels (TRP) present on afferent sensory trigeminal nerve fibers by environmental triggers. The released neuropeptides (substance P and other neuropeptides) activate the parasympathetic nerves that supply the nasal mucosal glands and vasculature. The triggers for this neural stimulation include many factors such as cold air, temperature change, and anxiety [53–55].

#### 14.5.2.2 Clinical Picture

Idiopathic rhinitis is diagnosed by exclusion. Clinical picture of vasomotor rhinitis is nonspecific and similar to that of allergic rhinitis. Vasomotor rhinitis may be associated with asthma but there is usually no ocular manifestations.

#### 14.5.2.3 Treatment

Treatment of NAR could be difficult due to the heterogenicity of the disease. In practice, treatment of a patient with NAR is rather trial-and-error. Several options are available.

Avoidance of triggers should be attempted whenever possible. Steroid nasal sprays are the most effective treatment. The response to antihistamines is generally poor or modest. Anticholinergic nasal sprays (ipratropium bromide) can be used when rhinorrhea is the prominent symptom.

Oral decongestants (sympathomimetics) can be used as a symptomatic treatment, but they may produce side effects such as dry mouth, constipation, and excitability. They should not be used long term, in patients with hypertension, glaucoma, or benign hypertrophy of the prostate, or in children.

Local nasal decongestants can temporarily relieve nasal blockage, but the relief may be followed by rebound congestion (rebound phenomenon). Prolonged excessive use of nasal decongestants may cause aggravation of nasal congestion, which eventually become unresponsive to the decongestant, and r**hinitis medicamentosa** may develop. Saline washes and topical steroids can help to reverse these changes.

Surgical measures to reduce nasal hyperreactivity include:

- Sphenopalatine block with botulinum toxin: This usually results in short-lived improvement of symptoms [56].
- Vidian Neurectomy: Section of the vidian nerve produces improvements for longer durations but there is risk of dry eye and numbness of the palate, and recurrence of symptoms is frequent [39].
- Posterior Nasal Neurectomy: Section of the posterior nasal nerves produces the same results as vidian neurectomy without the disadvantages of dryness of the eyes and palatal numbness. It is important not to miss any of the branches [41].

### 14.5.3 Non-Allergic Rhinitis with Eosinophilia Syndrome (NARES)

The other important form of NAR that may mimic allergic rhinitis is non-allergic rhinitis with eosinophilia syndrome (NARES). NARES is characteristically associated with eosinophilia (> 20%) in nasal smears. Patients with NARES have a higher tendency for nasal polyposis and aspirin sensitivity, and a better response to topical steroids and second-generation antihistamines than patients with VMR.

NARES is characterized by the presence of many eosinophils in nasal mucosa and secretions (10–20% on nasal smear). Allergy testing is typically negative. Patients with NARES have a higher tendency for nasal polyposis and a better response to topical steroids and second-generation antihistamines than patients with VMR [57, 58].

Treatment is like that of vasomotor rhinitis. Occasionally, short courses of steroids are needed for obstinate cases [47].

### 14.5.4 Other Types of Non-Allergic Rhinitis

#### 14.5.4.1 Irritant/Occupational-Induced Rhinitis

Environmental irritants usually induce symptoms via direct irritation rather than immunological way. Triggers such as perfumes, cleaning agents, smoke, and other irritants stimulate chemical irritant nociceptors of C sensory fibers leading to neuropeptide release. The neuropeptides produce vasodilation and edema independent of immune-mediated responses. The response to second-generation antihistamines in these cases is typically poor.

In occupational rhinitis, nasal symptoms are evoked in response to airborne agents present in the professional environment. Both high-molecular-weight (e.g., mites, adhesives, paints, insecticides flour, and dander) and low-molecular-weight agents (e.g., isocyanates, anhydrides, reactive dyes) can induce allergic inflammation. The latter can act as a hapten for immunologic interactions.

Symptoms are dependent on the exposure and can be perennially or seasonally present according to the work conditions. Daily PNIF measurements can be used as a diagnostic tool to confirm a temporal pattern related to working schedule. Provocation tests mimicking the workplace environment can also be performed to confirm the cause-effect relationship.

#### 14.5.4.2 Smokers' Rhinitis

Cigarette smoke is a mixture of pharmacologically active, toxic, mutagenic, and carcinogenic substances. A complex mixture of chemicals is generated from the burning and smoking of tobacco. Smoking whether active or passive (side stream smoking) has deleterious effects on the nasal mucosa including congestion of the mucosa and hyperplasia of the mucus-producing elements [49, 50]. Smoking also alters the glycoprotein content of the mucus and degrades its viscoelastic properties [59]. Moreover, it encourages the formation of biofilms on the nasal mucosa [60]. Quitting smoking reverses the nasal mucosal changes [61]. Smoking rhinitis may exist in combination with allergic rhinitis further complicating its treatment.

#### 14.5.4.3 Hormonal Rhinitis

Nasal symptoms can have hormonal causes. Estrogens induce nasal vasodilation and enhance eosinophil migration. Together with progesterone, estrogens induce eosinophil degranulation.

Hormonal rhinitis may be caused by contraceptive bills or occur in association with pregnancy, hypothyroidism, and acromegaly. Rhinopathy of pregnancy is a term used to describe appearance or exaggeration of nasal symptoms such as congestion, watery rhinorrhea, sneezing, and itching in pregnant females. Rhinopathy of pregnancy is probably multifactorial with female sex hormones playing part in its etiology [62–64]. In some females, the symptoms are related the menstrual cycle [65].

Hypothyroidism may induce submucosal edema and slowing down of mucociliary transport. Nasal obstruction and thick mucoid are the usual symptoms in these patients.

#### 14.5.4.4 Food-Induced Rhinitis (Gustatory Rhinitis)

In this type of rhinitis, eating hot or spicy foods lead to nasal obstruction and watery rhinorrhea may lead to nasal gustatory rhinitis which is thought to be neurogenic in origin. Spicy foods such as capsaicin stimulate type C trigeminal nerve endings in the oral cavity resulting in activation of the parasympathetic system. Usually, there is a clear temporal pattern with mealtime.

Food allergy uncommonly causes isolated rhinitis. However, rhinitis may occur due to hyperreactivity to preservatives or additives rather than the main food. The oral allergy syndrome describes irritation of oral cavity and nose due to association of food allergies with seasonal allergic rhinitis.

#### 14.5.4.5 Drug-Induced Rhinitis (Rhinitis Medicamentosa)

Drug-induced rhinitis can be divided into two pathophysiological groups: rhinitis induced by topical agents and rhinitis induced by oral drugs.

The most known form of drug-induced rhinitis is rebound congestion due to decreased vasomotor tone and refractoriness of sympathomimetic α receptors, following lengthy use of decongestant nasal drops. The vascular network of the nasal mucosa consists of both resistance vessels (arterioles), which contain α2-adrenoreceptors, and capacitance vessels (venous plexus) containing both α1- and α2-adrenoreceptors.

Topical decongestants typically contain α1-adrenergic β-phenylethylamine derivates, such as ephedrine or phenylephrine, or α2-adrenergic imidazoline derivates, such as naphazoline, oxymetazoline, or xylometazoline. Long-term use of these vasoconstrictors can lead to downregulation of α-receptors resulting in rebound congestion (tachyphylaxis). Chronic hypoxia of the nasal mucosa may lead to mucosal hypertrophy. The preservatives such as benzalkonium chloride have also been considered as causative factors in this type of rhinitis.

The usual symptoms are nasal obstruction and dryness. The patients usually complain from progressively decreasing efficacy of nasal drops and persistent nasal obstruction (Fig. 14.8).

Treatment: discontinuation of nasal decongestants; saline washes, and nasal steroid sprays. Short courses of oral corticosteroids may be needed [66, 67].

#### 14.5.4.6 Senile Rhinitis (Geriatric Rhinitis)

Senile rhinitis (rhinitis of the elderly) affects elderly patients. The patients typically complain of persistent clear rhinorrhea as the primary symptom. Loss of the physiological sympathetic predominance and relative parasympathetic overactivity activate the submucosal glands to secrete thin clear mucus.

With increasing age, additional physiological changes occur in the nose including dryness of the epithelium and weakness of mucociliary clearance leading to impaired humidification and warming of inhaled air and accumulation of mucus causing postnasal drip and cough. Topical anticholinergics are usually used to reduce the rhinorrhea.

## 14.6 Atrophic Rhinitis

Atrophic rhinitis is a chronic inflammation of the nasal mucosa characterized by atrophy of its epithelium and glands due to endarteritis and periarterial fibrosis. The functional ciliated respiratory nasal epithelium is replaced by a nonfunctional lining of non-ciliated squamous epithelium (squamous metaplasia), with a loss of mucosal glands and slowing down of mucociliary clearance.

There are two main types of atrophic rhinitis: primary and secondary.

### 14.6.1 Primary Atrophic Rhinitis (Ozena)

The main features of primary atrophic rhinitis include atrophy of the nasal mucosa, increased nasal patency, offensive odor, crust formation, and anosmia. The disease is more common in females around the age of puberty with a ratio of 5.6:1 [68].

Primary atrophic rhinitis (PAR) has been reported in families where females are affected with a positive family history in about 15–30% of the cases. Some studies have revealed either an autosomal dominant (67%) or autosomal recessive penetrance (33%).

The etiology of the disease is still unknown, and various theories (hormonal, infective…etc.) have been proposed. Bacteriologic cultures from the nasal cavity frequently reveal bacillus foetidus ozaenae which is thought to be responsible for the offensive odor that is not perceived by the patient due to anosmia [69, 70]. Other bacterial species such as *Pseudomonas aeruginosa*, *Diphtheroid bacillus*, *Bacillus mucosus*, and Proteus may be also present.

Progressive squamous metaplasia and atrophy of all mucosal components (epithelium, vessels, and glands) are the hallmarks of the disease. Increased osteoclastic activity results in a volumetric decrease of sinonasal structures and widening of the nasal cavities [69].

#### 14.6.1.1 Clinical Picture

The typical patient is a young adult female presenting with anosmia and offensive odor which is not perceived by the patient due to the associated anosmia. The anosmia is due to the atrophic process involving the olfactory epithelium as well as insufficient air reaching the olfactory areas due to crusting.

The patient usually complains of nasal obstruction despite the wide nasal cavities. This paradoxical nasal obstruction is due to accumulation of crusts and inability to sense the cooling effect of the inspired airflow due to loss of the trigeminal nerve endings in the nasal mucosa. Occasionally, there is mild epistaxis due to separation of crusts.

Anterior rhinoscopy/endoscopy shows wide nasal cavities and small turbinates. The mucus membrane looks pale, atrophic, and covered by thick yellowish or greenish crusts.

#### 14.6.1.2 Investigations

A full blood count may reveal a microcytic hypochromic picture (iron deficiency anemia). The serum protein and plasma vitamin level estimations are necessary to exclude malnutrition.

A raised erythrocyte sedimentation rate (ESR) as well as raised autoimmune markers (ANCA, angiotensin-converting enzyme, rheumatoid factor, anti-Ro, anti-La) may help to rule out other diagnoses (granulomatous conditions, Sjogren's).

#### 14.6.1.3 Imaging

CT scan may reveal widening of the nasal cavities with erosion and bowing of the lateral nasal wall. The middle and inferior turbinates appear small due to bony resorption and mucosal atrophy.

#### 14.6.1.4 Treatment

There is no curative treatment of the disease. Symptomatic measures include frequent cleaning of the nose by saline washes with or without moisturizing agents such as dexpanthenol spray or ointment. Lubricant drops, e.g., menthol paraffin drops and 25% glucose in glycerin may be also used. Intranasal injection of platelet-rich plasma (PRP) did not improve the histology of the nasal mucosa [71].

Local or systemic antimicrobial treatment is prescribed following nasal culture for bacteria or fungi. A nasal obturator can reduce nasal dryness with minimal cosmetic implications. These can be made from a material called dimethylpolysiloxane or from an acrylic resin [72].

Surgical treatment is also of limited value and includes:

1. Submucosal implantation of autogenous or synthetic implants to narrow the roomy nasal cavities. The implants may be autologous (bone, cartilage, muscle, fat), homologous (lyophilized bone, fat, human placenta extract), or synthetic (Teflon, acrylics, silicone, silastic). The major problems of their use are implant rejection, leakage, and chronic infection of the implant [73].
2. Young's Operation [74]: closure of the anterior nasal opening by mucocutaneous flaps. The flaps are sutured together in two layers. The nasal cavity is kept closed for a period of 6 months; then, the nasal cavity is reopened. Recurrence of atrophic changes after reopening has been reported. Modifications of the original procedure have been described without improvement of the outcome of surgery [75].

### 14.6.2 Secondary Atrophic Rhinitis

The most common cause of secondary atrophic rhinitis is aggressive resection of the inferior turbinates (iatrogenic atrophic rhinitis). The extreme form of it has been coined the name "empty nose syndrome" [76].

Other possible less common causes include:

1. Granulomatous diseases such as scleroma
2. Chronic cocaine abuse
3. Radiotherapy.

Treatment options are limited and may include irrigations, humidification to provide moisture, and experimental surgical procedures aiming at narrowing the nasal cavity with submucosal implants.

### 14.6.3 Rhinitis Sicca Anterior

An uncommon form of atrophic rhinitis is characterized by dry thin mucosa of the anterior part of the nasal cavity. The disease has been attributed to changes in temperature and humidity, frequent nose picking, and repeated exposure to dust.

The symptoms include dryness, crusting, nasal blockage, and mild epistaxis. Treatment is with saline irrigation, topical antibiotics, and oil based nasal ointments.

## 14.7 Sarcoidosis

Sarcoidosis is a chronic noncaseating granulomatous disease affecting the airway and other organs. Its exact etiology is still ill-defined. Sinonasal involvement occurs in about 1–5% of cases. The nasal mucosa usually appears dry, erythematous (strawberry-like appearance). Crusting is frequent and there may be septal perforation (Fig. 14.11). Ocular manifestations include uveitis, lacrimal gland enlargement, and conjunctivitis (Fig. 14.12). Other extra nasal manifestations include night sweats, weight loss, erythema nodosum, and peripheral lymphadenopathy.

### 14.7.1 Investigations

1. Plain chest radiograph typically shows showing bilateral hilar lymphadenopathy (butterfly pattern).
2. Angiotensin-converting enzyme (ACE) levels in serum are elevated.
3. Mucosal biopsies.

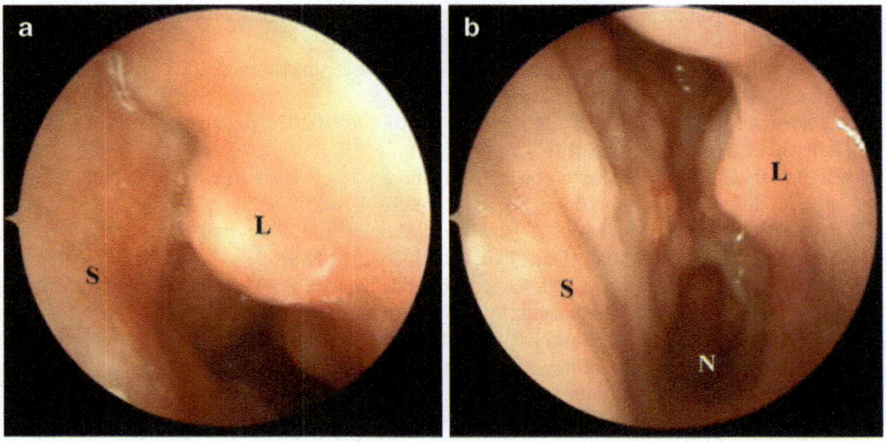


**Fig. 14.11** Sarcoidosis. The nasal mucosa appears dry and has strawberry-like appearance. S = Septum, L = lateral nasal wall, N = nasopharynx

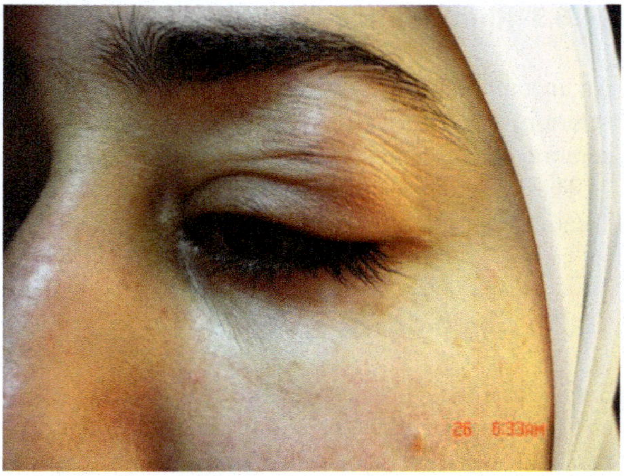


**Fig. 14.12** Sarcoidosis. The left upper lid appears swollen due to enlargement of the underneath lacrimal gland

### 14.7.2 Treatment

Oral steroids and immunosuppressants, such as methotrexate and azathioprine. Surgery for sinonasal sarcoidosis is controversial and is not recommended.

## References

1. Gaudin RA, Hoehle LP, Birkelbach M-A, Phillips KM, Beule AG, Caradonna DS, Gray ST, Sedaghat AR. The association between allergic rhinitis control and sleep quality. HNO. 2017;65:987–92.
2. Mims JW. Epidemiology of allergic rhinitis. Int Forum Allergy Rhinol. 2014;4(Suppl 2):S18–20.
3. Meltzer EO. Allergic rhinitis: burden of illness, quality of life, comorbidities, and control. Immunol Allergy Clin N Am. 2016;36:235–48.
4. Meltzer EO. The prevalence and medical and economic impact of allergic rhinitis in the United States. J Allergy Clin Immunol. 1997;99:S805–28.
5. Klain A, Indolfi C, Dinardo G, et al. United airway disease. Acta Biomed. 2021;92(S7):e2021526. https://doi.org/10.23750/abm.v92iS7.12399.
6. Dykewicz MS, Wallace DV, Amrol DJ, et al. Rhinitis 2020: a practice parameter update. J Allergy Clin Immunol. 2020;146:721–67.
7. Braunstahl G-J. United airways concept: what does it teach us about systemic inflammation in airways disease? Proc Am Thorac Soc. 2009;6:652–4.
8. Elwany S, Fattah HA, Mandour Z, Ismail AS, Abdelnabi M. A myriad of Scleroma presentations: the usual and unusual. Head Neck Pathol. 2020;14:588–92.
9. Ahmed ARH, El-Badawy ZH, Mohamed IR, Abdelhameed WAM. Rhinoscleroma: a detailed histopathological diagnostic insight. Int J Clin Exp Pathol. 2015;8:8438–45.
10. Hoffmann EO, Loose LD, Harkin JC. The Mikulicz cell in rhinoscleroma. Light, fluorescent and electron microscopic studies. Am J Pathol. 1973;73:47–58.
11. Singh CA, Sakthivel P. Rhinosporidiosis. N Engl J Med. 2019;380:1359.
12. Nagi K, Sekar R, Saxena SK, Stephen N. Naso-Bronchial Rhinosporidiosis. BMJ Case Rep. 2022;15(2):e247133. https://doi.org/10.1136/bcr-2021-247133.
13. Bousquet J, Anto JM, Bachert C, et al. Allergic rhinitis. Nat Rev Dis Primers. 2020;6:95.

14. Campbell AP, Hoehle LP, Phillips KM, Caradonna DS, Gray ST, Sedaghat AR. Depressed mood is associated with loss of productivity in allergic rhinitis. Allergy. 2018;73:1141–4.
15. Asher MI, Barry D, Clayton T, et al. The burden of symptoms of asthma, allergic rhinoconjunctivitis and atopic eczema in children and adolescents in six New Zealand centres: ISAAC phase one. N Z Med J. 2001;114:114–20.
16. Bousquet J, Khaltaev N, Cruz AA, et al. Review article allergic rhinitis and its impact on asthma ( ARIA ) 2008 * review group. Prim Care. 2008;63:8–160.
17. Kennedy JL, Hubbard MA, Huyett P, Patrie JT, Borish L, Payne SC. Sino-nasal outcome test (SNOT-22): a predictor of postsurgical improvement in patients with chronic sinusitis. Ann Allergy Asthma Immunol. 2013;111:246–251.e2.
18. Elwany S, Atef A, Ibrahim AA, Ismail AS, Hussein WK, Youssef AS, Elwany M, Bazak R. Arabic translation and validation of SNOT-22. Egy J Otolaryngol. 2017;33:611–5.
19. Ecevit MC, Özcan M, Haberal Can İ, et al. Turkish guideline for diagnosis and treatment of allergic rhinitis (ART). Turk Arch Otorhinolaryngol. 2021;59:1–157.
20. Campo P, Salas M, Blanca-López N, Rondón C. Local allergic rhinitis. Immunol Allergy Clin N Am. 2016;36:321–32.
21. Sonvico F, Colombo G, Quarta E, Guareschi F, Banella S, Buttini F, Scherließ R. Nasal delivery as a strategy for the prevention and treatment of COVID-19. Expert Opin Drug Deliv. 2023;20:1115–30.
22. Yang JM, Koh HY, Moon SY, Yoo IK, Ha EK, You S, Kim SY, Yon DK, Lee SW. Allergic disorders and susceptibility to and severity of COVID-19: a nationwide cohort study. J Allergy Clin Immunol. 2020;146:790–8.
23. Guvey A. How does allergic rhinitis impact the severity of COVID-19?: a case–control study. Eur Arch Otorrinolaringol. 2021;278:4367–71.
24. Xu C, Zhao H, Song Y, Zhou J, Wu T, Qiu J, Wang J, Song X, Sun Y. The association between allergic rhinitis and COVID-19: a systematic review and meta-analysis. Int J Clin Pract. 2022;2022:6510332. https://doi.org/10.1155/2022/6510332.
25. Fokkens WJ, Lund VJ, Hopkins C, et al. European position paper on rhinosinusitis and nasal polyps 2020. Rhinology. 2020;58:1–464.
26. Scadding GK, Kariyawasam HH, Scadding G, et al. BSACI guideline for the diagnosis and management of allergic and non-allergic rhinitis. (Revised Edition 2017; First edition 2007). Clin Exp Allergy. 2017;47:856–89.
27. Elwany S, Talaat M, Talaat M, Helmy A. Allergic nasal mucosa following topical treatment with beclomethasone dipropionate (Bdp) aerosol. Electron microscopic study. J Laryngol Otol. 1983;97:165–76.
28. Seth D, Kamat D. Intranasal steroid therapy for allergic rhinitis. Pediatr Ann. 2019;48:e43–8.
29. Berger WE, Meltzer EO. Intranasal spray medications for maintenance therapy of allergic rhinitis. Am J Rhinol Allergy. 2015;29:273–82.
30. Elwany SS, Stephanos WM. Rhinitis medicamentosa. An experimental histopathological and histochemical study. ORL J Otorhinolaryngol Relat Spec. 1983;45:187–94.
31. Mortuaire G, de Gabory L, François M, Massé G, Bloch F, Brion N, Jankowski R, Serrano E. Rebound congestion and rhinitis medicamentosa: nasal decongestants in clinical practice. Critical review of the literature by a medical panel. Eur Ann Otorhinolaryngol Head Neck Dis. 2013;130:137–44.
32. Cumbul A, Bulut F. The importance of vascular epithelial growth factor (VEGF) and inducible nitric oxide synthase (INOS) in rhinitis medicamentosa pathogenesis: an experimental rat model study. Histol Histopathol. 2022;37:261–7.
33. Head K, Snidvongs K, Glew S, Scadding G, Schilder AG, Philpott C, Hopkins C. Saline irrigation for allergic rhinitis. Cochrane Database Syst Rev. 2018;6:CD012597.
34. Pinto JM, Elwany S, Baroody FM, Naclerio RM. Effects of saline sprays on symptoms after endoscopic sinus surgery. Am J Rhinol. 2006;20:191–6.
35. Ji Z, Jiang F. Efficacy and safety of sublingual immunotherapy for allergic rhinitis: a network meta-analysis. Front Immunol. 2023;14:1144816.

36. Hoyte FCL, Nelson HS. Recent advances in allergic rhinitis. F1000Res. 2018;7:F1000 Faculty Rev-1333. https://doi.org/10.12688/f1000research.15367.1.
37. Soh JY, Thalayasingam M, Ong S, Loo EXL, Shek LP, Chao SS. Sublingual immunotherapy in patients with house dust mite allergic rhinitis: prospective study of clinical outcomes over a two-year period. J Laryngol Otol. 2016;130:272–7.
38. Harrison R. Inferior turbinectomy: comparison of four techniques. J Laryngol Otol. 1990;104:206–9.
39. Niu X, Chen Y, Zhou T, Xiao H. Endoscopic vidian and vidian-branch neurectomy for refractory allergic rhinitis: a systematic review. Int Forum Allergy Rhinol. 2023;14(3):679–94. https://doi.org/10.1002/alr.23259.
40. Qi Y, Liu J, Peng S, Hou S, Zhang M, Wang Z. Efficacy of selective Vidian Neurectomy for allergic rhinitis combined with chronic rhinosinusitis. ORL J Otorhinolaryngol Relat Spec. 2021;83:327–34.
41. Elwany S, Mandour Z, Ibrahim AA, Bazak R. Nasal reactivity after radiofrequency ablation of peripheral branches of posterior nasal nerve. Turk Arch Otorhinolaryngol. 2022;60:181–7.
42. Senanayake P, Wong E, McBride K, Singh N. Efficacy of Vidian Neurectomy and posterior nasal Neurectomy in the Management of Nonallergic Rhinitis: a systematic review. Am J Rhinol Allergy. 2022;36:849–71.
43. Rosi-Schumacher M, Abbas A, Young PR. Improvement in nasal symptoms of chronic rhinitis after Cryoablation of the posterior nasal nerve. OTO Open. 2023;7(4):e77. https://doi.org/10.1002/oto2.77.
44. Lee RU, Stevenson DD. Aspirin-exacerbated respiratory disease: evaluation and management. Allergy Asthma Immunol Res. 2011;3:3–10.
45. Kennedy JL, Stoner AN, Borish L. Aspirin-exacerbated respiratory disease: prevalence, diagnosis, treatment, and considerations for the future. Am J Rhinol Allergy. 2016;30:407–13.
46. Ellis AK, Keith PK. Nonallergic rhinitis with eosinophilia syndrome. Curr Allergy Asthma Rep. 2006;6:215–20.
47. Ellis AK, Keith PK. Nonallergic rhinitis with eosinophilia syndrome and related disorders. Clin Allergy Immunol. 2007;19:87–100.
48. Van Gerven L, Boeckxstaens G, Jorissen M, Fokkens W, Hellings PW. Short-time cold dry air exposure: a useful diagnostic tool for nasal hyperresponsiveness. Laryngoscope. 2012;122:2615–20.
49. Elwany S, Ibrahim AA, Mandour Z, Talaat I. Effect of passive smoking on the ultrastructure of the nasal mucosa in children. Laryngoscope. 2012;122:965–9.
50. Elwany S, Saeed YH, Talaat I. Effects of passive smoking on adult nasal respiratory mucosa. J Laryngol Otol. 2013;127:977–81.
51. Bachert C, Ganzer U. Nasal hyperreactivity. Allergic rhinitis and differential diagnoses—consensus report on pathophysiology, classification, diagnosis and therapy. Laryngorhinootologie. 1997;76:65–76.
52. Numata T, Konno A, Hasegawa S, Hanazawa T, Nagata H, Motosugi H, Terada N. Pathophysiological features of the nasal mucosa in patients with idiopathic rhinitis compared to allergic rhinitis. Int Arch Allergy Immunol. 1999;119:304–13.
53. Knipping S, Holzhausen HJ, Riederer A, Schrom T. Ultrastructural changes in allergic rhinitis vs. idiopathic rhinitis. HNO. 2008;56:799–807.
54. Sun S. Differentiation between allergic rhinitis and vasomotor rhinitis. Light and electron microscopic studies. Zhonghua Er Bi Yan Hou Ke Za Zhi. 1991;26:144–145,188.
55. Elwany SBR. Ultrastructural observations on vasomotor rhinitis. ORL. 1987;49:199–205.
56. Ozcan C, Ismi O. Botulinum toxin for rhinitis. Curr Allergy Asthma Rep. 2016;16:58.
57. Settipane GA, Klein DE. Non allergic rhinitis: demography of eosinophils in nasal smear, blood total eosinophil counts and IgE levels. N Engl Reg Allergy Proc. 1985;6:363–6.
58. Moneret-Vautrin DA, Hsieh V, Wayoff M, Guyot JL, Mouton C, Maria Y. Nonallergic rhinitis with eosinophilia syndrome a precursor of the triad: nasal polyposis, intrinsic asthma, and intolerance to aspirin. Ann Allergy. 1990;64:513–8.

59. Jeffery PK, Reid LM. The effect of tobacco smoke, with or without phenylmethyloxadiazole (PMO), on rat bronchial epithelium: a light and electron microscopic study. J Pathol. 1981;133:341–59.
60. Elwany S, Gamea MA, Talaat I. Passive smoking induces nasal biofilms in children. Int J Pediatr Otorhinolaryngol. 2021;146:110755.
61. Elwany S, Shewel Y, Bazak R, Talaat I, Elwany M. Quitting smoking reverses nasal mucosal changes. Eur Arch Otorrinolaringol. 2020;277:1691–8.
62. Baudoin T, Šimunjak T, Bacan N, Jelavić B, Kuna K, Košec A. Redefining pregnancy-induced rhinitis. Am J Rhinol Allergy. 2021;35(3):315–22. https://doi.org/10.1177/1945892420957490.
63. Toppozada H, Michaels L, Toppozada M, El-Ghazzawi I, Talaat M, Elwany S. The human respiratory nasal mucosa in pregnancy. An electron microscopic and histochemical study. J Laryngol Otol. 1982;96:613–26.
64. Toppozada H, Toppozada M, El-Ghazzawi I, Elwany S. The human respiratory nasal mucosa in females using contraceptive pills. An ultramicroscopic and histochemical study. J Laryngol Otol. 1984;98:43–51.
65. Toppozada H, Michaels L, Toppozada M, El-Ghazzawi E, Talaat AES. The human nasal mucosa in the menstrual cycle. A histochemical and electron microscopic study. J Laryngol Otol. 1981;95:1237–47.
66. Doshi J. Rhinitis medicamentosa: what an otolaryngologist needs to know. Eur Arch Otorrinolaringol. 2009;266:623–5.
67. Elwany S, Abdel-Salaam S. Treatment of rhinitis medicamentosa with fluticasone propionate—an experimental study. Eur Arch Otorrinolaringol. 2001;258:116–9.
68. Bist SS, Bisht M, Purohit JP. Primary atrophic rhinitis: a clinical profile, microbiological and radiological study. ISRN Otolaryngol. 2012;2012:404075.
69. Elwany S. Ultrastructural observations on primary atrophic rhinitis. Effect of partial closure of the nostril. ORL J Otorhinolaryngol Relat Spec. 1988;50:389–96.
70. Dutt SN, Kameswaran M. The aetiology and management of atrophic rhinitis. J Laryngol Otol. 2005;119:843–52.
71. Kim DH, Lee MH, Lee J, Song EA, Kim SW, Kim SW. Platelet-rich plasma injection in patients with atrophic rhinitis. ORL J Otorhinolaryngol Relat Spec. 2021;83:104–11.
72. Sajjad A. A new technique for nasal stent fabrication for atrophic rhinitis: a clinical report. J Prosthodont. 2011;20:326–8.
73. Goldenberg D, Danino J, Netzer A, Joachims HZ. Plastipore implants in the surgical treatment of atrophic rhinitis: technique and results. Otolaryngol Head Neck Surg. 2000;122:794–7.
74. Young A. Closure of the nostrils in atrophic rhinitis. J Laryngol Otol. 1971;85:715–8.
75. Poddar SK, Jagade MV. Modification of modified young's operation in the management of primary atrophic rhinitis. Indian J Otolaryngol Head Neck Surg. 2001;53:252–4.
76. Shah K, Guarderas J, Krishnaswamy G. Empty nose syndrome and atrophic rhinitis. Ann Allergy Asthma Immunol. 2016;117:217–20.

# Nasal Allergy

# 15

Matthew W. Ryan

**Key Points**

- Allergic rhinitis is a highly prevalent condition worldwide with substantial quality-of-life burden and particular importance for the rhinologist.
- Nasal allergy can be an important cofactor in sinonasal disease, and diagnosis and treatment of allergy may be necessary to achieve optimal patient outcomes.
- Both skin and in vitro testing are useful to confirm the diagnosis of allergy.
- Highly effective medications are now available for nasal allergy, and disease modification and immunomodulation may be achieved with allergen-specific immunotherapy.

## 15.1 Introduction

Allergic rhinitis is a nasal disorder characterized by irritative symptoms such as itching, sneezing, and rhinorrhea as well as nasal congestion and nasal airway obstruction induced by allergen exposure via an IgE-mediated inflammation of the nasal mucosa [1]. Allergic rhinitis is highly prevalent in industrialized nations. In some countries, the prevalence approaches 20% [2]. Allergy sufferers experience

M. W. Ryan (✉)
Department of Otolaryngology, UT Southwestern Medical Center, Dallas, TX, USA
e-mail: matthew.ryan@utsouthwestern.edu



S. Elwany (ed.), *Current Rhinology*,
https://doi.org/10.1007/978-3-031-70077-4_15

significant quality-of-life burden with lost work and school productivity, sleep disturbance, and comorbid ocular and respiratory disease. Comprehensive rhinology care includes assessment and treatment for nasal allergy.

Allergic rhinitis is an atopic disease with pathophysiologic similarities to asthma and atopic dermatitis (eczema). The susceptibility to atopic disease is hereditary and multifactorial. Genetic influences as well as early life childhood exposures to infectious disease can influence this susceptibility, and worldwide, the prevalence of allergic disease will vary based upon environmental exposures [3]. In countries with less industrial pollution and a higher prevalence of childhood infectious and parasitic disease, there appears to be a lower prevalence of allergy (hygiene hypothesis).

The pathophysiologic hallmark of allergy is allergen-induced IgE-mediated mast cell degranulation. Atopic individuals become sensitized after repeated exposure to various aeroallergens. These allergens are absorbed across respiratory mucosa, processed by dendritic cells and presented to lymphocytes within regional lymph nodes. The interaction of antigen-presenting cells with TH2 cells and B cells leads to the differentiation of allergen-specific plasma cells that then secrete allergen-specific IgE antibodies. These antibodies take up residence on the surface of mast cells and basophils primarily at epithelial and mucosal surfaces. (Only a small amount of IgE is unbound in the plasma.) This production of allergen-specific IgE constitutes the sensitization phase of allergy. The type I hypersensitivity reaction occurs when a repeat exposure to relevant aeroallergen causes cross-linking of surface-bound IgE molecules on mast cells and basophils. This cross-linking of membrane surface-bound IgE molecules triggers degranulation of the mast cell with release of histamine, tryptase, and other mediators that act as pro-inflammatory factors or chemotactic factors for eosinophils and other granulocytes. The early-phase response of allergy occurs within minutes after allergen exposure. Release of histamine results in nasal mucosal edema, pruritus, sneezing, and increased mucus production. The late-phase allergic response occurs hours later and is a result of influx of other granulocytes into the site of allergen exposure, with further cytokine elaboration that results in persisting inflammation. Historically, eosinophilia in tissue was equated with an allergic reaction. However, we now know that eosinophilic inflammation in the sinonasal mucosa may occur independent of any IgE-mediated reaction.

## 15.2 Diagnosis of Nasal Allergy

A presumptive diagnosis of nasal allergy can usually be made from information in the patient's history. Allergic rhinitis tends to be a disease of youth and is less likely in the geriatric population. Affected individuals will usually have a repeatable pattern of symptoms within minutes after allergen exposure in the environment, and patients often have an indication of which exposures trigger their symptoms. An example would be cat allergy, in which symptoms are reliably produced by entering a home with a cat. The classic nasal allergy symptoms include itchy nose, sneezing spells, stopped up or congested nose, postnasal drainage, and itchy, irritated, watery, or burning eyes. Irritative symptoms such as itching and sneezing are more likely in pollen sensitivity (seasonal allergic rhinitis) and are less common in individuals with "perennial rhinitis" triggered by exposure to dust mites, molds, or other non-seasonal allergens. Many patients with allergy are bothered by other head and neck symptoms including ear fullness or pressure, hyposmia, headache or facial pressure, palatal pruritus, and sleep disturbances. However, the most important symptoms to document are the cardinal symptoms of allergic rhinitis: nasal congestion/obstruction, nasal pruritus, and rhinorrhea [4].

Most chronic rhinitis is allergic in nature, but a variety of nonallergic triggers may precipitate classic allergic rhinitis symptoms. Also, some patients have "mixed" rhinitis with both allergic and nonallergic pathophysiologies. The likelihood of non-allergic rhinitis increases with patient age. In nonallergic rhinitis, nasal congestion, rhinorrhea, and postnasal drainage can be induced by triggers such as changes in temperature and humidity, particulate or pollution exposure, certain medications, and food and drink. The term idiopathic rhinitis is now favored in cases with no defined etiology.

A comprehensive history is our most valuable diagnostic tool. Patients should be asked to define their main symptoms. The total duration of symptoms can help differentiate allergy from other causes for symptoms (such as respiratory infection). Frequency of symptoms should be defined. Intermittent rhinitis is defined by symptoms less than 4 days a week or 4 weeks out of the year. In contrast, persistent allergic rhinitis is defined as symptoms occurring more than 4 days/week or more than 4 weeks/year [1]. An inventory of alleviating and exacerbating factors can help distinguish allergic versus nonallergic triggers. Associated head and neck, ocular, or pulmonary symptoms should be elicited. Other comorbid conditions such as eczema, asthma, oral allergy syndrome, or food allergy may point to an allergy diagnosis. Lifestyle factors are also important to review. Home and work environment, hobbies, sports, and occupation can all impact allergen exposures. Nasal allergy triggered by seasonal tree, grass, or weed pollens is denoted as seasonal allergic rhinitis. The term perennial allergic rhinitis is favored when symptoms are due to allergens that are present throughout the year such as animal danders, insects or mites, and molds. In the ARIA classification system for allergic rhinitis, the presence of sleep disturbance and/or impairment of daily activities at work or school help to define moderate/severe disease.

Physical examination and nasal endoscopy can provide supporting evidence for a diagnosis of nasal allergy [5]. Facial examination can show dark discoloration of the lower eyelids due to venous congestion (allergic shiners), and the medial lower eyelids may have fine creases or wrinkles (Dennie's lines). A horizontal nasal crease in the supratip region caused by excessive nasal manipulation is a hallmark of allergy. Intranasal examination may show edema, erythema, or a pale bluish hue to the nasal mucosa with clear exudates. Nasal endoscopy can identify adenoid hypertrophy, deviated septum, concha bullosa, turbinate hypertrophy, nasal polyps or other masses, or chronic sinusitis. A thorough intranasal examination serves primarily to exclude these other causes of chronic sinonasal symptoms.

The confirmation of an allergy diagnosis requires some form of testing [6]. Testing can be performed by measuring allergen-specific IgE concentrations in the blood or direct end-organ challenge with allergen (e.g., nasal provocation testing). However, the most commonly performed allergy test is skin testing. In allergy skin testing, allergen is introduced into the epidermis or dermis and the skin is observed for a type I immediate hypersensitivity reaction with cutaneous swelling, erythema, and pruritus (wheal and flare). Skin prick testing is the most common method. In skin prick testing, a needle or other sharp applicator device is used to deliver undiluted allergen extract into the epidermis. The skin is observed, and at 15 min, an assessment is made of the size of any resulting wheal as well as the surrounding erythema. The skin reaction induced by allergen is compared against positive (histamine) and negative (glycerin) control tests. By definition, an allergen-induced skin wheal that is ≥3 mm in diameter compared to the negative control is considered a positive result. Another skin test method that is commonly employed is intradermal testing. With intradermal testing, a needle is used to inject a small amount of diluted allergen extract into the dermis to create a 4-mm-diameter wheal. After waiting for 10 min, this wheal is again measured and compared against the negative control. With this method, a 7 mm or larger wheal is considered to be positive (again, utilizing positive and negative control tests.) Positive and negative controls are important to include in the testing procedure because there are a variety of variables that can impact skin test results. Some patients have sensitive skin that reacts to simple trauma with a wheal and flare reaction (dermatographism), and some patients may be taking medications such as antihistamines that can produce a false-negative result on skin testing. Thus, it is important at the outset of a skin testing session to place a positive control test with histamine to ensure that the patient's skin reacts appropriately. In situations where control tests do not yield the expected results, in vitro allergy testing may need to be performed. In vitro specific IgE testing is significantly more expensive than skin testing and is often reserved for special situations.

The selection of allergens for testing is based upon regionally important aeroallergens to which an individual is likely exposed. The clinically important aeroallergens include pollens from trees, grasses, or weeds, dust mites, molds, pets, and insects. The exact number of allergens to test is a matter of clinical judgment and may depend on your region of the world as well as commercial availability of allergen extracts. In the United States, respiratory aeroallergen testing panels can include 20–40 allergens [7].

Allergy tests are just like any other test in clinical medicine: The test result needs to be interpreted in the context of the patient's history. Allergic sensitization is much more common than true clinical allergy. For example, in the United States, the prevalence of allergic sensitization is greater than 50%, but the prevalence of physician diagnosed allergy is closer to 15% [8]. The astute clinician will take a patient's allergy test results and compare them to the history of symptoms during the seasons of the year, in certain environments, or after particular exposures to determine which positive allergy tests are clinically relevant. A positive result does not mean that an allergic disease is present, and some "allergy symptoms" may not be due to allergy. It is also the case that negative allergy tests do not definitively exclude allergy. In 1975, Huggins and Brostoff described a group of patients with a history suggesting dust mite allergy but negative dust mite allergy tests. However, these patients had dust mite-specific IgE in their nasal secretions [9]. In 2003, DG Powe coined the term "entopy" to describe local mucosal allergic disease in the absence of positive skin tests or detectable serum IgE [10]. Thus, some patients with rhinitis symptoms may have "local allergic rhinitis" with negative allergy tests.

The benefits of allergy testing are threefold: First, the diagnosis of allergy can be confirmed. Second, testing aids in the identification of clinically relevant allergic sensitivities. Finally, with testing the amount of pre-formed allergen-specific IgE can be qualitatively deduced and this aids in the selection of a safe starting dose for immunotherapy. The size of a skin test reaction correlates with the degree of sensitization but does NOT correlate with the severity of allergic symptoms. However, in general, the larger the skin reaction to an allergen, the more likely the sensitivity is clinically relevant. And the greater the degree of sensitization, the lower the starting dose of immunotherapy.

## 15.3 Allergy Treatment

Most allergic rhinitis is managed with a combination of allergen avoidance and pharmacotherapy. While allergen avoidance is sometimes impossible, we now have a wide array of effective pharmacologic treatments for allergic rhinitis [11]. Mild intermittent rhinitis may be treated with a second-generation oral antihistamine with or without an oral decongestant. Intranasal antihistamines have a rapid onset of action and are also a good choice for intermittent rhinitis. Persistent allergic rhinitis is best addressed with intranasal corticosteroid with or without an intranasal antihistamine, based on symptom severity. In general, oral antihistamines are only effective for pruritus and rhinorrhea (thus the frequent combination with an oral decongestant), while intranasal antihistamines and steroids alleviate all of the cardinal symptoms of rhinitis. Leukotriene receptor antagonists and injected corticosteroids are not recommended as first-line treatment for allergic rhinitis and should be reserved for special circumstances.

Immunotherapy is the one treatment that we have available that alters the natural course of allergic disease. The immunomodulation achieved with immunotherapy yields a durable reduction in symptoms that persists beyond the treatment period. With successful immunotherapy, there is a rapid desensitization of mast cells and basophils such that they are less likely to degranulate. Subsequently, immunotherapy induces an increase in regulatory T cells expressing IL-10 and TGF-beta. Immunotherapy also induces the production of antigen-specific IgG4 that acts as a blocking antibody. Finally, after a period of years the level of allergen-specific IgE in the serum decreases. These immunologic changes have been documented in multiple studies but are not used clinically. The assessment of success in immunotherapy is based upon improved symptoms and reduced medication require.

Allergy immunotherapy should be offered to patients with moderate/severe allergic rhinitis whose symptoms are not controlled with pharmacotherapy. Some patients may also choose immunotherapy due to a desire to avoid long-term pharmacotherapy and associated costs and adverse effects. Immunotherapy also has the potential benefit of preventing or reducing the severity of comorbid asthma [11]. Allergy immunotherapy can be administered sublingually or via subcutaneous injection. Both methods of administration are effective at reducing the symptoms of allergic rhinitis and are considered safe and effective [12]. However, the efficacy of immunotherapy depends on multiple factors. Clinically, relevant allergens must be correctly identified. Additionally, an adequate total administered dose of allergen is important to achieve clinical benefit. Low-dose immunotherapy is not recommended, though this was used extensively in the past. Sublingual immunotherapy (SLIT) is gaining in popularity because of its excellent safety profile and the ease of at-home administration. However, the total administered dose in SLIT is up to 60 times greater than with subcutaneous immunotherapy, and this increases the cost of treatment. Overall, allergy immunotherapy is underutilized worldwide due to the cost of treatment, the commitment required to complete a course of treatment, and a lack of access to commercial allergen extracts that are approved by regulatory bodies.

Allergy immunotherapy is a long-term treatment approach and success requires a commitment on the part of the patient to commit to years of treatment. Subcutaneous immunotherapy is initiated with a low-dose that is gradually increased until the effective maintenance dose is reached, usually with weekly injections. This escalation phase is required because of the risk of anaphylaxis with subcutaneous immunotherapy. (And this risk of anaphylaxis is the reason why office-based administration is recommended for subcutaneous immunotherapy.) The escalation phase may be abbreviated by using rush or cluster protocols that rapidly reach the effective maintenance dose. Injections are then performed biweekly or monthly for a period of 3–5 years. For sublingual immunotherapy, the allergen is administered at home daily (with minimal, if any, escalation phase) for a similar 3- to 5-year length of time. Sublingual immunotherapy is usually administered as monotherapy. In the United States, there are FDA-approved commercially available SLIT tablets for grass pollen, ragweed, and dust mite. In other regions of the world, there are aqueous and tablet-based SLIT preparations that are commercially available for a variety of allergens. Some clinicians in the United States will use commercially available SCIT extracts to make glycerinated SLIT drops. An advantage of this approach is that it is possible to treat multiple allergic sensitivities simultaneously. Sublingual immunotherapy is gaining in popularity because of its excellent safety profile and minimal risk of anaphylaxis. Immunotherapy continues to evolve and improve with novel delivery methods such as intralymphatic immunotherapy under development. Additionally, molecular alterations of allergen extracts may augment the tolerogenic effects of immunotherapy while minimizing anaphylactic adverse reactions.

## 15.4 Comorbidities

Allergic rhinitis is a risk factor for the development of asthma, and up to one-third of allergic rhinitis patients also have asthma [13]. The inflammation in asthma is like that seen in allergic rhinitis, with eosinophils, lymphocytes, and mononuclear cells elaborating an array of cytokines that are common to these two conditions. Because of this linkage, patients with allergic rhinitis should be screened for asthma and treated appropriately.

Patients with allergic rhinitis often experience ear symptoms. These symptoms include ear fullness and pressure, popping sounds during swallowing, transient hearing loss, and otalgia. The symptoms are manifestations of eustachian tube dysfunction (ETD). Inflammation of the nose can involve the eustachian tube, leading to negative middle ear pressure from inadequate eustachian tube opening. This clinical association is corroborated by studies showing that nasal instillation of histamine or allergens can induce eustachian tube dysfunction [14]. The association between allergic rhinitis and otitis media with effusion or acute otitis media is not so consistent. Cross-sectional studies have failed to demonstrate a clear and obvious association between allergic rhinitis and otitis, and interventional studies have failed to demonstrate that intranasal allergen challenge can cause otitis media [14]. The clinical importance of these distinctions is that medical therapy or immunotherapy for allergic rhinitis may improve ETD symptoms, but not otitis media.

Acute and chronic rhinosinusitis have historically been linked to allergic rhinitis. It is reasonable to assume that allergen-mediated inflammation in the nose can contribute to sinus obstruction and the development of secondary bacterial sinusitis. Additionally, the similar inflammatory milieu in allergic rhinitis and eosinophilic chronic rhinosinusitis makes such an association likely. However, we now understand that eosinophilic inflammation often occurs independent of a type I IgE-mediated allergen-driven inflammation. Extensive investigation has failed to demonstrate that chronic rhinosinusitis is more common in patients with allergic disease. It also does not appear to be the case that comorbid allergic rhinitis causes more severe or treatment refractory rhinosinusitis. Ultimately, the cross-sectional studies investigating this question have yielded widely divergent answers about the importance of allergy in CRS. Some of this confusion undoubtedly is the result of allergy test results being used as a surrogate marker of allergic rhinitis and the aggregation of multiple phenotypes of chronic rhinosinusitis into a single entity [15]. As our ability to categorize CRS phenotypes improves, so does our precision in associating allergy with chronic sinusitis. Allergic fungal rhinosinusitis (AFRS) is a phenotype of CRS with nasal polyposis that by definition requires type I hypersensitivity to fungus. A more recently described entity, central compartment atopic disease (CCAD), represents a clear association of nasal polyps with allergic rhinitis [16]. In CCAD, patients with allergic rhinitis develop polypoid edema of the middle turbinate, posterior septum, and sphenoethmoidal recess regions. Pedunculated nasal polyps may emanate from the middle turbinate. The bulk of polypoid inflammation is centrally located within the ethmoid region, often with sparing of the frontal, maxillary, and sphenoid sinuses. The EPOS 2020 categorization system for

CRS recognizes both of these conditions as distinct phenotypes of CRS [17]. What is the potential benefit of allergen-specific immunotherapy in these patients? To date, we do not have high-level interventional studies showing that allergen-specific immunotherapy alters the natural course of sinus disease, reduces symptom burden or medication requirements, or prevents the need for surgery. And so, for most forms of CRS, allergy should be considered a comorbid condition and be treated independent of sinus disease.

## 15.5 Conclusion

Complete rhinologic care includes the evaluation and treatment of allergic rhinitis and type I hypersensitivity. While a presumptive diagnosis of nasal allergy can often be made with a thorough history and physical examination, the ability to test for specific aeroallergen sensitivities allows the rhinologist to more thoroughly and completely treat chronic sinonasal symptoms. Allergy testing can be incorporated into the office evaluation of patients with minimal investment in supplies or equipment. Identification of aeroallergen sensitivities yields additional avenues of medical treatment, namely immunotherapy. Allergen-specific immunotherapy, whether administered via subcutaneous injections or sublingually, can induce host tolerance and reduce the hypersensitivity that contributes to chronic allergic head and neck symptoms.

## References

1. Bousquet J, Khaltaev N, Cruz AA, et al. Allergic rhinitis and its impact on asthma (ARIA) 2008 update (in collaboration with the World Health Organization, GA(2)LEN and AllerGen). Allergy. 2008;63(Suppl 86):8–160.
2. Mims JW. Epidemiology of allergic rhinitis. Int Forum Allergy Rhinol. 2014;4:s18–20.
3. Ege MJ, Mayer M, Normand AC, et al. Exposure to environmental microorganisms and childhood asthma. NEJM. 2011;364(8):701–9.
4. Schatz M. A survey of the burden of allergic rhinitis in the USA. Allergy. 2007;62(Suppl 85):9–16. https://doi.org/10.1111/j.1398-9995.2007.01548.x.
5. Wise SK, Damask C, Roland LT, et al. International consensus statement on allergy and rhinology: allergic rhinitis—2023. Int Forum Allergy Rhinol. 2023;13(4):293–859.
6. Bernstein IL, Li JT, Bernstein DI, et al. Allergy diagnostic testing: an updated practice parameter. Ann Allergy Asthma Immunol. 2008;100:s1–s148.
7. Ryan MW, Marple BF, Leatherman B, et al. Current practice trends in allergy: results of a United States survey of otolaryngologists, allergist-immunologists, and primary care physicians. Int Forum Allergy Rhinol. 2014;4:789–95.
8. Arbes S, Gergen PJ, Elliott L, Zeldin DC. Prevalences of positive skin test responses to 10 common allergens in the US population: results from the third National Health and nutrition examination survey. J Allergy Clin Immunol. 2005;116:377–83.
9. Huggins KG, Brostoff J. Local production of specific IgE antibodies in allergic-rhinitis patients with negative skin tests. Lancet. 1975;2:148–50.
10. Powe DG, Bonnin AJ, Jones NS. 'Entopy': local allergy paradigm. Clin Exp Allergy. 2010;40:987–97.

11. Dykewicz MS, Wallace DV, Amrol DJ, et al. Rhinitis 2020: a practice parameter update. J Allergy Clin Immunol. 2020;146:721–67.
12. Radulovic S, Calderon MA, Wilson D, Durham S. Sublingual immunotherapy for allergic rhinitis. Cochrane Database Syst Rev. 2010;12:Art. No.: CD002893. https://doi.org/10.1002/14651858.CD002893.pub2.
13. Meltzer EO. The relationships of rhinitis and asthma. Allergy Asthma Proc. 2005;26(5):336–40.
14. Wise SK, Lin SY, Toskala E, et al. International consensus statement on allergy and rhinology: allergic rhinitis. Int Forum Allergy Rhinol. 2018;8(2):108–352.
15. Halderman AA, Tully LJ. The role of allergy in chronic rhinosinusitis. Otolaryngol Clin N Am. 2017;50(6):1077–90.
16. Delgaudio JM, Loftus PA, Hamizan AW, et al. Central compartment atopic disease. Am J Rhinol Allergy. 2017;31(4):228–34.
17. Fokkens WJ, Lund VJ, Hopkins C, Hellings PW, Kern R, Reitsma S, et al. European position paper on rhinosinusitis and nasal polyps 2020. Rhinology. 2020;58(Suppl. S29):1–464.

# Surgical Treatment for Allergic Rhinitis 16

Omar El-Banhawy and Mohamed El-Banhawy

**Key Points**

- Allergic rhinitis (AR) affects 20–30% of the population. It confers a significant health burden upon the individual as it affects the patient's quality of life and is associated with serious comorbidities including asthma, sinusitis, and conjunctivitis.
- The mainstay of management is allergen identification and avoidance, pharmacotherapy with antihistamines, corticosteroids, nasal douching, immunotherapy, and a combination of the above.
- Some patients have symptoms of intractable AR in spite of adequate prolonged treatment. These patients want another adjuvant therapy for their severe discomfort.
- There are two major problems with intractable AR: Nasal obstruction and an increase in the secretory-motor activity of the nasal mucosa in the form of sneezing rhinorrhea.
- The objective of this chapter is to evaluate the effectiveness of surgical intervention on functional and symptomatic outcomes in patients with allergic rhinitis that have failed medical management. The primary aim is to improve the patient's quality of life.

**Supplementary Information** The online version contains supplementary material available at https://doi.org/10.1007/978-3-031-70077-4_16.

O. El-Banhawy (✉)
Department of Otolaryngology, Menofyia University, Shibin el Kom, Egypt

M. El-Banhawy
Department of Otolaryngology, Delta University, Cairo, Egypt


S. Elwany (ed.), *Current Rhinology*,
https://doi.org/10.1007/978-3-031-70077-4_16

## 16.1 Introduction

Allergic rhinitis (AR) is a chronic immune-mediated inflammatory nasal condition and is characterized by nasal mucosal inflammation in reaction to allergens, resulting in symptoms such as nasal congestion and pruritis, noninfectious sneezing, and watery rhinorrhea [1]. In children, AR has been associated with rhinosinusitis, Eustachian tube dysfunction, and conductive hearing loss affecting learning and development. The global spread of AR is a major public health concern. More than 500 million people reported experiencing AR symptoms, and their frequency has grown over the past few decades [2].

The mainstay of management is allergen identification and avoidance treatment with conventional pharmacotherapy such as antihistamines, decongestants, anticholinergic agents, mast cell stabilizers, intranasal steroid sprays, and allergen desensitization. In general, the goal of treatment for any medical condition is to achieve and maintain clinical control. Control is defined as a disease state in which the patients do not have symptoms anymore or the remaining symptoms are not regarded as bothersome. Despite guideline-directed pharmacotherapy, 10–20% of severe AR patients remain bothered by their symptoms [3]. Do such cases represent an "intractable" form of AR? However, some intractably allergic patients remain, as well as some inconvenience for those who have used these medicines over a long term.

There are two major problems with intractable AR: nasal obstruction and an increase in the secretory-motor activity of the nasal mucosa in the form of sneezing and rhinorrhea.

## 16.2 Surgical Intervention for Reduction of Nasal Obstruction

The most common applied surgical procedures are:

- Inferior turbinate surgery
- Septoplasty
- Endoscopic sinus surgery (ESS)
- Combination of the above

### 16.2.1 Inferior Turbinate Surgery

Hypertrophy of the inferior turbinate is common in allergic rhinitis. In many cases, the turbinate shrinks in size when nasal allergy is controlled with medical measures. However, in some patients, the turbinates remain hypertrophied, interfere with the patient's sleep and activities, and worsen the overall quality of life. Surgical reduction of the size of the inferior turbinates is indicated for those patients. Various techniques have been described in the literature. The details of these techniques are presented in the chapter on surgery of the inferior turbinates.

### 16.2.2 Septoplasty

Septoplasty is a surgical procedure performed to correct a deviated septum. It is one of the most commonly performed surgeries within otorhinolaryngology and plastic surgery. The primary indication for this functional (as opposed to purely esthetic) surgery is usually septal deviation resulting in significant and symptomatic nasal airway obstruction. Nonetheless, fixed septal deformities, such as bony spurs or cartilaginous deviation, may worsen subjective nasal obstruction in AR patients. In these cases, or in conjunction with endoscopic sinus surgery, septoplasty may be undertaken to improve the quality of life in patients with middle meatal edema and ostiomeatal complex obstruction in a patient with allergic rhinitis [4].

Nasal obstruction owing to septal deviation associated with allergic rhinitis mandates the use of septoplasty with or without inferior turbinate surgery technique. The use of this procedure has demonstrated improved quality of life, particularly when used in conjunction with other interventions. Many surgical techniques and approaches have been described; these include endonasal, endoscopic, and open procedures. Endoscopic septoplasty is an attractive alternative to traditional "headlight" approaches to septoplasty. The primary advantage of the technique is the ability to reduce morbidity and postoperative swelling in isolated septal deviations by limiting the dissection to the area of the deviation. This ability to markedly reduce the extent of subperichondrial dissection is particularly valuable in patients who have undergone prior septal cartilage resection [5].

- It is an alternative to conventional and/or microsurgical approaches.
- It allows:
  - Better visualization due to a wider, unobstructed visual field.
  - Less bleeding and reduced operation times.
  - Better view for posterior deviations.
  - Identification of the septal area to be corrected with a limited extent of the excision.
  - Possibility of using combined approaches.
  - Concurrent surgical endoscopy of paranasal sinuses.
  - Better assessment of nasal valve region during surgery.
- It is an effective teaching tool and allows excellent opportunity for recording and studying the procedures.

### 16.2.3 Endoscopic Sinus Surgery (ESS)

Endoscopic sinus surgery is considered as one of the most common otolaryngologic procedures for the treatment of nasal obstruction caused by many conditions as chronic sinusitis, paranasal and sinus polyposis, and allergic fungal sinusitis. Endoscopic sinus surgery does not have a primary role alone in treating AR, but is of benefit in patients who have comorbid diseases like chronic rhinosinusitis, allergic fungal disease, or nasal polyposis. These comorbidities are commonly seen and if maximal medical therapy proves ineffective in controlling their symptoms, then surgery may be indicated. Endoscopic sinus surgery may be combined with a turbinate reduction to provide relief to more refractory or advanced cases of AR, in which turbinoplasty alone may be inadequate [6].

Often, the recurrent edema and obstruction that is present in AR patients can lead to middle meatal swelling and blockage of the ostiomeatal complex. This in turn may predispose certain patients to recurrent infections or chronic sinusitis. The central goal of endoscopic surgery is to maximize nasal patency while alleviating the effects of edematous ostia [6].

#### 16.2.3.1 How ESS Addresses Nasal Allergies?

1. Treatment of Nasal Obstructions
   - ESS allows the surgeon to remove nasal polyps, which can be associated with allergic inflammation.
2. Widening Sinus Openings
   - The surgery can involve enlarging the natural openings of the sinuses, promoting better drainage and aeration of the sinuses.
3. Improved Medication Delivery
   - After surgery, topical medications such as nasal sprays may be more effective in reaching the sinus tissues.
4. Addressing Chronic Inflammation
   - ESS aims to reduce chronic inflammation in the sinuses, which is often a component of both chronic sinusitis and allergic rhinitis.

## 16.3 Surgery to Decrease the Secretory Motor Stimulus

Patients with intractable rhinitis often complain of persistent and severe nasal symptoms in spite of prolonged treatment and often have difficulties living ordinary lives and coping with different social situations. They want another adjuvant treatment for their discomfort without additional medications. In this respect, surgery to decrease the secretory-motor stimulus for the nasal mucosa can be considered the treatment of choice, because it is the only method that can permanently block the pathophysiological mechanism of intractable rhinitis. The aim of this surgical procedure is to overcome, excessive sneezing, rhinorrhea, and nasal itching.

### 16.3.1 Surgical Procedures to Decrease the Secretory-Motor Stimulus for Nasal Mucosa

- Vidian neurectomy
- Posterior nasal nerve resection
- Peripheral branches of the posterior nasal nerve

### 16.3.2 Vidian Neurectomy

The Vidian nerve (VN) supplies parasympathetic fibers to the nasal mucosa, palate, and lacrimal gland via the pterygopalatine ganglion. Overstimulation of this ganglion results in mucosal secretion causing rhinorrhea. The vidian nerve, along with the vidian artery, runs along the pterygoid canal—an osseous tunnel along the floor of the sphenoid sinus (hence also called the nerve of the pterygoid canal) [7]. It is located within the sphenoid bone, at the junction of the pterygoid plate and the sphenoid body; it carries the vidian nerve connecting the middle fossa to the pterygopalatine fossa. The greater superficial petrosal nerve (GSPN) branches off the geniculate ganglia via the hiatus and travels anteriorly along the base of the middle fossa [8]. The deep petrosal nerve joins the GSPN under the foramen lacerum, and, together, they become the vidian nerve which courses along the horizontal segment of the petrous carotid artery at the level of the foramen lacerum. The anterior end of the vidian nerve connects to the pterygopalatine ganglia in the pterygopalatine fossa where it branches off its terminal innervation [7].

The vidian nerve brings the parasympathetic fibers originating from the superior salivatory nucleus through the nervus intermedius, geniculate ganglia, and GSPN. The terminal fibers innervate the lacrimal gland, facilitating lacrimation as its main function. The deep petrosal nerve, the other root joining the vidian nerve, carries the sympathetic fibers from the superior cervical ganglion after branching off from the carotid plexus, the deep petrosal nerve courses through the pterygopalatine ganglia without synapsing which innervates the mucosa capillary along with the distribution of the trigeminal nerve branches [9].

Vidian neurectomy is typically performed for the management of conditions related to the autonomic nervous system, particularly, intractable allergic rhinitis, vasomotor rhinitis, intrinsic rhinitis, and crocodile tears. Golding-Wood [10] first introduced the concept of vidian neurectomy as definitive surgical management for vasomotor and allergic rhinitis in the 1960s. The theoretical basis of this surgery is an imbalance between parasympathetic and sympathetic innervation of the nasal cavity and the resultant stimulation of goblet cells and mucous glands. The aim of this surgical technique is to disrupt this imbalance and reduce nasal secretions. There are many surgical approaches for vidian neurectomy including transantral, transpalatal transnasal, and transsphenoidal [10].

With the revolution of various surgical procedures and instruments, including the microscope and endoscope, its surgical approach changed greatly. Transnasal endoscopic VN has become the main surgical approach. Ideal surgical view and exact localization of the vidian canal are the advantages of endoscope-guided VN compared with the traditional method [9].

Two different methods of surgical access have been used clinically through the sphenoid sinus and through the pterygopalatine fossa [11]. In the first case, the paper-thin vidian canal wall was often perforated with subsequent severing of the nerve. The key to this procedure is the anatomic protrusion of the vidian canal into the sphenoid sinus. If the canal is located deeply in the floor of the sinus, the procedure has to be modified accordingly. In the second situation, the vidian canal was exposed in the pterygopalatine fossa through the sphenopalatine foramen. The key to this procedure is the accurate location of the vidian canal on the posterior wall of the pterygopalatine fossa or between the sphenoid sinus and the pterygopalatine fossa [11].

However, many practitioners have abandoned vidian neurectomy due to technical difficulty, its transient effectiveness and reports of serious complications, such as visual loss, xerophthalmia (dry eye), trigeminal neuralgia, cheek and dental numbness, and disturbance of eye movements [12].

### 16.3.3 Long-Term Complications [13]

- Dry eye: This is the most commonly reported complication in nearly 50% of cases, ranging between 35 and 72%. Xerophthalmia is significantly more likely to occur after transsphenoidal/intrasphenoidal approaches. Most studies reported the resolution of dry eyes within 1–5 months of surgery.
- Palatal/Gingival/Cheek numbness (6.27%): Incidence is more likely after the pterygopalatine approach.
- Nasal crusting/dryness (3.7%)

With the advancement of endoscopic instrumentation and technique, identification and sectioning of the vidian nerve under direct visualization have become easier, resulting in fewer complications. Therefore, the effectiveness of vidian neurectomy needs to be reevaluated.

### 16.3.4 Posterior Nasal Nerve Resection

Over the last two decades, many endoscopic surgical techniques have been documented to alleviate nasal hyperreactivity accompanying intractable AR. Among them, posterior nasal neurectomy is an effective method to transect the neural networks surrounding the inferior turbinate that cause unregulated nasal hypersensitivity with excess secretion.

The posterior nasal nerve (PNN) is a peripheral branch of the sphenopalatine ganglion, entering the nasal cavity through separate foramen 4–5 mm below the sphenopalatine foramen/crista ethmoidalis after bifurcation of the nerve into the lacrimal nerve. The nerve bundles consist of parasympathetic and sympathetic components of the vidian nerve and somatosensory fibers from the maxillary branch of the trigeminal nerve and they are distributed in the nasal mucosa following the branches of the sphenopalatine vessels [13].

The reported surgical procedures for posterior nasal nerve neurectomy (PNNN) can be divided into three approaches. The first is selective resection of the posterior nasal nerve branches at the sphenopalatine foramen without resecting the sphenopalatine artery [14]. This approach is very difficult to keep a clear surgical field because of bleeding from the branches of the sphenopalatine artery and veins, and a few branches of the posterior nasal nerve remain. For example, Makihara et al. [15] only resected the anteroinferior branch toward the inferior turbinate and posterosuperior branch toward the middle meatus. The second approach resects the neurovascular bundle, which might cause serious intraoperative or postoperative nasal bleeding [16] The third is the resection of peripheral branches in the inferior turbinate, in which hypersecretion from the posterior part of the middle turbinate could not reduce [16]. In addition, the three methods do not resect the accessory posterior nasal nerve.

The mean distance between PNN and nasal sill (56.4 mm), maxillary sinus ostium (27 mm), posterior fontanel (12.5 mm), torus tubarius (13 mm), and crista ethmoidalis (8 mm) was determined. PNN was found consistently posterior to the sphenopalatine artery where the inferior turbinate attaches to the lateral nasal wall [17].

By resection of the posterior nasal nerve at this point, we can expect modifying the hyperreactivity of the neural network that augments the allergic reaction. In addition, this technique causes partial denervation of the middle turbinate and septum submucosal glands based on anatomical innervation. By denervating the nasal mucosa, one renders it unresponsive to any sort of allergen or allergic reaction.

Ogawa et al. [18] found out that PNN in allergic rhinitis patients significantly reduces levels of IL-5, eotaxin protein in nasal secretions. They also observed a reduction of infiltrated immuno-component cells in the subepithelial mucous layer, which are major sources of cytokine release.

As compared to vidian neurectomy, parasympathetic denervation of the nasal mucosa by posterior nasal nerve resection has an easier endoscopic surgical approach. It is minimally invasive and bypasses the ocular and dental complications of vidian neurectomy, thus reducing the scale of surgery. This procedure is usually combined with inferior turbinate surgery for drug therapy-resistant, intractable allergic rhinitis [19].

### 16.3.5 Resection of Peripheral Branches of the Posterior Nasal Nerve

Although posterior nasal nerve neurectomy denervates a wider area of the nasal mucosa, it is a more surgically demanding procedure that typically requires general anesthesia. In this approach, it is very difficult to keep a clear surgical field because of bleeding from the branches of the sphenopalatine artery and veins and often coagulation of the sphenopalatine artery. It is advisable to preserve the sphenopalatine artery as it has a positive effect on humidification inside the nose. Also, some of the branches arising through separate foramina may be missed [20]. The reported surgical procedures for posterior nasal nerve neurectomy all were selective resection of posterior nasal nerve branches, causing a residue of a few branches of the nerve. As a result, patients either do not achieve the best improvement of symptoms, or relapse and experience long-time failure after posterior nasal nerve neurectomy [20].

The peripheral branches of the posterior nasal nerves run within the tissues of the inferior turbinate close to the bony concha. Unintended surgical resection of these branches has been suggested as an explanation for the improvement of allergic symptoms following inferior turbinate reduction. Nevertheless, submucosal selective identification of all peripheral posterior nasal nerve branches within the inferior turbinate can be surgically demanding, and some branches may be frequently missed. Mori et al. [21] mentioned that surgically induced damage to peripheral posterior nasal nerve fiber during turbinoplasty might be a major factor in improving allergic symptoms after submucous turbinectomy. Kobayashi et al. [20] found that submucosal resection of peripheral branches of the posterior nasal nerve within the inferior turbinate had a good control of symptoms scores of AR. This is most likely due to the dominant role of the inferior turbinate in normal nasal breathing and reactivity [22].

In a study by Elwany et al. [23], they used the radiofrequency probe to coagulate the inferior turbinate tissue where the peripheral posterior nasal nerve branches normally pass submucosally close to the bony concha obviating the need for individual identification of the branches. This procedure was a short procedure that is technically easy, minimally invasive, and can be performed under local or general anesthesia. Furthermore, there is no risk of postoperative hemorrhage as may occur from the sphenopalatine artery and can be combined with complete radiofrequency turbinoplasty if needed.

Most recently, quantum molecular resonance (QMR) devices have been applied as energy-based devices to coagulate the peripheral posterior nasal nerve branches in inferior turbinate tissue. QMR devices are powered using electron energy quanta, which are generated by alternate current and high-frequency electron waves, and it is characterized by a well-defined dominant wave at 4 MHz, followed by waves at 8, 12, and 16 MHz with reduced amplitude [19]. As the quantum energy is delivered, cell molecular bonds in human tissue resonate, followed by subsequent bond breakage and a minimal temperature increase. The process also activates the physiological coagulation cascade without the need for necrotic plugs, which is contrary to methods that use other cauterization methods [24]. The mechanism of action is based on molecular bounds breaking: QMR generates frequencies that make bounds resonate and break keeping the surrounding tissues at a low temperature (<45 °C) [24].

Quantic molecular resonance treatment is an outpatient procedure that can be performed under minimally invasive local anesthesia, and it is a rapid (about 10 min of treatment) and accurate technique (the wound is extremely localized with minimal effects on the surrounding tissues). If necessary, this procedure can be repeated, and the rate of postoperative complications such as pain, early and late bleeding, synechiae, scabs, infections, and nasal dryness is substantially minimal [24].

## References


1. Brożek JL, Bousquet J, Agache I, et al. Allergic Rhinitis and its Impact on Asthma (ARIA) guidelines-2016 revision. J Allergy Clin Immunol. 2017;140:950–8.
2. Seidman MD, Gurgel RK, Lin SY, et al. Clinical practice guideline: allergic rhinitis. Otolaryngol Head Neck Surg. 2015;152:S1–43.
3. Bousquet PJ, Bachert C, Canonica GW, et al. Uncontrolled allergic rhinitis during treatment and its impact on quality of life: a cluster randomized trial. J Allergy Clin Immunol. 2010;126(3):666–8.

4. Karatzanis AD, Fragiadakis G, Moshandrea J, Zenk J, Iro H, Velegrakis GA. Septoplasty outcome in patients with and without allergic rhinitis. Rhinology. 2009;47(4):444–9.
5. Vandenbroeck S, Jorissen M. Endoscopic septoplasty: literature review, surgical techniques and retrospective analysis at the University Hospitals Leuven. J Laryngol Otol. 2019;133(4):262–8.
6. Ramadan HH, Hinerman RA. Outcome of endoscopic sinus surgery in children with allergic rhinitis. Am J Rhinol. 2006;20(4):438–40.
7. Osawa S, Rhoton AL Jr, Seker A, Shimizu S, Fujii K, Kassam AB. Microsurgical and endoscopic anatomy of the vidian canal. Neurosurgery. 2009;64(5, suppl 2):385–411. discussion 411–412
8. Tubbs RS, Menendez J, Loukas M, et al. The petrosal nerves: anatomy, pathology, and surgical considerations. Clin Anat. 2009;22(05):537–44.
9. Douglas R, Wormald PJ. Endoscopic vidian neurectomy. Oper Tech Otolaryngol Head Neck Surg. 2006;17(3):174–7. https://doi.org/10.1016/j.otot.2006.01.012.
10. Golding-Wood PH. Observations on petrosal and vidian neurectomy in chronic vasomotor rhinitis. J Laryngol Otol. 1961;75(3):232–47.
11. Zhao C, Ji Y, An Y, Xue J, Li Q, Suo L, Hou R, Zhang Y, Geng Z, Shen H, Ren J, Yang P. An alternative method of endoscopic intrasphenoidal vidian neurectomy. OTO Open. 2018;2(1):2473974X18764862.
12. Fernandes CM. Bilateral transnasal vidian neurectomy in the management of chronic rhinitis. J Laryngol Otol. 1994;108(7):569–73.
13. Balai E, Gupta KK, Jolly K, Darr A. Posterior nasal nerve neurectomy for the treatment of rhinitis: a systematic review and meta-analysis. Eur Ann Allergy Clin Immunol. 2023;55(3):101–14. https://doi.org/10.23822/EurAnnACI.1764-1489.268.
14. Ahilasamy N, Rajendran Dinesh K. Endoscopic posterior nasal neurectomy. J Laryngol Otol. 2019;133(9):825–9.
15. Takahara D, Takeno S, Hamamoto T, Ishino T, Hirakawa K. Management of intractable nasal hyperreactivity by selective resection of posterior nasal nerve branches. Int J Otolaryngol. 2017;2017:1907862.
16. Makihara S, Okano M, Miyamoto S, et al. Underwater posterior nasal neurectomy compared to resection of peripheral branches of posterior nerve in severe allergic rhinitis. Acta Otolaryngol. 2021;141(8):780–5.
17. Eren E, Zeybek G, Ecevit C, Arslanoğlu S, Ergur I, Kiray A. A new method of identifying the posterior inferior nasal nerve: implications for posterior nasal neurectomy. J Craniofac Surg. 2015;26(3):930–2.
18. Ogawa T, Takeno S, Ishino T, Hirakawa K. Submucous turbinectomy combined with posterior nasal neurectomy in the management of severe allergic rhinitis: clinical outcomes and local cytokine changes. Auris Nasus Larynx. 2007;34(3):319–26.
19. Ikeda K, Yokoi H, Saito T, Kawano K, Yao T, Furukawa M. Effect of resection of the posterior nasal nerve on functional and morphological changes in the inferior turbinate mucosa. Acta Otolaryngol. 2008;128(12):1337–41.
20. Kobayashi T, Hyodo M, Nakamura K, Komobuchi H, Honda N. Resection of peripheral branches of the posterior nasal nerve compared to conventional posterior neurectomy in severe allergic rhinitis. Auris Nasus Larynx. 2012;39(6):593–6.
21. Mori S, Fujieda S, Igarashi M, Fan GK, Saito H. Submucous turbinectomy decreases not only nasal stiffness but also sneezing and rhinorrhea in patients with perennial allergic rhinitis. Clin Exp Allergy. 1999;29:1542–8.
22. Feldman EM, Koshy JC, Chike-Obi CJ, Hatef DA, Bullocks JM, Stal S. Contemporary techniques in inferior turbinate reduction: survey results of the American Society for Aesthetic Plastic Surgery. Aesthet Surg J. 2010;30(5):672–9.
23. Elwany S, Mandour Z, Ibrahim AA, Bazak R. Nasal reactivity after radiofrequency ablation of peripheral branches of posterior nasal nerve. Turk Arch Otorhinolaryngol. 2022;60(4):1.
24. Vescovi P, Manfredi M, Merigo E, Fornaini C, Rocca J-P, Nammour S, et al. Quantic molecular resonance scalpel and its potential applications in oral surgery. Br J Oral Maxillofacial Surg. 2008;46(5):355–7.

# Acute Rhinosinusitis

# 17

Yasser Nour and Ahmed Thabet

**Key Points**

- Acute rhinosinusitis is a common problem with three identified phenotypes namely acute viral rhinosinusitis (AVRS), acute postviral rhinosinusitis, and acute bacterial rhinosinusitis (ABRS).
- Accurate diagnosis of each phenotype can be achieved through proper reviewing of the clinical symptoms with special emphasis on the duration and severity of symptoms.
- Diagnosis of ARS is mainly clinical with no need for additional imaging modalities except in selected situations.
- Tailoring of the treatment according to the diagnosed phenotype will prevent the misuse of antibiotics with its negative economic impact and the contribution to the emergence of resistant bacteria strains within the community.
- If antibiotic treatment is indicated, proper selection of the antibiotic with the most appropriate coverage for the prevalent bacteria causing ABRS is important. Certain factors should be considered to modify the selection of the antibiotic in certain situations, e.g., the usage of antibiotics within the community, the likelihood of bacterial resistance, or patient factors that increase the probability of antibiotic resistance.

Y. Nour (✉) · A. Thabet
Department of Otolaryngology, Alexandria University, Alexandria, Egypt


S. Elwany (ed.), *Current Rhinology*,
https://doi.org/10.1007/978-3-031-70077-4_17

Rhinosinusitis is an inflammatory condition affecting the lining of the sinuses and nasal passages that can be variable in its clinical presentation. Anatomically, the nasal mucosa is continuous with the sinus mucosa, and both are concomitantly involved in any inflammatory condition, therefore the term "rhinosinusitis" is more accurately used instead of "sinusitis." Recently rhinosinusitis has been classified into different phenotypes based on the etiology and the temporal pattern of inflammation. Proper understanding of those phenotypes is important as the prognosis and recommended treatment strategies can be different for each form of rhinosinusitis.

## 17.1 Classification

According to clinical practice guidelines of the American Academy of Otolaryngology-Head and Neck Surgery Foundation, acute rhinosinusitis (ARS) is defined as up to 4 weeks of purulent nasal drainage accompanied by nasal obstruction and/or facial pain/pressure/fullness. ARS is presumed to be caused by a viral infection when symptoms or signs are present in less than 10 days and not worsening in severity. ARS is presumed to be caused by bacterial infection when symptoms or signs fail to improve within 10 days or more beyond the onset of upper respiratory symptoms, or when symptoms or signs of acute rhinosinusitis worsen within 10 days after an initial improvement (double worsening) [1].

Recently the European Position Paper on Rhinosinusitis and Nasal Polyps 2020 (EPOS 2020) defined ARS as follows: [2]

Sudden onset of two or more symptoms, one of which should be either nasal blockage/obstruction/congestion or nasal discharge (anterior/posterior nasal drip) for less than 12 weeks:

- ± Facial pain/pressure
- ± Reduction or loss of smell

EPOS 2020 identified three phenotypes for ARS (Fig. 17.1) based on the duration and severity of the symptoms:

- Acute viral rhinosinusitis (AVRS, common cold).
- Post-viral rhinosinusitis.
- Acute bacterial rhinosinusitis (ABRS).

Common colds are defined as AVRS with the duration of symptoms of <10 days (but <12 weeks). When symptoms increase after 5 days, or when symptoms are persistent for more than 10 days, with <12 weeks duration, then EPOS classifies this as an acute postviral rhinosinusitis. Only a minority of ARS is of bacterial origin (Fig. 17.2). ABRS is diagnosed if at least three of the following symptoms/signs are fulfilled:

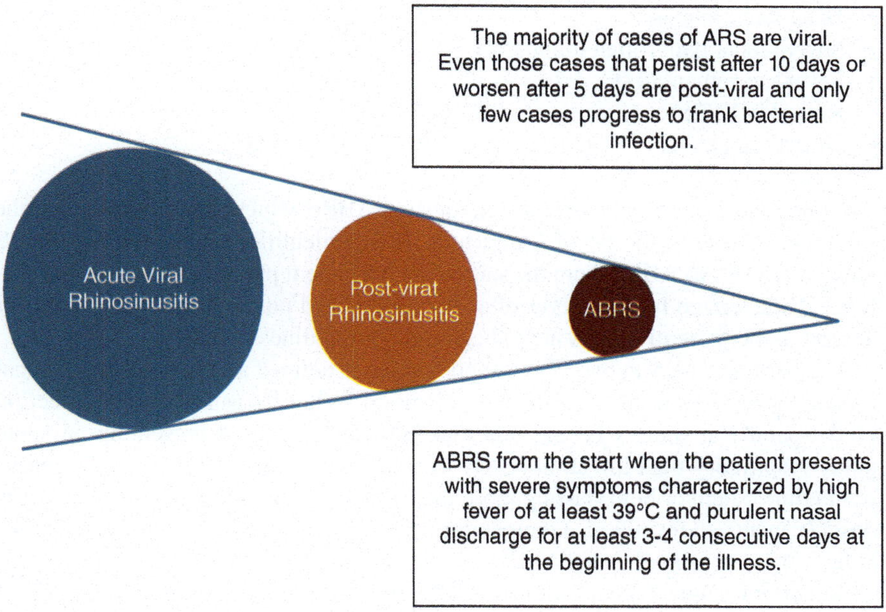


**Fig. 17.1** Different phenotypes of ARS

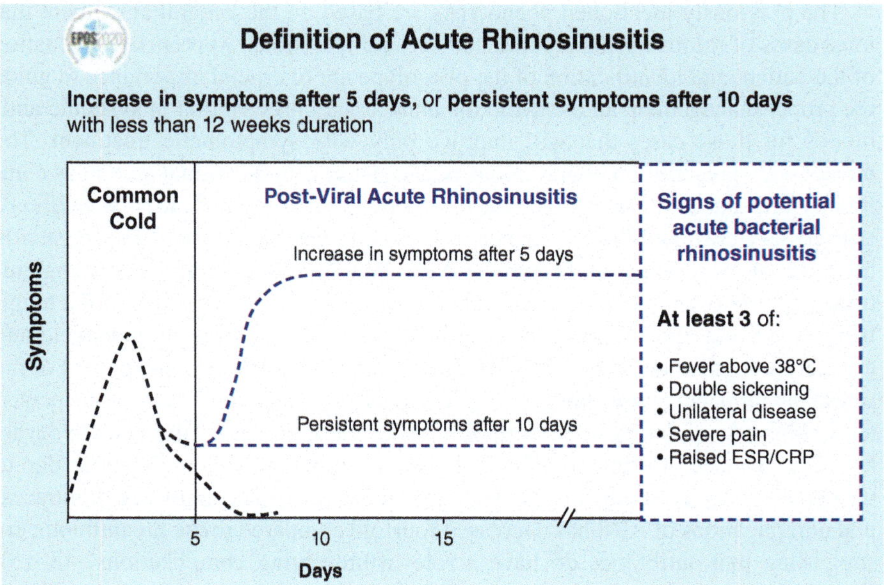


**Fig. 17.2** Definition of ARS

- Discolored mucus
- Severe local pain (often unilateral)
- Fever more than 38 °C
- Raised CRP/ESR
- Double sickening

There was a third guideline for diagnosing ABRS which was published by the Infectious Diseases Society of America in 2012; it identifies a special form of ARS which is known as ABRS from the start when the patient presents with severe symptoms characterized by high fever of at least 39 °C and purulent nasal discharge for at least 3–4 consecutive days at the beginning of the illness [3].

Furthermore, ARS in the pediatric population is defined according to the clinical practice guidelines of the American Academy of Pediatrics as follows: an infection of the paranasal sinuses lasting less than 30 days and often presenting an acute upper respiratory tract infection (URI) with persistent illness (i.e., nasal discharge or daytime cough or both) lasting more than 10 days, a worsening course, or severe onset (concurrent fever with a temperature ≥ 39 °C and purulent nasal discharge for at least three consecutive days) [4].

Recurrent acute rhinosinusitis (RARS) represents a unique clinical variant of rhinosinusitis and has an estimated incidence of 0.035% in the general population. RARS is clinically defined as the occurrence of greater than four ARS events within a 12-month period [5–7].

The previously mentioned phenotypes are based on the general agreement that most cases of rhinosinusitis are initiated by viral infections. Appropriate evaluation of the patient and identification of the phenotype are of crucial importance to guide the proper management and to avoid the unnecessary prescription of systemic antibiotics for those cases that will improve only with symptomatic treatment. The unnecessary prescription of antibiotics is associated with individual as well as community drawbacks including the risk for allergic reaction, medication side effects, unnecessary cost, and the emergence of resistant bacteria strains. The persistently high rate of prescribing antibiotics for ARS is likely multifactorial, reflecting cultural, economic, and microbiologic considerations [8, 9]. Patient desire for a tangible product of a clinical encounter, physician desire to satisfy patient demand and clinical throughput demands, and lack of information on behalf of the patient or the physician influence prescribing [9–11]. The most defensible rationale for the persistently high rate of antibiotic prescription for ARS is concern for the rare but devastating occurrence of septic, ophthalmologic, and intracranial complications due to the spread of bacterial infections beyond the sinuses [12]. The incidence of intracranial complications of ARS has decreased fourfold compared to the preantibiotic era suggesting that antibiotics do have a role in preventing complications [13–15]. However, recent studies suggest that ARS complications occur regardless of treatment in the modern era [16, 17]. In a multicenter study of patients with ARS complications, the majority of patients were started on antibiotics (59%) before admission, with similar complication rates in patients treated with and without antibiotics [16].

## 17.2 Epidemiology and Socioeconomic Burden

ARS is one of the most common diseases of the general population and generates an enormous number of visits to primary health care and specialized care physicians. In Europe, 1–2% of all patient visits to physicians in primary care are for suspected acute sinusitis [18]. The prevalence of ARS in the general population is variable depending on different studies, noted to be between 6% and 15% [3]. The high number of visits to physicians translates to a high burden on the healthcare system. In 2000, the direct costs in the United States were estimated to be nearly $6 billion [19, 20]. The mean total cost for an episode of acute mild to moderate rhinosinusitis in patients seeking primary care was approximately €1102 in May 2011. The direct costs (medications and visits to the physician) constituted only about 25% of the total costs, indicating that the main costs for acute rhinosinusitis are due to loss in productivity (indirect costs) [21]. ARS causes a high burden on the quality-of-life parameters. At baseline, pain/discomfort was reported by 88.4% of the patients, and problems with usual activities by 43.2%. Both dimensions showed improvement on day 15 [21]. In the British population, ARS is estimated to cause 6 million restricted working days per year [22].

The prevalence of the different phenotypes of ARS is highly variable. AVRS or common cold has a very high incidence, presenting two to five episodes per person a year [23]. In children, this incidence could be up to four times higher, with URTIs being one of the main causes of primary care consultations [24, 25]. Postviral ARS is less common, with an incidence of about three episodes per 100 inhabitants a year in adults (Iceland) with a lower frequency in pediatric populations and differences noted among different age groups (two cases per 100,000 in ≤4 years old, 4–7 cases per 100,000 in 5–14 years old, and 18 cases per 100,000 in 15–17 years old) [26, 27]. In a recent study in Germany, the incidence was found to be 18.8 episodes per 1000 inhabitants per year [28]. Classically, the incidence of bacterial ARS is estimated to be 0.5–2% of all ARS viral infections, although recent studies have suggested it to be higher. The rate of positive cultures is about 50% in patients with clinical suspicion of bacterial ARS [29].

## 17.3 Etiology and Pathogenesis

Irrespective of etiology, three key features characterize ARS: inflammatory edema of the sinus mucosa, obstruction of the sinus ostia, and decreased mucociliary activity. Impaired mucociliary transport fosters stagnation of secretions, decreases their pH, and lowers oxygen tension, thereby providing an environment favorable for bacterial growth.

The initial factor in the pathogenesis of ARS is mostly due to viral infection of the sinonasal passage. Evidence of the association of viral infection with sinusitis comes from studies reporting that seasonal exacerbations of sinusitis occur at the same time as the common cold, in the fall and in the late spring [30, 31]. Gwaltney et al. found that up to 87% of adults with a common cold develop sinus abnormalities seen on sinus computer-assisted tomography scan during their acute infection [32]. Viruses attach to the nasal epithelium and can spread from the nasal cavity to the paranasal sinuses. It has been previously reported that the pressure generated within the nasal cavity during nose blowing can reach 60 mm Hg which is enough pressure to propel mucous infected with a virus from the nose into the sinus cavities [33].

Viral infection leads to damage of the ciliary epithelium, release of proinflammatory cytokines, and swelling of the mucous membranes. Cytokines and mediators of the inflammatory response will cause the following: increase vascular permeability, induce edema of the mucous membrane, increased production of secretions, and disruption of mucociliary transport. This, in turn, leads to impairment of sinus passages' patency, impaired ventilation of the sinuses, and retention of secretions within the paranasal sinuses. The previous changes within the sinonasal cavity will provide a good environment for secondary bacterial infection resulting in ABRS in selected patients [30, 34].

The previously mentioned sinonasal mechanical obstruction induced by the inflammatory changes has been postulated for a long time as the sole mechanism by which viral infection induces a subsequent superadded bacterial infection. In recent years, more studies were showing the interaction between virus and bacteria with more complex mechanisms that explain the role of viral infection in promoting secondary bacterial infection. These include overexpression of cellular fibronectin and ICAM-1 that promote adhesion and internalization of bacteria, disruption of epithelial junctions that promote paracellular migration of bacteria and its epithelium invasion. Even more, bacterial exotoxins promote viral replication (Fig. 17.3) [35].

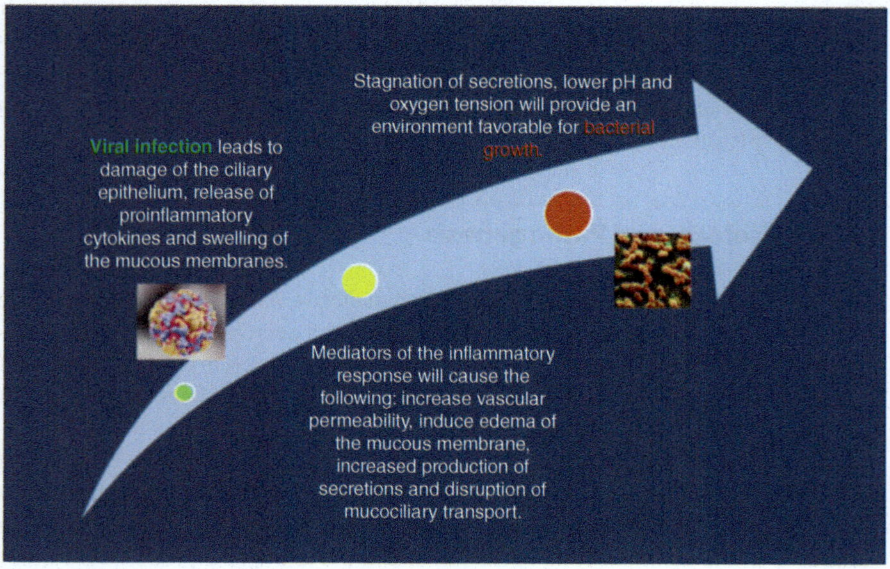


**Fig. 17.3** Pathogenesis or acute rhinosinusitis

The most common viruses that cause AVRS are rhinovirus, influenza virus, and coronavirus; others include parainfluenza virus, adenovirus, respiratory syncytial virus, and metapneumovirus [36–38].

The most common bacteria associated with ABRS are Streptococcus pneumoniae, Haemophilus influenzae, Moraxella catarrhalis, Group A beta-hemolytic Streptococci, and Staphylococcal aureus. Enteric bacteria are recovered less commonly. When a sinus culture is positive in a patient with ABRS, a single pathogen is usually found in high concentration, although in approximately 25% of the patients, two pathogens can be found in high concentration. The infection is polymicrobial in about one-third of the cases. The introduction of routine conjugated pneumococcal vaccination in children has changed the spectrum of bacterial infection. In both adults and children, the percentage of ABRS due to S. pneumoniae has decreased while the proportion due to H. influenzae has increased.

Microaerophilic Streptococci and anaerobic bacteria are commonly identified if the ABRS originates from an odontogenic source. Pseudomonas aeruginosa and other gram-negative rods are common in sinusitis of nosocomial origin (especially in patients who have nasal tubes or catheters), the immunocompromised, and patients who have HIV infection or cystic fibrosis. Anaerobic bacteria also can be recovered in these patients [39–41].

Although most episodes of acute sinusitis are caused by viral upper respiratory tract infections, they are also associated with asthma, allergic rhinitis, smoking, exposure to secondhand smoke or occupational irritants, odontogenic infections, and genetic factors such as immotile cilia syndrome or cystic fibrosis; certain systemic diseases or medical treatments that predispose individuals to bacterial infections.

The correlation between allergic rhinitis and the risk of recurrent ARS is still uncertain. In addition to the well-known mechanism of mechanical obstruction of the sinus ostia caused by inflammatory edema induced by allergic rhinitis and its predisposition to stagnation of secretions that favors secondary bacterial infection, several experimental studies showed that the allergic inflammation has a negative impact on the immunological function of the nasal cavity by different mechanisms. Allergic inflammation causes a reduction of tight junction proteins, overexpression of ICAM adhesion molecules which are the principal receptors for rhinovirus, and decreased production of interferon which is crucial for induction of apoptosis in virus-infected host cells because they prevent the establishment of viral replication and promote phagocytosis of infected cells. Recent study in Taiwan showed that pediatric patients with allergic rhinitis were significantly associated with a three times increased risk of developing acute rhinosinusitis [42, 43].

There is evidence that primary immunodeficiency disorders (PIDDs) such as common variable immunodeficiency (CVID), X-linked agammaglobulinemia, and selective immunoglobulin A (IgA) immunodeficiency are linked to sinusitis. However, there is a deficiency in evidence-based articles specific to diagnostic workup for PIDD in patients with RARS. Additional research is necessary to guide clinical practice recommendations [44].

Anatomic abnormalities such as large septal spurs and large paradoxical turbinates have been suggested to be associated with rhinosinusitis, but it is not currently clear whether a relation exists. The 2010 study by Alkire and Bhattacharyya [45] sought to assess sinonasal anatomic variants potentially associated with RARS by retrospectively comparing CT scans of RARS patients in a noninfected state with CT scans from a nonrhinosinusitis population. They found no statistically significant difference between concha bullosa and naso-septal spurs in the RARS population versus the comparison group but did find that the presence of Haller cells was significantly associated with the likelihood of RARS. Another study investigated additional anatomic variants including agger nasi cells, type 1–4 frontal cells, atelectatic uncinate processes, and maxillary sinus hypoplasia. There was no statistically significant correlation with RARS factors [46].

## 17.4 Diagnosis and Workup

Patients with acute rhinosinusitis typically complain of nasal congestion and obstruction, purulent nasal discharge, and facial pain or pressure that is worse when bending forward. Maxillary tooth discomfort may be present if the maxillary sinus is involved. Other less specific symptoms include fever, fatigue, cough, hyposmia, ear pressure, headache, and halitosis. The previously mentioned symptoms are similar in the different phenotypes of ARS and based on the clinical impression alone, physicians were estimated to diagnose bacterial sinusitis in only 50% of cases. There was a common belief among patients and physicians that the presence of purulent nasal discharge is highly suggestive of bacterial infection; however, this is considered a diagnostic fallacy. A particular emphasis on the duration, pattern, and/or severity of symptoms can help differentiate bacterial from viral illness. Acute viral rhinosinusitis will typically have partial or complete resolution of symptoms by 10 days, with a peak at 3–6 days. If symptoms persist beyond 10 days, or if symptoms improve but worsen again within 10 days ("double worsening"), there is a higher likelihood that the patient has ABRS [47, 48].

Past medical/surgical history, review of systems, allergies, social/work history, and family history are also essential elements of the evaluation. A history of recurring pneumonia, otitis media, and rhinosinusitis in an adult suggests the possibility of a CVID, other immunocompromised states, or ciliary dyskinesia. A family history of cystic fibrosis or allergy also has implications for additional diagnostic testing.

On physical examination, palpation of the facial skeleton might elicit tenderness over the involved sinus; however, this is not useful [49]. Anterior rhinoscopy which is the only tool available to the primary care physicians will provide a limited view for the anterior part of the nasal cavity. Findings may include purulent drainage in the nose or posterior pharynx. The routine usage of the endoscope during examination will provide more details through enhanced illumination and the magnified direct visualization of the nasal cavity, turbinates, septum, and drainage pathways of the paranasal sinuses. Findings include diffuse mucosal edema, narrowing of the

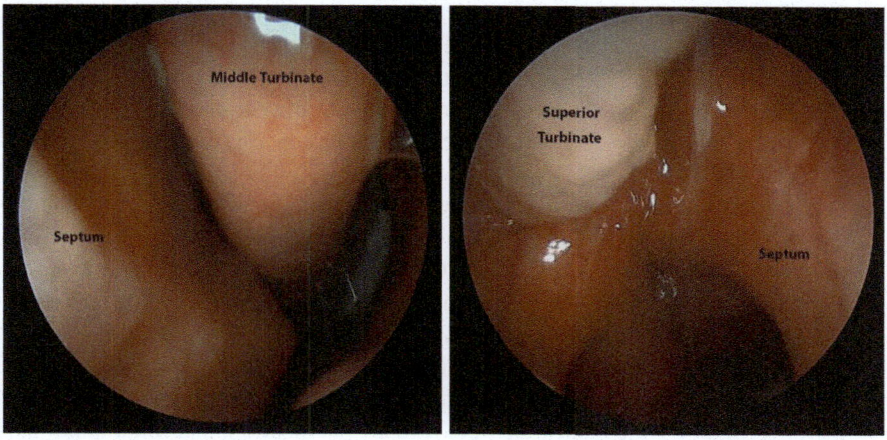


**Fig. 17.4** Endoscopic appearance of mucopurulent discharge in the middle meatus and spheno-ethmoidal recess

middle meatus, inferior turbinate hypertrophy, and purulence mainly in the middle meatus or in the sphenoethmoidal recess based on the involved sinus. (Fig. 17.4).

The differential diagnosis of ARS includes allergic rhinitis, headache or facial pain syndrome, dental conditions, orofacial pain syndromes, ocular pain syndromes, and glaucoma and chronic fatigue syndromes. Although diagnosis is most often possible solely on clinical grounds, additional testing may be helpful to differentiate ARS from other entities with overlapping symptoms [50].

### 17.4.1 Investigations

Diagnosis of ARS is mainly clinically based on the patient's medical history, symptoms, and physical findings. The need for further investigations is limited to certain selected clinical situations.

- Blood Workup: Complete blood count will show elevated white blood cell count in bacterial infection. A raised CRP/ESR increases the likelihood of bacterial infection. CRP is a more sensitive marker of acute phase inflammation than ESR. CRP rises within 24 h of inflammation and returns to normal within a day after resolution of inflammation. On the other hand, ESR increases days after the onset of inflammation and can remain elevated for several days after the cessation of inflammation. Some studies have shown that elevated CRP and ESR levels are associated with the presence of changes in computed tomography and that high levels can be considered predictive of positive bacterial culture [51–53].
- Culture and Sensitivity: Routine swabs and cultures are not indicated in uncomplicated ABRS. Culture is necessary in certain situations, e.g., complicated sinusitis, no response to antibiotic treatment, suspected resistant organisms as in

immunocompromised host. The site from which culture should be taken is very important. Direct nasal swab from the nasal cavity is not reliable and should not be done. The most sensitive site is from the maxillary sinus, and this can be done through antral puncture via the inferior meatus or the canine fossa. A less invasive alternative for maxillary puncture is the culture of endoscopic-guided swabs from the middle meatus [54].

- Imaging for ARS is not necessary unless there is a clinical concern for a complication or alternative diagnosis. Sinus plain films are generally not useful in detecting inflammation because of low sensitivity and specificity. They may show air-fluid levels. However, this does not help differentiate viral versus bacterial etiologies. Computed tomography is not indicated in the initial diagnosis of ARS. It is only indicated in certain situations such as unilateral symptoms and signs, suspected complications, and in cases of no response to maximal medical therapy. Sinus CT may show air-fluid levels, opacification, and inflammation. A thickened sinus mucosa over 5 mm is indicative of inflammation. It can also effectively assess bony erosion or destruction. However, these findings are also not helpful in differentiating viral versus bacterial etiologies. The use of contrast-enhanced CT scan is required to evaluate orbital and intracranial complications of ARS. Gadolinium-enhanced magnetic resonance imaging is superior to CT scan in evaluating soft tissue changes and can help in identifying the extent of orbital and intracranial complications.

## 17.5 Treatment

The treatment of ARS includes two pillars, first, symptomatic treatment, second, the use of antibiotics if indicated. If the clinical picture is suggestive of ABRS, the clinicians should decide the following: Which type of antibiotic? What is the appropriate dosing? What is the optimum duration? and when to consider an alternative based on the response to the initial treatment or the presence of risk for antibiotic resistance? The misuse of antibiotics should not be a replacement for spending time talking with and examining the patient and teaching the patient and or the patient's family the difference between viral and bacterial infections.

The challenge in discriminating bacterial from nonbacterial ARS often leads to an over-diagnosis of ABRS, which results in an overuse of diagnostic testing and early unnecessary prescription of antibiotics. In a study from the UK, 88% of the consultations for rhinosinusitis resulted in antibiotic prescription, while only 11% were deemed appropriate [55]. The same was true in the Netherlands where 34% of the interviewed primary care physicians chose an antibiotic as treatment for a patient with moderate severe acute rhinosinusitis [56]. In a study from Spain, even when ABRS patients were excluded, the use of antibiotics was found to be around 60% in patients with common cold and 70% in those with postviral ARS [57]. The American Rhinosinusitis guidelines highlight the fact that although effective in adults, the actual benefit of antibiotics is small, needing to treat between 11 and 15 patients to get one individual to improve [50].

Treatment depends on the phenotype of rhinosinusitis whether viral, postviral, or bacterial rhinosinusitis.

1. *Acute Viral Rhinosinusitis*

   Management of AVRS is primarily focused on symptomatic relief. The only required treatment is for the control of symptoms, this includes analgesics with either paracetamol or nonsteroidal anti-inflammatory drugs to treat pain, headache, or body aches, local or systemic decongestant for the control of nasal congestion which should not be used for more than 5–7 days to avoid rebound congestion. Topical ipratropium bromide nasal spray may reduce rhinorrhea if particularly troublesome. Nasal saline rinsing (also called nasal douching or irrigation), with or without sodium bicarbonate, mechanically washes out mucous secretion and debris from the nose and the middle meatus. It improves mucociliary function that may be helpful in reducing nasal blockage and clearing nasal discharge. Based on the data from a recent meta-analysis, patients with AVRS are recommended to perform a nasal rinse at least twice per day with isotonic saline using a high-volume device. The saline volume should be around 100–250 ml. Furthermore, the patients may wash until they get back to their premorbid status or 2 weeks at most, when nearly all patients are cured [58]. Vitamin C or zinc lozenges may reduce the length of symptoms in some patients. If the patient is having concurrent allergic rhinitis, the use of antihistaminic will reduce the symptoms of sneezing and rhinorrhea.
2. *Postviral Rhinosinusitis*

   Postviral ARS treatment is the same as for AVRS, although corticosteroid nasal sprays may help reduce postviral ARS symptoms [59]. Nasal saline treatment is recommended to improve the symptoms and to enhance the effects of intranasal corticosteroids (INCS) [58].

   It has been theorized that by decreasing the inflammatory response and reducing the mucosal swelling, an INCS steroid would promote drainage and increase the aeration of the sinuses, thus hastening the elimination of infectious organisms and decreasing the frequency and severity of recurrences [60]. Several studies produced results that suggest a clinically relevant, earlier resolution of symptoms in participants treated with INCS, without the risk of severe adverse events, even when higher doses in the therapeutic range were used [60].
3. *Bacterial Rhinosinusitis*

   There is a common belief among a considerable number of primary care physicians and otolaryngologists that once acute bacterial rhinosinusitis is diagnosed, antibiotics should be prescribed to reduce the duration and severity of symptoms, to prevent complications, and to minimize the risk of conversion to chronic sinusitis. Several randomized controlled trials did not show a clear superiority of antibiotics over placebo regarding, the duration of illness, the improvement in the severity of symptoms, or the prevention of complications [61–63]. Based on those findings, there is an increasing trend to provide the patient with a clinical diagnosis of ABRS and a period of watchful waiting without antibiotics provided that follow-up is guaranteed with the patient to ensure that antibiotic can be started if there is no improvement of symptoms within 7 days of diagnosis or if the condition worsens at any time. Wait-and-see policy requires adequate clarification of its benefits to the patient, and sometimes it is more helpful to prescribe antibiotics and ask the patient not to collect it unless indicated [1].

These guidelines differ from the 2012 IDSA guidelines, which recommend initiation of antibiotics for those with persistent symptoms or signs compatible with acute rhinosinusitis (ARS) lasting for ≥10 days without any evidence of clinical improvement **or** onset with severe symptoms or signs of high fever (≥39 °C [102 °F]) and purulent nasal discharge or facial pain lasting for at least three to four consecutive days at the beginning of the illness **or** worsening symptoms or signs for 3–4 days characterized by the new onset of fever, headache, or increase in nasal discharge following a typical viral upper respiratory infection that lasted 5–6 days and were initially improving ("double sickening") [3].

If an antibiotic is indicated, the physician should have answers to the following questions:

- *What Is the Most Appropriate Antibiotic?*

  In clinical practice, the choice of the antibiotic is based on the most common bacteria causing ABRS, and routine lab and culture for identification of the positive bacteria is not performed except in selected situations. Special consideration should be given to the resistant pattern of streptococcal pneumonia and H. influenzae within the community in order to select the most appropriate type and dosage of the antibiotic.

### 17.5.1 First-Line Therapy

- *Amoxicillin*

  Dosage: 500 mg orally three times daily or 875 mg orally twice daily.

  The justification for amoxicillin as first-line therapy for most patients with ABRS relates to its safety, efficacy, low cost, and narrow microbiologic spectrum. When used in sufficient doses, amoxicillin is effective against susceptible and intermediate-resistant pneumococci. It is ineffective against beta-lactamase-producing bacteria.
- *Amoxicillin-Clavulanate*

  Dosage: 500 mg/125 mg orally three times daily or 875 mg/125 mg orally twice daily.

  The addition of clavulanate to amoxicillin improves coverage for beta-lactamase-producing Haemophilus influenzae as well as Moraxella catarrhalis. Studies reported 46–52% beta-lactamase-positive strains of Hemophilus influenza. Across Canada, 19–92% of H influenzae and M catarrhalis isolates, respectively, were found to produce β-lactamase.

  Factors that would prompt clinicians to consider prescribing amoxicillin-clavulanate instead of amoxicillin are listed in Table 17.1 [64, 65].

**Table 17.1** Factors that would prompt clinicians to consider prescribing amoxicillin-clavulanate instead of amoxicillin

| Factor | Comment |
|---|---|
| Situations in which bacterial resistance is likely | Antibiotic use in the past month<br>Close contact with treated individuals, health care providers, or a health care environment<br>Failure of prior antibiotic therapy<br>Breakthrough infection despite prophylaxis<br>Close contact with a child in a daycare facility<br>Smoker or smoker in the family<br>High prevalence of resistant bacteria in community |
| Presence of moderate to severe infection | Moderate to severe symptoms of ABRS<br>Protracted symptoms of ABRS<br>Frontal or sphenoidal sinusitis<br>History of recurrent ABRS |
| Presence of comorbidity or extremes of life | Comorbid conditions, including diabetes and chronic cardiac, hepatic, or renal disease<br>Immunocompromised patient<br>Age older than 65 years |

- *High-Dose Amoxicillin with Clavulanate (2 g Orally Twice Daily or 90 mg/kg/d Orally Twice Daily)*

  To cover penicillin nonsusceptible (PNS) Streptococcus pneumoniae. This risk exists in those from geographic regions with high endemic rates (>10%) of invasive penicillin non-susceptible streptococcal pneumoniae, those with severe infection (e.g., evidence of systemic toxicity with temperature of 39 °C [102 °F] or higher, and threat of suppurative complications), age > 65 years, recent hospitalization, antibiotic use within the past month, or those who are immunocompromised [66].
- *Patients with Penicillin Allergy*

  For any patient with a penicillin allergy, **doxycycline** (100 mg orally twice daily or 200 mg orally daily) is a reasonable alternative to amoxicillin or amoxicillin-clavulanate for initial therapy.

Patients with nontype I hypersensitivity to penicillin, a **third-generation oral cephalosporin (cefixime 400 mg daily or cefpodoxime 200 mg twice daily)** can be used. The addition of **clindamycin (300 mg every 6 h)** is recommended to overcome the increasing rate of streptococcal pneumonia resistance to cephalosporines. Third- and fourth-generation cephalosporines are the preferred choice because of their potency and their lowest risk of cross-reactivity with penicillin.

A respiratory fluoroquinolone (levofloxacin 750 mg or 500 mg orally once daily or moxifloxacin 400 mg orally once daily) is another alternative for penicillin-allergic patients. However, fluoroquinolones should be reserved for those who have no alternative treatment options as the risk of serious adverse effects associated with fluoroquinolones generally outweighs the benefits for patients with acute sinusitis [67]. Fluoroquinolones are associated with a variety of adverse effects including central nervous system events (seizures, headaches, dizziness, sleep disorders), peripheral neuropathy, photosensitivity with skin rash, disorders of glucose homeostasis (hypoglycemia and hyperglycemia), prolongation of QT interval, hepatic dysfunction, and skeletomuscular complaints. Risk of Achilles tendon rupture is particularly high in the adult population (estimated prevalence rate, 15–20 per 100,000), particularly among those with advancing age and antecedent steroid therapy [3].

The high prevalence of macrolide-resistant S. pneumoniae in the US (>40%) and the high rates of resistance to trimethoprim-sulfamethoxazole among both S. pneumoniae (50%) and H. influenzae (27%) excludes these agents for the treatment of acute bacterial rhinosinusitis [68, 69].

### 17.5.2 What Is the Required Management in Case of Initial Treatment Failure of Presumed ABRS?

Failure is defined as worsening or no improvement of the clinical condition with the initial management option by the seventh day after diagnosis. The cut point of 7 days is based on clinical outcomes in multiple randomized controlled trials. Percentage of patients improving after receiving a placebo was 73–86% at 7–15 days and rising to 85–91% after antibiotic therapy. In such situation, the clinician should reassess the patient to confirm the diagnosis of ABRS, exclude other causes of illness and treatment failure, and detect complications including orbital or intracranial spread of infection. Special consideration should be given to acute severe frontal or sphenoid sinusitis. Acute frontal sinusitis typically causes severe headaches localized to the forehead over the orbits, with tenderness produced by pressure on the floor of the frontal sinus. Sphenoidal sinusitis typically causes a dull ache in the back of the head, specifically over the occiput with radiation to the frontal and retro-orbital regions. Imaging is only required if complications are suspected, if the clinical picture is not consistent with ABRS, or if the patient is not responding while taking fluoroquinolones [1].

When a change in antibiotic therapy is made, the clinician should consider the limitations in coverage of the initial agent and the choice of antibiotic should provide adequate coverage of anticipated bacteria. Beta-lactams, fluoroquinolones, and doxycycline-resistant S. pneumoniae, and beta-lactamase-producing H. influenzae and M. catarrhalis are more common following previous antibiotic exposure [70, 71]. Tables 17.2 and 17.3 summarize the antibiotic selection for ABRS in adults and children respectively [3].

### 17.5.3 What Is the Required Management in Case of Failure of Multiple Oral Antibiotic Courses?

Patients should respond to a second course of appropriate antibiotic therapy within 7 days of initiation. A noncontrast computed tomography (CT) scan is appropriate in the evaluation of treatment-resistant sinusitis to evaluate for anatomic blockage

**Table 17.2** Antibiotic therapy for ABRS in adults

| Indication | First-line (daily dose | Second-line (daily dose) |
|---|---|---|
| Initial empirical therapy | • Amoxicillin-clavulanate (500 mg/125 mg PO tid, or 875 mg/125 mg PO bid) | • Amoxicillin-clavulanate (2000 mg/125 mg PO bid) |
| B-lactam allergy | | • Doxycycline (100 mg PO bid or 200 mg PO qd)<br>• Doxycycline (100 mg PO bid or 200 mg PO qd)<br>• Levofloxacin (500 mg PO qd)<br>• Moxifloxacin (400 mg PO qd)<br>• Amoxicillin-clavulanate (2000 mg/125 mg PO bid) |
| Risk for antibiotic resistance or failed initial therapy | | • Levofloxacin (500 mg PO qd)<br>• Moxifloxacin (400 mg PO qd)<br>• Ampicillin-sulbactam (1.5–3 g N every 6 h)<br>• Launtinussin Emma Dharindi |
| Severe infection requiring hospitalization | | • Levofloxacin (500 mg PO or IV qd)<br>• Moxifloxacin (400 mg PO or IV qd)<br>• Ceftriaxone (1–2 g IV every 12–24 h)<br>• Cefotaxime (2 g V every 4–6 h) |

**Table 17.3** Antibiotic therapy for ABRS in children

| Indication | First-line (daily dose) | Second line (daily dose) |
|---|---|---|
| Initial empirical therapy | • Amoxicillin-clavulanate (45 mg/kg/day PO bid) | • Amoxicillin-clavulanate (90 mg/kg/day PO bid) |
| B-lactam allergy:<br>• Type I hypersensitivity<br>• Nontype I hypersensitivity | | • Levofloxacin (10–20 mg/kg/day PO every 12–24 h)<br>• Clindamycin* (30–40 mg/kg/day PO tid) plus cefixime<br>(8 mg/kg/day PO bid) or cefpodoxime (10 mg/kg/day PO bid)<br>• Amoxicillin-clavulanate (90 mg/kg/day PO bid) |
| Risk for antibiotic resistance or failed initial therapy | | • Amoxicillin-clavulanate (90 mg/kg/day PO bid)<br>• Clindamycin® (30–40 mg/kg/day PO tid) plus cefixime<br>(8 mg/kg/day PO bid) or cefpodoxime (10 mg/kg/day PO bid)<br>• Levofloxacin (10–20 mg/kg/day PO every 12–24 h) |
| Severe infection requiring hospitalization | | • Ampicillin/sulbactam (200–400 mg/kg/day IV every 6 h)<br>• Ceftriaxone (50 mg/kg/day IV every 12 h)<br>• Cefotaxime (100–200 mg/kg/day IV every 6 h)<br>• Levofloxacin (10–20 mg/kg/day IV every 12–24 h) |

[72]. Patients with anatomic abnormalities may require surgery. Patients should also be referred for sinus cultures either by direct aspirate or endoscopy of the middle meatus.

## References


1. Rosenfeld RM, Piccirillo JF, Chandrasekhar SS, Brook I, Kumar KA, Kramper M, et al. Clinical practice guideline (update). Otolaryngol Neck Surg. 2015;152(4):598–609.
2. Fokkens WJ, Lund VJ, Hopkins C, Hellings PW, Kern R, Reitsma S, et al. European position paper on rhinosinusitis and nasal polyps 2020. Rhinology. 2020;58(Supplement 29):1–464.
3. Chow AW, Benninger MS, Brook I, Brozek JL, Goldstein EL, Hicks LA, et al. IDSA clinical practice guideline for acute bacterial rhinosinusitis in children and adults. Clin Infect Dis. 2012;54:e72–e112.
4. Wald ER, Applegate KE, Bordley C, Darrow DH, Glode MP, Marcy SM, et al. Clinical practice guideline for the diagnosis and management of acute bacterial sinusitis in children aged 1 to 18 years. Pediatrics. 2013;132(1):e262–80.
5. Bhattacharyya N, Grebner J, Martinson NG. Recurrent acute rhinosinusitis: epidemiology and health care cost burden. Otolaryngol Head Neck Surg. 2012;146:307–12.
6. Rosenfeld RM, Andes D, Bhattacharyya N, Cheung D, Eisenberg S, Ganiatset TG, et al. Clinical practice guideline: adult sinusitis. Otolaryngol Head Neck Surg. 2007;137:S1–S31.
7. Bhattacharyya N, Lee KH. Chronic recurrent rhinosinusitis: disease severity and clinical characterization. Laryngoscope. 2005;115:306–10.
8. Avorn J, Harvey K, Soumerai SB, Herxheimer A, Plumridge R, Bardelay G. Information and education as determinants of antibiotic use: report of Task Force 5. Rev Infect Dis. 1987;9(suppl 3):S286–96.
9. Avorn J, Solomon DH. Cultural and economic factors that (mis)shape antibiotic use: the nonpharmacologic basis of therapeutics. Ann Intern Med. 2000;133:128–35.
10. Cals JW, Boumans D, Lardinois RJ, Gonzales R, Hopstaken RM, Butler CC, et al. Public beliefs on antibiotics and respiratory tract infections: an internet-based questionnaire study. Br J Gen Pract. 2007;57:942–7.
11. Wilson AA, Crane LA, Barrett PH, Gonzales R. Public beliefs and use of antibiotics for acute respiratory illness. J Gen Intern Med. 1999;14:658–62.
12. Fokkens WJ, Lund VJ, Mullol J, et al. European position paper on rhinosinusitis and nasal polyps 2012. Rhinology. 2012;50:1–307.
13. Betz CS, Issing W, Matschke J, Kremer A, Uhl E, Leunig A. Complications of acute frontal sinusitis: a retrospective study. Eur Arch Otorrinolaringol. 2008;265:63–72.
14. Bradley PJ, Manning KP, Shaw MD. Brain abscess secondary to paranasal sinusitis. J Laryngol Otol. 1984;98:719–25.
15. Mansfield EL, Gianoli GJ. Intracranial complications of sinusitis. J La State Med Soc. 1994;146:287–90.
16. Babar-Craig H, Gupta Y, Lund VJ. British Rhinological Society audit of the role of antibiotics in complications of acute rhinosinusitis: a national prospective audit. Rhinology. 2010;48:344–7.
17. Hansen FS, Hoffmans R, Georgalas C, Fokkens WJ. Complications of acute rhinosinusitis in The Netherlands. Fam Pract. 2012;29:147–53.
18. Lindbaek M. Acute sinusitis: guide to selection of antibacterial therapy. Drugs. 2004;64(8):805–19.
19. Slavin RG, Spector SL, Bernstein IL, et al. The diagnosis and management of sinusitis: a practice parameter update. J Allergy Clin Immunol. 2005;116(6 Suppl):S13–47.
20. Sande MA, Gwaltney JM. Acute community-acquired bacterial sinusitis: continuing challenges and current management. Clin Infect Dis. 2004;39(Suppl 13):S151–8.

21. Stjärne P, Odebäck P, Ställberg B, Lundberg J, Olsson P. High costs and burden of illness in acute rhinosinusitis: real-life treatment patterns and outcomes in Swedish primary care. Prim Care Respir J. 2012;21(2):174–9.
22. Ah-See K. Sinusitis (acute rhinosinusitis). BMJ Clin Evid. 2015;2015:0511.
23. Turner RB. Epidemiology, pathogenesis and treatment of the common cold. Ann Allergy Asthma Immunol. 1997;78:531–40.
24. Bachert C, Hormann K, Mosges R, Rasp G, Riechelmann H, Müller R, et al. An update on the diagnosis and treatment of sinusitis and nasal polyposis. Allergy. 2003;58:176–91.
25. Finley CR, Chan DS, Garrison S, Korownyk C, Kolber MR, Campbell S, et al. What are the most common conditions in primary care? Systematic review. Can Fam Physician. 2018;64:832–40.
26. Oskarsson JP, Halldorsson S. An evaluation of diagnosis and treatment of acute sinusitis at three healthcare centers. Laeknabladid. 2010;96:531–5.
27. Uijen JH, Bindels PJ, Schellevis FG, van der Wouden JC. ENT problems in Dutch children: trends in incidence rates, antibiotic prescribing and referrals 2002–2008. Scand J Prim Health Care. 2011;29:75–9.
28. Hoffmans R, Wagemakers A, van Drunen C, Hellings P, Fokkens W. Acute and chronic rhinosinusitis and allergic rhinitis in relation to comorbidity, ethnicity and environment. PLoS One. 2018;13:e0192330.
29. Smith SS, Ference EH, Evans CT, Tan BK, Kern RC, Chandra RK. The prevalence of bacterial infection in acute rhinosinusitis: a systematic review and metaanalysis. Laryngoscope. 2015;125:57–69.
30. Gwaltney JM. Acute community-acquired sinusitis. Clin Infect Dis. 1996;23:1209–23.
31. Osguthorpe JD, Hadley JA. Rhinosinusitis: current concepts inevaluation and management. Med Clin North Am. 1999;83:27–41.
32. Gwaltney JM, Phillips CD, Miller RD, Riker DK. Computed tomographic study of the common cold. N Engl J Med. 1994;330:25–30.
33. Gwaltney JM Jr, Hendley JO, Phillips CD, et al. Nose blowing propels nasal fluid into the paranasal sinuses. Clin Infect Dis. 2000;30:387–91.
34. Bakaletz LO. Viral potentiation of bacterial superinfection of the respiratory tract. Trends Microbiol. 1995;3:110–4.
35. Morgene MF, Botelho-Nevers E, Grattard F, Pillet S, Berthelot P, Pozzetto B, Verhoeven PO. Staphylococcus aureus colonization and non-influenza respiratory viruses: interactions and synergism mechanisms. Virulence. 2018;9(1):1354–63.
36. Heikkinen T, Järvinen A. The common cold. Lancet. 2003;361(9351):51–9.
37. Zou L, Ruan F, Huang M, Liang L, Huang H, Hong Z, Yu J, Kang M, Song Y, Xia J, Guo Q, Song T, He J, Yen HL, Peiris M, Wu J. SARS-CoV-2 viral load in upper respiratory specimens of infected patients. N Engl J Med. 2020;382(12):1177–9. https://doi.org/10.1056/NEJMc2001737.
38. Turner RB. The common cold. In: Bennett JE, Dolin R, Blaser MJ, editors. Mandell, Douglas, and Bennett's principles and practice of infectious diseases, vol. 8. Philadelphia: Elsevier (Saunders); 2015. p. 749–52.
39. Evans FO Jr, Sydnor JB, Moore WE, et al. Sinusitis of the maxillary antrum. N Engl J Med. 1975;293:735.
40. Brook I. Acute and chronic bacterial sinusitis. Infect Dis Clin N Am. 2007;21(2):427–48.
41. Gwaltney JM Jr, Scheld WM, Sande MA, et al. The microbial etiology and antimicrobialtherapy of adults with acute community-acquired sinusitis: a fifteen-year experience at the University of Virginia and review of other selected studies. J Allergy Clin Immunol. 1992;90:457–62.
42. De Corso E, Lucidi D, Cantone E, Ottaviano G, Di Cesare T, Seccia V, et al. Clinical evidence and biomarkers linking allergy and acute or chronic rhinosinusitis in children: a systematic review. Curr Allergy Asthma Rep. 2020;20(11):68.
43. Lin SW, Wang SK, Lu MC, Wang CL, Koo M. Acute rhinosinusitis among pediatric patients with allergic rhinitis: a nationwide, population-based cohort study. PLoS One. 2019;14(2):e0211547.

44. Mandava S, Lin J, Joshua C, Payne SC, Mattos JL. Evaluation and workup of immunodeficiencies in recurrent acute rhinosinusitis: a scoping review. Int Forum Allergy Rhinol. 2023;13(6):1017–23.
45. Alkire BC, Bhattacharyya N. An assessment of sinonasal anatomic variants potentially associated with recurrent acute rhinosinusitis. Laryngoscope. 2010;120:631–4.
46. Loftus PA, Lin J, Tabaee A. Anatomic variants of the paranasal sinuses in patients with recurrent acute rhinosinusitis. Int Forum Allergy Rhinol. 2016;6(3):328–33.
47. Rosenfeld RM, Piccirillo JF, Chandrasekhar SS, et al. Clinical practice guideline (update): adult sinusitis. Otolaryngol Head Neck Surg. 2015;152:S1–S39.
48. Gwaltney JM Jr, Hendley JO, Simon G, Jordan WS Jr. Rhinovirus infections in an industrial population. II. Characteristics of illness and antibody response. JAMA. 1967;202:494.
49. Bird J, Biggs TC, Thomas M, Salib RJ. Adult acute rhinosinusitis. BMJ. 2013;346:f2687.
50. Orlandi RR, Kingdom TT, Hwang PH, Smith TL, Alt JA, Baroody FM, et al. International consensus statement on allergy and rhinology: rhinosinusitis. Int Forum Allergy Rhinol. 2016;6(Suppl 1):S22–209.
51. Autio TJ, Koskenkorva T, Leino TK, Koivunen P, Alho OP. Longitudinal analysis of inflammatory biomarkers during acute rhinosinusitis. Laryngoscope. 2017;127(2):E55–61.
52. Hansen JG, Højbjerg T, Rosborg J. Symptoms and signs in cultureproven acute maxillary sinusitis in a general practice population. APMIS. 2009;117(10):724–9.
53. Savolainen S, Jousimies-Somer H, Karjalainen J, Ylikoski J. Do simple laboratory tests help in etiologic diagnosis in acute maxillary sinusitis? Acta Otolaryngol Suppl. 1997;529:144–7.
54. Vogan JC, Bolger WE, Keyes AS. Endoscopically guided sinonasal cultures: a direct comparison with maxillary sinus aspirate cultures. Otolaryngol Head Neck Surg. 2000;122:370–3.
55. Pouwels KB, Pouwels KB, FCK D, DRM S, Robotham JV, Smieszek T. Actual versus 'ideal' antibiotic prescribing for common conditions in English primary care. J Antimicrob Chemother. 2018;73:19–26.
56. Hoffmans R, Schermer T, van Weel C, Fokkens W. Management of rhinosinusitis in Dutch general practice. Prim Care Respir J. 2011;20:64–70.
57. Jaume F, Quintó L, Alobid I, Mullol J. Overuse of diagnostic tools and medications in acute rhinosinusitis in Spain: a population-based study (the PROSINUS study). BMJ Open. 2018;8(1):e018788.
58. Chitsuthipakorn W, Kanjanawasee D, Hoang MP, Seresirikachorn K, Snidvongs K. Benefits of nasal saline treatment in acute rhinosinusitis: systematic review and meta-analysis. Int Forum Allergy Rhinol. 2022 Aug;12(8):1006–17.
59. Keith PK, Dymek A, Pfaar O, Fokkens W, Kirby SY, Wu W, Garris C, Topors N, Lee LA. Fluticasone furoate nasal spray reduces symptoms of uncomplicated acute rhinosinusitis: a randomised placebo-controlled study. Primary Care Respir J. 2012;21(3):267–75.
60. Zalmanovici Trestioreanu A, Yaphe J. Intranasal steroids for acute sinusitis. Cochrane Database Syst Rev. 2013;2013(12):CD005149.
61. Ahovuo-Saloranta A, Rautakorpi UM, Borisenko OV, et al. Antibiotics for acute maxillary sinusitis in adults. Cochrane Database Syst Rev. 2014;2:CD000243.
62. Lemiengre MB, van Driel ML, Merenstein D, et al. Antibiotics for acute rhinosinusitis in adults. Cochrane Database Syst Rev. 2018;9:CD006089.
63. Harris AM, Hicks LA, Qaseem A. High value care task force of the American College of Physicians and for the Centers for Disease Control and Prevention. Appropriate antibiotic use for acute respiratory tract infection in adults: advice for high-value care from the American College of Physicians and the Centers for Disease Control and Prevention. Ann Intern Med. 2016;164:425.
64. Brook I, Foote PA, Hausfeld JN. Frequency of recovery of pathogens causing acute maxillary sinusitis in adults before and after introduction of vaccination of children with the 7-valent pneumococcal vaccine. J Med Microbiol. 2006;55:943–6.
65. Jenkins SG, Farrell DJ, Patel M, et al. Trends in anti-bacterial resistance among Streptococcus pneumoniae isolated in the USA, 2000-2003: PROTEKT US years 1-3. J Infect. 2005;51:355–63.

66. Brook I, Gober AE. Resistance to antimicrobials used for therapy of otitis media and sinusitis: effect of previous antimicrobial therapy and smoking. Ann Otol Rhinol Laryngol. 1999;108:645–7.
67. US Food and Drug Administration. FDA Drug Safety Communication: FDA advises restricting fluoroquinolone antibiotic use for certain uncomplicated infections; warns about disabling side effects that can occur together. Available at: http://www.fda.gov/Drugs/DrugSafety/ucm500143.htm. Accessed on 26 May 2016.
68. Jenkins SG, Farrell DJ. Increase in pneumococcus macrolide resistance, United States. Emerg Infect Dis. 2009;15:1260–4.
69. Zhang X, Wang R, Di X, Liu B, Liu Y. Different microbiological and clinical aspects of lower respiratory tract infections between China and European/American countries. J Thorac Dis. 2014;6:134–42.
70. Harrison CJ, Woods C, Stout G, Martin B, Selvarangan R. Susceptibilities of *Haemophilus influenzae, Streptococcus pneumoniae,* including serotype 19A, and *Moraxella catarrhalis* paediatric isolates from 2005 to 2007 to commonly used antibiotics. J Antimicrob Chemother. 2009;63:511–9.
71. Jansen WT, Verel A, Beitsma M, Verhoef J, Milatovic D. Surveillance study of the susceptibility of *Haemophilus influenzae* to various antibacterial agents in Europe and Canada. Curr Med Res Opin. 2008;24:2853–61.
72. Osguthorpe JD, Hadley JA. Rhinosinusitis. Current concepts in evaluation and management. Med Clin North Am. 1999;83:27.

# Complications of Sinusitis

# 18

Ahmed Thabet and Yasser Nour

**Key Points**

- The incidence of complications has declined significantly since the advent of antibiotics but has maintained a plateau over the past few decades.
- The complications of sinusitis can be broadly classified into three main categories in order of decreasing frequency: orbital complications; intracranial complications; and bony complications.
- The complications occur via one of two mechanisms, either through direct extension or through hematologic spread.
- Children under the age of 7 are more prone to the orbital complications of sinusitis. Conversely, intracranial and bony complications are more frequently observed in adolescent teenage patients, typically young men. A second smaller incidence peak occurs in the elderly.
- Several classification schemes for the orbital complications of sinusitis have been proposed over the years. They will be discussed in this chapter in the order described by Chandler et al., since his classification system is currently the most ubiquitous.
- The rarity of intracranial complications is problematic because their diagnosis is thus usually delayed.
- Bony complications are the least common of sinusitis complications, usually presenting as osteomyelitis of the frontal bone in adults.

**Supplementary Information** The online version contains supplementary material available at https://doi.org/10.1007/978-3-031-70077-4_18.

A. Thabet · Y. Nour (✉)
Department of Otolaryngology, Alexandria University, Alexandria, Egypt


S. Elwany (ed.), *Current Rhinology*,
https://doi.org/10.1007/978-3-031-70077-4_18

## 18.1 Introduction

Although acute bacterial sinusitis (ARS) is a common ailment with an often-predictable course and outcome, its complications are exceedingly rare and unpredictable (occurring once in every 95,000 pediatric hospital admissions) [1]. The incidence of complications has declined significantly since the advent of antibiotics but has maintained a plateau over the past few decades [2–4]. However, they are especially important because they can have devastating outcomes including blindness, neurologic morbidity, and even death. Therefore, early recognition of the signs and symptoms is critical as prompt medical and/or surgical treatment can lead to better outcomes [5].

The complications of sinusitis can be broadly classified into three main categories in order of decreasing frequency:

1. Orbital complications
2. Intracranial complications
3. Bony complications

This chapter reviews each of these complications in detail, providing a detailed discussion on their pathogenesis, presentation, diagnosis as well as medical and surgical interventions.

## 18.2 Relevant Orbital and Sinus Anatomy

The anatomy and embryology of the paranasal sinuses are crucial to the understanding of the pathogenesis of this disease process. Although both the maxillary and ethmoid sinuses are present at birth and are the first sinuses to develop and pneumatize, the ethmoid sinuses are far more commonly involved in the complications of sinusitis due to their precarious anatomy. In fact, the close proximity of the ethmoid sinuses to the orbit makes them the most commonly involved structure in complications of sinusitis, contributing to the higher propensity of orbital complications in younger children [6]. Conversely, the frontal sinus is the last sinus to pneumatize and is the most common source of intracranial complications of sinusitis followed by the ethmoid sinuses, hence the higher incidence of intracranial complications in adolescents [7–9]. The sphenoid sinuses are rarely involved in any complications of sinusitis [10].

The anatomy of the orbit foreshadows its potential for the development of complications. It is separated from the ethmoid sinuses medially by a thin and often dehiscent *lamina papyracea*, from the maxillary sinus by a similarly thin orbital floor, and from the frontal sinus by the horizontal orbital plate of the frontal bone—the thinnest wall of the frontal sinus.

The *orbital periosteum*, or the *periorbita*, is an important additional barrier between the orbital contents and the sinuses. It is a fibrous layer that is firmly adherent to the underlying bone at the orbital rims and suture lines, and as such can prevent the spread of infection into the orbit proper by limiting it to the potential subperiosteal space.

The *orbital septum* is another key feature in the classification of orbital complications. It is a reflection of the periorbita at the anterior orbital rim, fusing with the *levator aponeurosis* and the superior tarsal plate in the upper eyelid, and with the inferior tarsal plate in the lower eyelid. It forms an anterior anatomic barrier that prevents infection in the anterior part of the eye from spreading posteriorly. Based on the orbital septum, infections can therefore be divided into two groups: *preseptal* and *postseptal* infections.

Venous drainage of the ethmoid sinuses occurs via the ethmoid veins, which in turn drain into the superior ophthalmic vein. The superior ophthalmic vein—together with the inferior ophthalmic vein—represents the principal drainage system of the orbit, and both will ultimately drain into the cavernous sinus.

Venous drainage of the frontal sinus occurs via the valveless diploic veins *(veins of Breschet)* which pass through the multiple foramina of the anterior and posterior table of the frontal sinus *(Breschet's canals).* These veins coalesce into the frontal diploic vein that drains into the supraorbital vein. The supraorbital vein is one of the tributaries of the superior ophthalmic vein, and as such ultimately drains into the cavernous sinus as well. In addition, the small diploic veins that extend through the posterior table of the sinus directly contribute to the venous plexus of the dura.

## 18.3 Pathogenesis

Through the anatomical considerations described above, the routes of spread of infection from the sinuses can be gleaned. They occur via one of two mechanisms, either through direct extension or through hematologic spread.

1. *Direct Extension (Loss of an Anatomic Barrier)*:
   It occurs via preformed defects such as congenital or traumatic dehiscence of the lamina papyracea, sinus wall erosions, and fracture lines, as well as through existing fissures and foramina that transmit neurovascular structures into the sinuses.
2. *Hematogenous Spread*:
   Retrograde septic thrombophlebitis through the valveless diploic veins of the frontal and ethmoid bones, ethmoid veins, or other communicating veins is the most common route of spread. The superior and inferior ophthalmic veins in addition to the intracranial venous system are also valveless, allowing direct communication with the cavernous sinus. Subsequently, this permits further spread of thrombophlebitis leading to cavernous sinus thrombosis or superior sagittal sinus thrombosis, as well as septic emboli which can seed intracranial sites that are remote from the sinuses leading to meningitis, epidural or intracerebral abscesses, or subdural empyema [11, 12]. Involvement of the frontal diploic veins can also result in frontal bone osteomyelitis via their communications with the marrow cavity of the frontal bone, leading to *Pott's puffy tumor*.

## 18.4 Demographics

Orbital complications have a seasonal variation peaking around the winter months, indicating a possible viral role in the initiation of sinusitis [6]. Children under the age of 7 are more prone to the orbital complications of sinusitis, possibly because of their relatively higher rates of URTIs [13]. The majority of patients with orbital complications are within the pediatric age group, while intracranial complications are extremely rare under 7 years of age [13].

Conversely, intracranial and bony complications are more frequently observed in adolescent teenage patients, typically young men, correlating with the time of peak pneumatization of the frontal sinus [10]. A second smaller incidence peak occurs in the elderly [14]. Similarly, orbital complications of frontal sinusitis are most common in male patients in the second to third decades of life (average age of 25 years) and tend to involve the left eye more frequently than the right [15–18].

No gender predilection has been identified in preseptal infections. However, male gender has been identified as a risk factor in intracranial and postseptal infections in some case series, particularly in older children and adolescents, yet convincing explanations are lacking [19]. The majority of cases are sporadic, and as such do not have a predictable course of repeated infections.

## 18.5 Microbiology

Orbital complications do not have a bacterial profile that is particularly different from that of ARS. *Goytia et al* reported a 75% rate of polymicrobial cultures [20]. Similarly to ARS, the most commonly cultured organisms are *Streptococcus pneumoniae*, *Haemophilus influenzae*, *Moraxella catarrhalis*, *Streptococcus viridans*, *Staphylococcus aureus*, *Streptococcus pyogenes*, and less commonly anaerobes—the most common of which are Peptostreptococcus and Prevotella [21–24]. MRSA has also been increasingly found in some cultures [25]. Extensive sinus disease—especially that of the frontal sinus—leads to obstruction of the sinus ostia by inflammatory edema. The oxygen tension within the sinus is subsequently reduced, favoring the growth of microaerophilic and anaerobic bacteria [4].

*S. viridans*, especially the *S. anginosus* (formerly *S. milleri*) group organisms, as well as *S. aureus* have been implicated as the most common pathogens in serious orbital and intracranial complications of sinusitis in recent series [26, 27]. *S. aureus* and polymicrobial infections are found at a slightly higher frequency in cases of intracranial complications. Cultures from intracranial abscesses are often polymicrobial, including anaerobes. This shows that although anaerobes and *S. aureus* are not commonly cultured in ARS in children, they are associated with a higher incidence of complications of sinusitis. Contrarily, sinogenic meningitis is most commonly due to *S. pneumoniae* which is associated with a higher frequency of neurologic complications such as hearing loss [4, 7].

The incidence of bacteremia in patients with orbital complications is greatest in children and declines with age. *Schramm et al.* reported that the incidence is 33% in children under 4 years of age yet only 5% in adults [17]. In addition to the typical organisms, immunocompromised patients are also susceptible to some atypical pathogens and fungi leading to the development of invasive infections.

## 18.6 Classification

Several classification schemes for the orbital complications of sinusitis have been proposed over the years, the earliest of which was that of *Hubert's*—based on his experience with 114 patients in the preantibiotic era [28]. However, the most widely utilized classification system in clinical practice today is that of Chandler et al. in the 1970s, who classified patients into five categories based on the anatomical structures involved, perceived progression of the disease, treatment as well as prognosis [29] (Table 18.1 and Fig. 18.1).

The first complication proposed by *Chandler* is preseptal cellulitis which is a preseptal infection, while the latter four are postseptal [29]. Although commonly thought of as a continuum, each of these complications should be considered independently and the treatment thereof should be individualized. These complications are not sequential nor are they mutually exclusive and as such multiple complications can occur in the same patient and in differing orders.

Despite the practicality and universal use of the classification system proposed by Chandler et al., several other authors have modified his classification thenceforth. These modified schemes are useful because they shed light onto the gray areas between the five classical categories as well as highlight recent advances in diagnostic and therapeutic modalities.

Moloney et al. modified *Chandler's* classification to assign lower priority to orbital infections anterior to the orbital septum and then outlined the progression of postseptal intraorbital infections [30] (Table 18.2).

In the *Groote Schuur* hospital classification, the authors proposed a modification of *Moloney's* classification relying upon further stringent radiological differentiation to be made between cellulitis/phlegmon and abscess formation. The latter is of importance when a decision is made on whether surgical intervention is appropriate or not [15, 16] (Table 18.2).

On the other hand, intracranial complications do not have a classification system but include any infection implicating the central nervous system. This includes meningitis, epidural or subdural abscess/empyema, intracerebral abscess, and cavernous and superior sagittal sinus thrombosis. Conversely, bony complications primarily include just *Pott's puffy tumor* (frontal osteomyelitis with adjacent

**Table 18.1** Chandler's classification

| |
|---|
| Group 1 Inflammatory edema (preseptal cellulitis) |
| Group 2 Orbital cellulitis |
| Group 3 Subperiosteal abscess |
| Group 4 Orbital abscess |
| Group 5 Cavernous sinus thrombosis |

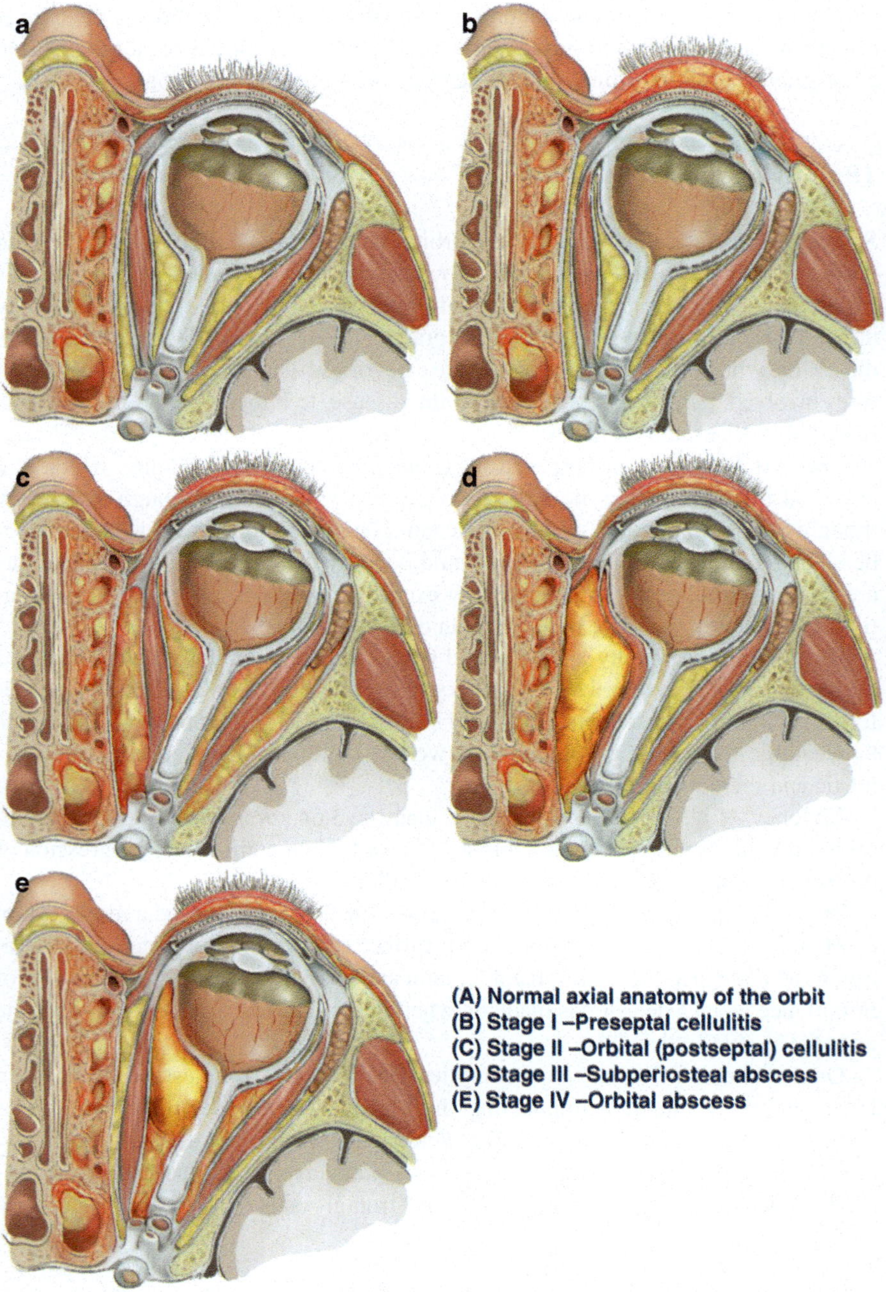


**Fig. 18.1** Diagram of Chandler's classification scheme stages I through IV. Stage V (Cavernous sinus thrombosis) is not shown here. (**a**) Normal axial anatomy of the orbit. (**b**) Stage I—preseptal cellulitis. (**c**) Stage II—orbital (postseptal) cellulitis. (**d**) Stage III—subperiosteal abscess. (**e**) Stage IV—orbital abscess

**Table 18.2** Moloney and Groote Schuur classifications

| Moloney | Groote Schuur modification |
|---|---|
| Preseptal cellulitis | Preseptal |
| Subperiosteal abscess | (a) Cellulitis |
| Orbital cellulitis | (b) Abscess |
| Orbital abscess | Postseptal (subperiosteal) |
| Cavernous sinus thrombosis | (a) Phlegmon/cellulitis |
| | (b) Abscess |
| | Postseptal (intraconal) |
| | (a) Cellulitis |
| | (b) Abscess |
| | Localized |
| | Diffuse |
| | Considered intracranial |

subperiosteal collection on the patient's forehead, which can occur secondary to ARS, CRS, or trauma) [31].

## 18.7 Diagnosis

### 18.7.1 History and Presentation

A detailed history underlining the duration and progression of the disease process is crucial for appropriate diagnosis and exclusion of other differential diagnoses. History of recent URTI, trauma (including insect bites), swimming, ear or dental infections, skin conditions, as well as systemic diseases should be obtained when evaluating a patient with orbital or intracranial findings.

Patients with orbital complications usually present with prior symptoms of acute sinusitis such as fever, cough, rhinorrhea, nasal congestion, facial pressure, anosmia, sore throat, and otalgia in addition to the periorbital swelling. Conversely, the majority of patients with intracranial complications do not have symptoms of sinusitis at the time of presentation but may provide a recent history of sinusitis symptoms and localizing frontal pressure or discomfort [31, 32]. Intracranial complications may be asymptomatic until late in their course, especially when silent areas of the brain are involved such as the frontal lobe. Consequently, a high index of suspicion should be maintained in any case with acute or progressive headache, fever, or behavioral changes along with any symptoms of increased intracranial pressure [31–33]. Symptoms that may indicate increased intracranial pressure include frontal or retro-orbital headache, lethargy, altered mental status, vomiting, seizures, and coma. In a small number of patients, there may be osteomyelitis of the anterior table of the frontal sinus, resulting in overlying edema of the forehead or even a pericranial abscess (*Pott's puffy tumor*).

Occasionally, the diagnosis of ABRS may have been made prior to presentation and some patients present after initiation of oral antibiotics. Nevertheless, it has been shown that despite prior antibiotic treatment, complications of ARS still seem to occur sporadically suggesting that oral antibiotics are of limited benefit in the primary care setting. Similar complication rates have been observed in patients with ARS treated with and without prior antibiotics. Hence, early treatment of URTIs solely with the aim of decreasing sinogenic complications is not supported by available clinical data [34].

### 18.7.2 Examination

Decongestion and examination with anterior rhinoscopy and nasal endoscopy should be performed in all patients, which may reveal polyposis or purulent rhinorrhea in the middle meatus.

In suspected orbital complications, the eye must be opened whenever possible and compared to the contralateral side. Visual acuity, extraocular muscle movements as well as any chemosis, or proptosis should be evaluated. If a postseptal infection is suspected clinically based on findings of proptosis and gaze restriction, an ophthalmologic consultation ought to be promptly obtained to accurately assess the visual status and determine the intraocular pressure as this may alter the modality of treatment.

In suspected intracranial complications, a neurosurgical consultation should be forthwith obtained. A full neurological examination should be performed including examination of signs of increased intracranial pressure (such as papilledema) as well as signs of meningismus (such as nuchal rigidity, photophobia, *Kernig's* and *Brudzinski's* signs). Late findings include hemiparesis, seizures, coma, and other focal neurologic deficits; these are usually associated with a poorer prognosis [32, 33].

### 18.7.3 Labs and Cultures

Standard lab workup for sepsis should be performed including a complete blood count with differential (CBC) and blood cultures, especially in cases of severe orbital or intracranial infections. In addition, endoscopically directed middle meatus cultures should be obtained whenever possible using a sterile swab or utilizing suction into a sterile trap device. Whenever intracranial infections are suspected, a lumbar puncture should also be considered. Imaging must be performed before lumbar puncture in the setting of increased intracranial pressure (ICP) so as to prevent brain herniation and further neurologic compromise.

### 18.7.4 Imaging

Imaging is often pivotal for the appropriate classification of orbital and intracranial complications. Contrast-enhanced computed tomography (CECT) is considered the gold standard for imaging of the orbit and the paranasal sinuses because of its superior delineation of the anatomy of the globe, retro-orbital tissues, sinuses, and cranium, as well as providing information for surgical planning. It is usually indicated when a postseptal or intracranial infection is suspected clinically, or when symptoms of preseptal infection progress within 24–48 h despite adequate antibiotic treatment. Uncomplicated preseptal infections do not require imaging studies [35, 36].

When intracranial complications are suspected based on clinical examination or CT findings, dedicated contrast-enhanced CT of the brain and/or magnetic resonance imaging (MRI) should also be performed. MRI offers superior soft tissue resolution and is most appropriate in the context of intracranial complications, while CT remains the standard initial, and often definitive, modality in the diagnosis and surgical treatment of sinusitis and its orbital extension. Furthermore, frontal sinus disease can be well delineated only on the basis of CT imaging [35, 36].

## 18.8 Orbital Complications

Orbital complications of sinusitis are the most common, especially preseptal cellulitis. They will be discussed in this chapter in the order described by Chandler et al., since his classification system is currently the most ubiquitous [29]. However, this should be taken with a grain of salt as this order is not chronological and does not always reflect the disease course. Therefore, the management of orbital complications should be tailored to each patient [6]. In addition to the five complications described by *Chandler*, other much rarer orbital complications may occur including superior orbital fissure and orbital apex syndromes, but they are out of the scope of this chapter [37, 38] (Fig. 18.1).

### 18.8.1 Preseptal Cellulitis

Preseptal cellulitis is the most commonly encountered orbital complication, constituting around 80% of all orbital complications [17, 35, 39]. It is usually a complication of ethmoid sinusitis; however, it can also occur secondary to skin conditions, eyelid infections such as styes and trauma (including insect bites). Immunodeficient patients such as those with diabetes, leukemia, and HIV are especially susceptible to preseptal cellulitis, unlike other orbital complications [5, 9]. It generally has a more favorable prognosis than other orbital complications.

*Presentation*: The infection is limited to the skin and subcutaneous tissues of the eyelids (especially the superior eyelid) anterior to the orbital septum, with associated inflammatory edema due to impaired venous drainage via the ethmoid veins. It typically presents with periorbital swelling, erythema, and tenderness, which may occasionally progress to a preseptal abscess. It is almost always unilateral. Visual acuity is usually preserved, and signs of postseptal involvement such as chemosis, proptosis, and gaze restriction are also typically not present [8, 29, 35] (Fig. 18.2a).

*CECT*: It is usually unnecessary unless symptoms progress within 24–48 h despite adequate antibiotic treatment or if a concomitant intracranial complication

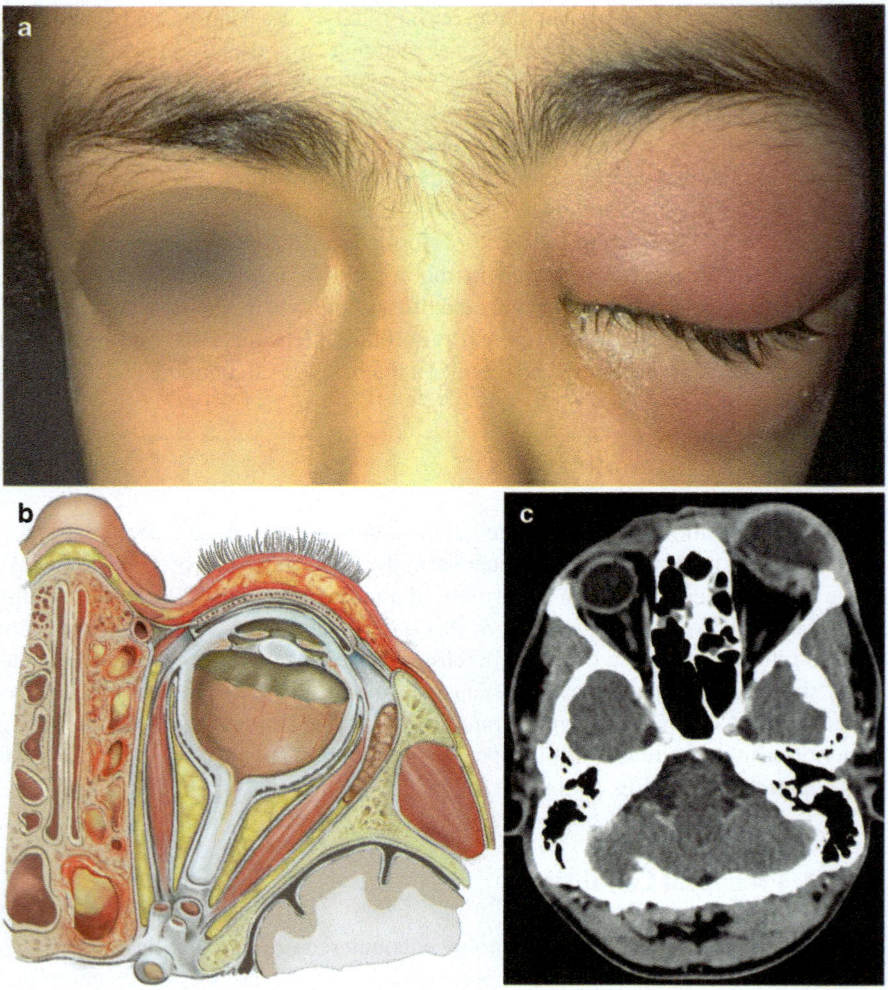

**Fig. 18.2** Preseptal cellulitis. (**a**) Preseptal cellulitis on the left side, particularly affecting the superior eyelid. (**b**) Diagram of preseptal cellulitis. (**c**) Axial CT scan of a left-sided lid abscess that is pushing the globe inferiorly

is suspected. CT would typically reveal diffuse thickening of the eyelids. A preseptal eyelid abscess may also be seen [6, 9] (Fig. 18.2c).

## 18.8.2 Orbital (Postseptal) Cellulitis

Orbital cellulitis is an infection that occurs within the orbit proper posterior to the orbital septum, but without discrete abscess formation. Orbital contents show diffuse swelling and edema, due to increased venous pressure resulting in transudation through vessel walls. It is most often a complication of ethmoid sinusitis, although it may occur following trauma or dental surgery. In immunocompromised individuals, other differential diagnoses must be excluded such as invasive fungal sinusitis. Orbital cellulitis is more concerning than preseptal cellulitis because it can evolve into an orbital abscess [6].

*Presentation*: It typically presents similar to preseptal cellulitis but with associated signs of postseptal involvement such as conjunctival injection, chemosis, proptosis, pain, and limited extraocular muscle movements (ophthalmoplegia). It is almost always unilateral. Visual acuity is not affected early in the disease process but may arise as the disease progresses, indicating optic neuritis and/or ischemia. Early visual acuity loss can present as color vision changes [36, 39, 40] (Fig. 18.3a).

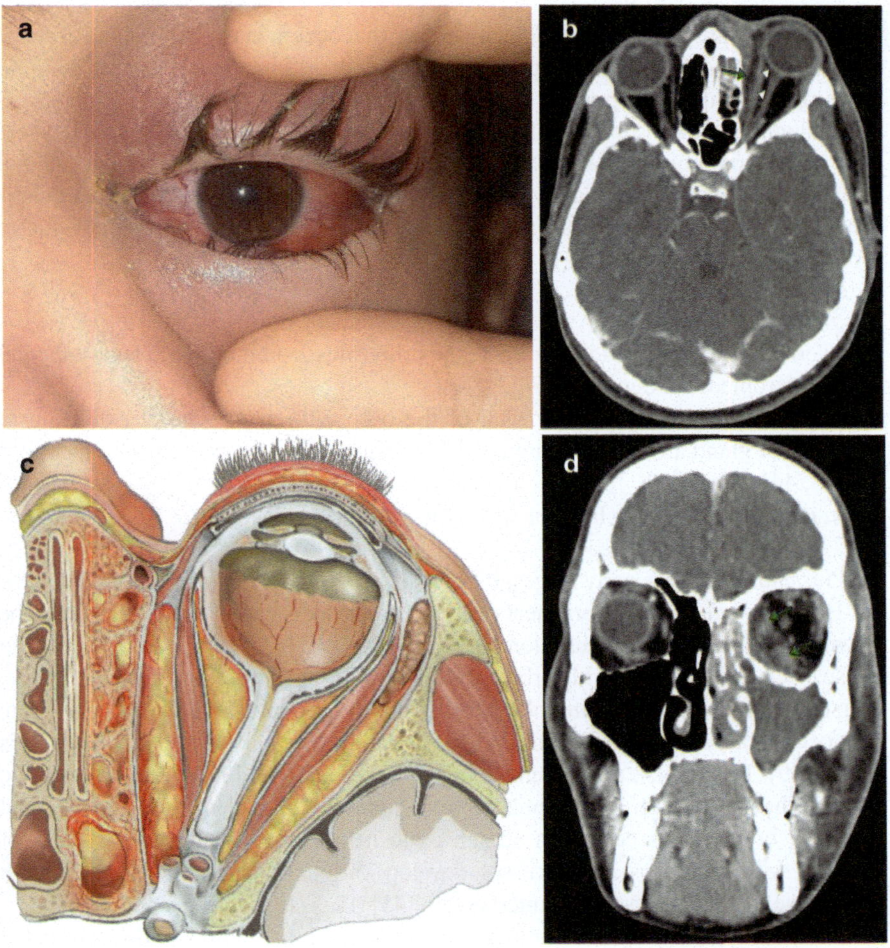


**Fig. 18.3** Orbital (postseptal) cellulitis. (**a**) Postseptal cellulitis on the left side, with evident conjunctival injection and chemosis. (**b**) Diagram of postseptal cellulitis. (**c**) Axial CT scan of left-sided postseptal cellulitis showing increased attenuation of medial orbital fat (green arrow) and thickening of the medial rectus muscle compared to the right side (white arrow heads). Additionally, the left eye is proptotic and the optic nerve is also visibly stretched. (**d**) Coronal CT scan of the same patient displaying displaced and thickened medial and inferior recti (green arrows)

*CECT*: It typically demonstrates a soft tissue density or enhancement of extraconal fat adjacent to the most severely affected sinus (usually at the site of the lamina papyracea), as well as enlargement and enhancement of the adjacent rectus muscle (usually the medial rectus), in addition to diffuse thickening of the eyelids. Discrete abscess formation should not be observed. Intraconal fat may be radiographically normal. It should be noted that the medial rectus muscle may be displaced, enhanced, or thickened in other orbital infectious or immunologic processes [41, 42] (Fig. 18.3c).

### 18.8.3 Subperiosteal Abscess

Subperiosteal abscess is an extraconal abscess that occurs in the subperiosteal space usually between the lamina papyracea and the periorbita, secondary to ethmoid sinusitis. The infection spreads through the lamina papyracea leading to subperiosteal phlegmon which subsequently progresses into a discrete abscess. It is the second most common orbital complication of sinusitis [6, 41]. Isolated medial subperiosteal abscesses typically occur in younger children due to ethmoid sinusitis but occur simultaneously with intracranial complications in teenage males due to frontal sinusitis [7, 31, 32].

*Sites*:

1. *In ethmoid sinusitis*: Medial wall of the orbit (most common) with superomedial or inferomedial extensions (Fig. 18.4).
2. *In frontal sinusitis*: Superior wall of the orbit with superolateral extension (a lacrimal gland abscess is a rare condition that may present in a similar location) [43, 44] (Fig. 18.5).
3. *In maxillary sinusitis*: Inferior wall of the orbit (Fig. 18.6).

*Presentation*: In the early stages, it typically presents similar to postseptal cellulitis. However, a medial subperiosteal phlegmon or abscess can also displace the globe downwards and laterally in addition to ophthalmoplegia. A subperiosteal abscess can be suspected in patients with orbital cellulitis who develop color vision changes, worsening proptosis, ophthalmoplegia, and decreasing visual acuity. An abscess may also occasionally break through the orbital septum and drain anteriorly in the eyelids [6, 36, 39]. It is almost always unilateral. It can rapidly lead to blindness via optic nerve ischemia through direct optic nerve compression, the elevation of intraorbital pressure, or proptosis causing a stretch optic neuropathy [6]. Nearly 15–30% of patients with subperiosteal abscesses develop various visual sequelae even with aggressive medical and surgical intervention [45] (Figs. 18.4d, 18.5a, and 18.6a).

*CECT*: It typically demonstrates a rim-enhancing hypodensity in the extraconal space adjacent to the lamina papyracea but can occur elsewhere along the orbital wall depending on the offending sinus. This hypodensity also exhibits mass-effect and lateral displacement and enlargement of the medial rectus muscle [6, 10]. Air-fluid levels, areas of cavitations, and gas formation may also be seen (Figs. 18.4b, c, 18.5b, c, 18.6b, c, 18.7a, b).

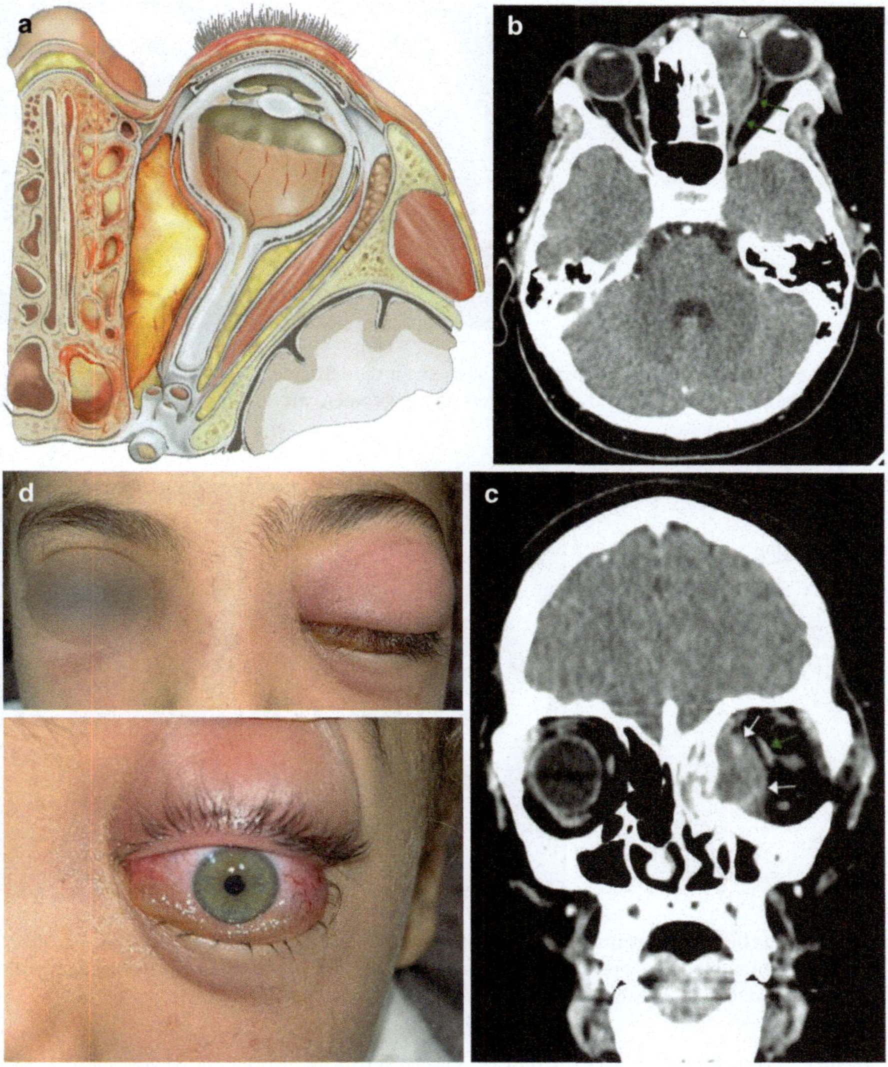


**Fig. 18.4** Medial subperiosteal abscess. (**a**) Diagram of medial subperiosteal abscess. (**b**, **c**) Axial and coronal CT scans of left-sided medial subperiosteal abscess (white arrows) that are displacing the medial rectus muscle laterally (green arrows) as well as displacing the globe inferolaterally. (**d**) Medial subperiosteal abscess on the left side, with extensive chemosis and proptosis

#### 18.8.3.1 Orbital Abscess

An orbital abscess is an intraconal abscess that occurs when orbital cellulitis coalesces into a discrete collection of pus within the intraconal orbital compartment. It is a serious complication which often leads to blindness even with treatment [29].

*Presentation*: It typically presents with similar but more profound manifestations of subperiosteal abscess such as severe pain, chemosis, and exophthalmos in

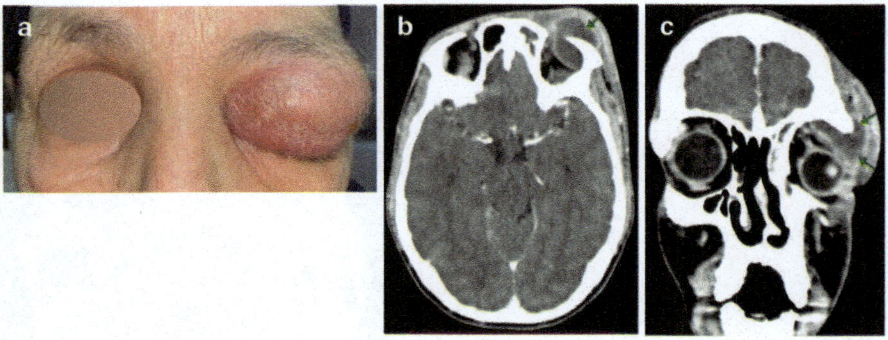


**Fig. 18.5** (**a**) Superolateral subperiosteal abscess on the left side. (**b**, **c**) Axial and coronal CT scans of left-sided superolateral subperiosteal abscess (green arrows) that is displacing the orbit inferomedially

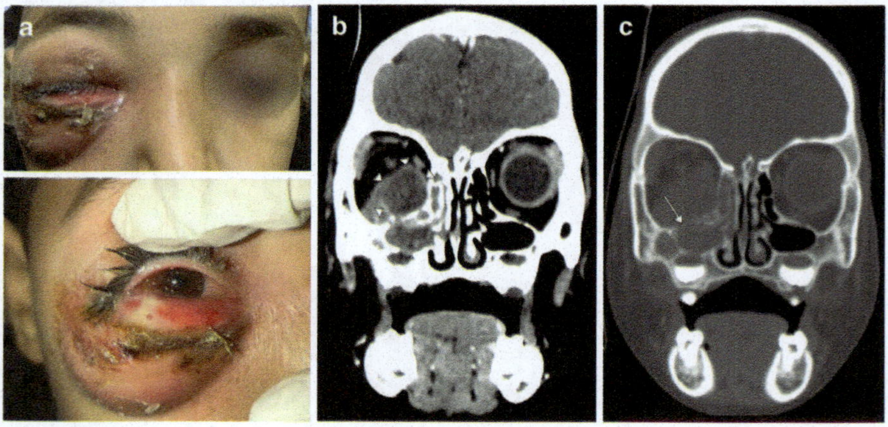


**Fig. 18.6** (**a**) Inferior subperiosteal abscess on the right side. (**b**, **c**) Axial and coronal CT scans of right-sided inferomedial subperiosteal abscess (white arrow heads) that is displacing the globe superiorly. A defect in the superior wall of the maxillary sinus can also be noted (white arrow)

addition to complete ophthalmoplegia. Visual acuity is almost always impaired, and blindness is occasionally observed at presentation [18, 39, 46] (Fig. 18.8a).

*CECT*: In the early stages, it typically demonstrates diffuse ill-defined infiltration of the intra and extraconal orbital fat with obliteration of the optic nerve and extra-ocular muscle enlargement. This is followed by the formation of a rim-enhancing hypodensity in the intraconal space [6].

*MRI Gad*: A definite orbital abscess would appear as an intraconal lesion displaying a hypointense signal on T1-weighted images and a hyperintense signal on T2-weighted images (Fig. 18.8b, c).

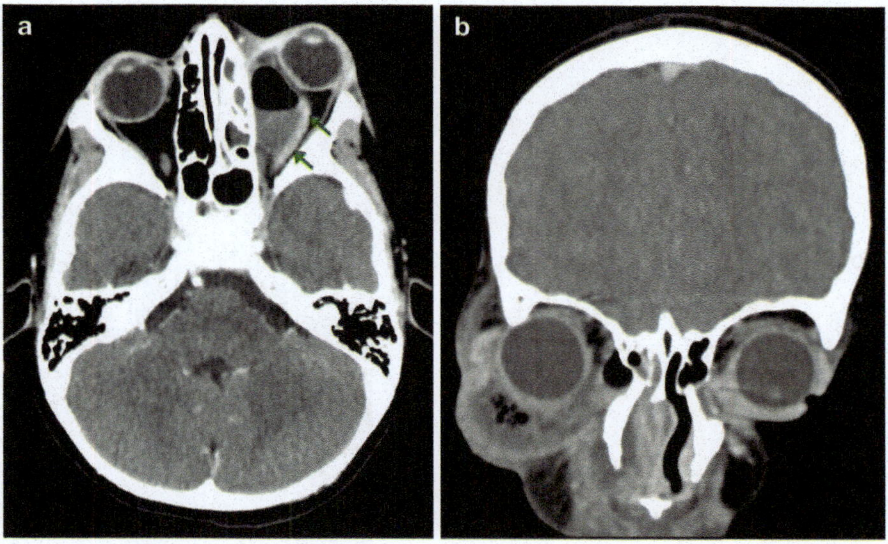


**Fig. 18.7** (**a**) Axial CT scan of left sided superomedial abscess showing an air-fluid level, in addition to lateral displacement of the superior rectus muscle (green arrows). (**b**) Coronal CT scan of right sided inferolateral subperiosteal abscess with evident areas of cavitations and gas formation denoting infection with a gas forming organism

### 18.8.4 Cavernous Sinus Thrombosis

Cavernous sinus thrombosis is both an orbital as well as an intracranial complication. It is the most serious orbital complication in *Chandler's* classification, with a very high mortality rate reaching up to 30% [47]. It results from retrograde septic thrombophlebitis through the valveless superior and inferior ophthalmic veins which are communicating with the cavernous sinus, which can spread further through the intercavernous sinuses to the contralateral cavernous sinus within 24–48 h of the initial presentation leading to the bilateral presentation (a hallmark feature of cavernous sinus thrombosis). Carotid thrombosis may ensue, with simultaneous strokes, intracranial abscesses, or meningitis. *Staphylococcus aureus* is the most common offending pathogen [6, 26, 27].

*Presentation*: Patients are usually septic and seriously ill. They typically present with unilateral or bilateral severe symptoms such as unbearable pain, severe chemosis, exophthalmos, and complete ophthalmoplegia. Trigeminal nerve branches may also be affected as they traverse the cavernous sinus. Papilledema usually occurs due to obstruction of retinal venous drainage, eventually leading to fixed dilated pupils. Blindness is very common [35, 36, 39] (Fig. 18.9a).

*CECT*: Cavernous sinus thrombosis is better demonstrated on MRI/MRV but may be suggested by poor venous enhancement on contrast CT. CT typically demonstrates thickening of the superior ophthalmic vein and irregular filling defects in

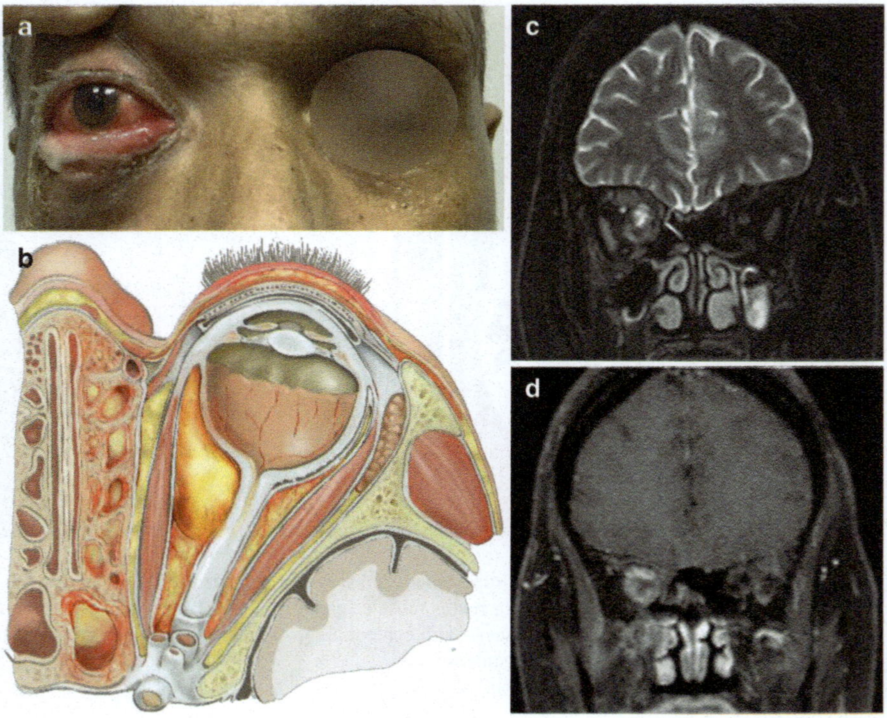

**Fig. 18.8** Orbital abscess. (**a**) Orbital abscess on the right side, with profound chemosis. (**b**) Diagram of the orbital abscess. (**c**, **d**) Coronal T1 and T2 MRI scans postcontrast of right-sided intraconal orbital abscess, which are completely encasing the right optic nerve

the cavernous sinus. Aneurysmal dilatation of the internal carotid artery may be observed in complicated cases [41, 42] (Fig. 18.9b, c).

*MRI Gad and MRV*: Typically demonstrate engorgement of the cavernous sinus and ophthalmic veins. A heterogenous intensity in the involved cavernous sinus is usually observed, along with a hyperintense signal of thrombosed vessels. The cavernous segment of the internal carotid artery is usually deformed/thrombosed, and occasionally complicated by aneurysmal dilatation. MRV is the gold standard method of diagnosis of cavernous sinus thrombosis [41, 42].

#### 18.8.4.1 Management of Orbital Complications

Orbital complications of sinusitis can be managed medically, surgically, or more commonly using a combination of both, depending on the stage of the disease process. The mainstay surgical treatment has traditionally been conventional external approaches such as *Lynch* or *Caldwell-Luc* approaches. However, in recent years, endoscopic sinus surgery (ESS) has effectively replaced them as the gold standard modality of treatment [6]. Although radiographic imaging is crucial for the diagnosis, staging, and surgical planning of orbital complications, it is not unerring. *Patt* and *Manning* described four cases of blindness in a series of 159 patients with

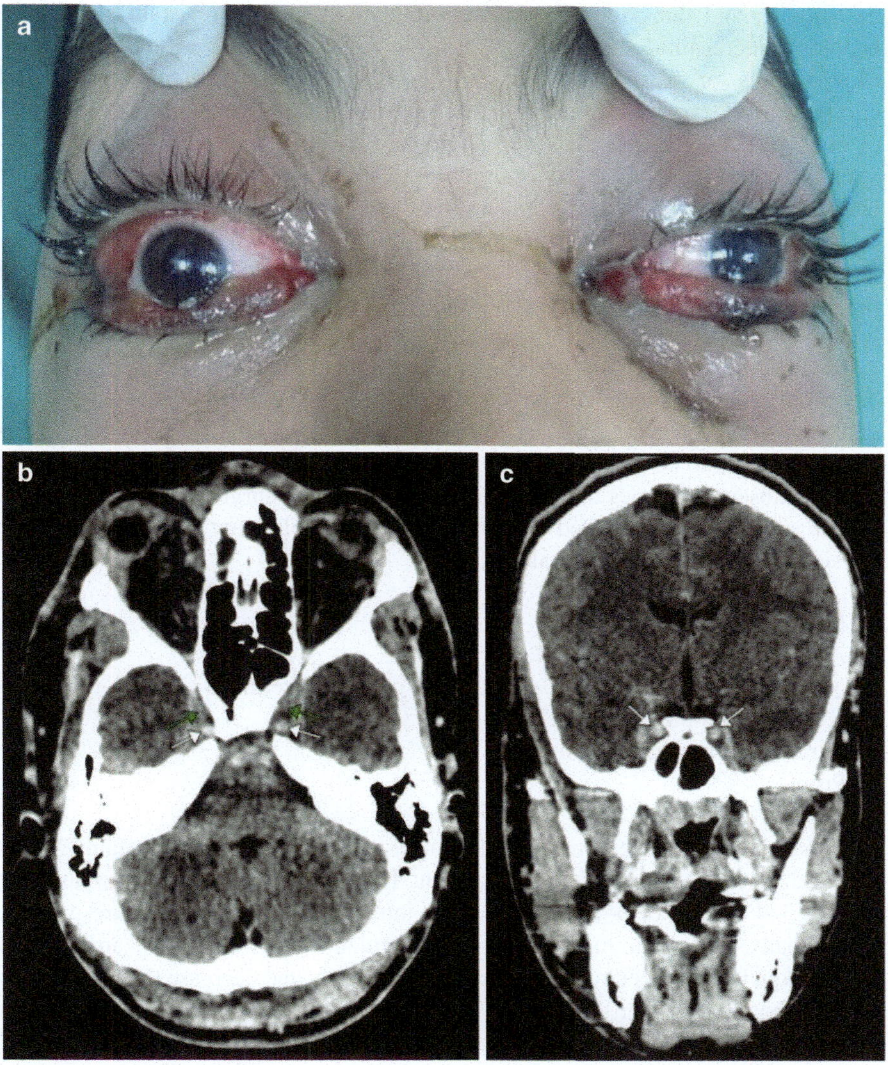


**Fig. 18.9** (**a**) Bilateral cavernous sinus thrombosis. (**b**, **c**) Axial and coronal CT scans of cavernous sinus thrombosis, showing filling defects within both cavernous sinuses in the venous phase (green arrows) with patent carotid arteries bilaterally (white arrows)

complicated acute sinusitis despite negative or equivocal CT scans which subsequently delayed surgical therapy. Hence, clinical decision-making should be individualized and not depend solely on radiology. Additionally, close follow-up of patients with orbital infections is needed as the infection may evolve or progress over the course of treatment with the development of new complications [48].

*Medical Management*: Consists of broad-spectrum IV antibiotics that can cross the blood-brain barrier, directed at the most common pathogens associated with the disease and considering prior antibiotic treatment as resistant strains are becoming increasingly ubiquitous. Antibiotic regimens include intravenous *fluoroquinolones* or a combination of 3rd-/4th-generation *cephalosporins* and *clindamycin/doxycycline*. *Vancomycin or Linezolid* can also be used if MRSA is of concern [49]. After clinical/radiological improvement of orbital findings, IV antibiotics may be switched to oral antibiotics which should be continued for at least another 2–3 weeks. Early oral antibiotics are appropriate only in adults with mild preseptal cellulitis and when daily follow-up can be ensured. Nasal decongestants, whether topical or oral, in addition to frequent saline irrigations may aid in sinus drainage. The use of systemic steroids in patients with orbital complications is controversial [50].

Medical therapy is typically sufficient to adequately treat patients with preseptal or orbital cellulitis, while in patients with subperiosteal abscesses, it is effective only in a subset of them. Todman et al. theorized the volume of the subperiosteal abscess seemed to be the most important criterion in determining surgical management, as abscess volumes of <1250 $mm^3$ did not require surgical intervention [51]. *Oxford* and *McClay* proposed fulfillment of all the following criteria in order to consider medical management alone [19]:

1. Medial subperiosteal abscess
2. Abscess width ≤4 mm on CT
3. Normal visual acuity (better than 20/40), pupil, and retina
4. No ophthalmoplegia
5. Intraocular pressure <20 mmHg
6. Proptosis ≤5 mm

In patients with cavernous sinus thrombosis, a multidisciplinary team (MDT) approach is required for proper management. IV antibiotics should be continued for at least 3–4 weeks, or 6–8 weeks if other intracranial complications are present. Additionally, early administration of anticoagulants, after excluding any hemorrhagic sequelae, has been reported to reduce morbidity and decrease the progression of thrombosis. However, the risk of a fatal hemorrhagic cerebral infarction or a subarachnoid hemorrhage should be considered [35, 46].

*Surgical Management*: It is the definitive treatment modality in most cases of subperiosteal abscess and orbital abscess in combination with medical therapy, as medical management alone would be inadequate. In patients with cavernous sinus thrombosis, sinus drainage should be performed once the patient has been stabilized. Preseptal cellulitis usually doesn't require any surgical intervention except incision and drainage of an eyelid abscess if present, while in patients with orbital cellulitis, surgical intervention is considered—despite the absence of a discrete abscess—if any of the following indications are present [6]:

1. Lack of improvement or progression of symptoms within 24–48 h despite adequate antibiotic treatment.
2. Visual acuity of 20/60 or worse on initial presentation.

3. Severe orbital complications, e.g., afferent pupillary defect on initial presentation.

Once indicated, surgical intervention should not be delayed as this may worsen the prognosis. The objectives of surgical intervention are the removal of the lamina papyracea to drain the abscess as well as decompress the optic nerve and opening of ethmoid/frontal air cells to facilitate sinus drainage. These objectives can be accomplished through any combination of the various techniques described below:

1. *Endoscopic Trans-nasal Approach (ESS)*: It is the gold standard approach for medial subperiosteal abscess, as well as some cases with superior or inferior subperiosteal abscesses. The periorbita should not be incised except in the case of an intraconal abscess, in which case the endoscopic approach could be combined with an external approach in order to adequately drain the intraconal abscess. Some authors have advocated for intraoperative measurement of intraocular pressure to dictate the extent of orbital decompression [52]. This approach avoids any facial scars while allowing the surgeon to remove intranasal polypoidal tissue and infectious debris. Nonetheless, it is technically more difficult as anatomical landmarks are obscured and the surgery is made cumbersome by the bleeding tendencies of acutely inflamed sinonasal mucosa. Additionally, there is a higher risk of postoperative synechia and stenosis especially in the frontal sinus ostium, but this can be mitigated through the use of stents (Fig. 18.10 and Video 18.1).
2. *External Frontoethmoidal Orbitotomy (Lynch) Approach*: It is indicated for superior or superomedial subperiosteal abscess if the endoscopic approach is not feasible. External ethmoidectomy may or may not be performed through this technique; however, a drain should be inserted if no ethmoidectomy is being performed. The main drawbacks of this approach are the presence of a facial

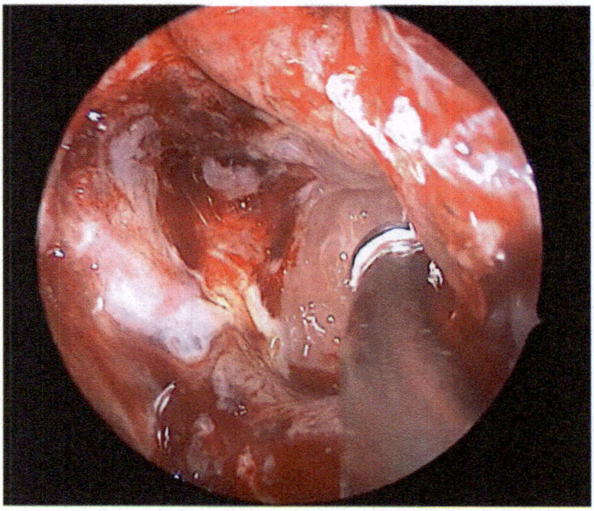

**Fig. 18.10** Drainage of medial subperiosteal abscess

scar, the potential risk of injury to the skull base with subsequent CSF leak as well as temporary diplopia [16].

3. *Lateral Eyebrow Orbitotomy*: It is mainly indicated for a superior subperiosteal abscess with any lateral extensions.
4. *Transcaruncular Medial Orbitotomy*: It is a relatively new oculoplastic technique, utilizing a medial transconjunctival incision. It is indicated for medial subperiosteal abscess if the endoscopic approach is not feasible. This approach avoids any facial scar while allowing easy access and visualization of the abscess cavity from the orbital side of the lamina papyracea especially when used in conjunction with ESS [53].

## 18.9 Intracranial Complications

Intracranial complications of sinusitis are even rarer than orbital complications and are estimated to occur, on average, in only three to four children per million [54]. The rarity of these complications is problematic because their diagnosis is thus usually delayed, and this rarity also makes prospective clinical research impractical. All intracranial complications are associated with significant morbidity and mortality and therefore warrant immediate attention. Moreover, multiple complications can occur in the same patient either concurrently or sequentially [7, 12, 43]. Management must be multidisciplinary including an otolaryngologist, neurosurgeon, pediatrician, internist, and critical care and infectious disease specialists.

### 18.9.1 Epidural Abscess

Epidural abscesses are the second most common intracranial complication of sinusitis. They are usually a complication of frontal sinusitis due to the loosely adherent dura in the frontal region. However, they tend to expand slowly because of the tight adherence of the dura to the cranium elsewhere. Patients usually have a prolonged period of nonspecific symptoms until the infection manages to penetrate the dura or the abscess becomes large enough to cause increased intracranial pressure [41, 42]. They have a more favorable prognosis than other intracranial complications [31].

*CECT*: It typically demonstrates an extra-axial biconvex (lentiform) hypodensity that is bounded by sutures and potentially crossing the midline, usually with strong peripheral contrast enhancement (Fig. 18.11d).

*MRI Gad*: It typically demonstrates a biconvex hypointense lesion on T1-weighted images that is hyperintense on T2-weighted images, with peripheral enhancement after administration of gadolinium (Fig. 18.11a–c).

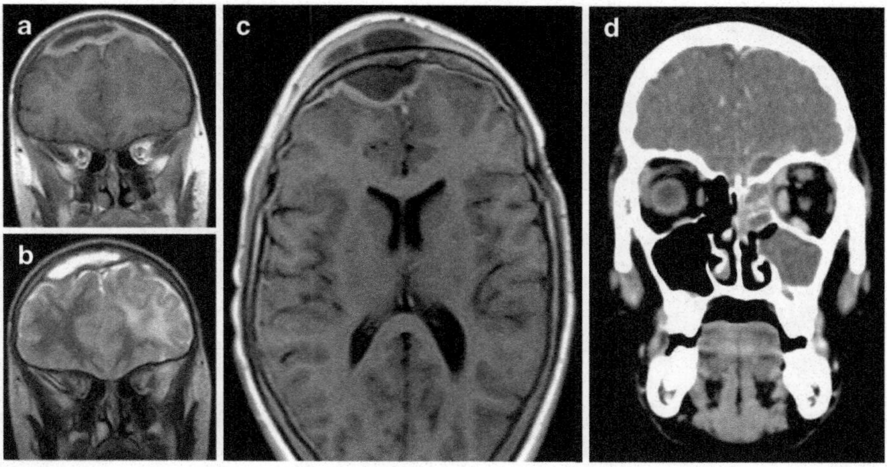


**Fig. 18.11** (**a**, **b**) Coronal T1 and T2 MRI scans post-contrast of an extradural abscess complicating frontal sinusitis. (**c**) Axial T1 MRI scan post-contrast of a different patient with an extradural abscess and Pott's puffy tumour complicating frontal sinusitis. (**d**) Coronal CT scan of another patient with an extradural abscess complicating ethmoid sinusitis

### 18.9.2 Sudural Abscess/Empyema

It is the most common intracranial complication of sinusitis, usually preceded by frontal sinusitis. It is usually unilateral. Due to the lack of anatomic barriers, pus can quickly dissect and disseminate through the subdural space over the cerebral convexities, interhemispheric fissure, tentorium, posterior fossa, and even the spinal canal, leading to subdural empyema. Patients usually deteriorate rapidly, hence the higher morbidity and mortality rates compared to other intracranial complications [20, 32].

*CECT*: It typically demonstrates an extra-axial concave (crescentic) hypodensity that is not bounded by sutures nor crossing the midline, and usually with strong peripheral contrast enhancement (Fig. 18.12a–c).

*MRI Gad*: It typically demonstrates a concave hypointense lesion on T1-weighted images that is hyperintense on T2-weighted images, with peripheral enhancement after administration of gadolinium.

### 18.9.3 Intracerebral Abscess

It is the third most common intracranial complication of sinusitis, usually preceded by frontal sinusitis. The most common locations are the frontal and frontoparietal lobes. The predominant route of parenchymal abscess formation is via implantation of septic emboli in areas of sluggish venous flow such as in the junction of white and gray matter. The presentation often depends on the location of the infection. In frontal lobe abscesses, for example, the only symptom may be a subtle change in personality [31, 55].

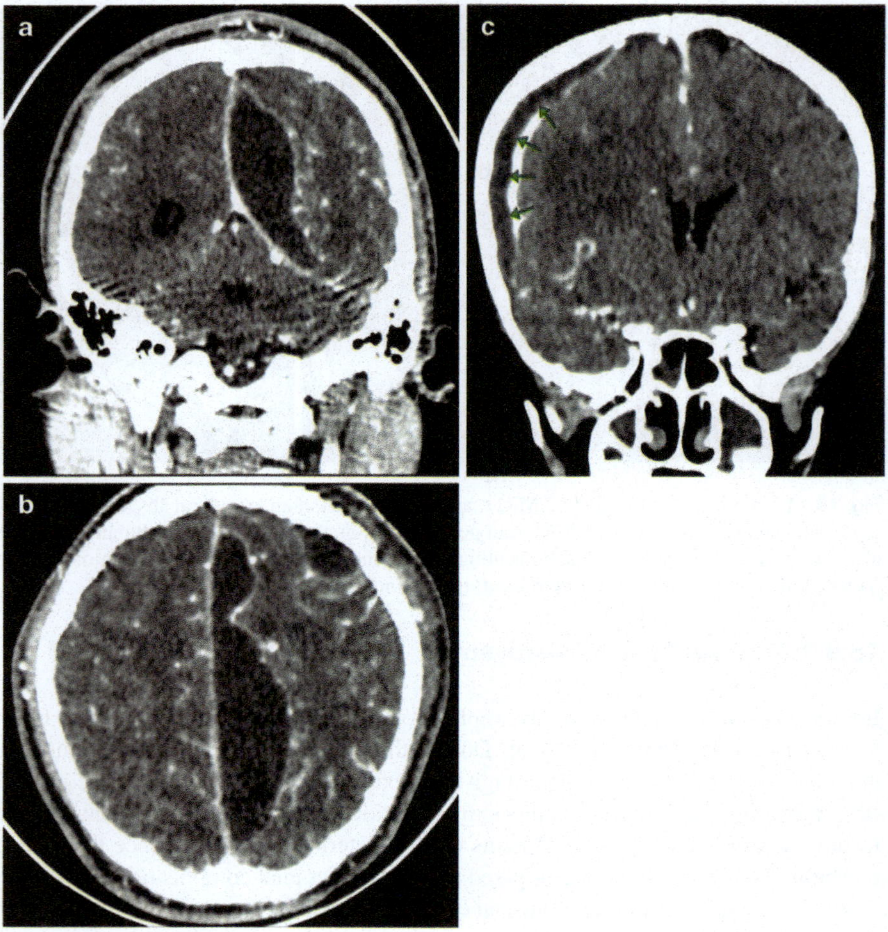


**Fig. 18.12** (**a**, **b**) Axial and coronal CT scans of extensive subdural empyema along the falx cerebri due to frontal sinusitis. (**c**) Coronal CT scan of a subtle right-sided subdural abscess also due to frontal sinusitis

*CECT*: It typically demonstrates an intracerebral hypodensity with strong peripheral contrast enhancement.

*MRI Gad*: It typically demonstrates a cystic hypointense lesion on T1-weighted images that is hyperintense with a distinct hypointense capsule on T2-weighted images. After administration of gadolinium, the capsule appears strongly enhanced (Fig. 18.13a, b).

#### 18.9.3.1 Meningitis

Meningitis is commonly associated with other complications of ARS and seldom occurs in isolation. Rhinosinusitis itself is an unusual cause of meningitis. However, focal dural enhancement (focal meningitis) in association with other complications

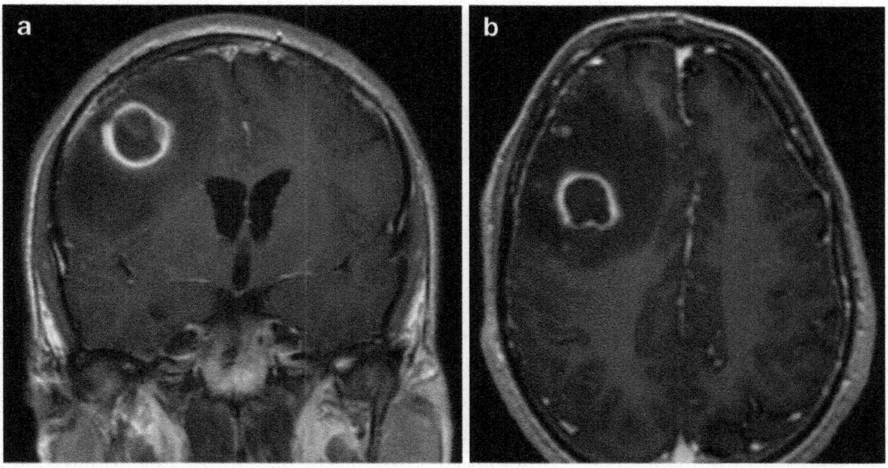


**Fig. 18.13** (**a**, **b**) Axial and coronal T1 MRI scans postcontrast showing right-sided frontoparietal intracerebral abscess with peripheral contrast enhancement

is somewhat more common [31]. It typically occurs subsequent to sphenoiditis or ethmoiditis [6].

*CECT*: Unremarkable.

*MRI Gad*: It typically demonstrates dural enhancement, most evidently along the falx cerebri, tentorium, and convexity dura.

*Lumbar Puncture*: It typically demonstrates turbid CSF with neutrophilia. It should be avoided in cases of increased intracranial pressure (ICP) so as to prevent brain herniation and further neurologic compromise.

### 18.9.4 Venous Sinus Thrombosis

Any dural venous sinus may be affected by rhinosinusitis. However, the superior sagittal sinus is the most commonly involved due to retrograde thrombophlebitis from frontal sinusitis. Acute occlusion of any dural sinus is not well tolerated and may lead to massive cerebral edema, venous congestion, and infarction. It is almost always found in association with other intracranial abscesses. Patients typically appear extremely ill, presenting with nausea and vomiting in addition to severe headaches [3, 6].

*CECT*: *Empty delta sign* is a sign specific to superior sagittal sinus thrombosis. It is a triangular area of enhancement with a relatively low-attenuating center, which is the thrombosed sinus (filling defect). It occurs due to recanalization around an organizing clot. Gyral enhancement and prominent intramedullary veins can also be found in some cases [56].

*MRI Gad and MRV*: Typically demonstrate focal defects of enhancement after gadolinium administration with decreased cavernous carotid artery flow void. The clot appears iso- to hyperintense on T1-weighted images, but hypointense on T2-weighted images. MRV studies can further delineate the clot [57].

#### 18.9.4.1 Management of Intracranial Complications

Due to the extensive nature of intracranial complications, a multidisciplinary team (MDT) approach is required for proper management. Furthermore, repeat CT scans of the brain and sinuses should be performed during treatment and prior to hospital discharge as patients may develop multiple intracranial complications at any time over the course of treatment [4, 14].

While intracranial complications are typically associated with acute or subacute sinusitis, underlying chronic sinusitis may be a factor in some patients as repeated cycles of infection and incomplete resolution often lead to mucosal scarring and polypoid changes which are theorized to result in hidden foci of infection with poor drainage and reduced antibiotic penetration [4].

*Medical Management*: It is the mainstay treatment modality in meningitis, and an essential adjunct modality in other intracranial complications. It consists of broad-spectrum IV antibiotics that can cross the blood-brain barrier, directed at the most common pathogens associated with the disease and considering prior antibiotic treatment as resistant strains are becoming increasingly ubiquitous. Antibiotic regimens include intravenous fluoroquinolones or a combination of 3rd-/4th-generation cephalosporins and clindamycin/doxycycline. Vancomycin or Linezolid can also be used if MRSA is of concern [49]. Antibiotics should be continued for at least 2–8 weeks postoperatively, depending on the presence of osteomyelitis. If indicated, anticonvulsant medications should also be used to reduce the risk of seizures [4].

The use of systemic steroids to treat secondary cerebral edema is controversial, as some authors argue that it impairs the abscess encapsulation process, reduces antibiotic penetration into the abscess as well as alters its appearance on imaging scans. In patients with dural venous sinus thromboses, anticoagulants may also be added to decrease the progression of thrombosis. However, the risk of a fatal hemorrhagic cerebral infarction or a subarachnoid hemorrhage should be considered [4, 6].

*Surgical Management*: It is the definitive treatment modality. Immediate neurosurgical drainage of epidural, subdural, and intracerebral abscesses is required in most cases. Nevertheless, patients with small abscesses and mild symptoms may be observed for 24–48 h while on medical therapy, only requiring drainage if they fail to improve or if symptoms worsen [14].

Additionally, sinus drainage can be achieved through endoscopic frontal sinusotomy (Draf 2a/Draf 2b), frontal sinus trephination, or combined approaches. This can be performed concurrently with neurosurgical drainage if the patient has been stabilized, or at a later stage as early sinus drainage may not improve outcome [14]. In patients with dural venous sinus thromboses, sinus drainage should be performed once the patient has been stabilized. In patients with isolated meningitis, most authors recommend sinus drainage to be performed if clinical improvement is not evident 24–28 h after the start of IV antibiotics [6].

## 18.10 Bony Complications

Bony complications are the least common of sinusitis complications, usually presenting as osteomyelitis of the frontal bone in adults [4]. Maxillary bone osteomyelitis can also occur following sinusitis especially in immunocompromised patients, albeit much rarer [58]. Distal bony complications in the form of septic arthritis—usually in the hip—have also been reported, even in immunocompetent patients [59].

Infection in the frontal sinus can spread beyond the confines of the sinus either by focal osteitis and osteomyelitis or through retrograde septic thrombophlebitis. Acute osteomyelitis of the posterior table of the frontal sinus can cause an epidural abscess, while transmural osteomyelitis of the anterior table often leads to either a periorbital subperiosteal abscess or a sub-pericranial abscess. Focal pitting/doughy forehead edema typically heralds the formation of a fluctuating forehead sub-pericranial abscess, hence the eponymous *Pott's "puffy" tumor*—after Sir *Percival Pott*. Left untreated, the soft tissue edema surrounding the sub-pericranial abscess will subsequently expand to involve the whole forehead and into the preseptal orbital space, and the abscess itself might drain anteriorly through the skin of the forehead, forming a fronto-cutaneous fistula [4, 60].

*Presentation*: A *Pott's puffy tumor* is the most common presentation of bony complications of sinusitis but can also occur following penetrating forehead trauma or surgery of the frontal sinus. It is associated with other intracranial complications in 60% of the cases, particularly epidural abscess [61]. It typically presents with a soft doughy forehead swelling, either as the sole presenting symptom or, more commonly, in association with symptoms of other intracranial complications such as headache and fever. Symptoms of acute sinusitis are occasionally present but are not usually prominent [4, 43] (Fig. 18.14).

*CECT*: It is essential for confirming the diagnosis, as well as for surgical planning; by defining the boundaries of the sub-pericranial abscess and delineating areas of osteomyelitis (Fig. 18.14).

*MRI Gad*: It is the best modality for excluding associated intracranial complications, especially when the CT scan is equivocal (Fig. 18.14).

### 18.10.1 Management of Bony Complications

Similar to other intracranial complications, a multidisciplinary team (MDT) approach is required for proper management.

*Medical Management*: Consists of broad-spectrum IV antibiotics that can cross the blood-brain barrier, directed at the most common pathogens associated with the disease, and considering prior antibiotic treatment as resistant strains are becoming increasingly ubiquitous. Antibiotic regimens include intravenous fluoroquinolones or a combination of 3rd-/4th-generation cephalosporins and clindamycin/doxycycline. Vancomycin or Linezolid can also be used if MRSA is of concern. Antibiotics should be continued for at least 6 weeks postoperatively, for adequate control of infection [43, 49].

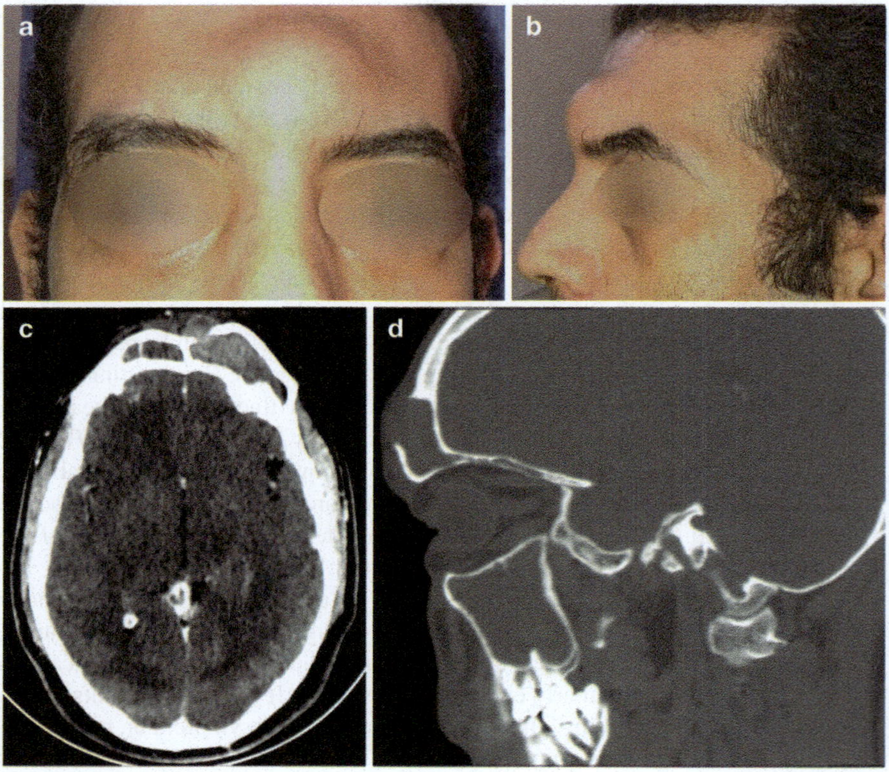


**Fig. 18.14** (**a**, **b**) Pott's puffy tumour presenting as a doughy forehead swelling complicating frontal sinusitis, with no orbital affection. (**c**) Axial CT scan of Potts puffy tumour extending through defective/necrotic anterior table of left frontal sinus. (**d**) Sagittal CT scan of another patient with Pott's puffy tumour showing large defect in anterior table of frontal sinus

*Surgical Management*: It is the definitive treatment modality. Surgical drainage of the abscess cavity and frontal sinus as well as debridement of osteomyelitic bone are the main objectives of surgical intervention. These objectives can be accomplished through an external approach to the frontal sinus in addition to ESS, e.g., through a bifrontal craniotomy incision, especially if concomitant intracranial complications are present [60].

Thorough debridement of infected bone is mandatory, and this may necessitate the removal of part of or even the entire anterior table of the frontal sinus, i.e., the *Riedel* procedure. For esthetic purposes, any defect in the anterior table of the frontal sinus should be reconstructed using autogenous grafts such as split calvarial bone grafts, or alloplastic materials such as titanium mesh. Reconstruction may be performed at the same setting or at a later stage, so as to give sufficient time for the original disease process to be eradicated. In order to prevent recurrence, the frontal sinus cavity can also be obliterated completely after fulguration of all sinus mucosa [62] (Fig. 18.15).

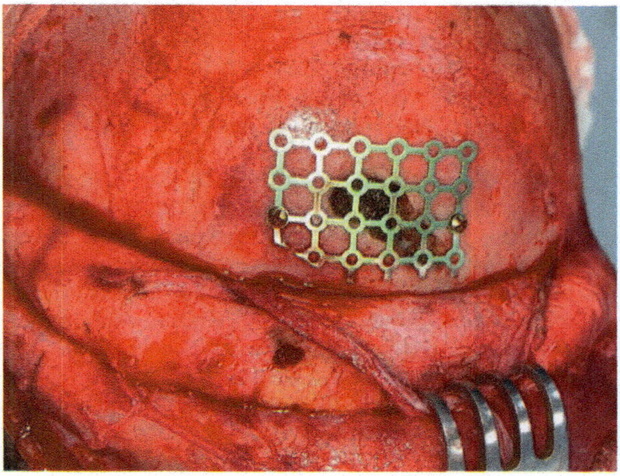

**Fig. 18.15** Pott's puffy tumor addressed through a bifrontal craniotomy incision, along with titanium mesh reconstruction

A minimally invasive approach has also been described, involving frontal sinus trephination and drainage of the sub-pericranial abscess through a small incision followed by endoscopic frontal sinus surgery [63]. The main drawback of this approach is that the surgeon will be unable to directly inspect the frontal bone and excise any necrotic bone. In addition, simple drainage of the abscess cavity and frontal sinus will be insufficient in the presence of an intracranial collection. Consequently, this approach should not be performed if intracranial complications are suspected and should generally be limited to the emergency setting followed by definitive management of the disease.

**Acknowledgment** We acknowledge Ms. Mayar Aboudy for drawing the medical illustrations.

## References

1. Conrad DA, Jenson HB. Management of acute bacterial rhinosinusitis. Curr Opin Pediatr. 2002;14:86–90.
2. Lerner DN, Choi SS, Zalzal GH, et al. Intracranial complications of sinusitis in childhood. Ann Otol Rhinol Laryngol. 1995;104(4 Pt 1):288–93.
3. Gallagher RM, Gross CW, Phillips CD. Suppurative intracranial complications of sinusitis. Laryngoscope. 1998;108:1635–42.
4. Kountakis SE, Senior BA, Draf W. The frontal sinus. Berlin: Springer; 2016. https://doi.org/10.1007/978-3-662-48523-1.
5. Botting AM, McIntosh D, Mahadevan M. Paediatric pre- and postseptal periorbital infections are different diseases: a retrospective review of 262 cases. Int J Pediatr Otorhinolaryngol. 2008;72(3):377–83.
6. Johnson J, Rosen CA, Bailey BJ. Bailey's head and neck surgery: otolaryngology. 5th ed. Philadelphia: Lippincott Williams & Wilkins; 2013.
7. Glickstein JS, Chandra RK, Thompson JW. Intracranial complications of pediatric sinusitis. Otolaryngol Head Neck Surg. 2006;134(5):733.
8. Goldberg AN, Oroszlan G, Anderson T. Complications of frontal sinusitis and their management. Otolaryngol Clin N Am. 2001;34(1):211–25.

9. Nageswaran S, Woods CR, Benjamin DK, et al. Orbital cellulitis in children. Pediatr Infect Dis J. 2006;25(8):695–9.
10. Flint PW, Haughey BH, Lund VJ, Robbins KT, Thomas JR, Lesperance MM, Francis HW. Cummings otolaryngology head and neck surgery, vol. 3. Amsterdam: Elsevier; 2020.
11. Remmler D, Boles R. Intracranial complications of frontal sinusitis. Laryngoscope. 1980;90:1814–24.
12. Herrmann BW, Chung JC, Eisenbeis JF, et al. Intracranial complications of pediatric frontal rhinosinusitis. Am J Rhinol. 2006;20(3):320–4.
13. Herrmann BW, Forsen JW. Simultaneous intracranial and orbital complications of acute rhino-sinusitis in children. Int J Pediatr Otorhinolaryngol. 2004;68:619–25.
14. DelGaudio JM, Evans SH, Sobol SE, et al. Intracranial complications of sinusitis: what is the role of endoscopic sinus surgery in the acute setting. Am J Otolaryngol. 2010;31(1):25–8.
15. Mortimore S, Wormald PJ. The Groote-Schuur hospital classification of the orbital complications of sinusitis. Laryngol Otol. 1997;111:719–23.
16. Mortimore S, Wormald PJ. Management of acute complicated sinusitis: a five year review. Otolaryngol Head Neck. 1999;121:639–42.
17. Schramm VL, Curtin HD, Kennerdell JS. Evaluation of orbital cellulites and results of treatment. Laryngoscope. 1982;92:732–8.
18. Younis RT, Lazar RH, Bustillo A, et al. Orbital infection as a complication of sinusitis: are diagnostic and treatment trends changing? Ear Nose Throat J. 2001;81:771–5.
19. Oxford LE, McClay J. Medical and surgical management of subperiosteal orbital abscess secondary to acute sinusitis in children. Int J Pediatr Otorhinolaryngol. 2006;70(11):1853–61.
20. Goytia VK, Giannoni CM, Edwards MS. Intraorbital and intracranial extension of sinusitis: comparative morbidity. J Pediatr. 2011;158(3):486–91.
21. Wald E. Sinusitis in children. N Engl J Med. 1992;326:319–23.
22. Brook I, Foote PA, Hausfeld JN. Frequency of recovery of pathogens causing acute maxillary sinusitis in adults before and after introduction of vaccination of children with the 7-valent vaccine. J Med Microbiol. 2006;55:943–6.
23. Brook I. Microbiology and antimicrobial treatment of orbital and intracranial complications of sinusitis in children and their management. Int J Pediatr Otorhinolaryngol. 2009;73:1183–6.
24. Olwoch IP. Microbiology of acute complicated bacterial sinusitis at the University of the Witwatersrand. S Afr Med J. 2010;100(8):529–33.
25. Huang WH, Hung PK. Methicillin-resistant Staphylococcus aureus infections in acute rhinosinusitis. Laryngoscope. 2006;116(2):288–91.
26. Wilson WR, Sande MA, editors. Current diagnosis and treatment in infectious diseases. New York: Lange Medical Books/McGraw-Hill; 2011.
27. Hwang SY, Tan KK. Streptococcus viridans has a leading role in rhinosinusitis complications. Ann Otol Rhinol Laryngol. 2007;116(5):381–5.
28. Hubert L. Orbital infections due to nasal sinusitis. N Y Med J. 1937;37:1559–64.
29. Chandler JR, Langenbrunner DJ, Stevens ER. The pathogenesis of orbital complications in acute sinusitis. Laryngoscope. 1970;80:1414–28.
30. Moloney JR, Badham NJ, McRae A. The acute orbit, preseptal (periorbital) cellulitis, subperiosteal abscess and orbital cellulitis due to sinusitis. J Laryngol Otol. 1987;101(12):1–18.
31. Germiller JA, Monin DL, Sparano AM, et al. Intracranial complications of sinusitis in children and adolescents and their outcomes. Arch Otolaryngol Head Neck Surg. 2006;132(9):969–76.
32. Giannoni CM, Sulek M, Friedman EM. Intracranial complications of sinusitis: a pediatric series. Am J Rhinol. 1998;12:173–8.
33. Giannoni CM, Stewart MG, Alford EL. Intracranial complications of sinusitis. Laryngoscope. 1997;107:863–7.
34. Young J, De Sutter A, Merenstein D, et al. Antibiotics for adults with clinically diagnosed acute rhinosinusitis: a meta-analysis of individual patient data. Lancet. 2008;371(9616):908–14.
35. Choi SS, Grundfast KM. Complications in sinus disease. In: Kennedy DW, Bolger WE, Zinreich SJ, editors. Diseases of the sinuses: diagnosis and management. Hamilton: B.C. Decker; 2001. p. 169–77.

36. Kendall KA, Senders CW. Orbital and intracranial complications of sinusitis in children and adults. In: Gershwin ME, Incaudo GA, editors. Diseases of the sinuses: a comprehensive textbook of diagnosis and treatment. Totowa: Humana Press; 1996. p. 247–72.
37. Pfeiffer ML, Merritt HA, Bailey LA, Richani K, Phillips ME. Orbital apex syndrome from bacterial sinusitis without orbital cellulitis. Am J Ophthalmol Case Rep. 2018;10:84–6. https://doi.org/10.1016/j.ajoc.2018.01.041. PMID: 29468204; PMCID: PMC5814374.
38. Pinna Fde R, Dutra DL, Neves MC, Ricci Romano F, Voegels RL, Botugan O. Superior orbital fissure syndrome due to sinusitis: report of two cases. Am J Rhinol. 2005;19(4):417–20.
39. Goodwin WJ. Orbital complications of ethmoiditis. Otolaryngol Clin N Am. 1995;18:139–47.
40. Davis JP, Stearns MP. Orbital complications of sinusitis: avoid delays in diagnosis. Postgrad Med J. 1994;70:108–10.
41. Mafee MF, Tran BH, Chapa AR. Imaging of rhinosinusitis and its complications: plain film, CT, and MRI. Clin Rev Allergy Immunol. 2006;30(3):165–86.
42. Vazquez E, Creixell S, Carreno JC, et al. Complicated acute pediatric bacterial sinusitis: imaging updated approach. Curr Probl Diagn Radiol. 2004;33(3):127–45.
43. Blumfield E, Misra M. Pott's puffy tumor, intracranial, and orbital complications as the initial presentation of sinusitis in healthy adolescents, a case series. Emerg Radiol. 2011;18(3):203–10.
44. Varshney S, Malhotra M, Kaur N, Goirala P. Lacrimal gland abscess leading to frontal bone chronic osteomyelitis: a rare case report. Clin Rhinol. 2020;9:102–4.
45. Rahbar R, Robson CD, Petersen RA, et al. Management of orbital subperiosteal abscess in children. Arch Otolaryngol Head Neck Surg. 2001;127(3):281–6. https://doi.org/10.1001/archotol.127.3.281.
46. Osguthorpe JD, Hochman M. Inflammatory sinus diseases affecting the orbit. Otolaryngol Clin N Am. 1993;26:657–71.
47. Absoud M, Hikmet F, Dey P, Joffe M, Thambapillai E. Bilateral cavernous sinus thrombosis complicating sinusitis. J R Soc Med. 2006;99(9):474–6. https://doi.org/10.1177/014107680609900921.
48. Patt BS, Manning SC. Blindness resulting from orbital complications of sinusitis. Otolaryngol Head Neck Surg. 1991;104:789–95.
49. Chow AW, Benninger MS, Brook I, Brozek JL, Goldstein EJC, Hicks LA, et al. IDSA clinical practice guideline for acute bacterial rhinosinusitis in children and adults. Clin Infect Dis. 2012;54:e72–e112. https://doi.org/10.1093/cid/cis370.
50. Kim BY, Bae JH. Role of systemic corticosteroids in orbital cellulitis: a meta-analysis and literature review. Braz J Otorhinolaryngol. 2022;88(2):257–62. https://doi.org/10.1016/j.bjorl.2021.02.003. Epub 2021 Mar 6. PMID: 33722520; PMCID: PMC9422736.
51. Todman MS, Enzer YR. Medical management versus surgical intervention of pediatric orbital cellulitis: the importance of subperiosteal abscess volume as a new criterion. Ophthalmic Plast Reconstr Surg. 2011;27(4):255–9. https://doi.org/10.1097/IOP.0b013e3182082b17.
52. Fakhri S. Endoscopic drainage of subperiosteal orbital abscesses. Oper Tech Otolaryngol Head Neck Surg. 2008;19:195–8. https://doi.org/10.1016/j.otot.2008.09.008.
53. Pelton RW, Smith ME, Patel BC, et al. Cosmetic considerations in surgery for orbital subperiosteal abscess in children: experience with a combined transcaruncular and transnasal endoscopic approach. Arch Otolaryngol Head Neck Surg. 2003;129:652–5.
54. Piatt JH. Intracranial suppuration complicating sinusitis among children: an epidemiological and clinical study. J Neurosurg Pediatr. 2011;7(6):567–74.
55. Hicks CW, Weber JG, Reid JR, et al. Identifying and managing intracranial complications of sinusitis in children: a retrospective series. Pediatr Infect Dis J. 2011;30(3):222–6.
56. Shinohara Y, Yoshitoshi M, Yoshii F. Appearance and disappearance of empty delta sign in superior sagittal sinus thrombosis. Stroke. 1986;17(6):1282–4. https://doi.org/10.1161/01.str.17.6.1282.
57. Tang PH, Chai J, Chan YH, Chng SM, Lim CC. Superior sagittal sinus thrombosis: subtle signs on neuroimaging. Ann Acad Med Singap. 2008;37(5):397–401.
58. Habib A, Sivaji N, Ashraf T. Maxillary osteomyelitis: a rare entity. Case Rep Otolaryngol. 2016;2016:9723806. https://doi.org/10.1155/2016/9723806.

59. Yan C, Chau WW, Ng B. Concomitant orbital subperiosteal abscess, sinusitis, and septic arthritis of the hip in a normal healthy adolescent patient. J Orthop Trauma Rehabil. 2018;26:1. https://doi.org/10.1016/j.jotr.2018.06.001.
60. Bambidakis NC, Cohen AR. Intracranial complications of frontal sinusitis in children: Pott's puffy tumor revisited. Pediatr Neurosurg. 2001;35:82–9.
61. Bannon PD, McCormack RF. Pott's puffy tumor and epidural abscess arising from pansinusitis. J Emerg Med. 2011;41(6):616–22. https://doi.org/10.1016/j.jemermed.2008.04.050. Epub 2008 Nov 20.
62. Kuttenberger JJ, Hardt N. Long-term results following reconstruction of craniofacial defects with titanium micro-mesh systems. J Craniomaxillofac Surg. 2001;29:75–81.
63. Sideris G, Delides A, Proikas K, Papadimitriou N. Pott puffy tumor in adults: the timing of surgical intervention. Cureus. 2020;12(11):e11781. https://doi.org/10.7759/cureus.11781. PMID: 33409028; PMCID: PMC7779183.

# Odontogenic Maxillary Sinusitis

# 19

Nelly Elwany and Samy Elwany

**Key Points**

- Odontogenic infections primarily involve the maxillary sinus; therefore, the term "Odontogenic Maxillary Sinusitis" (OMS) is more appropriate than "Odontogenic Sinusitis."
- Odontogenic maxillary sinusitis (OMS) is underdiagnosed and is frequently missed by rhinologists, dentists, and radiologists.
- Dental interventions and periapical infections are the primary causes of OMS. The incidence of implant-related maxillary sinusitis has increased especially after "sinus lift" procedures.
- Unilateral malodorous nasal discharge, nasal obstruction, and pain over the cheek are the most frequent clinical presentations.
- The doctor should explicitly ask the patients about their dental history because most patients do not volunteer this information and also because sinus infection may develop several months following dental treatment.
- CT scans and cone beam CT (CBCT) are the gold standard radiologic modality for diagnosing OMS.
- Treatment options include dental treatment, antibiotics, endoscopic sinus surgery, and closure of oroantral communication (OAC) or fistula (OAF).

N. Elwany (✉)
College of Dentistry, University of Kentucky, Lexington, KY, USA
e-mail: nmel228@uky.edu

S. Elwany
Department of Otolaryngology, Alexandria Faculty of Medicine, Alexandria, Egypt


S. Elwany (ed.), *Current Rhinology*,
https://doi.org/10.1007/978-3-031-70077-4_19

Odontogenic maxillary sinusitis (OMS) is a well-recognized but understudied form of sinusitis that requires a unique treatment regimen that differs from nonodontogenic sinusitis [1–3]. It is typically unilateral and is the most common cause of isolated maxillary sinusitis [3].

## 19.1 Anatomy

The maxillary sinus is the first of the paranasal sinuses to develop in fetal life and it reaches its full development with the eruption of permanent teeth between 12 and 14 years of age. The sinus has an average volume of 15–20 ml [4]. The roots of the maxillary second molars are in closest proximity to the sinus floor, followed in frequency by the roots of the first molar, third molar, second premolar, and first premolar. The roots of these teeth may be protruding into the maxillary sinus and are only separated from the sinus cavity by a thin mucoperiosteum (the Schneiderian membrane) (Fig. 19.1) [5]. The alveolar bone of the maxilla can become thinner with increasing age and with some diseases leaving the maxillary sinus in close proximity to the oral cavity.

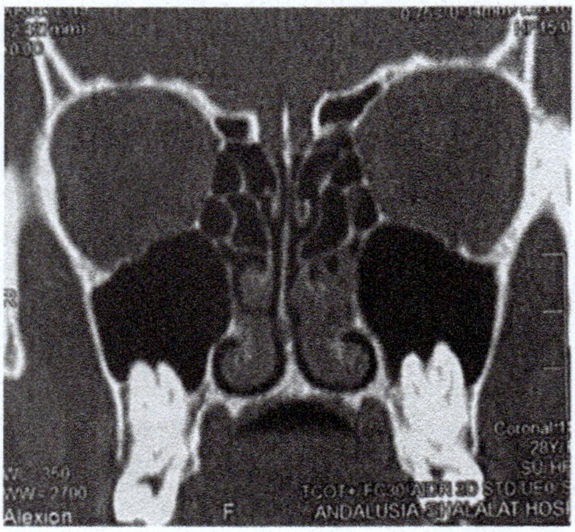


**Fig. 19.1** Roots of the first molar tooth into the maxillary sinus

## 19.2 Epidemiology

Before the 1970s, approximately 12% of maxillary sinusitis cases have been attributed to odontogenic infections [6]. Patel and Ferguson have reported that close to 30% of cases of unilateral maxillary sinusitis may have an underlying dental pathology [7]. Maillet et al., using cone beam CT, reported that the incidence can rise to 51.8% [8]. With the frequent use of dental implants, an increased incidence of OMS has been recorded over the last few decades [9].

## 19.3 Etiology

The most common etiology of OMS is dentoalveolar surgery or periapical dental infection (Fig. 19.2) through the Schneiderian membrane [3, 10]. Ferguson mentioned that the cause of OMS is usually periapical or periodontal infection defined as infections around the teeth [11]. Troeltzsch et al. reported that OMS due to oro-antral fistula (OAF) following surgical intervention was the commonest cause in their series [12].

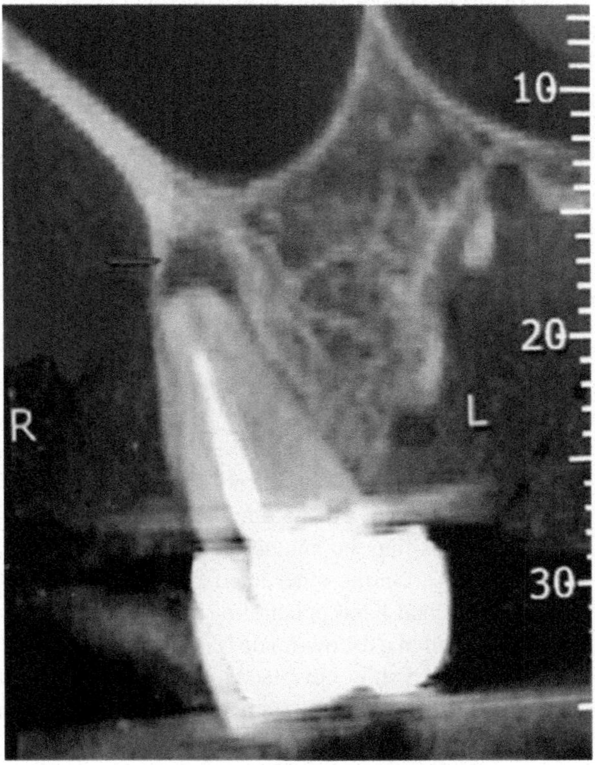


**Fig. 19.2** Periapical infection (arrow) in relation to root canal treatment

A recent systematic review studying the causes of OMS showed that iatrogenic etiology accounted for 65.7% of cases, apical periodontal pathologies for 25.5% (apical periodontitis for 18%, apical granulomas for 5%, and infected odontogenic cysts for 2.5%), and marginal periodontitis for 8.3% [13]. Iatrogenic causes included dental implants, artificial implants, dental amalgams, displaced teeth, and OAF. The teeth most affected were, in order of frequency, the first molar (35.6%), second molar (22%), third molar (17.4%), and second premolar (14.4%) [13]. In another systematic review, Akhlaghi et al. reported that OAF was the most common cause of OMS among all dental etiologies [14].

According to a meta-analysis based on articles published between 1986 and 2007, iatrogenic causes were responsible for 55.9% of OMS cases [15]. Other endodontic microtools and roots were reported to penetrate the apical foramen protruding into the maxillary sinus floor and resulting in OMC [16].

In a more recent study, Elwany et al. reported that the most frequently affected teeth in their series were the first molar (40.5%), second molar (25.7%), second premolar (21.6%), and third molar (12.2%). Odontogenic sinusitis followed dental procedures in 60.7% of the patients, periapical infections in 29.7%, and periodontal infections in 9.4% [3].

Odontogenic infections begin with the attachment of bacteria to the outer surface of teeth, eventually breaking down the outer enamel and inner dentin and making its way into the vital pulp [17]. Once the infection enters the pulp, it leads to necrosis and pus formation. Bacteria from the lesion can spread to the adjacent tissues and activate a reaction in the Schneiderian membrane epithelium which seems to be hypertrophic and inflamed [18]. When a periapical cyst, granuloma, or periapical infection is present, the surrounding bone becomes eroded and the bone separating the maxillary sinus from the oral cavity becomes thinner, resulting in exposure of the sinus mucoperiosteum [15].

OMS was associated with dentigerous cysts in two reports [19, 20]. Dentigerous cysts are odontogenic cysts that consist of a fluid-filled sac around an unerupted tooth. If untreated, the cyst can expand into the maxillary sinus.

Dental implants are increasingly used nowadays for partial or complete edentulous patients; moreover, before dental implantation, a sinus lift procedure may be needed to increase alveolar bone height [21–23]. However, during or after these procedures, local infections (peri-implantitis) may cause OMS, which may lead to implant failure or other complications [3].

The dislocation of a dental implant (Fig. 19.3) or broken roots (Fig. 19.4) into the maxillary sinus may be another cause of OMS. Even when no sinus lift was performed [3, 24]. On the other hand, Jung et al. evaluated nine patients with dental implants that had been penetrating the mucosa of the maxillary sinus floor more than 4 mm, and in a follow-up of 10 months, no clinical signs of OMS were reported [25]. Figure 19.5 shows displaced implant without a sinus infection. Amalgam and other dental materials may be also displaced inside the sinus during dental treatments (Fig. 19.6).

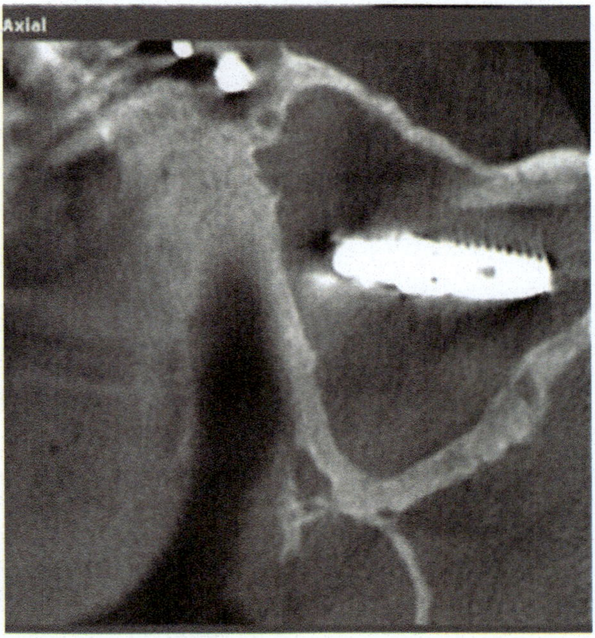


**Fig. 19.3** Odontogenic maxillary sinusitis following the displacement of the implant into the maxillary sinus

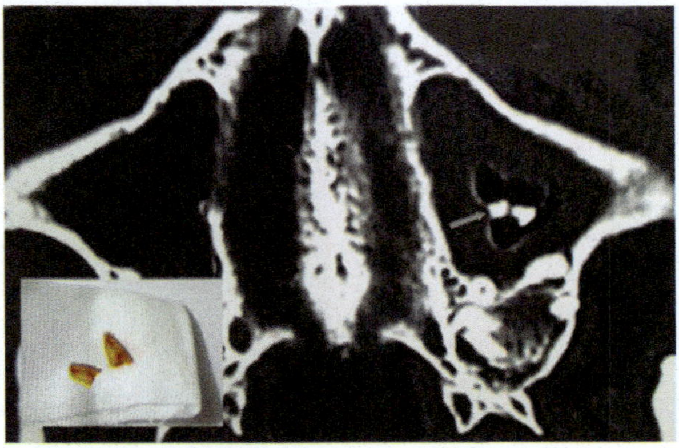

**Fig. 19.4** Broken roots (arrow) inside the left maxillary sinus

Oroantral communication (OAC) and epithelialized formation of OAF (Figs. 19.7 and 19.8) may occur during dental surgery and lead to sinus infection. OAC can occur with frequencies between 0.31% and 4.7% after the extraction of upper teeth [26]. A displacement of the dental root into the sinus may also occur following root fracture [14]. During tooth extraction, significant forces are exerted on the alveolar bone, especially in the presence of an impacted tooth or widely divergent roots, which makes this procedure more difficult. Elwany et al. reported nine cases of displaced roots and seven cases of implant-related OMS [3].

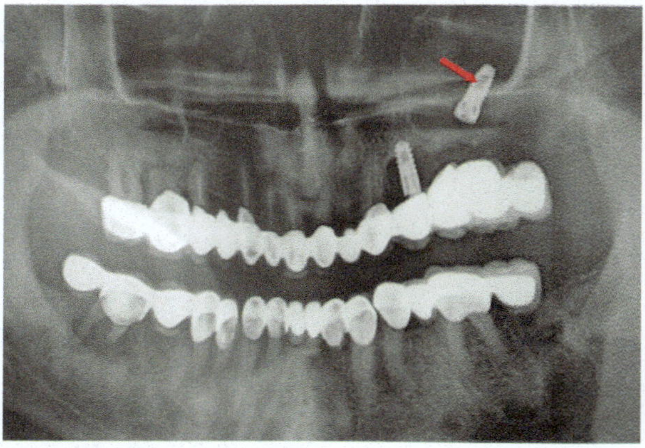

**Fig. 19.5** Displaced implant (arrow) without sinus infection

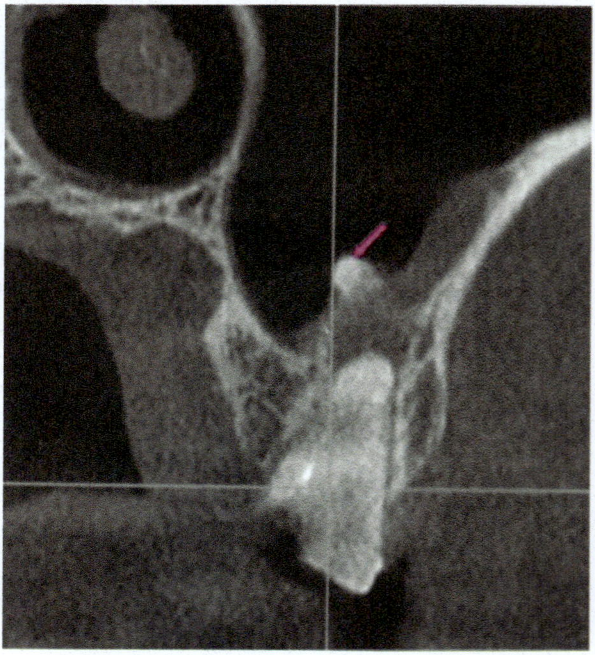

**Fig. 19.6** Displaced dental material inside the maxillary sinus (arrow) with secondary sinusitis

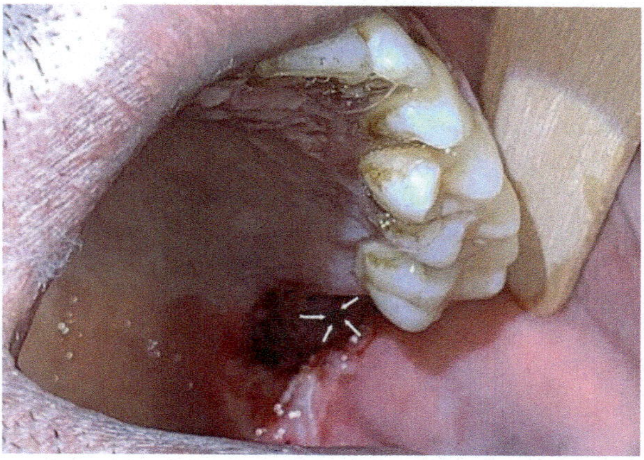

**Fig. 19.7** Oroantral fistula at the site of previous extraction (arrows)

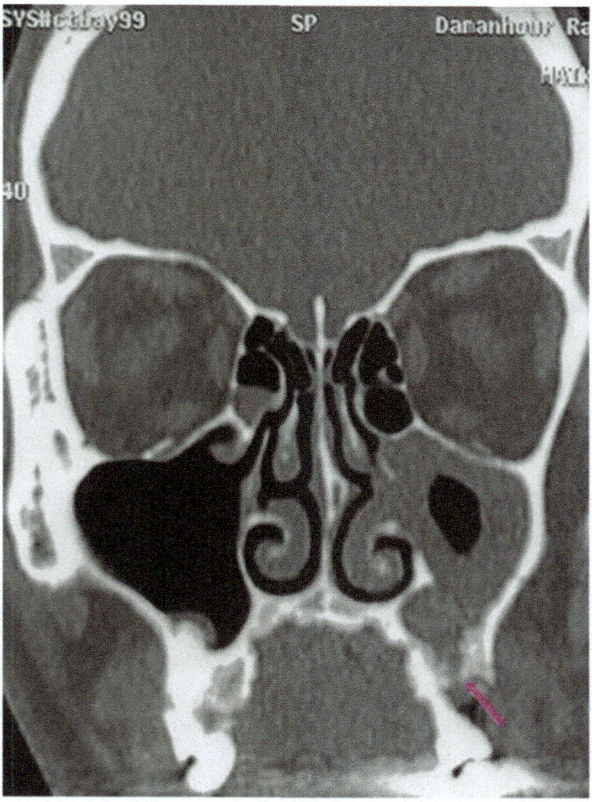


**Fig. 19.8** Left wide oroantral fistula (arrow)

## 19.4 Clinical Picture

The main symptoms related to OMS are unilateral nasal discharge with a bad odor and unilateral nasal obstruction. Facial pain and tenderness over the cheek may be reported [3]. Hoskison et al. reported that 21 (81%) and 19 (73%) out of 26 patients with OMS complained of unilateral nasal discharge and cacosmia [9]. In another study that included 27 patients with OMS, nasal discharge was found in 66.7% of cases, cheek pain in 33.3%, and cacosmia in 25.9% [27]. Two recent studies found that malodor was the most characteristic symptom of odontogenic sinusitis [28, 29].

In many cases, the diagnosis can be reached when the foul smell and unilateral nasal discharge are associated with unilateral maxillary opacification and a recent history of dental infection or treatment. However, Longhini and Ferguson [30] reported that dentists did not diagnose a dental infection causing OMS in six (85%) out of seven cases; similarly, 56 (55%) out of 99 OMS cases were missed on routine dental examinations including dental X-ray [31].

In fact, the diagnosis of odontogenic sinusitis may not be easy in all cases for several reasons. First, dental pain may not be present in all cases [6, 7, 32]. Second, the diagnosis of odontogenic sinusitis may be missed by radiologists, especially if they are not given enough clinical information [3, 33]. Third, many patients do not report their previous dental procedures or treatments voluntarily without being asked about it [3, 12]. Fourth, in implant-associated sinusitis, there may be a long latent period between implant surgery and the development of nasal symptoms [12]. Troeltzsch et al. confirmed that OMS may occur after a latency period of almost 4 years as a late complication of dental implantology due to progressive peri-implantitis [12].

## 19.5 Diagnosis

The diagnosis of OMS is based on the evaluation of patient's symptoms and past medical history followed by rhinologic and dental and medical examination. Both OAC and OAF can most of the time be diagnosed clinically, with the Valsalva test or by examining the extraction site with a blunt probe. In many cases, a small amount of purulent discharge may drip through the OAF. Air or fluids may leak from a large OAF.

Paranasal CT is the "gold standard" for diagnosis of odontogenic sinusitis because of its high resolution and ability to discern bone and soft tissue and then to detect sinonasal inflammation. Axial and coronal sinus CT views can show the relationship between periapical abscess with sinus floor defect and determine the exact location of a foreign body within the maxillary sinus. Careful evaluation of a sinus CT or cone beam CT scans may show a lucency around a tooth root adjacent to the maxillary sinus floor (halo sign) (Fig. 19.9) indicating periapical abscess [33].

Intraoral radiographs and panoramic radiographs provide suboptimal information about the maxillary sinus although they can be helpful in determining the size of periapical lesions or visualization of pseudocysts, displaced roots, teeth, or

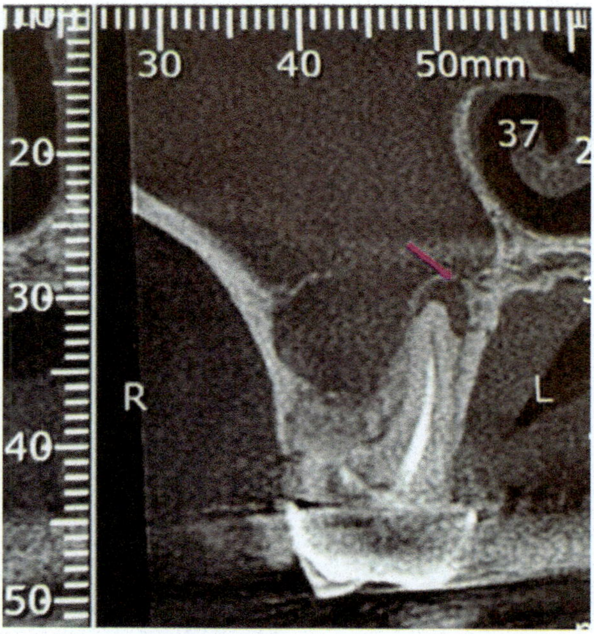


**Fig. 19.9** Halo sign (arrow)

foreign bodies inside the maxillary sinus [34]. However, panoramic radiography has lower sensitivity than periapical radiography for the detection of apical periodontitis due to anatomical superimposition [35].

More recently, cone beam computed tomography (CBCT) was increasingly used in dental practice. CBCT consumes approximately 10% of the radiation dose of conventional thin-slice CT, focusing on image- bony details, although soft tissue quality is reduced. Compared to a panoramic dental radiograph, the radiation dosage for CBCT is approximately tenfold higher [36, 37]. However, the CBCT is actually preferred in the field of implant dentistry, in order to assess the thickness of the floor of the maxillary sinus before implantation [7, 37]. Likewise, periapical lesions are better detected by CBCT compared to periapical radiography, which can only spot approximately 40% of apical periodontitis on posterior maxillary teeth and 3% of all apical infections extending on the sinuses [34].

Mucosal thickening and granuloma formation in relation to dental infection are common radiologic findings (Figs. 19.10 and 19.11). It has been shown that the majority of unilateral maxillary sinusitis cases (more than 70%) are of odontogenic origin [3]. OMS has most commonly been identified on CT radiographs (axial, coronal planes) as mucosal thickening greater than 2mm of the maxillary sinus membrane, associated with a dental focus responsible for sinus pathology, such as OAC, foreign bodies (dental fillings, teeth roots), periapical abscess, granulomas, or extraction site [38, 39].

Vidal et al. supported that the mucosal thickening could be limited to the area of a tooth presenting one or more of the following pathological findings: caries, defective restoration, periapical lesion, or an extraction site [40]. Mehra and Jeong have

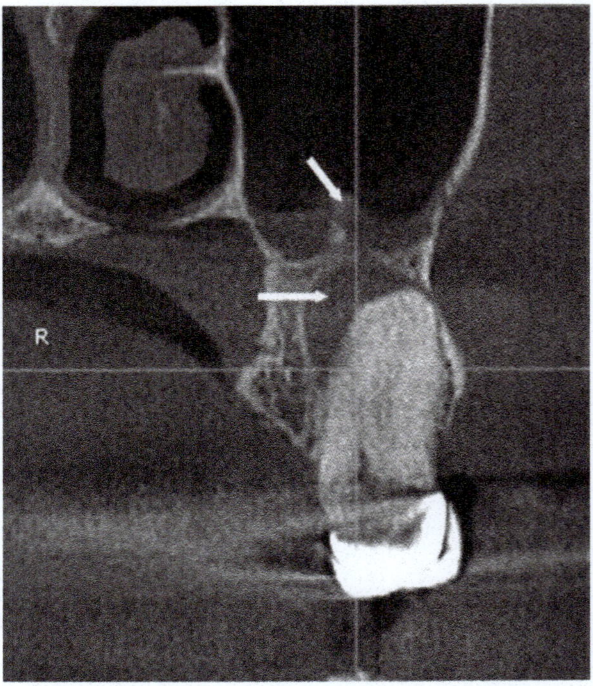


**Fig. 19.10** Mucosal thickening greater than 2 m (upper arrow) in relation to dental focus (lower arrow)

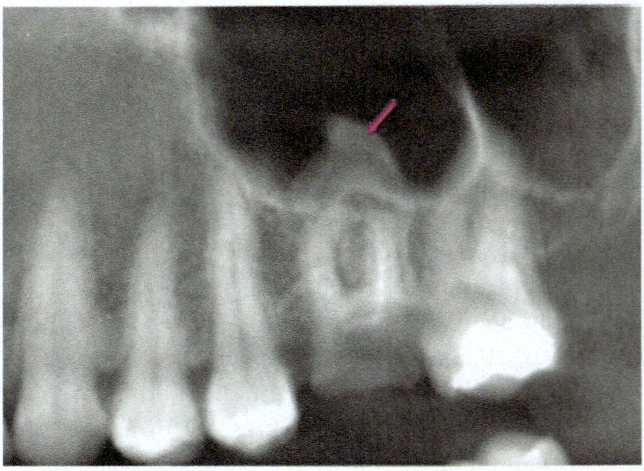

**Fig. 19.11** Granuloma in relation to periapical infection

extensively described the process of transition from endodontic pulpal necrosis to periapical osteitis and finally to periapical abscess that is radiographically detected [4]. Pokorny and Tataryn found that approximately two-thirds (64%) of the OMS cases showed evident periapical infection on CT imaging; in the remaining 36%, there was no obvious dental disease on CT, including cases with failure of root canal therapy and loss of bone [32].

Unilateral partial or total opacification of the maxillary sinus was observed in 82.4% of Elwany et al. patients [3]. This finding supports other reports indicating that unilateral opacification of the maxillary sinus on imaging is dental in origin until proven otherwise [33, 41]. Whyte and Boeddinghaus reported that extension from the maxillary sinus to other sinuses may be seen in up to 60–70% of cases [33].

In a retrospective study, Saibene et al. [42] reported bilateral involvement of the sinuses in 18.7% of their cases. However, the authors did not comment on the incidence of allergies and chronic sinusitis Elwany et al., on the other hand, found that all patients who had bilateral or multisinus opacifications gave a positive history of nasal allergies and/or chronic rhinosinusitis [3].

Mucosal thickening along the floor of the maxillary sinus is usually the first radiological sign seen in patients with periapical infection. The severity of mucosal thickening is related to both the extent of periapical inflammation and the proximity of the roots to the sinus floor [39, 43]. However, retrospective reviews of sinus CT or cone beam CT images of asymptomatic patients showed mucosal thickening in 29–53% [41, 44]. Moreover, mucosal thickening is more common with advancing age [40] and after dental restorations [33]. Therefore, mucosal thickening in the absence of symptoms and other radiological signs suggestive of odontogenic sinusitis should not be considered as a definite sign of dental sinus infection. Likewise, maxillary retention cysts (Figs. 19.12 and 19.13) that are not related to dental

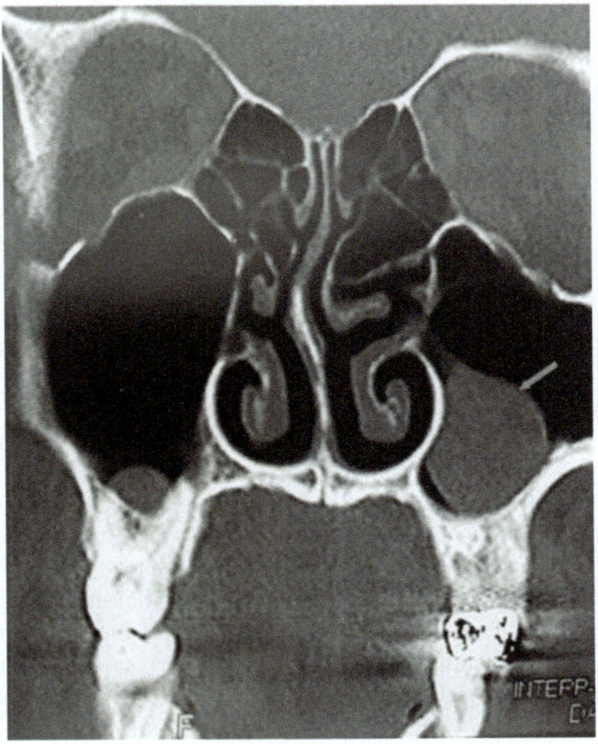

**Fig. 19.12** Big asymptomatic retention cyst in the left maxillary sinus (arrow). No treatment required

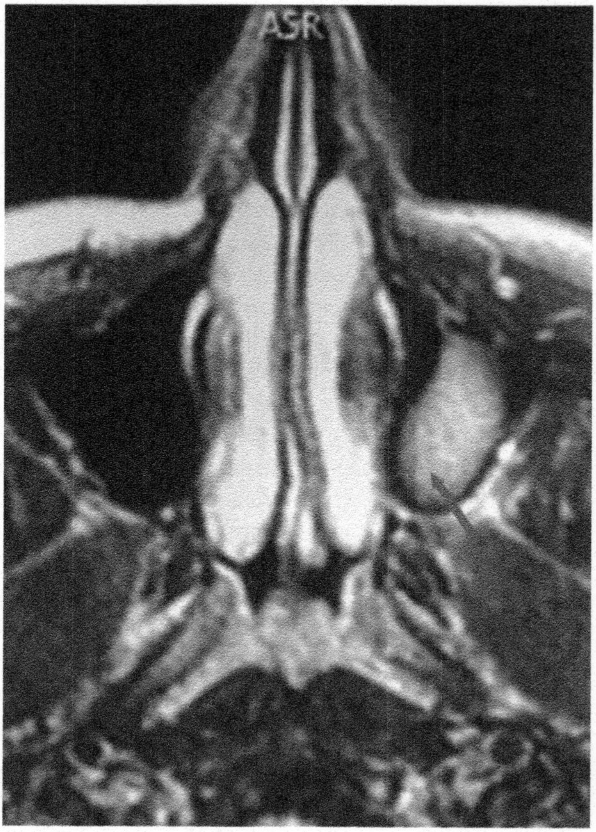


**Fig. 19.13** MRI showing retention cyst in the maxillary sinus (arrow). The cyst is clearly separated from the sinus wall except at its site of origin from the anterior wall of the sinus

pathology or treatment should be differentiated from cysts of dental origin. Periodontitis is a less frequent cause of odontogenic sinusitis, although it may be associated with mucosal thickening in up to 40% cases [45, 46]. Periodontitis was encountered in only 9.4% of Elwany et al. series [3].

## 19.6 Treatment

Identification of the dental cause is key to successful treatment of odontogenic sinusitis. However, to date, there is no consensus about the ideal treatment protocol for odontogenic sinusitis. In many cases, treatment of dental causative factors and appropriate antibiotics are sufficient to control the infection.

The decision to perform endoscopic sinus surgery (ESS) was based on two criteria: (1) persistence of symptoms; and (2) objective evidence of disease on posttreatment sinus CT scans or nasal endoscopy after the completion of dental treatment and a full antibiotic course. Patients with displaced foreign bodies or roots inside the maxillary sinus cavity needed only ESS to extract the displaced material. Some studies recommend ESS when the osteomeatal complex is blocked [47] and/or the height of the thickened mucosa is more than one-half of the maxillary sinus [22]. In all cases, the dental source of the infection (complicated root canal therapy of causative tooth, periapical or periodontal infection, etc.) must be eliminated in order to prevent the recurrence of sinusitis.

Implant-related OMS should initially be treated with antibiotics, such as amoxicillin-clavulanate associated with clindamycin, or fourth-generation quinolones which cover anaerobes. If OMS persists, an ESS is indicated, consisting of wide middle antrostomy to allow the removal of inflammatory mucosa, granulation tissue, or foreign bodies located in the maxillary sinus; lesions in the ethmoid, frontal, and sphenoid sinuses were equally eliminated, depending on the diseased sinus [21, 23, 48]. Intraoral intervention is not necessary except for the presence of OAC, a local buccal or palatal flap could then be performed [23, 49]. In the case of implant-related OMS, it is not clear whether the dental implant should be removed or not. Felisati et al. [49] proposed a combined approach with the removal of the implant dislocated into the sinus, while other authors [22, 23] preserve the implant, even after sinus lift [21]. Chen et al. [22] suggested that dental implants should be removed if they are mobile or present with severe peri-implantitis.

Since dental implantation or maxillary sinus lift may involve the maxillary sinus, it is recommended to check the status of the maxillary sinuses beforehand since the success rate of dental implants may be affected by the status of the sinus [50].

The management of OAC depends on the size of the defect, time of diagnosis, and presence of OMS. If OAF is present for more than 3 weeks, it should be surgically closed and ESS may be required to eliminate granulation tissue and to keep osteomeatal complex patent in order to achieve OAC closure [51]. If OAC is smaller than 3 mm and without epithelization, it generally closes spontaneously or with primary suturing in the absence of infection [52, 53]. When OAC is larger than 3mm, surgical closure is indicated with buccal advancement flaps Palatal flaps are recommended for large bony defects [51, 54]. Buccal flaps are easier to fashion but they are thin and care should be taken not to damage Stensen's duct. Also, they may interfere with dentures. Palatal flaps are thick and vascularized, but the palatal raw area needs more time to heal. They are more suitable for large fistulae. When the fistula is large, a buccal fat plug can be used to close the bony defect [3].

## References


1. Han S-J. The role of oral and maxillofacial surgeons in maxillary sinus diseases related to dental implants. J Korean Assoc Oral Maxillofac Surg. 2023;49:241–2.
2. Rangics A, Répássy GD, Gyulai-Gaál S, Dobó-Nagy C, Tamás L, Simonffy L. Management of odontogenic sinusitis: results with single-step FESS and dentoalveolar surgery. J Pers Med. 2023;13(9):1291. https://doi.org/10.3390/jpm13091291.
3. Elwany S, Ibrahim AA, Hussein WKA, Medra AM. Ten-year experience with multidisciplinary diagnosis and treatment of odontogenic sinusitis. J Laryngol Otol. 2021;135:987–92.
4. Mehra P, Jeong D. Maxillary sinusitis of odontogenic origin. Curr Allergy Asthma Rep. 2009;9:238–43.

5. Hauman CHJ, Chandler NP, Tong DC. Endodontic implications of the maxillary sinus: a review. Int Endod J. 2002;35:127–41.
6. Brook I. Sinusitis of odontogenic origin. Otolaryngol Head Neck Surg. 2006;135:349–55.
7. Patel NA, Ferguson BJ. Odontogenic sinusitis: an ancient but under-appreciated cause of maxillary sinusitis. Curr Opin Otolaryngol Head Neck Surg. 2012;20:24–8.
8. Maillet M, Bowles WR, McClanahan SL, John MT, Ahmad M. Cone-beam computed tomography evaluation of maxillary sinusitis. J Endod. 2011;37:753–7.
9. Hoskison E, Daniel M, Rowson JE, Jones NS. Evidence of an increase in the incidence of odontogenic sinusitis over the last decade in the UK. J Laryngol Otol. 2012;126:43–6.
10. Gaudin RA, Hoehle LP, Smeets R, Heiland M, Caradonna DS, Gray ST, Sedaghat AR. Impact of odontogenic chronic rhinosinusitis on general health-related quality of life. Eur Arch Otorrinolaringol. 2018;275:1477–82.
11. Ferguson M. Rhinosinusitis in oral medicine and dentistry. Aust Dent J. 2014;59:289–95.
12. Troeltzsch M, Pache C, Troeltzsch M, Kaeppler G, Ehrenfeld M, Otto S, Probst F. Etiology and clinical characteristics of symptomatic unilateral maxillary sinusitis: a review of 174 cases. J Craniomaxillofac Surg. 2015;43:1522–9.
13. Lechien JR, Filleul O, Costa de Araujo P, Hsieh JW, Chantrain G, Saussez S. Chronic maxillary rhinosinusitis of dental origin: a systematic review of 674 patient cases. Int J Otolaryngol. 2014;2014:1–9.
14. Akhlaghi F, Esmaeelinejad M, Safai P. Etiologies and treatments of odontogenic maxillary sinusitis: a systematic review. Iran Red Crescent Med J. 2015;17:e25536.
15. Arias-Irimia O, Barona-Dorado C, Santos-Marino JA, Martínez-Rodriguez N, Martínez-González JM. Meta-analysis of the etiology of odontogenic maxillary sinusitis. Med Oral Patol Oral Cir Bucal. 2010;15:e70–3.
16. Liston PN, Walters RF. Foreign bodies in the maxillary antrum: a case report. Aust Dent J. 2002;47:344–6.
17. Abrahams JJ, Glassberg RM. Dental disease: a frequently unrecognized cause of maxillary sinus abnormalities? AJR Am J Roentgenol. 1996;166:1219–23.
18. Taschieri S, Torretta S, Corbella S, Del Fabbro M, Francetti L, Lolato A, Capaccio P. Pathophysiology of sinusitis of odontogenic origin. J Investig Clin Dent. 2017;8:e12202.
19. López-Carriches C, López-Carriches I, Bryan RB-P. Odontogenic sinusitis caused by an inflammation of a dentigerous cyst and subsequent finding of a fibrous dysplasia. A case report. Open Dent J. 2016;10:647–55.
20. Prabhu SP, Padwa BL, Robson CD, Rahbar R. Dentigerous cyst associated with a displaced tooth in the maxillary sinus: an unusual cause of recurrent sinusitis in an adolescent. Pediatr Radiol. 2009;39:1102–4.
21. Jiam NT-L, Goldberg AN, Murr AH, Pletcher SD. Surgical treatment of chronic rhinosinusitis after sinus lift. Am J Rhinol Allergy. 2017;31:271–5.
22. Chen Y-W, Huang C-C, Chang P-H, Chen C-W, Wu C-C, Fu C-H, Lee T-J. The characteristics and new treatment paradigm of dental implant-related chronic rhinosinusitis. Am J Rhinol Allergy. 2013;27:237–44.
23. Kim SJ, Park JS, Kim HT, Lee CH, Park YH, Bae JH. Clinical features and treatment outcomes of dental implant-related paranasal sinusitis: a 2-year prospective observational study. Clin Oral Implants Res. 2016;27:e100–4.
24. Galindo-Moreno P, Padial-Molina M, Avila G, Rios HF, Hernández-Cortés P, Wang H-L. Complications associated with implant migration into the maxillary sinus cavity. Clin Oral Implants Res. 2012;23:1152–60.
25. Jung J-H, Choi B-H, Jeong S-M, Li J, Lee S-H, Lee H-J. A retrospective study of the effects on sinus complications of exposing dental implants to the maxillary sinus cavity. Oral Surg Oral Med Oral Pathol Oral Radiol Endod. 2007;103:623–5.
26. Gacic B, Todorovic L, Kokovic V, Danilovic V, Stojcev-Stajcic L, Drazic R, Markovic A. The closure of oroantral communications with resorbable PLGA-coated beta-TCP root analogs, hemostatic gauze, or buccal flaps: a prospective study. Oral Surg Oral Med Oral Pathol Oral Radiol Endod. 2009;108:844–50.

27. Lee KC, Lee SJ. Clinical features and treatments of odontogenic sinusitis. Yonsei Med J. 2010;51:932–7.
28. Goyal VK, Ahmad A, Turfe Z, Peterson EI, Craig JR. Predicting odontogenic sinusitis in unilateral sinus disease: a prospective, multivariate analysis. Am J Rhinol Allergy. 2021;35:164–71.
29. Simuntis R, Vaitkus J, Kubilius R, Padervinskis E, Tušas P, Leketas M, Šiupšinskienė N, Vaitkus S. Comparison of sino-nasal outcome test 22 symptom scores in rhinogenic and odontogenic sinusitis. Am J Rhinol Allergy. 2019;33:44–50.
30. Longhini AB, Ferguson BJ. Clinical aspects of odontogenic maxillary sinusitis: a case series. Int Forum Allergy Rhinol. 2011;1:409–15.
31. Melén I, Lindahl L, Andréasson L, Rundcrantz H. Chronic maxillary sinusitis. Definition, diagnosis and relation to dental infections and nasal polyposis. Acta Otolaryngol. 1986;101:320–7.
32. Pokorny A, Tataryn R. Clinical and radiologic findings in a case series of maxillary sinusitis of dental origin. Int Forum Allergy Rhinol. 2013;3:973–9.
33. Whyte A, Boeddinghaus R. Imaging of odontogenic sinusitis. Clin Radiol. 2019;74:503–16.
34. Shahbazian M, Vandewoude C, Wyatt J, Jacobs R. Comparative assessment of periapical radiography and CBCT imaging for radiodiagnostics in the posterior maxilla. Odontology. 2015;103:97–104.
35. Estrela C, Bueno MR, Leles CR, Azevedo B, Azevedo JR. Accuracy of cone beam computed tomography and panoramic and periapical radiography for detection of apical periodontitis. J Endod. 2008;34:273–9.
36. Nair UP, Nair MK. Maxillary sinusitis of odontogenic origin: cone-beam volumetric computerized tomography-aided diagnosis. Oral Surg Oral Med Oral Pathol Oral Radiol Endod. 2010;110:e53–7.
37. Schulze D, Heiland M, Thurmann H, Adam G. Radiation exposure during midfacial imaging using 4- and 16-slice computed tomography, cone beam computed tomography systems and conventional radiography. Dentomaxillofac Radiol. 2004;33:83–6.
38. Maska B, Lin G-H, Othman A, Behdin S, Travan S, Benavides E, Kapila Y. Dental implants and grafting success remain high despite large variations in maxillary sinus mucosal thickening. Int J Implant Dent. 2017;3:1.
39. Capelli M, Gatti P. Radiological study of maxillary sinus using CBCT: relationship between mucosal thickening and common anatomic variants in chronic rhinosinusitis. J Clin Diagn Res. 2016;10:MC07–10.
40. Vidal F, Coutinho T, CarvalhoFerreira D, Souza R, Gonçalves L. Odontogenic sinusitis: a comprehensive review. Acta Odontol Scand. 2017;75(8):623–33. https://doi.org/10.1080/00016357.2017.1372803.
41. Matsumoto Y, Ikeda T, Yokoi H, Kohno N. Association between odontogenic infections and unilateral sinus opacification. Auris Nasus Larynx. 2015;42:288–93.
42. Saibene AM, Pipolo GC, Lozza P, Maccari A, Portaleone SM, Scotti A, Borloni R, Messina F, Di Pasquale D, Felisati G. Redefining boundaries in odontogenic sinusitis: a retrospective evaluation of extramaxillary involvement in 315 patients. Int Forum Allergy Rhinol. 2014;4:1020–3.
43. Eggmann F, Connert T, Bühler J, Dagassan-Berndt D, Weiger R, Walter C. Do periapical and periodontal pathologies affect Schneiderian membrane appearance? Systematic review of studies using cone-beam computed tomography. Clin Oral Investig. 2017;21:1611–30.
44. Shanbhag S, Karnik P, Shirke P, Shanbhag V. Association between periapical lesions and maxillary sinus mucosal thickening: a retrospective cone-beam computed tomographic study. J Endod. 2013;39:853–7.
45. Phothikhun S, Suphanantachat S, Chuenchompoonut V, Nisapakultorn K. Cone-beam computed tomographic evidence of the association between periodontal bone loss and mucosal thickening of the maxillary sinus. J Periodontol. 2012;83:557–64.
46. Ren S, Zhao H, Liu J, Wang Q, Pan Y. Significance of maxillary sinus mucosal thickening in patients with periodontal disease. Int Dent J. 2015;65:303–10.
47. Mattos JL, Ferguson BJ, Lee S. Predictive factors in patients undergoing endoscopic sinus surgery for odontogenic sinusitis. Int Forum Allergy Rhinol. 2016;6:697–700.

48. Saibene AM, Collurà F, Pipolo C, et al. Odontogenic rhinosinusitis and sinonasal complications of dental disease or treatment: prospective validation of a classification and treatment protocol. Eur Arch Otorrinolaringol. 2019;276:401–6.
49. Felisati G, Chiapasco M, Lozza P, Saibene AM, Pipolo C, Zaniboni M, Biglioli F, Borloni R. Sinonasal complications resulting from dental treatment: outcome-oriented proposal of classification and surgical protocol. Am J Rhinol Allergy. 2013;27:e101–6.
50. Kim Y-K, Hwang J-Y, Yun P-Y. Relationship between prognosis of dental implants and maxillary sinusitis associated with the sinus elevation procedure. Int J Oral Maxillofac Implants. 2013;28:178–83.
51. Workman AD, Granquist EJ, Adappa ND. Odontogenic sinusitis: developments in diagnosis, microbiology, and treatment. Curr Opin Otolaryngol Head Neck Surg. 2018;26:27–33.
52. Yalçın S, Oncü B, Emes Y, Atalay B, Aktaş I. Surgical treatment of oroantral fistulas: a clinical study of 23 cases. J Oral Maxillofac Surg. 2011;69:333–9.
53. Kiran Kumar Krishanappa S, Eachempati P, Kumbargere Nagraj S, Shetty NY, Moe S, Aggarwal H, Mathew RJ. Interventions for treating oro-antral communications and fistulae due to dental procedures. Cochrane Database Syst Rev. 2018;8:CD011784.
54. Borgonovo AE, Berardinelli FV, Favale M, Maiorana C. Surgical options in oroantral fistula treatment. Open Dent J. 2012;6:94–8.

# Chronic Rhinosinusitis (CRS) 20

Samy Elwany

**Key Points**

- Chronic rhinosinusitis (CRS) ranks as one of the most prevalent chronic diseases. It represents an inflammatory process of the sinonasal mucosa that persists for a period of at least 12 weeks.
- CRS phenotypes are based upon differences in physical characteristics of disease expression and are considered as a preliminary step toward a directed treatment strategy. The two major phenotypes are CRS with nasal polyps (CRSwNP) and CRS without nasal polyps (CRSsNP).
- Criteria have been recently established for the diagnosis of CRSwNP and CRSsNP. The diagnosis of CRS requires the presence of at least two or more recognized symptoms, as well as evidence of inflammation as demonstrated by endoscopic or radiologic examination.
- There are several triggers, modifiers, and common inflammatory mediators that contribute to the pathogenesis of CRS.
- The clinical picture and management of CRSsNP are distinct from CRSwNP.
- Treatment-resistant CRSsNP might point to an underlying cause (secondary CRS) which warrants further workup.
- Better intranasal delivery of medication may further reduce the need for both surgery and systemic treatments.

S. Elwany (✉)
Department of Otolaryngology, Alexandria Faculty of Medicine, Alexandria, Egypt
e-mail: samy.elwany@alexmed.edu.eg


S. Elwany (ed.), *Current Rhinology*,
https://doi.org/10.1007/978-3-031-70077-4_20

CRS ranks as one of the most prevalent chronic diseases. Given the worldwide prevalence of CRS, the disease is commonly encountered within the practice of many medical specialties [1, 2]. Gliklich and Metson found that the impact of CRS in the domains of societal functioning and bodily pain is greater than other chronic diseases [3].

## 20.1 Pathogenesis of CRS

CRS is divided into two phenotypes based upon the presence or absence of polyps on examination, as supported by histologic and inflammatory cytokine findings [4]. This clinical classification of CRS is also supported by differences in treatment responses and recurrence rates [5]. Generally speaking, CRSsNP has lower recurrence rates and better response to standard therapies than CRSwNP.

There is no definite comprehensive theory addressing the etiology and pathogenesis of CRS. In many cases individually proposed lines of research may appear to compete or conflict with one another. The etiology and underlying pathogenesis of CRS, therefore, remain controversial. Initial hypotheses broadly focused upon either the role of exogenous factors or that of the host response to these factors as potential explanations for CRSwNP with and without polyps.

Allergens, viruses, fungi [6, 7], bacterial biofilms [8], and Staphylococcus aureus endotoxins [9] have been suggested as such potential exogenous factors that are capable of initiating inflammation within the sinonasal mucosa. While there are objective evidences that support a potential role for each of these as a contributor to the pathogenesis of CRS, no single factor has proven to be universally causative [10].

The association between nasal polyps and allergic rhinitis is complex. Nasal polyps are reported to be less common in those with allergic rhinitis and childhood-onset allergic asthma than in the general population. Allergic rhinitis and childhood asthma are strongly correlated with central compartment allergic disease, where polyps may be seen growing from the middle turbinate and surrounding mucosa [11].

Biofilms, existing as a protective bacterial adaptation against host defenses and antibiotics, have been observed in CRS and have been associated with poorer outcomes following surgery [8].

Cigarette smoking has been associated with higher prevalence and odds of CRS [12]. Studies have shown that smoking can enhance bacterial biofilm formation [13–15] and this may explain the recalcitrance of CRS in smokers. Reversal of nasal mucosal changes to normal after quitting smoking has been also reported [16].

The "fungal hypothesis of CRS" is perhaps the best example of the frailty that underlies the concept of external pathogens serving a sole causative role in CRS. Initial enthusiasm for the fungal hypothesis began to wane when results could not be duplicated at other institutions. In the end, a large multi-institutional, blinded, randomized, controlled trial using intranasal amphotericin failed to show any evidence of efficacy [7].

The "immune barrier hypothesis" suggested that defects in the barrier function of the sinonasal epithelium are implicated in the pathogenesis of CRSwNP [17].

Innate interactions between the host and its environment may also play a role in the progression of mucosal inflammation [18]. Epithelial cells can interact with surface microbes leading to the release of several cytokines. Mucus production is increased in the presence of IL-4 and IL-13 and serves to decrease mucociliary function [19].

Eicosanoids are signaling molecules generated through the metabolism of arachidonic acid present within the cell membranes of a wide range of cells. Several families of eicosanoids with differing properties exist. This class of inflammatory mediators has immunologic properties critical to local regulation of inflammation [20]. Leukotrienes exhibit pro-inflammatory properties and are generated by lipoxygenase (5-LO). Prostaglandins and prostacyclins are generated by the cyclooxygenase enzyme (Cox-1, Cox-2). Defects within the eicosanoid pathway are associated with aspirin intolerance, asthma, and CRSwNP [21–23]. The relationship between *S. aureus* colonization and defects in the eicosanoid pathway has been suggested as important in the etiology of nasal polyposis [20].

## 20.2 Phenotypes of CRS

A strategy based on clinically available disease characteristics was adopted. Polyps, and their correlation with the histologic presence of eosinophils, were proposed as a clinical surrogate for eosinophilic inflammation [24].

CRS phenotypes are primarily based upon the presence (CRSwNP) or absence (CRSsNP) of nasal polyposis, which serves as a general surrogate for the type of underlying inflammation. The following phenotypes have been described [25]:

- CRSsNP
- CRSWNP
- Allergic fungal sinusitis
- CRS with aspirin-exacerbated respiratory disease
- Infectious CRS
- CRS with cystic fibrosis
- CRS with immune deficiencies such as common variable immunodeficiency and specific antibody deficiency
- CRS with immotile cilia syndrome
- CRS with anatomical abnormalities
- Biomarker based (endotypes)
  - Eosinophilic CRS versus noneosinophilic CRS (Th-2 versus Th-1 CRS)
  - Allergic CRS versus nonallergic CRS
  - Type 2 high versus Type 2 low
  - High IgE versus normal IgE

Broadly speaking, CRSsNP (Fig. 20.1) mainly has a nontype 2 inflammatory endotype, whereas in the majority of CRSwNP, it is type 2 (Fig. 20.2). This has important implications for clinical practice and patient management. Although there is similar prevalence of CRSwNP in Europe and Asia, their inflammatory endotypes

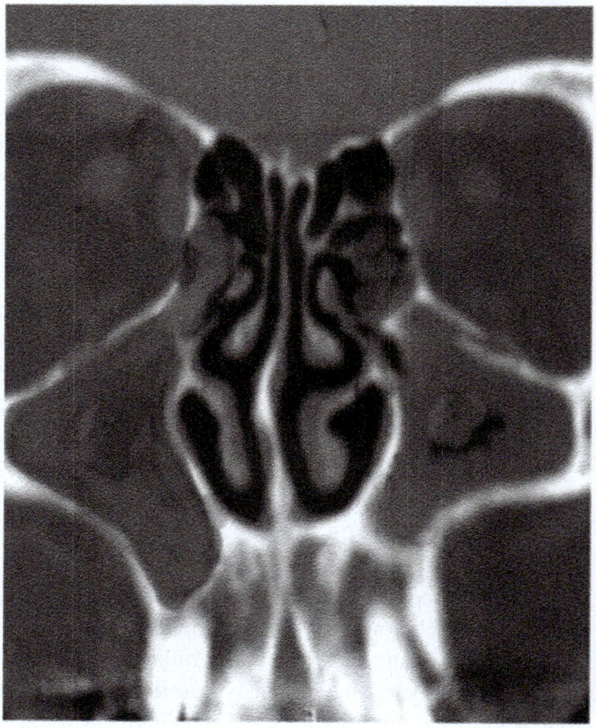

**Fig. 20.1** CRSsNP. Note the involvement of several sinuses

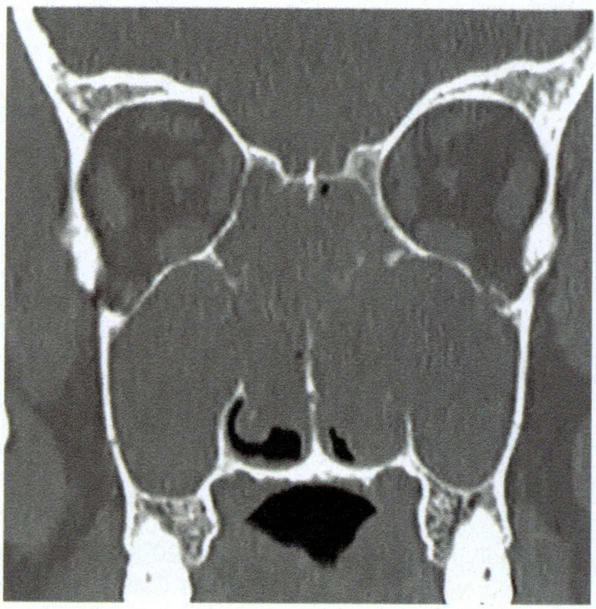

**Fig. 20.2** CRSwNP. The polyps are bilateral and fill the nasal cavity (grade 4 polyps) and the sinuses

are distinct. CRSwNP in Western countries commonly presents with type 2 inflammation, whereas type 1 and 3 inflammations are more frequent in Asian countries despite polyposis [11].

There is conflicting literature regarding gender, age, and smoking differences between CRSsNP and CRSwNP. Generally, CRSsNP patients tend to be younger. Male gender is associated with an increased risk for CRS in general, but no definitive conclusions about gender differences between CRSsNP and CRSwNP can be found [17].

Further refinement of CRS phenotypes can be accomplished through consideration of other comorbid conditions associated with an individual patient. Asthma and CRS recurrence appear to be predictive of the presence of Staphylococcus aureus enterotoxin-specific IgE and high levels of tissue IL-5. Aspirin-exacerbated respiratory disease (ARED) and CRS combination is highly associated with underlying tissue eosinophilia [26, 27].

## 20.3 Central Compartment Allergic Disease (CCAD)

CCAD may occur in patients with allergic rhinitis. The polyps arise from the middle turbinates and surrounding mucosa. CCAD is distinct from the pattern of polyposis seen in CRSwNP [28]. Skin prick testing or measurement of specific IgE can help identify potential targets for immunotherapy (Figs. 20.3 and 20.4).

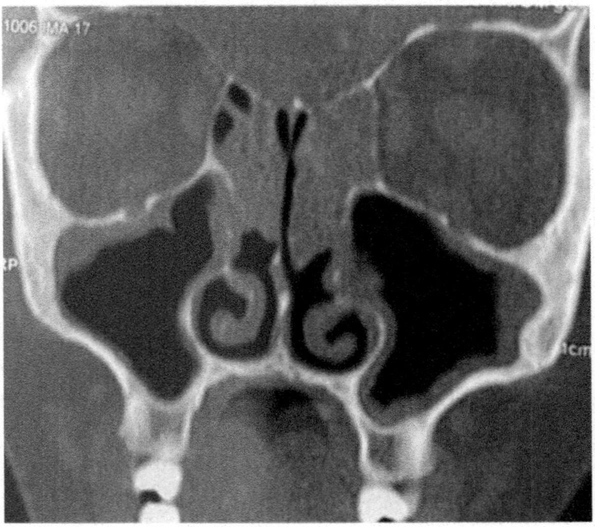

**Fig. 20.3** CCAD. The polyps occupy the central compartment of the nasal cavity. They arise from the middle turbinates and surrounding mucosa. The patient is typically atopic

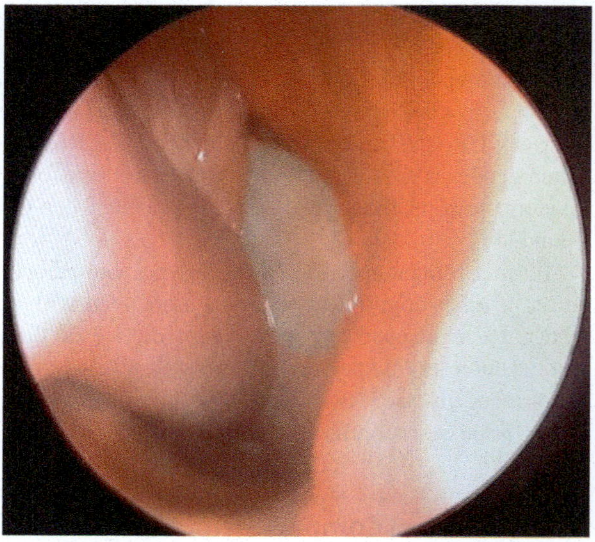

**Fig. 20.4** CCAD. The polyps arise from the middle turbinate and fill the central compartment of the nasal cavity

## 20.4 Secondary CRS

It is of utmost importance to consider a secondary etiology in CRS in patients who do not respond (properly) to therapy or have symptoms in other organ systems. Secondary etiologies include vasculitis, immunodeficiencies, and rarely midline or natural killer/T-cell lymphoma. Further investigations are required for those patients to address the hidden secondary etiology [29, 30].

## 20.5 NSAID-Exacerbated Respiratory Disease (N-ERD)

N-ERD usually begins in the third decade and is characterized by the triad of CRS with severe eosinophilic nasal polyps, asthma, and respiratory reactions triggered by the ingestion of substances that inhibit cyclooxygenase (Fig. 20.5). The disease is usually recalcitrant to treatment than CRSwNP and is more rapidly recurrent after intervention [31].

A diagnosis of N-ERD can be made with a history of two clear reactions to NSAIDs. When the diagnosis is uncertain, the patient could be considered for an aspirin provocation test which is done in an outpatient setting under medical supervision with capacity for resuscitation [32].

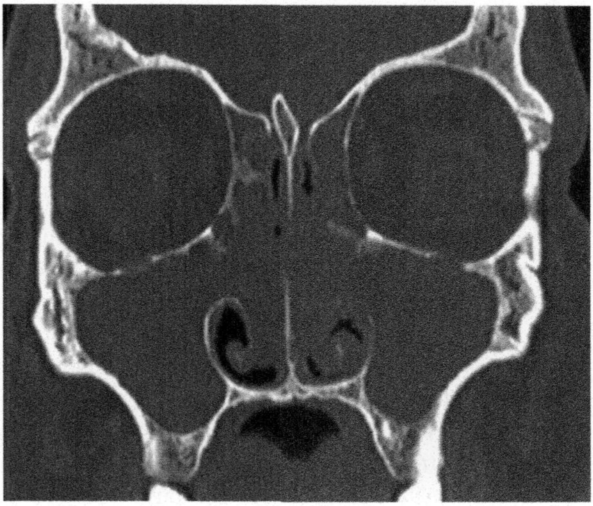

**Fig. 20.5** NSAID-exacerbated respiratory disease (N-erd)

## 20.6 Diagnosis of CRS

Interpreting an accurate diagnosis of CRS can be challenging. In many cases, a patient may present with a chief complaint of "chronic sinusitis." Given the lack of specificity of the individual symptoms in isolation, care should be taken to ensure the correct estimation of the patient's complaints.

Because of the overlap of many of the symptoms of CRSsNP and other common symptoms, such as headache and nasal congestion or blockage, it can be difficult to differentiate from other diseases. Appropriate use of nasal endoscopy, allergy evaluation, and radiologic examination are employed to ensure proper diagnosis [33].

The clinical history is focused on the duration, frequency, and severity of sinonasal symptoms and their impact on quality of life. Primary complaints (duration ≥12 weeks) may include facial pain, congestion, nasal obstruction, discolored nasal drainage more often postnasal into the pharynx, hyposmia, foul smell or taste, etc.

Both CRSsNP and CRSwNP patients complain most of the nasal obstruction. Patients with CRSsNP complain more of headache/facial fullness/facial pain. Patients with CRSwNP suffer from more loss of sense of smell than those with CRSwNP. Facial pain and pressure can be present but are not alone enough to make a clinical diagnosis.

Quantification of symptoms using a patient-rated outcome measure may facilitate assessment. The SNOT-22 is a widely used clinical scoring system considering common sinonasal and associated symptoms. The test determines the quality-of-life impact of the condition and response to interventions and also can be used to predict the likelihood of benefit from them [34, 35].

The Nasal Polyp Score is a grading system for nasal polyps: Zero is no polyp, 1 = small polyps in the middle meatus not reaching below the inferior border of the middle turbinate, 2 = polyps reaching below the lower border of the middle turbinate, 3 = large polyps reaching the lower border of the inferior turbinate or polyps medial to the middle turbinate, and 4 = large polyps causing complete obstruction of the inferior nasal cavity [36].

Comorbid conditions such as asthma, allergy, sensitivity to nonsteroidal anti-inflammatory medications, recurrent infections, immune deficiency, cystic fibrosis, etc. are important factors that further help in the process of understanding the patient [37]. Comorbidities suggesting a type 2 inflammatory propensity, such as adult-onset or late-onset asthma and atopic dermatitis, are more common in CRSwNP.

Anterior rhinoscopy is inadequate for evaluation of CRS due to its limited visualization of the middle meatus and depth of the nasal cavity, and is therefore of limited value for CRS. A comprehensive endoscopic examination is essential during the evaluation of all patients under evaluation for CRS. The hallmark difference between CRSsNP and CRSwNP obviously is the appearance of polyps in the middle meatus and beyond. The presence of mucopurulent discharge in the middle meatus is a good indication of CRSsNP. There can be also other mucosal changes such as mucosal edema, cobblestone mucosa, and localized or generalized congestion. Endoscopic examination may also reveal a complication such as mucoceles.

Several studies have demonstrated a correlation between normal endoscopic examination and normal CT scan, indicating that properly performed nasal endoscopy can result in more judicious use of CT scans [38].

## 20.7 Radiology

Computed tomography (CT) has been the modality of choice for the evaluation of CRS since it offers high-resolution, multiplanar imaging of bony structures and soft tissue. CT also provides semi-quantitative analysis of inflammatory mucosal disease [38].

Computed tomography correlates poorly with symptoms, a fact that is particularly true when CT scans are obtained prior to assessment and treatment [20]. Therefore, it is not considered as a primary step in the assessment of CRS, except in the case of unilateral findings or suspicion of suppurative complications of rhinosinusitis [39].

Several CT staging systems have been described, but the Lund-MacKay system remains a validated rating system that is commonly used and referenced. The Lund-MacKay system relies upon sinus(es) involved and the degree of opacification:

- Opacification 0 = normal
- Opacification 1 = partial
- Opacification 2 = total pacification

These ratings are then applied separately to the frontal, anterior ethmoid, posterior ethmoid, maxillary, and sphenoid sinuses. The infundibulum is graded as either a score of 0 (no involvement) or 2 (involved). A maximum score of 12 per side can be achieved [40, 41].

Computed tomography may correlate poorly with symptoms, and therefore it is not considered as a primary step in the assessment of CRS, except in the case of unilateral findings or suspicion of complications [39]. Also, given the potential reversibility of several findings on CT after medical treatment, it is recommended to perform the study following an appropriate course of medical therapy in order to separate medical from surgical disease [10].

## 20.8 Other Tests

Clinically, the distinction can be made on the level of serum eosinophils (with cutoffs ranging from 150 to 300 cells/μL) or tissue eosinophils (with cutoffs ≥10 per high-powered field) [17]. A serum total IgE of ≥100 is indicative of a type 2 endotype. Although there is no clear link between allergic sensitization and CRS, a skin prick test or blood test (RAST or ISAC) may be needed in some patients.

Other tests are needed when secondary etiology is suspected. For example, if there is suspicion of vasculitis, the presence of antinuclear or antineutrophil cytoplasmic antibodies should be measured, as well as organ-specific tests depending on patient history. In case of a suspected underlying immunodeficiency, a full blood count, erythrocyte sedimentation rate, and serum levels of IgA, IgG, and IgG subclasses should be determined. Nasal tissue biopsies may be needed in some patients both from the suspected mucosa as well as from areas with apparent normal mucosa.

## 20.9 Diagnostic Criteria of CRS

Chronic rhinosinusitis (CRS) is defined as an inflammatory process involving the mucosa of the nasal cavity and paranasal sinuses that persists for greater than 12 weeks. It also requires the presence of at least two or more of the following symptoms, as well as evidence of inflammation as shown by radiologic or endoscopic examination [17, 24, 37, 42]. The phenotype determines the required criteria as follows:

**CRSsNP**

- Duration ≥12 weeks
- ≥2 of the following symptoms:
  - Mucopurulent drainage
  - Nasal obstruction
  - Facial pressure, fullness, or pain

- Endoscopic evidence of inflammation as demonstrated by:
  - Discolored mucus
  - Middle meatus mucosal edema
  - Ethmoid mucosal edema
- CT evidence of rhinosinusitis

**CRSwNP**

- Duration ≥12 weeks
- ≥2 of the following symptoms:
  - Mucopurulent drainage
  - Nasal obstruction
  - Hyposmia
- Endoscopic evidence of inflammation as demonstrated by nasal polyps
- CT evidence of rhinosinusitis

## 20.10 Medical Management of CRS

Although there is a clear distinction between CRSsNP and CRSwNP, the first line of treatment is similar for both. The initial "basic" medical therapy for both consists of nasal rinsing and intranasal corticosteroids (INCS). Xylitol may be used as a rinsing additive (limited evidence). There is very limited evidence supporting the use of short-term or long-term macrolide in CRSsNP. Systemic steroids are not indicated in CRSsNP.

Saline rinsing is a cornerstone treatment of CRS next to intranasal corticosteroids. There is solid enough evidence for nasal rinsing with isotonic saline or Ringer's lactate in CRS in spite of the great variability between the studies regarding the concentration of NaCl, use of additives, rinsing volume, rinsing pressure, devices used, frequency, etc. [17].

Many studies have addressed the value of INCS for CRS in general, more often for CRSwNP. The studies support the use of INCS in CRS, although the effects are much more pronounced in CRSwNP patients [17].

The effectiveness of topical steroids is believed to be enhanced after surgery, likely owing to improved access. The delivery of glucocorticoids with high-volume nasal irrigation has been shown as more effective in reducing endoscopic evidence of recurrence than delivery of an equivalent dose by means of nasal spray after sinus surgery [43]. Other modes of delivery, such as breath-activated exhalation delivery devices, may also enhance the effectiveness [29]. Nasal steroids are widely underutilized with a database study showing only 20% of CRS patients regularly use a nasal steroid. Patients should be educated regarding appropriate delivery techniques and the need for long-term adherence to therapy.

Steroid-eluting stents have been developed for use before and after sinus surgery, with the aim of delivering higher local concentrations of steroids than other delivery methods and overcoming compliance issues [30]. Their use has been investigated postoperatively where improvement has been demonstrated in endoscopic and imaging scores but not in terms of symptoms of quality of life.

Xylitol is a naturally occurring sugar alcohol with the ability to reduce biofilms. The use of Xylitol is especially when thick, sticky discharge is found upon nasal endoscopy, which is a sign of biofilm formation [44].

Although short courses (<4 weeks) of antibiotics are prescribed frequently for (exacerbations of) CRS, there is a lack of high-quality studies justifying their routine use in CRS. Short-term doxycycline has demonstrated a small but statistically significant reduction in nasal polyp endoscopic scores and rhinorrhea in one study [30].

There is limited evidence supporting the use of long-term macrolides in CRSwNP [17]. The use of long-term antibiotics/macrolides is not advised in CRSsNP [9]. There is also the risk of cardiovascular morbidity with long-term use of some antibiotics.

Oral steroids have a long history of use in airway inflammation. They are effective in the management of CRSwNP reducing symptoms at least in the short term. Short courses of oral corticosteroids are often used in CRSwNP and have proven to be effective, albeit for short periods of time only. This is in line with the steroid responsiveness of the type 2 inflammatory endotype [17]. However, it is not advised to use them regularly for CRSsNP, especially given the adverse effects [45].

However, the immediate benefits of systemic glucocorticoid therapy need to be balanced with the long-term potential adverse effects. Therefore, systemic steroids should not be considered as a first line of treatment for CRSwNP. They can be used in a short course for 2–3 weeks as a last resort of treatment when combinations of other medications are ineffective [30].

Antileukotriene medications target the inflammatory pathway driven by leukotrienes. They have little added benefit in terms of symptom improvement when used as an add-on to intranasal corticosteroids [46]. Some may have a role in NSAID-exacerbated respiratory disease (N-ERD) but have not been formerly evaluated in RCTs. Neuropsychiatric adverse effects were described, and so their use is not currently recommended [31].

## 20.11 Biological Therapy in CRSwNP

Biologic therapy using monoclonal antibodies (Mabs) that block the action of interleukins (IL) or other targets central to type 2 inflammation now plays an important role in the management of difficult-to-treat asthma. Many of these treatments have also been shown to be useful in the management of severe CRSwNP [47].

Consensus guidelines are available and suggest they should be considered for patients with at least moderate symptoms or a moderate Lund-MacKay score who fail conventional medical and surgical treatment. Their role in specific subsets of CRSwNP, such as AFRS and N-ERD, is still undefined.

IL4/IL13 pathway activation is targeted by dupilumab, an IL4 receptor subunit Mab. It has been shown to improve symptom and imaging scores, nasal polyp scores, and olfaction. Dupilumab seems well tolerated in available trials [47]. The most commonly reported adverse events include nasopharyngitis, headache, injection-site erythema, worsening nasal polyps, and asthma.

Anti-IgE therapy with omalizumab has shown improvements in nasal polyp burden and symptom scores. Associated adverse effects include anaphylaxis, arterial and venous thromboembolic events, and frequent common colds.

Both dupilumab and omalizumab have been approved by regulatory bodies for use in severe CRSwNP. Head-to-head comparisons are not available, but indirect comparison data presently favors dupilumab [48].

IL5 is targeted by mepolizumab, benralizumab, and reslizumab. Only mepolizumab currently has available evidence for reduced symptoms and decreased revision surgery in CRSwNP patients. There are no serious noted adverse effects [47].

The high costs of biologics and the need for long-term treatment make them unlikely to be the most cost-effective treatment of CRSwNP, but in the future, they may be given much earlier in the disease process in an attempt to alter the natural history of the disease, or in combination with surgery [47].

Patients with CRS can have comorbidities and/or traits that contribute to a worse disease course. These include allergic rhinitis [49], asthma, occupational exposure [50, 51], and smoking [16, 52]. Appropriate treatment of the CRS component should include addressing these comorbidities/traits.

## 20.12 Surgical Management of CRS

Surgery for uncomplicated CRSWNP is usually restricted to those patients who fail to achieve adequate symptomatic benefit from a trial of adequate medical therapy [32]. What constitutes failed medical therapy is debatable in the literature but at a minimum requires a sustained 12-week trial of intranasal saline and topical steroid, usually in conjunction with a trial of systemic corticosteroid [28].

The aim of surgical intervention is to reduce the volume of inflammatory tissue, remove obstruction, and facilitate the delivery of topical medication [35]. The impact of surgery is especially noticed in those patient groups with high baseline symptom and imaging scores. Older patients benefit more but asthmatic and aspirin-sensitive patients having less improvement [53].

There is some data that earlier intervention with surgery relative to when symptoms started leads to better outcomes [30]. There is also some evidence that earlier surgery reduces the subsequent development of asthma [32].

In a large systematic review, Smith et al. found 45 studies reporting on the effect of ESS for CRS. Nearly all of them support the fact that ESS improves symptom scores and/or quality of life [54]. There is evidence that endoscopic sinus surgery improves mucociliary clearance in CRS patient [55].

The goal of surgery, especially in CRSsNP, is to create a more open paranasal sinus cavity to which medical therapy can be more effectively distributed. It is said that ESS resets the polyp clock. ESS is generally indicated if the patient needs >2–3 courses of oral steroids/year. Patient counseling should include the expected reduction in symptom burden, the risk of complications, the rationale for surgery, postoperative follow-up and therapy, and the possibility of revision surgery.

The extent of primary surgery for CRSwNP is debated. The balance of extent of surgery must be discussed with and tailored to each individual patient. Approaches range from minimally invasive to complete or extensive. A functional approach based on the ostial drainage pathways is well established as beneficial [30]. Heterogeneity between the studies makes assessment difficult, but there is some evidence for more extensive sinus surgery, especially in revision cases surgery [13, 56]. Lower revision rates and greater improvements in symptoms have been demonstrated in complete sinus surgery cohorts such as those by Masterson and Deconde [57] (Figs. 20.6 and 20.7). Recently, there has been a proposal for the removal of diseased mucosa, described as a sinonasal mucosal reboot, as opposed to mucosal

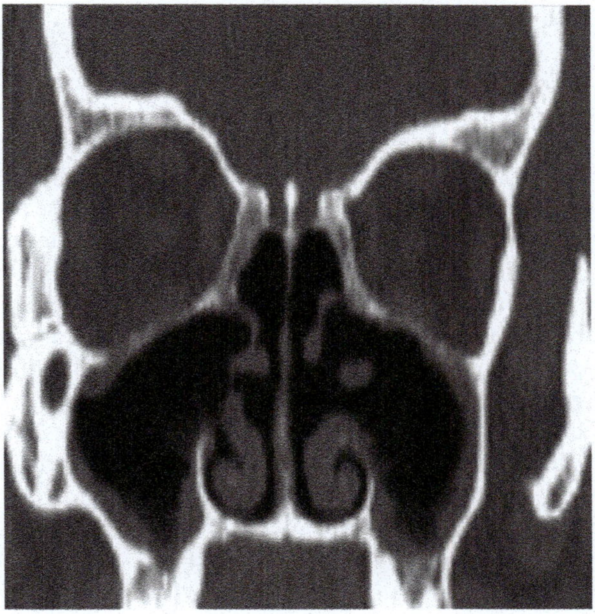

**Fig. 20.6** Better results may be achieved by complete endoscopic sinus surgery. For a significant polyp disease, it is recommended to do complete surgery the very first time

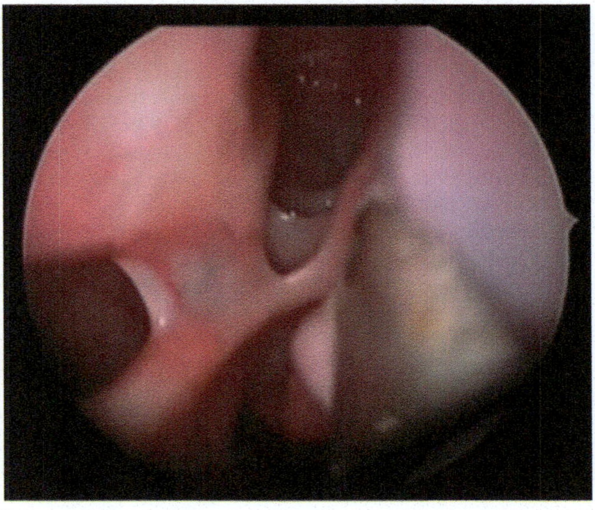

**Fig. 20.7** Postoperative endoscopic view of the same case shown in Fig. 20.6

sparing techniques, but further evidence is required to support efficacy [58]. The balance of extent of surgery must be discussed with and tailored to each individual patient.

Management of specific subgroups such as allergic fungal sinusitis and N-erd usually includes more extensive surgery and adjunctive treatments. Those with cystic fibrosis and ciliary dyskinesia require a multidisciplinary systemic treatment paradigm. Allergic fungal rhinosinusitis requires early and extensive surgical treatment of the affected compartments [30].

## 20.13 Postoperative Care

Postoperative care of patients with CRSwNP undergoing endoscopic sinus procedures is important for the optimization of outcomes. Nasal saline irrigation 24–48 h after surgery has low risk and a good evidence base for improving postoperative symptoms and medium-term symptomatic outcomes [7]. Budesonide added to postoperative irrigation has an increasing evidence base to support its use [21].

Postoperative debridement has been shown to reduce granulation and synechiae formation but increases postoperative pain. This is especially true in patients with significant mucosa and bone removal with extended approaches. Postoperative antibiotics have not demonstrated a benefit, and oral steroids have shown improved polyp scores but not symptom scores to date [30]. Management of specific subgroups requires a tailored treatment protocol and sometimes a multidisciplinary treatment paradigm. In the N-ERD group, there is some support for the use of adjunctive treatments such as aspirin desensitization and leukotriene modifiers [31, 59].

## References


1. Rosenfeld RM, Piccirillo JF, Chandrasekhar SS, et al. Clinical practice guideline (update): adult sinusitis. Otolaryngol Head Neck Surg. 2015;152:S1–S39.
2. Albu S. Chronic rhinosinusitis-an update on epidemiology, pathogenesis and management. J Clin Med. 2020;9(7):2285. https://doi.org/10.3390/jcm9072285.
3. Gliklich RE, Metson R. The health impact of chronic sinusitis in patients seeking otolaryngologic care. Otolaryngol Head Neck Surg. 1995;113:104–9.
4. Lasso A, Masoudian P, Quinn JG, Cowan J, Labajian V, Bonaparte JP, Kilty S. Long-term low-dose macrolides for chronic rhinosinusitis in adults - a systematic review of the literature. Clin Otolaryngol. 2017;42:637–50.
5. Schwartz JS, Tajudeen BA, Cohen NA. Medical management of chronic rhinosinusitis - a review of traditional and novel medical therapies. Expert Opin Investig Drugs. 2017;26:1123–30.
6. Sasama J, Sherris DA, Shin S-H, Kephart GM, Kern EB, Ponikau JU. New paradigm for the roles of fungi and eosinophils in chronic rhinosinusitis. Curr Opin Otolaryngol Head Neck Surg. 2005;13:2–8.
7. Orlandi RR, Marple BF. Fungus and chronic rhinosinusitis: weighing the evidence. Otolaryngol Head Neck Surg. 2010;143:611–3.
8. Psaltis AJ, Weitzel EK, Ha KR, Wormald P-J. The effect of bacterial biofilms on post-sinus surgical outcomes. Am J Rhinol. 2008;22:1–6.

9. Zhang N, Holtappels G, Claeys C, Huang G, van Cauwenberge P, Bachert C. Pattern of inflammation and impact of Staphylococcus aureus enterotoxins in nasal polyps from southern China. Am J Rhinol. 2006;20:445–50.
10. Marple BF, Stankiewicz JA, Baroody FM, et al. Diagnosis and management of chronic rhinosinusitis in adults. Postgrad Med. 2009;121:121–39.
11. Wang X, Zhang N, Bo M, Holtappels G, Zheng M, Lou H, Wang H, Zhang L, Bachert C. Diversity of T(H) cytokine profiles in patients with chronic rhinosinusitis: a multicenter study in Europe, Asia, and Oceania. J Allergy Clin Immunol. 2016;138:1344–53.
12. Tan CJ-W, Leow BHW, Tan BKJ, Tan SF-J, Teo NWY, Charn TC. Association between smoking and chronic rhinosinusitis: a systematic review and meta-analysis. Laryngoscope. 2023;134(6):2513–24. https://doi.org/10.1002/lary.31223.
13. Elwany S, Saeed YH, Talaat I. Effects of passive smoking on adult nasal respiratory mucosa. J Laryngol Otol. 2013;127:977–81.
14. Elwany S, Gamea MA, Talaat I. Passive smoking induces nasal biofilms in children. Int J Pediatr Otorhinolaryngol. 2021;146:110755.
15. Elwany S, Ibrahim AA, Mandour Z, Talaat I. Effect of passive smoking on the ultrastructure of the nasal mucosa in children. Laryngoscope. 2012;122:965–9.
16. Elwany S, Shewel Y, Bazak R, Talaat I, Elwany M. Quitting smoking reverses nasal mucosal changes. Eur Arch Otorrinolaringol. 2020;277:1691–8.
17. Fokkens WJ, Lund VJ, Mullol J, et al. EPOS 2012: European position paper on rhinosinusitis and nasal polyps 2012. A summary for otorhinolaryngologists. Rhinology. 2012;50:1–12.
18. Tam A, Wadsworth S, Dorscheid D, Man SFP, Sin DD. The airway epithelium: more than just a structural barrier. Ther Adv Respir Dis. 2011;5:255–73.
19. Seshadri S, Lu X, Purkey MR, et al. Increased expression of the epithelial anion transporter pendrin/SLC26A4 in nasal polyps of patients with chronic rhinosinusitis. J Allergy Clin Immunol. 2015;136:1548–58.
20. Soyka MB, Wawrzyniak P, Eiwegger T, Holzmann D, Treis A, Wanke K, Kast JI, Akdis CA. Defective epithelial barrier in chronic rhinosinusitis: the regulation of tight junctions by IFN-γ and IL-4. J Allergy Clin Immunol. 2012;130:1087–96.
21. Van Crombruggen K, Zhang N, Gevaert P, Tomassen P, Bachert C. Pathogenesis of chronic rhinosinusitis: inflammation. J Allergy Clin Immunol. 2011;128:728–32.
22. Okano M, Fujiwara T, Haruna T, Kariya S, Makihara S, Higaki T, Nishizaki K. Prostaglandin E(2) suppresses staphylococcal enterotoxin-induced eosinophilia-associated cellular responses dominantly through an E-prostanoid 2-mediated pathway in nasal polyps. J Allergy Clin Immunol. 2009;123:868–74.
23. Pérez-Novo CA, Waeytens A, Claeys C, Van Cauwenberge P, Bachert C. Staphylococcus aureus enterotoxin B regulates prostaglandin E2 synthesis, growth, and migration in nasal tissue fibroblasts. J Infect Dis. 2008;197:1036–43.
24. Meltzer EO, Hamilos DL, Hadley JA, et al. Rhinosinusitis: establishing definitions for clinical research and patient care. Otolaryngol Head Neck Surg. 2004;131:1–62.
25. Bayar Muluk N, Cingi C, Scadding GK, Scadding G. Chronic rhinosinusitis-could phenotyping or endotyping aid therapy? Am J Rhinol Allergy. 2019;33:83–93.
26. Dennis SK, Lam K, Luong A. A review of classification schemes for chronic rhinosinusitis with nasal polyposis endotypes. Laryngosc Investig Otolaryngol. 2016;1:130–4.
27. Bachert C, Akdis CA. Phenotypes and emerging endotypes of chronic rhinosinusitis. J Allergy Clin Immunol Pract. 2016;4:621–8.
28. Bousquet J, Khaltaev N, Cruz AA, et al. Allergic rhinitis and its impact on asthma (ARIA) 2008 update (in collaboration with the World Health Organization, GA(2)LEN and AllerGen). Allergy. 2008;63(8):8–160.
29. Hopkins C. Chronic rhinosinusitis with nasal polyps. N Engl J Med. 2019;381:55–63.
30. Fokkens WJ, Lund VJ, Hopkins C, Hellings PW, Kern R, Reitsma S, Toppila-Salmi S, Bernal-Sprekelsen M, Mullol J. Executive summary of EPOS 2020 including integrated care pathways. Rhinology. 2020;58:82–111.

31. Li KL, Lee AY, Abuzeid WM. Aspirin exacerbated respiratory disease: epidemiology, pathophysiology, and management. Med Sci. 2019;7(3):45. https://doi.org/10.3390/medsci7030045.
32. Adappa ND, Ranasinghe VJ, Trope M, Brooks SG, Glicksman JT, Parasher AK, Palmer JN, Bosso JV. Outcomes after complete endoscopic sinus surgery and aspirin desensitization in aspirin-exacerbated respiratory disease. Int Forum Allergy Rhinol. 2018;8:49–53.
33. Kennedy DW, Wright ED, Goldberg AN. Objective and subjective outcomes in surgery for chronic sinusitis. Laryngoscope. 2000;110:29–31.
34. Elwany S, Atef A, Ibrahim AA, Ismail AS, Hussein WK, Youssef AS, Elwany M, Bazak R. Arabic translation and validation of SNOT-22. Egyptian J Otolaryngol. 2017;33:611–5.
35. Hopkins C, Slack R, Lund V, Brown P, Copley L, Browne J. Long-term outcomes from the English national comparative audit of surgery for nasal polyposis and chronic rhinosinusitis. Laryngoscope. 2009;119:2459–65.
36. Gevaert P, Calus L, Van Zele T, et al. Omalizumab is effective in allergic and nonallergic patients with nasal polyps and asthma. J Allergy Clin Immunol. 2013;131:110–6.
37. Cho SH, Bachert C, Lockey RF. Chronic rhinosinusitis phenotypes: an approach to better medical care for chronic rhinosinusitis. J Allergy Clin Immunol Pract. 2016;4:639–42.
38. Stankiewicz JA, Chow JM. Nasal endoscopy and the definition and diagnosis of chronic rhinosinusitis. Otolaryngol Head Neck Surg. 2002;126:623–7.
39. Fokkens WJ, Lund VJ, Mullol J, et al. European position paper on rhinosinusitis and nasal polyps 2012. Rhinol Suppl. 2012;23(3):1–298.
40. Metson R, Gliklich RE, Stankiewicz JA, Kennedy DW, Duncavage JA, Hoffman SR, Ohnishi T, Terrell JE, White PS. Comparison of sinus computed tomography staging systems. Otolaryngol Head Neck Surg. 1997;117:372–9.
41. Lund VJ, Mackay IS. Staging in rhinosinusitus. Rhinology. 1993;31:183–4.
42. Benninger MS, Ferguson BJ, Hadley JA, et al. Adult chronic rhinosinusitis: definitions, diagnosis, epidemiology, and pathophysiology. Otolaryngol Head Neck Surg. 2003;129:1–32.
43. Harvey RJ, Snidvongs K, Kalish LH, Oakley GM, Sacks R. Corticosteroid nasal irrigations are more effective than simple sprays in a randomized double-blinded placebo-controlled trial for chronic rhinosinusitis after sinus surgery. Int Forum Allergy Rhinol. 2018;8:461–70.
44. Weissman JD, Fernandez F, Hwang PH. Xylitol nasal irrigation in the management of chronic rhinosinusitis: a pilot study. Laryngoscope. 2011;121:2468–72.
45. Hox V, Lourijsen E, Jordens A, et al. Benefits and harm of systemic steroids for short- and long-term use in rhinitis and rhinosinusitis: an EAACI position paper. Clin Transl Allergy. 2020;10:1.
46. Fokkens WJ, Viskens A-S, Backer V, et al. EPOS/EUFOREA update on indication and evaluation of biologics in chronic rhinosinusitis with nasal polyps 2023. Rhinology. 2023;61:194–202.
47. Kim C, Han J, Wu T, Bachert C, Fokkens W, Hellings P, Hopkins C, Lee S, Mullol J, Lee JT. Role of biologics in chronic rhinosinusitis with nasal polyposis: state of the art review. Otolaryngol Head Neck Surg. 2021;164:57–66.
48. Peters AT, Han JK, Hellings P, et al. Indirect treatment comparison of biologics in chronic rhinosinusitis with nasal polyps. J Allergy Clin Immunol Pract. 2021;9:2461–71.
49. Bousquet J, Pfaar O, Togias A, et al. 2019 ARIA care pathways for allergen immunotherapy. Allergy. 2019;74:2087–102.
50. Dietz de Loos DAE, Ronsmans S, Cornet ME, Hellings PW, Hox V, Fokkens WJ, Reitsma S. Occupational exposure influences control of disease in patients with chronic rhinosinusitis. Rhinology. 2021;59:380–6.
51. Velasquez N, Moore JA, Boudreau RM, Mady LJ, Lee SE. Association of air pollutants, airborne occupational exposures, and chronic rhinosinusitis disease severity. Int Forum Allergy Rhinol. 2020;10:175–82.
52. Reh DD, Higgins TS, Smith TL. Impact of tobacco smoke on chronic rhinosinusitis: a review of the literature. Int Forum Allergy Rhinol. 2012;2:362–9.
53. DeConde AS, Mace JC, Levy JM, Rudmik L, Alt JA, Smith TL. Prevalence of polyp recurrence after endoscopic sinus surgery for chronic rhinosinusitis with nasal polyposis. Laryngoscope. 2017;127:550–5.

54. Smith TL, Batra PS, Seiden AM, Hannley M. Evidence supporting endoscopic sinus surgery in the management of adult chronic rhinosinusitis: a systematic review. Am J Rhinol. 2005;19:537–43.
55. Elwany S, Hisham M, Gamaee R. The effect of endoscopic sinus surgery on mucociliary clearance in patients with chronic sinusitis. Eur Arch Otorrinolaringol. 1998;255:511–4.
56. Bassiouni A, Wormald P-J. Role of frontal sinus surgery in nasal polyp recurrence. Laryngoscope. 2013;123:36–41.
57. Masterson L, Tanweer F, Bueser T, Leong P. Extensive endoscopic sinus surgery: does this reduce the revision rate for nasal polyposis? Eur Arch Otorrinolaringol. 2010;267:1557–61.
58. Alsharif S, Jonstam K, van Zele T, Gevaert P, Holtappels G, Bachert C. Endoscopic sinus surgery for type-2 CRS wNP: an endotype-based retrospective study. Laryngoscope. 2019;129:1286–92.
59. Morrissey DK, Bassiouni A, Psaltis AJ, Naidoo Y, Wormald P-J. Outcomes of modified endoscopic Lothrop in aspirin-exacerbated respiratory disease with nasal polyposis. Int Forum Allergy Rhinol. 2016;6:820–5.

# Biologics in Rhinology

# 21

Samy Elwany

**Key Points**

- Biologics are monoclonal antibodies that represent a new option for the treatment of recalcitrant CRSwNP.
- The current guidelines advise the use of biologics in patients fulfilling certain criteria. The currently available biologics for CRSwNP are Omalizumab, Benralizumab, Mepolizumab, Reslizumab, and Dupilumab.
- Omalizumab and Dupilumab have been used for selected cases of allergic rhinitis.
- An important issue that should be considered is the cost of biologics therapy compared to other options.
- There is still a lack of head-to-head studies to provide real-life comparisons of the effectiveness of different biological drugs.

The European Medical Agency (EMA) defines biologics as biopharmaceutical medicinal products that are applied in vivo as biological medicinal substances and will usually be applied as therapeutic agents. Also, they include biotechnologically produced active substances such as therapeutic antibodies and recombinant proteins. In the daily language of life science and medicine, the term biologics was established mainly for therapeutic antibodies and rarely also for recombinant therapeutic proteins [1].

S. Elwany (✉)
Department of Otolaryngology, Alexandria Faculty of Medicine, Alexandria, Egypt
e-mail: samy.elwany@alexmed.edu.eg


S. Elwany (ed.), *Current Rhinology*,
https://doi.org/10.1007/978-3-031-70077-4_21

## 21.1 Monoclonal Antibodies

The use of biological agents such as monoclonal antibodies (MAb) in treatment is called **biological therapy** or **biotherapy**. Monoclonal antibodies are produced by animals (i.e., mouse) cell sequences/clones that are immunized to a specific antigen. Their structure can also be chimeric, which contains a part of the antibody obtained from the mouse in the variable region and part of the human antibody in the rest of the regular part. Humanized ones contain only the antibody part obtained from the mouse in the hypervariable region. Human ones contain only human antibodies.

The naming of the monoclonal antibodies is performed according to the syllables used before the last appendix—mab:

- If the last appendix—"o" arrives before—mab (-omab), it is considered that it is a mouse antibody.
- If there is a "u" before—mab (-umab), it is considered that it is a human antibody.
- If there is a "xi" before—mab (-ximab), it is considered that it is a chimeric antibody.
- If there is "zu" before—mab (-zumab), it is necessary to consider that it is humanized antibody.

## 21.2 Biologics in Chronic Rhinosinusitis (CRS)

Chronic rhinosinusitis (CRS) is defined as an inflammatory disease of the mucosa of the nose and sinuses that lasts for more than 12 weeks without resolution of symptoms and signs. It is estimated that CRS affects about 5–12% of the general population. The treatment of CRS can be pharmacological, surgical, or immunological.

For many years, CRS was divided into CRS with nasal polyps (CRSwNP) and CRS without nasal polyps (CRSsNP). Other classifications divide CRS into primary and secondary forms and localized and diffuse types.

New ways of classifying CRS by endotypes appeared after the most recent understanding of the pathophysiology of the disease. CRSwNP can be classified into eosinophilic CRSwNP (eosCRSwNP) or noneosinophilic CRSwNP (noneosCRSwNP) based on the extent of eosinophilic inflammation in the polyp tissues. Consequently, a new type of treatment has been administered in the last years, biologics [2].

For the moment, biologics are indicated just in the cases of the patients who have undergone ESS or have contraindications for surgery and have bilateral polyps and meet a minimum of three of the following criteria: the necessity for systemic corticosteroids or contraindications to systemic steroids, significant loss of smell, impaired QoL score, comorbid asthma, and type 2 inflammation [3].

Pathogenesis of CRS includes a complex interplay between immunity, airway epithelium, genetics, and environmental factors. External factors (bacteria, viruses, and fungi) and environmental factors (air pollution, dust, allergens) will activate several processes. These processes include: TLRs (Toll-like receptors) and solitary chemosensory cell activation. It will be also associated with epithelial proinflammatory cytokines and epithelial defense molecules production as well as mucociliary clearance impairment [2].

These factors activate innate immune cells and adaptative immune cells. The resultant chronic inflammation will be associated with apparition of tissue remodeling, goblet cell hyperplasia, tight junction disruption, activation of solitary chemosensory cells, and bacteria dysbiosis. These modifications will translate into symptoms like nasal congestion and discharge, facial pressure, and olfactory dysfunction.

Chronic diseases have been classified by their genotype, phenotype, and endotype. Endotype classification subdivides CRS based on the underlying pathobiological mechanisms.

T1 endotype is characterized by the preferential expression of IFN-$\gamma$, produced from Th1 cells, cytotoxic T cells, NK cells, and group 1 innate lymphoid cells (ILC1s). Other biomarkers: include CXCL9, CXCL11, GZMH, ZNF683, FCRL6, and SLCO1B3.

T2 endotype is characterized by the IL-4, IL-5, and IL-13 produced from Th2 cells, mast cells, and ILC2s and eosinophils. Other biomarkers include: EPX, CCL18, CCL26, CCR3, CST1, CST2, CLCA1, FCER2, POSTIN, PTGDR2, and SIGLEC8. Type 2 endotype is predominantly displayed in patients with CRSwNP in Western countries, whereas a mixed type 2 endotype is predominantly displayed on the Asian continent [4].

T3 endotype is characterized by IL-17A and IL-17F that are produced from Th17 cells and ILC3. Other biomarkers include: IL1B, IL8, CXCL1, CXCL2, CXCL6, CCL20, CHI3L1, SAA1, SAA2, and NOX1 [5].

Patients may fit in one of these endotypes or can present mixed mechanisms. Few do not express elevated levels of any kind of biomarker genes. On the other hand, the T1,2,3 endotype comprises a group of patients that have elevated levels of all three sets of biomarker genes with none of them being the most relevant [6].

Another way to endotype CRS is to use histopathology: eosinophilic, neutrophilic, and mixed granulocytic [7]. Phenotypic classification is determined by the presence or absence of nasal polyps [8].

Grayson et al. proposed some years ago, a simple and practical system of classification. They suggested that the functional anatomical compartments involved in CRS could be a diagnostic tool for the first level of separation into local and diffuse (pansinusitis) CRS. Either of them can have unilateral or bilateral distribution [9].

The pathogenesis of the nontype 2 endotype in CRS is currently not definitely known. This varies with race, geography, and environment [10].

Biologics are monoclonal antibodies that are used to treat some immune system dysfunctions. Common Th2 immune pathway is the reason for most of the biologics developed for asthma being effective in CRSwNP.

Biologic treatment can be used in CRSwNP patients meeting the eligibility criteria [11]. EPOS 2020 has made indications for the biological treatment of CRSsNP and established the criteria used for the evaluation of its efficiency [12].

Currently, patients who underwent endoscopic sinus surgery or have contraindications for surgery receive biologic treatment if they meet a minimum of three of the following criteria (Box 21.1):

1. A need for systemic corticosteroids or contraindications to its use
2. Significantly impaired quality of life
3. Hyposmia
4. Comorbid asthma
5. Type 2 inflammation

The criteria used to evaluate the efficiency of biologic therapy are [12]:

1. Reduced NP size
2. Reduced need for systemic corticosteroids
3. Improved QoL
4. Improved sense of smell

**Box 21.1 EPOS 2020 Criteria for Biologic Treatment in Patients with CRSwNP**

EPOS 2020 Criteria for Biologic Treatment in Patients with CRSwNP

Presence of bilateral nasal polyps in a patient who had endoscopic sinus surgery

AND

**3** of the following criteria:

Evidence of type 2 inflammation (tissue EOS ≥10/hpf OR blood EOS ≥250 OR total IgE ≥100)

Need for systemic corticosteroids (SCS) or contraindications to SCS (22 courses in the past year OR long-term [>3 months])

Significant impaired quality of life (SNOT-22 ≥40)

Significant loss of smell (anosmic on smell test [score depending on test)

Diagnosis of comorbid asthma (asthma needing regular inhaled corticosteroids)

## 21.3 Side Effects of Biological Therapies

Hypersensitivity and anaphylaxis have been reported in all biological agents. Common problems with Omalizumab are urticaria, headaches, and problems at the injection site. Anaphylaxis (0.2%) has been warned by FDA. It is emphasized that after the first three injections of omalizumab, the patient should wait for at least 2 h, and in subsequent injections, patients should wait at least 1/2 h.

Dupilumab uncommonly may cause hypersensitivity and serum disease-like reactions [13].

Some concerns about omalizumab safety have been raised as its use has been recently linked to potential increased cancer risk. Nevertheless, literature evidence does not support this statement, and clinical studies and evidence from real-world registries and surveillance analysis have consistently reported drug safety. Also, real-world life data do not support any association between anti-IL-5 and anti-IL-4Ra biologics and cancer. Since these biologicals have only been available for a short period, the effect may be underestimated, and a larger period may be needed to better assess cancer incidence [14].

### 21.3.1 Anti-IgE (Omalizumab)

IgE is an antibody that is produced by specialized cells and is involved in several human pathologies. A growing body of evidence shows that IgE has an important role in the diagnosis and prognostication of CRS. Total serum IgE was observed to present significantly higher levels in recurrent CRS patients when compared with controls [15]. Tissue IgE concentrations were increased in eosCRS polyps as compared to controls [16]. High nasal IgE as well as high nasal IL-5 levels were found to be specific to CRSwNP [17].

**Omalizumab** is a recombinant DNA-derived humanized (IgG1k) monoclonal antibody that connects to free human immunoglobulin E (IgE) in the blood and interstitial fluid, and to the membrane-bound form of IgE (mIgE) present on the surface of cells with mIgE.

The main effect of Omalizumab is reducing the levels of IgE in serum and tissues, with a later blocking of the IgE-mediated inflammatory cascade with subsequent reduction of blood and tissue eosinophil counts, nasal polyp size, and sinus opacification [18–22].

Omalizumab proved to be an effective treatment in 17 patients with CRSwNP with or without concomitant asthma. Sinonasal outcome parameters significantly improved: SNOT-22, NOSE score, and VAS [23, 24]. After patients stopped omalizumab, the scores gradually decreased over the 4 months of follow-up but remained better than pretreatment levels [25].

The FDA has approved Xolair for the add-on maintenance treatment of nasal polyps in adult patients 18 years of age and older with an inadequate response to nasal corticosteroids (November 2020) [5].

The Committee for Medicinal Products for Human Use (CHMP) of the European Medicine Agency approved Xolair (omalizumab) as an add-on therapy with intranasal corticosteroids (INC) for the treatment of adults (18 years and above) with severe CRSwNP for whom therapy with INC does not provide adequate disease control [5].

### 21.3.2 Anti-IL5 (Benralizumab, Mepolizumab, and Reslizumab)

IL-5 promotes eosinophil development and survival. Anti-IL-5 is intended to reduce blood and tissue eosinophil counts [17]. Patients who have CRSwNP with elevations in serum and mucosal eosinophils tend to present more severe NP disease. Blood and tissue eosinophils may be associated with increased disease severity and recurrence rates postsurgery and they may remain elevated in spite of systemic corticosteroid use [26].

Three monoclonal antibodies have been approved until now: Mepolizumab, reslizumab, and benralizumab. These are human monoclonal (IgG1) antibodies targeting interleukin 5 (IL-5) or the IL-5 receptor α subunit on the surface of eosinophils and are administered subcutaneously or intravenously [17].

## 21.4 Benralizumab

Benralizumab is a humanized IL-5 receptor alpha-effective cytolytic monoclonal antibody (IgG1, kappa). Like Mepolizumab and Reslizumab, it is a monoclonal antibody that binds to the IL-5 receptor α (IL-5Rα) unit located on the surface of eosinophils. It shows pro-eosinophilic action. It also binds to natural killer cells, leading to cellular cytotoxic action and apoptosis on eosinophils [27, 28]. Benralizumab improved CRS with improvements in total SNOT-22 score in patients with severe, eosinophilic asthma and nasal polyps. The antibody was well tolerated and improved symptoms and sensation of smell for patients with CRS. Subsequent studies extended the safety and efficacy profile of benralizumab in cases with nasal polyps [29].

A phase 2, randomized, double-blinded, placebo-controlled study in patients with eosinophilic chronic sinusitis showed a reduction of the nasal polyps score in the benralizumab group compared with the placebo group over the entire study period especially in patients with high levels of blood eosinophils [30].

A phase 3 study (OSTRO) enrolled patients with severe symptomatic CRSwNP, despite treatment with intranasal corticosteroids, a history of systemic corticosteroid use, and/or surgery for nasal polyps. Benralizumab reduced nasal polyps score and reduced problems with sense of smell compared to placebo in patients with CRSwNP [31].

Benralizumab also improved asthma control and lung function and sinonasal quality of life in a case series of patients with severe eosinophilic asthma and CRSwNP [27, 28].

Fasenra (benralizumab) has been officially indicated in Europe as an add-on maintenance treatment in adult patients with severe eosinophilic asthma inadequately controlled despite high-dose inhaled corticosteroids plus long-acting β-agonist (updated 21 September 2023) [5].

## 21.5 Mepolizumab

Mepolizumab is a humanized Anti-IL-5, a monoclonal antibody (IgG1 kappa). Interleukin 5 (IL-5) is produced by Th2 lymphocytes, innate lymphoid cells (ILC-2), and mast cells. It is the basic cytokine involved in eosinophils' activation, regeneration, and life process. Anti-IL-5 agents suppress eosinophilic airway inflammation [32].

Mepolizumab prevents IL-5 from connecting to its receptor on eosinophils and thus selectively inhibits eosinophilic inflammation [33].

A randomized, double-blind, placebo-controlled trial that recruited adult patients with recurrent nasal polyposis requiring surgical intervention showed the administration of mepolizumab in addition to daily topical corticosteroid treatment. Reduced the severity of nasal polyposis, VAS score, endoscopic nasal polyp score, and sinonasal outcome with an important reduction in the need for surgery [34].

SYNAPSE is a randomized, double-blind, placebo-controlled, parallel-group, phase 3 trial that has been conducted in 11counteries. According to the trial, Mepolizumab reduced polyp size and nasal obstruction and reduced the risk of recurrent sinus surgery in chronic rhinosinusitis with NP regardless of the presence of comorbid asthma or AERD [35].

Several other studies showed that treatment with mepolizumab reduced sinonasal symptoms, polyp scores, blood eosinophils, and systemic corticosteroid use [36].

The FDA has approved the monoclonal antibody mepolizumab as a treatment for patients with chronic rhinosinusitis with nasal polyps (CRSwNP (July 2021)) [5].

The Committee for Medicinal Products for Human Use (CHMP) of the European Medicine Agency approved Nucala (mepolizumab) as an add-on therapy with intranasal corticosteroids for the treatment of adult patients with severe CRSwNP for whom therapy with systemic corticosteroids and/or surgery does not provide adequate disease control [5].

## 21.6 Reslizumab

Reslizumab is a humanized IL-5 antagonist monoclonal antibody (IgG4κ), an anti-IL-5 agent. IL-5 contributes to eosinophil activation, maturation, and survival. Therefore, anti-IL-5 treatment can suppress inflammation of eosinophil origin. The drug directly targets IL-5, reducing circulating eosinophils [37].

A phase 1, single-dose, randomized, double-blind, placebo-controlled, three-arm, parallel-group study of reslizumab in patients with nasal polyps showed that a single injection of anti-IL-5 reslizumab reduced the size of nasal polyps in half of the patients, and the response to anti-IL-5 treatment was predicted using nasal IL-5 levels [38].

Cinqaero (reslizumab) has been officially indicated in Europe as an add-on therapy in adult patients with severe eosinophilic asthma inadequately controlled despite high-dose inhaled corticosteroids plus another medicinal product for maintenance treatment (updated 26 May 2023) [5].

### 21.6.1 Anti-IL4/IL13 (Dupilumab)

Dupilumab is a human IgG monoclonal antibody that connects specifically to IL-4Rα, disrupting the activity of both IL-4 and IL-13.

The cytokines IL-4 and IL-13act on the same receptors in type 2 inflammation. Type 1 receptor has an IL-4Rα subunit, and type 2 receptor has IL-4Rα and IL-13Rα1 subunits. The two cytokines play an essential role in T2 inflammation including:

- Differentiation of T cells to Th2 cells.
- IgE production from B cells (IL-4).
- Remodeling the airways.
- Production of mucus from the Goblet cells.
- Causes effects such as flat muscle contractility (IL-13).
- IL-13 directly affects the production of exhaled nitric oxide fraction (Fe-NO) in the airway epithelium and plays an essential role in eosinophil migration by activating vascular adhesion molecules [39, 40].

Dupilumab has been used to treat moderate to severe atopic dermatitis, asthma, and nasal polyps accompanied by chronic rhinosinusitis in adolescents and adults [41].

Dupilumab reduced Eotaxin-3, total IgE, eosinophilic cationic protein, eotaxin-2, and IL-13 in CRSwNP patients receiving 300 mg dupilumab weekly for 16 weeks [41].

Dupilumab (600 mg loading dose, then 300 mg once weekly for 15 weeks or matched placebo) reduced disease severity and significantly improved HRQoL in adults with CRSwNP refractory to intranasal corticosteroids (INCS) [42, 43].

In the SINUS-24 study, patients were assigned to receive 300 mg dupilumab or placebo every 2 weeks for 24 weeks. In SINUS-52, the patients received 300 mg dupilumab every 2 weeks for 52 weeks or dupilumab every 2 weeks for 24 weeks and then every 4 weeks for the remaining 28 weeks. In both studies, Dupilumab was well tolerated and reduced sinus opacification, polyp size, and the severity of clinical symptoms [44]. Several other studies reported similar results [45–51].

A recent study concluded that dupilumab should be the first choice when switching biologic agents, based on the fact that most patients who failed with omalizumab and/or an anti-IL-5 treatment were well controlled on dupilumab. It was ineffective to switch to a second anti-IL5 treatment if the first one was not successful [43].

The US Food and Drug Administration approved Dupixent (dupilumab) to treat adults with nasal polyps accompanied by chronic rhinosinusitis (prolonged inflammation of the sinuses and nasal cavity), being the first treatment approved for inadequately controlled chronic rhinosinusitis with nasal polyps (26 June 2019) [5].

The Committee for Medicinal Products for Human Use (CHMP) of the European Medicine Agency approved Dupixent (dupilumab) as an add-on therapy with intranasal corticosteroids for the treatment of adults with severe CRSwNP for whom therapy with systemic corticosteroids and/or surgery does not provide adequate disease [5].

### 21.6.2 Biologics for CRS in Real Life

Currently, the guidelines for managing allergic chronic rhinosinusitis focus on symptomatic treatment and eventually surgical solutions. The presence of a strong mucosal disease raises the question of when biological treatment should be initiated? There are still debates about whether biologic treatment could be initiated before surgical removal or after surgical removal of the polyps [52].

The focus of the research is preventing recurrence after surgical removal [53]. Among the factors responsible for recurrence after endoscopic sinus surgery are high levels of eosinophil cationic protein, high antidouble-stranded DNA IgG, high IL-5, high-modified Lund-Mackay radiographic score, and asthma [54].

There is still the question regarding the size of the polyps and the level of polyposis that is still responding to the action of biological treatments [55, 56].

EPOS2020 (The European Position Paper on Rhinosinusitis and Nasal Polyps) advised on the use of biologics in the treatment of CRSwNP. The authors considered that patients who have the proof of presence of bilateral polyps and have ESS in their medical history if they present evidence of type 2 inflammation, the need for systemic corticosteroids or contraindication of systemic steroids, significantly impaired quality of life, significant loss of smell and diagnosis of comorbid asthma, are suitable candidates for biologics. Five criteria were suggested to be evaluated for defining response: reduced nasal polyp size, a reduced need for systemic corticosteroids, improved quality of life and sense of smell, and reduced impact of comorbidities at 16 and 48 weeks [57].

ESS and dupilumab offered comparable improvement in smell identification at 24 weeks. ESS offered significantly greater reductions in polyp size compared to omalizumab, dupilumab, and mepolizumab therapies in 111 patients suffering from CRSwNP [58].

ESS showed comparable improvement in quality of life and symptoms to omalizumab, mepolizumab, and benralizumab. Dupilumab seemed to be more effective than ESS in selected items in a network meta-analysis [59].

In the last years, authors from different countries have studied the differences between biologics and between surgery and biologics.

Olfaction (anosmia, hyposmia) was improved in a real-world study of patients with CRSwNP with four monoclonal antibodies (omalizumab [35.8%], mepolizumab [35.4%], reslizumab [35.7%], and benralizumab [39.1%]), with no differences between the groups [60].

Soyka et al. collected data from 2014 to 2020 from 48 treatments in 29 patients. A correlation between biomarkers and treatment success could not be found [61].

Solano J and colleagues conducted an observational study of adults on anti-IL5 m-AB treatment and reported a statistically significant difference in the ACT and

SNOT-22 scores before and after mAb treatment with no significant differences between mAb groups [62].

Ulrike Förster-Ruhrmann et al. conducted a monocentric study that included 115 adult patients with CRSwNP who received one of the four biologics (mepolizumab; benralizumab; dupilumab; and omalizumab). The most significant differences in pre/postscores were observed in the patients receiving dupilumab [63].

As a result of the conflicting conclusions, a recent review analyzed from a critical point of view the methodology of research in this field. Borish et al. pointed out some aspects that need more attention in the future including accurate and clinically meaningful characterization of baseline CRSwNP, different enrollment criteria for phase 3 clinical trials, and differences in treatment populations. They also pointed to the need to use head-to-head comparisons, comparable patient populations, and standardized outcome measures [64].

## 21.7 Biologics in Allergic Rhinitis

Biologics, especially Omalizumab and Dupilumab, may be used more in allergic rhinitis. Omalizumab treatment led to an improvement in the Daily Nasal Rescue Medication Score (DNSSS) and reduced allergic reactions associated with allergen immunotherapy, such as anaphylaxis. Dupilumab treatment led to significant improvement of SNOT-22 total scores in perennial allergic rhinitis [65].

A meta-analysis that included 11 randomized controlled trials (2870 patients with seasonal and perennial allergic rhinitis and rhino-conjunctivitis) reported that Omalizumab treatment improved the Daily Nasal Rescue Medication Score (DNSSS) and decreased the use of antiallergic drugs [66].

In a study called "SOLAR," the authors tried the effectiveness of Omalizumab treatment in adults and adolescents with moderate-severe perennial allergic rhinitis lasting for 2 years and concomitant uncontrolled persistent allergic asthma. For 28 weeks, the patients were given Omalizumab every four weeks at a dose of 0.016 mg/kg per IgE I.U./mL. In the posttreatment evaluation, asthma exacerbations were lower, asthma and rhinitis symptom scores were lower, and quality of life scores were better. Patients and researchers have described the treatment effectiveness of omalizumab in asthma-rhinitis as good or flawless [67].

Omalizumab was also used in selected immunotherapy patients with allergic rhinitis for the following reasons to reduce the side effects of specific immunotherapy [68].

## 21.8 Conclusions

Biologics represent a new option for the treatment of recalcitrant CRSwNP. The present guidelines advise the use of biologics in patients fulfilling certain criteria. An important issue that should be considered is the cost of biologics therapy compared to surgery. There is still a lack of head-to-head studies to provide real-life comparisons of the effectiveness of different biologics drugs.

## References


1. Chaker AM. Biologics in rhinology - forthcoming personalized concepts: the future starts today. Laryngorhinootologie. 2018;97:S142–84.
2. Seah JJ, Thong M, Wang DY. The diagnostic and prognostic role of biomarkers in chronic rhinosinusitis. Diagnostics. 2023;13(4):715. https://doi.org/10.3390/diagnostics13040715.
3. Rank MA, Chu DK, Bognanni A, et al. The Joint Task Force on Practice Parameters GRADE guidelines for the medical management of chronic rhinosinusitis with nasal polyposis. J Allergy Clin Immunol. 2023;151:386–98.
4. Yao Y, Zhu H-Y, Zeng M, Liu Z. Immunological mechanisms and treatable traits of chronic rhinosinusitis in Asia: a narrative review. Clin Otolaryngol. 2023;48:363–70.
5. Cergan R, Berghi ON, Dumitru M, Vrinceanu D, Manole F, Serboiu CS. Biologics for chronic rhinosinusitis—a modern option for therapy. Life. 2023;13:2165.
6. Kato A, Peters AT, Stevens WW, Schleimer RP, Tan BK, Kern RC. Endotypes of chronic rhinosinusitis: relationships to disease phenotypes, pathogenesis, clinical findings, and treatment approaches. Allergy. 2022;77:812–26.
7. Chapurin N, Wu J, Labby AB, Chandra RK, Chowdhury NI, Turner JH. Current insight into treatment of chronic rhinosinusitis: phenotypes, endotypes, and implications for targeted therapeutics. J Allergy Clin Immunol. 2022;150:22–32.
8. Kim SD, Cho KS. Treatment strategy of uncontrolled chronic rhinosinusitis with nasal polyps: a review of recent evidence. Int J Mol Sci. 2023;24(5):5015. https://doi.org/10.3390/ijms24055015.
9. Grayson JW, Hopkins C, Mori E, Senior B, Harvey RJ. Contemporary classification of chronic rhinosinusitis beyond polyps vs no polyps: a review. JAMA Otolaryngol Head Neck Surg. 2020;146:831–8.
10. Cui N, Zhu X, Zhao C, Meng C, Sha J, Zhu D. A decade of pathogenesis advances in non-type 2 inflammatory endotypes in chronic rhinosinusitis: 2012-2022. Int Arch Allergy Immunol. 2023;184:1237–53.
11. Brzost J, Czerwaty K, Dżaman K, Ludwig N, Piszczatowska K, Szczepański MJ. Perspectives in therapy of chronic rhinosinusitis. Diagnostics. 2022;12(10):2301. https://doi.org/10.3390/diagnostics12102301.
12. Fokkens WJ, Lund VJ, Hopkins C, Hellings PW, Kern R, Reitsma S, Toppila-Salmi S, Bernal-Sprekelsen M, Mullol J. Executive summary of EPOS 2020 including integrated care pathways. Rhinology. 2020;58:82–111.
13. Sitek A, Chiarella SE, Pongdee T. Hypersensitivity reactions to biologics used in the treatment of allergic diseases: clinical features, diagnosis and management. Front Allergy. 2023;4:1219735.
14. Bagnasco D, Canevari RF, Del Giacco S, Ferrucci S, Pigatto P, Castelnuovo P, Marseglia GL, Yalcin AD, Pelaia G, Canonica GW. Omalizumab and cancer risk: current evidence in allergic asthma, chronic urticaria, and chronic rhinosinusitis with nasal polyps. World Allergy Organ J. 2022;15:100721.
15. Wei B, Liu F, Zhang J, Liu Y, Du J, Liu S, Zhang N, Bachert C, Meng J. Multivariate analysis of inflammatory endotypes in recurrent nasal polyposis in a Chinese population. Rhinology. 2018;56:216–26.
16. Baba S, Kondo K, Toma-Hirano M, Kanaya K, Suzukawa K, Ushio M, Suzukawa M, Ohta K, Yamasoba T. Local increase in IgE and class switch recombination to IgE in nasal polyps in chronic rhinosinusitis. Clin Exp Allergy. 2014;44:701–12.
17. Riechelmann H, Deutschle T, Rozsasi A, Keck T, Polzehl D, Bürner H. Nasal biomarker profiles in acute and chronic rhinosinusitis. Clin Exp Allergy. 2005;35:1186–91.
18. Kobayashi Y, Kanda A, Van BD, Yun Y, Nguyen LM, Chu HH, Mitani A, Suzuki K, Asako M, Iwai H. Omalizumab restores response to corticosteroids in patients with eosinophilic chronic rhinosinusitis and severe asthma. Biomedicine. 2021;9(7):787. https://doi.org/10.3390/biomedicines9070787.

19. Chong L-Y, Piromchai P, Sharp S, Snidvongs K, Webster KE, Philpott C, Hopkins C, Burton MJ. Biologics for chronic rhinosinusitis. Cochrane Database Syst Rev. 2021;3:CD013513.
20. Tajiri T, Matsumoto H, Hiraumi H, et al. Efficacy of omalizumab in eosinophilic chronic rhinosinusitis patients with asthma. Ann Allergy Asthma Immunol. 2013;110:387–8.
21. Pinto JM, Mehta N, DiTineo M, Wang J, Baroody FM, Naclerio RM. A randomized, double-blind, placebo-controlled trial of anti-IgE for chronic rhinosinusitis. Rhinology. 2010;48:318–24.
22. Zhu R, Owen R, Wilkins J, et al. Pharmacokinetics and exposure-efficacy relationships of omalizumab in patients with nasal polyps. Pulm Pharmacol Ther. 2021;71:102080.
23. Damask C, Chen M, Holweg CTJ, Yoo B, Millette LA, Franzese C. Defining the efficacy of omalizumab in nasal polyposis: a POLYP 1 and POLYP 2 subgroup analysis. Am J Rhinol Allergy. 2022;36:135–41.
24. Tat TS. Omalizumab is effective in nasal polyposis with or without asthma, a real-life study. World Allergy Organ J. 2022;15:100670.
25. Gevaert P, Saenz R, Corren J, et al. Long-term efficacy and safety of omalizumab for nasal polyposis in an open-label extension study. J Allergy Clin Immunol. 2022;149:957–65.
26. DeConde AS, Mace JC, Levy JM, Rudmik L, Alt JA, Smith TL. Prevalence of polyp recurrence after endoscopic sinus surgery for chronic rhinosinusitis with nasal polyposis. Laryngoscope. 2017;127:550–5.
27. Canonica GW, Harrison TW, Chanez P, Menzella F, Louis R, Cosio BG, Lugogo NL, Mohan A, Burden A, Garcia Gil E. Benralizumab improves symptoms of patients with severe, eosinophilic asthma with a diagnosis of nasal polyposis. Allergy. 2022;77:150–61.
28. Lombardo N, Pelaia C, Ciriolo M, Della Corte M, Piazzetta G, Lobello N, Viola P, Pelaia G. Real-life effects of benralizumab on allergic chronic rhinosinusitis and nasal polyposis associated with severe asthma. Int J Immunopathol Pharmacol. 2020;34:2058738420950851.
29. Tversky J, Lane AP, Azar A. Benralizumab effect on severe chronic rhinosinusitis with nasal polyps (CRSwNP): a randomized double-blind placebo-controlled trial. Clin Exp Allergy. 2021;51:836–44.
30. Takabayashi T, Asaka D, Okamoto Y, et al. A phase II, multicenter, randomized, placebo-controlled study of benralizumab, a humanized anti-IL-5R alpha monoclonal antibody, in patients with eosinophilic chronic rhinosinusitis. Am J Rhinol Allergy. 2021;35:861–70.
31. Bachert C, Han JK, Desrosiers MY, et al. Efficacy and safety of benralizumab in chronic rhinosinusitis with nasal polyps: a randomized, placebo-controlled trial. J Allergy Clin Immunol. 2022;149:1309–17.
32. Varricchi G, Bagnasco D, Borriello F, Heffler E, Canonica GW. Interleukin-5 pathway inhibition in the treatment of eosinophilic respiratory disorders: evidence and unmet needs. Curr Opin Allergy Clin Immunol. 2016;16:186–200.
33. Fokkens WJ, Mullol J, Kennedy D, et al. Mepolizumab for chronic rhinosinusitis with nasal polyps (SYNAPSE): in-depth sinus surgery analysis. Allergy. 2023;78:812–21.
34. Bachert C, Sousa AR, Lund VJ, et al. Reduced need for surgery in severe nasal polyposis with mepolizumab: randomized trial. J Allergy Clin Immunol. 2017;140:1024–31.
35. Bachert C, Sousa AR, Han JK, et al. Mepolizumab for chronic rhinosinusitis with nasal polyps: treatment efficacy by comorbidity and blood eosinophil count. J Allergy Clin Immunol. 2022;149:1711–21.
36. Domínguez-Sosa MS, Cabrera-Ramírez MS, Marrero-Ramos MDC, Dávila-Quintana D, Cabrera-López C, Carrillo-Díaz T, Del Rosario JJB. Real-life effectiveness of mepolizumab in refractory chronic rhinosinusitis with nasal polyps. Biomedicine. 2023;11(2):485. https://doi.org/10.3390/biomedicines11020485.
37. Castro M, Zangrilli J, Wechsler ME, Bateman ED, Brusselle GG, Bardin P, Murphy K, Maspero JF, O'Brien C, Korn S. Reslizumab for inadequately controlled asthma with elevated blood eosinophil counts: results from two multicentre, parallel, double-blind, randomised, placebo-controlled, phase 3 trials. Lancet Respir Med. 2015;3:355–66.

38. Gevaert P, Lang-Loidolt D, Lackner A, Stammberger H, Staudinger H, Van Zele T, Holtappels G, Tavernier J, van Cauwenberge P, Bachert C. Nasal IL-5 levels determine the response to anti-IL-5 treatment in patients with nasal polyps. J Allergy Clin Immunol. 2006;118:1133–41.
39. Bachert C, Mannent L, Naclerio RM, et al. Effect of subcutaneous dupilumab on nasal polyp burden in patients with chronic sinusitis and nasal polyposis: a randomized clinical trial. JAMA. 2016;315:469–79.
40. Pelaia C, Vatrella A, Gallelli L, Terracciano R, Navalesi P, Maselli R, Pelaia G. Dupilumab for the treatment of asthma. Expert Opin Biol Ther. 2017;17:1565–72.
41. Bhatt SP, Rabe KF, Hanania NA, et al. Dupilumab for COPD with type 2 inflammation indicated by eosinophil counts. N Engl J Med. 2023;389:205–14.
42. Bachert C, Hellings PW, Mullol J, et al. Dupilumab improves patient-reported outcomes in patients with chronic rhinosinusitis with nasal polyps and comorbid asthma. J Allergy Clin Immunol Pract. 2019;7:2447–9.
43. Otten J, van der Lans R, de Corso E, et al. Evaluation of switching or simultaneous use of biologic treatment in patients with severe chronic rhinosinusitis with nasal polyps and severe asthma. Considerations in clinical decision making. Expert Rev Clin Immunol. 2023;19:1041–9.
44. Bachert C, Han JK, Desrosiers M, et al. Efficacy and safety of dupilumab in patients with severe chronic rhinosinusitis with nasal polyps (LIBERTY NP SINUS-24 and LIBERTY NP SINUS-52): results from two multicentre, randomised, double-blind, placebo-controlled, parallel-group phase 3 trials. Lancet. 2019;394:1638–50.
45. Fujieda S, Matsune S, Takeno S, et al. The effect of dupilumab on intractable chronic rhinosinusitis with nasal polyps in Japan. Laryngoscope. 2021;131:E1770–7.
46. Albrecht T, Sailer MM, Capitani F, van Schaik C, Löwenheim H, Becker S. Real-world evidence for the effectiveness and safety of dupilumab in patients with CRSwNP after 1 year of therapy. World Allergy Organ J. 2023;16:100780.
47. Hopkins C, Wagenmann M, Bachert C, et al. Efficacy of dupilumab in patients with a history of prior sinus surgery for chronic rhinosinusitis with nasal polyps. Int Forum Allergy Rhinol. 2021;11:1087–101.
48. Desrosiers M, Mannent LP, Amin N, et al. Dupilumab reduces systemic corticosteroid use and sinonasal surgery rate in CRSwNP. Rhinology. 2021;59:301–11.
49. Chuang C-C, Guillemin I, Bachert C, et al. Dupilumab in CRSwNP: responder analysis using clinically meaningful efficacy outcome thresholds. Laryngoscope. 2022;132:259–64.
50. Berger P, Menzies-Gow A, Peters AT, et al. Long-term efficacy of dupilumab in asthma with or without chronic rhinosinusitis and nasal polyps. Ann Allergy Asthma Immunol. 2023;130:215–24.
51. Galletti C, Barbieri MA, Ciodaro F, Freni F, Galletti F, Spina E, Galletti B. Effectiveness and safety profile of dupilumab in chronic rhinosinusitis with nasal polyps: real-life data in tertiary care. Pharmaceuticals. 2023;16(4):630. https://doi.org/10.3390/ph16040630.
52. Thamboo A, Kilty S, Witterick I, et al. Canadian Rhinology Working Group consensus statement: biologic therapies for chronic rhinosinusitis. J Otolaryngol Head Neck Surg. 2021;50:15.
53. Rizzi A, Gammeri L, Cordiano R, et al. Therapeutic strategies to prevent the recurrence of nasal polyps after surgical treatment: an update and in vitro study on growth inhibition of fibroblasts. J Clin Med. 2023;12(8):2841. https://doi.org/10.3390/jcm12082841.
54. Bai J, Huang JH, Price CPE, et al. Prognostic factors for polyp recurrence in chronic rhinosinusitis with nasal polyps. J Allergy Clin Immunol. 2022;150:352–61.
55. Gelardi M, Bocciolini C, Notargiacomo M, et al. Chronic rhinosinusitis with nasal polyps: how to identify eligible patients for biologics in clinical practice. Acta Otorhinolaryngol Ital. 2022;42:75–81.
56. Mullol J, Azar A, Buchheit KM, Hopkins C, Bernstein JA. Chronic rhinosinusitis with nasal polyps: quality of life in the biologics era. J Allergy Clin Immunol Pract. 2022;10:1434–53.
57. Fokkens WJ, Viskens A-S, Backer V, et al. EPOS/EUFOREA update on indication and evaluation of biologics in chronic rhinosinusitis with nasal polyps 2023. Rhinology. 2023;61:194–202.

58. Miglani A, Soler ZM, Smith TL, Mace JC, Schlosser RJ. A comparative analysis of endoscopic sinus surgery versus biologics for treatment of chronic rhinosinusitis with nasal polyposis. Int Forum Allergy Rhinol. 2023;13:116–28.
59. Chen J, Wang H, Zhang C, Shi L, Zhang Q, Song X, Wang D, Hu L, Yu H, Sun X. Comparative short-term efficacy of endoscopic sinus surgery and biological therapies in chronic rhinosinusitis with nasal polyps: a network meta-analysis. Clin Transl Allergy. 2023;13:e12269.
60. Barroso B, Valverde-Monge M, Alobid I, et al. Improvement in olfaction in patients with CRSwNP and severe asthma taking anti-IgE and anti-IL-5 biologics: a real-life study. J Investig Allergol Clin Immunol. 2023;33:37–44.
61. Meier EC, Schmid-Grendelmeier P, Steiner UC, Soyka MB. Real-life experience of monoclonal antibody treatments in chronic rhinosinusitis with nasal polyposis. Int Arch Allergy Immunol. 2021;182:736–43.
62. Maza-Solano J, Calvo-Henríquez C, Alobid I, Álvarez-Cendrero M, Palomares Ó, Moreno-Luna R, Santos-Perez J, González-García J, Sánchez-Gómez S. Nasal symptoms in asthmatic patients under treatment with anti-IL-5 monoclonal antibodies. A real-life cohort study. J Clin Med. 2022;11(23):7056. https://doi.org/10.3390/jcm11237056.
63. Förster-Ruhrmann U, Stergioudi D, Szczepek AJ, Fluhr JW, Zuberbier T, Olze H, Bergmann K-C. A real-life comparison of pulmonary and nasal outcomes in patients with severe asthma and nasal polyposis treated with T2-biologics. World Allergy Organ J. 2023;16:100746.
64. Borish L, Cohen NA, Chupp G, et al. Evaluating enrollment and outcome criteria in trials of biologics for chronic rhinosinusitis with nasal polyps. Ann Allergy Asthma Immunol. 2022;129:160–8.
65. Geng B, Dilley M, Anterasian C. Biologic therapies for allergic rhinitis and nasal polyposis. Curr Allergy Asthma Rep. 2021;21:36.
66. Tsabouri S, Tseretopoulou X, Priftis K, Ntzani EE. Omalizumab for the treatment of inadequately controlled allergic rhinitis: a systematic review and meta-analysis of randomized clinical trials. J Allergy Clin Immunol Pract. 2014;2:332–40.
67. Vignola AM, Humbert M, Bousquet J, Boulet L-P, Hedgecock S, Blogg M, Fox H, Surrey K. Efficacy and tolerability of anti-immunoglobulin E therapy with omalizumab in patients with concomitant allergic asthma and persistent allergic rhinitis: SOLAR. Allergy. 2004;59:709–17.
68. Stock P, Rolinck-Werninghaus C, Wahn U, Hamelmann E. The role of anti-IgE therapy in combination with allergen specific immunotherapy for seasonal allergic rhinitis. BioDrugs. 2007;21:403–10.

# Fungal Sinusitis

# 22

Kamal Ebeid

**Key Points**

- Fungal ball is a noninvasive form of fungal rhinosinusitis. The treatment of choice for fungal ball is surgery, systemic antifungal therapy is not indicated.
- Surgical and medical treatment with surgical treatment as the first stage of treatment is the optimal management for allergic fungal rhinosinusitis.
- A high suspicion is required for the diagnosis of acute invasive fungal rhinosinusitis, which is suggested by the aggressive nature of this disease in the immunocompromised patient.
- Urgent medical treatment and aggressive surgical debridement may enhance the prognosis of acute invasive fungal rhinosinusitis.

## 22.1 Background

Fungi are present normally in our breathed air, thus they can be found in the mucous of every healthy and diseased nasal sinus. Not the fungi itself but the host immunity is the factor determining whether the fungi become a pathogen developing the pathological process or not. Based on that, the state of the host immunity is used in the classification of patients with fungal rhino sinusitis dividing them into the immune-competent group and immune-deficient group [1, 2].

K. Ebeid (✉)
Otorhinolaryngology Department, Tanta University, Tanta, Egypt
e-mail: kamal.ebeid@med.tanta.edu.eg


S. Elwany (ed.), *Current Rhinology*,
https://doi.org/10.1007/978-3-031-70077-4_22

For immune-competent individuals, the fungi become pathological when inhaled fungi debris can't be cleared from the sinus resulting in fungi deposition inside the sinus and multiplying forming a fungal ball with normal foreign body reaction from sinus mucosa. The pathology may arise from the abnormal hyper response of nasal mucosa from the inhaled fungi present normally in the air in an immune-competent patient resulting in what is known as Allergic fungal rhinosinusitis. For immune-compromised individuals, fungi acquire the ability to invade the mucosal lining of the sinus resulting in what is known as invasive fungal rhinosinusitis which may be acute or has a more chronic or indolent course depending on the degree of immunity deficiency [3].

## 22.2 Classification

1. Noninvasive fungal rhinosinusitis:
   (a) Fungal colonization
   (b) Fungal ball
   (c) Allergic fungal rhinosinusitis (AFRS)
   (d) Eosinophilic fungal rhinosinusitis (EFRS)
2. Invasive fungal rhinosinusitis:
   (a) Acute invasive fungal sinusitis
   (b) Granulomatous invasive fungal sinusitis
   (c) Chronic invasive fungal sinusitis

## 22.3 Fungal Colonization

Fungal colonization is commonly present in patients having nasal crusts due to other diseases. Fungal colonization per se is asymptomatic. Symptoms and treatment are those of the original disease.

## 22.4 Fungal Ball

Fungal ball is a collection of fungal debris inside usually one sinus without any invasion of the sinus mucosal lining by the fungal hyphae. Fungal ball may cause an inflammatory reaction inside the affected sinus which may extend to the other sinuses in the same functional unit as to the frontal and anterior ethmoid sinuses in case of maxillary sinus affection. This inflammatory response is a result of a foreign body reaction elected by the sinus mucosa toward the retained fungal mass inside the sinus [4].

Fungal ball is more common in females and elderly patients at the age of 50–60 years old. It affects mostly the maxillary sinus and less commonly the sphenoid sinus. Fungal ball can present without a prior diagnosis for up to 17 years in some documented cases. Although fungal ball usually is an incidental finding in a review study of 70 radiologically observed fungal balls, only 22–26% of cases were asymptomatic [5, 6].

Many studies demonstrated receiving dental treatment as a risk factor for developing maxillary sinus fungal ball. This increased incidence may be due to impaired mucociliary clearance due to inflamed mucosa because of periapical pathology, the procedure itself, or the extrusion of the filling material as zinc and copper are found in both dental filling materials and fungal ball. Other studies showed that the incidence of developing fungal ball isn't affected by the presence of different anatomical variants such as septal deviation, concha bullosa, and infraorbital Haller cell. Primary osteomeatal complex (OMC) occlusion has no role in developing fungal ball as fungal ball patients are less likely to have OMC occlusion in comparison with patients with CRS and there are a lot of reported cases in patients with patent OMC [6].

The predominance of the fungal ball in female gender may support the idea that the hormonal factors may be involved in the pathogenesis [7]. Another observation, first reported by Dufour et al. [8] indirectly confirmed a possible hormonal influence is the absence of fungal ball in children before puberty. It can be also hypothesized that the absence of fungal ball in young patients may be due to the rarity of endodontic treatments in this age group [7].

The presenting symptoms of fungal ball are nonspecific. Maxillary and ethmoid localizations frequently mimic chronic rhinosinusitis. Patients complain of longstanding unilateral nasal obstruction, purulent rhinorrhea with cacosmia, and facial pain scarcely responsive to anti-inflammatory or antibiotic agents. The most common presenting symptoms of the sphenoid fungal ball are vertex headache, sometimes associated with postnasal drip [4, 7–9].

Despite the long indolent course of the disease, the low-grade inflammation and expansible nature of the disease may cause orbital or intracranial infective complications. In some studies, 16% of cases of sphenoid sinus fungal developed orbital complications due to loss of bone wall architecture [10, 11].

One of the cornerstones of preoperative diagnostic workup is imaging studies. Both CT and MR findings of fungal ball are strictly related to the content of heavy metals (iron and manganese) and calcium within fungal hyphae. As a result, fungal balls appear spontaneously hyperdense at CT; microcalcifications, possibly scattered within the lesion, may also be observed. Though extremely specific, these signs lack sensitivity. The MRI pattern may often be misleading; in reality, the magnetic susceptibility of iron and manganese, combined with the reduced water content of fungal ball, accounts for the shortening of both T1 and T2. Consequently, on both sequences, MRI may show a sinus filled with a hypointense content bordered by hyperintense (T2) and enhancing (T1, after contrast administration) mucosa. In some cases, T1 and T2 signal shortening may be so marked that it results in a signal void, making discrimination between fungal ball and intrasinus air very difficult, particularly if improper windowing (brightness and contrast) is used. Chronically infected sinuses often show bony changes (focal or diffuse) that encompass both remodeling or erosion and areas of thickened, osteitic-like bone [7, 12].

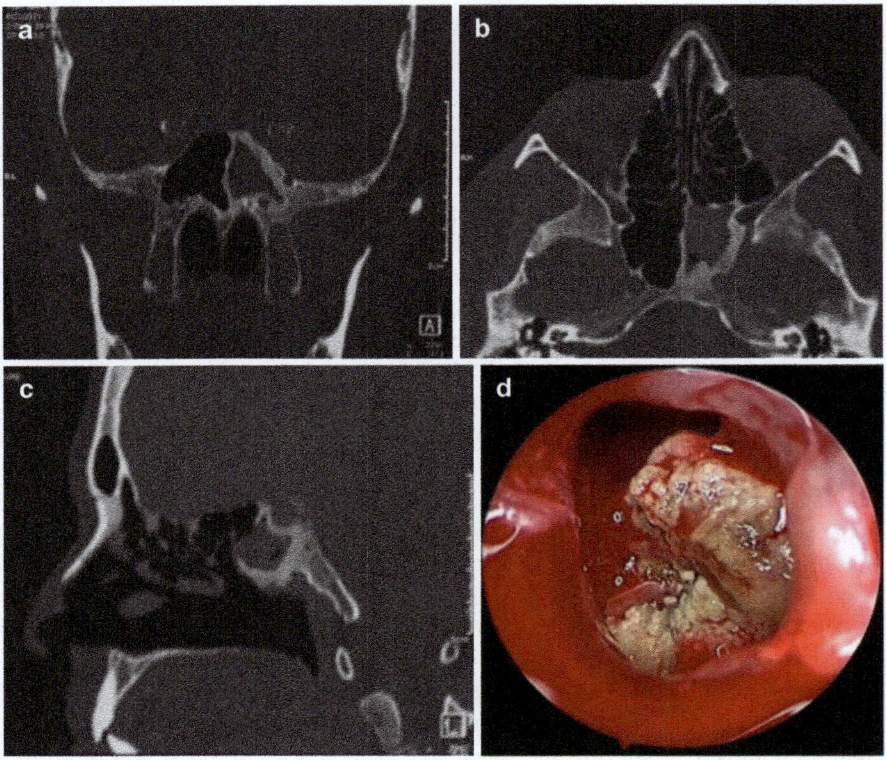


**Fig. 22.1** CT scan of the paranasal sinuses showing left-sided isolated sphenoidal opacity with sclerotic bony wall. (**a**) Coronal cuts, (**b**) axial cuts, (**c**) sagittal cuts, (**d**) endoscopic view of the left sphenoidal cavity filled with fungal debris

The treatment of choice for fungal ball is surgery, which removes fungal debris from the affected sinus and reestablishes proper ventilation and drainage. Pure endoscopic approach should be considered the gold standard in the treatment of paranasal sinus fungal ball (Figs. 22.1 and 22.2) [7, 13].

Endoscopy may be combined with a canine fossa approach to better visualization of the anteroinferior part of the maxillary sinus and the lacrimal recess and to remove residual fungal elements. The canine fossa approach may cause persistent facial numbness, pain, and/or tingling due to the damage to the anterior superior alveolar nerve and its branches [14, 15].

Moreover, the use of a 70-angled scope, angled suction tube, and curved antrum forceps also allows visualization of the anterior wall of the maxillary sinus and removal of residual fungal debris, respectively, without the need for other approaches [7].

Chao and Liu [16] proposed combining endoscopy with a so-called gauze-assisted technique, which attempts to expel fungal debris from the anterior corner of the maxillary sinus by pushing gauze into it.

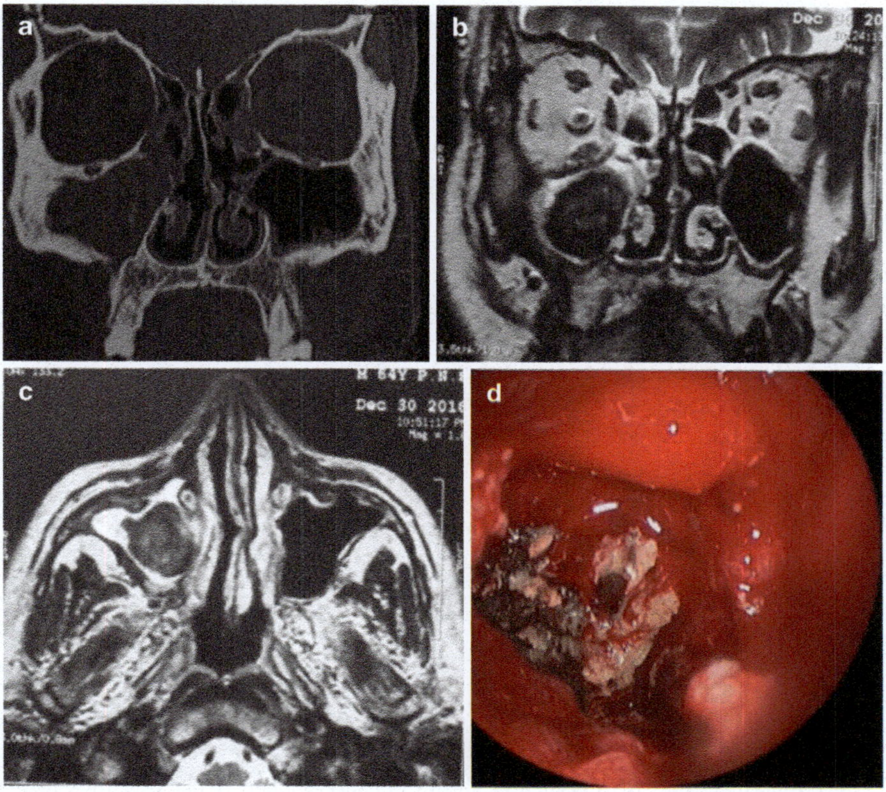


**Fig. 22.2** (**a**) CT scan (coronal cuts) of the paranasal sinuses showing right-sided maxillary sinus opacity with sclerotic bony wall. (**b**, **c**) Coronal and axial cuts of MRI of the paranasal sinuses showing hypointensity lesion surrounded with hyperintensity of the inflamed maxillary sinus mucosa. (**d**) Endoscopic view of the left sphenoidal cavity filled with fungal debris

Histologic examination, by assessing the presence of fungal hyphae in the concretions and excluding mucosal invasion, is essential for the diagnosis of fungal ball. Microbiological evaluation is useful to identify fungal species. It is, however, well known that, upon culture, growth of fungal elements is difficult to obtain, with a positivity rate ranging between 23% and 50% [17].

Long- term postoperative mucostasis occurred in 17.9% of patients following an adequate maxillary antrostomy for the treatment of a fungal ball with a greater need for further surgery (modified medial maxillectomy) [18].

## 22.5 Allergic Fungal Rhinosinusitis

Allergic fungal rhinosinusitis (AFRS) is a type I IgE-mediated hypersensitivity of the sinus mucosal lining against fungal debris deposited on the sinus mucosa. AFRS is considered a special type of polypoid chronic rhinosinusitis which is characterized by the presence of allergic or eosinophilic mucin without invasion of the fungal hyphae into the sinus mucosa. Although other types of polypoid CRS may have allergic sensitization against fungi, AFRS is distinct from those types with higher IgE levels. AFRS is more common in females and young adults with an incidence as common as 5% of all chronic rhinosinusitis cases [19–21].

The Bent-Kuhn diagnostic criteria postulated five major criteria to diagnose AFRS [22], those criteria are:

1. Nasal polyps
2. Presence of fungi identified by staining
3. The presence of eosinophilic mucin
4. Type I hypersensitivity against fungi
5. CT finding of unilaterality, anatomical discrete sinus involvement, and soft tissue differential densities

All those five criteria should be met for the optimal diagnosis of AFRS as at least three of them are common findings in most types of polypoid CRS.

The other minor criteria include:

1. The presence of bone erosions
2. Unilateral pathology
3. Charcot-Leyden crystals
4. Peripheral eosinophilia

CT imaging of AFRS classically shows densely packed hyper densities in the paranasal sinuses along with expansion and erosion of the affected sinus wall. Those hyper densities are the result of the high-level proteins and low levels of the free water content of allergic mucin along with air, calcium deposits, and metals such as iron, magnesium, and manganese. Those are the same reasons for the signal voids in both T1 and T2 found in the MRI scan of AFRS [23].

Most of the clinical studies indicate that the combination of endoscopic sinus surgery and perioperative systemic steroids as the first stage of treatment is the optimal management for AFRS. Almost all cases of AFRS require surgical debridement of the affected sinuses to remove the antigenic stimulation, promoting sinus drainage and for easier access to topical treatment (Fig. 22.3) [24, 25].

Systemic corticosteroids can play an important role in both pre- and postoperative treatment regimes of AFRS. Intranasal Corticosteroids may play an important role in controlling AFRS [26].

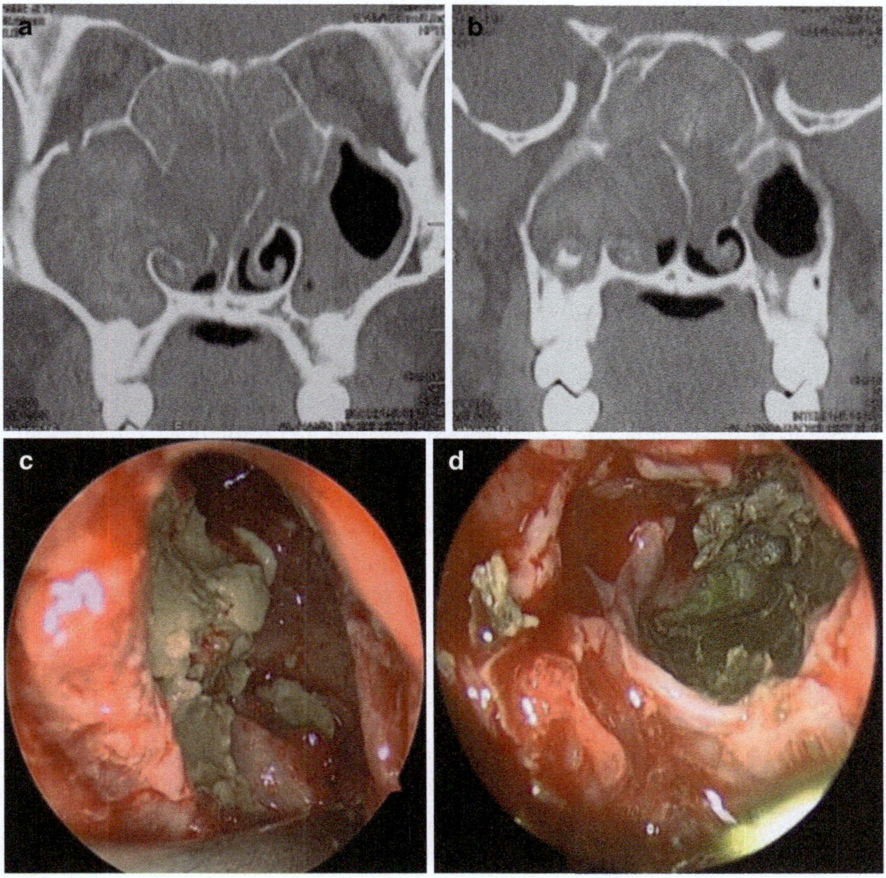


**Fig. 22.3** (**a**, **b**) CT scan (coronal cuts) of the paranasal sinuses showing expansion of the paranasal sinus walls by heterogenic opacity. (**c**, **d**) Endoscopic view of the right maxillary and sphenoidal cavity filled with fungal debris respectively

## 22.6 Eosinophilic Fungal Rhinosinusitis (EFRS)

Eosinophilic fungal rhinosinusitis (eosinophil-related fungal rhinosinusitis) is a less recognized noninvasive eosinophilic inflammation of the sinonasal mucosa. It is non-IgE-mediated inflammation, and it is commonly associated with nasal polyps. The fungi trigger cytokine-driven eosinophilic inflammation in the sinuses independent from IgE-mediated allergy. Treatment is the same as allergic fungal sinusitis.

## 22.7 Acute Invasive Fungal Sinusitis

Invasive fungal rhinosinusitis, also known as mucormycosis (black fungus), describes fungal infection to paranasal sinuses where the fungal hyphae can be seen within the mucosal tissue demonstrating angioinvasion or other infiltrative patterns. Mucormycosis is an acute, often fatal infection caused by fungi of the family Mucoraceae. The principal pathogens in this family are Rhizopus, Mucor, and Absidia species. Often, mucormycosis attacks immunocompromised patients, notably poorly controlled diabetes mellitus, blood dyscrasias, severe burns, renal diseases, sepsis, severe dehydration, and liver cirrhosis [27–37].

The clinical presentation of mucormycosis is highly variable, making early diagnosis challenging. Clinical signs are nonspecific and include fever, headache, nasal congestion, facial numbness, ophthalmoplegia, and vision loss. Neurologic manifestations arise secondary to vascular inflammation and thrombosis by angioinvasion with the fungal hyphae. Intracranial extension of the fungi into the cavernous sinus, brain parenchyma, and meninges represents the most ominous disease course and results in a dramatically worse prognosis [38–41].

Sudden onset and rapid progression of mucormycosis-like symptoms in an immunosuppressed individual should raise a clinician's suspicion of a fungal infection [40].

Signs of mucormycosis on MRI include obliteration or infiltration of perimaxillary fat, inflammatory changes in orbital fat and extraocular muscles, and leptomeningeal enhancement. MRI is preferred over CT for its superior soft tissue visualization. CT is better able to detect bone erosion, which occurs later in acute invasive fungal infections and is unlikely to contribute to an earlier diagnosis (Figs. 22.4 and 22.5) [42, 43].

Nasal endoscopy allowed for rapid, minimally invasive biopsy. Visualizing hyphae from frozen sections of the biopsied specimen can shorten the time to diagnosis, guide surgical debridement, and allow for rapid medical intervention (Figs. 22.6 and 22.7) [42].

Reversal of the immunosuppressed state is considered critical for eradicating mucormycosis. Early aggressive surgical resection with clear margins and systemic antifungal therapy are paramount in this life-threatening condition. Considering the severity of this disease, an aggressive surgical approach is required, often including orbital exenteration [39, 40].

Orbital exenteration may improve a patient's prognosis but the indications for doing so remain unclear [44]. A review of 179 AIFS cases found that orbital exenteration may be required in the case of retinal artery thrombosis, orbital apex

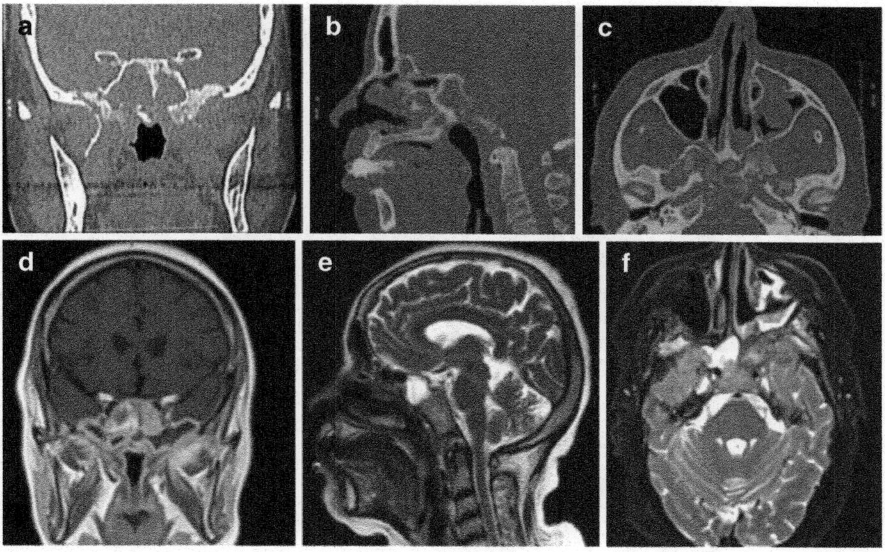


**Fig. 22.4** (**a**–**c**) CT scan (coronal, sagittal, and axial cuts) of the paranasal sinuses showing sphenoid bone fungal osteomyelitis. (**d**–**f**) MRI (coronal, sagittal, and axial cuts) of the paranasal sinuses of the same patient demonstrating mucosal changes of the sphenoid sinus with osteomyelitis of the sphenoid bone

necrosis, or ocular invasion [45]. A second review of 292 mucormycosis patients found that exenteration improved survival only in those who had a fever [46]. The objective of orbital exenteration is to remove fungal infections showing signs of spread to the orbit. There are no standard treatment guidelines for either traditional or globe-sparing orbital exenteration in treating AIFRS (Figs. 22.8 and 22.9) [47].

The medical treatment consists mainly of a low-toxicity Lyophilized Amphotericin-B, it is less nephrotoxic than Amphotericin-B, allowing the drug to be administered at higher doses, and even 20-fold doses, for a longer duration [48].

The new triazole Cresemba is an isavuconazole prodrug that is approved for use in invasive mucormycosis and aspergillosis. It has fewer serious adverse effects and drug-drug interactions compared to Posaconazole and voriconazole [49].

During COVID-19 pandemic, acute invasive fungal rhinosinusitis may be a fatal complication of critically ill COVID-19 patients and its early diagnosis and initiation of appropriate antifungal therapy together with surgical debridement is essential to reduce high mortality rate [50].

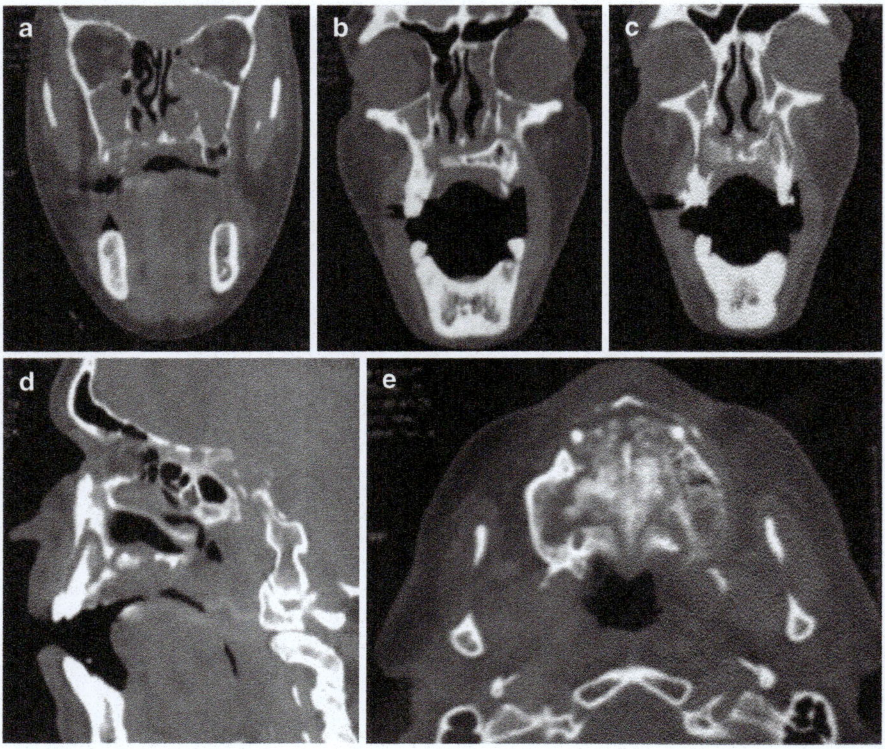


**Fig. 22.5** (**a**–**c**) CT scan coronal cuts, (**d**, **e**) sagittal and axial cuts of the paranasal sinuses showing alveolar bone, palate, medial and lateral maxillary walls resorption consistent with maxillary bone fungal osteomyelitis. Also, there are mucosal polypoidal changes in both maxillary sinuses and ethmoidal air cells

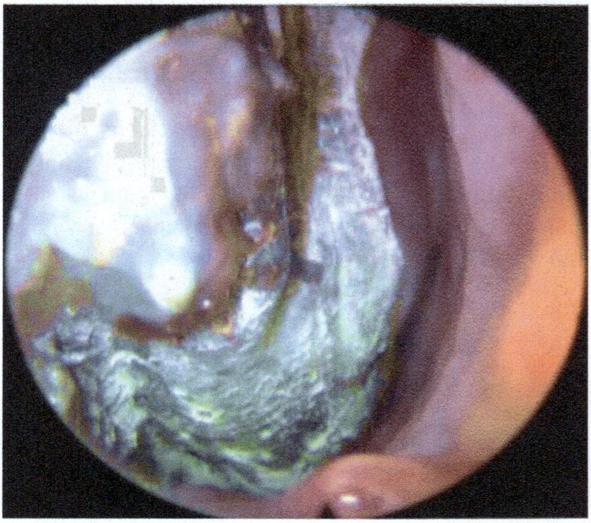

**Fig. 22.6** Endoscopic view of a patient presented with acute invasive fungal rhinosinusitis showing marked gangrene of the right middle turbinate tissues

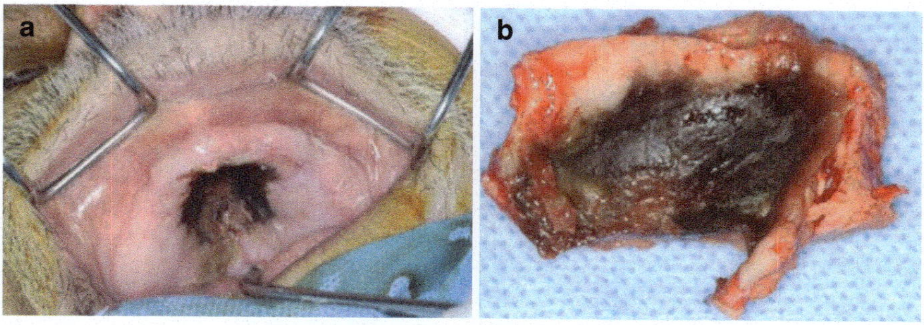


**Fig. 22.7** (**a**) Intraoral view of a patient with acute invasive fungal rhinosinusitis showing gangrene of the hard palate, (**b**) surgical specimen of the patient after surgical debridement

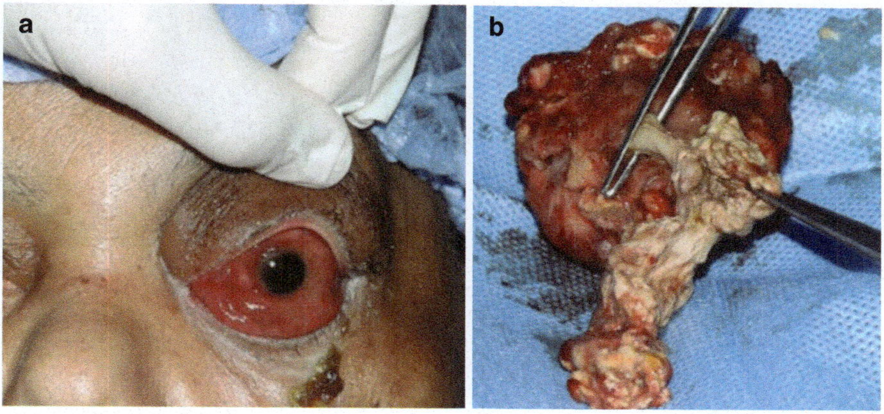


**Fig. 22.8** (**a**) A patient with acute invasive fungal rhinosinusitis presented with left orbital apex syndrome together with severe conjunctival edema and proptosis, (**b**) surgical specimen of the patient after orbit exenteration and surgical debridement showing necrosis of the optic nerve and adnexal tissues

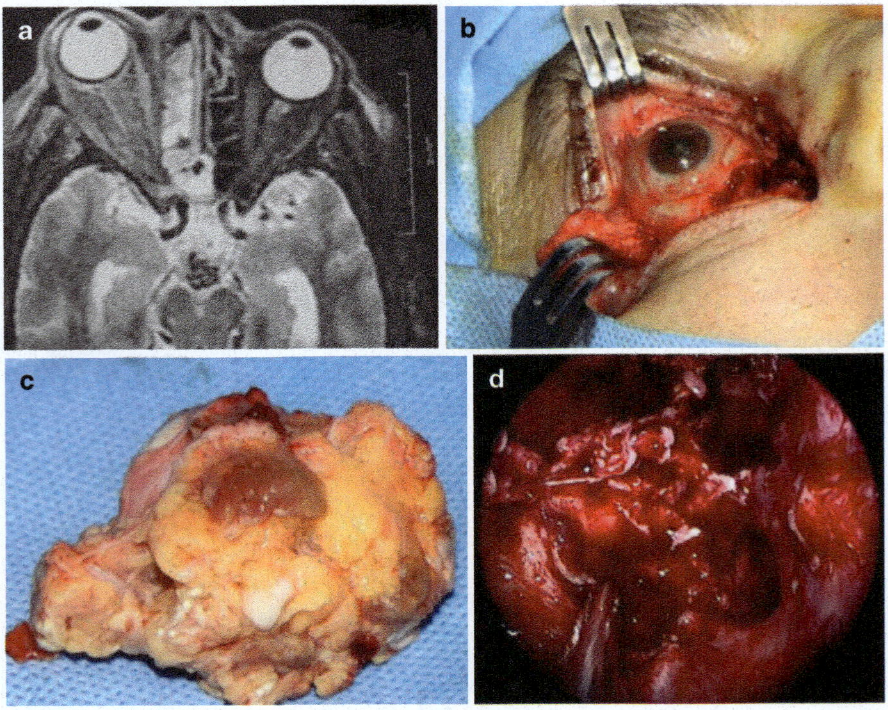


**Fig. 22.9** A 61-year-old female patient presented with right orbital apex syndrome and extensive necrosis of the right nasal cavity. (**a**) MRI T2-weighted image showing extensive fungal invasion of the right orbital tissues with evident proptosis. (**b**) Open approach for orbit exenteration and debridement of the right nasal cavity. (**c**) Orbit eventration specimen showing evident necrotic orbital tissues. (**d**) View of the operative cavity after orbit exenteration and extensive debridement

## 22.8 Granulomatous Invasive Fungal Rhinosinusitis

Chronic granulomatous invasive fungal rhinosinusitis and chronic invasive fungal rhinosinusitis have a longer time course than acute invasive rhinosinusitis. The main differences between chronic and granulomatous invasive fungal rhinosinusitis are the histopathological characteristics and the immune status of the patients [51].

Granulomatous invasive fungal rhinosinusitis is a noncaseating granuloma around a few fungal hyphae with Langhans-type giant cells, vasculitis, vascular proliferation, and perivascular fibrosis. It is most associated with *Aspergillus flavus* infection in immunocompetent patients. The disease occurs more commonly in hot humid countries.

CT shows soft tissue mass within one or more sinuses, bone destruction, and infiltration of surrounding tissues. The lesion may be a mistaken malignancy.

T1-weighted MRI with contrast shows variable hypointensity and T2-weighted MRI usually shows low signal intensity.

The mortality rate is about 5–20%. Treatment is the same as acute invasive fungal sinusitis [52].

## 22.9 Chronic Invasive Fungal Rhinosinusitis

Chronic invasive fungal rhinosinusitis is a nongranulomatous, slowly destructive process which is more commonly in diabetics and acquired immunodeficiency syndrome (AIDS). The disease is characterized by the dense accumulation of the hyphae, occasional invasion of the blood vessels, and destructive involvement of adjacent tissues. The disease is usually associated with *Aspergillus fumigatus*. The Mortality rate is about 20–40%. Treatment is the same as acute invasive fungal sinusitis [53].

## References


1. Buzina W, Braun H, Freudenschuss K, Lackner A, Habermann W, Stammberger H. Fungal biodiversity–as found in nasal mucus. Med Mycol. 2003;41:149–61.
2. Chakrabarti A, Denning DW, Ferguson BJ, et al. Fungal rhinosinusitis: a categorization and definitional schema addressing current controversies. Laryngoscope. 2009;119:1809–18.
3. Toussain G, Botterel F, Alsamad IA, et al. Sinus fungal balls: characteristics and management in patients with host factors for invasive infection. Rhinology. 2012;50:269–76.
4. Grosjean P, Weber R. Fungus balls of the paranasal sinuses: a review. Eur Arch Otorrinolaringol. 2007;264:461–70.
5. Yoon YH, Xu J, Park SK, Heo JH, Kim YM, Rha KS. A retrospective analysis of 538 sinonasal fungus ball cases treated at a single tertiary medical center in Korea (1996-2015). Int Forum Allergy Rhinol. 2017;7:1070–5.
6. Seo MY, Lee SH, Ryu G, et al. Clinical pattern of fungal balls in the paranasal sinuses: our experience with 70 patients. Eur Arch Otorrinolaringol. 2019;276:1035–8.
7. Nicolai P, Lombardi D, Tomenzoli D, Villaret AB, Piccioni M, Mensi M, Maroldi R. Fungus ball of the paranasal sinuses: experience in 160 patients treated with endoscopic surgery. Laryngoscope. 2009;119:2275–9.
8. Dufour X, Kauffmann-Lacroix C, Ferrie JC, Goujons JM, Rodier MH, Klossek JM. Paranasal sinus fungus ball: epidemiology, clinical features, and diagnosis. A retrospective analysis of 173 cases from a single medical center in France, 1989–2002. Med Mycol. 2006;44:61–7.
9. Klossek JM, Serrano E, Peloquin L, Percodani J, Fontanel JP, Pessey JJ. Functional endoscopic sinus surgery and 109 mycetomas of paranasal sinuses. Laryngoscope. 1997;107:112–7.
10. Bowman J, Panizza B, Gandhi M. Sphenoid sinus fungal balls. Ann Otol Rhinol Laryngol. 2007;116:514–9.
11. Jung JH, Cho GS, Chung YS, Lee BJ. Clinical characteristics and outcome in patients with isolated sphenoid sinus aspergilloma. Auris Nasus Larynx. 2013;40:189–93.
12. Lee TJ, Huang SF, Chang PH. Characteristics of isolated sphenoid sinus aspergilloma: report of twelve cases and literature review. Ann Otol Rhinol Larynges. 2009;118:211–7.
13. Pagella F, Matti E, De Bernardi F, et al. Paranasal sinus fungus ball: diagnosis and management. Mycoses. 2007;50:451–6.

14. Feng LR, Tang CQ, Guo QM. Treatment of non-invasive aspergillosis of maxillary sinus by functional endoscopic sinus surgery. Lin Chuang Er Bi Yan Hou Ke Za Zhi. 2000;14:554–5.
15. Robinson S, Wormald PJ. The incidence of complications after canine fossa puncture performed during endoscopic sinus surgery. Am J Rhinol. 2005;19:203–6.
16. Chao TK, Liu CM. Gauze-assisted technique in endoscopic removal of fungus ball of the maxillary sinus. Am J Rhinol. 2006;20:417–20.
17. Ferreiro JA, Carlson BA, Cody DT. Paranasal sinus fungus balls. Head Neck. 1997;19:481–6.
18. Cavada MN, Wong E, Orgain CA, Grayson JW, Alvarado R, Campbell RG, Kalish L, Harvey RJ. Fungal ball of the maxillary sinus and the risk of persistent sinus dysfunction after simple antrostomy. Am J Otolaryngol. 2020;41(4):102541.
19. Kuhn FA, Javer AR. Allergic fungal rhinosinusitis: perioperative management, prevention of recurrence, and role of steroids and antifungal agents. Otolaryngol Clin N Am. 2000;33:419–33.
20. Bakhshaee M, Fereidouni M, Nourollahian M, Movahed R. The presence of fungal-specific IgE in serum and sinonasal tissue among patients with sinonasal polyposis. Eur Arch Otorrinolaringol. 2014;271:2871–5.
21. Lu-Myers Y, Deal AM, Miller JD, et al. Comparison of socioeconomic and demographic factors in patients with chronic rhinosinusitis and allergic fungal rhinosinusitis. Otolaryngol Head Neck Surg. 2015;153:137–43.
22. Bent JP, Kuhn FA, Bent JP, Kuhn FA. Diagnosis of allergic fungal sinusitis. Otolaryngol Head Neck Surg. 1994;111:580–8.
23. Aribandi M, McCoy VA, Bazan C. Imaging features of invasive and noninvasive fungal sinusitis: a review. Radiographics. 2007;27:1283–96.
24. Hoyt AEW, Borish L, Gurrola J, Payne S. Allergic fungal rhinosinusitis. J Allergy Clin Immunol Pract. 2016;4:599–604.
25. Marple BF, Mabry RL. Allergic fungal sinusitis: learning from our failures. Am J Rhinol. 2000;14:223–6.
26. Ikram M, Abbas A, Suhail A, Onali MA, Akhtar S, Iqbal M. Management of allergic fungal sinusitis with postoperative oral and nasal steroids: a controlled study. Ear Nose Throat J. 2009;88:8–11.
27. Ribes JA, Vanover-Sams CL, Baker DJ. Zygomycetes in human disease. Clin Microbiol Rev. 2000;13:236–301.
28. Blitzer A, Lawson W. Fungal infections of the nose and paranasal sinuses. Part I. Otolaryngol Clin N Am. 1993;26:1007–35.
29. Fairley C, Sullivan TJ, Bartley P, Allworth T, Lewandowski R. Survival after rhino-orbital-cerebral mucormycosis in an immunocompetent patient. Ophthalmology. 2000;107:555–8.
30. Naussbaum ES, Holl WA. Rhinocerebral mucormycosis: changing patterns of disease. Surg Neurol. 1994;41:152–6.
31. Harill WC, Stewart MG, Lee AG, Cernoch P. Chronic rhinocerebral mucormycosis. Laryngoscope. 1996;106:1292–7.
32. Yohai RA, Bullock JD, Aziz AA, Markert RJ. Survival factors in rhino-orbital-cerebral mucormycosis. Surv Ophthalmol. 1994;39:3–22.
33. Thajeb P, Thajeb T, Dai D. Fatal strokes in patients with rhino-orbito-cerebral mucormycosis and associated vasculopathy. Scand J Infect Dis. 2004;36:643–8.
34. McDevitt GR Jr, Brantley MJ, Cawthon MA. Rhinocerebral mucormycosis: a case report with magnetic resonance imaging findings. Clin Imaging. 1989;13:317–20.
35. Luna JD, Ponssa XS, Rodriguez SD, Luna NC, Juarez CP. Intraconal amphotericin B for the treatment of rhinoorbital mucormycosis. Ophthalmic Surg Lasers. 1996;27:706–8.
36. Lee BL, Holland GN, Glasgow BJ. Chiasmal infarction and sudden blindness caused by mucormycosis in AIDS and diabetes mellitus. Am J Ophthalmol. 1996;122:895–6.
37. Georgopoulou S, Kounougeri E, Katsenos C, Rizos M, Michalopoulos A. Rhinocerebral mucormycosis in a patient with cirrhosis and chronic renal failure. Hepato-Gastroenterology. 2003;50:843–5.
38. Peterson KL, Wang M, Canalis RF, et al. Rhinocerebral mucormycosis: evolution of the disease and treatment options. Laryngoscope. 1997;107:855–62.

39. Spellberg B, Edwards J Jr, Ibrahim A. Novel perspectives on mucormycosis: pathophysiology, presentation, and management. Clin Microbiol Rev. 2005;18:556–69.
40. Turner JH, Soudry E, Nayak JV, et al. Survival outcomes in acute invasive fungal sinusitis: a systematic review and quantitative synthesis of published evidence. Laryngoscope. 2013;123:1112–8.
41. Lee DH, Yoon TM, Lee JK, et al. Invasive fungal sinusitis of the sphenoid sinus. Clin Exp Otorhinolaryngol. 2014;7:181–7.
42. Groppo ER, El-Sayed IH, Aiken AH, et al. Computed tomography and magnetic resonance imaging characteristics of acute invasive fungal sinusitis. Arch Otolaryngol Head Neck Surg. 2011;137:1005–10.
43. Shaban E, Saleh RA, Ammar MI, et al. post-COVID-19 acute invasive fungal rhinosinusitis: a systematic radiological approach in the light of clinico-surgical characteristics. Egypt J Radiol Nucl Med. 2022;53:206.
44. Plowes Hernandez O, Prado Calleros HM, Soberon Marmissolle Daguerre GS, et al. Rhino-orbito-cerebral mucormycosis. Management strategies to avoid or limit intracraneal affection and improve survival. Acta Otorrinolaringol Esp. 2015;66:348–52.
45. Blitzer A, Lawson W, Meyers BR, et al. Patient survival factors in paranasal sinus mucormycosis. Laryngoscope. 1980;90:635–48.
46. Hargrove RN, Wesley RE, Klippenstein KA, et al. Indications for orbital exenteration in mucormycosis. Ophthalmic Plast Reconstr Surg. 2006;22:286–91.
47. Colon-Acevedo B, Kumar J, Richard MJ, et al. The role of adjunctive therapies in the management of invasive sino-orbital infection. Ophthalmic Plast Reconstr Surg. 2015;31:401–5.
48. Jung SH, Kim SW, Park CS, Song CE, Cho JH, Lee JH, Kim NS, Kang JM. Rhinocerebral mucormycosis: consideration of prognostic factors and treatment modality. Auris Nasus Larynx. 2009;36(3):274–9.
49. Miceli MH, Kauffman CA. Isavuconazole: a new broad-spectrum triazole antifungal agent. Clin Infect Dis. 2015;61:1558–65.
50. Ebeid K, Gamea M, Allam AA, Shehata E. Impact of COVID-19 on acute invasive fungal rhinosinusitis: a comparative study. Egypt J Ear Nose Throat Allied Sci. 2021;22:1–7.
51. Stringer SP, Ryan MW. Chronic invasive fungal rhinosinusitis. Otolaryngol Clin N Am. 2000;33(2):375–87.
52. Chakrabarti A, Denning DW, Ferguson BJ, Ponikau J, Buzina W, Kita H. Fungal rhinosinusitis: a categorization and definitional schema addressing current controversies. Laryngoscope. 2009;119(9):1809–18.
53. Nakaya K, Oshima T, Kudo T, Aoyagi I, Katori Y, Ota J. New treatment for invasive fungal sinusitis: three cases of chronic invasive fungal sinusitis treated with surgery and voriconazole. Auris Nasus Larynx. 2010;37(2):244–9.

# Allergic Fungal Rhinosinusitis

# 23

Rayan AlFallaj and Saad Alsaleh

**Key Points**

- Allergic fungal rhinosinusitis (AFRS) is a subtype of chronic sinusitis with nasal polyps that exhibits type 2 inflammation, characterized by the distinct presence of eosinophilic mucin, along with fungal hyphae.
- The diagnosis of AFRS primarily follows the diagnostic criteria established by Bent and Kuhn, as AFRS is characterized by unique clinical and radiological features.
- The current gold standard for managing AFRS cases consists of functional endoscopic sinus surgery and postoperative steroid nasal rinses, focusing on eliminating mucin and fungal debris.
- Biologic therapies are emerging as promising treatment options for AFRS cases.

## 23.1 Introduction

Chronic rhinosinusitis (CRS) can be classified into two types: localized or diffuse, based on the type of inflammation present, which can also be categorized as either T-helper 2 (Th2) or non-T-helper 2 (non-Th2). For instance, allergic fungal rhinosinusitis (AFRS) is characterized by chronic inflammation that is dependent on the Th2 immune response [1], and it is considered a specific subtype of CRS that can be distinguished from others according to the presence of hypersensitivity, sinus

**Supplementary Information** The online version contains supplementary material available at https://doi.org/10.1007/978-3-031-70077-4_23.

R. AlFallaj · S. Alsaleh (✉)
Department of Otolaryngology–Head and Neck Surgery, King Saud University, Riyadh, Kingdom of Saudi Arabia


S. Elwany (ed.), *Current Rhinology*,
https://doi.org/10.1007/978-3-031-70077-4_23

expansion, nasal polyps, and the characteristic occurrence of eosinophilic mucin, along with fungal hyphae [1, 2]. Fungal rhinosinusitis can be categorized into two main types: invasive and noninvasive, where invasive types include acute invasive fungal sinusitis (AIFRS), chronic invasive fungal sinusitis (CIFRS), and chronic granulomatous fungal rhinosinusitis (CGFRS). Conversely, noninvasive types include fungus ball, saprophytic fungal infection, and allergic fungal rhinosinusitis (AFRS) [1], the latter of which is a type of noninvasive AFS associated with an allergic reaction to fungi within the nasal cavity [1] and which accounts for approximately 5–10% of CRS cases [3].

## 23.2 Epidemiology of AFRS

AFRS is primarily observed in regions with high humidity, where mold counts are notably elevated. In these specific locations, AFRS can account for up to 32% of CRS cases that undergo functional endoscopic sinus surgery (FESS). The onset of AFRS tends to occur at a younger age, typically between 21 and 33 years, and it is more frequently diagnosed in African Americans, with a higher incidence among males (with a male-to-female ratio ranging from 1.5 to 2.6:1) [4]. AlQahtani et al. conducted a global ecological study, revealing that regions experiencing higher temperatures had a greater occurrence of AFRS [5]. Conversely, cities characterized by a humid continental climate exhibited a significantly lower prevalence of AFRS. Surprisingly, areas with a higher prevalence of AFRS were found to have lower humidity levels, but the study found no significant impact of socioeconomic factors on the prevalence of AFRS [5]. Meanwhile, retrospective studies have revealed that individuals with AFRS often exhibit more complex and advanced stages of the disease than other forms of CRS [4].

## 23.3 Molecular and Immune Profile

Carney et al. conducted immunohistochemistry analysis on AFRS tissue for comparison with nonallergic eosinophilic fungal sinusitis (NEFS) and CRS. The study found similar quantitative measures of mast cells, eosinophils, and IgE cells between AFRS and NEFS [6]. However, Tyler et al. performed microarray analysis on 130 patients with various subtypes of CRS, revealing that AFRS and AERD tissue exhibited higher levels of local IgE compared to other subtypes. Furthermore, all subtypes of CRS, including CRSwNP, AERD, AFRS, and CRSsNP, demonstrated markers of type 2 inflammation, such as IL-13 and IL-5, but IL-5 was specifically associated with AFRS and CRSwNP. Gene expression clusters related to eosinophilic inflammation, such as CCL13, CCL18, CCL26, and periostin, were overexpressed in all subtypes examined [4]. Additionally, AFS has been linked to class II major histocompatibility (MHC) with the beta chains of human leukocyte antigens (HLAs)—DQB1*0301* and *DQB1*0302 [7].

## 23.4 Pathogenesis of AFRS

Understanding the pathogenesis of AFRS fully remains a topic of debate, but it has been observed that AFRS shares similar pathophysiological mechanisms with allergic bronchopulmonary aspergillosis (ABPA). Additionally, the development of AFRS is believed to be influenced by the dysregulation of innate immunity.

The epithelial barrier of the sinonasal mucosa acts as the primary defense mechanism against microbial and allergenic challenges. It serves as an initial protective layer consisting of diverse cells, peptides, and proteins involved in the adaptive immune response. AFRS is also characterized by a defective and diminished epithelial barrier, distinguishing it from other forms of CRS inflammation. As such, this compromised barrier is believed to be a contributing factor to the persistent type 2 inflammation triggered by fungal antigens in AFRS. Analysis using microarrays on AFRS samples revealed increased levels of IL-33, believed to contribute to the development of type 2 inflammation. Further, it was found that fungal antigens can stimulate the production of IL-33 and stimulate the allergic response in predisposed individuals [8–10].

Certain types of fungal organisms, such as Aspergillus, and dematiaceous fungi, including Bipolaris, Curvularia, and Alternaria, have been associated with the development of AFRS. However, unlike invasive fungal sinusitis, their role in AFRS is primarily allergenic rather than pathogenic [11]. Yet, there is controversy regarding the fungal theory and its contributory role in AFRS. One side of the debate, supported by Braun et al., states that fungi can be found in the sinus secretions of both diseased patients and healthy individuals [12]. However, Porter et al. found that fungi are more prevalent in CRS with nasal polyps (CRSwNP) and even more so in AFRS. Thus, they propose that the development of phenotypic AFRS is due to host factors, such as the hypersensitivity response and immunologic memory of the fungi. They further suggest that altered mucosal barrier physiology, fungi-activated molecular signaling, and an exaggerated type 2 immune response are primary drivers of airway inflammation in response to fungi, which are not present in non–TH2-associated disease [13].

Conversely, the opposing side of the debate, known as Ponikau theory, suggests that fungi are the drivers of all CRS inflammation, inducing type 2 inflammation. However, a key argument against this theory is the lack of a clear therapeutic response to antifungal treatment in individuals with CRS [14].

In sum, the debate primarily concerns the role of fungi in AFRS and CRS, with different perspectives regarding the presence of fungi, their association with specific subtypes of sinusitis, and the effectiveness of antifungal therapies.

## 23.5 Diagnosis and Clinical Features

The diagnosis of AFRS relies primarily on a clinical assessment using the Bent and Kuhn criteria, which are definitively established during surgery [4]. These criteria include (1) type I IgE-mediated hypersensitivity, (2) nasal polyposis, (3) characteristic computed tomography (CT) findings, as shown in (Fig. 23.1), (4) eosinophilic mucus, and (5) positive fungal smear [15]. In the Bent and Kuhn criteria, specific features function as minor criteria, but while inessential to confirming

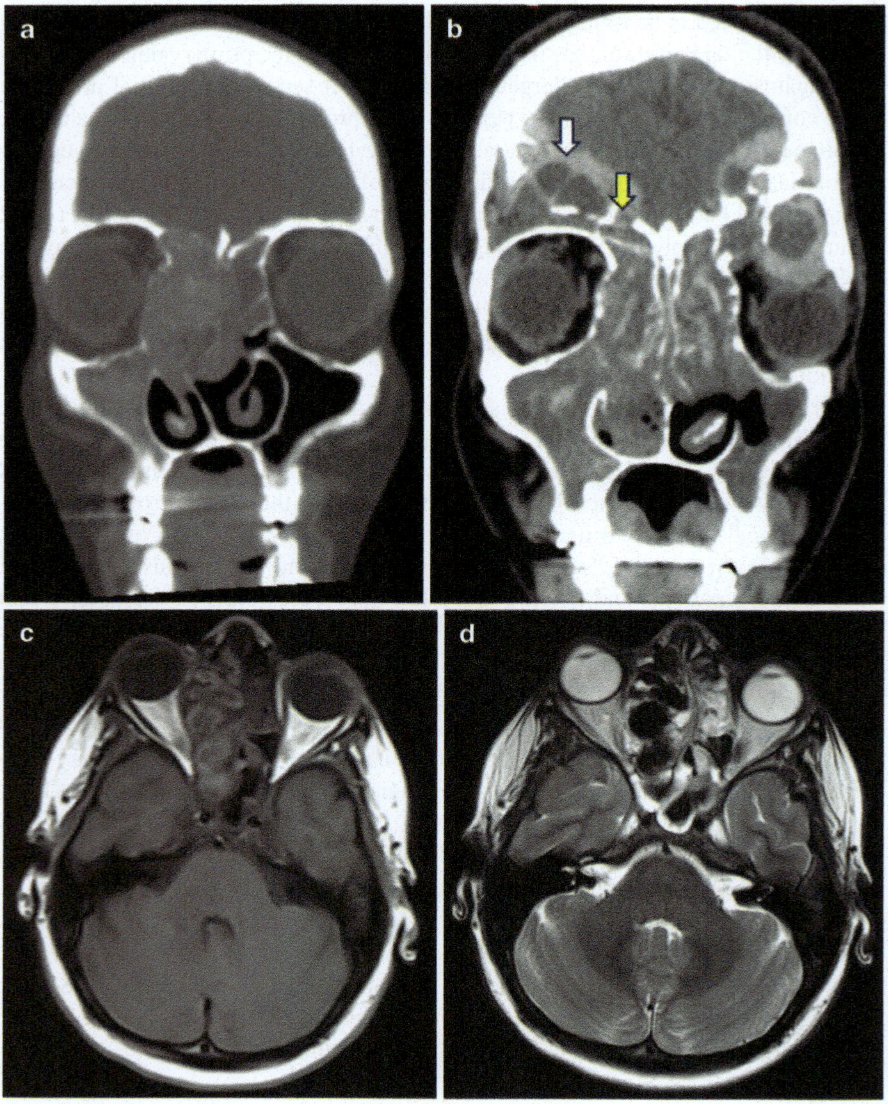


**Fig. 23.1** (**a**) Expansion of the right ethmoidal sinuses. Right maxillary and bilateral ethmoid showing complete inhomogeneous opacification with hyperdense material. (**b**) Complete opacification of all sinuses with hyperdense material associated with erosion of right side fovea ethmoidalis (yellow arrow) and posterior frontal sinus wall and concomitant intracranial expansion (white arrow). (**c**) Axial MRI demonstrates internal high signal at TIWI. (**d**) Signal void at T2WI with contrast enhancement of mucosal lining

**Table 23.1** Bent and Kuhn criteria for allergic fungal rhinosinusitis (AFRS)

| Major criteria | Minor criteria |
|---|---|
| Type I IgE-mediated hypersensitivity | Presence of asthma |
| Nasal polyposis | Unilateral disease |
| Characteristic computed tomography (CT) findings | Presence of bone erosion |
| Eosinophilic mucus | Charcot–Leyden crystals |
| Positive fungal smear | Serum eosinophilia |
| | Positive fungal culture |

an AFRS diagnosis, their presence primarily serves as additional support for the diagnosis, including the presence of asthma, unilateral disease, bone erosion, positive culture of fungus organisms, and eosinophil degradation products, including Charcot–Leyden crystals and serum eosinophilia, as shown in Table 23.1 [16].

AFRS can exhibit the gradual development of clinical symptoms, which commonly include nasal obstruction, facial pressure, hyposmia or anosmia, and postnasal drip. Additionally, patients may experience symptoms associated with bony remodeling, such as proptosis or telecanthus [15]. Bozeman and colleagues proposed a system for classifying the complications of AFRS into distinct groups, including ophthalmic complications, sinobronchial allergic mycosis, bony erosion with or without intracranial extension, cavernous venous thrombosis with ophthalmoplegia and cranial nerve (CN) palsy, and ear (otic) involvement. The most common complications are ophthalmic, including proptosis, decreased visual acuity, blurred vision, diplopia (double vision), CN palsy, and lacrimal duct obstruction [16]. Meanwhile, orbital complications associated with AFRS are considered uncommon, with a prevalence of 18.3–34%. These complications primarily manifest as proptosis, potentially affecting the extraocular muscles and leading to diplopia. In more severe cases, vision impairment can occur, which can be attributed in AFRS to two mechanisms. First, there is bony expansion and sinus remodeling, which can result in compression of the optic nerve or optic chiasm. Second, there is irritation and inflammation of the optic nerve triggered by a hyperimmune response to fungal antigens, and mechanical compression of the optic nerve can occur due to various suggested reasons, including conduction blockage, ischemic injury, demyelination, and retrograde or anterograde degeneration [17]. The duration of visual impairment and the timing of intervention are crucial factors influencing the recovery of visual impairment, where a shorter period of vision loss and prompt surgical intervention have been observed to have a beneficial effect [17]. To summarize, poorer outcomes are linked to delayed presentation and sudden onset of visual impairment. Additionally, complete visual loss is considered to carry a higher risk and presents challenges in reversing vision loss [17, 18]. Rare cases have been reported of cranial neuropathies, believed to be caused by external compression and vascular compromise resulting from the mass effect of fungal disease, rather than direct involvement of the nerves. However, if these manifestations are promptly addressed and decompressed, they appear to be reversible. The extrinsic compression of neural structures, such as the optic nerve, abducens nerve, and optic chiasm, initially leads to venous occlusion, causing tissue edema and further compression of the nerve fibers. Over time, the pressure exerted on these structures surpasses arterial pressure, leading to infarction and irreversible nerve damage. However, according to a case series review by Illing et al., most patients who underwent nerve decompression experienced complete recovery within 5 weeks of intervention [19]. Thus, it is believed that those with partial or no recovery may have experienced partial nerve ischemia and infarction due to the pressure effect on the nerve [19].

Several indicators can provide physicians with clues suggestive of AFRS, including the occurrence of CRS in immunocompetent individuals who are young to middle-aged and have a history of atopy. In addition, the presence of unilateral disease and an incomplete response to courses of antibiotics can raise further suspicions of AFRS [20]. Furthermore, histopathological examination of mucosal samples from AFRS patients using hematoxylin-eosin (H&E) staining plays a crucial role in confirming the diagnosis by revealing specific features indicative of AFRS, including the presence of inflammatory infiltration by eosinophils, lymphocytes, and plasma cells. In addition, it shows mucosal hypertrophy or hyperplasia without any signs of tissue invasion, granulomas, necrosis, or giant cells, which, if observed, may suggest an alternative diagnosis, such as invasive fungal sinusitis [20]. Moreover, it is crucial to have a thorough understanding of the fungal mucin examination during the diagnostic procedure, as shown in Fig. 23.2. Fungal mucin is characterized by its thickness, high viscosity, and diverse coloration, resembling the texture and appearance of peanut butter or axle grease [20]. Thus, differentiating between allergic mucin and fungal debris is important due to their contrasting endoscopic characteristics, including the thick, adhesive nature of allergic mucin, whereas fungal debris appears as a thickened putty-like material [21]. Furthermore, distinguishing between AFRS and eosinophilic mucus rhinosinusitis (EMRS) can be challenging due to the clear similarities and shared features between the two conditions. Even more, reliance on severity of CRS symptoms, as well as macroscopic and microscopic features, CT scan findings, and immunological studies, does not always enable definitive differentiation. However, it is worth noting that individuals with EMRS generally exhibit more severe disease symptoms, and the presence of bone erosion is not exclusively limited to allergic individuals or those with a positive fungal culture [22]. In contrast to AFRS, EMRS displays features that can help

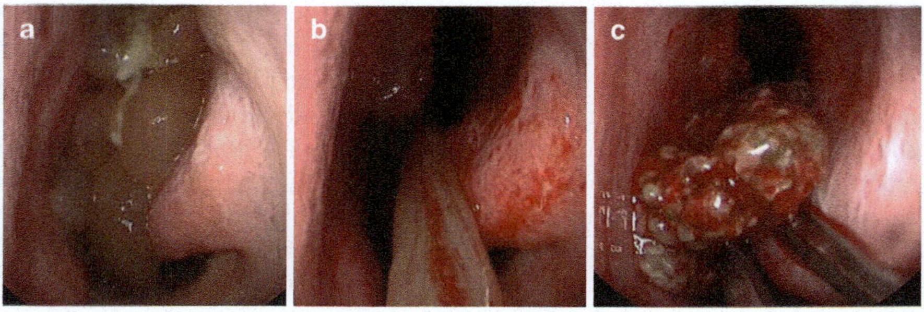


**Fig. 23.2** Intraoperative picture of (**a**) Polyps. (**b**) Allergic mucin. (**c**) Fungal debris

differentiate it from AFRS. These features include the mean patient age, which is 30 years in the AFRS group and 48 years in the EMRS group. In addition, bilateral disease is more common in EMRS (91.6%) compared to AFRS (62.5%), though EMRS is also more strongly associated with asthma and has an increased incidence of aspirin sensitivity. Despite having a similar radiological appearance to AFRS, EMRS tends to exhibit a bilateral distribution and has a significantly lower percentage of orbital involvement at presentation. Furthermore, during surgery, typical mucoid material is observed in both conditions, but fungal cultures are negative in EMRS [23].

Regarding pathophysiology, it is believed that the two conditions follow different pathways, with AFRS thought to result from an immunological response to fungi in predisposed individuals, while EMRS is characterized by a local immune reaction secondary to an underlying systemic disorder. Both conditions may present with similar initial clinical symptoms, but they have different clinical courses [23]. Noneosinophilic chronic sinusitis, a form of CRS with polyps, primarily affects middle-aged, obese women, Although its clinical and radiological characteristics resemble those of the eosinophilic type, the noneosinophilic variant lacks eosinophilic mucin during endoscopy. Instead, patients exhibit thick, discolored secretions and sinus obstruction. Furthermore, compared to the eosinophilic type, individuals with the noneosinophilic variant generally show a suboptimal response to intranasal corticosteroids [24].

## 23.6 Imaging

CT findings in AFRS can vary among patients, and not all individuals will exhibit the same imaging characteristics. Nevertheless, certain common radiological features are often associated with this condition, including unilateral involvement, which is more common than bilateral, and near-complete opacification of the sinuses, and CT hyperattenuation of the sinuses greater than that of muscle, in addition to the presence of bone thinning or thickening [25]. Furthermore, reports have indicated the presence of sinus expansion, bone erosion, and intracranial and intraorbital involvement in cases of this condition, as shown in Fig. 23.1a, b [26]. Additionally, when observed on MRI, AFRS typically exhibits signal voids on T2-weighted images that are then attributed to the presence of dense fungal elements or debris within the sinuses [3]. The Lund–Mackay CT staging system is commonly used to grade the severity of sinus opacification in cases of CRS, including AFRS. However, one drawback of this system is that it does not address bone erosion. To address this limitation, Wise et al. developed a novel radiological staging system in which each paranasal sinus wall with expansion/erosion is assigned one point, with a maximum of three points for each frontal sinus, two points for each ethmoid complex, three points for each sphenoid sinus, three points for each maxillary sinus, and one point each for the frontal and sphenoid intersinus septa. This system allows for a maximum score of 24 points [27].

## 23.7 Surgical Management

Endoscopic sinus surgery is the standard treatment method for managing AFRS, and its importance lies in its ability to eliminate fungal debris and eosinophilic mucin successfully, thus reducing the likelihood of disease recurrence and related complications. Furthermore, surgery for AFRS not only helps prevent complications but can also reverse certain complications, such as proptosis. The primary goal of surgery is thus to eradicate the disease by effectively removing fungal debris and mucin. As such, it is noteworthy that the utilization of image guidance during the procedure is exceptionally valuable, as it ensures precise and accurate surgical intervention, particularly in cases with distorted anatomy [28]. Further, there are concerns about the probability of recurrence in instances of unilateral AFRS and about the most effective surgical approach. The recurrence rates of AFRS are observed to be high, with instances of recurrence affecting the unaffected sinuses on the opposite side in cases of unilateral AFRS. Thus, the significant likelihood of recurrence in the nondiseased sinuses can be attributed to numerous factors, such as the presence of subclinical contralateral disease or early-stage disease in the unilateral sinus [29]. A multicenter study conducted by AlQahtani et al. involved 68 patients in total exclusively diagnosed with unilateral AFRS, and it identified a recurrence rate of 55.8%, with most occurring on the same (ipsilateral) side [30]. Conversely, and interestingly, 30.8% of these recurrences involved the nondiseased sinuses, suggesting that unilateral AFRS may be an early manifestation of an eventual bilateral disease. Regarding surgery, the study indicated that ipsilateral endoscopic sinus surgery, whether performed using conservative or conventional FESS (a regular sinusotomy that preserves the middle turbinate) or extended FESS (maximum opening of the sinus ostia and/or partial middle/superior turbinectomy), did not show statistically significant evidence in the development of contralateral disease. However, the authors emphasized the importance of examining the noninvolved side during postoperative follow-up to assess the need for further intervention and raised a question about the necessity of prophylactic surgery to prevent such occurrences [30].

## 23.8 Medical Management

Systemic steroids have demonstrated effectiveness when used in conjunction with surgery for AFRS, playing a role in stabilizing the disease, preventing recurrence, and positively impacting endoscopic and radiologic findings, as well as subjective symptoms reported by patients. However, there is controversy in the literature regarding the optimal duration and timing of systemic steroid administration—whether it should be used only preoperatively or postoperatively. Both approaches have shown benefits; thus, a suggested and widely accepted approach is to administer oral steroids for 7–14 days postoperatively, followed by a tapered course, transitioning to topical steroids [21, 31–34]. The use of high-volume intranasal steroid irrigation, specifically budesonide at a concentration of 2 ml of 0.5 mg/ml in 240 ml, for postoperative treatment, has demonstrated effectiveness and safety without impacting the hypothalamic–pituitary–adrenal (HPA) axis [35, 36]. The available evidence for using antifungal therapy in the treatment of AFRS is limited, primarily centered on the azole class of antifungals, including Posaconazole, itraconazole, and others, which specifically target the fungal genus commonly associated with AFRS. However, it is important to note that antifungal therapy does not replace the role of steroids or surgery in AFRS treatment. Their use is typically justified in cases of disease recurrence or when there is no response to maximal medical and surgical therapy [37–40]. Regarding immunotherapy (IT), there is a lack of evidence from well-designed studies to draw sufficient conclusions about its effectiveness and safety in the treatment of AFRS [28]. Biologic therapy is an emerging and innovative treatment for CRSwNP, as its mechanism of action primarily involves targeting mediators of type 2 inflammation. Examples of biologic therapies that specifically target type 2 inflammation in CRS include dupilumab, which binds to the IL-4R alpha, whereas other monoclonal antibodies, such as mepolizumab and reslizumab, target IL-5, benralizumab targets the IL-5 a-chain receptor, and omalizumab targets IgE [28]. Although studies have not provided conclusive evidence of the benefits of biologics in treating AFRS, there is a belief that these treatments may be effective in halting the disease process and potentially serve as steroid-sparing agents due to the shared immunopathologic mechanism in Type 2 inflammation. Limited studies have explored the role of Omalizumab in AFRS, suggesting potential superiority in subjective tests compared to intranasal steroid therapy. However, studies that are more extensive and robust are required to draw definitive conclusions on this matter [41]. Retrospective case series studies were conducted to evaluate the efficacy of dupilumab in managing difficult cases of AFRS, focused on patients who had undergone multiple sinus surgeries and received extensive medical treatment. The results revealed a remarkable improvement in symptoms, endoscopy scores, SNOT-22, olfaction scores, asthma control test, and serum eosinophilia after a biweekly course of 300 mg dupilumab over a period of 6 months, though some minor side effects associated with the use of dupilumab were reported, including nasopharyngitis, injection-site reactions, and headaches [42, 43].

## 23.9 Follow-Up

The follow-up of AFRS cases play a significant role in identifying features that may predict recurrence. Although there is no definitive period for how long patients should be monitored, the literature indicates that the longest reported periods of recurrence without prednisone treatment were 29 and 34 months. Nasal endoscopic examination is the most practical method of monitoring these cases, as it often remains a silent disease during recurrence. Also, total serum IgE levels serve as an important marker for confirming genuine disease recurrences. In certain instances, obtaining an endoscopic culture can be useful, as bacterial infections can sometimes mimic an AFRS recurrence. Further, regarding the endoscopic examination and follow-up of AFRS, the widely used mucosal staging system proposed by Kupferberg et al. consists of the following stages: 0, which indicates the absence of mucosal

**Table 23.2** Kupferberg mucosal scoring system

| Grading | State of mucosa |
|---|---|
| Stage 0 | Absence of mucosal edema or allergic mucin |
| Stage 1 | Mucosal edema with or without allergic mucin |
| Stage 2 | Polypoid edema with or without allergic mucin |
| Stage 3 | Presence of sinus polyps with fungal debris/mucin |

**Table 23.3** Philpott–Javer endoscopic staging system for AFRS[a]

| Grading | State of mucosa |
|---|---|
| 0 | No edema |
| 1–3 | Mucosal edema (mild/moderate/severe) |
| 4–6 | Polypoid edema (mild/moderate/severe) |
| 7–9 | Frank polyps (mild/moderate/severe) |

[a] +1 point for each sinus that contains mucin

edema or allergic mucin; 1, which involves mucosal edema with or without allergic mucin; 2, characterized by polypoid edema with or without allergic mucin; and 3, indicating the presence of sinus polyps with fungal debris or mucin, as shown in Table 23.2 [21]. Meanwhile, the Philpott–Javer postoperative endoscopic mucosal staging system is a modified version that builds on the Kupferberg scoring system, and it was specifically designed for endoscopic follow-up of patients with AFRS. One key difference in this system is that it provides more detailed grading for mucosal edema, polypoid edema, and frank polyps, categorizing them as mild, moderate, or severe. In addition, the system assigns points to each sinus cavity and includes additional points for the presence of allergic mucin, as outlined in Table 23.3 [44]. Surprisingly, when it comes to the follow-up process in the treatment of AFRS, it has been observed that patients, particularly young males, are more prone to loss to follow-up after surgery compared to patients with CRSwNP [45].

## References


1. Kokoszka M, Stryjewska-Makuch G, Kantczak A, Górny D, Glück J. Allergic fungal rhinosinusitis in Europe: literature review and own experience. Int Arch Allergy Immunol. 2023;184(9):856–65. https://doi.org/10.1159/000531017.
2. Cameron BH, Luong AU. New developments in allergic fungal rhinosinusitis pathophysiology and treatment. Am J Rhinol Allergy. 2023;37(2):214–20. https://doi.org/10.1177/19458924231152983.
3. Fokkens WJ, Lund VJ, Hopkins C, Hellings PW, Kern R, Reitsma S, et al. European position paper on rhinosinusitis and nasal polyps 2020. Rhinology. 2020;58(29):1–464.
4. Tyler MA, Luong AU. Current understanding of allergic fungal rhinosinusitis. World J Otorhinolaryngol Head Neck Surg. 2018;4(3):179–85. https://doi.org/10.1016/j.wjorl.2018.08.003.
5. AlQahtani A, Alim B, Almudhaibery F, Mulafikh D, Almutairi S, Almohanna S, Alfawwaz F. The impact of climatic, socioeconomic, and geographic factors on the prevalence of allergic

fungal rhinosinusitis: a worldwide ecological study. Am J Rhinol Allergy. 2022;36(4):423–31. https://doi.org/10.1177/19458924211069226.
6. Carney AS, Tan LW, Adams D, Varelias A, Ooi EH, Wormald PJ. Th2 immunological inflammation in allergic fungal sinusitis, nonallergic eosinophilic fungal sinusitis, and chronic rhinosinusitis. Am J Rhinol. 2006;20(2):145–9.
7. Schubert MS. Allergic fungal sinusitis: pathophysiology, diagnosis, and management. Med Mycol. 2009;47(Suppl 1):S324–30. https://doi.org/10.1080/13693780802314809.
8. Shaw JL, Fakhri S, Citardi MJ, Porter PC, Corry DB, Kheradmand F, Liu Y-J, et al. IL-33–responsive innate lymphoid cells are an important source of IL-13 in chronic rhinosinusitis with nasal polyps. Am J Respir Crit Care Med. 2013;188(4):432–9. https://doi.org/10.1164/rccm.201212-2227oc.
9. Tieu DD, Kern RC, Schleimer RP. Alterations in epithelial barrier function and host defense responses in chronic rhinosinusitis. J Allergy Clin Immunol. 2009;124(1):37–42. https://doi.org/10.1016/j.jaci.2009.04.045.
10. Den Beste KA, Hoddeson EK, Parkos CA, Nusrat A, Wise SK. Epithelial permeability alterations in an in vitro air–liquid interface model of allergic fungal rhinosinusitis. Int Forum Allergy Rhinol. 2013;3(1):19–25. https://doi.org/10.1002/alr.21077.
11. Torres C, Ro JY, El-Naggar AK, Sim SJ, Weber RS, Ayala AG. Allergic fungal sinusitis: a clinicopathologic study of 16 cases. Hum Pathol. 1996;27(8):793–9.
12. Braun H, Buzina W, Freudenschuss K, Stammberger H, Beham A. 'Eosinophilic fungal rhinosinusitis': a common disorder in Europe? Laryngoscope. 2003;113(2):264–9. https://doi.org/10.1097/00005537-200302000-00015.
13. Porter PC, Lim DJ, Maskatia ZK, Mak G, Tsai C-L, Citardi MJ, et al. Airway surface mycosis in chronic TH2-associated airway disease. J Allergy Clin Immunol. 2014;134(2):325–31. https://doi.org/10.1016/j.jaci.2014.04.028.
14. Tyler MA, Lam K, Marino MJ, Yao WC, Schmale I, Citardi MJ, et al. Revisiting the controversy: the role of fungi in chronic rhinosinusitis. Int Forum Allergy Rhinol. 2021;11(11):1577–87. https://doi.org/10.1002/alr.22826.
15. Loftus PA, Wise SK. Allergic fungal rhinosinusitis: the latest in diagnosis and management. Rhinology. 2016;54(1):13–9. https://doi.org/10.4193/Rhin15.064.
16. Bozeman SA, Moak JS, deShazo R, Stringer S, Arnold J. Complications of allergic fungal sinusitis. J Allergy Clin Immunol. 2010;125(2):AB101.
17. Alhussien A, Alghulikah A, Albaharna H, Alserhani A, Alromaih S, Aloulah M. Loss of vision outcome for allergic fungal sinusitis: case report and literature review. Ther Adv Allergy Rhinol. 2023;14:27534030231176774.
18. Allami H, Alarfaj HM, Almousa H, Aldhahri RA, Alfallaj R, Alharbi A, et al. Acute vision loss in patients with allergic fungal rhinosinusitis: a case series. Ther Adv Allergy Rhinol. 2023;14:27534030231214400.
19. Illing EA, Dunlap Q, Woodworth BA. Outcomes of pressure-induced cranial neuropathies from allergic fungal rhinosinusitis. Otolaryngol Head Neck Surg. 2015;152(3):541–5.
20. Glass D, Amedee RG. Allergic fungal rhinosinusitis: a review. Ochsner J. 2011;11(3):271–5.
21. Kuhn FA, Javer AR. Allergic fungal sinusitis: a four-year follow-up. Am J Rhinol. 2000;14(3):149–56.
22. Pant H, Kette FE, Smith WB, Macardle PJ, Wormald PJ. Eosinophilic mucus chronic rhinosinusitis: clinical subgroups or a homogeneous pathogenic entity? Laryngoscope. 2006;116(7):1241–7.
23. Uri N, Ronen O, Marshak T, Parpara O, Nashashibi M, Gruber M. Allergic fungal sinusitis and eosinophilic mucin rhinosinusitis: diagnostic criteria. J Laryngol Otol. 2013;127(9):867–71.
24. Grayson JW, Cavada M, Harvey RJ. Clinically relevant phenotypes in chronic rhinosinusitis. J Otolaryngol Head Neck Surg. 2019;48(1):1–10.
25. Ilica AT, Mossa-Basha M, Maluf F, Izbudak I, Aygun N. Clinical and radiologic features of fungal diseases of the paranasal sinuses. J Comput Assist Tomogr. 2012;36(5):570–6.
26. Al-Dousary SH. Allergic fungal sinusitis: radiological and microbiological features of 59 cases. Ann Saudi Med. 2008;28(1):17–21.

27. Wise SK, Rogers GA, Ghegan MD, Harvey RJ, Delgaudio JM, Schlosser RJ. Radiologic staging system for allergic fungal rhinosinusitis (AFRS). Otolaryngol Head Neck Surg. 2009;140(5):735–40.
28. Tyler MA, Luong AU. Current concepts in the management of allergic fungal rhinosinusitis. Immunol Allergy Clin. 2020;40(2):345–59.
29. Bitner BF, John MAS, Kennedy DW, Kuan EC. What is appropriate management for the contralateral uninvolved side in unilateral allergic fungal rhinosinusitis? Curr Opin Otolaryngol Head Neck Surg. 2023;31(1):53–6.
30. AlQahtani A, Alshaikh N, Alzarei A, Musleh A, Alamri A, Alqahtani A, Alfawwaz F, Alshammari F, Aloulah M, Marglani O, Alsaleh S, Alandejani T, Mokarbesh H. Contralateral sinus involvement of surgically treated unilateral allergic fungal rhinosinusitis. Eur Arch Otorrinolaringol. 2017;274(8):3097–101. https://doi.org/10.1007/s00405-017-4604-x.
31. Kupferberg SB, Bent JP III, Kuhn FA. Prognosis for allergic fungal sinusitis. Otolaryngol Head Neck Surg. 1997;117(1):35–41.
32. Woodworth BA, Joseph K, Kaplan AP, Schlosser RJ. Alterations in exotoxin, monocyte chemoattractant protein-4, interleukin-5, and interleukin-13 after systemic steroid treatment for nasal polyps. Otolaryngol Head Neck Surg. 2004;131(5):585–9.
33. Landsberg R, Segev Y, DeRowe A, Landau T, Khafif A, Fliss DM. Systemic corticosteroids for allergic fungal rhinosinusitis and chronic rhinosinusitis with nasal polyposis: a comparative study. Otolaryngol Head Neck Surg. 2007;136(2):252–7.
34. Joe SA, Thambi R, Huang J. A systematic review of the use of intranasal steroids in the treatment of chronic rhinosinusitis. Otolaryngol Head Neck Surg. 2008;139:340–7.
35. Soudry E, Wang J, Vaezeafshar R, Katznelson L, Hwang PH. Safety analysis of long-term budesonide nasal irrigations in patients with chronic rhinosinusitis post endoscopic sinus surgery. Int Forum Allergy Rhinol. 2016;6:568–72.
36. Smith KA, French G, Mechor B, Rudmik L. Safety of long-term high-volume sinonasal budesonide irrigations for chronic rhinosinusitis. Int Forum Allergy Rhinol. 2016;6:228–32.
37. Rojita M, Samal S, Pradhan P, Venkatachalam VP. Comparison of steroid and itraconazole for prevention of recurrence in allergic fungal rhinosinusitis: a randomized controlled trial. J Clin Diagn Res. 2017;11:MC01–3.
38. Rains BM, Mineck CW. Treatment of allergic fungal sinusitis with high-dose itraconazole. Am J Rhinol. 2003;17:1–8.
39. Chan KO, Genoway KA, Javer AR. Effectiveness of itraconazole in the management of refractory allergic fungal rhinosinusitis. J Otolaryngol Head Neck Surg. 2008;37:870–4.
40. Seiberling K, Wormald PJ. The role of itraconazole in recalcitrant fungal sinusitis. Am J Rhinol Allergy. 2009;23:303–6.
41. Luong AU, Chua A, Alim BM, Olsson P, Javer A. Allergic fungal rhinosinusitis: the role and expectations of biologics. J Allergy Clin Immunol Pract. 2022;10(12):3156–62.
42. Bulkhi AA, Mirza AA, Aburiziza AJ, Marglani OA. Dupilumab: an emerging therapy in allergic fungal rhinosinusitis. World Allergy Organ J. 2022;15(3):100638.
43. Alotaibi NH, Zahlan AM, Alali S, Alzarei AH, Arnaout RK, Khouqeer R, et al. Dupilumab as a treatment for allergic fungal rhinosinusitis: a case series. Rhinol Online. 2023;6:18–24.
44. Parhar HS, Thamboo A, Habib AR, Chang B, Gan EC, Javer AR. The interrater and intrarater reliability of the Philpott–Javer staging system based on level of training. Otolaryngol Head Neck Surg. 2014;150(4):538–41.
45. Gutierrez JA, Khan S, Chapurin N, Schlosser RJ, Soler ZM. Factors impacting follow-up care in allergic fungal rhinosinusitis. Otolaryngol Head Neck Surg. 2023;170(2):577–85. https://doi.org/10.1002/ohn.575.

# Basic Endoscopic Sinus Surgery (ESS): Performing a Safe ESS and Minimizing Potential Complications

24

Usamah El Hadi, Nadine El Hadi, and Zeina Kurban

**Key Points**
- Functional endoscopic sinus surgery (FESS) is now accepted as the standard approach for the surgical management of chronic rhinosinusitis.
- Minimalistic endoscopic approaches and the Ostiomeatal Complex evolved as a major concept in FESS for the treatment of diseased sinus.
- CT scan of the sinuses allowed understanding and comprehension of the detailed anatomical structure of the sinuses as well as all of its variations in order to perform safe FESS.
- The endoscopic sinus surgeon should recognize and be aware of important anatomical landmarks to minimize and avoid complications.

## 24.1 Surgical Anatomy

Over the past two decades, there has been a major shift in the concept of managing chronic sinus disease. Dr. Stammberger [1] and Dr. Kennedy were the pioneers in advancing the notion of moving away from major open sinus surgery toward the minimalistic endoscopic approaches targeting the opening of the natural sinus ostium of the diseased sinus. FESS is now accepted as the standard approach for the surgical management of chronic rhinosinusitis with and without nasal polyposis. This could not have been possible without the advancement in radiologic evaluation with the evolution of a high-resolution CT scan of the sinuses that allowed the detailed anatomical study of the sinuses as well as all of their variations. This has

**Supplementary Information** The online version contains supplementary material available at https://doi.org/10.1007/978-3-031-70077-4_24.

U. El Hadi (✉) · N. El Hadi · Z. Kurban
Department of Otolaryngology Head and Neck Surgery, American University of Beirut, Beirut, Lebanon


S. Elwany (ed.), *Current Rhinology*, https://doi.org/10.1007/978-3-031-70077-4_24

paved the way for executing and planning detailed surgery of the sinus. As such, otolaryngologist acquired the knowledge and training to understand and be able to read the CT scans of their patient before embarking on any surgical procedures.

Endoscopic, endonasal visualization of the sinonasal tract became common practice and mainstay of any clinical evaluation of the region either preoperatively or postoperatively. It is important to observe the nasal septum to decide whether there is a need to correct a deviated septum to improve access to the sinuses (Figs. 24.1 and 24.2).

The lamina papyracea should be evaluated for any dehiscences or abnormalities in order not to confuse it with ethmoid sinus disease (Fig. 24.3).

The middle meatus has been recognized as the center where the maxillary sinus, the frontal sinus, and the anterior and middle ethmoidal cells drain. Relevant anatomical structures of the region that are crucial for performing safe endoscopic surgery are the uncinate process, the infundibulum, and the ethmoidal bulla. The recognition of such anatomical structures and understanding of the variation that exists will improve surgical outcomes and reduce the complication of FESS (Fig. 24.4) [1].

The second most important region that needs to be comprehended by the endoscopist is the Ostiomeatal Complex. The OMC (Fig. 24.4) is a practical concept. It is considered the hypothetical site for the drainage and ventilation of the ethmoidal, maxillary, and frontal sinuses.

The exact confines of the OMC are not well outlined. It comprises structures between the medial orbital wall and the middle turbinate. The OMC encompasses the uncinate process, ethmoidal infundibulum, hiatus semilunaris, anterior ethmoidal cells, and the ostia of the anterior ethmoidal, maxillary, and frontal sinuses.

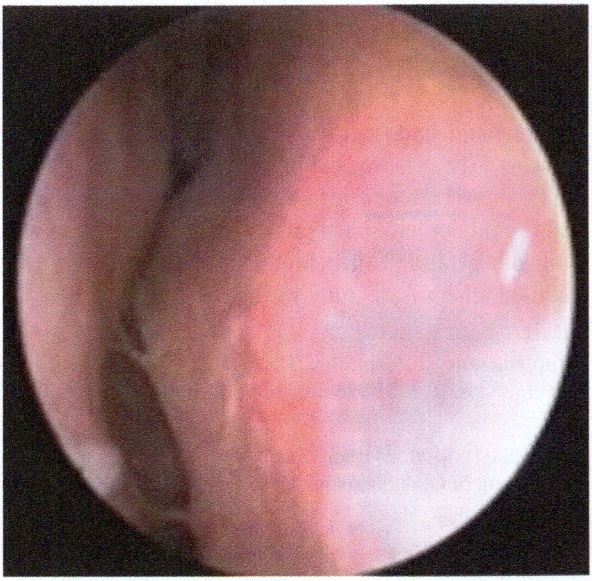

**Fig. 24.1** Septal spur impinging on the lateral nasal wall and middle meatus

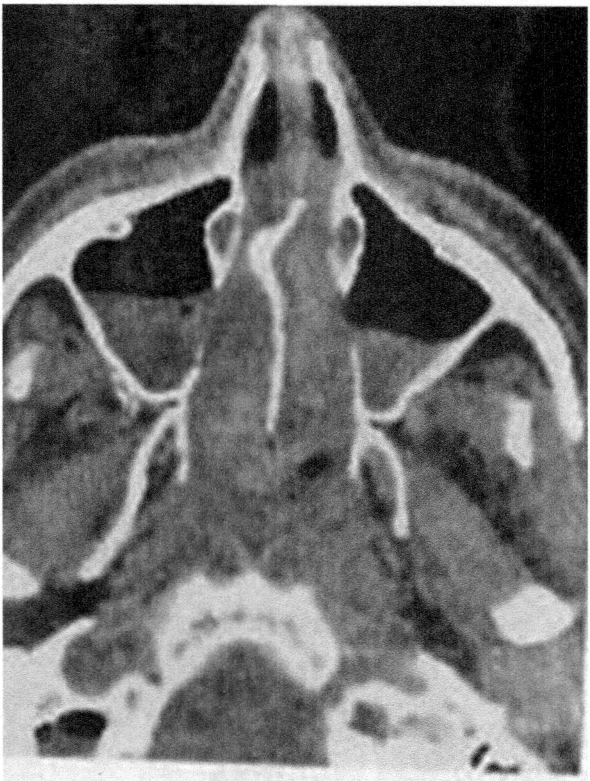

**Fig. 24.2** A spur that impinges on the lateral nasal wall and middle meatus

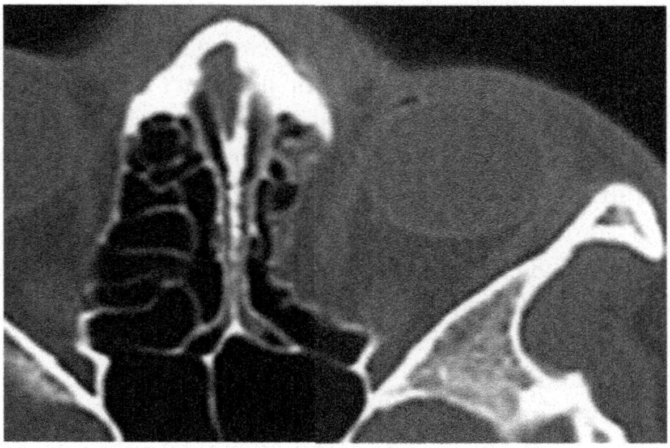

**Fig. 24.3** Dehiscence in the right lamina papyracea

The uncinate process is a bony curvilinear structure that the endoscopist first encounters as the middle meatus is approached. The ethmoidal infundibulum is a three-dimensional space between the uncinate process medially and the lamina papyracea laterally. Most of the anterior ethmoid sinus as well as the frontal sinus and maxillary sinus drain either superiorly or inferiorly into the infundibulum (Fig. 24.4).

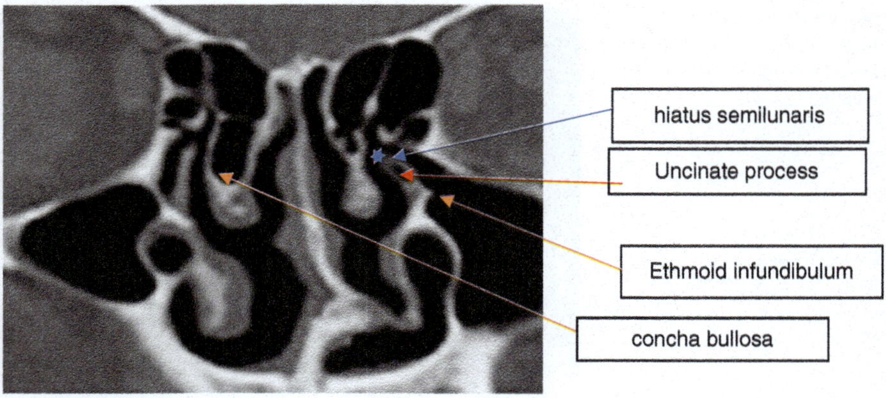


**Fig. 24.4** Conceptual OMC unit. Uncinate process, the infundibulum, and the ethmoidal bulla, concha bullosa

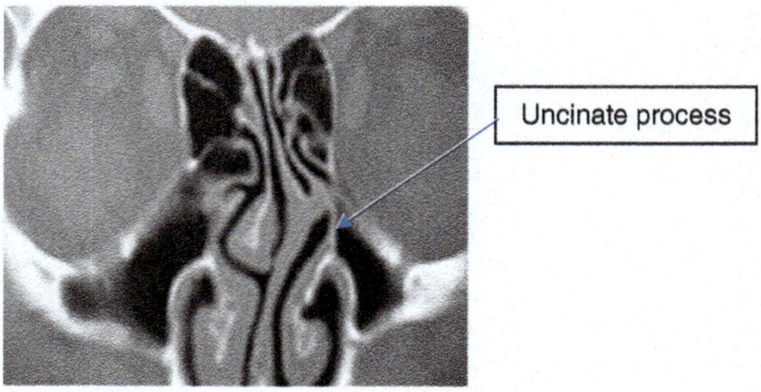


**Fig. 24.5** Uncinate process and its proximity to the orbital wall

Position of the uncinate process and its proximity to the orbital wall should be noted in especially hypoplastic maxillary sinus to avoid inadvertent penetration of the orbit while performing an uncinectomy during FESS (Fig. 24.5).

The uncinate process may be inserted on the lamina papyracea (Fig. 24.6), the skull base (Fig. 24.7), and the middle turbinate (Fig. 24.8).

The hiatus semilunaris, is a two-dimensional space that occupies the area between the free edge of the uncinate process and the ethmoidal bulla. The drainage of the frontal sinus into or out of the infundibulum is determined by the superior attachments of the uncinate process either to the lamina papyracea skull base or middle turbinate.

The ethmoidal complex is divided by the basal lamella of the middle turbinate into the anterior and posterior ethmoidal cells into the anterior and posterior ethmoidal cells.

The ethmoidal bulla is a major and the most bulging cell of the ethmoid complex. It is apparent just posterior to the uncinate process and drains into the sinus lateralis that compromises the suprabullar or retrobullar recess.

The agger nasi cell is a bony most constant protuberance of the ethmoid complex and is located at the shoulder of the middle turbinate attachment onto the lateral nasal wall [2] (Fig. 24.9).

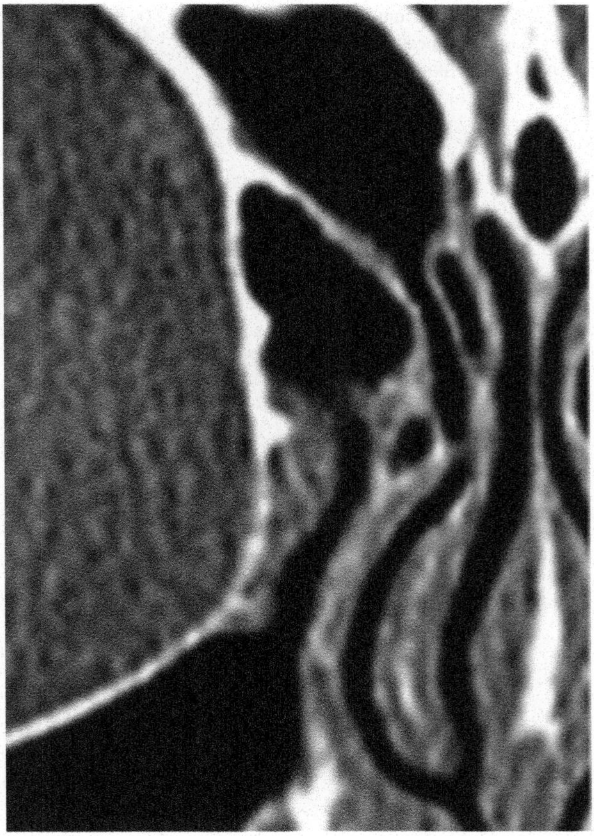

**Fig. 24.6** Attachment of the uncinate process to the lamina papyracea

Haller cell is a special cell from the anterior ethmoid complex group of cells that creeps under the floor of the orbit and tends to narrow the maxillary sinus ostium (Fig. 24.10). Failure to recognize such an anomaly will lead to accidental penetration of the orbit.

The posterior ethmoidal complex comprises one to five cells. In highly pneumatized cells, it might extend above the orbit and lie posterior and lateral to the frontal sinus and form what is known supraorbital ethmoidal air cell.

It might also extend superior and lateral to the sphenoid sinus. This cell is called the Onodi cell. It needs to be recognized on CT scan so that it will not be penetrated inadvertently on the assumption that it is the sphenoid as both the optic nerve and internal carotid artery might be exposed in the cell and can be injured with drastic complications (Fig. 24.11).

The Maxillary Sinus is the largest sinus and is considered as an important landmark to safely navigate to other sinuses as well as to other sites to the skull base [3]. Its ostium is located below the orbital floor in the medial wall of the sinus and drains into the ethmoid infundibulum [3]. It is found upper one-third of the infundibulum in around 10%, in the middle third in around 25%, and mostly in the lower third in 65% of the patients [4]. It is elliptical in shape whereas the accessory ostium is

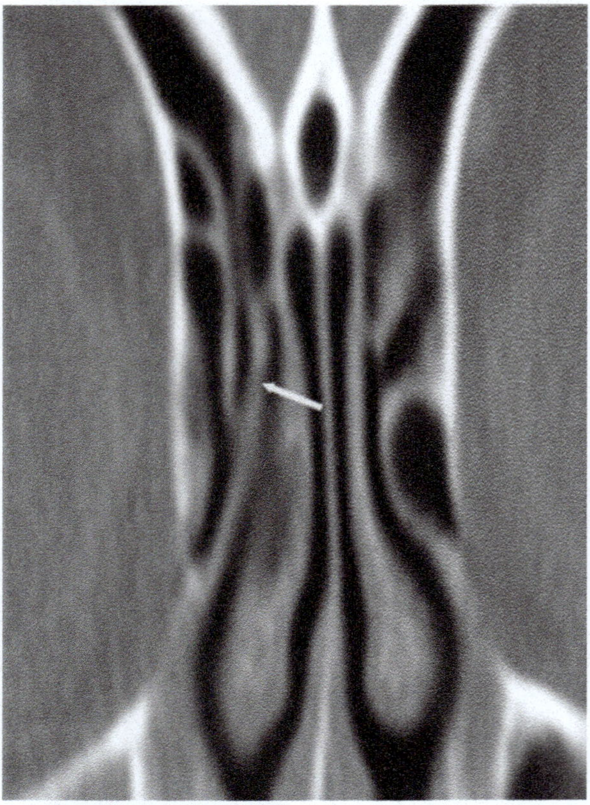

**Fig. 24.7** Attachment of the uncinate process (arrow) to the skull base

round and usually found in either the anterior or the posterior fontanelles [3] (Fig. 24.12).

Accessory ostia must not be confused with the natural ostium thus missing the natural ostium and hence leading to recirculation phenomena and persistent sinus infection [5]. Ostia seen by endoscopy in the presence of an intact uncinate process should always be considered as accessory ostia rather than the natural ostium which is typically hidden behind the uncinate process.

The sphenoid sinus is the furthermost posterior paranasal sinus [6]. Its ostium drains into a sphenoethmoid recess that is located medial to the superior turbinate, lateral to the nasal septum, and just anterior to the anterior face of the sphenoid sinus around 50% up to 75% up the surface of the sphenoid sinus and is always lower than the level of the maxillary roof [7] as envisioned by a horizontal virtual line drawn from the roof of the maxillary sinus all the way back to anterior face of sphenoid sinus wall [8, 9].

The sphenoid sinus can be partitioned by single or multiple septations [8]. These can be inserted on the optic nerve and carotid artery (Fig. 24.13) and should be identified on CT scan to avoid causing injury to these vital structures during dissection within the sinus cavity. At times, the carotid artery within the sphenoid sinus is dehiscent and extra care should be implemented while performing surgeries within

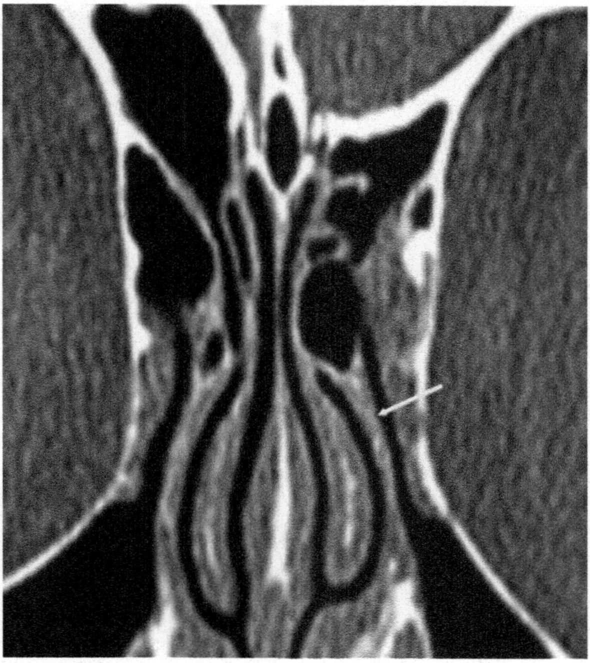

**Fig. 24.8** Attachment of the uncinate process (arrow) to the middle turbinate

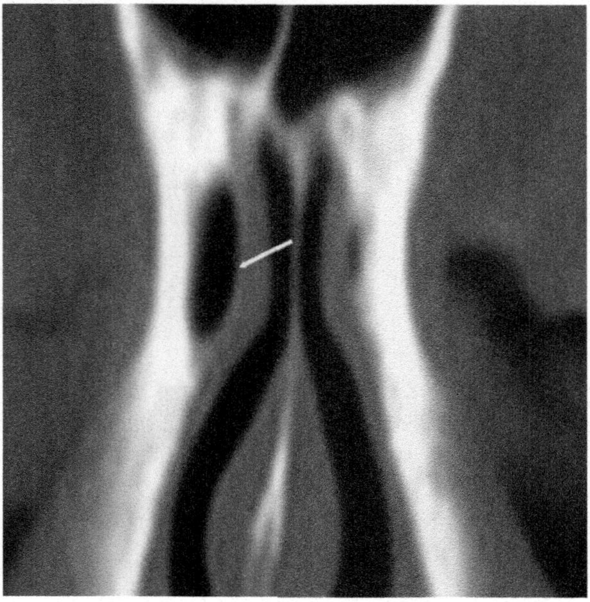

**Fig. 24.9** Agger cell (arrow)

the sinus to avoid accidental injury to the carotid artery (Fig. 24.10). The optic nerve can also be floating in the sphenoid sinus and can accidentally be injured (Figs. 24.14, 24.15, and 24.16) or in an Onodi cell (Fig. 24.17).

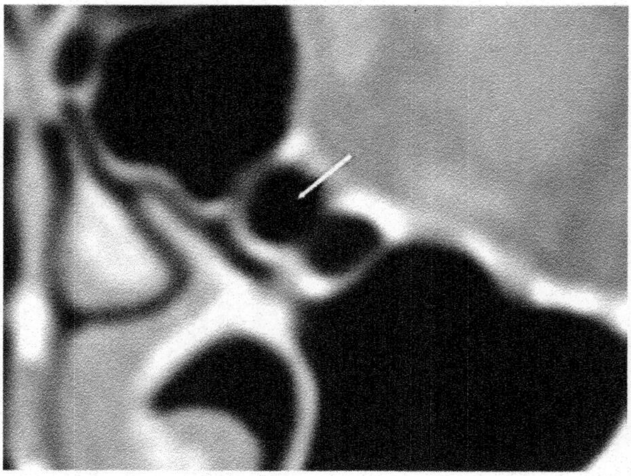

**Fig. 24.10** Haller cell (arrow)

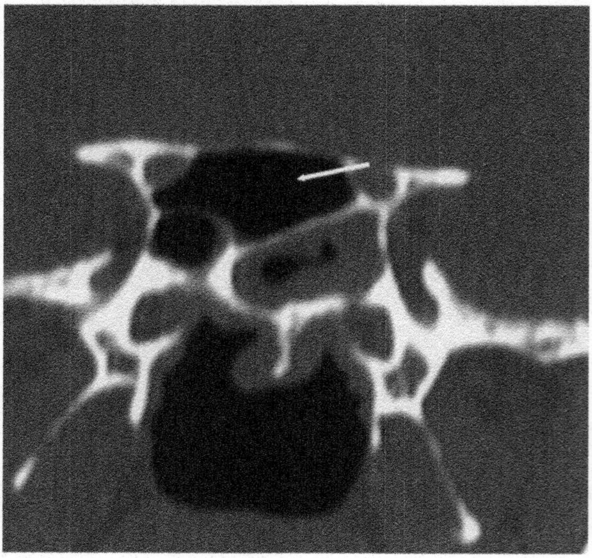

**Fig. 24.11** Onodi cell (arrow) superior to the diseased sphenoid sinus

The sphenoid sinus is always located inferior and medial to the Onodi cell. This should be noticed by careful analysis of the CT scan of the patient to avoid injuring vital structures such as the optic nerve and carotid artery or penetrating the skull base [6] (Fig. 24.8).

The carotid artery in the sphenoid sinus can be dehiscent macroscopically or microscopically (Fig. 24.18) or bulge excessively into the sphenoid cavity (Fig. 24.19) placing it at high risk for injury. Occasionally, the carotid artery can be dehiscent and should be identified to avoid inadvertent injury with catastrophic sequelae.

The Frontal Sinus drainage into the anterior ethmoid sinus is not a tube or a bony canal but forms an hourglass shaped by spaces or recess. Though not an ostium but

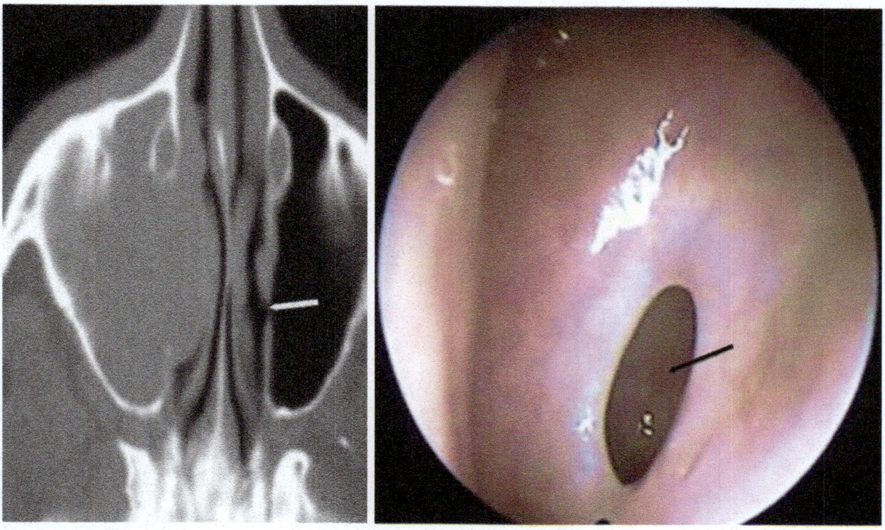

**Fig. 24.12** Accessory ostium of the maxillary sinus

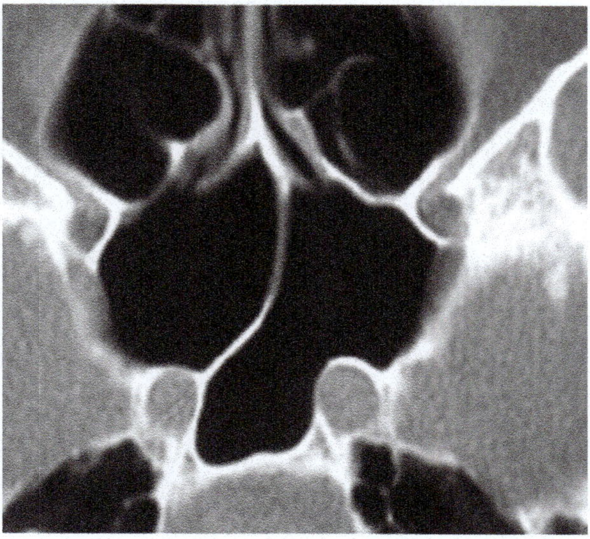

**Fig. 24.13** Intersinus septum that attaches to the carotid artery

has been labeled as a frontal sinus ostium and is considered as the narrowest part of the drainage tract [2] (Fig. 24.20).

The shape of the frontal sinus drainage pathway is determined by single or multiple frontal recess cells originating from the anterior ethmoid cells.

Kuhn [2] described four types of cells that tend to narrow or shape the drainage pathway to different configurations and sizes (Fig. 24.21).

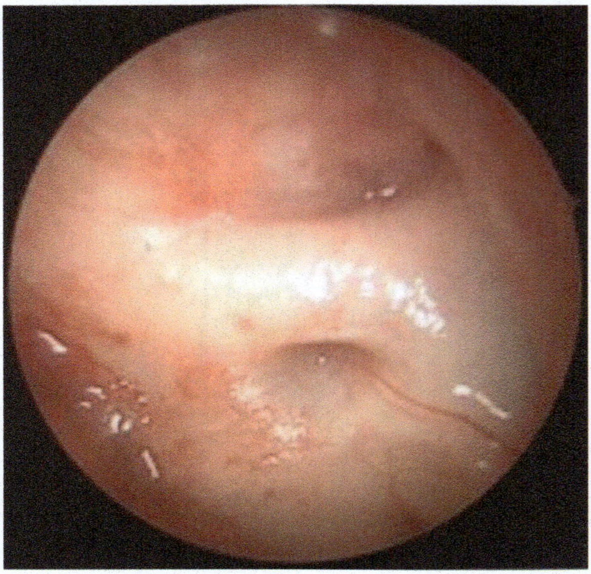

**Fig. 24.14** Optic nerve in sphenoid sinus

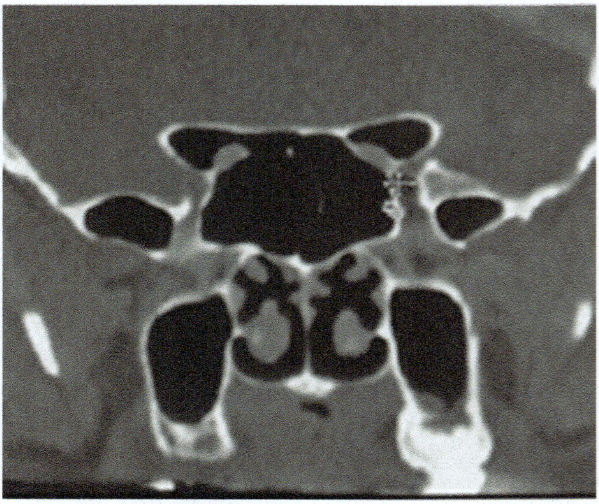

**Fig. 24.15** Optic nerve in sphenoid sinus

Wormald [10] suggested that a type 4 cell is a cell whose height extends up to 50% of the height of the frontal sinus, whereas a type 3 cell extends to less than 50% of the frontal sinus height.

Another classification by the international consensus document in 2016 [11] states that cells that are located anterior to the frontal sinus drainage pathway are labeled as agger nasi cells, the supra agger nasi cells (older classification as Kuhn type 1 and Kuhn type 2 cells), and the supra agger frontal cells (older classification Kuhn type 3 or Kuhn type 4 cells) [2, 10, 11]. Cells posterior to the frontal recess are the ethmoidal bulla, suprabullar cell, and suprabullar frontal cell [12, 13].

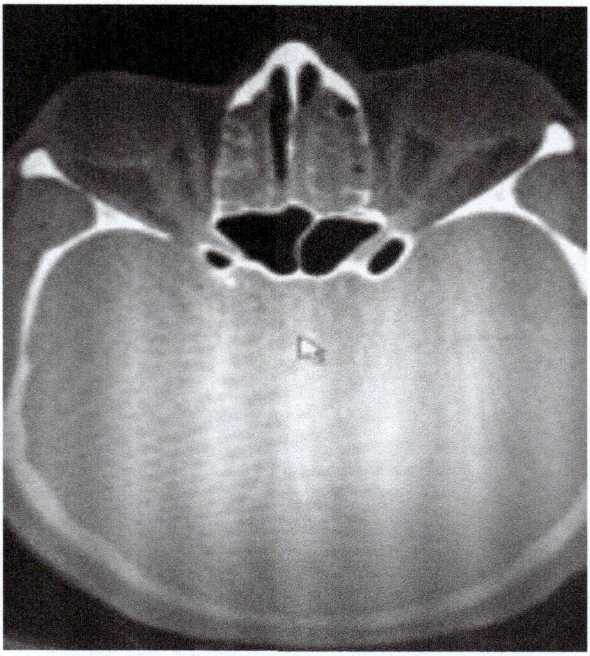

**Fig. 24.16** Optic nerve floating in an onodi cell

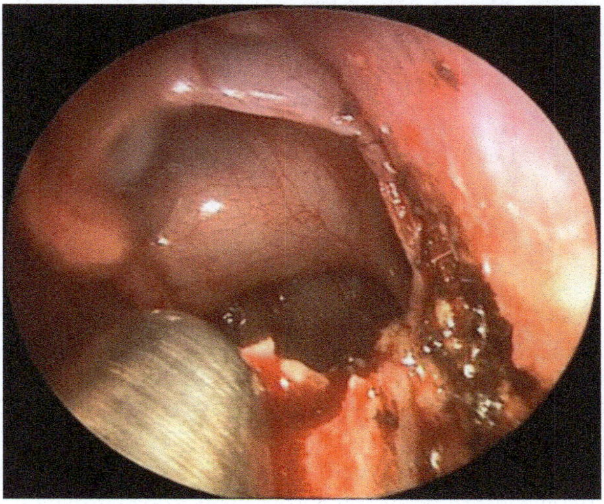

**Fig. 24.17** Optic nerve in an onodi cell

The anterior skull base is formed by the cribriform plate medially and the ethmoidal roof laterally which is formed by the frontal sinus bone. The cribriform plate is thin measuring around 0.1–0.2 mm thick and may lie much lower than the ethmoidal roof whereas the frontal bone forming the ethmoid roof is much thicker.

Keros [14] suggested a classification for the skull base. He described it into three configurations that were labeled as type 1–3 and classified the skull base into three types, according to the depth (Shallow, medium, or deep) of the olfactory groove:

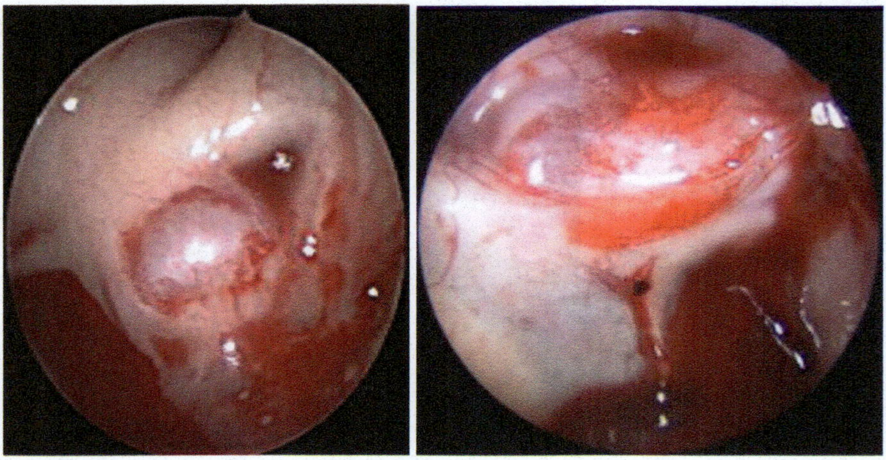

**Fig. 24.18** Dehiscent carotid artery in sphenoid sinus

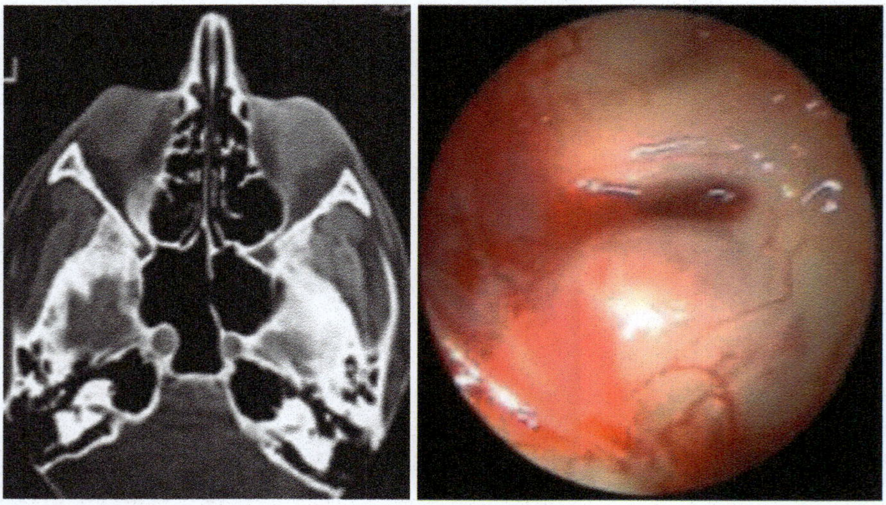

**Fig. 24.19** Prominent carotid artery and optic nerve

type 1 is 1–3 mm, type 2 is 4–7 mm, and type 3 is 8–16 mm. Type 3 is considered the riskiest for violation during FESS due to its height and being the thinnest part of the roof. Besides, the slope of the roof may also put the patient at a higher risk for penetration during dissection of the ethmoid sinuses. It is also important to state that the roof between both sides is not always symmetrical and should be noted during FESS to avoid any inadvertent injury to the skull base (Figs. 24.22, 24.23, 24.24, and 24.25).

There are three types of olfactory fossa according to Keros. The length of the lateral lamella of the cribriform increases from type I 1–3 mm to type 2 4–7 mm to

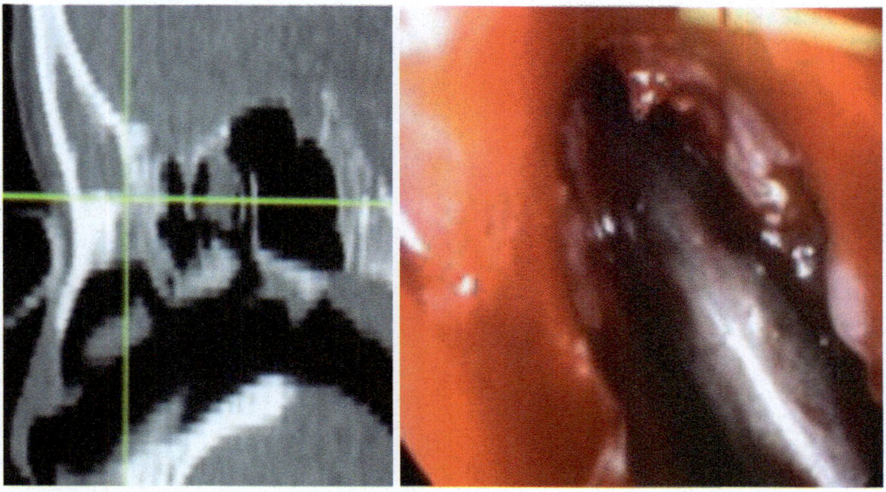

**Fig. 24.20** Frontal recess

**Fig. 24.21** Frontal cells encroaching into the frontal sinus recess

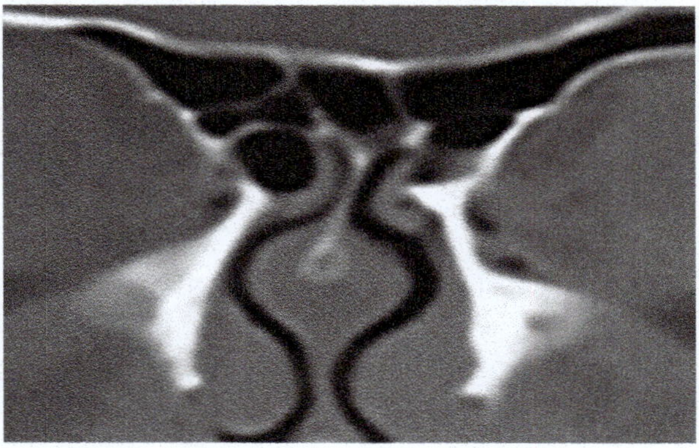

type III 8–16 mm. Note the asymmetry in the roof of the last image (Figs. 24.22, 24.23, 24.24, and 24.25) [15, 16].

It should be noted that an anomaly of the fovea ethmoidal might occur and should be noted to avoid injury to the skull base during FESS [15] (Fig. 24.26).

The anterior ethmoidal artery lies posterior to the frontal recess, and usually posterior to the basal lamella of the bulla ethmoidalis. It can either traverse the skull base or hang downward from the skull base in a mesentery placing it at a higher risk of injury resulting in hemorrhage and interorbital hematoma with a potential risk for the blindness of the nipple sign or indentation artery at the orbital wall and into the ethmoid sinus indicates the location of the artery (see Figs. 24.27, 24.28, and 24.29) [13].

On the other hand, the posterior ethmoid artery can be identified in the bony roof of the posterior ethmoid sinus just anterior to the face of the sphenoid sinus wall.

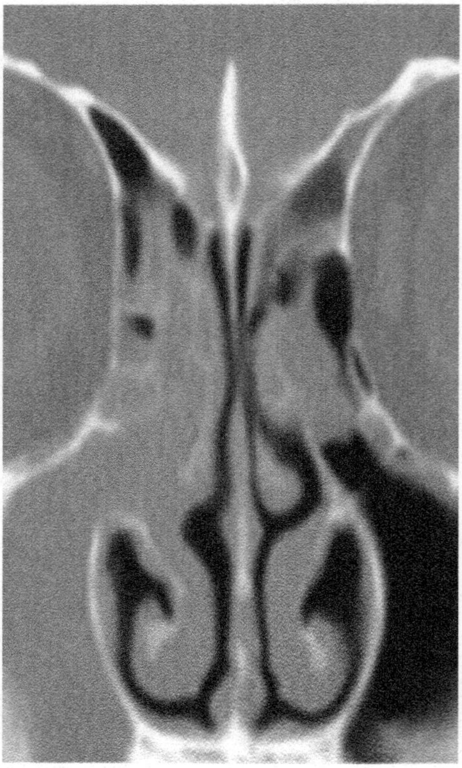

**Fig. 24.22** Keros type 1

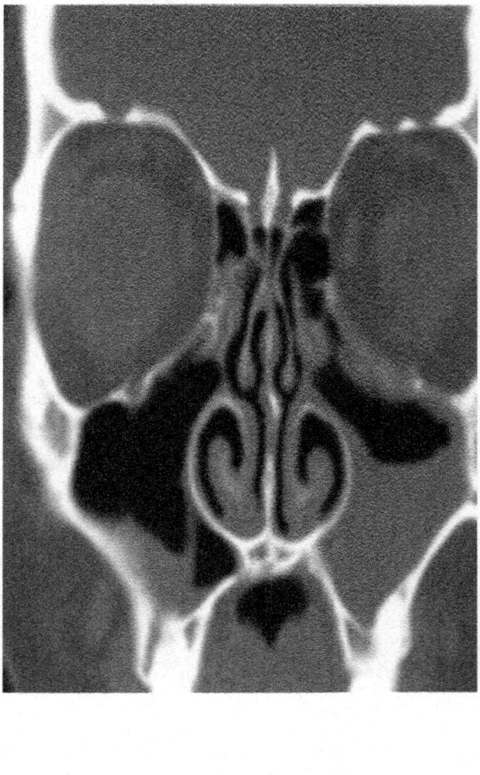

**Fig. 24.23** Keros type 2

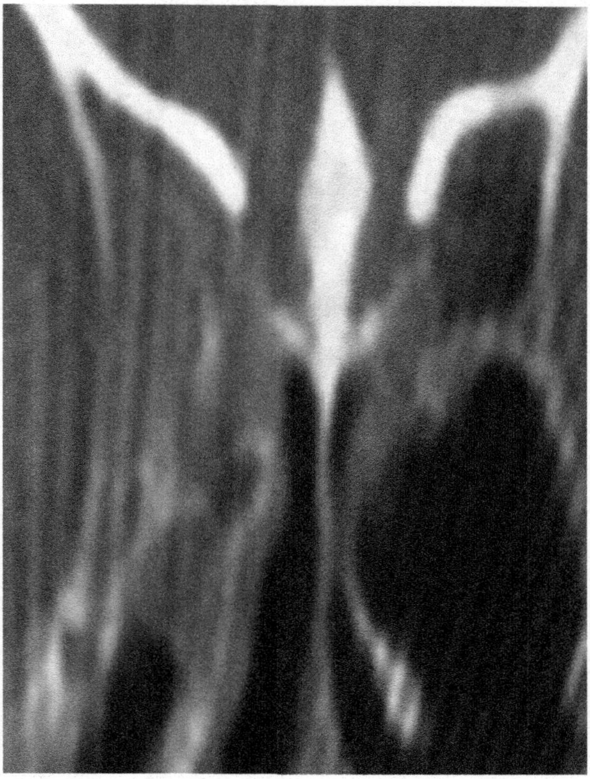

**Fig. 24.24** Keros type 3

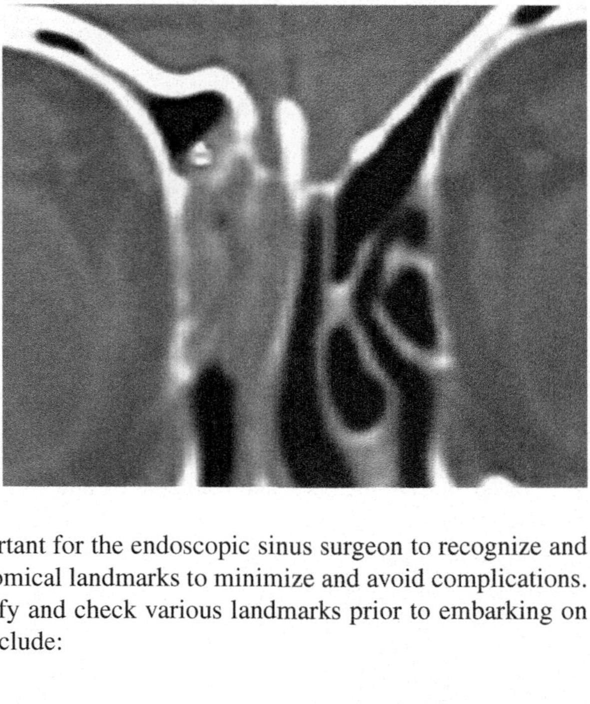

**Fig. 24.25** Keros asymmetric roof

In conclusion, it is important for the endoscopic sinus surgeon to recognize and be aware of important anatomical landmarks to minimize and avoid complications. It prudent for him to identify and check various landmarks prior to embarking on any FESS surgery. These include:

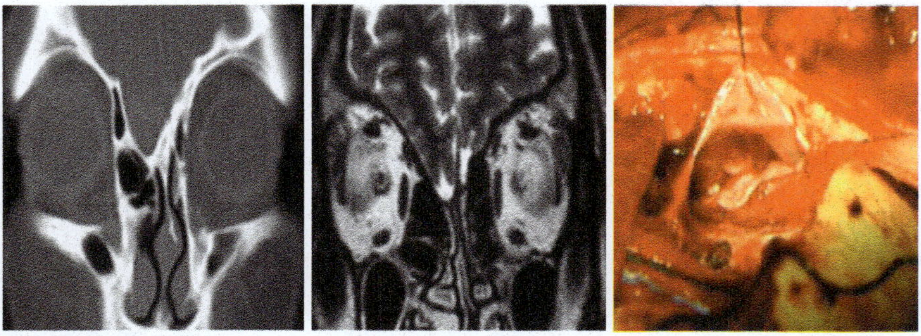

**Fig. 24.26** Anomaly in the cribriform plate and fovea ethmiodalis. An encephalocele rather than an ethmoid sinus disease

**Fig. 24.27** Anterior ethmoid artery (nipple sign)

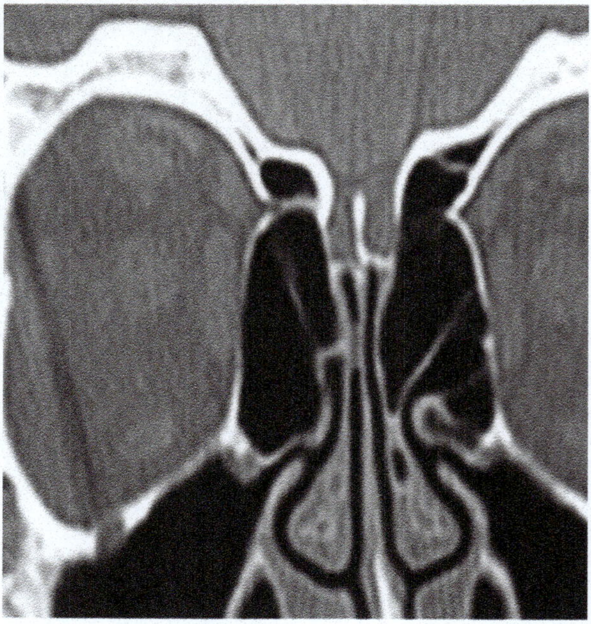

1. The level of the skull base in relation to the maxillary sinus roof.
2. The lamina papyracea with dehiscences or defects within it, prior orbital fracture, or iatrogenic injuries from previous surgeries.
3. The sphenoid sinus pneumatization, intersinus septum, and its attachments to either the optic nerve or the carotid artery.
4. The presence of Onodi cells.
5. The location of the optic nerve and the carotid artery.
6. The slope of the skull base and the height of the lateral lamella (Keros classification).
7. The anterior ethmoid artery (nipple sign).
8. The anatomy of the frontal recess.

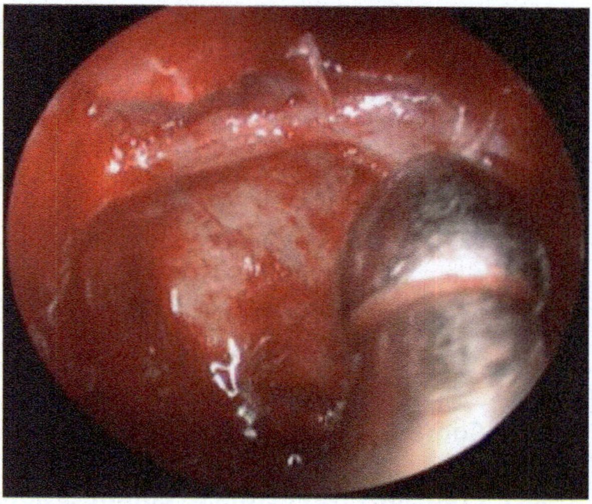

**Fig. 24.28** Dehiscent anterior ethmoid artery

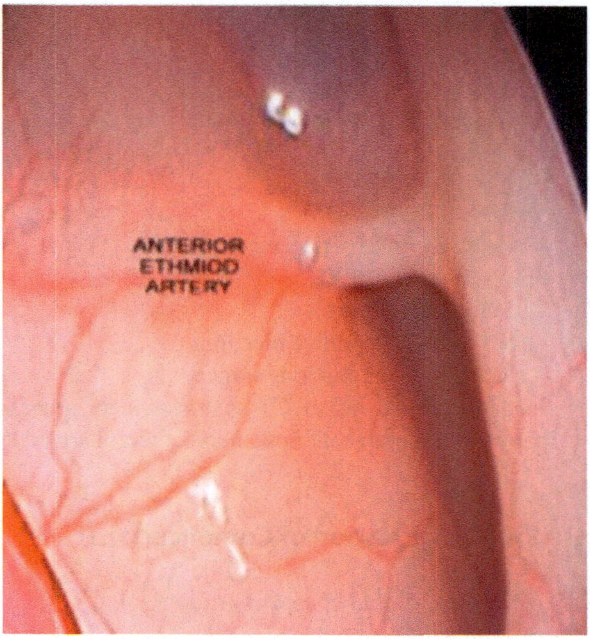


**Fig. 24.29** Anterior ethmoid artery hanging from the roof by a mesentery

## 24.2 Indications of Endoscopic Sinus Surgery

The basic indications for Sinonasal Surgery include a variety of conditions:

1. Inflammatory sinonasal disease such as:
   (a) Chronic rhinosinusitis (with or without nasal polyposis)
   (b) Recurrent acute rhinosinusitis

   (c) Antrochoanal polyps as well as mucoceles
   (d) Fungal ball, invasive fungal rhinosinusitis
   (e) Complications of rhinosinusitis
2. Noninflammatory diseases
   (a) Intractable epistaxis with ligation of the sphenopalatine artery
   (b) Endoscopic repair of meningoencephaloceles with or without cerebrospinal fluid rhinorrhea
   (c) Endoscopic repair of choanal atresia
   (d) Endoscopic resection of sinonasal tumors
   (e) Endoscopic resection of orbital tumors as well as approaches via the orbit to the skull base

## 24.3 Complications of Endoscopic Sinus Surgery

### 24.3.1 Predisposing Factors to Complications

- **3A**
  - Anatomic variation
  - Advanced disease
  - Absence of anatomic landmarks
- **3R**
  - Revision surgery
  - Right-handed
  - Relatively inexperienced surgeon
- **3S**
  - Sinonasal polyposis
  - Severe intraoperative bleeding
  - Scarring from previous surgery
- Inadequate analysis of CT scan (uncinate process, fovea ethmoidalis, lamina papyracea, Onodi cell, optic nerve, carotid artery)

### 24.3.2 Classification of Complications

1. According to time of appearance:
   (a) Immediate
   (b) Delayed
2. According to the seriousness of the complications:
   (a) Minor complications
      Minor epistaxis
      Hyposmia
      Adhesions
      Headache
      Periorbital ecchymosis or emphysema

Dental or facial pain

(b) Major complications

Major epistaxis
Anosmia
Nasolacrimal trauma
Carotid injury, intracranial hemorrhage, and stroke
Orbital hematoma, diplopia, decreased visual acuity
Blindness
Cerebrospinal fluid leak, pneumocephalus, and meningitis [17]

### 24.3.3 How to Avoid Complications

- Train the surgeon on how to perform diagnostic endoscopies and to manipulate intranasal instruments.
- Supervised Cadaver dissection/surgery
- Supervised surgery
- Staged surgery
- Follow-up Cadaver dissection courses for advanced surgery [18, 19]

## 24.4 Clinical Cases

### 24.4.1 Case 1

Clinical case of periorbital fat herniation during FESS. Proceed with care and removal of remaining ethmoid sinus disease without manipulation of the periorbital fat (Fig. 24.30).

### 24.4.2 Case 2 (Fig. 24.31)

Complications in patients undergoing FESS with periorbital and intraorbital emphysema due to violation of the lamina papyracea, treated conservatively with removal of nasal packs.

### 24.4.3 Case 3 (Fig. 24.32)

A patient undergoing FESS complicated by injury to the anterior ethmoid artery resulting in periorbital ecchymosis treated by medication and canthotomy and cantholysis (Fig. 24.32).

**Fig. 24.30** Periorbital fat

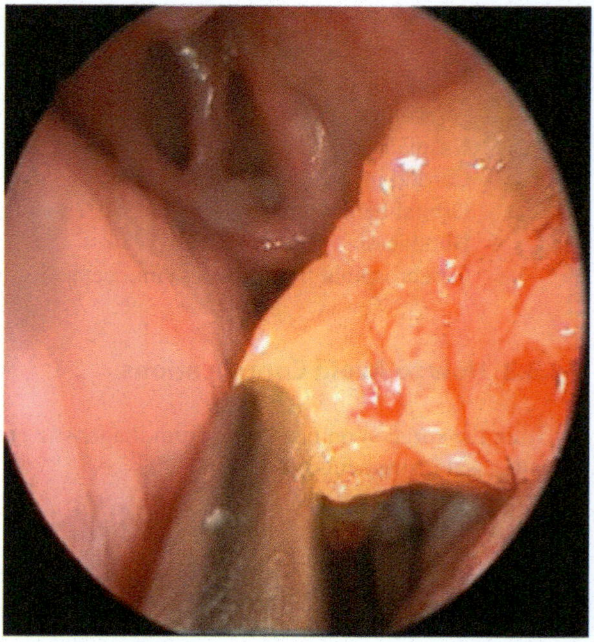

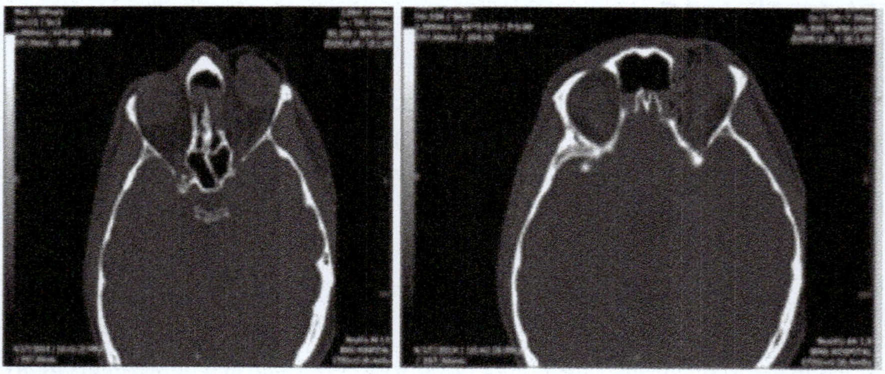

**Fig. 24.31** Periorbital ecchymosis or emphysema

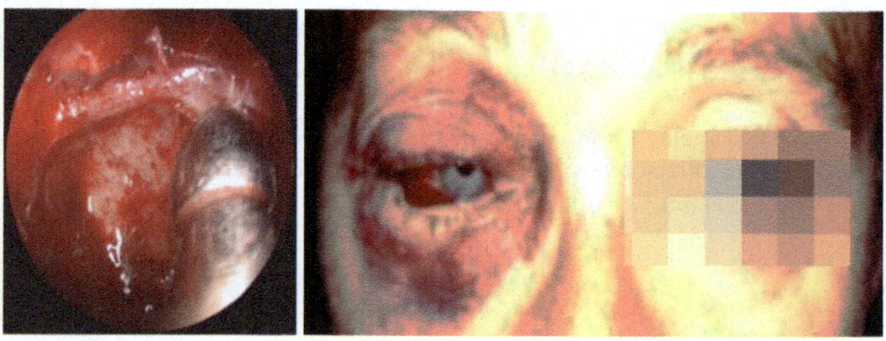

**Fig. 24.32** Periorbital ecchymosis or emphysema

### 24.4.4 Case 4 (Fig. 24.33)

Orbital emphysema due to injury lamina papyracea secondary to shaver violation of posterior lamina papyracea and injury to medial rectus muscles.

### 24.4.5 Case 5 (Fig. 24.34)

Diplopia secondary to medial rectus injury by cold instruments

### 24.4.6 Case 6 (Fig. 24.36)

Patients presented with blindness due to iatrogenic transection optic nerve and violation of the roof of the sphenoid sinus resulting in CSF leak and transection of the optic nerve (Fig. 24.35). Figure 24.36 shows another patient with an optic nerve in the Onodi cell.

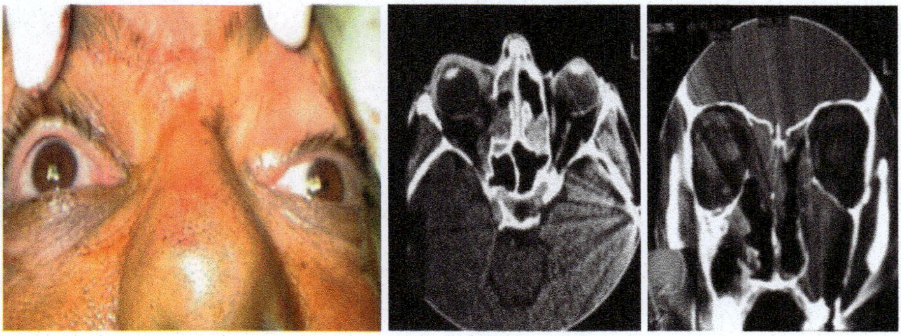

**Fig. 24.33** Diplopia secondary to shaver injury to medial rectus

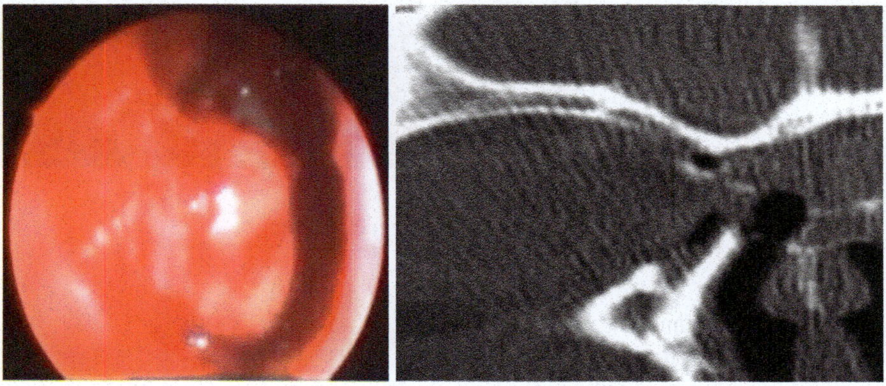

**Fig. 24.34** Diplopia secondary to medial rectus injury

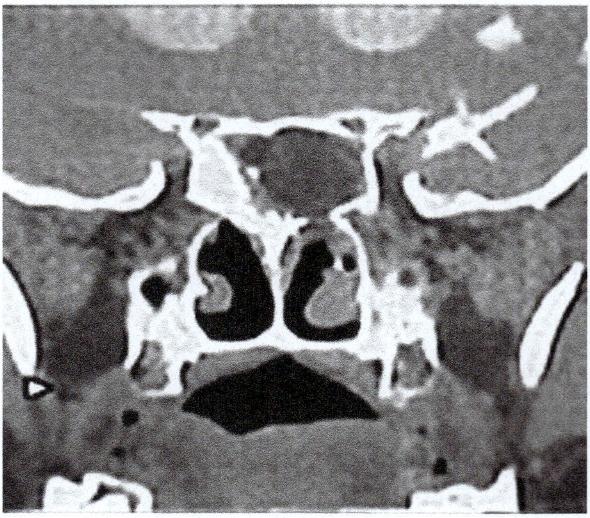

**Fig. 24.35** Optic nerve in onodi cell

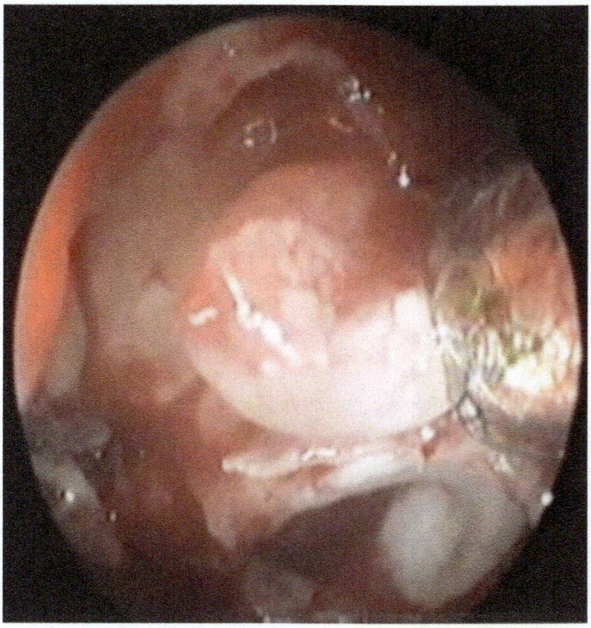

**Fig. 24.36** Transected optic nerve in onodi cell

Blindness following endoscopic sinus surgery can be:

1. Temporary (if treated early)
   (a) Orbital hematoma
2. Permanent due to
   (a) Direct injury to optic nerve (Fig. 24.36)
   (b) Indirect injury to optic nerve: Use of forceps or electrocautery in superior–lateral sphenoid sinus or posterior ethmoid sinus (onodi cell)

### 24.4.7 Case 7 (Fig. 24.37)

Patient presented with an injury to the orbit during orbital decompression for Graves' disease.

### 24.4.8 Case 8

A patient with intraoperative bleeding due to injury of the sphenopalatine artery branch during transnasal endoscopic pituitary surgery controlled by suction cautery.

### 24.4.9 Case 9

A patient with an injury to the anterior ethmoid artery during FESS. Initial attempt at control using suction cautery resulted in further injury to the vessel. Appropriate control was achieved using bipolar cautery.

### 24.4.10 Case 10

A patient with intraoperative bleeding due to injury to cavernous sinus during transnasal endoscopic pituitary surgery. Controlled by pressure packs and Surgicel as well as Gelfoam.

### 24.4.11 Case 11

A patient with intraoperative bleeding due to injury to a branch of the internal carotid artery during transnasal endoscopic pituitary surgery. Initially controlled by pressure packs and Surgicel as well as Gelfoam followed by application of muscle plug together with pressure packs and Surgicel as well as Gelfoam. After stabilization, interventional angiography was performed with coiling of the injured vessel.

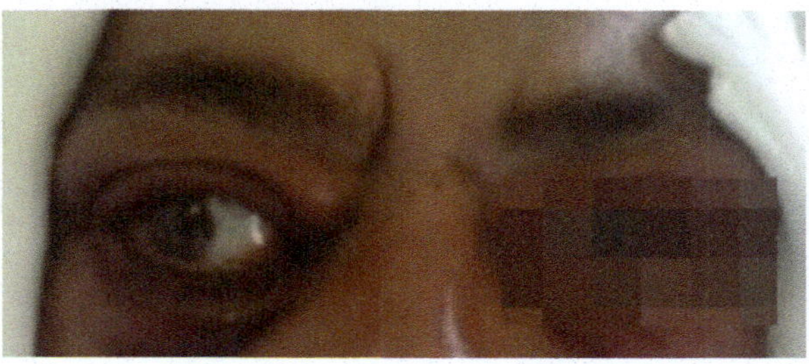

**Fig. 24.37** Injuries to the medial rectus muscle as well as oculomotor nerve. Notice dilation of the pupil

## 24.5 Accessory Ostia

### 24.5.1 Case 12 (Figs. 24.38 and 24.39)

A patient suffering from persistent and recurrent sinusitis due to iatrogenic accessory ostia resolved by revision FESS and joining the ostia with the natural ostium.

### 24.5.2 Case 13

Recirculation. A patient with iatrogenic ostium and secondary recirculation of mucous resulting in persistent sinusitis (Figs. 24.40 and 24.41).

### 24.5.3 Case 14

The typical patient with CSF leak with drippling of unilateral clear fluid from the nostril.

### 24.5.4 Case 15 (Figs. 24.42 and 24.43)

Two patients were referred for repair of iatrogenic cribriform, anterior ethmoid roof defect associated with CSF leak.

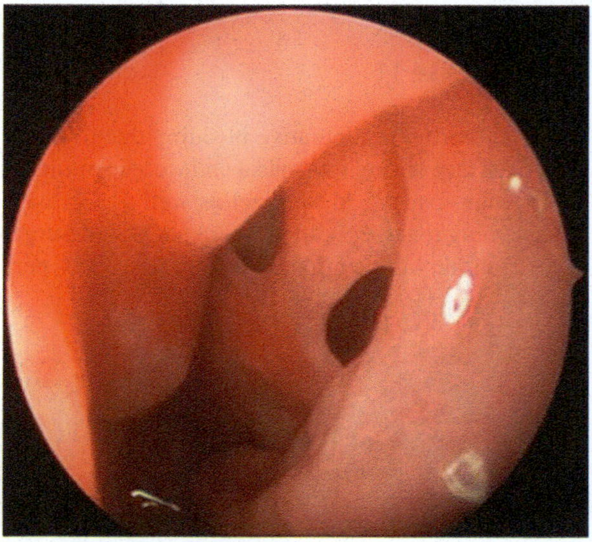

**Fig. 24.38** Accessory ostia

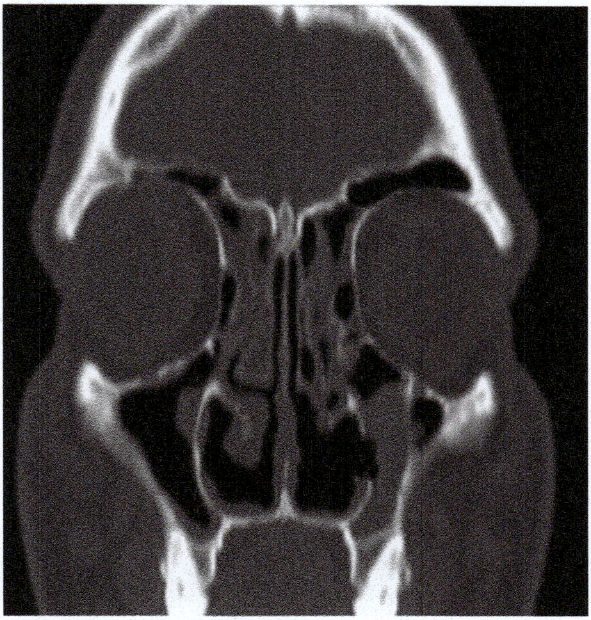

**Fig. 24.39** Persistent sinusitis due to accessory ostia

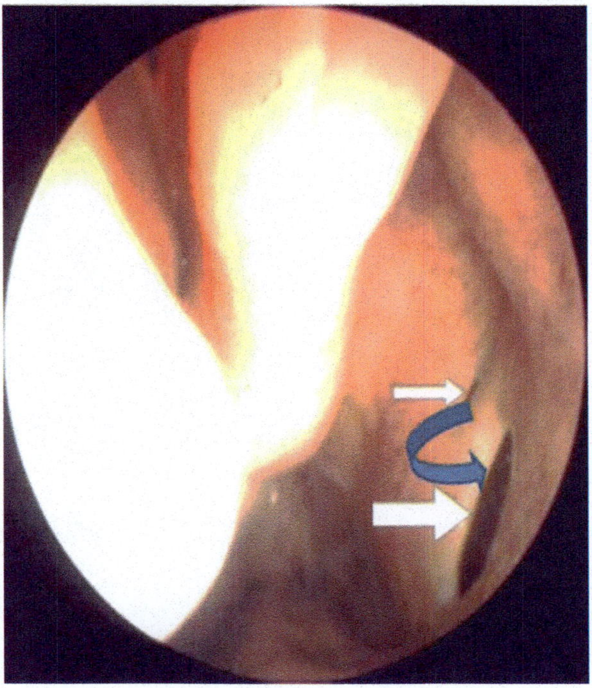

**Fig. 24.40** Bule arrow signifying recirculation of mucous from the accessory ostium to the natural ostium

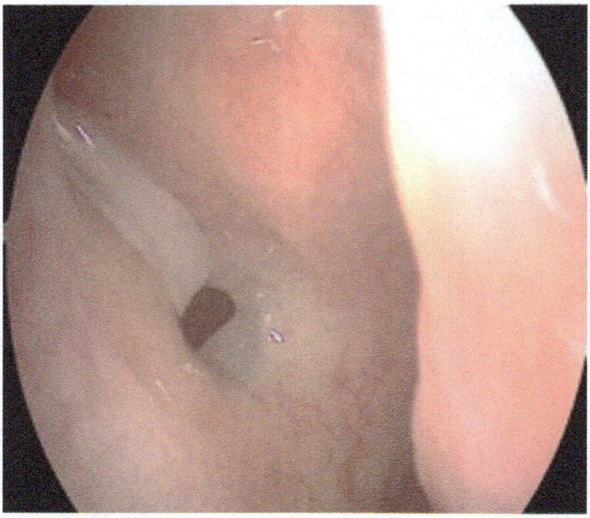

**Fig. 24.41** Recirculation

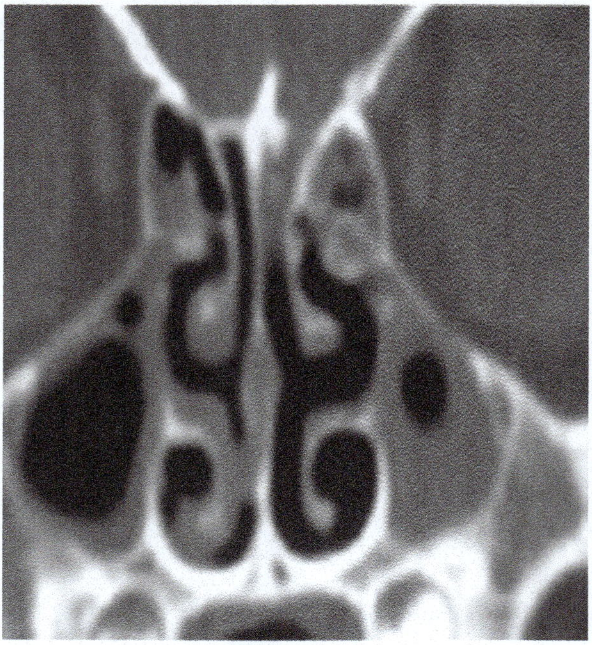

**Fig. 24.42** Iatrogenic cribriform plate defect

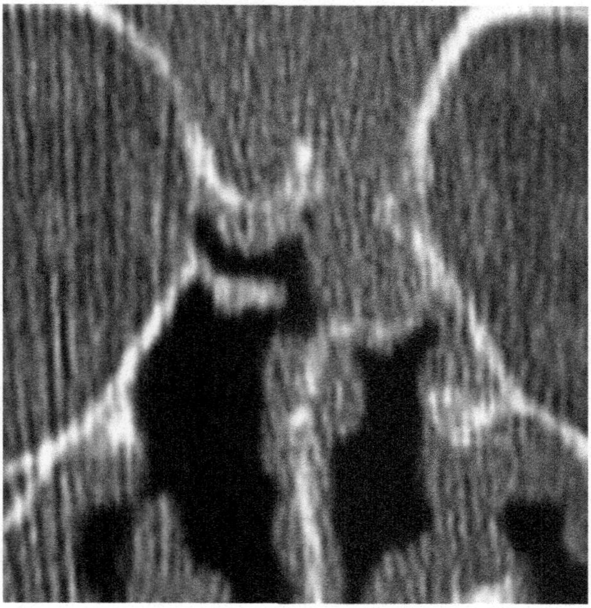

**Fig. 24.43** Iatrogenic ethmoid sinus roof defect

### 24.5.5 Case 16 (Fig. 24.44)

A patient presented with sphenoid sinus violation with CSF leak and pneumocephalus.

### 24.5.6 Case 17 (Fig. 24.45)

A patient referred with an Iatrogenic CSF leak might be associated with Tension Pneumocephalus. Iatrogenic anterior ethmoid roof violation with Intradural air indicates disruption of the dura with the potential occurrence of tension Pneumocephalus.

### 24.5.7 Case 18

An intraoperative consultation for a patient who sustained an ethmoid roof violation with a CSF leak that was repaired immediately.

### 24.5.8 Case 19 (Figs. 24.46, 24.47, and 24.48)

A consultation for the management of a patient with massive violation of the skull base with intracerebral bleeding following FESS.

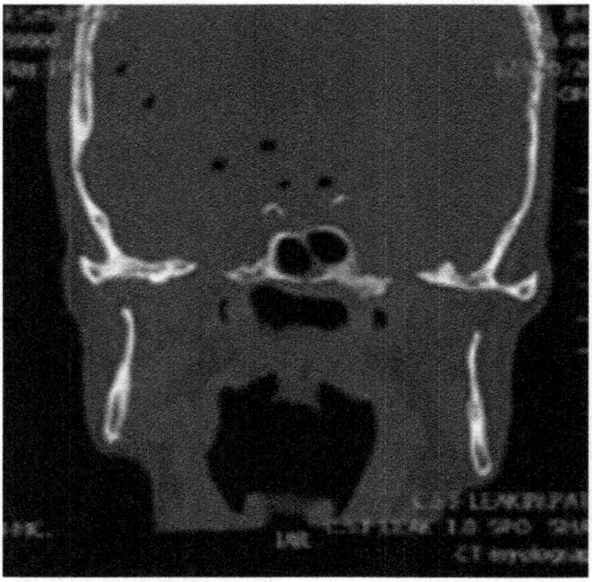

**Fig. 24.44** Sphenoid sinus violation with CSF leak and pneumocephalus

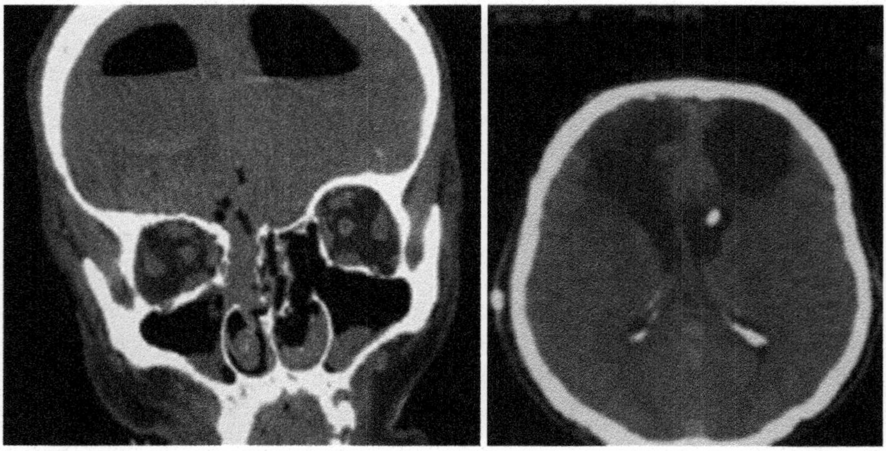

**Fig. 24.45** Iatrogenic CSF leak might be associated with tension pneumocephalus

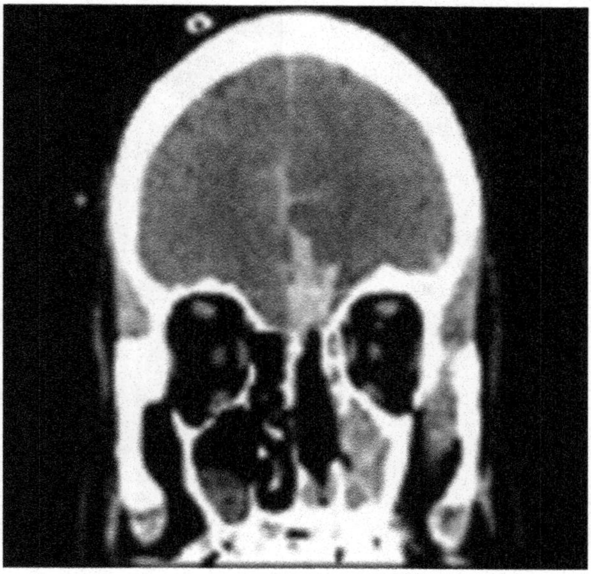

**Fig. 24.46** Coronal CT. Massive violation of skull base with resultant CSF leak as well as intracerebral injury and hematoma

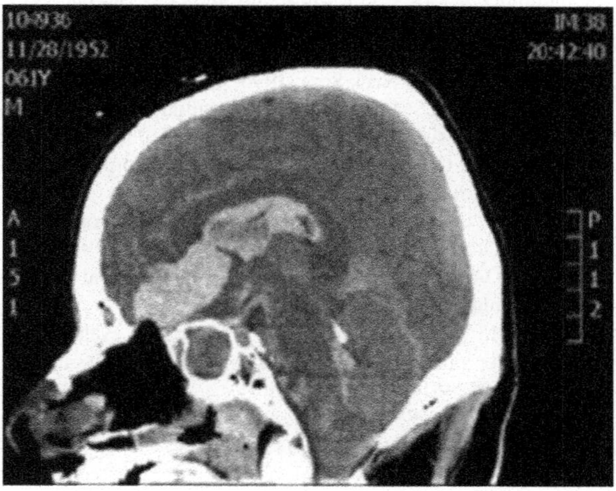


**Fig. 24.47** Sagittal view. Massive violation of skull base with resultant CSF leak as well as intracerebral injury and hematoma

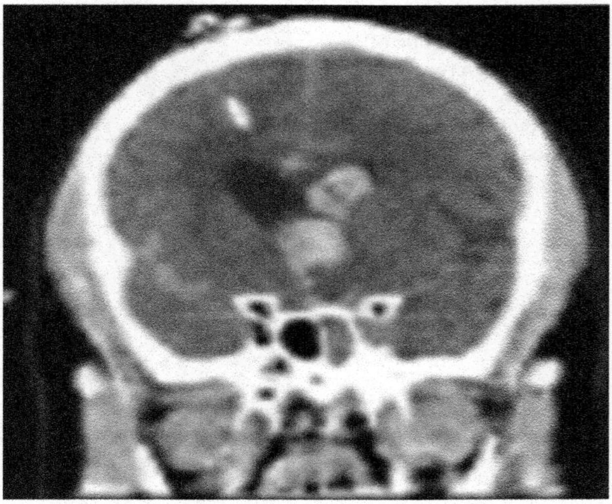

**Fig. 24.48** Coronal CT. Massive violation of skull base with resultant CSF leak as well as intracerebral injury and hematoma

## References


1. Stammberger H. FESS: uncapping the egg. The endoscopic approach to frontal recess and sinuses. Tuttlingen: Storz GmbH; 2015.
2. Kuhn FA. Chronic frontal sinusitis: the endoscopic frontal recess approach. Oper Tech Otolayngol Head Neck Surg. 1996;7:222–9.
3. May M, Sobol SM, Korzec K. The location of the maxillary os and its importance to the endoscopic sinus surgeon. Laryngoscope. 1990;100(10):1037–42.
4. Van Alyea OE. The ostium maxillare: anatomic study of its surgical accessibility. Arch Otolaryngol. 1936;24:553–69.
5. Turgut S, Gumusalan Y, Arifoglu Y, et al. Endoscopic anatomic distances on the lateral nasal wall. J Otolaryngol. 1996;25:371–4.
6. Millar DA, Orlandi RR. The sphenoid sinus natural ostium is consistently medial to the superior turbinate. Am J Rhinol. 2006;20(2):180–1.
7. Lee JM, Woods T, Grewal A. Preoperative evaluation of the maxillary sinus roof as a guide for posterior ethmoid and sphenoid sinus surgery. J Otolaryngol Head Neck Surg. 2012;41(5):361–9.
8. Kim HU, Kim SS, Kang SS, et al. Surgical anatomy of the natural ostium of the sphenoid sinus. Laryngoscope. 2001;111:1599–602.
9. Lee JM, Woods T, Grewal A. Preoperative evaluation of the maxillarysinus roof as a guide for posterior ethmoid and sphenoid sinus surgery. J Otolaryngol Head Neck Surg. 2012;41(5):361–9.
10. Wormald PJ. Surgery of the frontal recess and frontal sinus. Rhinology. 2005;43(2):82–5.
11. Pianta L, Ferrari M, Schreiber A, et al. Agger-bullar classification (ABC) of the frontal sinus drainage pathway: validation in a preclinical setting. Int Forum Allergy Rhinol. 2016;6(9):981–9. https://doi.org/10.1002/alr.21756.
12. Wormald PJ, Hoseman W, Callejas C, et al. The international frontal sinus anatomy classification (IFAC) and classification of the extent of endoscopic frontal sinus surgery (EFSS). Int Forum Allergy Rhinol. 2016;6(7):677–96.
13. Sjogren P. Phayvanh International Frontal Sinus Anatomy Classification and anatomic predictors of low-lying anterior ethmoidal arteries. Am J Rhinol Allergy. 2017;31(3):174–6.
14. Keros P. Über die praktische Bedeutung der Niveauunterschiede de Lamina cribrosa des Ethmoids. Laryngol Rhinol Otol. 1965;41:808–13.

15. Elwany S, Medanni A, Eid M, Aly A, El-Daly A, Ammar SR. Radiological observations on the olfactory fossa and ethmoid roof. J Laryngol Otol. 2010;124(12):1251–6.
16. Harvey RJ, Shelton W, Timperley D, et al. Using fixed anatomical landmarks in endoscopic skull base surgery. Am J Rhinol Allergy. 2010;24(4):301–5.
17. Levine HL. Endoscopic diagnosis and management of cerebrospinal fluid rhinorrea. Oper Tech Otolaryngol Head Neck Surg. 1991;2(4):282–4.
18. Levine HL, May M. Endoscopic sinus surgery. New York: Thieme Medical Publishers; 1993.
19. Stammberger H. Functional endoscopic sinus surgery. Philadelphia: Mosby Year Book; 1991.

# Complications of Endoscopic Sinus Surgery

# 25

Apostolos Karligkiotis, Gianluca Dalfino,
Paolo Castelnuovo, and Giacomo Gravante

**Key Points**

- The proper assessment of complication risk can be structured into three temporal periods: preoperative, intraoperative, and postoperative.
- Preoperative radiological studies are essential for accurate surgical planning and enable the identification of any anatomical variations and potential sites of vulnerability in formulating a surgical roadmap.
- Endoscopic surgical training prepares for the correct management of major complications during operations.

## 25.1 Background

During endoscopic sinus surgery (ESS), several complications may arise. These complications encompass a spectrum from potential intraoperative issues to postoperative concerns [1]. Properly assessing and mitigating these risks across the *preoperative*, *intraoperative*, and *postoperative periods* is crucial to ensure optimal surgical outcomes and patient safety. For this reason, the aim of this chapter is not only to outline the complications that may arise in this surgery but also to recognize and manage them according to the three aforementioned steps.

A. Karligkiotis (✉) · G. Dalfino · P. Castelnuovo · G. Gravante
Division of Otorhinolaryngology, Department of Surgical Specialties, ASST Sette Laghi, Ospedale di Circolo, University of Insubria, Varese, Italy


S. Elwany (ed.), *Current Rhinology*,
https://doi.org/10.1007/978-3-031-70077-4_25

## 25.2 Epidemiology and Classification

The ESS is a routine procedure performed by otolaryngologists worldwide for the treatment of sinonasal pathology as well as in many extended approaches through the nasal cavity, to the periorbital region, infratemporal fossa, and anterior, middle, and posterior skull base [2].

Based on the investigations carried out by the European Rhinologic Society (ERS), complications of endonasal endoscopic sinus surgery could be classified into two severity levels of minor and major complications (Table 25.1) [3, 5]. However, the overall classifications contain four degrees of severity ranging from harmful side effects to death (Grade C) [5]:

1. Harmful side effects, which would be treated spontaneously, and could be managed easily.
2. Complication of grade A; minor complications which require further surgical therapy without any permanent injuries.
3. Complications of grade B; major complications which could cause irreversible damages.
4. Complication of grade C; disastrous complication which could cause death.

The rate of complications during the past decade has been reduced globally [6]. In the literature, the overall complication rate for ESS ranged from 0.3 to 22.4%, with minor and major complication rates ranging from 1.1 to 20.8% and 0 to 1.5%, respectively [7–9]. Anyway, complication risk would increase within the following situations [5, 10, 11]:

- Advanced inflammatory disease of the paranasal sinuses which requires a broader surgical procedure.
- Revision endoscopic sinus surgery.
- Patient with serious comorbidities.
- The presence of anatomical abnormalities and variations.
- Increased risk of acute bleeding during the operation procedure.
- The absence of a sufficiently experienced surgeon.

**Table 25.1** Complications of endoscopic sinonasal surgery, divided into major and minor according to severity. Data extracted from "European position paper on rhinosinusitis and nasal polyposis" with additions [3, 4]

| | Complications | |
|---|---|---|
| Location | Minor | Major |
| Orbit and nasolacrimal duct | Orbital emphysema<br>Eyelid ecchymosis | Orbital hematoma<br>Loss of visual acuity/blindness (optic nerve damage)<br>Diplopia<br>Enophthalmia<br>Papyracea damage with intraorbital fat herniation<br>Nasolacrimal duct trauma (with epiphora) |
| Intracranial | Uncomplicated CSF leak | Cranial CSF leak<br>Encephalocele<br>Pneumocephalus (tension)<br>Meningitis<br>Cerebral abscess<br>Direct brain trauma<br>Subarachnoid and intracerebral hemorrhage |
| Vascular network (bleeding) | Minor hemorrhage without any need for blood transfusion and stoppable with nasal packing | Anterior ethmoid artery (AEA) injury<br>Posterior ethmoid artery (PEA) injury<br>Sphenopalatine artery (SPA) injury<br>Internal carotid artery (ICA) injury<br>Major bleeding which needs a blood transfusion |
| Other | Synechiae and stenosis<br>Slight exacerbation of preexistent asthma<br>Septal perforation<br>Hyposmia<br>Paraffinoma<br>Local infection (osteitis, inferior turbinate necrosis, etc.)<br>Atrophic rhinitis<br>Myospherulosis<br>Temporary irritation of the infraorbital nerve<br>Teeth or lip hypo-/hyperesthesia | Toxic shock syndrome (TSS)<br>Anosmia<br>Severe exacerbation of preexistent asthma or bronchospasm<br>Death |

*CSF* cerebrospinal fluid

## 25.3 How to Manage Complications

### 25.3.1 Preoperative Period

A thorough preoperative assessment and detailed knowledge of the anatomical structures are essential to prevent potential complications. Awareness is crucial: the study of possible variations in the patient's sinonasal anatomy and the assessment of disease extension facilitates the most appropriate choice in surgical planning.

#### 25.3.1.1 Medical History Collection and Endoscopic Findings

It is of paramount importance to clarify symptoms characteristics, investigate any previous conservative or surgical treatments, and the outcomes of therapies administered. Comorbidities such as hypertension, diabetes mellitus, lifestyle habits, coagulopathies, or antiplatelet/anticoagulant therapies constitute a pivotal aspect of the medical history evaluation. The collected elements present a clinical picture with intricate contours [12]. Endoscopic examination defines anatomy and guides the judgment toward a diagnostic hypothesis, whether inflammatory or neoplastic in nature [13].

#### 25.3.1.2 Radiological Imaging

Maxillofacial computed tomography (CT) scan without contrast medium is now considered the gold standard for surgical planning: it is advisable to perform it in axial, sagittal, and coronal projections with bone algorithm. The acquisition of different planes provides an opportunity to identify and analyze in detail the anatomical structures, volumes, and spaces that define themselves. Implementing this method in daily practice, through practice and consistency, offers the possibility of a "three-dimensional" view of the ethmoid labyrinth and forming a mental roadmap of the surgical steps [14, 15]. Concerning inflammatory pathology of the lacrimal pathways, when possible, performing a radiological study with dacryo-CT is always recommended [16]. An adjunct to CT is magnetic resonance imaging (MRI), performed with a contrast medium. This method is highly useful in characterizing the extension, nature, and biological behavior of the pathology. Often underestimated, the necessity of this examination is indispensable in revealing skull base defects, revision surgery, staging tumors, defining the suspicion of invasive mycosis, and for many other differential diagnoses where MRI sequences provide valuable information in the diagnostic workup [14]. Some authors have proposed the acronym "CLOSE" in order to define a mental checklist of the structures to be looked for and analyzed during the study of preoperative radiological anatomy. It stays for Cribriform plate depth, symmetry, and slope of lateral lamella; Lamina papyracea integrity; Onodi cells and Optic nerve dehiscence; Sphenoid pneumatization and Skull base integrity; Ethmoid artery position. They recommend analyzing the points described in the first preoperative period and reviewing every aspects at the end of the surgery: the comparison between the expectations collected in the preparatory period and the experience acquired during the surgery will guide the surgical training [17].

#### 25.3.1.3 Nasal Biopsy

When facing a doubt about tumor—benign or malignant—it is recommended to perform a biopsy (after evaluating the vascular supply to the lesion and/or the possible presence of meningocele/meningoencephaloceles) [18, 19].

**Checklist: "Clinical Risk" Assessment**

- "Exogenous" risk
- Surgical technique adopted
- Surgical experience of the operator
- "Endogenous" risk
  - Extent and degree of sinonasal pathology
  - Previous surgery (subverted anatomy, loss of anatomical findings, aberrant scarring)
  - Anatomical variants at risk
  - Intraoperative bleeding (most expected in revision surgery, in patients with chronic liver disease, alcoholism, chronic renal failure, malnutrition, or vitamin K deficiency)
  - Age
  - Preoperative assessment of olfactory function
  - Comorbidities
  - Other (Cystic fibrosis, connective tissue disorders, Kartagener syndrome, vasculitis, sarcoidosis, Samter's triad, fungal pathology...)

### 25.3.2 Intraoperative Period

The preparatory steps before the surgical procedure are as crucial as the intervention itself. It is a prudent practice to ensure the patient is optimally prepared and to carefully study the radiological images in all three projections to identify any anatomical variations. The perioperative anesthetic management will be pivotal for the success of the procedure. The major anesthetic objectives include (a) airway management; (b) adequate hemodynamic support; (c) absence of movements on the surgical field; (d) prompt awakening without coughing, straining, or tension; (e) facilitated discharge by adequate pain control, potential bleeding management, hemodynamic parameters control, and nausea and vomiting management [20, 21]. In particular, regarding (b), the need for visibility and reduced bleeding in the surgical field are paramount in endoscopic surgery. Anesthetic strategies involve maintaining superior hemodynamic stability, preference for total intravenous anesthesia (TIVA) using propofol and remifentanil, controlled moderate hypotension, relative bradycardia, elevating the patient's head by 15–20°, monitoring the depth of sedation, and optimizing inspiratory pressure during controlled ventilation [22]. Endoscopic endonasal surgery requires adequate, updated, and complete instrumentation. It involves a broad array of forceps and aspirators of various sizes and angles, as well as endoscopes, high-definition acquisition systems, recording systems, hemostasis materials, cutting drills, endoscopic navigation, and more. The success of a safe surgery relies on a combination of solid anatomical knowledge and technological support [23, 24]. The radiological imaging-guided navigation (IGN) system is a widespread technology that provides detailed information about the complex nasal and paranasal anatomy during a surgical procedure. A statistically significant reduction in the complication rate has been demonstrated over time [25]. However, it is important to note that the navigator's localization is based on a predefined set of preoperative images. As the surgical procedure alters the anatomical spaces, the precision and accuracy offered by the navigator diminish. Therefore, IGN is considered an additional tool in selected cases and cannot substitute inadequate knowledge of endoscopic anatomy by the operator. Table 25.2 displays the surgical steps of functional endoscopic sinus surgery (FESS) with potential complications in relation to the surgical maneuver performed.

### 25.3.3 Postoperative Period

Endoscopic sinus surgery, especially for inflammatory conditions, follows standardized steps (Table 25.2). However, repetition or automation does not safeguard against complications; managing them correctly is a significant part of mastering this surgery. A thorough anatomical understanding of the region, supported by dissection practice and surgical training, is deemed essential. The biological variability and unpredictability are considered the sole independent variable in the realm of complications. It is important to note that the severity of complications, barring gross errors, generally aligns with the difficulty level of the performed endoscopic surgery. Different publications stress the need to recognize one's limitations: when excessive bleeding or disorientation from the absence of surgical landmarks don't permit to conduct safe surgical procedure, the best decision may be to conclude the surgery and reschedule it, or refer the patient to an experienced sinus/skull base center. Focusing on chronic sinusitis which is the most commonly treated pathology, major complications involve the orbit, skull base, and uncontrolled arterial bleeding. Detailed postoperative management of major and minor complications is described in the following paragraphs.

**Table 25.2** Surgical steps of functional endoscopic sinus surgery (FESS) with potential complications in relation to the surgical maneuver performed

| Surgical step | Anatomical variant | Surgical maneuver | Possible complications |
|---|---|---|---|
| Retrograde uncinectomy | – Insertion of uncinate process on the nasolacrimal duct<br>– Lateralization of the uncinate process<br>– Pneumatization of the uncinate process<br>– Concha bullosa of the middle turbinate<br>– Haller's cells | Endonasal endoscopy starts with a rigid 0° optic. To access the middle meatus and visualize the free edge of the uncinate process, it is sometimes necessary to resect the anterior free portion of the middle turbinate. This is followed by an uncinectomy by using backbiter forceps to engage the free posterior margin of the uncinate process in the area between the vertical and horizontal portions under the floor of the ethmoidal bulla, progressively cutting forward to the bony portion (thicker and more consistent) of the frontal process of the maxillary bone | – CSF leak for fracture of the cranial portion of the middle turbinate where it articulates with lateral lamella during the middle turbinate plastic procedure<br>– Papyracea and orbit lesion for engagement with backbiter forceps very lateral or above the floor of the bulla<br>– Nasolacrimal duct injury due to excessive forward cut with backbiter forceps |
| Inferior partial uncinectomy and maxillary sinusotomy | – Accessory ostium<br>– Infraorbital nerve dehiscence | With a rigid 45° angled optic, it is possible to assess the correct exposure of the natural ostium of the maxillary sinus. The inferior partial uncinectomy is completed by removing the horizontal portion of the uncinate process with sharp forceps. The Mackay-Grünwald forceps allow anterior-posterior cutting by engaging the posterior edge of the ostium; Stammberger side-cutting antrum punch forceps allow the top-bottom widening by engaging the lower edge of the ostium | – Infraorbital nerve injury due to its canal dehiscence on the roof of the maxillary sinus<br>– Injury of the posterior lateral branch of the sphenopalatine artery due to excessive cut behind the posterior border of the ostium<br>– Lesion of the upper margin of the inferior turbinate during inferior calibration of antrostomy with Stammberger side-cutting antrum punch forceps |
| Upper partial uncinectomy | – Variants of uncinate process insertion according to Landsberg and Friedman's classification [26]<br>– Pneumatization of agger nasi | With 0° optic, after frontalization of the vertical portion of the uncinate process, the uncinectomy is completed with angled cutting forceps, taking care to preserve its most cranial portion, an important reference point in the identification of the frontal recess (vertical bar) | – Lesion of the nasolacrimal duct during the removal of the uncinate process<br>– CSF leak due to inexperience in cranial disarticulation of the uncinate process |

(continued)

**Table 25.2** (continued)

| Surgical step | Anatomical variant | Surgical maneuver | Possible complications |
|---|---|---|---|
| Frontal sinusotomy | – Relation between agger nasi and bulla ethmoidalis<br>– AEA<br>– Kuhn cells<br>– Lateral lamella<br>– Supraorbital recess | With 45° angled optic, the cranial portion of the uncinate process (vertical bar) is visualized: depending on its insertion, it can lead toward the frontoethmoidal recess or end laterally on the lamina papyracea, taking the name of agger nasi. Once the vertical bar has been removed, the ostium of the frontal sinus can be visualized in its entirety, and it is possible to appreciate the posterior wall of the sinus itself. The posterior wall of the frontal sinus is an important reference point, as it is the most anterior portion of the anterior skull base. The landmark for finding the AEA is the posterior wall of the first foveola. It is recommended to use sharp forceps at this stage to avoid tearing the AEA | – CSF leak due to lateromedial or anteroposterior movements at the level of the frontal recess in the search for the frontal sinus<br>– Lesion of the lamina papyracea due to aggressive lateral movements in search for the frontal sinus<br>– Hemorrhage of the AEA with risk of its retraction in the orbital cavity and subsequent retrobulbar hemorrhage/hematoma due to stripping and rupture of the AEA |
| Ethmoidal bullectomy | – Pneumatization of bulla ethmoidalis<br>– Supra- and retrobullar recesses<br>– Lamina papyracea dehiscence | With 0° optic, the bulla ethmoidalis is opened with the aid of a J curette, engaging its inferomedial angle, and first removing its anterior wall and then adjusting the inferior and medial walls with the aid of a Mackay-Grünwald forceps. At this point, the posterior wall of the bulla will be visualized, which can have a retrobullar space or correspond to the basal lamella, which represents the second portion of the middle turbinate and the boundary between the anterior and posterior ethmoid | – Lesion of the lamina papyracea due to engagement of the bulla with J curette laterally and not in its inferomedial angle of safety<br>– CSF leak due to engagement of the bulla with J curette superiorly and not in its inferomedial angle of safety |
| Basal lamella | | The opening of the basal lamella or second portion of the middle turbinate, to access the posterior ethmoid, occurs in the carrefour between the first, second, and third portions of the middle turbinate, with J curette | – Same risks as ethmoidal bullectomy<br>– Destabilization of the first portion of the middle turbinate by abatement of the third portion in the carrefour research |

| | | | |
|---|---|---|---|
| Posterior ethmoidectomy | – Onodi cells<br>– Orbital apex procidence | The dissection of the posterior ethmoid involves the opening of the ethmoidal cells with the aid of J curette, Mackay-Grünwald forceps, and straight circular cutting punch forceps having as reference limits: laterally the lamina papyracea, inferiorly the third portion of the middle turbinate, superiorly the ethmoidal roof and medially the first portion of the middle turbinate and the superior turbinate. The latter represents the key structure in the detection of the sphenoid ostium by transethmoidal route and therefore the posterior limit of the posterior ethmoid, i.e., the anterior wall of the sphenoid sinus. If the posterior ethmoidal cell is pneumatized and extends into the sphenoid sinus, it is then called the Onodi cell, and within its lateral wall, it is possible to identify the bony canal of the optic nerve and sometimes the internal carotid artery (ICA) | – CSF leak, lamina papyracea lesion, orbital injury, middle turbinate destabilization, PEA lesion, for exceeding the limits described in the procedure<br>– Optic nerve or ICA injury due to lesions of the bone boundaries of the Onodi cell |
| Sphenoidotomy | – Types of sphenoid pneumatization (sellar, presellar, conchal)<br>– Rostrum pneumatization<br>– Intersphenoid septal insertion on ICA/optic nerve<br>– Lateral recess pneumatization | With the aid of Mackay-Grünwald forceps, the tail of the superior turbinate is dissected, taking care not to direct the instrumentation upwards due to the risk on the common lamella and the skull base. At this point, the natural ostium of the sphenoid sinus will be visible, which, depending on the rostral pneumatization, may be medial to the superior turbinate (the most common case) or lateral to it. With the help of a straight circular cutting punch forceps, the ostium is engaged and the anterior wall of the sphenoid sinus is completely removed. At this point, the sphenoid landmarks will be clearly visible on the posterior wall of the sphenoid sinus in a sellar pneumatized sinus | – CSF leak, optic nerve injury, ICA hemorrhage, pituitary lesion due to lesion of the posterior wall of the sphenoid sinus |

## 25.4 Major Complications

### 25.4.1 Orbital Complications

The involved anatomical structures include (1) Nasolacrimal duct; (2) Intraorbital or retrobulbar spaces; (3) Lamina papyracea; (4) Extraocular muscles; (5) Optic nerve.

The injury to the nasolacrimal duct typically occurs during the uncinectomy to approach the maxillary sinus; conservative treatment involves the intraoperative immediate marsupialization of the damaged duct and the use of corticosteroids and antibiotics. Persistent epiphora may require a dacryocystorhinostomy [27].

Any orbital fat herniation due to a small breach in the lamina papyracea can be effectively treated with bipolar cauterization [28]. Intraorbital hemorrhage or retrobulbar hematoma results from iatrogenic injury to the ethmoidal arteries, often caused by damage to the anterior ethmoidal artery, majorly when it is dehiscent within a pneumatized ethmoid labyrinth mesentery. The damaged arterial vessel may retract into the orbital cavity especially if it gets pulled or striped with a Blakesley forceps. Bleeding within the rigid orbital cavity leads to an orbital compartmental syndrome, representing an ophthalmologic emergency. Manifestations include rapid and progressive vision loss, orbital edema, proptosis, eyelid ecchymosis, diplopia, decreased extraocular motility, and severe pain. The increased intraorbital pressure raises intraocular pressure, compressing the optic nerve and its vascular bundle. If left untreated, this heightened pressure leads to permanent vision loss. Recognizing and promptly treating this complication is crucial: actions taken immediately can minimize the duration of retinal ischemia. An ophthalmological consultation is always recommended, but it should not delay an operative approach: relieving pressure on the eye through lateral canthotomy and cantholysis is necessary. The medial and lateral canthal ligaments secure the eye within the orbit and eyelids. Lateral canthotomy is the surgical exposure of the lateral canthal tendon. Cantholysis involves incising the branch (crus), usually the lower one, of the tendon. This allows the globe to expand outside the orbit. The procedure is painful and requires the patient's cooperation or sedation. The maneuvers executed so far constitute a gradual process aimed at achieving intraorbital pressure reduction; they also provide valuable time for the urgent execution of endoscopic orbital decompression. Attaining this goal involves complete uncinectomy, extensive maxillary antrostomy identifying the orbital floor, up to the posterior wall of the maxillary sinus, complete sphenoethmoidectomy, and frontal recess opening. Upon completing these steps, there is wide illumination of the nasal lateral wall, lamina papyracea in its entirety, orbital floor, and posterior wall of the maxillary sinus. The described preparation also aims to prevent potential frontal or maxillary sinusitis: excessive orbital fat herniation could obstruct sinus ostia. Subsequently, the entire lamina papyracea is removed—from the orbital floor to the ethmoidal roof—proceeding ventrodorsally toward the sphenoid sinus while preserving the orbital periosteum at this stage (excessive fat herniation may obscure the field, making dissection more challenging). Decompression of the medial wall is completed by incising the periorbita. If further reduction of intraorbital pressure is necessary, bone removal can extend to the orbit floor. Endoscopically, only the posterior half of the orbital floor is accessible through maxillary antrostomy; the lateral limit of dissection is the infraorbital nerve. A superior eyelid approach extends decompression to the anterior half of the orbital floor and lateral wall. A breach in the lamina papyracea may cause subtle, delayed venous bleeding hours later, typically presenting with pain and visual decline. Optic nerve injury, though rare, mostly results from unrecognized Onodi cells, leading to iatrogenic damage. Treatment involves systemic corticosteroids, ophthalmologic evaluation, and endoscopic optic nerve decompression as a final option [29].

### 25.4.2 Cerebrospinal Fluid (CSF) Leak

The upper limit of the nasal cavities is defined by the base of the anterior cranial fossa. This plane is a composite of several structures: paranasal sinus mucosa, skull base bones and their periosteum, dura mater, and arachnoid. While the skull base offers some resistance to trauma and inadequate iatrogenic maneuvers, there are intrinsic points of fragility where a disruption in this plane can occur. The resultant discontinuity is termed a cerebrospinal fluid (CSF) leak or rhinoliquorrhea, creating a communication between the intracranial space and the sinonasal region, which in turn can lead to endocranial complications such as migraines, pneumocephalus, meningitis, meningoencephalitis, sepsis, intracranial hypotension, and coma. Surgical maneuvers within the ethmoidal roof, sphenoid, and frontal sinus must be carefully considered. Areas of higher risk include (1) lateral ethmoid lamella (Fig. 25.1); (2) cribriform plate; (3) transition area between the ethmoid roof and the posterior table of the frontal sinus; (4) sphenoid sinus. The eventual iatrogenic leak must be accurately recognized and addressed during the surgery (Fig. 25.2). Three factors are critical in determining the most suitable procedure: the size of the defect, the location of the discontinuity, and the speed of the CSF flow through the fistulous tract. Generally, a large defect and/or high CSF flow necessitate a more comprehensive sealing technique. This goal can be achieved using a gasket seal technique or alternatively with a multilayer approach (employing grafts of fascia lata and autologous fat, intracranially; pedunculated local intranasal flaps, as overlay). Conversely, a small defect and/or low CSF flow may benefit from a pedunculated local flap alone or an overlay fascia lata graft on the defect. After the procedure, several measures should be taken to reduce CSF pressure and prevent infectious complications. These include laxatives, antihistamines, broad-spectrum antibiotic therapy, bed rest with gradual head elevation (at 0° for the first postoperative day, then 30° on the second, 45° on the third with the possibility of sitting up for main meals, then 45° on the fourth day with the option of sitting in a chair, and finally unrestricted mobilization on the fifth day, with discharge possible on the sixth day). Among conservative treatments, continuous lumbar drainage (150 ml/day) is mentioned; however, it is important to note that it may increase the risk of tension pneumocephalus and infectious and neurological complications like meningitis [30]. Diagram 25.1 provides a decision-making algorithm regarding the assessment and recognition of a potential CSF leak following sinonasal surgical procedures.

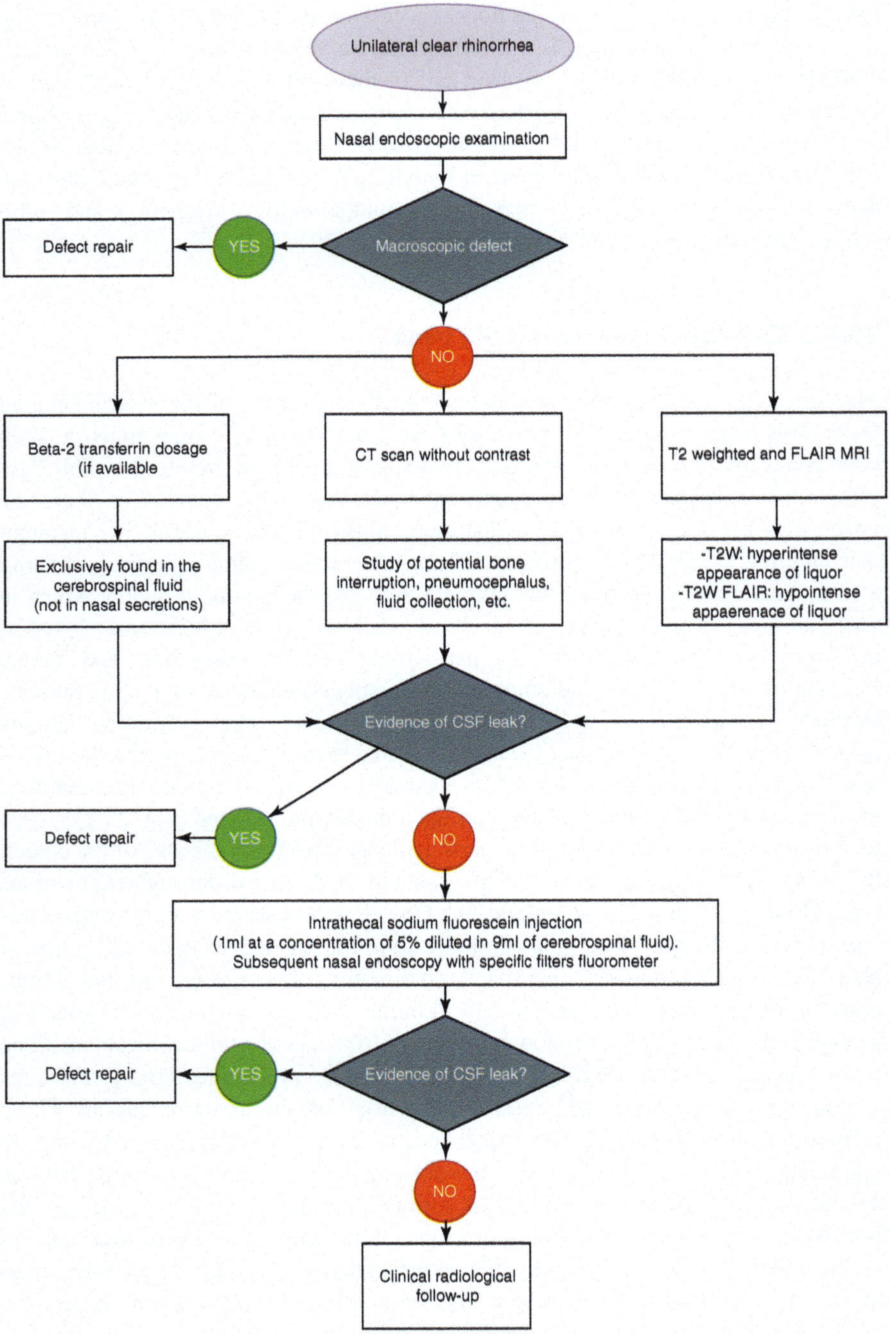


**Diagram 25.1** Diagnostic-decisional algorithm in the suspicion of CSF leak

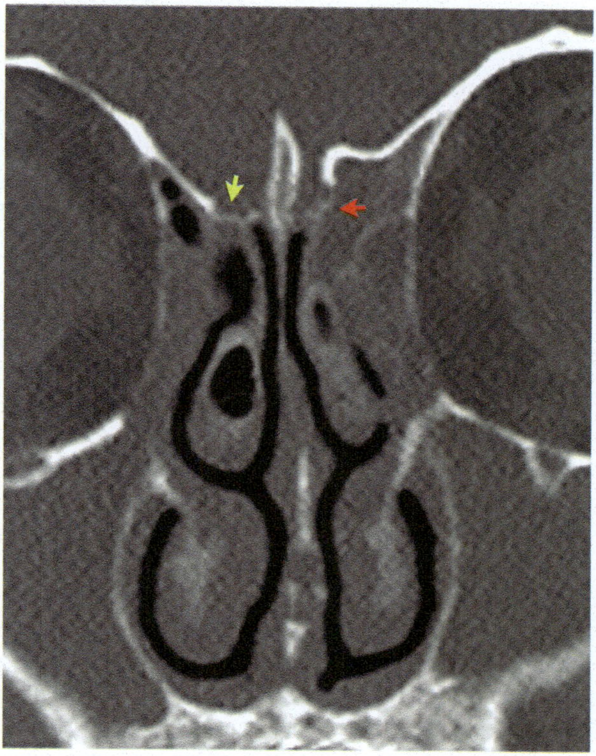

**Fig. 25.1** Ethmoidal lateral lamella on CT scan: note the two different inclinations, placing more at risk of damage on the right side (yellow arrow) than on the left side (red arrow)

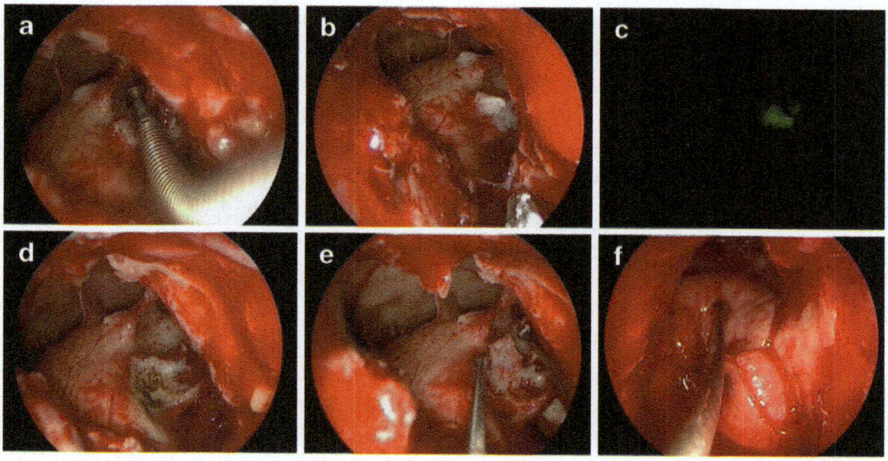


**Fig. 25.2** Clinical case of iatrogenic CSF fistula. In the intraoperative image, widening of the frontal sinusotomy is shown, using the STAMMBERGER curved frontal sinus punch (**a**); evidence of the following iatrogenic fistula with CSF leak from the bone breach (**b**) also confirmed by the fluorescein test (**c**); smoothing of the edges of the defect to get a surfactant effect for the graft/flap (**d**); positioning of septal cartilage fragment to seal the defect (**e**); apposition of a septal mucoperichondrial flap to cover the defect (**f**)

### 25.4.3 Hemorrhagic Complications

Hemorrhagic complications related to sinonasal surgery can manifest within the first postoperative hours or occur days later—generally between 1–3 weeks—and, in such cases, are more frequently related to the sphenopalatine region. The highly vascularized region within the nasal cavities is known as Kiesselbach's plexus (also called Little's area) at the level of the anterior nasal septum. Although it is the source of most spontaneous nosebleeds, its contribution to postbleeding complications appears negligible. During surgical maneuvers, the major arteries at risk of iatrogenic injury include the nasolabial artery (NLA), anterior ethmoidal artery (AEA), posterior ethmoidal artery (PEA), sphenopalatine artery (SPA), and internal carotid artery (ICA). The NLA might be severed during a septoplasty intervention. Regarding the ethmoidal arteries (AEA and PEA), correct identification using preoperative CT scans helps avoid inadvertently disrupting them during the ethmoidectomy procedure. Tearing these vessels and their retraction into the orbital cavity can lead to retrobulbar hemorrhage/hematoma. Hence, near the ethmoidal arteries, it is essential to proceed cautiously with sharp forceps and cauterize the severed vessel edges. The SPA and its branches account for most postoperative bleeding. Specifically, the nasoseptal artery and the posterolateral nasal artery, with its branches to the turbinates, are commonly involved. Surgical maneuvers that risk injuring these structures include inferior widening of a sphenoidotomy and volume reduction of the middle turbinate tail. Finally, utmost care must be taken to avoid injuring the ICA during surgical maneuvers involving the sphenoid sinus. There are anatomical conditions at higher risk, primarily involving three aspects: (1) the degree of sphenoid sinus pneumatization (more challenging in presellar and conchal variants); (2) variations in the intersphenoid sinus septum (when lateralized, it can insert at the internal carotid artery bony canal or the optic nerve); (3) dehiscence or prolapse of the ICA. In a sellar-type sphenoid sinus, ICA typically exhibits a distinctive prominence on the posterior wall of the sphenoid sinus making it identifiable. However, in a presellar-type sphenoid sinus, recognition is more challenging, and the risk of injury is higher. Preoperative imaging through a maxillofacial CT scan allows the examination of the sphenoid tract in its paraclival and parasellar components, facilitating the identification of ICA dehiscence, its close distance from the anterior wall of the sphenoid sinus, and potential intersphenoid septum insertion, or bony septa on the paraclival carotid prominence.

The management of epistaxis involves assessing the bleeding extent, the opportunity to visualize and control the bleeding area, patient compliance, hemodynamic stability, and airway management. These factors are crucial in deciding whether to resolve the bleeding under local anesthesia or to return the patient to the operating room. In both cases, under endoscopic vision with a 0° rigid endoscope, the nasal cavities are decongested using cotton pads soaked in oxymetazoline. This technique selectively packs and maps the territory of the described vessels, reducing active bleeding by vasoconstriction. Using bipolar forceps (straight Dessi type), the active bleeding point is cauterized, often resolving the issue. Bleeding sustained from SPA branches can be insidious, sometimes necessitating the isolation and cauterization of the internal maxillary artery's terminal branch. Bleeding due to ICA injury is a dramatic, challenging, and potentially fatal event. Addressing this emergency requires a variety of measures: sphenoid packing with hemostatic gauze and resuscitative support, followed by urgent angiography and embolization or flow diverter endovascular stent placement using interventional neuroradiology techniques (Fig. 25.3) [31].

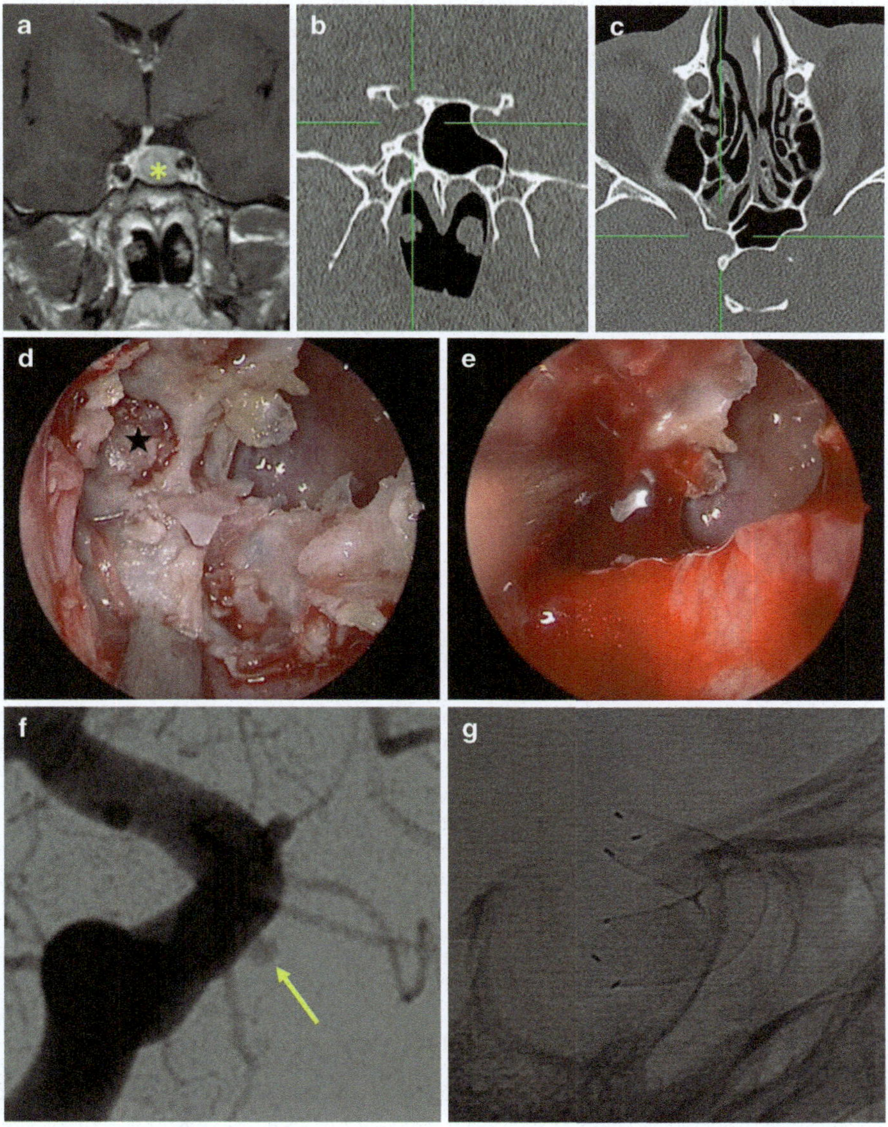


**Fig. 25.3** Clinical case of ICA bleeding. Preoperative coronal contrast-enhanced MRI (**a**) of a GH-secreting pituitary adenoma indicated with yellow asterisk; preoperative coronal (**b**) and axial (**c**) radiological study with CT scan with focus on the cavernous tract of the right ICA (area outlined by green lines); exposure of the right ICA at the previously reported point (black star) during widening of the sphenoidotomy (**d**); onset of ICA bleeding (**e**); angiography with evidence (yellow arrow) of cavernous ICA (anterior genu) pseudoaneurysm (**f**); pseudoaneurysm exclusion using an endovascular flow diverter stent (**g**)

## 25.5 Minor Complications

Minor complications are more commonly encountered and easily resolved compared to major ones. The mean rate of these complications is reported to be around 6% in the literature [32]. In the context of functional endoscopic sinus surgery, they include scarring, delayed wound healing, mild bleeding, necrosis of the inferior turbinate, small septal perforations, periorbital ecchymosis or emphysema, and lip or teeth hypoesthesia/hyperesthesia. Scars can lead to stenosis or closure of paranasal sinus drainage pathways, potentially causing inflammatory complications such as mucoceles and abscesses. If medical therapy does not improve symptoms and clinical status, revision surgery may be considered. Mild bleeding can be managed with nasal packing for 48 h or cauterization of the bleeding vessel. Necrosis of the inferior turbinate might occur due to excessive heat from cauterizing instruments during decongestion; any necrotic portion should be promptly removed to prevent more significant complications like osteitis. Small septal perforations, if nonfunctional, usually do not require surgical treatment. Periorbital ecchymosis or emphysema of mild/moderate extent generally requires observation; if they pose a risk of major ocular complications due to their size, drainage may be necessary. Lip or teeth hypoesthesia/hyperesthesia in the perinasal innervation territories are usually temporary and do not lead to long-term effects [33].

## References

1. Battaglia P, Lambertoni A, Castelnuovo P. Transnasal endoscopic surgery: surgical techniques and complications. In: Nicolai P, Bradley PJ, editors. Advances in oto-rhino-laryngology, vol. 84. Basel: Karger; 2020. p. 46–55. https://doi.org/10.1159/000457924.
2. Hosemann W, Draf C. Danger points, complications and medico-legal aspects in endoscopic sinus surgery, vol. 12. GMS Curr Top Otorhinolaryngol Head Neck Surg; 2013. p. Doc06. https://doi.org/10.3205/cto000098.
3. Fokkens WJ, et al. European position paper on rhinosinusitis and nasal polyps 2020. Rhinology. 2020;58(S29):464. https://doi.org/10.4193/Rhin20.600.
4. Fokkens W, Lund V, Mullol J, European Position Paper on Rhinosinusitis and Nasal Polyps Group. European position paper on rhinosinusitis and nasal polyps 2007. Rhinol Suppl. 2007;20:136.
5. Khademi S, Kazemi A, Divanbeigi R, Afzalzadeh M. A review of the revisions and complications management procedure in sinus surgery. J Family Med Prim Care. 2022;11(3):887–95. https://doi.org/10.4103/jfmpc.jfmpc_897_21.
6. Ramakrishnan VR, Kingdom TT, Nayak JV, Hwang PH, Orlandi RR. Nationwide incidence of major complications in endoscopic sinus surgery. Int Forum Allergy Rhinol. 2012;2(1):34–9. https://doi.org/10.1002/alr.20101.
7. Suzuki S, Yasunaga H, Matsui H, Fushimi K, Kondo K, Yamasoba T. Complication rates after functional endoscopic sinus surgery: analysis of 50,734 Japanese patients. Laryngoscope. 2015;125(8):1785–91. https://doi.org/10.1002/lary.25334.
8. Dalziel K, Stein K, Round A, Garside R, Royle P. Endoscopic sinus surgery for the excision of nasal polyps: a systematic review of safety and effectiveness. Am J Rhinol. 2006;20(5):506–19. https://doi.org/10.2500/ajr.2006.20.2923.

9. Alharbi A, et al. Complications of endoscopic sinus surgery for chronic rhinosinusitis in a tertiary care teaching hospital in Saudi Arabia. Saudi Med J. 2023;44(6):601–6. https://doi.org/10.15537/smj.2023.44.6.20230911.
10. Siedek V, Pilzweger E, Betz C, Berghaus A, Leunig A. Complications in endonasal sinus surgery: a 5-year retrospective study of 2,596 patients. Eur Arch Otorrinolaringol. 2013;270(1):141–8. https://doi.org/10.1007/s00405-012-1973-z.
11. Stankiewicz JA, Lal D, Connor M, Welch K. Complications in endoscopic sinus surgery for chronic rhinosinusitis: a 25-year experience. Laryngoscope. 2011;121(12):2684–701. https://doi.org/10.1002/lary.21446.
12. Stankiewicz JA. Complications of endoscopic sinus surgery. Otolaryngol Clin N Am. 1989;22(4):749–58. https://doi.org/10.1016/S0030-6665(20)31395-5.
13. Smith LF, Brindley PC. Indications, evaluation, complications, and results of functional endoscopic sinus surgery in 200 patients. Otolaryngol Head Neck Surg. 1993;108(6):688–96. https://doi.org/10.1177/019459989310800610.
14. Labruzzo SV, Aygun N, Zinreich SJ. Imaging of the paranasal sinuses: mitigation, identification, and workup of functional endoscopic surgery complications. Otolaryngol Clin N Am. 2015;48(5):805–15. https://doi.org/10.1016/j.otc.2015.05.008.
15. Varshney H, Varshney J, Biswas S, Ghosh SK. Importance of CT scan of paranasal sinuses in the evaluation of the anatomical findings in patients suffering from sinonasal polyposis. Indian J Otolaryngol Head Neck Surg. 2016;68(2):167–72. https://doi.org/10.1007/s12070-015-0827-6.
16. Alañón Fernández FJ, Alañón Fernández M, Alañón Cárdenas F, Marín González B, Cueva-López V. Improvements in planning lacrimal surgery using DICOM Horos® viewer 3D images. Arch Soc Esp Oftalmol. 2021;96(10):509–14. https://doi.org/10.1016/j.oftale.2020.12.010.
17. O'Brien WT, Hamelin S, Weitzel EK. The preoperative sinus CT: avoiding a "CLOSE" call with surgical complications. Radiology. 2016;281(1):10–21. https://doi.org/10.1148/radiol.2016152230.
18. López F, et al. Nasal juvenile angiofibroma: current perspectives with emphasis on management. Head Neck. 2017;39(5):1033–45. https://doi.org/10.1002/hed.24696.
19. Xue L, Gehong D, Ying W, Jianhua T, Hong Z, Honggang L. Nasal meningoencephalocele: a retrospective study of clinicopathological features and diagnosis of 16 patients. Ann Diagn Pathol. 2020;49:151594. https://doi.org/10.1016/j.anndiagpath.2020.151594.
20. Amorocho MC, Fat I. Anesthetic techniques in endoscopic sinus and skull base surgery. Otolaryngol Clin N Am. 2016;49(3):531–47. https://doi.org/10.1016/j.otc.2016.03.004.
21. Carlton DA, Govindaraj S. Anesthesia for functional endoscopic sinus surgery. Curr Opin Otolaryngol Head Neck Surg. 2017;25(1):24. https://doi.org/10.1097/MOO.0000000000000322.
22. Moffatt DC, McQuitty RA, Wright AE, Kamucheka TS, Haider AL, Chaaban MR. Evaluating the role of anesthesia on intraoperative blood loss and visibility during endoscopic sinus surgery: a meta-analysis. Am J Rhinol Allergy. 2021;35(5):674–84. https://doi.org/10.1177/1945892421989155.
23. Castelnuovo P, Dallan I, Battaglia P, Bignami M. Endoscopic endonasal skull base surgery: past, present and future. Eur Arch Otorrinolaringol. 2010;267(5):649–63. https://doi.org/10.1007/s00405-009-1196-0.
24. Tajudeen BA, Kennedy DW. Thirty years of endoscopic sinus surgery: what have we learned? World J Otorhinolaryngol Head Neck Surg. 2017;3(2):115–21. https://doi.org/10.1016/j.wjorl.2016.12.001.
25. Dalgorf DM, et al. Image-guided surgery influences perioperative morbidity from endoscopic sinus surgery: a systematic review and meta-analysis. Otolaryngol Head Neck Surg. 2013;149(1):17–29. https://doi.org/10.1177/0194599813488519.
26. Landsberg R, Friedman M. A computer-assisted anatomical study of the nasofrontal region. Laryngoscope. 2001;111(12):2125–30. https://doi.org/10.1097/00005537-200112000-00008.

27. Singh GB, Rana N, Tomar S, Malhotra S, Kumar S. Radiological evaluation of lacrimal apparatus injury after functional endoscopic sinus surgery. J Laryngol Otol. 2021;135(3):229–33. https://doi.org/10.1017/S0022215121000384.
28. Westfall E, Fridirici Z, El-Kouri N, McSpadden R, Loochtan M, Stankiewicz J. Diagnosis and management of orbital fat exposure during endoscopic sinus surgery. Ear Nose Throat J. 2023;102(9):573–9. https://doi.org/10.1177/01455613211015438.
29. Seredyka-Burduk M, Burduk PK, Wierzchowska M, Kaluzny B, Malukiewicz G. Ophthalmic complications of endoscopic sinus surgery. Braz J Otorhinolaryngol. 2017;83:318–23. https://doi.org/10.1016/j.bjorl.2016.04.006.
30. Castelnuovo P, Valentini M, Sileo G, Battaglia P, Bignami M, Turri-Zanoni M. Management of recurrent cerebrospinal fluid leak, current practices and open challenges. A systematic literature review. Acta Otorhinolaryngol Ital. 2023;43(Suppl 1):S14–27. https://doi.org/10.14639/0392-100X-suppl.1-43-2023-02.
31. Halderman AA, Sindwani R, Woodard TD. Hemorrhagic complications of endoscopic sinus surgery. Otolaryngol Clin N Am. 2015;48(5):783–93. https://doi.org/10.1016/j.otc.2015.05.006.
32. Hopkins C, et al. Complications of surgery for nasal polyposis and chronic rhinosinusitis: the results of a national audit in England and Wales. Laryngoscope. 2006;116(8):1494–9. https://doi.org/10.1097/01.mlg.0000230399.24306.50.
33. Stankiewicz JA. Complications of endoscopic intranasal ethmoidectomy. Laryngoscope. 1987;97(11):1270–3. https://doi.org/10.1288/00005537-198711000-00004.

# Image Guidance in Endoscopic Sinonasal Surgery

# 26

Paresh P. Naik, Louis Luke, and Ajit Mishra

**Key Points**

- Image guidance (IG) offers real-time information during surgery, potentially enhancing accuracy, decreasing complications, and improving outcomes.
- Increased accessibility to IG in educational centers has proved as a useful tool for learning.
- Technologies like augmented and virtual reality have a wider scope in future.
- Future improvements should aim to enhance the surgeon's procedural & teaching experience.

## 26.1 Introduction

Messerklinger revolutionized the management of chronic rhinosinusitis by enhancing the understanding of drainage pathways of the sinuses and how they are affected by anatomical variations [1]. This subsequently led to the development of functional endoscopic sinus surgery (FESS) in the late 1980s as a modality to better treat chronic inflammation of the sinonasal cavity by aiming to restore the natural mucociliary

**Supplementary Information** The online version contains supplementary material available at https://doi.org/10.1007/978-3-031-70077-4_26.

P. P. Naik (✉)
University of Northamptonshire, Cliftonville, UK
e-mail: pareshnaikp@gmail.com

L. Luke
ENT Department, University Hospitals, Northamptonshire NHS Trust, Cliftonville, Northampton, UK

A. Mishra
HCG Hospital, Borivali/Coloba, Mumbai, India


S. Elwany (ed.), *Current Rhinology*,
https://doi.org/10.1007/978-3-031-70077-4_26

drainage and ventilation of the sinuses by resecting localized disease [2]. Computed tomography (CT) imaging of the paranasal sinuses is an essential prerequisite before surgery as it delineates the presence and extent of disease in addition to highlighting important anatomical variations that could potentially predispose to complications [3–5].

### 26.1.1 Definition

**Image-guided surgery (IGS) is defined** as an invasive surgery performed with the assistance of or guided by images of the treated organ using either fluoroscopy, endoscopy, intraoperative CT or magnetic resonance imaging (MRI), ultrasound or stereotaxis [6]. It is a passive system which is aimed at tracking the surgical tool with respect to the patient's body by combining preoperative imaging modality and a tracking system.

Conventionally, the use of image guidance in surgery refers to stereotactic surgery. The three-dimensional position of the surgical instrument is accurately mapped onto a patient's preoperative imaging through the use of reference markers, fiducials, and a tracking device in the surgical field [7].

This chapter will outline the principles of image guidance in endoscopic sinus surgery, the evolution of technology, and its utilization in rhinology.

### 26.1.2 Evolution

The advent of image-guided stereotactic surgery started in neurosurgery in the late 1970s using an acrylic plastic head frame attached to the patient by screws that was compatible with the CT scanner [8]. It further evolved in the 1980s with the advent of computers to enable three-dimensional volumetric reconstructions of CT and MRI images [9]. Rods attached to the frame produce fiducial points on the CT image which enables the position of a probe to be transposed from the frame to the CT slice [8].

The use of stereotactic image guidance systems in otorhinolaryngology has become increasingly popular in endoscopic sinus surgery since its introduction in the late 1990s. This is for a multitude of reasons including, improved safety, reduction of complication rates by highlighting key anatomical landmarks and vital structures intraoperatively, its value in training, and its role in improving clinical outcomes [10, 11].

The application of image guidance in sinus surgery was initiated in the mid-1990s, with the primary objective of enhancing both efficiency and safety in surgical procedures [12]. Historically, the first use of Image guidance surgery was started in Germany in 1986 [13].

### 26.1.3 Suggestive Indications of Use of Image Guidance (IG)

In simpler terms, IGS is like a GPS (Global Positioning Satellite) in the car. It is used as an aid for the surgeon to confirm the anatomical location.

The American Academy of Otolaryngology-Head and Neck Surgery formulated a consensus of expert opinion on indications for image-guided surgery [14] that

**Table 26.1** Indications can be classified to anatomy involved or access to the anatomy [14]

| |
|---|
| Indications can be classified as anatomy involved or access to the anatomy |
| Revision cases |
| Complications of infective sinusitis |
| Surgery to the frontal sinus |
| Lesions abutting skull base, orbit, carotid, optic nerve |
| Endonasal cranial/brain surgery |
| Transnasal transsphenoidal endoscopic skull base and brain surgery |
| Transpterygoid fossa approach surgery |
| Transnasal endoscopic repair of CSF leak |
| Osteoplastic frontal sinus surgery |
| Pediatric skull base surgery |
| Extensive sinonasal pathology |
| Expanded endoscopic endonasal surgery |

include revision surgery, distorted anatomy, skull base defects, and sinonasal neoplasms (Table 26.1).

## 26.2 Fundamentals

The utilization of technology to enhance surgical precision by providing real-time anatomical localization during surgery is referred to as image guidance (Fig. 26.1).

### 26.2.1 What Is Registration

Image registration is a process which is defined as the integration of digital radiological images with the actual patient surface anatomy to calibrate the exact location of the surgical landmark.

The steps involved in registration are preoperative imaging, intraoperative image acquisition via PACS software, and uploading the images in the image guidance system. Identifying the surface anatomy using a tracker and probe.

At the end of registration, the system generates an "Error" or "Target Registration Error" (TRE)—which can be a few millimeters to cm. It is ideal to keep the error as low as possible and under 5 mm.

The principles across IGS systems are similar. The general steps are image acquisition, planning, registration, instrument tracking, and visualization [7] (Fig. 26.2). Firstly, acquiring preoperative cross-sectional images from the hospital's picture archiving and communication system (PACS) using an ethernet connection or using a storage device such as a USB drive or CD with Digital Imaging and Communications in Medicine (DICOM) formatted images is required to be loaded onto a computer workstation that uses the image guidance software. Depending on the purpose of surgery, CT and MRI images can be used alone or in combination. CT imaging of sinuses is helpful in delineating sinus and skull base anatomy whilst MRI imaging can be useful in defining blood vessels and soft tissue masses such as tumors on a contrasted T1 sequence whereas T2-weighted images are used for visualizing cerebrospinal fluid.

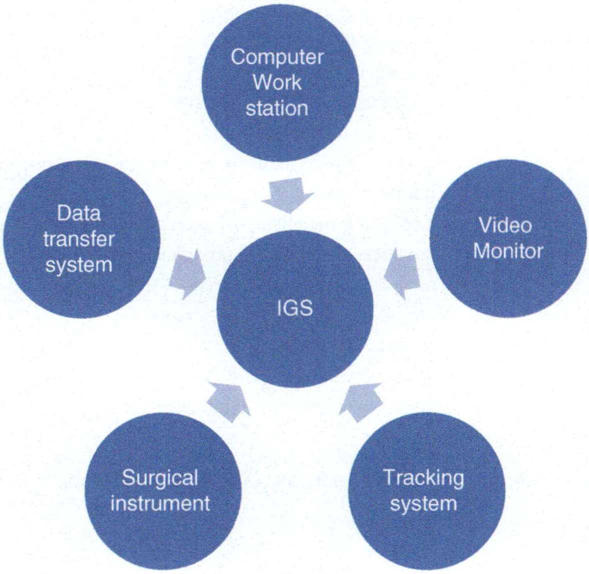


**Fig. 26.1** Elements of IGS

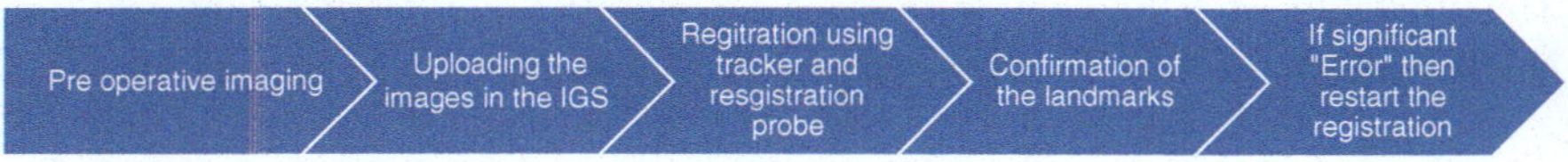
Pre operative imaging
Uploading the
images in the IGS
Regitration using
tracker and
resgistration
probe
Confirmation of
the landmarks
If significant
"Error" then
restart the
registration

**Fig. 26.2** Setting up image guidance

Image guidance software allows the merging of CT and MRI images and blending to varying degrees depending on user preference. Depending on the image guidance software, various planning packages can be used. These can include creating 3D reconstructions and highlighting important anatomical landmarks in the field [7]. The original operating systems use a UNIX platform but newer workstations either use Microsoft Windows or LINUX systems. Most image guidance systems have a video monitor attached that allows the output of the image guidance system superimposed on preoperative imaging typically in the three anatomical planes of coronal, axial, and sagittal views with visual output of the endoscope. They use high-resolution screens to ensure high-quality visuals [15].

Registration is the next step in setup. It involves creating specific coordinates on a volumetric reconstruction of the patient's images and linking this together with the real patient in the operating theater. Registration is crucial for ensuring the highest degree of accuracy and reliability of the IGS [7]. There are three methods of one-to-one mapping between the surgical field and image data volume, contour-based registration (the most commonly used), paired-point registration, and automatic registration (the least commonly used) [16, 17]. In contour-based registration, the IGS builds a 3D model from the preoperative data. Next, the user identifies corresponding points on the surgical field by moving the registration probe along the surgical field. This helps the system register multiple points at varying contours on the surgical volume and map this with the preoperative imaging volume [17]. Conversely, paired-point registration starts with identifying fiducial points or anatomical landmarks using external marks that are selected by the user or automatically by the software The user then uses a registration probe to localize to each point and then the software aligns the corresponding points on the images and surgical field [13].

Following the completion of the registration process, it is essential to evaluate the *target registration error (TRE)*. The *TRE* is defined as the distance between the measured position of a tracked instrument tip, as observed on the IGS computer monitor, and the actual position of the instrument tip in the physical world.

In general, a target registration error (TRE) of 2.0 mm or less is deemed clinically acceptable. Presently, contemporary Image-Guided Surgery (IGS) platforms typically achieve mean TREs ranging from 1.5 to 2.0 mm in real-world scenarios (Table 26.2). Higher the error, lesser is the efficiency of accurately localizing anatomical landmarks (Fig. 26.3).

**Table 26.2** Common anatomical landmarks used for registration

| Common anatomical landmarks used for registration | |
|---|---|
| 1. | Nasion |
| 2. | Tragus |
| 3. | Medial canthus |
| 4. | Lateral canthus |
| 5. | Nasal tip |

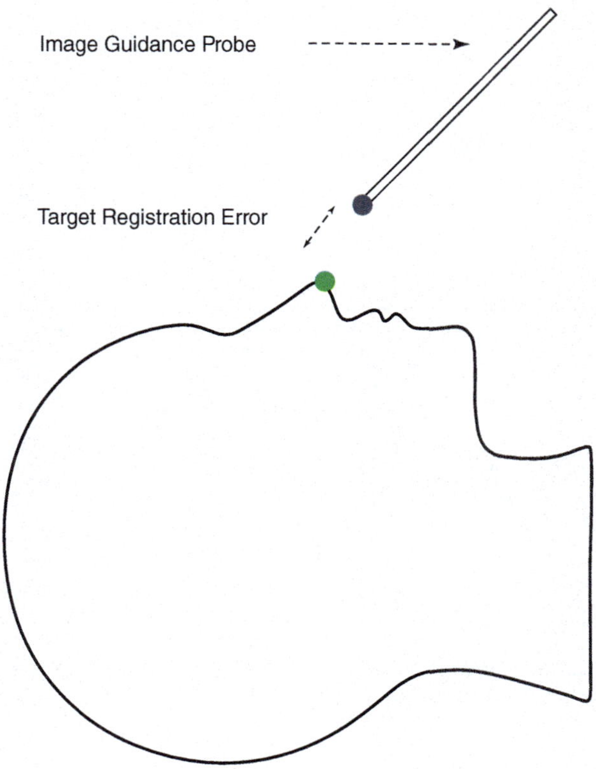


**Fig. 26.3** Showing "error" or "target registration error"

## 26.3 Tracking System

There are two different types of tracking systems used for determining the orientation of probes or instruments in the surgical field for IGS (Fig. 26.4).

Optical tracking
Electromagnetic Technology

Both require the use of an intraoperative localization device that is placed and fixed onto the patient's head or operating table. This is to allow compensation for the movements of the surgical field during surgery.

Optical tracking systems use light-emitting diodes or reflective spheres tracked via infrared waves by an overhead camera array that maps the intraoperative localization device and instruments. Optical Tracking Systems (OTSs) work within the optical spectrum to track the position and orientation, i.e., the pose of target surgical instruments. OTSs are characterized by high accuracy and robustness to environmental conditions. Optical tracking system is mainly used where large anatomical volume is needed to be tracked like brain. The main limitation of OTSs is the need for a direct line-of-sight between the optical markers and the camera sensor, rigidly fixed into the operating theater [18].

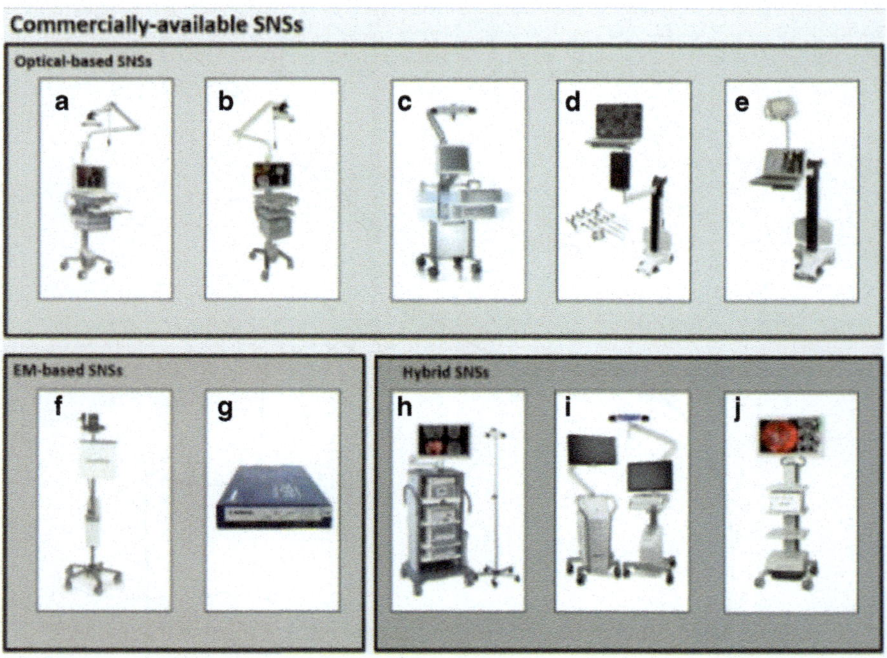


**Fig. 26.4** Types of tracking system [12] showing (**a-e**) optical based Surgical Navigation System (SNS); (**f, g**) Electromagnetic based (SNS); (**h-j**) Hybrid SNS

**Table 26.3** Examples of tracking system in ENT

| Examples of tracking system in ENT [12] | |
|---|---|
| Optical based | Stryker Corp |
| | Masmec S.p.A.-Orion |
| | ClaroNav-NaviENT |
| Electromagnetic tracking based | BrainLab |
| Hybrid | Karl Storz-Nav 1 |
| | Medtronics Corp-Stealth station |

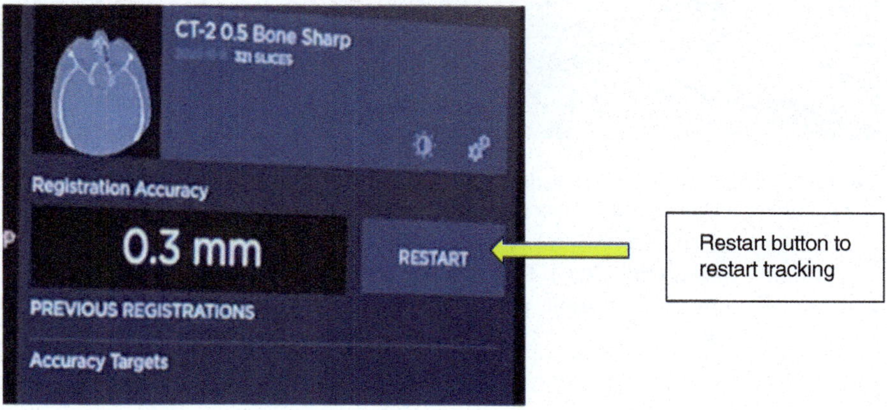


**Fig. 26.5** Showing registration showing accuracy and restart button to recalibrate

Whereas, the electromagnetic system uses an electromagnetic field generator and sensors that track instruments in the field [12]. Electromagnetic Tracking Systems (EMTSs) use electromagnetic field generators to detect the pose of electromagnetic sensors. EMTSs do not require such a direct line-of-sight; however, the presence of metal or ferromagnetic sources in the operating workspace can significantly affect the measurement accuracy. EMTs are employed in surgeries where a small volume is needed to be tracked like Endoscopic sinus surgery [18]. The advantage of this is that instruments do not have to be within the direct line of sight during tracking [19].

Nowadays, there are hybrid tracking systems which can use both EMT and OTS, e.g., Stealth Medronic®, Scopic® Karl Storz Nav1® (Table 26.3)

### 26.3.1 Factors Influencing TRE

There are three factors that influence the degree of TRE. Firstly, the degree of error from the IGS to sense instrument position is generally less than 1 mm in modern systems. The quality of the imaging data uploaded onto the system influences TRE with a lower limit TRE of 0.5 mm with high-resolution CT images with a thickness of 0.5 mm (Fig. 26.5). Lastly, TRE can be influenced by the user variability of the

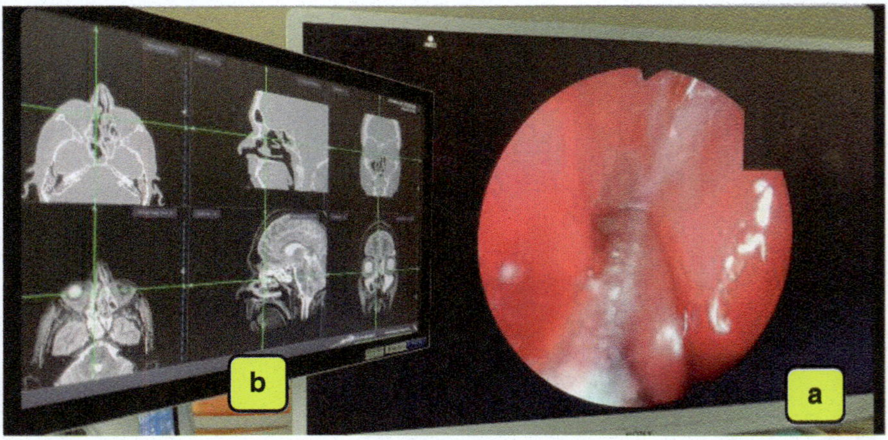


**Fig. 26.6** (**a**) Showing instrument in the nasal cavity intra op view. (**b**) Showing real-time position of the instrument with respect to other preoperative scan

registration process (Fig. 26.6). Ensuring the registration probe remains in contact with the skin covering multiple fiducial points minimizes errors in contour-based registration [20].

## 26.4 Benefits of IGS

Assistance in defining landmarks
Reduction of complications
Increasing surgeon's confidence
R0 resection of the lesion
Identifying variations in the sinonasal skull base anatomy
Medicolegal point of view
Image-guided biopsy

## 26.5 Future of Image Guidance in Rhinology

Intraoperative imaging technologies in skull-base surgeries started in the 1990s in the form of intraoperative CT scans.

Target-guided surgeries have been developed where planned pathways are laid in real time. This system developed by Scopis® by Stryker Corp® provides the surgeon with unique augmented reality technology. A road map is created to assist the surgeon in guiding the instruments on the pathways directly to the targets.

Augmented reality (AR) enhances the surgical experience by integrating virtual information with a live surgical view. After annotating images during preoperative planning, AR software enables surgeons to visualize this information on the video monitor. The augmented data is presented as an overlay of the actual anatomy, providing real-time guidance within the surgeon's endoscopic view.

Registration of intraoperative imaging can be used to access the residual lesion and targeted precise excision can be done.

## 26.6 Integrated Live Image Guidance Surgery

In an era characterized by a dependence on swiftly advancing computer artificial intelligence, the field of robotics emerges as a captivating dimension introduced to humanity. Its purpose is to aid in diverse tasks.

The idea of robotic surgery in cooperation with the Image Guidance navigation system will revolutionize the field of minimal invasive surgery, offering unparalleled precision, control and safety.

The AI-integrated system makes Image guidance very user-friendly, most of the systems come with intuitive user interfaces with touch screens and multitouch gestures.

## 26.7 Image Guidance in Pediatrics

Skull and sinus surgery in children poses many risks and challenges. The sinus and nasal anatomy changes continuously as the child grows. IGS can be safely applied in pediatric cases with a broad range of pathologies.

General indications include:

Complications of chronic rhinosinusitis
Tumors
Mucoceles
Skull base cases
As an approach to endonasal neurosurgery cases

Special cases as in pediatric Juvenile angiofibroma, postartery embolization scans enable accurate identification of the extent of the tumor postembolization, allowing the surgeon to use intraoperative surgical navigation to reach the embolization coils and the main feeding arteries to the tumor. IG will play a crucial role in expanded endoscopic transpterygoid surgery. Use of preoperative CT angiography will increase precision.

This ultimately facilitates the more radical resections required for this condition.

## 26.8 Image Guidance in Frontal Sinus

Cases like where approach is advised with the aid of image guidance.

Remnant agger nasi
Samter's triad requiring DRAF III procedures
Bone erosion in invasive frontal sinus surgery

Revision cases
Frontal sinusitis complicated with frontal lobe abscess or orbital involvement
Osteoplastic flap procedure for frontal sinus

## 26.9 Image Guidance in Sphenoid Surgery

Sphenoid sinus is surrounded by vital structures. Because of close association with the optic nerve, optic chiasma, pituitary gland, carotid artery, and cavernous sinus, surgery to the sphenoid sinus requires high surgical precision:

IG can be used to localize the functioning pituitary adenoma and excise.
Helpful in addressing supra-sellar lesions.
Helpful in expanded transsphenoidal approach which includes, transplanum, transclival, transodontoid approach.

| Tips for beginners |
|---|
| Start with easier cases |
| Assist at least 50 cases before starting independently |
| Do not overbook the list as setup can take time |
| Avoid the use of image guidance if the disease is limited to the maxillary sinus and anterior ethmoids |
| Use in medicolegal aspect |
| Use of three-dimensional images and angiography |

## 26.10 Conclusion

As advancements in image guidance and intraoperative imaging systems continue to progress, their utilization in sinus and skull base surgery has broadened. These technologies provide crucial real-time information regarding ongoing surgery, contributing to the potential enhancement of surgical thoroughness and overall outcomes. The recent strides in technologies like augmented and virtual reality signify a glimpse into the prospective developments in image-guided surgery (IGS). The forthcoming improvements should strive to elevate the surgeon's procedural experience, focusing on augmenting user satisfaction, and ultimately fostering superior surgical outcomes.

## 26.11 Limitations

Image guidance is not meant for every surgeon or every surgery. The system can distract the surgeon or scrub team and has a learning curve. One must understand that the use of IGS is not a replacement for knowledge and surgical experience. Cost of the setup and instruments which are compatible with the image guidance increases operating time.

1. Cost and surgeon and scrub team learning curve
2. Lack of familiarity

## References


1. Kane KJ. The early history and development of endoscopic sinonasal surgery in Australia: 1985–2005. Austr J Otolaryngol. 2018;1:7. Available from: https://www.theajo.com/article/view/3997.
2. Stammberger H, Posawetz W. Functional endoscopic sinus surgery. Concept, indications and results of the Messerklinger technique. Eur Arch Otorrinolaringol. 1990;247(2):63–76.
3. Fokkens WJ, Lund VJ, Hopkins C, Hellings PW, Kern R, Reitsma S, et al. European position paper on rhinosinusitis and nasal polyps 2020. Rhinology. 2020;58(S29):1–464.
4. Zinreich SJ, Kennedy DW, Rosenbaum AE, Gayler BW, Kumar AJ, Stammberger H. Paranasal sinuses: CT imaging requirements for endoscopic surgery. Radiology. 1987;163(3):769–75.
5. Tewfik MA, Wormald PJ. Ten pearls for safe endoscopic sinus surgery. Otolaryngol Clin N Am. 2010;43(4):933–44.
6. Bucholz RD. Introduction to Journal of Image Guided Surgery. Comput Aided Surg. 1995;1(1):1–3.
7. Azagury DE, Dua MM, Barrese JC, Henderson JM, Buchs NC, Ris F, et al. Image-guided surgery. Curr Probl Surg. 2015;52(12):476–520.
8. Brown RA. A stereotactic head frame for use with CT body scanners. Investig Radiol. 1979;14(4):300–4.
9. Jacques S, Shelden CH, McCann GD. A computerized microstereotactic method to approach, 3-dimensionally reconstruct, remove and adjuvantly treat small CNS lesions. Appl Neurophysiol. 2007;43(3–5):176–82.
10. Freysinger W, Gunkel AR, Thumfart WF. Image-guided endoscopic ENT surgery. Eur Arch Otorrinolaringol. 1997;254(7):343–6.
11. Fried MP, Kleefield J, Gopal H, Reardon E, Ho BT, Kuhn FA. Image-guided endoscopic surgery: results of accuracy and performance in a multicenter clinical study using an electromagnetic tracking system. Laryngoscope. 1997;107(5):594–601.
12. Metson R. Image-guided sinus surgery: lessons learned from the first 1000 cases. Otolaryngol Head Neck Surg. 2003;128:8–13. https://doi.org/10.1067/mhn.2003.40.
13. Anon JB. Computer-aided endoscopic sinus surgery. Laryngoscope. 1998;108(7):949–61.
14. Schmale IL, Vandelaar LJ, Luong AU, Citardi MJ, Yao WC. Image-guided surgery and intraoperative imaging in rhinology: clinical update and current state of the art. Ear Nose Throat J. 2021;100(10):475–86.
15. Sorriento A, Porfido MB, Mazzoleni S, Calvosa G, Tenucci M, Ciuti G, Dario P. Optical and electromagnetic tracking systems for biomedical applications: a critical review on potentialities and limitations. IEEE Rev Biomed Eng. 2020;13:212–32. https://doi.org/10.1109/RBME.2019.2939091. Epub 2019 Sep 2.
16. Citardi MJ, Batra PS. Image-guided sinus surgery: current concepts and technology. Otolaryngol Clin N Am. 2005;38(3):439–52.
17. Knott PD, Batra PS, Citardi MJ. Computer aided surgery: concepts and applications in rhinology. Otolaryngol Clin N Am. 2006;39(3):503–22.
18. Cleary K, Peters TM. Image-guided interventions: technology review and clinical applications. Annu Rev Biomed Eng. 2010;12(1):119–42.
19. [Internet]. [cited 2024 Feb 18]. Available from: https://www.stryker.com/content/dam/stryker/navigation/products/target-guided-surgery/images/Scopis-Product-Catalog.pdf.
20. Citardi MJ, Yao W, Luong A. Next-generation surgical navigation systems in sinus and skull base surgery. Otolaryngol Clin N Am. 2017;50(3):617–32.

# Surgery of the Maxillary Sinus

# 27

Mohamed Ossama Tomoum

**Key Points**

- Understanding the anatomic variation of the maxillary sinus and related structures is important to avoid complications during surgery.
- CT and MRI are complementary to each other for proper diagnosis and preoperative planning of the maxillary sinus lesions and adequate surgery.
- The goals of endoscopic maxillary sinus surgery are the complete removal of the maxillary sinus pathology and the restoration of its physiological functions.
- Angled endoscopes and instruments are mandatory for adequate exploration and management of the maxillary sinus pathology during endoscopic middle meatal antrostomy.
- Due to the significant morbidity of the Caldwell-Luc approach to the maxillary sinus, it should be reserved for patients who failed aggressive medical and surgical therapy.
- The prelacrimal recess approach, maxillary sinus trephination, and Caldwell-Luc approach are options for the management of anterior and lateral maxillary sinus pathology combined with the middle meatal antrostomy.
- Recirculation of mucus and retained pathology within the maxillary sinus, e.g., fungal remnants, and scarring are the main causes of failure of surgery.

**Supplementary Information** The online version contains supplementary material available at https://doi.org/10.1007/978-3-031-70077-4_27.

M. O. Tomoum (✉)
Department of Otolaryngology, Tanta University, Tanta, Egypt


S. Elwany (ed.), *Current Rhinology*,
https://doi.org/10.1007/978-3-031-70077-4_27

## 27.1 Embryology of the Maxillary Sinus

A group of five to six ridges known as ethmoturbinals form in the seventh to eighth week of development. Through differential growth and development, only three to four ridges eventually remain. The ascending part of the first ethmoturbinal develops into the Agger nasi, whereas the descending part develops into the uncinate process. The middle turbinate is formed by the second ethmoturbinal, the superior turbinate by the third, and the supreme turbinate by the fusion of the fourth and fifth ethmoturbinals. The maxilloturbinal is a ridge of maxillary origin that is inferiorly directed and eventually forms the inferior turbinate [1].

At around 6 weeks of age, the maxilla begins to ossify. There is conflicting evidence regarding the precise mechanism of osteogenesis of the maxillary sinus. Two ossification foci, one in the maxilla proper and the other in the premaxilla, may be the sites where bone formation begins. Alternatively, Vacher et al. [2] showed that a single layer of ossification located cranially in relation to the dental lamina is where the maxillary ossification begins on either side. Then, the ossification extends medially to the whole palate with preservation of the median transverse mesenchymal septum that separates the primary and secondary palate.

Nasal meatuses and recesses are formed by the major furrows that are located in between the ethmoturbinals. The ethmoid infundibulum, hiatus semilunaris, and middle meatus are formed by the descending portion of the first furrow that is situated between the first and second ethmoturbinals. The ascending part likely contributes to the frontal recess. At around 16 weeks, the inferior part of the ethmoidal infundibulum gives rise to the primordial maxillary sinus [1]. The superior meatus is formed by the second primary furrow, and the supreme meatus is created by the third primary furrow [3, 4].

The maxillary sinus continues to grow from the maxillary infundibulum throughout the second and third trimesters. At birth, the maxillary sinus is approximately 7 millimeters (mm) in anteroposterior depth, 4.0 mm in height, and 2.7 mm in width [5].

The maxillary sinus continues to pneumatize most quickly between ages 1 and 8 years, by which time it has expanded inferiorly to the mid-inferior meatus and laterally past the infraorbital canal. Initially, the maxillary sinus floor is positioned higher than the nasal floor. Following exfoliation and replacement of the primary dentition, pneumatization of the maxillary sinus reaches the level of the nasal floor. The maxillary sinus roof slopes inferolaterally during development, but as pneumatization advances, it progressively assumes the more horizontal orientation seen during adulthood [6].

## 27.2 Anatomy of the Maxillary Sinus

In adults, the maxillary sinus is pyramidal in shape, its base at the medial face and its vertex directed toward the zygomatic process of the maxilla [7]. The orbital floor is formed by the roof of the maxillary sinus. The infraorbital canal, which may be dehiscent, passes through it. The posterior superior alveolar nerve is related to the posterior wall. The floor of the maxillary sinus is thicker and related to the roots of teeth (the second premolar and first molar teeth) [8].

The lacrimal groove, which lies just behind the frontal process of the maxilla, is transformed into the nasolacrimal canal by the lacrimal bone and the lacrimal process of the inferior nasal concha. The nasolacrimal duct is transmitted by this canal, which enters the inferior meatus of the nose [9]. The greater palatine canal, which transmits the greater palatine nerve and arteries, is developed posteriorly between the perpendicular plate of the palatine bone and maxilla [8]. The infraorbital foramen is located in the anterior wall of the maxillary sinus in the mid-superior part. The canine fossa is the thinnest part of the anterior maxillary wall that is situated above the canine tooth. The posterior wall of the maxillary sinus forms the anterior boundary of the pterygomaxillary fossa.

### 27.2.1 Recesses of the Maxillary Sinus [10]

1. **Palatine recess:** Inferomedial pneumatization of the sinus into the hard palate.
2. **Infraorbital recess:** Anterior pneumatization of the maxillary sinus adjacent to the infraorbital canal in the roof of the maxillary sinus.
3. **Alveolar recess:** Inferior pneumatization of the maxillary sinus in the area of the molar and premolar dentition.
4. **Zygomatic recess:** Anterolateral pneumatization of the maxillary sinus in the direction of the infratemporal fossa.
5. **Prelacrimal recess:** Anteromedial pneumatization of the maxillary sinus anterior to the nasolacrimal duct as presented in Fig. 27.1.

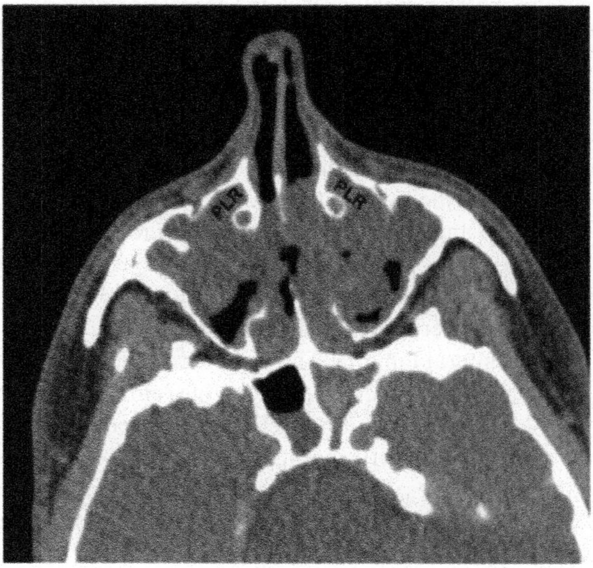


**Fig. 27.1** Computed tomography scan "axial view" of the paranasal sinus shows the prelacrimal recess of the maxillary sinus anterior to the nasolacrimal duct. *PLR* prelacrimal recess

## 27.2.2 Anatomy of Related Structures

### 27.2.2.1 Anatomy of the Lateral Nasal Wall

The frontal process of the maxilla and the lacrimal bone make up the lateral nasal wall's anterior portion. The ethmoid labyrinth, the maxilla, and the inferior turbinate make up the middle portion. The perpendicular plate of the palatine bone and the medial pterygoid plate of the sphenoid bone make up the posterior portion of the lateral nasal wall [11].

There are three turbinates and three meatuses, on each side. The maxillary, frontal, and anterior ethmoidal sinuses all drain into the middle meatus. The superior meatus drains the posterior ethmoid cells. Postero-superior to the superior turbinate is the sphenoethmoid recess, into which the sphenoid sinus drain. The nasolacrimal duct opens in the inferior meatus [11].

### 27.2.2.2 Inferior Turbinate

The inferior turbinate is made of a separate bone, and it has an irregular surface, perforated and grooved by vascular channels to which the mucoperiosteum is tightly attached. It has a maxillary process that articulates with the inferior margin of the maxillary hiatus. It also articulates with the ethmoid, palatine, and lacrimal bones to form the medial wall of the nasolacrimal duct [11].

In males, the inferior turbinate measures 40–48 mm in length, whereas in females, it is 38–42 mm. The inferior turbinate height varies, reaching its maximum height in the plane of the lacrimal sac and decreasing progressively toward its anterior and posterior ends [12].

### 27.2.2.3 Inferior Meatus

The part of the nasal lateral wall that is lateral to the inferior turbinate is known as the inferior meatus. It is the largest meatus and nearly fills the entire nasal cavity. The meatus is highest at the junction of the anterior and middle thirds. The nasolacrimal duct opens into the inferior meatus just anterior to its highest point [11].

### 27.2.2.4 Middle Turbinate

Anteriorly, the middle turbinate is attached to the ethmoid crest of the maxillary bone and Agger nasi. Posteriorly, it is attached to the ethmoid crest of the perpendicular plate of the palatine bone. The middle turbinate consists of three parts. Its first part lies sagittally in an anterior and medial position and is attached vertically to the skull base superiorly between the cribriform plate and the lateral lamella. The second middle part, basal lamella, lies in a coronal plane and is attached laterally to the lamina papyracea obliquely, superiorly to the skull base at the fovea ethmoidal, medially to the first part, and inferiorly to the third part, it separates the anterior ethmoid sinuses from the posterior ethmoid sinuses. The third part lies in an axial plane posteriorly and is attached laterally to the perpendicular plate of the palatine bone just anterior to the sphenopalatine foramen [7].

#### 27.2.2.5 Ethmoidal Infundibulum

The uncinate process, the lamina papyracea, the frontal process of the maxilla, and the lacrimal bone encircle the three-dimensional space known as the ethmoidal infundibulum, which is situated in the anterior ethmoid region. Through the hiatus semilunaris, the ethmoidal infundibulum communicates with the middle meatus as shown in Fig. 27.2 [1, 11].

#### 27.2.2.6 Superior Hiatus Semilunaris

Superior hiatus semilunaris is a sickle-shaped cleft between the posterior wall of the ethmoidal bulla and the basal lamella of the middle turbinate [8].

#### 27.2.2.7 Inferior Hiatus Semilunaris

Inferior hiatus semilunaris is a two-dimensional sagittal cleft between the concave free posterior border of the uncinate process and the convex anterior surface of the ethmoidal bulla.

#### 27.2.2.8 Uncinate Process

The uncinate process is a sagittal-oriented structure that forms the anteromedial boundary of the ethmoid infundibulum. Antero-superiorly, the uncinate process attaches to the ethmoidal crest of the maxilla just inferior to the middle turbinate attachment and the Agger nasi cell, and it fuses with the posterior aspect of the lacrimal bone. Postero-inferiorly, it articulates with the ethmoidal process of the inferior turbinate.

The superior part of the uncinate process has several patterns of attachment [13]:

1. Most commonly, it attaches to the lamina papyracea, where the ethmoid infundibulum is closed superiorly by a blind pouch called the recessus terminalis.

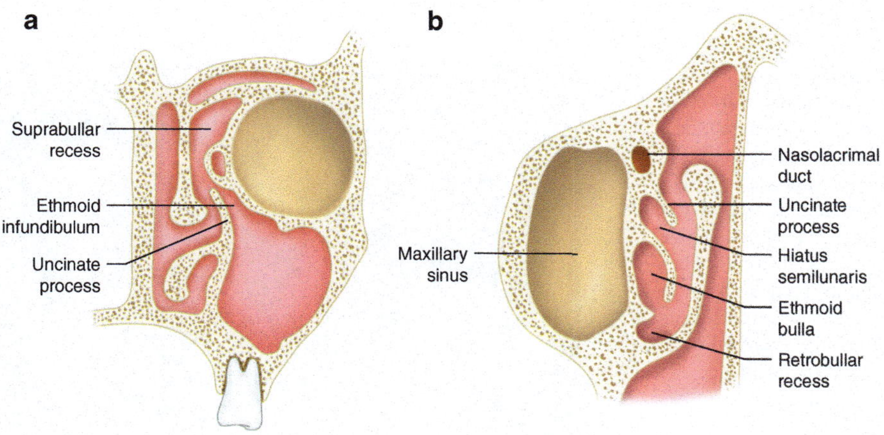


**Fig. 27.2** Diagrams of (**a**) coronal view of the left maxillary sinus. (**b**) Axial view of the right maxillary sinus, demonstrating the uncinate process, the ethmoid infundibulum that open into the middle meatus through hiatus semilunaris, the nasolacrimal duct, ethmoid bulla, retrobullar recess

2. It may attach centrally to the skull base or medially to the superior aspect of the vertical lamella of the middle turbinate near the turbinate's insertion to the cribriform plate.
3. It can also fuse with an anterior ethmoidal cell, e.g., the Agger nasi cell.
4. Rarely, the superior portion of the uncinate process can split to attach to the lamina papyracea, skull base, and middle turbinate.

#### 27.2.2.9 Ethmoid Bulla

Bulla ethmoidalis is the largest anterior ethmoid air cell based on the lamina papyracea and lies posterior to the uncinate process and anterior to the basal lamella of the middle turbinate. Superiorly, it forms the posterior boundary of the frontal recess. Suprabullar and retrobullar recesses are two spaces that may be present above and behind the ethmoid bulla, respectively.

#### 27.2.2.10 Haller Cell

It is an anterior ethmoidal cell that pneumatizes along the medial part of the roof of the maxillary sinus and the inferomedial part of the lamina papyracea [14].

## 27.3 Silent Sinus Syndrome

Silent sinus syndrome is a rare anatomic abnormality characterized by hypoplasia or atelectasis of the maxillary sinus as demonstrated in Fig. 27.3 [15, 16]. It is mostly a unilateral and asymptomatic condition. The pathophysiology of silent sinus syndrome may be due to obstruction of the natural ostium by a lateralized uncinate process [17, 18] which may result in negative pressure with consequent remodeling and involution of the maxillary bony walls. The atelectatic maxillary sinus is filled with thick mucus, and the condition is often asymptomatic. The

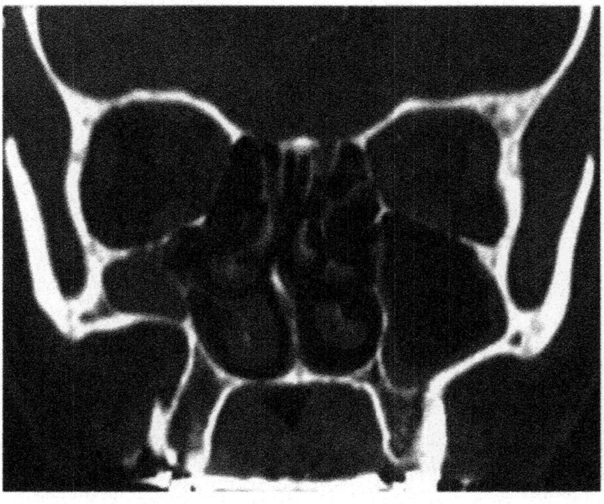

**Fig. 27.3** Computed tomography scan "coronal view" of the paranasal sinus shows complete opacification of the right hypoplastic maxillary sinus and a very thin uncinate process adherent to the lamina papyracea with a downward displacement of the inferior orbital wall (right silent sinus syndrome)

**Table 27.1** Clinical and radiographic characteristics of silent sinus syndrome

| Clinical findings of silent sinus syndrome | Radiographic findings of silent sinus syndrome |
|---|---|
| 1. Spontaneous, gradual enophthalmos (eye recession into the globe) | 1. Ipsilateral hypoplastic "atelectatic" maxillary sinus |
| 2. Spontaneous, gradual hypoglobus (inferior descent of eye) | 2. Inferior displacement of ipsilateral orbital floor |
| 3. Ocular asymmetry | 3. Partial to complete opacification of affected maxillary sinus |
| 4. Absence of sinus-related symptoms | 4. Increased orbital volume on the affected side |

presenting symptom is often enophthalmos due to the descent of the orbital floor [19]. Table 27.1 represents the clinical and radiographic characteristics of silent sinus syndrome.

## 27.4 Endoscopic Maxillary Sinus Surgery

### 27.4.1 The Most Common Indications of Endoscopic Maxillary Sinus Surgery

1. Chronic and/or recurrent maxillary sinusitis, unresponsive to prior medical treatment.
2. Complicated acute maxillary sinusitis.
3. Isolated fungal maxillary sinusitis with the formation of the fungal ball.
4. Antrochoanal polyp.
5. Maxillary sinus mucocele.
6. Extraction of a migrated tooth within the maxillary sinus.
7. Excision of dental cyst, e.g., dentigerous cyst.
8. Sphenopalatine artery ligation.
9. Resection of small benign tumors, especially inverted papillomas.
10. Resection of selected malignant tumors.

### 27.4.2 Preoperative Evaluation

The patient must be thoroughly questioned regarding their symptoms, paying particular attention to their frequency, duration, and time of occurrence. The most common symptoms of chronic sinusitis are nasal obstruction, hyposmia, headache and facial pain, recurrent facial swelling, and postnasal drip.

#### 27.4.2.1 Past Medical and Surgical History

It is mandatory to ask all patients about:

- Previous sinus surgery, if the patient was symptom-free after surgery.

- Previous medical therapy, e.g., antibiotics, corticosteroids, anticoagulant therapy.
- History of asthma, and aspirin intolerance.
- History of dental problems.

#### 27.4.2.2 Physical Examination and Endoscopy

Endoscopic examination of the nasal cavities with the observation of septal deviation, size and shape of the inferior and middle turbinates (concha bullosa and paradoxical middle turbinate), and the extent and size of any polyps as shown in Fig. 27.4.

### 27.4.3 Imaging

#### 27.4.3.1 Computerized Tomography (CT)

Computerized tomography in coronal, axial, and sagittal planes (soft tissue and bony windows) is necessary for the proper diagnosis of the patients and preoperative planning for surgery [20].

Computerized tomography enables the surgeon to evaluate the followings before endoscopic surgery of the maxillary sinus: the anatomical landmarks of the maxillary sinus, general overview of the other paranasal sinuses, assessment of the ostiomeatal complex, superior attachment of the uncinate process, possible dehiscent areas in the lamina papyracea, and anatomical variations of middle turbinate, e.g., concha bullosa.

The extension of the disease, in unilateral maxillary sinus opacification, the following pathologies should be suspected:

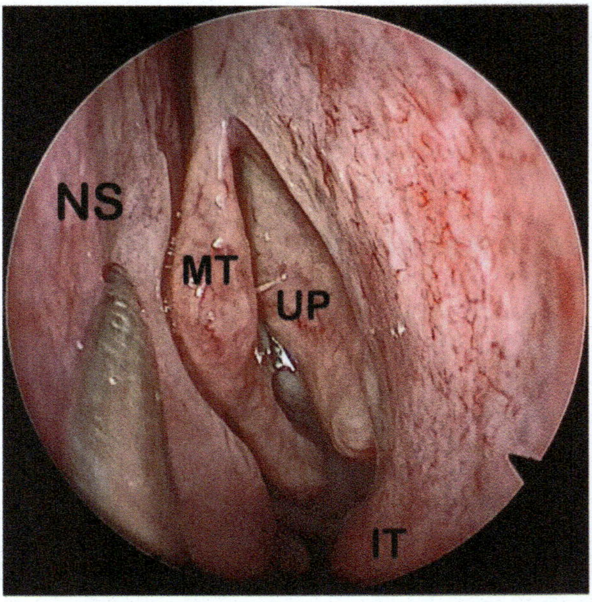


**Fig. 27.4** Endoscopic view of the left nasal cavity demonstrating nasal septum "NS," middle turbinate "MT," uncinate process "UP," and inferior turbinate "IT"

1. Odontogenic sinusitis and oroantral fistula
2. Isolated fungal ball (Fig. 27.5)
3. Antrochoanal polyp
4. Inverted papilloma
5. Dental cysts, e.g., dentigerous cyst (Fig. 27.6)

**The coronal view** of computerized tomography better demonstrates the following about the maxillary sinus [21]:

1. The degree and shape of pneumatization of the maxillary sinus (in vertical and transverse planes)
2. The orientation and superior attachment of the uncinate process
3. Presence and size of palatine, alveolar, and infraorbital recesses
4. Site and abnormalities of the infraorbital nerve
5. Presence and size of Haller cell
6. Detection of the extent of previous sinus surgery
7. Detection of foreign body (e.g., missed dental filling, migrated tooth)

**The axial view** of a computerized tomography reveals the following about the maxillary sinus:

1. The location of the nasolacrimal duct, the presence of the prelacrimal recess, and its size
2. Presence and size of zygomatic recess
3. Assessment of sphenopalatine foramen and pterygopalatine fossa

#### 27.4.3.2 Magnetic Resonance Imaging (MRI)

Magnetic resonance imaging (MRI) has many advantages in the assessment of maxillary sinus pathologies including:

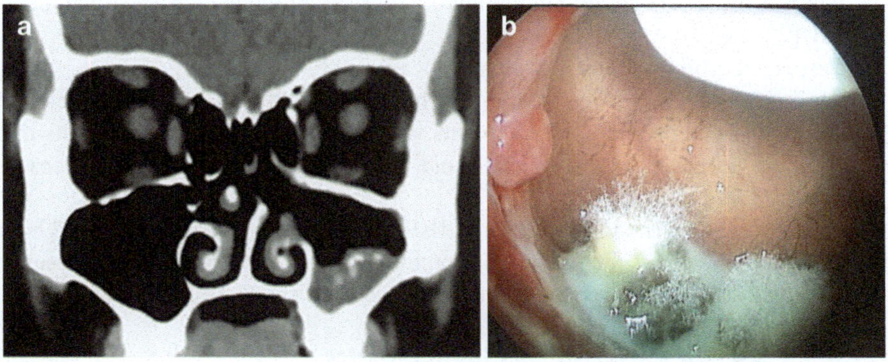


**Fig. 27.5** (**a**) Computed tomography scan "coronal view" of the paranasal sinus shows partial opacification with hyperdense signal in the floor of the left maxillary sinus. (**b**) Endoscopic view by 45-degree endoscope shows a fungal ball in the floor of the left maxillary sinus

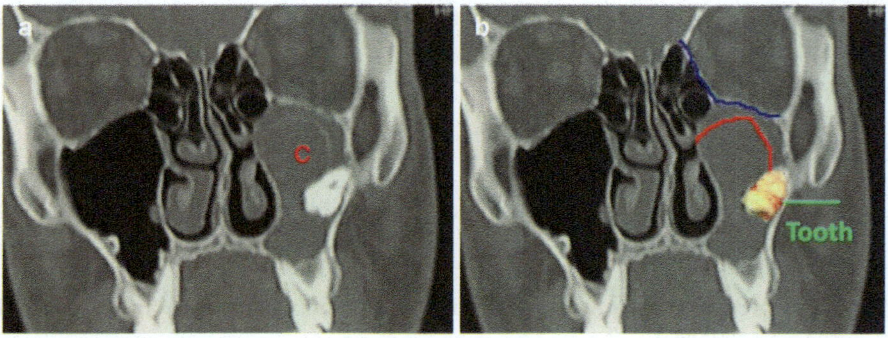


**Fig. 27.6** (**a**, **b**) Computed tomography scans "coronal view" of the paranasal sinus shows a left sided dentigerous cyst (**C**) with a tooth inside the cyst. The blue line represents the inferior and medial orbital wall, and the red line represents the wall of the cyst

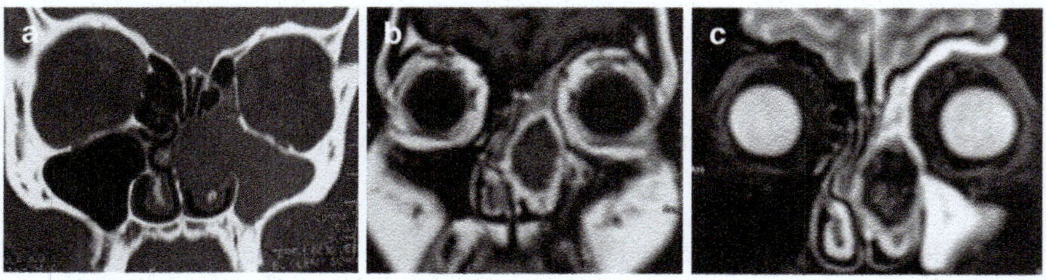


**Fig. 27.7** (**a**) Computed tomography scan "coronal view" of the paranasal sinus demonstrates complete opacification of the left maxillary sinus, and the osteomeatal complex. (**b**, **c**) T1-weighted image and T2-weighted image MRI, respectively, reveal the signal void sign within the left concha bullosa characteristic for fungal ball with hypertense signal in the T2-weighted image of the left maxillary sinus suggesting retained secretion within it

1. Ability to differentiate retained mucus from soft tissue masses based on signal intensity characteristics: Neoplasms display an intermediate T2 signal intensity, whereas bacterial and viral inflammatory diseases produce high T2 signal intensity [22, 23].
2. Suspected orbital or intracranial complications of sinusitis [24].
3. Chronic non-invasive localized fungal rhinosinusitis "fungal ball": The presence of calcium and paramagnetic elements within the fungal concretion results in a very low to absent signal "signal void" on T2-weighted image sequences as demonstrated in Fig. 27.7 [25].
4. Mucoceles: The usual signal characteristics for a mucocele are low T1 and high T2 signal intensities, but variations commonly occur depending on the presence of blood and the water content of the mucoceles as shown in Fig. 27.8.

#### 27.4.3.3 Specific Radiological Characteristics

- **Antrochoanal Polyp**: Computerized tomography shows complete or near-complete opacification of the maxillary sinus. Widening of the maxillary sinus

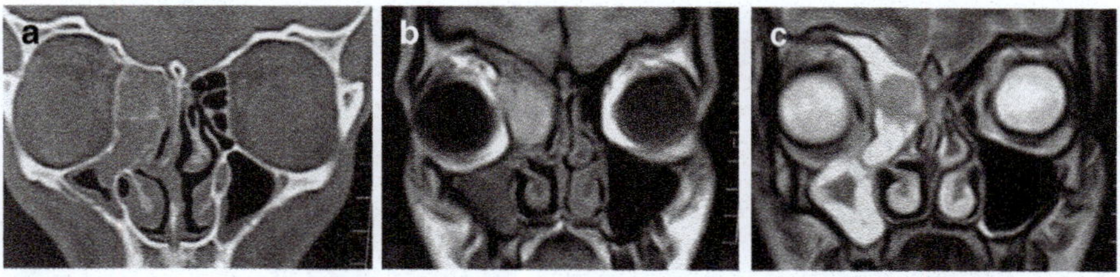


**Fig. 27.8** (**a**) Computed tomography scan "coronal view" of the paranasal sinus demonstrates partial opacification of the right maxillary sinus and complete opacification of the anterior ethmoid sinus. (**b**, **c**) T1-weighted image and T2-weighted image MRI, respectively, reveal hypertense signal in T2-weighted image of the left frontal recess, and the mucosal lining the right maxillary sinus with isotense signal of the right ethmoid sinus "increase of the protein content," picture suggesting mucocele formation

**Fig. 27.9** Computed tomography scan "axial view" of the paranasal sinus shows complete opacification of the left maxillary sinus with a smooth border polyp extending to the nasopharynx suggesting the diagnosis of antrochoanal polyp

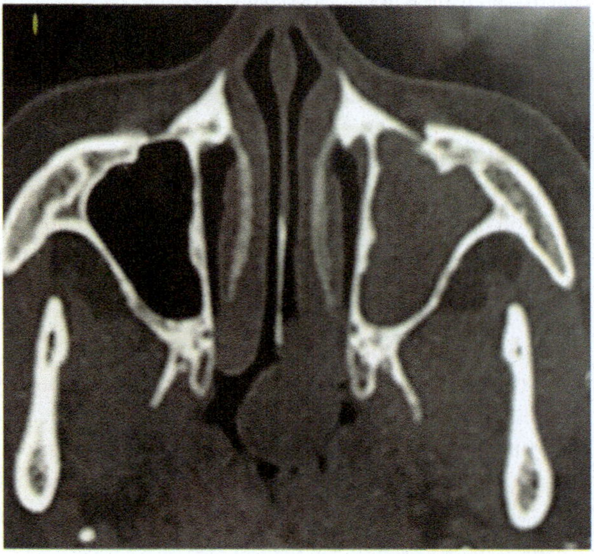

natural or accessory ostium, medial bulging of the medial maxillary sinus wall, and backward extension of the polyp toward the posterior choana as demonstrated in Fig. 27.9.

- **Allergic Fungal Rhinosinusitis (AFRS)**: The CT scan may show expansion of the maxillary sinus with remodeling and thinning of its bony wall. Areas of a hyperdense signal can be observed especially in the soft tissue window settings as shown in Fig. 27.10. The MRI T2-weighted images show a signal void within the sites of allergic fungal sinusitis, while the surrounding, inflamed mucosa shows high-signal intensity on T2-weighted images.

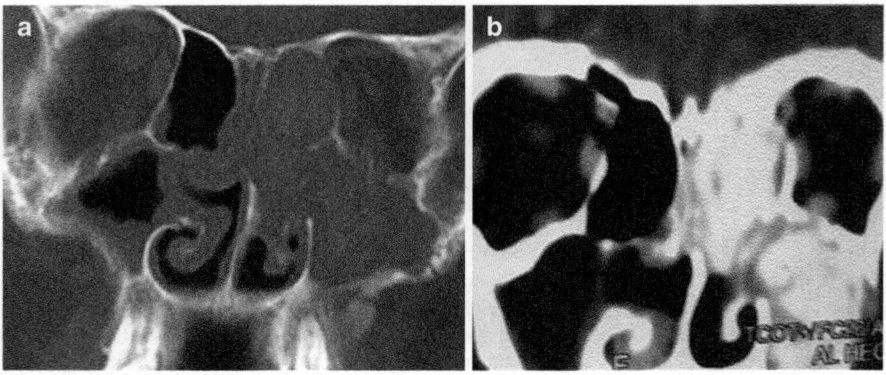


**Fig. 27.10** Computed tomography scan "coronal view" of the paranasal sinus. (**a**) Bony window and (**b**) soft tissue window show complete opacification of the left maxillary and anterior ethmoid sinuses with the hyperdense signal more evident in the soft tissue window

## 27.4.4 Surgical Techniques

### 27.4.4.1 Anesthesia

Endoscopic sinus surgery is performed under general anesthesia. We inject a combination of 1% lidocaine and 1/100,000 to 1/200,000 epinephrine into the agger nasi and the uncinate process area. Cotton pledgets soaked in oxymetazoline can be placed at the level of the inferior turbinate and lateral to the middle turbinate.

### 27.4.4.2 Endoscopic Uncinectomy

Using a zero-degree endoscope, uncinectomy is done by gentle medialization of the middle turbinate; then, the uncinate process is resected to expose the ethmoid bulla. The uncinectomy can be done in a posterior-to-anterior direction with backbiting forceps, or an anterior-to-posterior direction with a sickle knife or a Freer elevator. The most cranial portion of the uncinate process should be left intact to preserve the integrity of mucosa in the frontal recess area. Once the uncinate process is incised, it can be excised with straight thru-cutting forceps to avoid stripping the nasal mucosa. The uncinate process is resected anteriorly till the thick lacrimal crest is reached, and we should not go further anteriorly to avoid injury to the nasolacrimal duct [26].

### 27.4.4.3 Endoscopic Middle Meatal Antrostomy

Following uncinectomy, the maxillary sinus ostium can be visualized. To see the maxillary cavity more clearly, we switch to a 45-degree endoscope. Widening of the natural maxillary sinus ostium to the posterior fontanel by anterior thru-cutting forceps and side-biting punch forceps. Dissections extended too far posteriorly may result in injury of the sphenopalatine artery branches, which can be controlled by electrocautery. We explore the maxillary sinus cavity utilizing 45- and 70-degree endoscopes. We use 45-degree grasping forceps, 90-degree grasping forceps, and

Heuwieser forceps to remove any pathology within the maxillary sinus. We also use a curved shaver to remove large polyps within the maxillary sinus.

#### 27.4.4.4 Endoscopic-Modified Medial Maxillectomy

Endoscopic-modified medial maxillectomy is another option that entails the removal of the medial wall of the maxillary sinus, and widening of the antrostomy to its anatomic limits may be down to the nasal cavity floor inferiorly and to the posterior wall of the maxillary sinus posteriorly and medial orbital floor superiorly with preservation of the nasolacrimal duct and a portion of the inferior turbinate. It allows proper access to the maxillary sinus, including difficult-to-reach areas such as the lateral recesses, the anterior wall of the maxillary sinus, and the floor of the maxillary sinus; in addition, it creates a wide opening into the maxillary sinus that may allow improved mucus clearance and better penetration of topical medication and nasal douches [27].

#### 27.4.4.5 Endoscopic Medial Maxillectomy

It is an extended endoscopic endonasal technique that is indicated for the resection of benign and, in special circumstances, malignant tumors that are restricted to the lateral nasal wall. Endoscopic medial maxillectomy was described originally for the management of inverted papilloma [28]. The following structures may be resected in medial maxillectomy: the medial wall of the maxillary sinus including the inferior turbinate, the nasolacrimal duct, beside the middle turbinate, and anterior and posterior ethmoid sinuses. Endonasal medial maxillectomy enables us to visualize all the tumor margins to achieve total removal of the tumor.

#### 27.4.4.6 Extended Endoscopic Medial Maxillectomy

Endoscopic medial maxillectomy can be extended to resect the posterior wall of the maxillary sinus to get better access to the pterygopalatine fossa. It can also be extended to resect the medial portion of the anterior wall of the maxillary sinus including the piriform crest (Denker operation) as demonstrated in Fig. 27.11 [29, 30].

#### 27.4.4.7 Endoscopic Inferior Meatal Antrostomy

The need for an inferior antrostomy has significantly reduced as a result of the success of functional endoscopic sinus surgery. Nowadays, the inferior meatal antrostomy is indicated in persistent or recurrent isolated maxillary sinusitis with cysts, polyps, or fungal ball within the maxillary sinus. Inferior meatal antrostomy may be also indicated in patients without functional mucociliary clearance, such as in Kartagener's syndrome, cystic fibrosis, or even secondary ciliary dysfunction due to chronic sinus disease, gravity-dependent drainage facilitated by an inferior meatal antrostomy may be of benefit. It provides better exposure to the floor and anterior wall of the maxillary sinus. We use 90-degree curved J-curette to puncture the lateral nasal wall about one centimeter posterior to Hasner valve, midway between the nasal floor and the genu of the inferior turbinate; then, we can enlarge the created

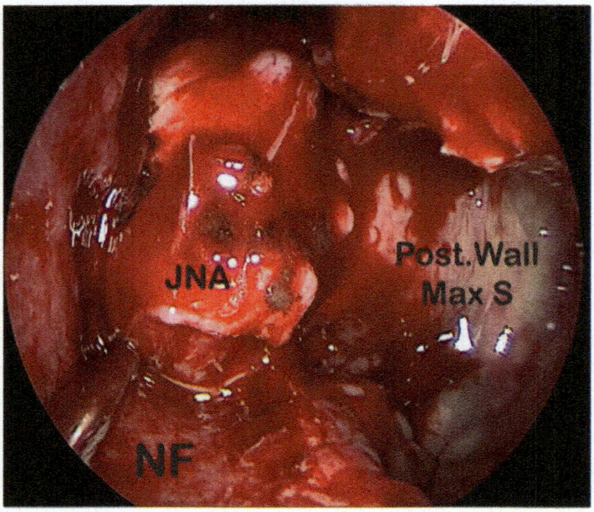


**Fig. 27.11** Extended medial maxillectomy with resection of the medial part of the left pyriform aperture, all the medial wall of the maxillary sinus including the inferior turbinate and nasolacrimal duct to get better access to the pterygopalatine fossa and infratemporal fossa for complete exposure and resection of juvenile nasopharyngeal angiofibroma. *JNA* juvenile nasopharyngeal angiofibroma, *Post.Wall Max S* posterior wall of the maxillary sinus, *NF* nasal floor

opening with a backbiter forceps anteriorly, anterior thru-cut forceps posteriorly, and down-biter forceps inferiorly [31].

#### 27.4.4.8 Postoperative Care

Postoperative antibiotics, systemic and local corticosteroids, and nasal irrigation are indicated for patients according to the pathology, and their duration is tailored to each patient according to the endoscopic follow-up of the patients.

Endoscopic surveillance for removal of crustations and blood, separation of synechiae, and suction of nasal secretion should be performed twice per week for one month; following this, patients were followed up according to endoscopic findings of the paranasal sinus cavities postoperatively.

#### 27.4.4.9 Complications of Endoscopic Maxillary Sinus Surgery

- Injury of the lamina papyracea during sinus surgery can lead to periorbital emphysema and ecchymosis "Injury of the periorbita usually occurs during uncinectomy."
- Injury of the nasolacrimal duct may result in epiphora.
- Injury of the infraorbital nerve.
- Bleeding from injury of sphenopalatine artery branches.
- Recirculation of mucus due to failure of identification of the natural maxillary sinus ostium as demonstrated in Fig. 27.12.

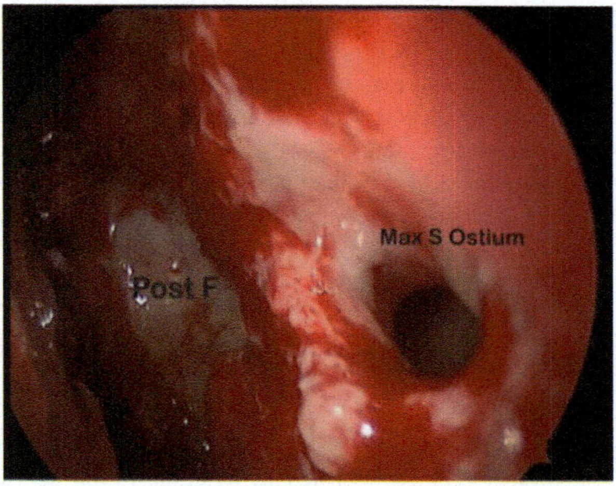


**Fig. 27.12** Endoscopic view by 45-degree endoscope shows the left natural maxillary sinus ostium anteriorly and posterior fontanelle [Post F] posteriorly, and connection between both openings is necessary to avoid recirculation of the mucus

#### 27.4.4.10 Balloon Sinuplasty of the Maxillary Sinus

Balloon catheter dilatation is a minimally invasive tool for remolding the anatomy of the paranasal sinus ostium without removing bone or tissue. The balloon system consists of several guide catheters, a pumping bomb, a guide wire, and a balloon. Maxillary balloon sinuplasty is contraindicated in chronic rhinosinusitis with nasal polyps, allergic fungal rhinosinusitis, and extensive osteogenesis.

The sinus ostium is dilated by the insertion of the balloon catheters under fluoroscopic guidance and high-pressure inflation of the balloon [32–34]. Due to its location behind the uncinate process, the maxillary sinus ostium is regarded as the trickiest for the introduction of surgical catheters. Utilizing 45-degree endoscope, the uncinate process is gently displaced with a 90-degree maxillary guiding catheter during catheter insertion. After positioning the balloon, it is inflated with about 8–10 atmospheres of pressure, resulting in the dilation of the ostium. A catheter may also be used to provide suction and irrigation. No need for nasal packing after balloon dilatation and the patient can be discharged on the same day [33, 34].

## 27.5 Anterior Approaches to the Maxillary Sinus

### 27.5.1 Caldwell-Luc Procedure

The Caldwell-Luc procedure was first described in 1893 [35]. The Caldwell-Luc surgery involves opening the maxillary sinus through the anterior wall through a gingival-labial incision, in adjunct with inferior meatal antrostomy to ensure adequate drainage of the maxillary sinus.

#### 27.5.1.1 Indications for Caldwell-Luc Surgery

The Caldwell-Luc approach through the anterior antral window is recommended in cases involving [36]:

1. Malignant tumors of the maxillary sinus extend to the lateral wall of the nasal fossa and the pterygomaxillary space.
2. Benign tumor, e.g., inverted papilloma.
3. Foreign objects within the maxillary sinus.
4. Orbital floor fractures.
5. Expanded access to the pterygopalatine fossa.
6. When aggressive medical and surgical interventions to treat persistent maxillary sinusitis have failed, the Caldwell-Luc operation with removal of the sinus mucosa should be taken into consideration.

#### 27.5.1.2 Surgical Technique of the Caldwell–Luc Procedure

A gingival incision is made in the mucosa above the canine tooth and is carried laterally to the level of the first molar with caution to retain enough vertical height of the inferior mucosal cuff for sufficient tension-free wound closure at the end of the surgery. The incision is carried down to the periosteum with dissection in the subperiosteal plane to the level of the infraorbital nerve to expose the anterior face of the maxilla. Attention should be paid to avoid injury of the infraorbital nerve and the anterior superior alveolar nerve.

To decrease the incidence of injury of the infraorbital and anterior superior alveolar nerve branches, the transantral opening is positioned just superolateral to the canine fossa. Opening of the anterior face of the maxilla can be carried out using a trocar, then enlarging it with a Kerrison punch, or by using a high-speed drill as it is less traumatic and more accurate. After the entrance into the maxillary sinus, the diseased mucosa and the pathology within the maxillary sinus can be removed with various instruments.

Complications of Caldwell–Luc surgery include a delayed recovery period in comparison with the endoscopic approach, facial edema and pain, bleeding and hematoma, numbness in the infraorbital and anterior superior alveolar nerve distributions, dacryocystitis and persistent epiphora, devitalized teeth and oro-antral fistulae, and facial hypoesthesia. More serious, though extremely rare, complications include inadvertent entrance into the orbit and damage to the ocular contents.

### 27.5.2 Canine Fossa Trephination

The posterior lateral wall of the maxillary sinus, the posterior area of the roof of the maxillary sinus, and the posterior wall of the maxillary sinus are accessible through the middle meatal antrostomy. Endoscopic treatment for maxillary sinus disease particularly in the anterior and inferior parts of the maxillary sinus may be difficult and requires access through the anterior maxillary wall of the maxillary sinus [37]. One such method is the Caldwell–Luc approach. The canine fossa puncture is an alternative method of getting access to the maxillary sinus through the anterior wall [38].

A Description of the Standard Technique of the Canine Fossa Trephination [39]:

Elevation of the upper lip of the patient, then trace the root of the canine tooth superiorly till the canine fossa is reached. We inject 2% lidocaine with 1:100,000 of adrenalin into the canine fossa. A small incision is made in the gingivobuccal sulcus above and lateral to the apex of the canine tooth, and the soft tissue is dissected off the anterior face of the maxilla. We open the anterior wall of the maxillary sinus with a trocar in the canine fossa and directed posteriorly, to create an opening of about 4 mm. This sublabial mucosal incision is small enough to close spontaneously and is not sutured. Now, we have two ports (middle meatal antrostomy and the opening of the anterior wall) to the maxillary sinus, one port for the endoscope and the other port for the instruments.

Complications of the canine fossa puncture technique include cheek swelling, tooth injury, facial pain, facial numbness, cheek pain, dental numbness, gingival complications, facial tingling, and injury to the orbit [39]. Most of these complications resolve within the first month after surgery; however, some patients have persistent complications with facial tingling, numbness, or continued pain [40].

### 27.5.3 Prelacrimal Recess Approach (Fig. 27.13)

The prelacrimal recess approach was first described by Zhou et al. [41] as a minimally invasive approach to certain maxillary sinus lesions with complete preservation of the nasolacrimal duct and the inferior turbinate [42]. Prelacrimal recess approach allows for the assessment of the entire maxillary sinus including the anterior wall, alveolar recess, palatine recess, and zygomatic recess of the maxillary sinus with adequate eradication of the pathology within the maxillary sinus.

All patients have surgery under general anesthesia. A middle meatal antrostomy is performed at the beginning of surgery. Following an injection of 1% lidocaine and 1:100,000 epinephrine in the submucosal plane of the lateral nasal wall, a horizontal mucosal incision is made on the lateral nasal wall starting from the anterior edge of the antrostomy, a few millimeters above the anterior insertion of the inferior turbinate, to the edge of the pyriform aperture. A freer elevator is used to elevate the mucoperiosteal flaps to expose the bone of the lateral nasal wall. A window through the lateral nasal wall, anterior to the nasolacrimal duct, is formed using a drill or an osteotome, and it can be widened by Kerrison forceps or a drill.

The lacrimal bone may be resected, and the nasolacrimal duct is released from its bony canal and medialized to get wide access to the maxillary sinus [43]. Depending on the size of the prelacrimal recess, either the endoscope and an instrument can be inserted together, or the endoscope can only be inserted while curved instruments are inserted through the middle meatal antrostomy to remove the pathology (two ports technique) [44]. The mucosal flap is re-draped and approximated by one or two absorbable sutures at the end of the surgery, without nasal packing.

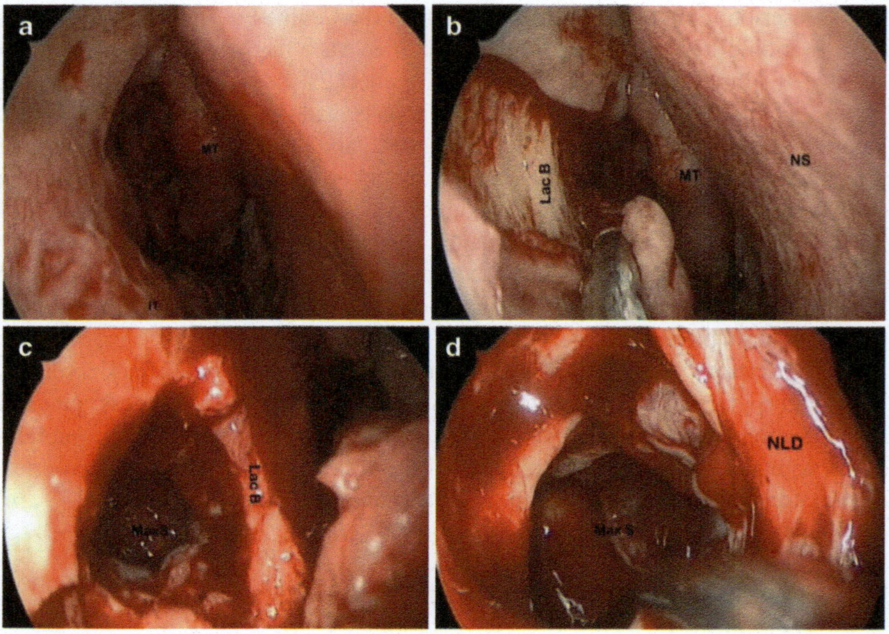


**Fig. 27.13** Prelacrimal recess approach. (**a**) Endoscopic view of the right nasal cavity after middle meatal antrostomy. *MT* middle turbinate, *IT* inferior turbinate. (**b**) Horizontal incision from the right pyriform aperture anteriorly to the lacrimal bone posteriorly with an elevation of the mucoperiosteal flap to expose the underlying bone. *Lac B* lacrimal bone, *MT* middle turbinate, *NS* nasal septum. (**c**) Creation of an opening to get access to the prelacrimal recess of the maxillary sinus. *Max S* maxillary sinus, *Lac B* lacrimal bone. (**d**) Endoscopic view by a 0-degree endoscope with the removal of the bone over the nasolacrimal duct (NLD) and medial displacement of the NLD to get wide access through the prelacrimal recess to the floor and anterior wall of the maxillary sinus. *Max S* maxillary sinus, *NLD* nasolacrimal duct

## 27.6 Causes of Failed Maxillary Sinus Surgery

Middle turbinate lateralization was described by Musy and Kountakis [45] as the most common finding in revision cases. Other findings included incomplete anterior ethmoidectomy, scarred frontal recess, retained agger nasi cell, incomplete posterior ethmoidectomy, retained uncinate process, middle meatal antrostomy stenosis, and recurrent polyposis. Ramadan [46] reviewed 52 cases and reported that the most common cause of failure was residual air cells and adhesions in the ethmoid area (31%), followed by maxillary sinus ostial stenosis (27%) and frontal recess stenosis (25%).

Richtsmeier [47] reported that the most common causes of failed endoscopic sinus surgery of the maxillary sinus were as follows: obstructed natural ostium, disease in the anterior ethmoid or frontal sinus, resistant organisms, intrasinus foreign body, incurable mucosal disease, noncompliant patient, wrong primary diagnosis, maxillary osteitis, mucus recirculation, and immunodeficiency.

Cohen and Kennedy [48] showed that the causes of failed endoscopic maxillary sinus surgery were as follows: infection draining into the maxillary sinus from

**Table 27.2** Causes of failure of endoscopic maxillary sinus surgery

| | |
|---|---|
| 1. Recirculation of the mucus | |
| 2. Infection draining into the maxillary sinus from elsewhere | |
| 3. Retained disease or foreign material | For example, dental filling material, fungal concretions, or bone chips |
| 4. Failure of mucociliary transport | For example, cystic fibrosis or Kartagener syndrome |
| 5. Scar formation | It may result from the striping of sinus mucosa with a circumferential mucosal injury that leads to obstruction of the sinus outflow tract, osteitis with significant bony hypertrophy, and mucocele formation |
| 6. Osteitis | Thru-cutting instruments and powered microdebrider prevent excessive mucosal stripping and decrease bone exposure, which lower the risk of osteitis |
| 7. Biofilm formation | |
| 8. Other causes | For example, smoking, immune deficiency, connective tissue disorder, cigarette smoking, or a genetic disorder such as cystic fibrosis or primary ciliary dyskinesia |

elsewhere, recirculation of mucus, failure of mucociliary transport, retained foreign material (including dental filling material), and local osteitis.

Recirculation of the mucus results from a partially resected uncinate process, failure of identification of natural maxillary sinus ostium, and scarring at the anterior aspect of the antrostomy. Parsons et al. [49] described the "missed ostium sequence" that occurs due to incomplete removal of the anterior part of the uncinate process, concealing the natural maxillary sinus ostium, which prevents the middle meatal antrostomy from communicating with the natural ostium, resulting in a recirculation phenomenon. Table 27.2 summarizes the causes of failure of endoscopic maxillary sinus surgery.

## 27.7 Maxillectomy (Fig. 27.14)

### 27.7.1 Types of Maxillectomy (Table 27.3)

1. Limited maxillectomy involves the resection of one wall: There are three types of limited maxillectomy: medial maxillectomy, infrastructure maxillectomy or alveolectomy, and anterolateral maxillectomy.
2. Subtotal maxillectomy has two walls resected: This involves complete resection of the maxilla except for the roof of the maxillary sinus.
3. Total maxillectomy has all walls of the maxilla resected.

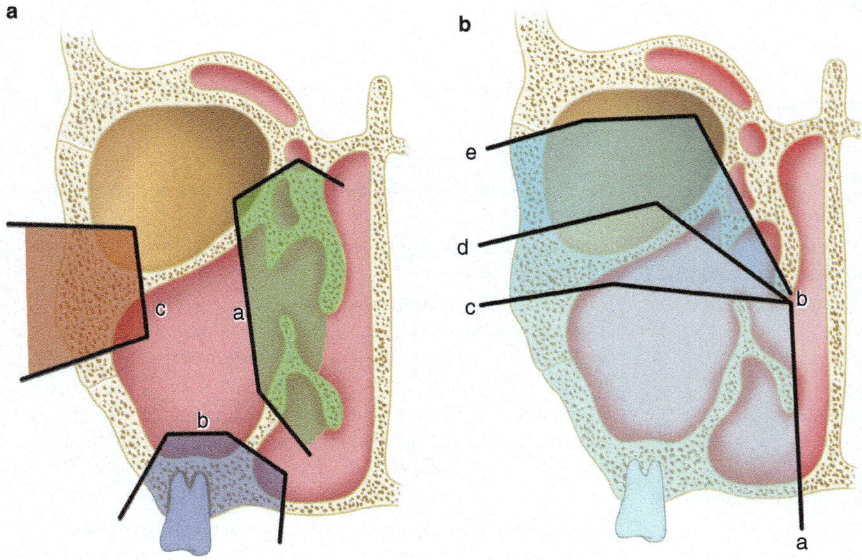


**Fig. 27.14** (**A**) A diagram illustrating the limits of limited maxillectomy: (a) Medial maxillectomy "green." (b) Infrastructure maxillectomy "blue." (c) Anterolateral maxillectomy "red." (**B**) A diagram illustrating the limits of maxillectomy: subtotal maxillectomy "a-b-c," total maxillectomy with orbital preservation "a-b-d," total maxillectomy with orbital exenteration "a-b-e"

**Table 27.3** Types, indications, the extent of resection, and incisions of maxillectomy operation

| | Indications | Extent of resection | Incision |
|---|---|---|---|
| Medial maxillectomy | Management of lesions of the lateral nasal wall, most commonly inverting papilloma [50] | – Removal of the lateral nasal wall from the floor to the ethmoid roof and from the pyramidal aperture to the plane defined by the most posterior aspect of the maxilla<br>– The inferior turbinate and portions of the ethmoid, the lacrimal bones, may be resected | – Transnasal endoscopic medial maxillectomy [50]<br>– Lateral rhinotomy approach<br>– Midface degloving approach may also be employed to increase surgical exposure |
| Infrastructure Maxillectomy, alveolectomy | Diseases originating in the oral cavity or those of odontogenic origin | – Resect the involved alveolar segment and/or hard palate<br>– Resection can encompass as little as a segment of the hard palate to varying degrees of alveolectomy, to total bilateral alveolectomy and palatectomy | – Sublabial incision for small lesions—extended<br>– Lateral rhinotomy or a midface degloving approach for more extensive pathologies |
| Anterolateral maxillectomy | Lesions originating from the facial skin, the parotid gland, or the bucco-alveolar sulcus that involves the maxilla secondarily | | – Facial incisions designed to manage the primary location of the tumor<br>– Extended lateral rhinotomy approach with a lip split or a midface degloving approach |

(continued)

**Table 27.3** (continued)

| | Indications | Extent of resection | Incision |
|---|---|---|---|
| Subtotal maxillectomy | Neoplasms arise in the maxillary sinus sparing the bone of the orbital floor or for more extensive pathology of the oral cavity | Complete resection of the maxilla except for the roof of the maxillary sinus | Midface degloving or extended lateral rhinotomy approaches |
| Total maxillectomy with orbital preservation | Tumor involves the bony orbital floor, for those patients whose periorbita has not been invaded by the tumor | | A midface or an extended lateral rhinotomy approach |
| Total maxillectomy with orbital exenteration | Maxillary tumor invasion extending into the orbit | Orbital exenteration is generally subdivided into two groups: preservation of the eyelid and resection of the eyelid | A lateral rhinotomy is commonly used with a supraorbital extension, upper and lower lid incisions, or transconjunctival incisions, depending on the intention to spare or sacrifice the eyelids |

## References


1. Stammberger H, Posawetz W. Functional endoscopic sinus surgery. Concept, indications and results of the Messerklinger technique. Eur Arch Otorrinolaringol. 1990;247:63–76.
2. Vacher C, Copin H, Sakka M. Maxillary ossification in a series of six human embryos and fetuses aged from 9 to 12 weeks of amenorrhea: clinical implications. Surg Radiol Anat. 1999;21:261–6.
3. Bingham B, Wang RG, Hawke M, Kwok P. The embryonic development of the lateral nasal wall from 8 to 24 weeks. Laryngoscope. 1991;101:992–7.
4. Wang RG, Jiang SC, Gu R. The cartilaginous nasal capsule and embryonic development of human paranasal sinuses. J Otolaryngol. 1994;23:239–43.
5. Barghouth G, Prior JO, Lepori D, Duvoisin B, Schnyder P, Gudinchet F. Paranasal sinuses in children: size evaluation of maxillary, sphenoid, and frontal sinuses by magnetic resonance imaging and proposal of volume index percentile curves. Eur Radiol. 2002;12:1451–8.
6. Chrcanovic BR, Freire-Maia B. Maxillary sinus aplasia. Oral Maxillofac Surg. 2010;14(3):187–91.
7. Yoon JH, Kim KS, Jung DH, Kim SS, Koh KS, Oh CS, et al. Fontanelle and uncinate process in the lateral wall of the human nasal cavity. Laryngoscope. 2000;110:281–5.
8. Lund VJ, Stammberger H, Fokkens WJ, Beale T, Bernal-Sprekelsen M, Eloy P, et al. European position paper on the anatomical terminology of the internal nose and paranasal sinuses. Rhinol Suppl. 2014;24:1–34.
9. Ozcelik Erdem R, Dundar MA, Arbag S, Arbag H, Seker M. Endoscopic anatomy of the lacrimal sac: a cadaveric study. Acta Med Acad. 2022;51:175–80.
10. Iwanaga J, Wilson C, Lachkar S, Tomaszewski KA, Walocha JA, Tubbs RS. Clinical anatomy of the maxillary sinus: application to sinus floor augmentation. Anat Cell Biol. 2019;52:17–24.
11. Stammberger HR, Kennedy DW. Paranasal sinuses: anatomic terminology and nomenclature. Ann Otol Rhinol Laryngol Suppl. 1995;167:7–16.
12. Sargi ZB. Surgical anatomy of the paranasal sinuses. In: Kountakis SE, editor. Rhinologic and sleep apnea surgical techniques. Berlin: Springer; 2007. p. 17–26.
13. Landsberg R, Friedman M. A computer-assisted anatomical study of the nasofrontal region. Laryngoscope. 2001;111:2125–30.
14. Stackpole SA, Edelstein DR. The anatomic relevance of the Haller cell in sinusitis. Am J Rhinol. 1997;11:219–23.
15. Bolger WE, Woodruff WW, Morehead J, Parsons DS. Maxillary sinus hypoplasia: classification and description of associated uncinate process hypoplasia. Otolaryngol Head Neck Surg. 1990;103:759–65.
16. Stryjewska-Makuch G, Kokoszka M, Goroszkiewicz K, Karłowska-Bijak O, Kolebacz B, Misiołek M. What may surprise a rhinologist in everyday clinical practice: silent sinus syndrome or pneumosinus dilatans/pneumocele? Literature review and own experience. Eur Arch Otorrinolaringol. 2023;2023(280):519–27.
17. Annino DJ, Goguen LA. Silent sinus syndrome. Curr Opin Otolaryngol Head Neck Surg. 2008;16:22–5.
18. Virgin F, Ling FT, Kountakis SE. Radiology and endoscopic findings of silent maxillary sinus atelectasis and enophthalmos. Am J Otolaryngol. 2008;29:167–70.
19. Nivean PD, Sayee TS, Nivean M. Silent sinus syndrome: a missed entity? Oman J Ophthalmol. 2023;16:133–5.
20. Min YG, Lee JW, Shin JS. Radiologic assessment of diseased mucosa of the maxillary sinus after functional endoscopic sinus surgery. Acta Otolaryngol. 1994;114:657–62.
21. Chiu AG, Vaughan WC. Revision endoscopic frontal sinus surgery with surgical navigation. Otolaryngol Head Neck Surg. 2004;130:312–8.
22. Bernhardt TM, Rapp-Bernhardt U, Fessel A, Ludwig K, Reichel G, Grote R. CT scanning of the paranasal sinuses: axial helical CT with reconstruction in the coronal direction versus coronal helical CT. Br J Radiol. 1998;71:846–51.
23. Ludwick JJ, Taber KH, Manolidis S, Sarna A, Hayman LA. A computed tomographic guide to endoscopic sinus surgery: axial and coronal views. J Comput Assist Tomogr. 2002;26:317–22.

24. Branstetter BF, Weissman JL. Role of MR and CT in the paranasal sinuses. Otolaryngol Clin N Am. 2005;38:1279–99.
25. Aygun N, Uzuner O, Zinreich SJ. Advances in imaging of the paranasal sinuses. Otolaryngol Clin N Am. 2005;38:429–37.
26. Schauss F, Weber R, Draf W, Keerl R. Surgery of the lacrimal system. Acta Otorhinolaryngol Belg. 1996;50:143–6.
27. Woodworth BA, Parker RO, Schlosser RJ. Modified endoscopic medial maxillectomy for chronic maxillary sinusitis. Am J Rhinol. 2006;20:317–9.
28. Sadeghi N, Al-Dhahri S, Manoukian JJ. Transnasal endoscopic medial maxillectomy for inverting papilloma. Laryngoscope. 2003;113:749–53.
29. Lim SC, Lee JK, Yoon TM. Extended endoscopic medial maxillectomy for sinonasal neoplasms. Otolaryngol Head Neck Surg. 2008;139:310–2.
30. Smith W, Lowe D, Leong P. Resection of pyriform aperture: a useful adjunct in nasal surgery. J Laryngol Otol. 2009;123:123–5.
31. Landsberg R, Masalha M, Margulis A, Rosman Y, Schneider S. Endoscopic inferior meatal antrostomy for antrochoanal polyps: a long-term follow-up. ORL. 2022;84:336–41.
32. Vaughan WC. Review of balloon sinuplasty. Curr Opin Otolaryngol Head Neck Surg. 2008;16:2–9.
33. Christmas DA, Mirante JP, Yanagisawa E. Endoscopic view of balloon catheter dilation of sinus ostia (balloon sinuplasty). Ear Nose Throat J. 2006;85:698–700.
34. Siow JK, Al Kadah B, Werner JA. Balloon sinuplasty: a current hot topic in rhinology. Eur Arch Otorrinolaringol. 2008;265:509–11.
35. Macbeth R. Caldwell, luc, and their operation. Laryngoscope. 1971;81:1652–7.
36. Barzilai G, Greenberg E, Uri N. Indications for the Caldwell-Luc approach in the endoscopic era. Otolaryngol Head Neck Surg. 2005;132:219–20.
37. Seresirikachorn K, Kondo M, Png LH, Kalish L, Campbell RG, Alvarado R, et al. Prelacrimal approach to maxillary sinus pathology. Am J Rhinol Allergy. 2023;37:369–73.
38. Byun JY, Lee JY. Canine fossa puncture for severe maxillary disease in unilateral chronic sinusitis with nasal polyp. Laryngoscope. 2013;123:79–84.
39. Robinson SR, Baird R, Le T, Wormald PJ. The incidence of complications after canine fossa puncture performed during endoscopic sinus surgery. Am J Rhinol. 2005;19:203–6.
40. Robinson S, Wormald PJ. Patterns of innervation of the anterior maxilla: a cadaver study with relevance to canine fossa puncture of the maxillary sinus. Laryngoscope. 2005;115:1785–8.
41. Zhou BHD, Cui SJ, Huang Q, Wei YX, Liu HC. Endoscopic nasal lateral wall dissection approach to maxillary sinus. Chin J Otorhinolaryngol Head Neck Surg. 2007;42:743–8.
42. Arosio AD, Valentini M, Canevari FR, Volpi L, Karligkiotis A, Terzakis D, et al. Endoscopic endonasal prelacrimal approach: radiological considerations, morbidity, and outcomes. Laryngoscope. 2021;131:1715–21.
43. Lock PSX, Siow GW, Karandikar A, Goh JPN, Siow JK. Anterior maxillary wall and lacrimal duct relationship in Orientals: CT analysis for prelacrimal access to the maxillary sinus. Eur Arch Otorhinolaryngol. 2019;276:2237–41.
44. Tomoum MO, Askar MH, Hamad AH, El-Naggar A, Amer M. Third window approach assisted middle meatal antrostomy: prospective cohort study of the two ports technique in management of hard to reach maxillary sinus pathology. J Laryngol Otol. 2020;134:636–41.
45. Musy PY, Kountakis SE. Anatomic findings in patients undergoing revision endoscopic sinus surgery. Am J Otolaryngol. 2004;25:418–22.
46. Ramadan HH. Surgical causes of failure in endoscopic sinus surgery. Laryngoscope. 1999;109:27–9.
47. Richtsmeier WJ. Top 10 reasons for endoscopic maxillary sinus surgery failure. Laryngoscope. 2001;111:1952–6.
48. Cohen NA, Kennedy DW. Revision endoscopic sinus surgery. Otolaryngol Clin N Am. 2006;39:417–35.
49. Parsons DS, Stivers FE, Talbot AR. The missed ostium sequence and the surgical approach to revision functional endoscopic sinus surgery. Otolaryngol Clin N Am. 1996;29:169–83.
50. Liu Q, Weng C, Zheng H, Wu L, Huang S. Endoscopic modified medial maxillectomy for inverted papilloma of the maxillary sinus. J Craniofac Surg. 2022;33:71–3.

# Endoscopic Approaches to Maxillary Sinus

28

Veerasigamani Narendrakumar, Aarthi Sundararajan, and Febin James

**Key Points**

- Maxillary pathologies are unique and common, dealing with them and to avoid recurrence is always challenging.
- Selection of approach to reach maxillary sinus is essential.
- Angled endoscopes and instruments are a must for maxillary sinus surgeries.

## 28.1 Embryology and Anatomy

Maxillary sinus was first described by Nathaniel Highmore (1613–1685), a British physician and anatomist [1]. Maxillary sinuses are embryologically the first to develop, starting at around tenth week, and are almost always present at the time of birth [2]. The growth patterns of the maxillary sinus indeed undergo significant changes during childhood and adolescence. The most extensive growth of the maxillary sinus occurs until the end of the eighth year. By the age of 16, the maxillary sinus achieves its maximum values for all its diameters and its volume [3]. At

**Supplementary Information** The online version contains supplementary material available at https://doi.org/10.1007/978-3-031-70077-4_28.

V. Narendrakumar (✉)
Pragathi ENT & Endocrine Clinic, Chennai, India

A. Sundararajan
MS ENT DNB ENT, Chennai, India

F. James
IQRAA Hospital, Elittil Hospital, Calicut, India


S. Elwany (ed.), *Current Rhinology*,
https://doi.org/10.1007/978-3-031-70077-4_28

maturity, the typical volume of a fully developed maxillary sinus ranges from 15 to 20 ml on average [3].

The maxillary sinus is a pyramidal-shaped cavity with the base adjacent to the nasal cavity and the apex towards the zygoma. Maxillary sinus walls have six walls, the superior, anterior, lateral and medial walls which are broad and posterior and inferior walls which are narrower. The sinus has several recesses namely, the alveolar recess pointing inferiorly, the zygomatic recess pointing laterally, the palatine recess which lies between the floor of the nasal cavity and the roof of the oral cavity and the infraorbital recess pointing superiorly. The natural ostium of the maxillary sinus is situated on the superior aspect of the medial wall of the sinus. Accessory ostia are seen in 20–40% of the population, arise in the thin, membranous portion of the medial wall of the maxillary sinus and usually lie posteroinferior to the main ostium. They are mostly acquired rather than developmental, as a result of infection of the sinus and obstruction of its main natural ostium. The cilia that line the mucosa of the sinus move in the direction of the natural ostium, effectively clearing the secretions out of the sinus [4].

Maxillary sinus can be affected by a wide range of pathologies ranging (Fig. 28.1) from infection and allergy to benign and malignant conditions which needs surgical management. With the introduction of endoscopic sinus surgery and the development of advanced angled endoscopes and surgical instruments, approaches to sinus surgeries have evolved significantly, rendering the traditional open approaches largely obsolete.

According to Harvey et al., the maxillary sinus is divided into five zones of access [5]:

1. Nasal cavity (zone 1)
2. Medial to the infraorbital nerve (zone 2)
3. Lateral to the infraorbital nerve (zone 3)
4. Anterior maxilla (zone 4)
5. Premaxillary tissue (zone 5)

Of which, zones 3, 4 and 5 are considered the most difficult areas to access endoscopically.

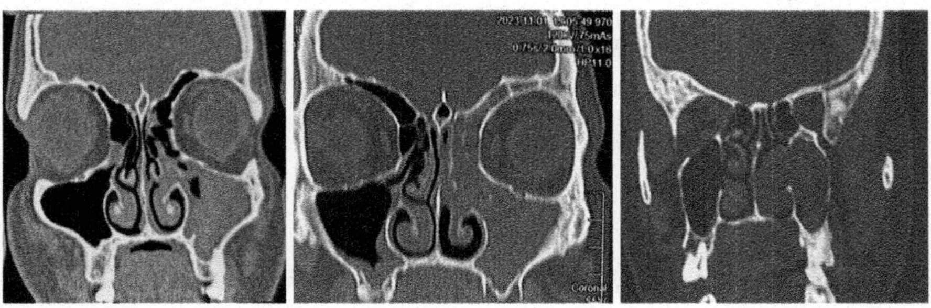

**Fig. 28.1** Examples of maxillary sinus pathologies

In addition to conventional endoscopic approaches to the maxillary sinus, several newer modifications of endoscopic sinus surgery (ESS) have been introduced to target inaccessible and challenging-to-reach zones within the maxillary sinus.

This chapter delves into the diverse endoscopic approaches currently utilized for accessing the maxillary sinus, outlining key procedural steps, indications and limitations associated with each approach.

## 28.2 Uncinectomy and Infundibulotomy

The maxillary sinus ostium opens into the inferior aspect of the infundibulum which lies lateral to the free edge of the uncinate process, which is usually not visible with a 0° endoscope. Thus, dissection and removal of the entire uncinate process allows visualization of the natural maxillary ostium, especially with an angled endoscope.

This procedure commonly involves the resection of uncinate, exposure of the infundibulum and preservation of the mucosa around the natural ostium.

**Indications**

It is done for isolated purulent maxillary sinusitis to establish drainage, irrigation of maxillary contents. To improve delivery of therapeutic agents to the sinuses.

**Key Steps [6]**

The uncinectomy can be done by either antegrade or retrograde technique [5] of which Retrograde is a safer option.

The retrograde approach is done using a backbiter to divide the uncinate at the junction of the inferior third and superior two-thirds. The superior component and inferior components can then be removed separately with a down-biting antral punch.

For the anterograde approach, a sickle knife or Freer's elevator is used to incise and separate the uncinate process from the lateral wall at its attachment with the lacrimal bone. Once the uncinate is removed, an angled endoscope can be used for clear visualization of the natural ostium.

**Complication**

Risk of injury to orbit and nasolacrimal duct (NLD).

**Limitation**

It cannot be used in conditions that need wider exposure into sinus cavity to remove the actual pathology.

## 28.3 Middle Meatal Antrostomy

Middle meatal antrostomy is nothing but the enlargement of the natural ostium of the maxillary sinus, and if accessory ostium is present, it is connected to the natural ostium to prevent the recirculation of the mucus secretions.

There are **3 types** described [7].

**Type I**: The natural ostium is enlarged posteriorly to a limited extent, not more than 1 cm (Fig. 28.2).
**Type II**: Enlarging the ostium posteriorly and inferiorly approximately up to 2 cm (Fig. 28.3).
**Type III**: Posteriorly, the ostium is extended close the level of the posterior wall of the maxillary sinus, inferiorly till the base of the inferior turbinate and anteriorly up to lacrimal sac. (Fig. 28.4).

**Indications**

- To drain mucopus.
- In the presence of accessory ostium as a result of infection
- To treat minor inflammatory disease and infective pathologies like chronic rhinosinusitis (CRS)
- To remove postero-medially based tumours/pathologies;
- Type III is also called as the mega antrostomy which is used in conditions like extensive polyposis, allergic fungal rhinosinusitis (AFRS) and antrochoanal (AC) polyp, where removal of the stalk is very crucial in avoiding recurrence
- Conditions like cystic fibrosis, recalcitrant maxillary sinusitis and Samter's triad where there is a need for extending the natural ostium to clear the troublesome contents.

**Key Steps**

Following initial standard steps of uncinectomy and identification of natural ostium of maxillary sinus is done, enlargement of the ostium is usually done posteriorly and

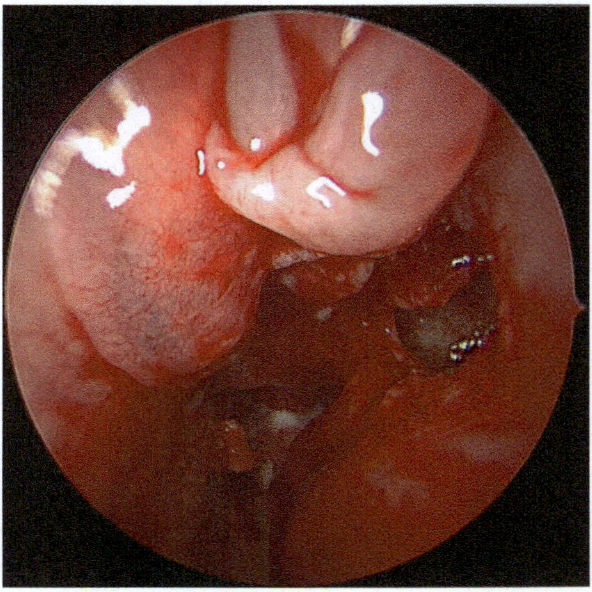

**Fig. 28.2** Middle meatal antrostomy type I

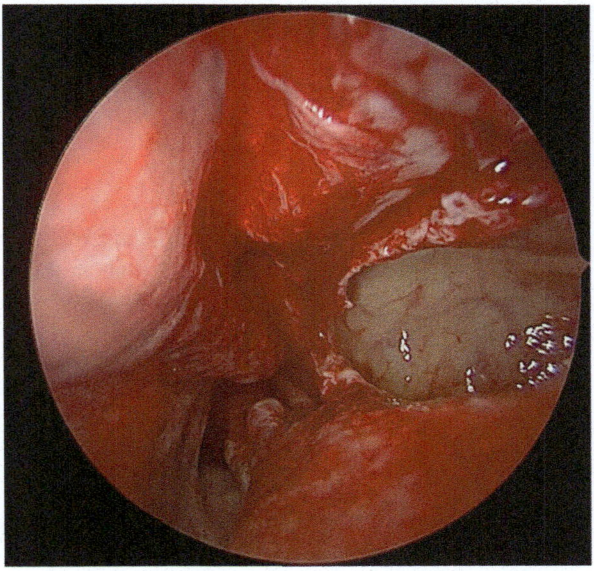

**Fig. 28.3** Middle meatal antrostomy type II

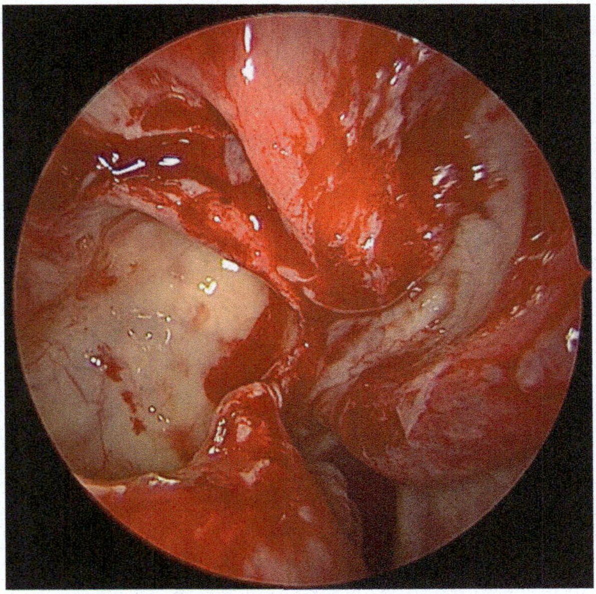

**Fig. 28.4** Middle meatal antrostomy type III

inferiorly using straight through cutting forceps, and anterior enlargement can be done with a back biter carefully to avoid injury to the NLD. The size of enlargement depends on the disease and pathology. Using angled endoscope and instruments, pathology can be cleared from the maxillary sinus.

**Complications**

- Injury to orbit and NLD
- In case of type III, the drying effect of nasal airflow which in turn predisposes to biofilm formation [8]
- The loss of protective nitric oxide concentration within the maxillary sinus [9]

**Limitation**

This procedure may not always be sufficient for addressing more substantial disease. In 2010, a cadaveric study found that middle meatal antrostomy provides access to only 24–34% of the total sinus volume and rarely offered access to the anterior wall and sinus floor, regardless of the angulation of the instruments used [10].

## 28.4 Endoscopic Medial Maxillectomy

Conventional endoscopic medial maxillectomy consists of complete removal of the lateral nasal wall of the nasal cavity, including the inferior turbinate and the nasolacrimal duct [11].

**Indication**

- Benign and malignant tumours of the nasal turbinate, maxillary sinus
- Fungal invasion like mucormycosis and aspergillosis

**Key Steps**

Following uncinectomy, ostium is widened posteriorly until the posterior wall of the maxillary sinus is visualized. Inferior turbinate is medialized and crushed, and turbinectomy is done in flush with the lateral wall. Nasal floor mucosal flap is created, and bone cuts are made along the mucosal incision lines along the floor of the nose to the maxillary sinus.

The medial maxillary wall is mobile now, only tethered anteriorly with NLD. NLD is visualized and transected. The specimen can now be removed entirely, allowing excellent visualization into the maxillary sinus (Fig. 28.5).

**Complications**

Atrophic rhinitis, epiphora and recurrent dacryocystitis may occur due to complete removal of the inferior turbinate and of the nasolacrimal duct.

In order to reduce the above-said complications, several modifications were developed in order to preserve the anatomy and physiology of the sinonasal cavity: preservation of inferior turbinate while NLD sacrificed [12], preservation of both inferior turbinate and NLD by medialization [13].

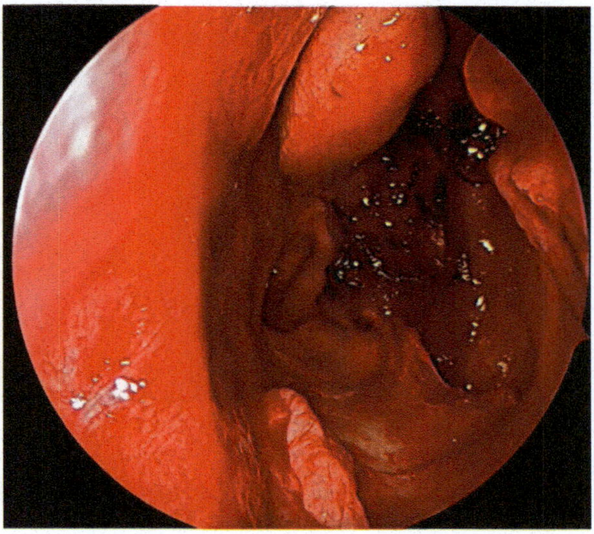

**Fig. 28.5** Endoscopic medial maxillectomy

## 28.5 Prelacrimal Approach

The prelacrimal recess is a concave area situated in the medial and anterosuperior portion of the maxillary sinus. It is situated in front of the lacrimal passage eminence on the medial sinus wall [14].

The endoscopic prelacrimal recess approach (PLRA) is a minimally invasive, which gives clear view and easy access for removal of benign maxillary sinus lesions. This surgery is both physiological and functional, offering significant advantages in the treatment of nasal and paranasal sinus diseases [15].

**Indications**

- Removal of recurrent antrochoanal polyps
- Benign and malignant tumours of maxillary sinus
- Refractory fungal infections
- Useful in approaching to the pterygopalatine and infratemporal fossae

**Key Steps**

This approach entails making a vertical incision along the lateral nasal wall, just behind the piriform aperture, followed by medialization of a mucosal flap to expose the bone of the anteromedial maxillary wall. Utilizing sharp osteotomies or a drill, the bone covering the pre lacrimal recess is excised, enabling identification of the lacrimal apparatus and providing direct access into the maxillary sinus (Fig. 28.6). The mucosal flap is then replaced back and sutured.

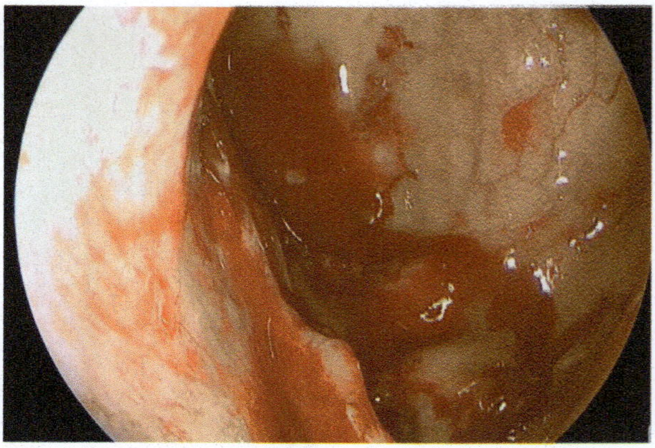

**Fig. 28.6** Prelacrimal approach

**Complication**

Facial numbness, facial pain, facial swelling, epiphora, IT-NLD flap disturbance [16].

**Limitation**

There occurs a great variation in the prelacrimal recess anatomy. Even if the prelacrimal recess is narrow, the nasolacrimal apparatus can be mobilized and pushed medially to accommodate appropriate instrumentation, without compromising its long-term function.

## 28.6 Endoscopic Inframeatal Antrostomy

This approach is done to fully expose the medial and inferior aspect of the maxillary sinus. It involves creation of permanent window through which the maxillary sinus and the nasal cavity communicate so that the secretions of the maxillary are drained into the nasal cavity.

**Indication**

- Pathologies like mucoceles or antrochoanal polyps located in the posterolateral wall and floor of the maxilla.

**Key Steps [17]**

Mucosal incision is made vertically below and 0.5 cm posterior to the anterior end of the inferior turbinate to the nasal floor; the whole mucosal flap is raised and exposing the bony medial wall of the maxillary sinus, using a chisel and bone forceps a window of size 10 mm × 10 mm created. Care was taken to avoid stripping the mucosa and injuring Hasner's valve.

The antrostomy can be widened anteriorly using backbiting forceps and an irrigated diamond burr even till the edge of the pyriform aperture to achieve proper exposure.

Through this fenestration using straight or angled endoscopes, pathologies inside the maxillary sinus are visualized, instruments like straight and upturned Blakesley forceps and a powered microdebrider, the pathology can be cleared. At the end of the procedure, the flap was repositioned and the incision sutured.

Depending on anatomical conditions and location of the tumour attachment, this procedure can be combined with middle meatal antrostomy, which can be used for sinus inspection and/or easy instrumentation.

**Complication**

Injury to Hasner's valve.

**Limitation**

The anterior wall of the maxillary sinus is a blind spot in this approach [17].

## 28.7 Endoscopic Denker's

This is a novel approach which provides a direct access to the anterior, inferior and lateral recesses of the maxillary sinus. Furthermore, the entire posterior wall of the maxillary sinus can be made exposed, thus affording access to both pterygopalatine and infratemporal fossae.

Avoidance of sublabial or transseptal incisions, as well as the requirement for highly angled endoscopes and instrumentation, is also possible [18]. It provides a straight trajectory, which facilitates four-handed surgery.

**Indications**

Benign and malignant conditions of maxillary sinus, infratemporal fossa, pterygopalatine fossa.

**Key Steps**

This procedure involves first mucosal incision placed inferiorly at the junction of the nasal floor and lateral nasal wall, and a second mucosal incision is then made superiorly along the lateral nasal wall and which is carried antero-inferiorly to lie in front of the anterior end of the inferior turbinate overlying the edge of the pyriform aperture.

Subperiosteal dissection is done to expose the lateral and the anterior aspect of the maxilla, the infraorbital foramen, with its contents. A bony window is drilled into the anterior wall of the maxillary sinus, cautiously staying inferior to the infraorbital nerve.

This procedure is usually combined with middle meatal antrostomy, thereby allowing access to the anteroinferior corner of the maxillary sinus through which pathology can be removed.

**Complication**

- Damage to the infraorbital nerve (ION) and anterior superior alveolar nerve (ASAN) during creation of the antral window.

- Alar collapse secondary to loss of the pyriform ridge [19]
- Check pain and swelling [20]
- Nasolacrimal duct stenosis

## 28.8 Endoscopic Reverse Denkers

This procedure provides a proper exposure, visualization and clearance of the pathology involving the anterolateral and anterior wall of the maxillary sinus. Since less bone is removed, olfaction is preserved and crusting is less with no atrophic nasal changes. It also prevents alar collapse by preserving the pyriform aperture with faster healing and less morbidity [21].

**Indications**

- Clearance of benign and malignant conditions and invasive fungal infections like mucormycosis of maxillary sinus present in the antrolateral and anterior wall of the maxillary sinus.
- Infratemporal fossa pathologies

**Key Steps [21]**
The sequence of steps involves performing inferior turbinectomy, uncinectomy and followed by a mega middle meatal antrostomy. Drilling begins from the anterior edge of the middle meatal antrostomy, extending towards the pyriform aperture anteriorly until the anterior wall of the maxilla is visualized and the nasolacrimal duct becomes visible for transection. This method preserves the pyriform aperture and anterior wall. An angled endoscope helps in proper exposure, visualization and clearance of the pathology (Fig. 28.7).

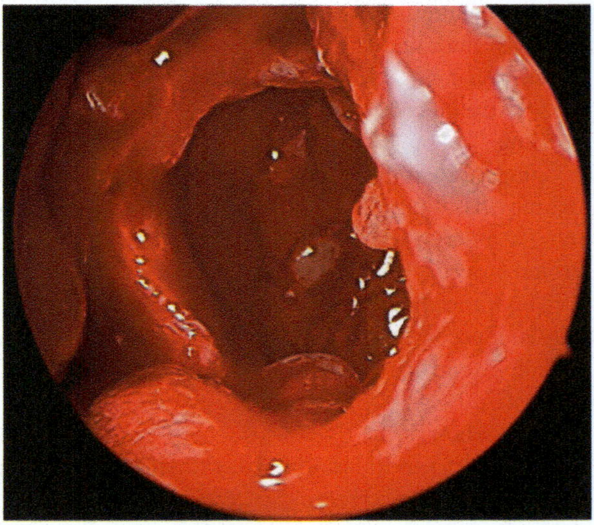

**Fig. 28.7** Endoscopic reverse Denker's approach

**Complication**
Crusting, epiphora, epistaxis [21].

**Limitation**
This approach may be challenging in certain anatomical variations of the maxillary sinus [21].

## 28.9 Pyriform Turbinoplasty and Lateral Nasal Wall Lateralization

Simmen and Jones described pyriform turbinoplasty (PT) as an option for the management of inferior turbinate hypertrophy [22].

PT with lateral nasal wall lateralization (LNWL) along with an extended maxillary sinusotomy can be done without damaging the lacrimal duct by removing the bone in this area which allows the visualization of maxillary sinus and management of pathologies with a zero-degree endoscope [23].

**Indications**
This procedure provides a way of entering the maxilla at the level of inferior turbinate (IT) as a start of a medial maxillectomy.

**Key Steps [22, 23]**
Pyriform turbinoplasty involves a horizontal incision which is performed at the base of the inferior turbinate where its "shoulder" is situated at the level of maxillary ostium to the pyriform aperture. A flap is elevated from below, extending upward to expose the attachment of the bone of the inferior turbinate onto the lateral nasal wall. A gentle osteotomy is done to remove the bone which overlies the lacrimal duct by placing the osteotome at the inferior portion of the "shoulder" of the inferior turbinate and the bone removed avoiding injury to the lacrimal duct.

After pyriform turbinoplasty, the lacrimal duct can be identified. Dissection is done to expose the attachment of the lacrimal bone to the maxilla. The exposed bone posterior, lateral and inferior to lacrimal duct is removed by osteotomy. This bone comprises the junction of the lacrimal bone and uncinate process, lying just behind the lacrimal duct, the base of the IT and the portion of the maxilla that lies at the pyriform aperture. After this procedure, the entire inferior turbinate can be lateralized, the level of middle meatal antrostomy is reduced below the middle turbinate, mobilizing mucosa of maxillary sinus ostium with an ant and post-cutting to design a flap from maxillary sinus that will overlap the inferior turbinate; after this procedure, the middle turbinate will not close the middle meatal antrostomy; and with a straight instrument, we can reach maxillary sinus without any need for angled instruments and scope.

**Complications**
1. Bleeding from the lacrimal artery,
2. Numbness, given that the area is innervated by the anterior superior alveolar nerve,
3. Crusting and epiphora if the resection compromises the tear sac [24].

## 28.10 Sturman-Canfield Procedure

The extended endoscopic maxillectomy, also known as the Sturman-Canfield procedure, provides complete visualization of the maxillary sinus by excision of the medial portion of the anterior maxillary wall and transection of the lacrimal duct [26].

**Indications**
Sturman-Canfield operation for benign tumours like inverted papilloma involving the mucosa of the alveolar recess or of the anterolateral corner of the maxillary sinus [26].

**Complications and Limitations**
Mucocele formation, lacrimal pathway obstruction, paraesthesia and hypoesthesia in malar region [25].

## 28.11 PliENT [27]

PliENT is a recent innovation which is a slender and a steerable endoscope. This endoscope can be used for maxillary sinus surgeries through a classical medial antrostomy. Due to its small size and the flexibility, removal of additional functional structures like the nasolacrimal duct or the inferior turbinate is avoided. Moreover, its flexibility allows a wide range of angles of view without necessitating the removal of the endoscope from the operative field.

## References

1. Prideaux de C. A Note on Nathaniel Highmore, M.D. [1613–1685], and his Memorial Tablet in Purse Caundle Church, Dorset. Proc R Soc Med. 1914;7(Sect Hist Med):106–8. PMID: 19978163; PMCID: PMC2003558.
2. Lorkiewicz-Muszyńska D, Kociemba W, Rewekant A, Sroka A, Jończyk-Potoczna K, Patelska-Banaszewska M, Przystańska A. Development of the maxillary sinus from birth to age 18. Postnatal growth pattern. Int J Pediatr Otorhinolaryngol. 2015;79(9):1393–400. https://doi.org/10.1016/j.ijporl.2015.05.032. Epub 2015 Jun 30.
3. Cho SH, Kim TH, Kim KR, Lee JM, Lee DK, Kim JH, Im JJ, Park CJ, Hwang KG. Factors for maxillary sinus volume and craniofacial anatomical features in adults with chronic rhinosinusitis. Arch Otolaryngol Head Neck Surg. 2010;136(6):610–5. https://doi.org/10.1001/archoto.2010.75.
4. Gosau M, Rink D, Driemel O, Draenert FG. Maxillary sinus anatomy: a cadaveric study with clinical implications. Anat Rec (Hoboken). 2009;292:352–4.
5. Harvey RJ, Sheehan PO, Debnath NI, Schlosser RJ. Transseptal approach for extended endoscopic resections of the maxilla and infratemporal fossa. Am J Rhinol Allergy. 2009;23(4):426–32. https://doi.org/10.2500/ajra.2009.23.3333.
6. Philpott C, Sama A. Endonasal approaches to maxillary sinus. Int J Head Neck Surg. 2018;9(1):26–31.

7. Simmen D, Jones N. Manual of endoscopic sinus surgery and its extended applications, How? Operative procedures: a step -by- step safe and logical approach. Thieme; 2005.
8. Kennedy DW, Adappa ND. Endoscopic maxillary antrostomy: not just a simple procedure. Laryngoscope. 2011;121(10):2142–5.
9. Kirihene RK, Rees G, Wormald PJ. The influence of the size of the maxillary sinus ostium on the nasal and sinus nitric oxide levels. Am J Rhinol. 2002;16(5):261–4.
10. Robey A, O'Brien EK, Leopold DA. Assessing current technical limitations in the small-hole endoscopic approach to the maxillary sinus. Am J Rhinol Allergy. 2010;24:396–401.
11. Nakayama T, Asaka D, Okushi T, Yoshikawa M, Moriyama H, Otori N. Endoscopic medial maxillectomy with preservation of inferior turbinate and nasolacrimal duct. Am J Rhinol Allergy. 2012;26(05):405–8.
12. Weber RK, Werner JA, Hildebrand T. Endonasal endoscopic medial maxillectomy with preservation of the inferior turbinate. Am J Rhinol Allergy. 2010;24:132–5.
13. Gras-Cabrerizo JR, Massegur-Solench H, Pujol-Olmo A, MontserratGili JR, Adema-Alcover JM, Zarraonandia-Andraca I. Endoscopic medial maxillectomy with preservation of inferior turbinate. How do we do it? Eur Arch Otorrinolaringol. 2011;268:389–92.
14. Hosemann W, Scotti O, Bentzien S. Evaluation of telescopes and forceps for endoscopic transnasal surgery on the maxillary sinus. Am J Rhinol. 2003;17:311–6.
15. Chen Y, Zhang H, Ge P, Wei T, Luo X, Huang P. Combined middle meatus and expand prelacrimal recess-maxillary sinus approach for endoscopic maxillary sinus surgery. Chin Mid J. 2012;26:1070–2.
16. Kamel SB, Gad HA, Abdelazeem HM, Mohammed GA, Elnem S. Prelacrimal versus canine fossa approach for anterior maxillary sinus lesions. Pan Arab J Rhinol. 2020;10:118–26.
17. Zhao Y, Cheng J, Yang J, Li P, Zhang Z, Wang Z. Modified endoscopic inferior meatal fenestration with mucosal flap for maxillary sinus diseases. Videosurg Other Miniinv Tech. 2018;13(4):533–8. https://doi.org/10.5114/wiitm.2018.77556.
18. Lee JT, Suh JD, Carrau RL, Chu MW, Chiu AG. Endoscopic Denker's approach for resection of lesions involving the anteroinferior maxillary sinus and infratemporal fossa. Laryngoscope. 2017;127(3):556–60.
19. Prosser JD, Figueroa R, Carrau RI, et al. Quantitative analysis of endoscopic endonasal approaches to the infratemporal fossa. Laryngoscope. 2011;121:1601–5.
20. Upadhyay S, Dolci RLL, Buohliqah L, et al. Endoscopic endonasal anterior maxillotomy. Laryngoscope. 2015;125:2668–271.
21. Ahilasamy N, Narendrakumar V, Kumar RD, et al. How I do it:- endoscopic reverse Denker's approach. Indian J Otolaryngol Head Neck Surg. 2023;75(Suppl 1):781–4. https://doi.org/10.1007/s12070-022-03330-8.
22. Simmen D, Jones N. Manual of endoscopic sinus and skull base surgery. Stuttgart: Georg Thieme Verlag; 2014. https://doi.org/10.1308/rcsann.2014.96.3.252a.
23. De Sousa Machado A, Briner HR, Simmen D. Pyriform turbinoplasty and lateral nasal wall lateralization: practical hints on how we do it. Cureus. 2022;14(12):e32584. https://doi.org/10.7759/cureus.32584.
24. Simmen D, Veerasigamani N, Briner HR, Jones N, Schuknecht B. Anterior maxillary wall and lacrimal duct relationship - CT analysis for prelacrimal access to the maxillary sinus. Rhinology. 2017;55:170–4. https://doi.org/10.4193/Rhino16.318.
25. Bertazzoni G, Accorona R, Schreiber A, Pietrobon G, Karligkiotis A, Fazio E, Castelnuovo P, Nicolai P. Postoperative long-term morbidity of extended endoscopic maxillectomy for inverted papilloma. Rhinology. 2017;55(4):319–25. https://doi.org/10.4193/Rhin17.035.
26. Tomenzoli D, Castelnuovo P, Pagella F, Berlucchi M, Pianta L, Delù G, Maroldi R, Nicolai P. Different endoscopic surgical strategies in the management of inverted papilloma of the sinonasal tract: experience with 47 patients. Laryngoscope. 2004;114:193–200. https://doi.org/10.1097/00005537-200402000-00003.
27. Legrand J, Ourak M, Van Gerven L, Vander Poorten V, Vander PE. A miniature robotic steerable endoscope for maxillary sinus surgery called PliENT. Sci Rep. 2022;12(1):2299. https://doi.org/10.1038/s41598-022-05969-3. PMID: 35145155; PMCID: PMC8831515.

# Endoscopic Surgery of the Frontal Sinus

# 29

Magdy Eisa Saafan and Mohamed Ossama Tamom

**Key Points**

- A graduated approach for endoscopic surgical management of frontal sinus diseases is advocated. This approach is individualized to the particular patient and the extent of the disease present.
- Factors to be considered include the patient's history, nasal endoscopy, and CT scan findings.
- The extent of surgery performed is based on the tenet, "Do as little as possible, but as much as necessary."
- Inflammatory frontal sinusitis can be considered a spectrum of disease; minimal disease requires minimal surgery, severe disease requires advanced surgery, and absence of disease requires that no surgery be performed.
- The integrated approach to endoscopic frontal sinus surgery includes the following: endoscopic frontal sinuplasty, endoscopic frontal sinusotomy, modified intranasal endoscopic Lothrop, endoscopic trans-septal frontal sinusotomy, and above-and-below approaches (trephine and endoscopic, osteoplastic flap and endoscopic).

## 29.1 Frontal Sinus Development

The frontal sinus begins to develop during the fourth fetal month, after the development of the frontal recess. Initially, this recess is a pocket found medial to the very cephalic or superior aspect of the uncinate process and

**Supplementary Information** The online version contains supplementary material available at https://doi.org/10.1007/978-3-031-70077-4_29.

M. E. Saafan (✉) · M. O. Tamom
Department of Otolaryngology, Tanta University, Tanta, Egypt
e-mail: magdy.saafan@med.tanta.edu.eg


S. Elwany (ed.), *Current Rhinology*,
https://doi.org/10.1007/978-3-031-70077-4_29

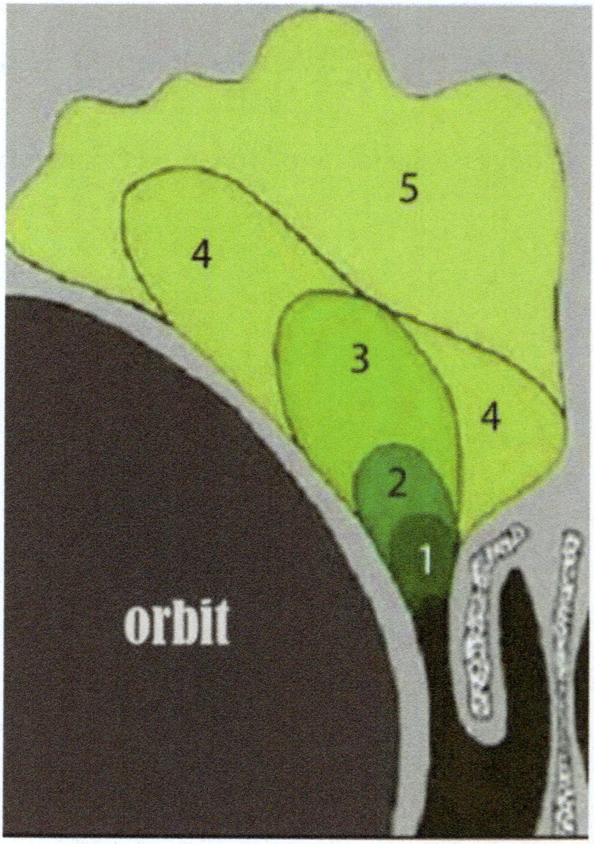


**Fig. 29.1** Coronal view of the right frontal sinus noting its progressive secondary pneumatization, (1) 4 years of age. (2) 4–8 years of age. (3) age of 8 years. (4) early adolescence, (5) 18 years of age

expands into the thick nasal capsule mesenchyme. The fetal frontal recess is found between the uncinate process and the anterior attachment of the middle turbinate [1].

Secondary pneumatization occurs postnatally. Initially, the secondary pneumatization occurs laterally toward the orbital side of the frontal bone, but during the second year of life, pneumatization has a more vertical direction. However, by definition, a frontal sinus is not present until the cell enters the vertical (ascending) portion of the frontal bone. During its development, the superior extremity of the frontal sinus reaches the mid-vertical height of the orbit at 4 years of age and the level of the superior orbital rim at 8 years. It grows into the frontal squama at 10 years of age. The frontal sinus continues its growth at a slow rate into adolescence, when it may reach its final size. The expansion into the vertical frontal bone occurs closer to the cranial cavity, and consequently, the external table of the frontal bone is thicker than the inner table. The left and the right frontal sinuses develop independently, and asymmetry between the frontal sinus is more the rule than the exception (Fig. 29.1) [1].

## 29.2 Anatomy of the Frontal Sinus

The frontal sinus is contained within the frontal bone. The frontal bone makes a major contribution to the floor of the anterior cranial fossa and, in doing so, forms the roof of the orbits. The frontal bone articulates with the ethmoid, sphenoid, parietal, and nasal bones, as well as with the zygoma and the maxilla [2].

The frontal sinus is a triangular, pyramid-shaped cavity extending between the anterior and posterior tables of the ascending portion of the frontal bone. The apex of the pyramid is superior, and the base lies inferiorly [1].

There are two frontal sinuses separated by a bony septum. Bilateral asymmetry is a frequent anatomical finding. Each sinus is further divided into incomplete chambers by a bony intrasinus septation, which creates deep recesses of the sinus. Thus, the interior surface of the frontal sinus is often irregular because of the bony projections from the different walls [2].

The anterior wall of the sinus forms the forehead and is by far the thickest of all sinus walls, measuring up to 12 mm [1]. The posterior wall is a plate of thin, compact bone (1–2 mm) whose upper part is vertical. It gradually curves downward and posteriorly until it is almost horizontal. The posterior wall of the frontal sinus is also the anterior wall of the anterior cranial fossa. The thin posterior wall of the frontal sinus is attached to the dura of the anterior cranial fossa. The medial wall of the frontal sinus is represented by the intersinus septum. The inferior wall of the frontal sinus is formed by the orbital roofs on the lateral side and the nasoethmoid floor on the medial side. The most anterior area of the sinus floor is directly above the roof of the nose. It consists of a very thick bony mass of the nasal spinous process of the frontal bone, or internal nasal spine (spina nasalis interna).

At the frontal sinus, floor close to the anteromedial aspect of the intersinus septum rests the frontal sinus ostium. The frontal sinus ostium marks the site where pneumatization of the sinus began. The frontal sinus drainage pathway has an hourglass shape composed of three distinct segments: The top part of the hourglass is the frontal infundibulum, which is the inferior portion of the frontal sinus cavity narrowing like an upright funnel toward the second segment, the frontal ostium (Fig. 29.2). The third segment is the inferior air chamber named the frontal recess. This functional unit for frontal sinus drainage has been referred to as the frontal sinus outflow tract [2].

**N.B.** Sinus lateralis: Refers to both the suprabullar (green shadow) and retrobullar recesses (yellow shadow).

**Frontal Recess**

The frontal recess is the most anterosuperior aspect of the anterior ethmoid sinus that forms the connection with the frontal sinus. The boundaries of the frontal recess are the lamina papyracea laterally, the middle turbinate medially, the posterosuperior wall of the agger nasi cell (when present) anteriorly, and the anterior wall of the ethmoid bulla posteriorly. If the anterior wall of the ethmoid bulla does not reach the

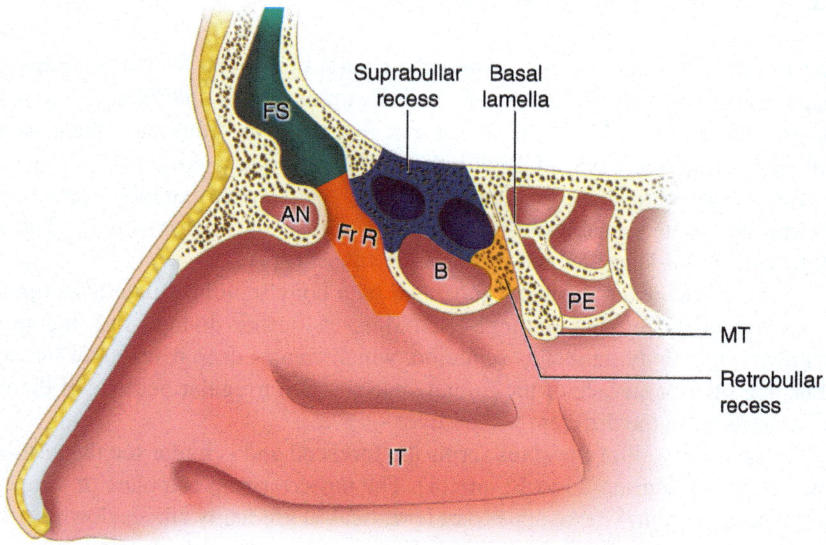


**Fig. 29.2** A diagram demonstrating the frontal recess (Fr R) bounded posteriorly by anterior face of the bulla ethmoidalis (B) and suprabullar recess and bounded anteriorly by the posterior surface of agger nasi cell (AN). FS: frontal sinus, MT: middle turbinate,

skull base and form a complete posterior wall, the frontal recess may communicate with the suprabullar recess. The frontal recess tapers as it approaches the superiorly located internal os of the frontal sinus; above the os, it again widens, as the anterior and posterior tables diverge to their respective positions [2].

**Nasal Process of the Frontal Bone (Spina Nasalis Interna)**
During frontal sinusotomy (Draf type I-II procedure, nasofrontal approach type II), an individual dense bone is encountered anteriorly and (mostly) medially that limits the enlargement of the natural frontal ostium by means of a slender sharp spoon. This piece of bone has been called spina nasalis interna by Halle [3], and spina nasalis (anterior) ossis frontalis by Lang [4] (Fig. 29.3). The spina nasalis interna may be defined in clinical terms as a medially and anteriorly situated significant thickening of the frontal sinus floor resistant to ablation with a sharp spoon [5]. The anterior-posterior diameter of the basal anterior wall of the frontal sinus averaged 3.5 mm (2.0–6.0 mm), while that of the spina was 6.1 mm (0–11 mm) on an average.

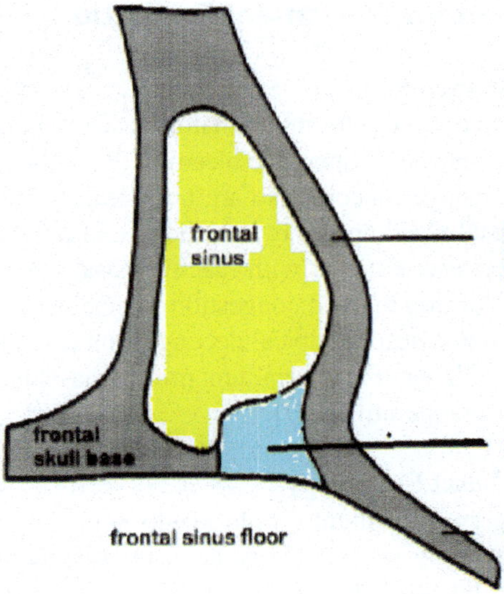


**Fig. 29.3** Scheme of left-sided anatomic specimen showing major spina nasalis interna

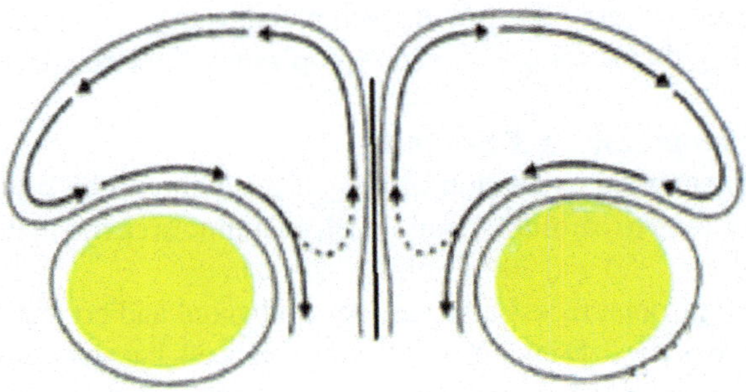

**Fig. 29.4** Frontal sinus mucociliary flow and clearance pattern

## 29.3 Physiological Considerations of Frontal Sinus

Frontal sinus ciliary beat pattern and therefore mucus flow are up the interfrontal sinus septum, lateral across the frontal sinus roof, and then medial over the frontal sinus floor to the ostium (Fig. 29.4).

Mucus clearance out of the sinus is active by ciliary action down the lateral aspect of the frontal recess, whether it is directly down the medial orbital wall, or over the medial or posterior aspect of a frontal recess cell, such as an agger nasi cell. If this mucus membrane is damaged or removed, the sinus may not function properly after healing. As Moriyama [6] demonstrated in 1996, pseudostratified ciliated columnar epithelium does not regenerate well after being stripped off of bone. Only 40% to 60% of the frontal sinus mucus is swept out of the frontal sinus on any given circuit of the mucus around the interior of the frontal sinus. The other 60% to 40% recirculates around the sinus (Fig. 29.4).

## 29.4 Preoperative Patient Evaluation

**Medical Treatment**

Prior to elective surgery for inflammatory disease, infection should be minimized, if possible, to reduce intraoperative bleeding. Patients with severe polyposis or markedly hyper-reactive mucosa also are best treated with a course of oral steroids to reduce mucosal bleeding and reduce the size of polypi, unless there is a contraindication to their use. Patients with reactive nasal mucosa can be identified by their tendency to develop marked congestion, sneezing, and hypersecretion during diagnostic endoscopy, despite topical decongestion and anesthesia. If untreated, a similar tendency will result in intermittent profuse nasal bleeding in response to mucosal stimulation intraoperatively [7].

**Diagnostic Nasal Endoscopy**

Prior to surgery, the patient should ideally undergo diagnostic nasal endoscopy to review the anatomy and pathology, to ensure that there has been no acute exacerbation, and, if indicated, to take cultures to guide intraoperative and postoperative antibiotic therapy. During the preoperative endoscopy, access to the ethmoid cavity is re-evaluated. If the 4 mm 0° endoscope cannot be introduced to the anterior attachment of the middle turbinate because of septal deviation, then it will be evident that at least a limited septoplasty will be required at the time of surgery [7].

**Preoperative CT Scanning**

Presurgical evaluation of the CT scan should be performed in a routine checklist fashion to carefully review each anatomic area for anatomic variations [7] Table 29.1 (Figs. 29.5 and 29.6).

The frontal recess also requires both axial and coronal views to achieve understanding of the 3-D anatomy of the area. Indeed, because of the complexity of the anatomy in this area, the sagittal reconstruction provided by intraoperative surgical navigation is frequently invaluable in providing a complete understanding of the anatomic relationships, particularly concerning the anteroposterior diameter of the frontal sinus, as well as the relationship to adjacent agger nasi and supraorbital ethmoid cells [7].

**Table 29.1** Preoperative CT evaluation

| Site | Evaluation |
|---|---|
| Skull base | Slope, height, erosions, areas of relative thickening and thinning |
| Medial orbital wall | Integrity, erosion, shape, infundibular size, and uncinate position |
| Ethmoid vessels | Position of anterior and posterior ethmoid vessels relative to skull base |
| Posterior ethmoid | Vertical height |
| Frontal recess and Frontal sinus | Frontal sinus pneumatization, frontal recess size, agger nasi and supraorbital ethmoid pneumatization, frontal sinus drainage |

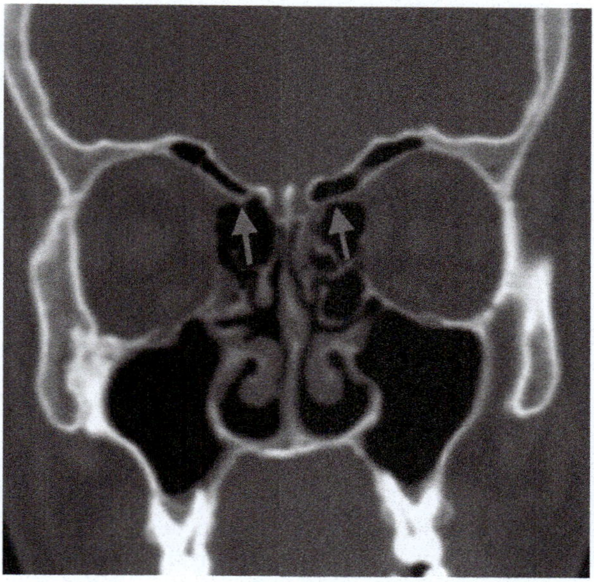

**Fig. 29.5** CT scan demonstrating the site of the anterior ethmoidal artery (arrows). The vessel can usually be identified by a "nipple" pointing medially from the medial orbital wall

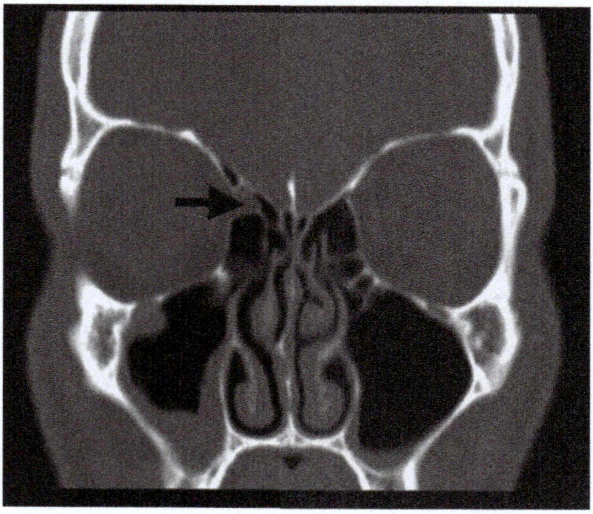

**Fig. 29.6** CT showing lamina papyracea dehiscence with orbital fat protrusion (arrow)

## 29.5 Indications of Endoscopic Frontal Sinus Surgery: [8]

A) Absolute indications:
1. Acute or chronic frontal sinusitis with complications.
2. Frontal sinus mucocele.
3. Invasive or allergic fungal rhinosinusitis affects the frontal sinus.
4. Circumscribed benign frontal sinus tumors.
5. Frontal sinus C.S.F leaks.

B) Relative indications:
Chronic or recurrent frontal sinusitis after adequate and appropriate medical treatment.

**Contraindications of Endoscopic Frontal Sinus Surgery: [9]**

1. Frontal sinus lesions are located in the extreme lateral portion of the frontal sinus (relative contraindication depending upon the available instrumentation and experience of the surgeon).
2. If there is evidence of osteitis or osteomyelitis of the frontal bone with sequestration.

## 29.6 The Endoscopic Frontal Sinus Surgery Approaches

A graduated approach for endoscopic surgical management of frontal sinus diseases is advocated [10]. This approach is individualized to the particular patient and the extent of the disease present. Factors to be considered include the patient's history, nasal endoscopy, and CT scan findings. The extent of surgery performed is based on the tenet, "Do as little as possible, but as much as necessary." Inflammatory frontal sinusitis can be considered a spectrum of disease; minimal disease requires minimal surgery, severe disease requires advanced surgery, and absence of disease requires that no surgery be performed.

**The integrated approach to endoscopic frontal sinus surgery: [11]**

I) Endoscopic frontal sinuplasty
II) Endoscopic frontal sinusotomy
III) Modified intranasal endoscopic Lothrop
IV) Endoscopic trans-septal frontal sinusotomy
V) Frontal sinus rescue procedure
VI) Above-and-below approach (trephine and endoscopic)
VII) Above-and-below approach (osteoplastic flap and endoscopic)

### 29.6.1 Endoscopic Frontal Sinuplasty

**Introduction**

The balloon catheter system has recently been introduced as a potentially minimally invasive, ambulatory strategy for the treatment of chronic rhinosinusitis (CRS). What this system accomplishes specifically for CRS is the dilatation of the sinus ostia by advancing balloon catheters under fluoroscopic guidance to the narrowed segment, and inflating them with high pressure [12].

**Indications: [12]**

1. In patients with a history of chronic or recurrent rhinosinusitis
2. Access to the sinuses and direct cultures by sinus irrigation can be performed with sinuplasty.

3. The frontal ostia can be dilated so that fluoroscopic-guided biopsies of sinus neoplasms are also possible.

**Contraindications**

- History of previous sinus surgery.
- Diagnosed sinonasal polyps, mucopyocele or pyocele, allergic fungal rhinosinusitis, sinonasal osteoneogenesis, sinonasal tumors, or obstructive lesions.
- History of facial trauma that distorts sinus anatomy (relative contraindication)
- Severe rhinosinusitis with Lund–McKay scores above 10 (relative contraindication).

**Instruments**

Standard endoscopic sinus instruments (including 0°, 30°, and 45° endoscopes) are used in the procedure. Additionally, balloon dilatation requires sinus guiding catheters, flexible sinus guide wires, sinus balloon catheters, sinus lavage catheters, and a sinus balloon inflation device with a manometer [12].

The inflation device consists of a high-pressure syringe barrel with a piston handle and a gauge used to monitor the pressure inside the balloon at the tip of the catheter. The solution used for injection into the balloon consists of iodine contrast medium, diluted in sterile saline or water at a concentration of approximately 150–180 mg/ml. Contrast medium is used so that the balloon can be visualized fluoroscopically as it is inflated. The standard balloon size is 5 ml, although there are 7 ml and 3 ml balloons, depending on the size of the target sinus ostium and the surgeon's judgment. The maximum pressure recommended by the manufacturer is 16 atm, although usually pressures of 10–12 atm are used with satisfactory results (Fig. 29.7) [12].

The C-arm is positioned at the head of the table, in order to provide fluoroscopic guidance when cannulating the involved sinuses and performing balloon catheter insertion and inflation at the sinus ostia. Unlike FESS, which is usually performed on all involved sinuses on one side, followed by the involved sinuses on the contralateral side, endoscopic sinuplasty is best performed on each set of involved sinuses bilaterally (when indicated), in order to minimize the need to reposition the C-arm [12].

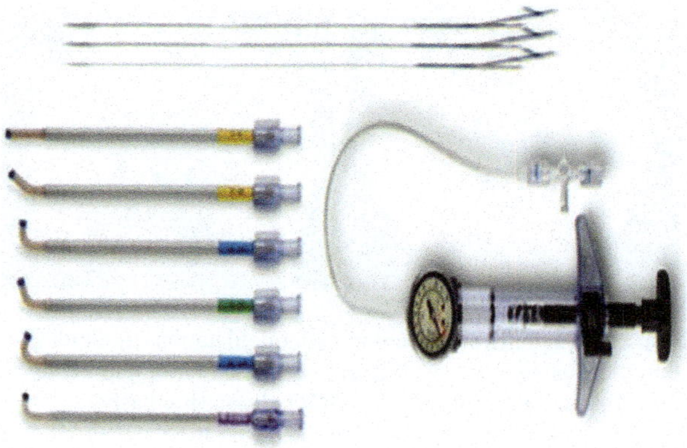

**Fig. 29.7** Balloon sinuplasty equipment: sinus guiding catheters, sinus balloon catheters, inflation device, consisting of a high-pressure piston syringe and a manometer

**Surgical Technique (Fig. 29.8)**

The procedure, like FESS, can be performed under general anesthesia, or with local anesthesia with sedation. Since the procedure is very short, local anesthesia is more commonly used than it is with FESS [12].

To limit radiation exposure during fluoroscopy, it is better to place a lead apron over the patient's chest and place a protective collar around the patient neck. A mobile fluoroscopy unit with a C-arm is placed to the left of the patient neck. The fluoroscopy monitor and a standard endoscopic tower are placed at the head of the bed. All personnel in the theater wore appropriate lead aprons [13].

Under endoscopic visualization, a guiding catheter is placed in the region of sinus ostia. A guidewire then is introduced through guiding catheter. Under fluoroscopic guidance, the guidewire is advanced through the sinus ostia into the sinus. If any resistance is met, gentle manipulation of the guiding catheter and guidewire is performed until the guidewire successfully cannulated the sinus. The guidewire is then further advanced into the sinus in such a way that it curled upon itself and formed a loop within the sinus.

Then, an uninflated balloon catheter is threaded over the guidewire and through the guiding catheter. Under fluoroscopy, the uninflated balloon is advanced into position until it straddled the sinus ostium. The balloon is then inflated with a contrast medium to a maximum of 16 atmospheric pressure. A pressure gauge attached to the end of the balloon catheter recorded the incremental rise in balloon pressure. The balloon was then deflated and removed. The dilated sinus ostial region is examined with sinonasal endoscopy.

The final ostial size with balloon catheter ostial dilation is another important consideration to discuss. As expected, dilated ostia appeared to be slightly smaller than the maximal balloon diameter used. It is important to note that the optimal ostial size to achieve with surgery has never been scientifically established. Although balloon catheter ostial dilation achieves a smaller final ostial size than that achieved with FESS, the reduced mucosal trauma and improved mucosal preservation may prove advantageous.

Since the frontal outflow tract is not a true "ostium," two overlapping dilatations should be performed to ensure that the entire outflow tract is dilated. A confirmatory fluoroscopic image of the deflated balloon is obtained before pulling the balloon

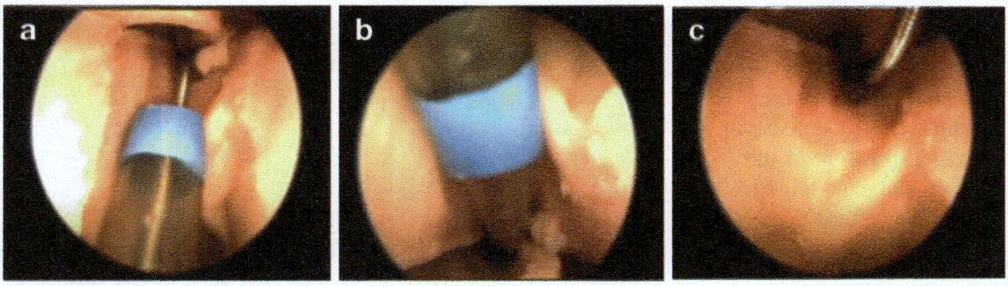


**Fig. 29.8** Frontal sinus ostium balloon dilatation (**a**) Guiding catheter in position, wire advanced into the frontal sinus. (**b**) Inflated sinuplasty balloon in the frontal recess. (**c**) Dilated frontal sinus drainage pathway immediately after balloon sinuplasty

catheter out through the guiding catheter. The dilated ostium is visualized again with an endoscope, to confirm adequate dilatation of the ostium, and to assess the sinus interior.

**Morbidity and Complications**

Sinuplasty morbidity and complications are the same as with FESS; however, owing to the less invasive nature of the procedure, they are likely to be less common. Vascular or nerve injuries, the inability to identify the natural ostium, and inadvertent injury to the orbit or brain are all possible [12].

**Outcomes**

The procedure is relatively new. As the number of patients treated with sinuplasty increases, the number of complications may increase as well, until a learning curve is established. Increasing experience and proper patient selection will likely keep complications at a minimum so that outcomes are not compromised by technical difficulties [12].

**Cost**

The cost of the balloon system (approximately $1200) and the use of the C-arm (approximately $500) must be included [12].

### 29.6.2 Endoscopic Frontal Sinusotomy

After performing a standard uncinectomy with maxillary antrostomy, anterior ethmoidectomy, and posterior ethmoidectomy (if indicated), the skull base is identified following the skull base from posterior to anterior, its upward change of direction forming the posterior wall of frontal recess that can be recognized just anterior to the anterior ethmoidal artery [14].

Loury [15] advocated preserving the bulla lamella before performing frontal sinusotomy to avoid injury of the anterior ethmoidal artery. However, the technique has been criticized as the supraorbital ethmoidal cell can be overlooked during surgery; also, removal of the bulla lamella firstly widens the frontal recess making instrumentation within this area easier [16].

The angled curettes are passed up the posterior frontal recess wall behind the cells, such as agger nasi cells or frontal cells (Fig. 29.9). The cell walls are fractured forward and inferiorly. The bony fragments can then be removed with through-cutting punches if attached to the mucosa or with giraffe's forceps if free of bony attachments. If bone fragments are pushed into the frontal sinus, the different frontal ostium seekers facilitate easy removal. This process is repeated until the internal frontal ostium is visualized. Forward movement is the safest because there are no vital structures anteriorly, only the dense anterior buttress bone. The instruments should not be used in an anterior-to-posterior direction or lateral to medial, because of the risk of skull base penetration or injury to the thin lateral cribriform plate lamella. Both of these bony walls are thin and highly prone to fracture with subsequent CSF leaks [14].

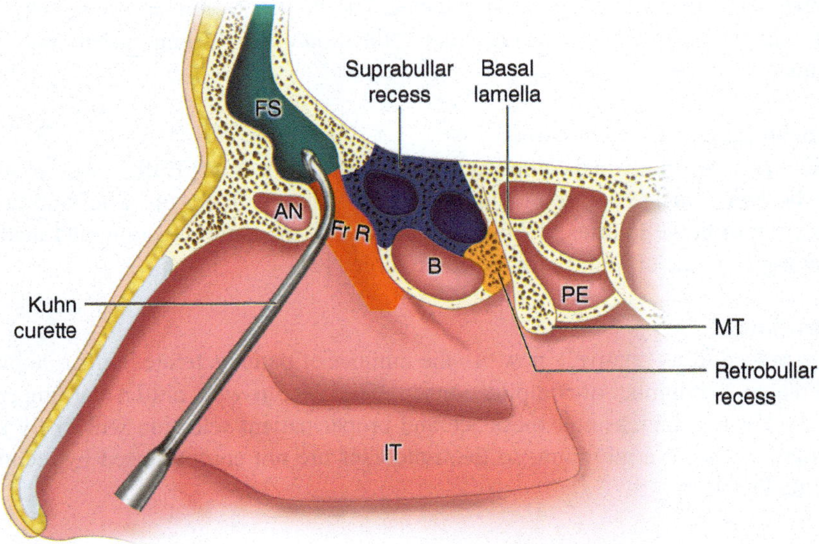


**Fig. 29.9** Frontal sinus ostium balloon dilatation (**a**) Guiding catheter in position, wire advanced into the frontal sinus. (**b**) Inflated sinuplasty balloon in the frontal recess. (**c**) Dilated frontal sinus drainage pathway immediately after balloon sinuplasty

***Uncapping the Egg***

The ethmoidal bulla, uncinate process, and agger nasi (or other cells of the anterior ethmoid, for instance, so-called infundibular cells) may expand into the frontal recess thus with their cranial cap of bone may fill the frontal recess; thus, the access to the frontal sinus is blocked by a paper-thin cap of bone with its two mucosal layers. The technical challenge is to identify carefully and remove this cap of bone. Simple but delicate instruments are required as curved curettes, giraffe forceps, and upturned circular cutting punches (Fig. 29.10) [17].

In the sagittal section, the transition from frontal sinus down to frontal recess has an hourglass shape, and one might as well say: The shape of an egg holder. The waist corresponds to the level of frontal sinus ostium. If one now puts a breakfast-egg into the egg holder, opens and empties it, the lower portion of the "cap of the egg" remains in the egg holder. If this now is turned upside down, the situation is now analogous to the frontal recess: The superior "empty" part of the egg holder represents the frontal sinus infundibulum; and the inferior part of the egg holder with the cap of the egg represents the frontal recess (Fig. 29.11). The task now is to remove the eggshell (Fig. 29.12) sitting tightly in the frontal recess. The parietal mucosa should remain intact, and areas of denuded bone must be minimized [17].

**Extension of Endoscopic Frontal Sinusotomy "Draf Procedures"**

The least extensive of the Draf procedures, the Draf I, opens the frontal recess within the defined boundaries by removing the ethmoid bulla and any other ethmoidal cells directly obstructing the outflow tract. The Draf IIa expands the frontal

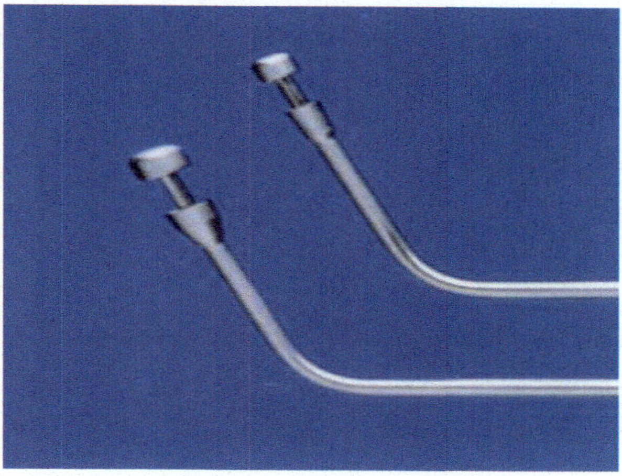

**Fig. 29.10** Upturned circular cutting punches

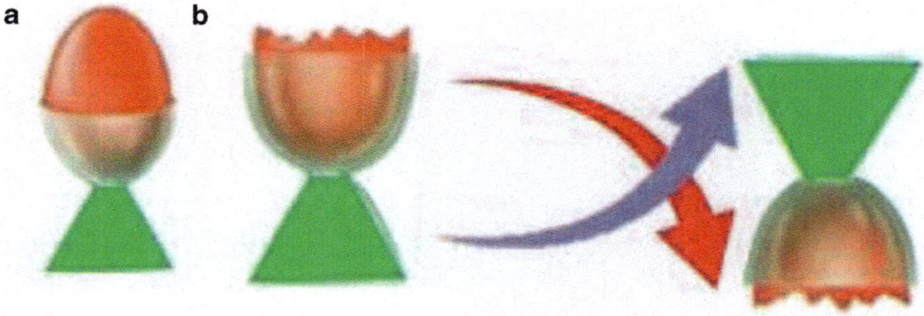


**Fig. 29.11** Uncapping of the egg. (**a**) "The egg" in an egg holder. (**b**) The egg is uncapped, the contents removed, and the egg holder turned upside down

recess by removing the agger nasi cell and ethmoid bulla completely as well as removing any partitions lateral to the edge of the middle turbinate. The Draf IIb extends the recess medially to the nasal and intersinus septum, often by using a drill or other frontal sinus instruments. The Draf III is the most extensive and involves bilateral Draf IIb procedures combined with a superior septectomy and removal of the intersinus septation to create a common frontal sinus cavity. The Draf III "endoscopic-modified Lothrop procedure" limits of resection are the external periosteum of the frontal process of the maxilla anteriorly, the lamina papyracea of the orbit laterally, and the first olfactory fibers posteriorly (Fig. 29.13) [18].

## Identification of Frontal Sinus

1. Trans-illumination of the frontal sinus which is a reliable indicator in differentiating it from neighboring cells [19].
2. Frontal sinus can also be identified by the presence of convexity and lobulation of its posterior wall [20].

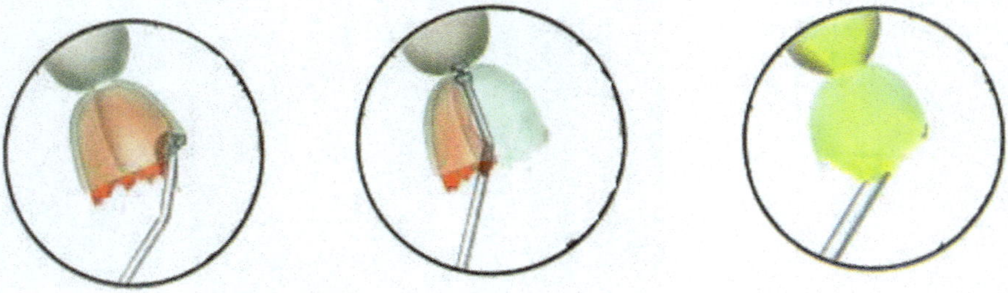

**Fig. 29.12** Challenge to remove the remaining "cap of the egg" from frontal recess to reach the frontal sinus ostium

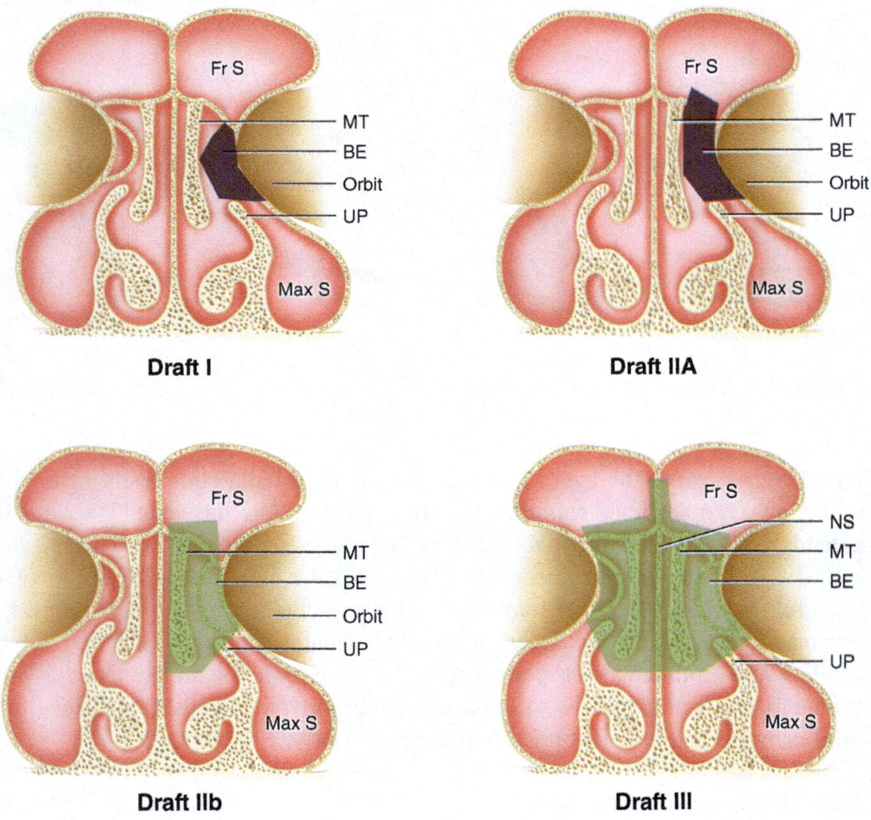


**Fig. 29.13** Extension of Draf procedures. Red areas denote extent of removal of tissue. Frs: frontal sinus, MT: middle turbinate, BE: bulla ethmoidalis, UP: uncinate process. Max S:maxillary sinus, NS: nasal septum

3. In order to make sure that you have entered the frontal recess and are into the frontal sinus, grip the shaft of the ball probe between the thumb and the index finger next to the nasal spine, noting the angle of the instrument at the same time. The instrument is then withdrawn and placed alongside the outside of the nose, placing it at the same angle with the pinch grip placed alongside the nasal spine. If the end of the ball probe is then higher than the eyebrow line, it is likely that the instrument is in the frontal sinus. If it is around or just above the medial canthus, then it is likely that the ball probe is not within the frontal recess but is within an agger nasi air cell. If the handle of the ball probe is noted to have been turned laterally when the instrument is passed up what is thought to be the frontal recess, then it may have been channeled in this direction by a bulla frontalis or a supraorbital cell [21].
4. Irrigation of the frontal sinus through the trephine in the anterior wall. The endoscope is used within the middle meatus to visualize the draining irrigation fluid (this can be colored with methylene blue) [22].

**The Axillary Flap Approach to the Frontal Recess**

The axillary flap technique is suitable for patients who have not had extensive previous dissection in the frontal recess and who still have agger nasi and frontal cells present [23].

**Surgical Technique**

An uncinectomy is performed. No attempt to clear the frontal recess with traditional techniques is made. The first step of the axillary flap approach to the frontal recess is to raise a posteriorly based full-thickness mucosal flap. Using a scalpel blade, a superior incision is made approximately 8 mm above the axilla (insertion of the anterior middle turbinate into the lateral nasal wall) of the middle turbinate. This incision is continued vertically to the level of the axilla. The inferior incision runs around the axilla onto the middle turbinate and is continued for 2 mm posteriorly along the medial aspect of the middle turbinate. A suction Freer is used to elevate the mucosal flap. The flap usually adheres to the junction of the middle turbinate and lateral nasal wall and is freed with a sickle knife until the vertical anterior bone of the middle turbinate is visible. Then, the flap is tucked between the middle turbinate and septum using the sickle knife. The flap should not be seen in the surgical field again until it placed over the newly created axilla at the completion of the operation. The medial wall, roof, and posterior wall of the agger nasi cell are visualized and removed with a 45° curette. If there are frontal cells present, these are visualized and removed. Depending on how these are situated with relation to the agger nasi cell, each frontal cell is entered and identified and its posterior wall and roof removed. Complete clearance of the frontal recess is achieved, and the frontal ostium is identified [23].

The frontal ostium is not instrumented unless a frontal cell or polyp is blocking it. If this occurs, the frontal cell or polyp is removed until complete clearance of the ostium is achieved. If the frontal ostium cannot be identified with this technique, a minitrephine is placed through the anterior table of the frontal sinus and the sinus irrigated with fluorescein-stained saline. This allows the flow of stained saline to be followed until the ostium is identified and cleared. The final step is to replace the axillary flap so that the raw bone which was created with removal of the anterior face of the agger nasi cell is covered [23].

### 29.6.3 Endoscopic-Modified Lothrop Procedure (EMLP) = Draf III

**Introduction**

The remote location and anatomic complexity of the frontal recess along with its proximity to the lamina papyracea and anterior skull base led Lothrop [24] to state that an intranasal approach for frontal sinus drainage was too dangerous to perform. Instead, he described an external approach, which consisted of external ethmoidectomy to enlarge the nasofrontal drainage pathway. This included the removal of the frontal sinus floors that were connected through a large nasal septectomy, and bilateral removal of the lacrimal bone and portion of the lamina papyracea that caused medial orbital fat collapse, with later stenosis of the newly created nasofrontal outflow communication [25].

As endoscopic advances continued, the Lothrop procedure was revisited as an alternative to the open destructive techniques. The endoscopic-modified Lothrop procedure offers several distinct advantages over open techniques and is slowly displacing the osteoplastic flap approach as the procedure of choice in persistent frontal disease after failure of medical therapy and more conservative endoscopic surgery [25].

**Indications of EMLP: [26]**

- Revision cases when scarring or persistent disease in the frontal recess and internal frontal ostium interfere with frontal sinus drainage.
- Patients with underlying extensive mucosal disease such as sarcoidosis, Wegener's granulomatosis, and Samter's triad.
- Frontal sinus mucoceles
- Inverted papilloma
- Osteoma

The total anterior-posterior dimension at the cephalad margin of the frontal recess between the nasal bones at the root of the nose and the anterior skull base should be at least 1.5 cm. The anterior-posterior thickness of the nasal beak should not exceed 1 cm [27].

**Contraindications of EMLP: [25]**

- Hypoplastic frontal sinus and frontal recess.
- Sinus disease is located in a supraorbital ethmoid air cell and not in the frontal sinus.

**Surgical Technique**

It has the same surgical concept as Draf type III but instead, it is performed totally under endoscopic guidance. Surgery is performed with the patient under general anesthesia. If the maxillary, ethmoid, and sphenoid sinuses are diseased, these are dealt with before the EMLP [28].

The middle turbinate or remnant is medialized, and the superior attachment of the uncinate process remnant is resected using a microdebrider. In the most common configuration, the uncinate process attaches to the lamina papyracea forming the recessus terminalis. The frontal ostium is identified posterior and medial to the recessus terminalis. Computer image guidance may be used to help with the identification of the internal frontal sinus ostium. Drilling is initiated in an anterior direction through the anterior insertion of the middle turbinate to enlarge the frontal sinus ostium until the level of the nasal bone is reached. Similarly, drilling is performed in a lateral direction until the level of the plane of the lamina papyracea is reached. Care is taken not to remove the mucosa over the lateral wall of the frontal recess at the plane of the lamina papyracea to preserve the ciliated epithelium responsible for transporting secretions out of the frontal sinus. Care is also taken to prevent mucosal injury at the posterior margin of the frontal sinus and ostium to prevent circumferential mucosal injury with possible postoperative ostial stenosis and to avoid injury to the skull base with possible CSF rhinorrhea [25].

Once the level of the nasal bones is reached anteriorly, drilling is directed medially until the plane of the nasal septum is reached. In the process, part of the nasal beak is removed. To avoid going through the nasal bones and causing soft tissue injury over the nasal root at the glabella, two fingertips are placed over the nasal root to feel and sense the closeness of the drill to the nasal bones. Once the nasal septum is reached, a partial septectomy necessary for the creation of a large common nasofrontal drainage pathway is performed. The center of the surgical septal perforation is located under the floors of the frontal sinuses. The size of the septectomy should be approximately 2 cm. Smaller septal perforations accumulate crusting despite aggressive nasal saline irrigation and thus cause inflammation and delayed healing. Drilling then is continued through the nasal beak, removing the frontal sinus floor on the opposite side and continued until the opposite lamina papyracea is reached [25].

In the process, the posterior wall of the frontal sinus is protected to prevent injury to the skull base and to avoid circumferential mucosal scarring with stenosis. With successful surgery, the common frontal sinus cavities can be easily inspected using a nasal endoscope (Fig. 29.14). [25].

### 29.6.4 Endoscopic Trans-septal Frontal Sinusotomy

**Introduction**

The novel technique of endoscopic trans-septal frontal sinusotomy (TSFS) augments the management of refractory frontal sinus disease. TSFS is a unique endoscopic surgical approach that utilizes the relationship of the nasal septum to the

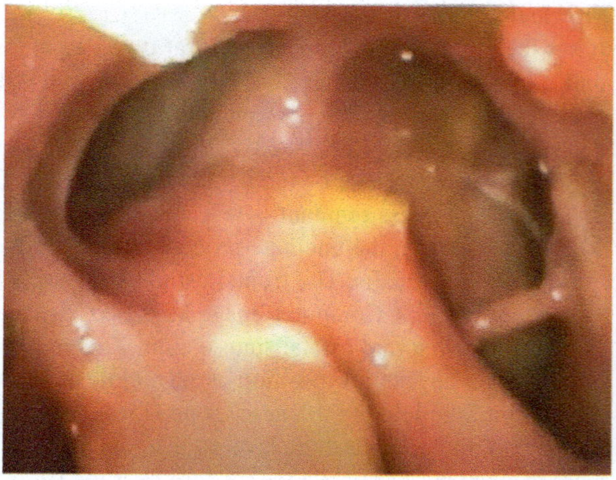

**Fig. 29.14** Endoscopic view of the common frontal sinus cavities two years after the endoscopic

midline floor of the frontal sinus. Like the Draf III or modified Lothrop procedure, the trans-septal approach provides good access to the midline floor of the frontal sinus and permits but does not require intersinus septum removal [29].

**Indications: [29]**

- Chronic frontal sinusitis after failed endoscopic sinus surgery, especially in the setting of "neo-osteogenesis" or middle turbinate resection
- Frontal sinus mucocele formation
- Inverted papilloma
- Fibro-osseous lesions
- Trauma

**Operative Technique**

An endoscopic septoplasty approach is usually done, the septum is typically approached from the left side, and a hemitransfixion incision is done. The bony cartilaginous junction is then fractured, and the septum is mobilized off of the maxillary crest. Quadrangular cartilage mobilization in addition to resection of any deviated portions of septal cartilage can significantly improve surgical exposure, aid in ease of instrumentation, and minimize the need for large septal perforations [30].

An iatrogenic septal perforation is created just below the skull base to allow for exposure, aeration and drainage, future endoscopic inspection, and debridement of the sinus through the nasal cavity. The perforation is created just below the frontal sinus with an approximate diameter of 1.5–2 cm. Through-cutting forward and backward endoscopic forceps help to complete the perforation.

After careful inspection of the roof of the nasal vault, the frontal sinus is entered from below using a combination of drilling with a large cutting burr and angled instruments. Depending upon the thickness of the floor of the sinus, curetting may be sufficient to enter the frontal sinus in some cases. Concurrent saline irrigation while drilling is applied through a 5 FR ureteral catheter with the help of an assistant. The catheter is positioned through the contralateral nares and positioned away from the operative field of view. Concurrent irrigation is essential to avoid inadvertent heat injury to bone and surrounding tissue. Drilling without irrigation allows intense heat build-up (Fig. 29.15).

After entry into the lumen of the frontal sinus has been visually confirmed, the opening of the frontal sinus can be enlarged by drilling anteriorly and laterally. Dissection is carried out laterally to include the natural ostium. The inferior aspect of the intersinus septum may be resected to provide a common outlet for both the right and left frontal sinuses at the midline. Additionally, angled "giraffe" forceps may be used to remove bone fragments and enlarge the opening. In general, all efforts are made to preserve the mucosa throughout the procedure. This minimizes bone exposure and may reduce the risk of delayed stenosis [30].

The hemitransfixion septal incision is closed with an interrupted chromic suture. An important distinguishing feature between the endoscopic TSFS and the modified Lothrop procedure is the exposure that is obtained by septal translocation. Obstructions resulting from septal deviations that may be prominent in a narrow nasal cavity are easily managed with this approach. In addition, the translocation of the septum affords the ability to minimize the size of the superiorly based septal perforation necessary for exposure and safe instrumentation [30].

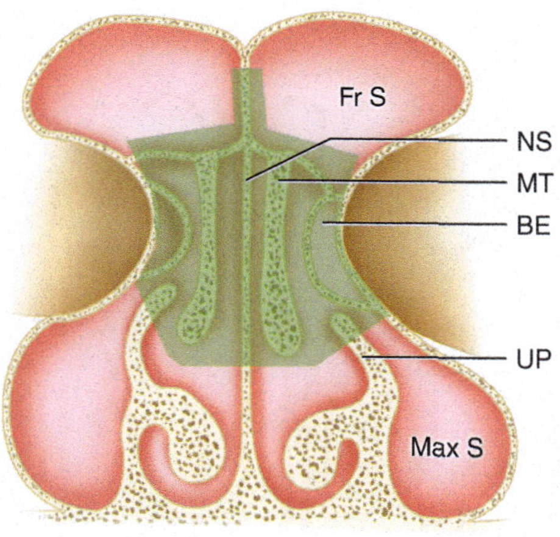


**Fig. 29.15** Coronal illustration demonstrates drilling of the frontal sinus floor through a superiorly-created septal perforation

### 29.6.5 Frontal Sinus Rescue

**Introduction**
If a frontal recess boundary is not fixed, then it may collapse into the frontal recess and cause secondary frontal recess/ostium stenosis. Because the middle turbinate remnant that remains after middle turbinate resection is often destabilized, it may fall laterally and compromise frontal recess patency. Revision endoscopic frontal sinusotomy with mucoperiosteal flap advancement termed the frontal sinus rescue procedure (FSR) has been developed as a modification of the standard endoscopic frontal sinusotomy technique [31].

**Technique: (Fig. 29.16) [32]**

**Advantages: [32]**
FSR offers several distinct advantages:

- Because the lateral frontal recess mucosa is not disturbed by the procedure, mucociliary clearance is restored.
- FSR compensates for both bony and soft tissue stenosis induced by middle turbinate resection.
- FSR mucoperiosteal flap minimizes the tendency for granulation tissue and stenosis.
- FSR is truly minimally invasive; in contrast, the alternative procedure of frontal sinus obliteration is quite extensive with significant morbidity.

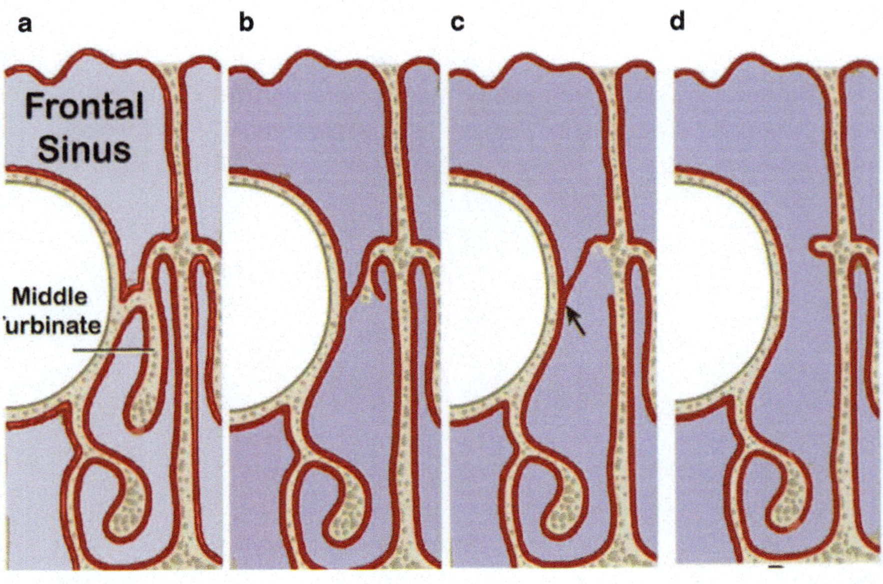


**Fig. 29.16** Fundamental principles of the frontal sinus rescue procedure

- FSR is also a truly functional procedure; in contrast, the alternative procedure of modified endoscopic Lothrop causes significant frontal recess trauma that may ultimately compromise the final surgical result.
- Because FSR is not destructive to the frontal recess, surgical revision under endoscopic visualization is reasonably easy to pursue.

### 29.6.6 Above-and-Below Approach (Trephine and Endoscopic)

**Indications for "Above-and-Below" Approach: [33]**

- Electively, for visualization to facilitate endoscopic frontal sinusotomy
- Inability to completely address disease endoscopically:
- Laterally based frontal sinus lesions/
- Type III or IV frontal cell, which cannot be addressed endoscopically
- Large tumors or inflammatory lesions involving frontal sinus, including:
- Osteoma
- Inverted papilloma
- Fibrous dysplasia
- Trauma with distorted frontal recess or need to evaluate posterior frontal wall
- Revision cases with extensive scarring or neo-osteogenesis
- Distorted anatomy in the frontal recess
- Pott's puffy tumor

**Technique**
Once the endonasal frontal sinusotomy has been completed to its full extent, then the external approach is begun. Lidocaine with epinephrine is used to infiltrate the eyebrow incision. A 1–2 cm incision is carried through the medial eyebrow. The incision should be beveled to parallel the hair shafts of the eyebrow. [33].

A self-retaining retractor is placed into the incision. The incision is carried down to bone. Next, a 4 mm drill bit is used to perform the external trephine through the anterior table. The trephine may be enlarged using Kerrison rongeurs. Angled endoscopes (adult or pediatric) along with curved instruments are used to visualize the frontal sinus through the trephine and manage the remaining pathology of the frontal sinus. If the frontal sinus outflow tract is still not seen endonasally, the frontal sinus can be irrigated through the trephine (this can be colored with methylene blue). If necessary, a stent may be placed upon completion of the above-and-below procedure from below and visualized from above. The external incision is closed in layers using absorbable suture for deep tissues and permanent 5–0 sutures for the skin [33].

### 29.6.7 Above and Below (Osteoplastic and Endoscopic)

When there are frontal sinus problems beyond the reach of the trephine or that are too large to be corrected through the small opening, there is still an alternative to frontal sinus obliteration. The frontal sinus may be opened via an osteoplastic flab, the lesion repaired or removed, and the frontal recess opened under direct vision from above and endoscopically from below. The osteoplastic flab can then be replaced without removing the mucous membrane or obliterating the sinus [34].

## References


1. Clemente MP. Surgical anatomy of the paranasal sinus. In: Levine HL, Clemente MP, editors. Sinus surgery endoscopic and microscopic approaches. 333 Seventh Ave. New York: Thieme Medical Publishers, Inc; 2005. p. 1–56.
2. Bolger WE. Anatomy of the paranasal sinuses. In: Kennedy DW, Bolger WE, Zinreich SJ, editors. Diseases of the sinuses diagnosis and treatment. Hamilton London: B.C. Decker; 2001. p. 1–11.
3. Halle M. Die intranasale Eröffnung und Behandlung der chronisch kranken Stirnhöhlen. Arch Laryngol Rhinol. 1911;24:249–59.
4. Lang J. Clinical anatomy of the nose, nasal cavity and paranasal sinuses. Stuttgart, New York: Thieme; 1989. p. 32.
5. Hosemann W, Gross R, Goede U, Kuehnel T. Clinical anatomy of the nasal process of the frontal bone (spina nasalis interna). Otolaryngol-Head Neck Surg. 2001;125(1):60–5.
6. Moriyama H, Yanagi K, Ohtori N. Healing process of sinus mucosa after endoscopic sinus surgery. Am J Rhinol Allergy. 1996;10:61–6.
7. Kennedy DW. Functional endoscopic sinus surgery: concepts, surgical indication, and instrumentation. In: Kennedy DWBW, Zinreich SJ, editors. Diseases of the sinuses diagnosis and management. Hamilton London: B.C. Decker Inc.; 2001. p. 197–210.
8. Becker DG. The minimally invasive, endoscopic approach to sinus surgery. J Long-Term Eff Med Implants. 2003;13(3):207–21.
9. Stammberger H. Indications for endoscopic surgery. In: Stammberger H, Hawke M, Kopp W, editors. Functional endoscopic sinus surgery: Messerklinger technique. Philadelphia: B.C Decker; 1991. p. 273–81.
10. Metson R, Sindwani R. Endoscopic surgery for frontal sinusitis – a graduated approach. Otolaryngol Clin N Am. 2004;37(2):411–22.
11. Kuhn FA. An integrated approach to frontal sinus surgery. Otolaryngol Clin N Am. 2006;39(3):437–61.
12. Kuhn FA, Melroy CT, Dubin MG, et al. Functional endoscopic dilatation of the sinuses patient selection and surgical technique. In: Kountakis SEOM, editor. Rhinologic and sleep apnea surgical techniques. Verlag Berlin Heidelberg: Springer; 2007. p. 243–52.
13. Brown CL, Bolger WE. Safety and feasibility of balloon catheter dilation of paranasal sinus ostia: a preliminary investigation. Ann Otol Rhinol Laryngol. 2006;115(4):293–9; discussion 300–1.
14. Karanfilov BI, Kuhn FA. The endoscopic frontal recess approach. In: Kountakis SE, Senior BA, Draf W, editors. The frontal sinus. Verlag Berlin Heidelberg: Springer; 2005. p. 179–89.
15. Loury MC. Endoscopic frontal recess and frontal sinus ostium dissection. Laryngoscope. 1993;103(4 Pt 1):455–8.
16. Khun FA. Surgery of the frontal sinus. In: Kennedy DW, Bolger WE, Zinreich SJ, editors. Diseases of the sinuses diagnosis and management. Hamilton London: B.C. Decker; 2001. p. 281–301.
17. Stammberger H. "Uncapping the egg" the endoscopic approach to frontal recess and sinuses. Tuttlingen, Germany: Endopress; 2002. p. 15–6.
18. Draf W. Endonasal micro-endoscopic frontal sinus surgery: the Fulda concept. Oper Tech Otolaryngol Head Neck Surg. 1991;2(4):234–40.

19. Friedman M, Landsberg R, Tanyeri H. Intraoperative and postoperative assessment of frontal sinus patency by transillumination. Laryngoscope. 2000;110(4):683–4.
20. Friedman M, Landsberg R, Schults RA, Tanyeri H, Caldarelli DD. Frontal sinus surgery: endoscopic technique and preliminary results. Am J Rhinol. 2000;14(6):393–403.
21. Simmen D, Jones N. Operative procedures: a step-by-step safe and logical approach. In: Simmen D, Jones N, editors. Manual of endoscopic sinus surgery. 333 Seventh Ave. New York: Thieme; 2005. p. 50–105.
22. Kaplan S, Schwartz A, Metson BF. Mucocele of the frontal and ethmoid sinuses; evaluation of the use of acrylics and tantalum in the surgical treatment. Arch Otolaryngol. 1950;51(2):172–87, illust.
23. Wormald PJ. The axillary flap approach to the frontal recess. Laryngoscope. 2002;112(3):494–9.
24. Lothrop HA. Frontal sinus suppuration: the establishment of permanent nasal drainage; the closure of external fistulae; Epidermization of Sinus. Ann Surg. 1914;59(6):937–57.
25. Kountakis SE. Endoscopic modified Lothrop procedure. In: Kountakis SE, Senior BA, Draf W, editors. The frontal sinus. Verlag Berlin Heidelberg: Springer; 2005. p. 234–41.
26. Shirazi MA, Silver AL, Stankiewicz JA. Surgical outcomes following the endoscopic modified Lothrop procedure. Laryngoscope. 2007;117(5):765–9.
27. Close LG, Lee NK, Leach JL, Manning SC. Endoscopic resection of the intranasal frontal sinus floor. Ann Otol Rhinol Laryngol. 1994;103(12):952–8.
28. Wormald PJ. Salvage frontal sinus surgery: the endoscopic modified Lothrop procedure. Laryngoscope. 2003;113(2):276–83.
29. Batra PS, Lanza DC. Endoscopic trans-septal frontal sinusotomy. In: Kountakis SE, Senior BA, Draf W, editors. The frontal sinus. Springer: Verlag Berlin Heidelberg; 2005. p. 251–9.
30. McLaughlin RB, Hwang PH, Lanza DC. Endoscopic trans-septal frontal sinusotomy: the rationale and results of an alternative technique. Am J Rhinol. 1999;13(4):279–87.
31. Citardi MJ, Javer AR, Kuhn FA. Revision endoscopic frontal sinusotomy with mucoperiosteal flap advancement: the frontal sinus rescue procedure. Otolaryngol Clin N Am. 2001;34(1):123–32.
32. Citardi MJ, Batra BS, Kuhn FA. Frontal Sinus Rescue. In: Kountakis SE, Senior BA, Draf W, editors. The frontal sinus. Verlag Berlin Heidelberg: Springer; 2005. p. 243–9.
33. Karanfilov BI, Kuhn FA. "Above and below" FESS: simple trephine with endoscopic sinus surgery. In: Kountakis SE, Senior BA, Draf W, editors. The frontal sinus. Verlag Berlin Heidelberg: Springer; 2005. p. 211–8.
34. Bent JPSR, Kuhn FA, et al. Combined endoscopic intranasal and external frontal sinusotomy (the above and below approach to chronic frontal sinusitis: alternatives to obliteration). Am J Rhinol Allergy. 1997;11:349–54.

# Endoscopic Surgery of the Sphenoid Sinus

30

Ahmed A. Ibrahim, Ahmed G. Sholkamy, Haitham Morsi, and Shimaa Ibrahim

**Key Points**

- The sphenoid sinus is a paired mucosal-lined air cell within the body of the sphenoid with a variable degree of pneumatization posteriorly, laterally, and inferiorly.
- Vital structures such as the optic nerve, internal carotid artery, cavernous sinuses, and other cranial nerves are closely related to the sphenoid sinus.
- The most common sphenoid sinus pathology according to the literature is inflammatory.
- There are several factors affecting the selection of the approach to the sphenoid sinus.
- The approach should be tailored to allow excision of the pathology or to provide a wide corridor to the skull base lesions and keeps the sinus drained and ventilated.

A. A. Ibrahim (✉)
Alexandria University, Alexandria, Egypt

A. G. Sholkamy · S. Ibrahim
ORL Department, Assiut University, Asyut, Egypt

H. Morsi
Alexandria University Hospital/Canadian Hospital, Dubai, UAE


S. Elwany (ed.), *Current Rhinology*,
https://doi.org/10.1007/978-3-031-70077-4_30

## 30.1 Introduction

The sphenoid bone is the skull base's central skeleton and the main corridor to the skull base lesions. It consists of a body, four lateral arms (2 lesser and 2 greater wings), and two inferior bony projections (pterygoid bodies). The sphenoid sinus is a paired mucosal-lined air cell within the body of the sphenoid with a variable degree of pneumatization posteriorly, laterally, and inferiorly. It is bounded by an ethmoidal air cell anteriorly with variable extended pneumatization posteriorly to form a sphenoethmoidal (Onodi) air cell. It is bordered superiorly by the pituitary gland and the planum sphenoidale, inferiorly by the choanae, posteriorly by the clivus, and laterally by the cavernous sinuses and the cavernous carotid arteries [1]. Vital structures such as the optic nerve, internal carotid artery, cavernous sinuses, maxillary nerves, and Vidian bundle may be injured during endoscopic sphenoidal surgery. So, surgeons should have excellent anatomical knowledge and experience before navigating into the sphenoid sinus and the skull base.

## 30.2 Preoperative Radiological Assessment

A meticulous preoperative radiological evaluation should be done for the degree of sinus pneumatization, presence of Onodi cell, anatomy of the optic and carotid canal in the lateral wall, and presence of any bony dehiscence. The course of the inter-sphenoid sinus septum\septa and its\their attachment to a vital structure should be assessed. The presence of an Onodi cell is variable with its prevalence ranging from 10% to 98% [2, 3].

### 30.2.1 Degree of the Sinus Pneumatization

*In the sagittal plane*, the sphenoid sinus pneumatization is classified into [4]: type I (conchal) in which there are no or minimal air cells (Fig. 30.1), type II (presellar): the posterior sinus wall is anterior to the anterior wall of the sella, type III (Sellar) the posterior sinus wall lies in between the anterior and posterior wall of the sella, type IVa (postsellar) where the posterior sinus wall lies posterior to the posterior sellar wall with no pneumatization dorsal to it, and type IVb (postsellar) where the posterior sinus wall lies posterior to the posterior sellar wall with pneumatization of the dorsum sellae.

*In the coronal plane,* the sphenoid sinus pneumatization is classified into [5]: type I (pre-Vidian) the pneumatization extends to the medial edge of the Vidian canal, type II (pre-rotundum) pneumatization extends to the medial edge of the foramen rotundum, and type III (post-rotundum) extends beyond the medial border of the foramen rotundum.

The anterior clinoid process (ACP) has a variable degree of pneumatization with an associated high incidence of optic canal dehiscence when present [6].

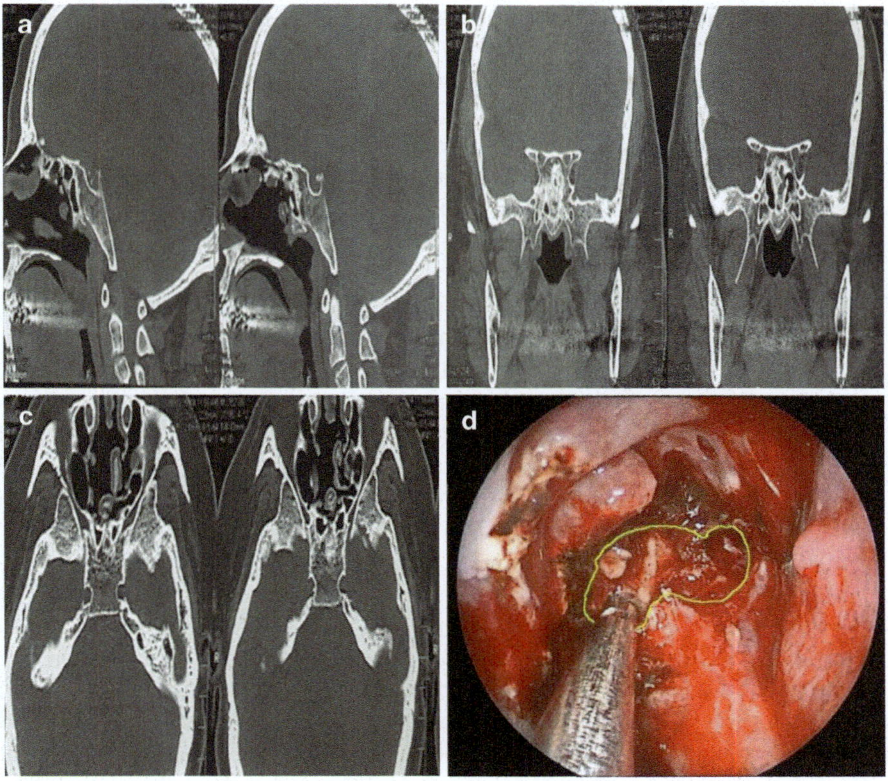


**Fig. 30.1** Radiological (**a**, **b**, **c**) and endoscopic view (**d**) of the conchal sphenoid

### 30.2.2 The Course of the Optic Nerve

Delano et al. [6] described the relation of the optic canal to the sinus wall and classified it into: type 1 where the optic nerve passes adjacent to the sinus wall without any bony indentation, type 2 where there is a bony indentation, type 3 where the nerve passes through the sphenoid sinus, and type 4 where the course of the optic nerve passes immediately lateral to the posterior ethmoid and sphenoid sinus. The optic canal may be dehiscent in 4–30% [6, 7] with a great risk of being injured during surgery, and the dehiscence should be suspected when there is pneumatization of ACP.

### 30.2.3 The Course of the Internal Carotid Artery (ICA)

The course of the ICA should be identified preoperatively to avoid its injury and fatal intraoperative bleeding. The incidence of protrusion of the ICA into the sphenoid sinus may be present up to 40% [7] with the incidence of bony wall dehiscence up to 35% [8]. The inter-sphenoid sinus septum may be deviated to one side and attached to the canal wall of the ICA.

### 30.2.4 Identification of the Sphenoid Ostium

The different sphenoidal approaches aim to have a safe surgery with a good lifelong patency with subsequent fair ventilation and drainage. During endoscopic sinus surgery, the location of the sphenoid sinus ostium is of great importance in the assessment of different sphenoidal lesions such as mucocele, isolated sphenoid sinusitis, allergic fungal sinusitis, and different tumors. Additionally, the natural ostium is considered an important landmark during endoscopic approaches to excise different pituitary and skull base lesions. Sometimes, it may be difficult even for the expert surgeon to localize the natural ostium because of anatomical variations, the nature of the pathology, and ill-defined landmarks during revision surgeries. Even after localization of the ostium, there is still a risk during sphenoidotomy to injure: the skull base upon widening the ostium superiorly, cavernous sinus laterally, and posterior septal branches of the sphenopalatine artery (SPA) inferiorly [9]. The natural ostium is located about 7–8 cm with an angle of 25–30° relative to the horizontal plane of the anterior nasal spine [10] and 5.5–8 cm from the limen nasi with an angle of 26–34° which is considered a more practical landmark in endoscopic approaches [11].

In relation to the anterior wall of the sphenoid sinus, the natural ostium can be visualized nearly halfway between the top of the choana and skull base [9, 12–14]. Other studies divided the anterior wall into three parts with most of the ostia lying at the upper third [11, 15]. The distance between the natural ostium and the roof of the choana ranges from 1 to 1.5 cm in most studies [12–14]. Wigand [16] described a simple technique to find the sphenoid ostium by insertion of a blunt instrument 10–15 mm above the roof of the choana and 2–4 mm lateral to the septum. The ostium is located mostly medial to the superior turbinate but may be lateral or partially covered by the superior turbinate. It usually presents within 1 cm from the posteroinferior end of the superior turbinate [11] so cutting of the lower third of the superior turbinate may facilitate localization of the natural ostium. The variable degree of sphenoid pneumatization is the main factor affecting the position of the sphenoid sinus ostium which affects the technique to safely widen the ostium. Pneumatization of the Onodi air cell, rostrum, and pterygoid body can shift the location of the sphenoid ostium [17]. When the landmarks are obscured as in revision cases and extensive pathology, the posterior wall of the maxillary sinus as well as the medial part of the maxillary roof may be used as reliable landmarks in addition to the choana to do sphenoidotomy safely [18].

## 30.3 Sphenoid Sinusotomy

Simmen and Jones [19] classified sphenoidotomy into 3 types: Type I includes the identification of the natural sphenoid ostium without further instrumentation. Type II sphenoidotomy describes the widening of the ostium to the skull base superiorly and to half its height inferiorly. Type III sphenoidotomy is done by extending the opening to the sinus floor inferiorly and to the vital structures laterally. The extension of the pathology is the main factor that determines the approach to the sphenoid sinus. Regardless of *the approach,* localization of the natural ostium is an important landmark to enter the sphenoid sinus and avoid injury of the vital structures [20]. To be safe during sphenoidotomy, it is wise to start close to the vomer and 1–1.5 cm from the choana. Then, the ostium could be widened inferomedially using the straight curette or even the microdebrider with its blade facing down. If a wide sphenoidotomy is needed, the mucosa over the anterior face of the sphenoid is incised at the lower margin of the ostium and the mucosa is dissected and elevated. This allows the extension of the sphenoidotomy to the sinus floor and preservation of the septal branch of the SPA where the nasoseptal flap may be needed for skull base repair [20].

## 30.4 Endoscopic Endonasal Approaches to the Sphenoid Sinus

There are several factors affecting the selection of the approach to the sphenoid sinus. The approach is tailored to facilitate the excision of the pathology or to have a wide corridor to the skull base lesions and keeps the sinus drained and ventilated. The main factor is the extension of the pathology. *Other* factors including anatomical variations and previous nasal surgery are also considered (Fig. 30.2).

The patient is placed in a supine position with a slight hyperextension of the head. The table head should be elevated for 30° with the placement of the endotracheal tube to the left mouth corner to allow fair access of the anesthesiologist to the airway and prevent interference with the main surgeon's hand during instrumentation. The middle third of the face with perioral area is prepped and draped in a

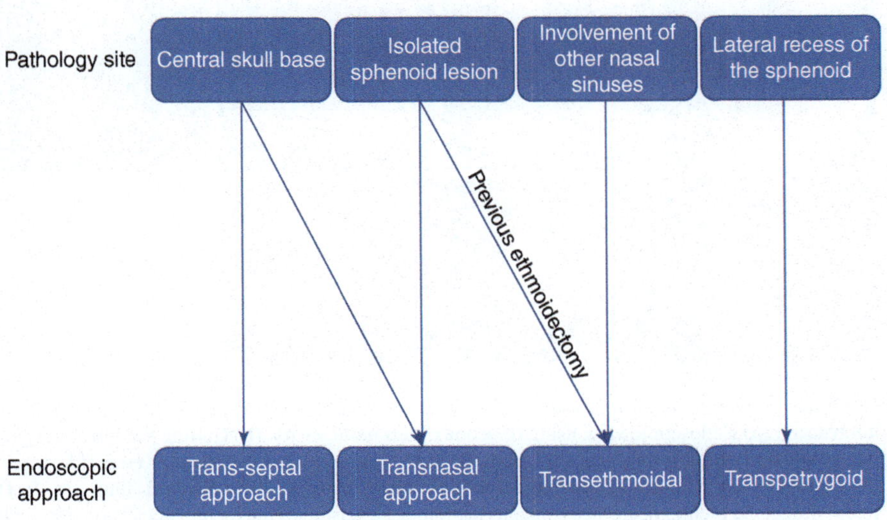


**Fig. 30.2** Approaches to the sphenoid sinus according to pathology extension

sterile fashion. Cottonoids soaked in 0.1% oxymetazoline are applied to achieve vasoconstriction and improve intraoperative visualization. A 0° scope allows good visualization for all approaches.

### 30.4.1 Endoscopic Trans-ethmoidal Sphenoidotomy

This approach should be selected when there is extensive pathology involving different nasal sinuses. Uncinectomy followed by identification of the maxillary sinus ostium, then middle meatal antrostomy should be done widely to identify the posterior wall and the medial part of the maxillary roof. Complete ethmoidectomy with skeletonization of the medial orbital wall will delineate the safe lateral extension of the sphenoidotomy. Identification of the natural sphenoid ostium should be done before starting the posterior ethmoidectomy. The removal of the lower third of the superior turbinate could be helpful. Identification of the sphenoid roof could be a good landmark as the posterior ethmoids could not be below that level. Then, the basal lamella is opened infero-medially 2–3 mm above the junction of the second and third part of the middle turbinate to enter the posterior ethmoids. It is important to identify the Onodi cell during the meticulous reading of the preoperative CT *if present*. Once the Onodi is opened, a blunt instrument could be used to complete the sphenoethmoidectomy by starting from the most superolateral point and then directed vertically toward the previously widened sphenoid ostium [21]. In this approach, the middle turbinate instability is avoided as there is no need to fracture the middle turbinate. Another advantage is that the ethmoid sinuses allow a wide corridor to the sphenoid sinus [22] (Fig. 30.3).

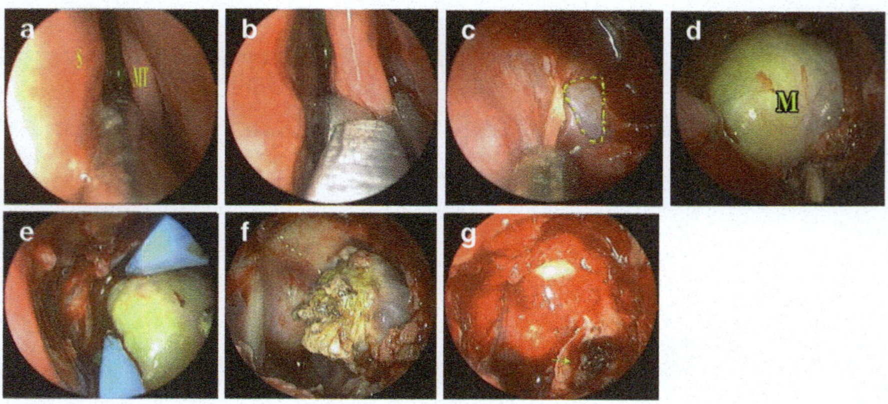


**Fig. 30.3** Trans-ethmoidal approach to a lateral recess meningocele injected with intrathecal 10% fluorescein. (**a**) Endoscopic view using 0° scope of left nasal cavity. (**b**) Cutting the lower third of the middle and superior turbinate (**c**) Localization of sphenoid sinus ostium after ethmoidectomy. (**d**) Type III sphenoidotomy: meningoencephalocele occupying the sphenoid sinus. (**e** & **f**) Reduction of the meningocele size by cauterization. (**g**) Excision of the meningocele from the neck leaving a defect in the lateral recess of the sphenoid. MT: middle turbinate, S: nasal septum, M: meningoencephalocele, Dashed line: sphenoid ostium, Yellow arrow: skull base defect

### 30.4.2 Endoscopic Trans-nasal Approach Sphenoidotomy

This approach is used to access the sphenoid when there is an isolated sphenoid lesion or use the sphenoid as a corridor to the skull base. The middle turbinate is fractured laterally to gain access to the sphenoethmoidal recess. The superior turbinate is then identified, cutting the lower third could be helpful to allow easy identification of the natural ostium. Coagulation of the mucosa surrounding the ostium may be helpful when there is excessive mucosal bloody ooze. Then, sphenoidotomy is done as previously described. Posterior septectomy and removal of the sphenoid rostrum may be done to allow binostril approach and a wide access to the skull base. This allows exposing of both optic\carotid protuberances and opticocarotid recesses (OCR) laterally, clivus or clival recess inferiorly, and planum sphenoidale superiorly [23]. The advantage of this approach is that it allows medial access to the sphenoid sinus away from any vital structures, i.e., optic nerve, carotid artery, and cavernous sinus. It gives direct access to the sphenoid sinus without disruption of the ethmoid sinus anatomy so it is considered to be a more physiologic approach [22] (Fig. 30.4).

### 30.4.3 Endoscopic Trans-septal Approach to the Sphenoid Sinus

It is considered the standard approach to skull base lesions, especially pituitary adenomas. After examination of the nasal cavity and choosing the wider side, a

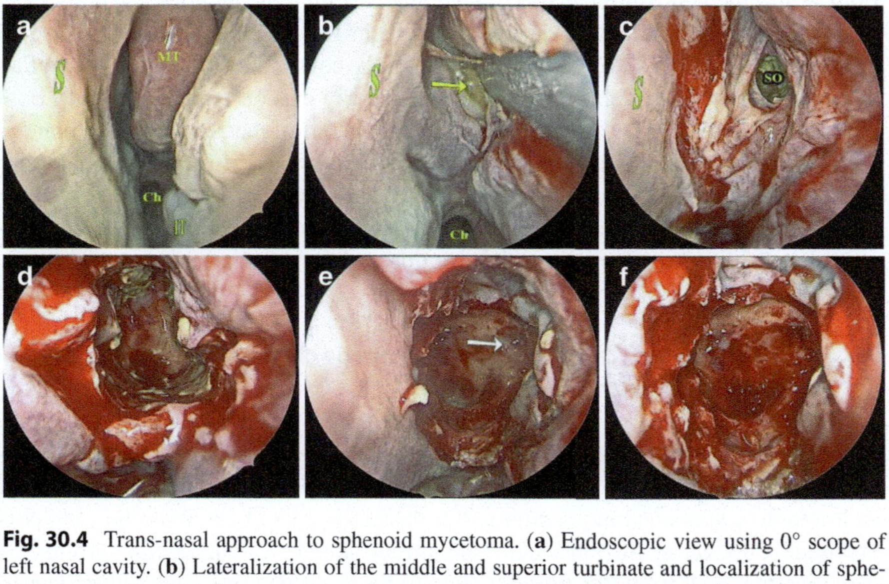


**Fig. 30.4** Trans-nasal approach to sphenoid mycetoma. (**a**) Endoscopic view using 0° scope of left nasal cavity. (**b**) Lateralization of the middle and superior turbinate and localization of sphenoid sinus ostium. (**c**) Sphenoidotomy: Fungal ball occupying the sphenoid sinus. (**d**), (**e**) & (**f**) Wide sphenoidotomy and sinus clearance. MT: middle turbinate, S: nasal septum, Ch: choana, yellow arrow: polyp obstructing the sphenoid ostium and white arrow: lateral OCR

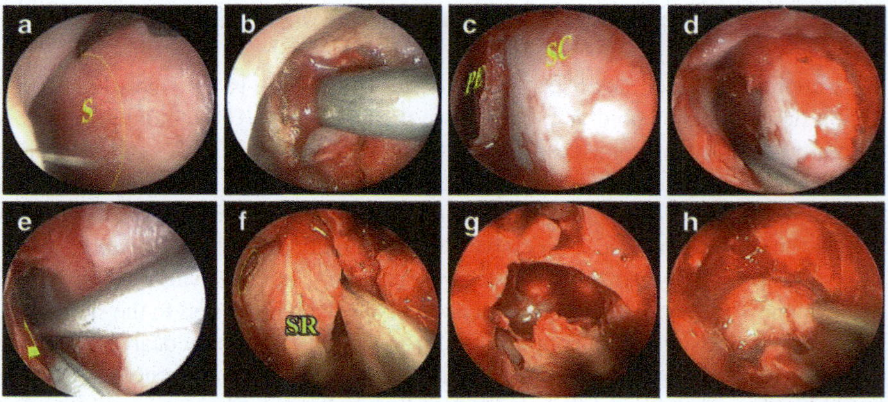


**Fig. 30.5** Trans-septal approach to the sphenoid sinus. (**a**) Endoscopic view using 0° scope of right nasal cavity anterior incision of the septal mucosa. (**b**) Elevation of the mucoperichondrial flap. (**c**) Disarticulation of the septal cartilage from the perpendicular plate of ethmoid bone (PE) and the vomer (V). (**d**) Elevation of the mucoperiosteal flap of the contralateral side. (**e**) Removal of the lower part of the PE and V. (**f**) Localization of both sphenoid ostia. (**g**) & (**h**): Removal of the anterior sphenoid wall. S: nasal septum, SC: septal cartilage, PE: perpendicular plate of ethmoid bone, V: vomer, SR: sphenoid rostrum

Killian incision is done, then dissecting in a subperichondrial plane superiorly and inferiorly to elevate the ipsilateral septal flap. The dissection of this plane is continued posteriorly along the bony cartilaginous junction to the anterior phase of the sphenoid. It is important to extend the dissection to the nasal floor to widen the corridor or use the neurosurgical speculum. Once reaching the anterior sphenoid face, the quadrangular cartilage is disarticulated from the maxillary crest, vomer, and perpendicular plate of the ethmoid bone. Then, the contralateral mucoperiosteal flap is elevated. The dissection is carried out posteriorly on both sides to identify both sphenoid ostia. After that, the vomer and the lower part of the perpendicular plate of the ethmoid bone are resected using the bone nibbler. The rostrum and the anterior wall of the sphenoid sinus are resected using a high-speed drill [24, 25].

This approach allows less experienced surgeons to have direct access to the sphenoid sinus with minimal anatomical disruption and fewer complications (Fig. 30.5).

### 30.4.4 Endoscopic Trans-pterygoid Approach to the Sphenoid Sinus

This approach is ideal to have access to the lateral recess pathology. As in trans-ethmoidal approach to the sphenoid, uncinectomy wide middle meatal antrostomy, and complete sphenoethmoidectomy, the posterior wall of the maxillary sinus is exposed by dissecting the mucosa till the infraorbital nerve. The middle turbinate is then disarticulated from the ethmoid crest of the palatine bone, and a blunt instrument may be used to dissect the periosteum anterior to the sphenopalatine foramen.

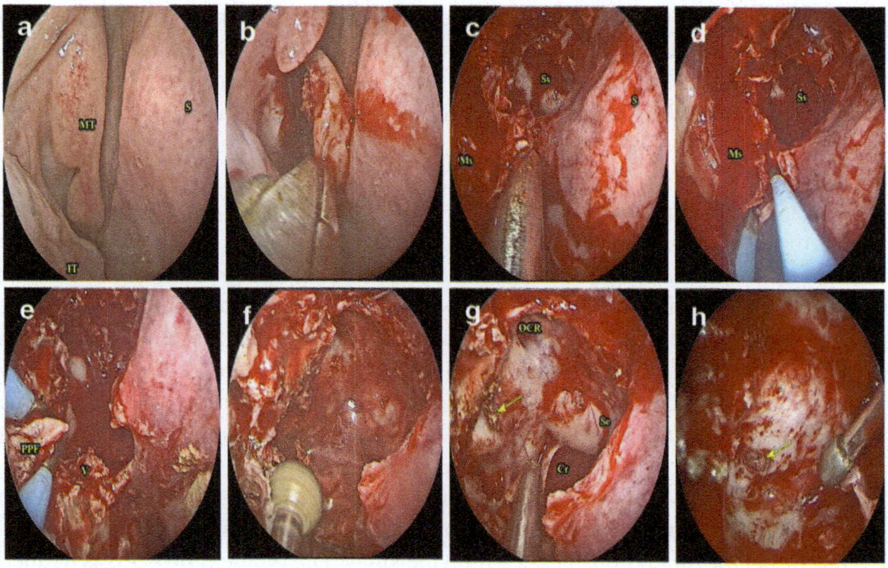


**Fig. 30.6** Trans-pterygoid approach to lateral recess skull base defect. (**a**) Endoscopic view using 0° scope of the right nasal cavity. (**b**) Cutting the lower part of the middle and superior turbinate to have a wider corridor. (**c**) Exposure of the sphenoid sinus after ethmoidectomy and wide opening of the maxillary sinus. (**d**) Cauterization of the sphenopalatine artery. (**e**) Mobilization of pterygopalatine fossa content. (**f**) Drilling of the pterygoid body to expose the defect. (**g**) & (**h**) Exposure of the defect. MT: middle turbinate, S: nasal septum, IT: inferior turbinate, Ms.: maxillary sinus, Ss: sphenoid sinus, PPF: pterygopalatine fossa content, V: Vidian nerve, OCR: opticocarotid recess, Se: sella, Cr: clival recess, yellow arrow: skull base defect

A high-speed drill or Kerrison rongeur is used to remove the perpendicular plate of the palatine bone and the upper part of the posterior maxillary wall. The periosteum of the pterygopalatine fossa is incised, after that the underlying fat is bluntly dissected with coagulation of the small blood vessels. Then, the terminal branches of the maxillary artery are mobilized or ligated. It is important to preserve the pterygopalatine ganglion, its lacrimal branch, Vidian, and the infraorbital bundles. After mobilization of the pterygopalatine fossa content, a second periosteal layer is found and incised to expose the pterygoid process; then, the pterygoid muscle attachment is defined. Drilling the bone medial to the muscle attachment to enter the lateral recess. A Kerrison forceps may be used to enlarge this opening [26, 27] (Fig. 30.6).

## 30.5 Endoscopic Anatomy of the Sphenoid Sinus

Once sphenoidotomy is done, great care should be taken while advancing any instrument inside the sinus as the posterior wall could be within 6–22 mm from the ostium. The carotid artery is located approximately 25 mm inferolateral to the ostium at an angle of 45°, and the optic canal is present at approximately 15 mm from the ostium in a lateral to superolateral direction at an angle of 60° [14]. Any inter-sphenoid septum should be removed carefully by a high-speed drill or cutting instrument and not fractured to avoid injury of any vital structure. *This allows a wide corridor for skull base* surgery. After all the septa are flattened, the following landmarks should be identified:

- *The sphenoid rostrum* or its remnant should be used as an anatomical landmark for the midline.
- *The sellar prominence* presents in the midline posterosuperiorly related to the pituitary gland; in the sellar and postsellar types of pneumatization, the sella is well-defined and protrudes into the sphenoid sinus. In the presellar and conchal types, it is ill-defined and neuronavigation system and micro-Doppler probe may be helpful for identification of the midline and the cavernous segment of the ICA. *The bone thickness in this region is* variable ranging from 0.1 mm to 0.7 mm with a thinner bone on the undersurface of the sella [28].
- *The planum sphenoidale* is located anterosuperior to the sella. Its junction with the sella corresponds to the tuberculum sella and the chiasmatic sulcus intracranially and *the tubercular recess* within the sinus. *The tubercular recess* is defined as a horizontal depression between the sella inferiorly and the planum sphenoidale in the sinus wall. *The medial opticocarotid recess (OCR)* has been described as the lateral edge of the tubercular recess [29].
- *The clival recess* is present as an indentation below the sella when the sphenoid is well-pneumatized. It is the junction of the middle third of the clivus and sellar region. The para clival part of the ICA bounded the recess laterally [30].
- *Carotid prominence* is located in the lateral wall of the sinus lateral to the sella. It corresponds to the cavernous part of the ICA and to a lesser extent to the clinoid segment of the ICA. The bony covering of the artery is variable and is often thinner than that covering the sella [31]. It is reported that the carotid dehiscence may be up to 22.8% [32]. The distance of the different parts of the ICA is variable. The mean intercarotid distance reported at the sella ranged from 17 to 18 mm [12, 28, 33], at the tuberculum sella 13.3–14 mm [28, 33, 34], and at the clivus 17.1–19.7 mm [28, 33, 35, 36].
- *Optic prominence* is located laterally and related to the optic nerve within its canal. The optic chiasma does not have any impression within the sinus wall but in a good pneumatized sinus the tubercular recess is related to the chiasmatic sulcus intracranially [31]. Optic canal dehiscence is reported at a rate up to 23% [32], and the distance between both optic nerves at the entrance of the carotid canal ranges from 9 to 24 mm. According to sinus pneumatization, supraoptic and infraoptic recesses may be present [34].
- *Opticocarotid recesses* are small spaces present in a direct relation to the optic and carotid prominences depending on the degree of the sphenoid pneumatization. The medial OCR is located medial to the carotid prominence where it is bounded by the optic nerve superiorly, the sella inferiorly, and the carotid prominence laterally. It is considered a lateral extension of the tubercular recess [29]. The lateral OCR is a triangular-shaped depression lateral to the carotid promi-

nence bounded by the optic canal superiorly and the carotid prominence medially. The lateral OCR is an important landmark for the optic strut.

- *The Vidian canal* is located on the floor of a well-pneumatized sphenoid sinus inferior and medial to the trigeminal nerve. It is a landmark for the site of the horizontal and lacerum segments of the ICA [37]
- *Trigeminal prominence* may be seen in the lateral wall of the sphenoid depending on the degree of pneumatization. The second division of the trigeminal nerve—the maxillary nerve—is running in the inferolateral aspect of the cavernous sinus and produces this ridge [31].

## 30.6 Pathologies of the Sphenoid Sinus

The most common cause of sphenoid sinus lesions according to the literature is inflammatory in up to 65–72% of cases, followed by neoplasms which account for 18% (in benign) and 10.9% (in malignant) of the cases, respectively [38]. There are many important and vital structures that are located adjacent to the sphenoid sinus, including optic nerve and chiasma, cranial nerves (3rd, 4th, 5th, and 6th) [39], middle cranial fossa, and cavernous sinus. Thus, the advancement of the disease of the sphenoid sinus may lead to life-threatening complications. Common presentations in these patients include headache (33–81%), visual disturbance (24–50%), nasal obstruction and discharge, and ptosis and may be asymptomatic [38].

**Differential Diagnosis of Isolated Sphenoid Sinus Lesions Includes the Following:**

A. *Inflammatory*
   (a) Bacterial sphenoid sinusitis (acute and chronic).
   (b) Allergic fungal sinusitis.
   (c) Fungal ball.
   (d) Invasive fungal sinusitis.
   (e) Mucocele, mucopyocele
   (f) Sphenochoanal polyp.

B. *Tumors:*
   (a) *Benign*
      (i) Inverted papilloma.
      (ii) Juvenile angiofibroma
      (iii) Fibrous dysplasia.
      (iv) Osteoma.
   (b) *Malignant*
      (i) Lymphoma
      (ii) Squamous cell carcinoma
      (iii) Adenoid cystic carcinoma
      (iv) Metastatic carcinoma
      (v) Sarcoma

(c) *Tumors originating from the sella turcica and invading the sphenoid sinus*
    (i) Pituitary adenoma
    (ii) Chordoma
    (iii) Meningioma
    (iv) Craniopharyngioma

C. *CSF and meningocele*
    (a) CSF leaks
    (b) Meningocele

## References


1. García-Garrigós E, et al. Transsphenoidal approach in endoscopic endonasal surgery for skull base lesions: what radiologists and surgeons need to know. Radiographics. 2015;35(4):117085.
2. Pérez P, et al. Anatomical variations in the human paranasal sinus region studied by CT. J Anat. 2000;197(Pt 2):221–7.
3. Meyers RM, Valvassori G. Interpretation of anatomic variations of computed tomography scans of the sinuses: a surgeon's perspective. Laryngoscope. 1998;108(3):422–5.
4. Güldner C, et al. Analysis of pneumatization and neurovascular structures of the sphenoid sinus using cone-beam tomography (CBT). Acta Radiol. 2012;53(2):214–9.
5. Vaezi A, et al. Classification of sphenoid sinus pneumatization: relevance for endoscopic skull base surgery. Laryngoscope. 2015;125(3):577–81.
6. DeLano MC, Fun FY, Zinreich SJ. Relationship of the optic nerve to the posterior paranasal sinuses: a CT anatomic study. AJNR Am J Neuroradiol. 1996;17(4):669–75.
7. Elwany S, Elsaeid I, Thabet H. Endoscopic anatomy of the sphenoid sinus. J Laryngol Otol. 1999;113(2):122–6.
8. Asal N, et al. Carotid canal and optic canal at sphenoid sinus. Neurosurg Rev. 2019;42(2):519–29.
9. Kim HU, et al. Surgical anatomy of the natural ostium of the sphenoid sinus. Laryngoscope. 2001;111(9):1599–602.
10. Davis WE, Templer J, Parsons DS. Anatomy of the paranasal sinuses. Otolaryngol Clin N Am. 1996;29(1):57–74.
11. Gupta T, Aggarwal A, Sahni D. Anatomical landmarks for locating the sphenoid ostium during endoscopic endonasal approach: a cadaveric study. Surg Radiol Anat. 2013;35(2):13742.
12. Abuzayed B, et al. Endoscopic endonasal transsphenoidal approach to the sellar region: results of endoscopic dissection on 30 cadavers. Turk Neurosurg. 2009;19(3):237–44.
13. Hidir Y, et al. Optimum height from the roof of the choana for seeking the sphenoid ostium. J Craniofac Surg. 2011;22(3):1077–9.
14. Enatsu K, et al. Surgical anatomy of the sphenoid sinus on the CT using multiplanar reconstruction technique. Otolaryngol Head Neck Surg. 2008;138(2):182–6.
15. Lanzu DC. Clinical Anatomy of the Nose, Nasal Cavity, and Paranasal Sinuses, by Johannes Lang. 144 pages with illustrations. Thieme Medical Publishers, Inc., New York, 1989. Otolaryngol–Head Neck Surg. 1991;105(5):762.
16. Wigand ME, Iro H, Birkholz T. *Endoscopic surgery of the paranasal sinuses and anterior skull base*. New York: Thieme Stuttgart; 2008.
17. Doubi A, et al. Location of the sphenoid sinus ostium in relation to adjacent anatomical landmarks. Ear Nose Throat J. 2021;100(10_suppl):961s–8s.
18. Lee SJ. The relationship of the medial roof and the posterior wall of the maxillary sinus to the sphenoid sinus: a radiologic study. Braz J Otorhinolaryngol. 2017;83(4):375–80.
19. Balakrishnan K, et al. In: Simmen D, Jones N, editors. Manual of endoscopic sinus and Skull Base surgery. Stuttgart: Georg Thieme Verlag KG; 2014. p. 91–165.

20. Gibbons MD, Sillers MJ. Minimally invasive approaches to the sphenoid sinus. Otolaryngol–Head Neck Surg. 2002;126(6):635–41.
21. Schlosser RJ, Bolger WE. Endoscopic transethmoidal sphenoidotomy. Oper Tech Otolaryngol Head Neck Surg. 2003;14(3):178–84.
22. Youssef TA. Endoscopic approaches to the sphenoid: how I do it? Egypt J Otolaryngol. 2013;29(4):284–9.
23. Carrau RL, Jho H-D, Ko Y. Transnasal-Transsphenoidal endoscopic surgery of the pituitary gland. Laryngoscope. 1996;106(7):914–8.
24. Hinohira Y, Hyodo M, Gyo K. Endoscopic endonasal transseptal approach for localized sphenoid sinus diseases. Auris Nasus Larynx. 2009;36(4):411–5.
25. Papay FA, et al. Transnasal transseptal endoscopic approach to the sphenoid sinus. J Craniofac Surg. 1997;8(3):159–63.
26. Al-Nashar IS, et al. Endoscopic transnasal transpterygopalatine fossa approach to the lateral recess of the sphenoid sinus. Laryngoscope. 2004;114(3):528–32.
27. Bolger WE. Endoscopic transpterygoid approach to the lateral sphenoid recess: surgical approach and clinical experience. Otolaryngol Head Neck Surg. 2005;133(1):20–6.
28. Fujii K, Chambers SM, Rhoton AL Jr. Neurovascular relationships of the sphenoid sinus. A microsurgical study. J Neurosurg. 1979;50(1):31–9.
29. Elwany S, Elsaeid I, Thabet H. Endoscopic anatomy of the sphenoid sinus. J Laryngol Otol. 1999 Feb;113(2):122–6.
30. Chan Y, Goddard JC. *Endoscopic Skull Base surgery*. In: *K.J. Lee's essential otolaryngology: head and neck surgery, 12e*. New York: McGraw-Hill Education; 2019.
31. Baskin JZ, Kuriakose MA, Lebowitz RA. The anatomy and physiology of the sphenoid sinus. Oper Tech Otolaryngol Head Neck Surg. 2003;14:168–72.
32. Şirikci A, et al. Variations of sphenoid and related structures. Eur Radiol. 2000;10(5):844–8.
33. Perondi GE, et al. Endoscopic anatomy of sellar region. Pituitary. 2013;16(2):251–9.
34. Lang J. Clinical anatomy of the nose, nasal cavity, and paranasal sinuses. George Thieme Verlag; 1989.
35. Wang Q, Lan Q, Lu XJ. Extended endoscopic endonasal transsphenoidal approach to the suprasellar region: anatomic study and clinical considerations. J Clin Neurosci. 2010;17(3):3426.
36. Unlu A, et al. Endoscopic anatomy of sphenoid sinus for pituitary surgery. Clin Anat. 2008;21(7):627–32.
37. Fortes FS, et al. Endonasal endoscopic exposure of the internal carotid artery: an anatomical study. Laryngoscope. 2012;122(2):445–51.
38. Knisely A, et al. Isolated sphenoid sinus opacification: a systematic review. Am J Otolaryngol. 2017;38(2):237–43.
39. Martin TJ, et al. Evaluation and surgical management of isolated sphenoid sinus disease. Arch Otolaryngol Head Neck Surg. 2002;128(12):1413–9.

# Endoscopic Hypophysectomy

# 31

Ahmed A. Ibrahim, Mustafa Wagdy, and Mohamed K. Taha

**Key Points**

- Endoscopic endonasal transsphenoidal approach become the gold standard for most pituitary lesions.
- Good experience with endoscopic anatomy of sellar, presellar, and suprasellar anatomy must be achieved.
- Proper instrumentations and usage of angled endoscopes are useful to confirm complete removal and decrease rate of complications.
- For large tumors or tumors with suprasellar and cavernous sinus extension, complete drill-out of the anterior sphenoid wall and the face of the sella (extending, as required, to the tuberculum sella and planum sphenoidale) is vital.
- Arachnoid membrane rent must be avoided but if it happens graduated reconstruction must be performed to avoid CSF rhinorrhea.
- A multidisciplinary approach (including outpatient clinics, patient selection, planning of approach, the operation, and postoperative care) can improve safety and overall quality of care.

**Supplementary Information** The online version contains supplementary material available at https://doi.org/10.1007/978-3-031-70077-4_31.

A. A. Ibrahim (✉)
Alexandria University, Alexandria, Egypt

M. Wagdy · M. K. Taha
Alexandria University Hospital, Alexandria, Egypt


S. Elwany (ed.), *Current Rhinology*,
https://doi.org/10.1007/978-3-031-70077-4_31

## 31.1 Surgical Anatomy

The pituitary gland is situated within the hypophyseal fossa near the center of the cranial base. This fossa is demarcated laterally and superiorly by reflections of dura in the body of the sphenoid bone. In that location, the gland has proximity to several important cranial nerves and vascular structures.

### 31.1.1 Sellar Anatomy

The pituitary fossa is limited anteriorly, posteriorly, and inferiorly by bony constituents of the sella turcica. The anterior wall is called the tuberculum sellae, and its posterior wall is named the dorsum sellae. Superior to the tuberculum lies the sulcus chiasmaticus, which terminates on each side in the optic foramen. The superolateral margins of the dorsum sellae are formed by the posterior clinoid processes, which provide attachment for dural folds.

The degree of pneumatization of the sphenoid bone and the thickness of bone separating the sphenoid sinus from the hypophyseal fossa are both highly variable. The pattern of bony trabeculae that divide the sphenoid sinus is also quite inconstant [1, 2].

The diaphragma sellae, a fold of dura with a central defect, forms an incomplete roof above the sella turcica. The diaphragma separates the anterior lobe from the overlying optic chiasm [1]. The central aperture of the diaphragma is of variable size, ranging from a small foramen in an otherwise complete barrier to a large hole surrounded by a tenuous membrane of tissue. The central aperture transmits the pituitary stalk and its blood supply [3].

### 31.1.2 Para-sellar and Suprasellar Anatomy

The folds of dura matter that form the lateral walls of the hypophyseal fossa contain the cavernous sinuses. The two sinuses communicate with one another by means of the anterior and posterior intercavernous sinuses, also known as the circular sinuses. The oculomotor nerve and trochlear nerve are embedded in the lateral wall of the cavernous sinus, whereas the abducens nerve is contained within the sinus itself. The cavernous sinus also envelops a portion of the internal carotid artery (ICA) and the sympathetic nerve plexus encircling it [1, 4].

## 31.2 Pituitary Surgery (Hypophysectomy)

### 31.2.1 History and Evolution of Pituitary Surgeries

Over the past century, surgical approaches to pituitary adenomas have undergone significant adaptation since the first attempted transcranial and transsphenoidal decompression operations of the early nineteenth century. Microscopic transsphenoidal surgery has long been considered the "gold standard" in surgical treatment of pituitary tumors. The use of rigid endoscopes for sinus surgery provided the inspiration for their application to pituitary surgery [5]. In 1992, Jankowski provided the first description of fully endoscopic trans-nasal technique [6].

Over the last two decades, endoscopic endonasal surgery has gradually gained favor as a primary approach for sellar and para-sellar lesions, primarily due to the wide panoramic, up-close visualization offered by the endoscope. Angled endoscopes allow for complete resection of high-grade (invasive) tumors, visualizing para-sellar and suprasellar tumor extension, and allowing for rapid decompression of the optic chiasm [7]. Minimally invasive endoscopic endonasal trans-sphenoidal surgery provides easy and quick recovery; therefore, this procedure is recommended for sellar and para-sellar lesions in children. It is essential to keep children's anatomical and functional integrity to ensure their normal growth and nasosphenoidal ventilation [8].

The differential diagnosis of sellar lesions includes primary and metastatic tumors, cysts, and inflammatory and vascular lesions. The most common are pituitary adenomas, craniopharyngiomas, meningiomas, Rathke cleft cysts, and pituitary apoplexies.

### 31.2.2 Indications

The main aims of surgery for pituitary adenomas are

1. Normalization of excess hormone secretion
2. Elimination of mass effect
3. Preservation or restoration of normal neurologic function, including visual acuity and fields
4. Preservation or restoration of normal pituitary function
5. Prevention of tumor recurrence
6. Achievement of a complete pathologic diagnosis

### 31.2.3 Preoperative Evaluation

Preoperatively, all patients should undergo clinical examination, endocrine testing, ophthalmological (visual field and acuity) (Fig. 31.1) and rhinological assessment, and radiological investigations. MRI is the investigation of choice, because it provides better definition of tumors. Gadolinium is given to help identify the tumor, as well as to delineate adjacent vessels, indicating the proximity to the tumor of such para-sellar structures such as optic nerves, cavernous sinuses, and internal carotid arteries (Fig. 31.2).

CT scanning (with bone window, high-resolution coronal and axial scans, intravenous contrast, and three-dimensional reconstruction) is performed for sellar and

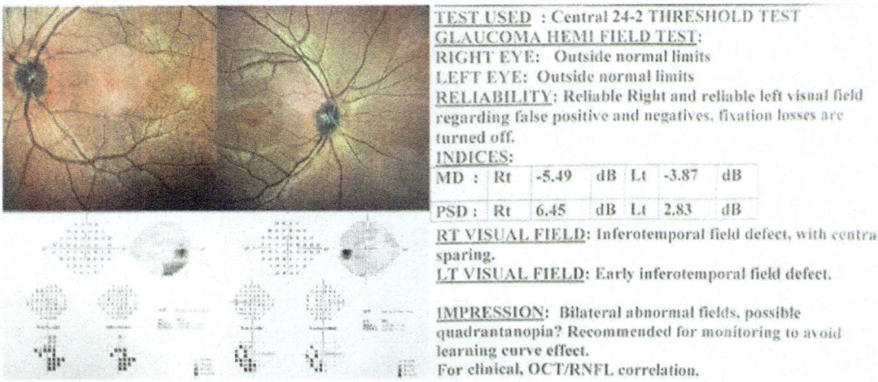


**Fig. 31.1** Preoperative fundus examination and perimetric assessment

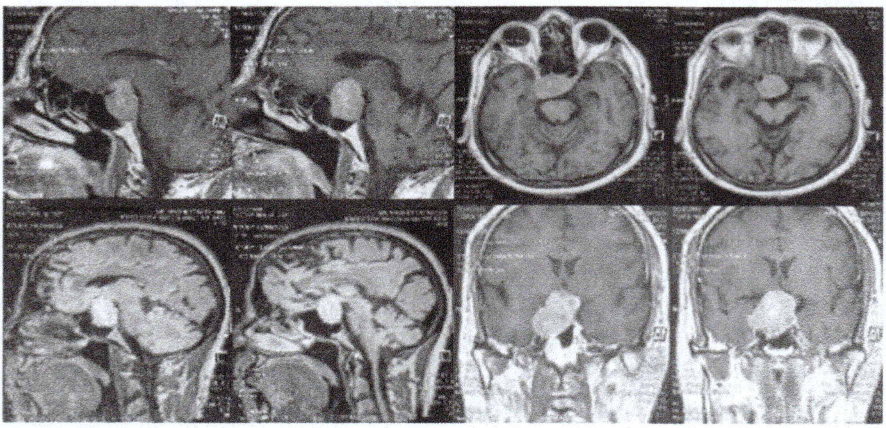

**Fig. 31.2** MRI assessment of sella

para-sellar surgery to view nasal cavities and paranasal sinuses. Also, CT scan images are useful to select the approach (right or left), to assess the pneumatization of the sphenoid, and the position of its septae.

### 31.2.4 Equipment

These require proper endoscopic equipment and specifically designed surgical tools. Endoscopes are rigid with 4 mm wide angle, 18 cm in length, and zero-, 30-, and 45-degree lenses, according to different steps of the surgical operation. High-definition camera monitor system. The use of the neuro-navigation system can be helpful to assist in the identification of the anatomic landmarks, particularly in patients with recurrent tumors [9, 10]. Surgical instruments including bayonet and straight instruments and curettes with different angled tips such that surgeons can manage all areas that become visible as a result of the wider view afforded by the endoscope (Fig. 31.3).

### 31.2.5 Standardized Surgical Technique

The operation is performed under general anesthesia with orotracheal intubation. Patients are placed supine, and their torso is elevated about 10–20° to reduce the venous pressure in the cavernous sinus. Patient's head is turned 10–20° in a horizontal plane toward the surgeon. Change of the head position and patient position may vary according to the extension and site of the lesion. We prepare the thigh or the abdomen for any fat graft needed for skull base repair [11]. The surgery is divided into 3 phases: nasal, sphenoid, and sellar.

#### 31.2.5.1 Nasal Phase

Adequate nasal vasoconstriction prior to surgery to ensure a minimal bleeding from nasal mucosa. The middle turbinate, the anterior wall of the sphenoid, and the rostrum are infiltrated with 1:200000 adrenaline. Cottonoids soaked in 1:10000 adrenaline or any topical nasal vasoconstrictor are then placed in the nose both sides [12]. Start with the wider side of the nasal cavity. Gentle lateral displacement or partial removal of the middle and superior turbinates is necessary to improve access (Fig. 31.4) [13].

#### 31.2.5.2 Sphenoid Phase

Once the sphenoid ostium is identified, coagulation of the mucosa of the anterior wall of the sphenoid sinus is performed. This serves to avoid arterial bleeding originating from septal branches of the sphenopalatine artery. The vomer is the landmark for the midline. Wide sphenoidotomy, removal of the anterior face of the sphenoid sinus on both sides, partial posterior septectomy, and removal of the rostrum. This is made with a microdrill or with Kerrison punches to allow a wide exposure and approach to work by both nostrils (4 hands technique). The

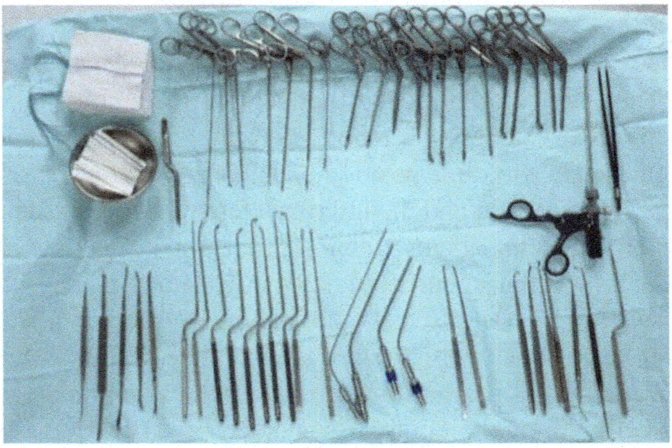

**Fig. 31.3** Equipment set

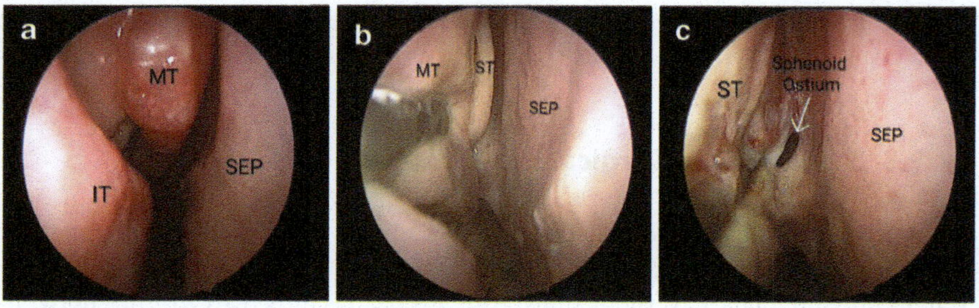


**Fig. 31.4** (**a**) Endoscopic view of nasal cavity showing inferior turbinate (IT), middle turbinate (MT), and septum (SEP), (**b**) Lateral displacement of MT to show superior turbinate (ST), (**c**) Lateralization of SP to show sphenoid ostium

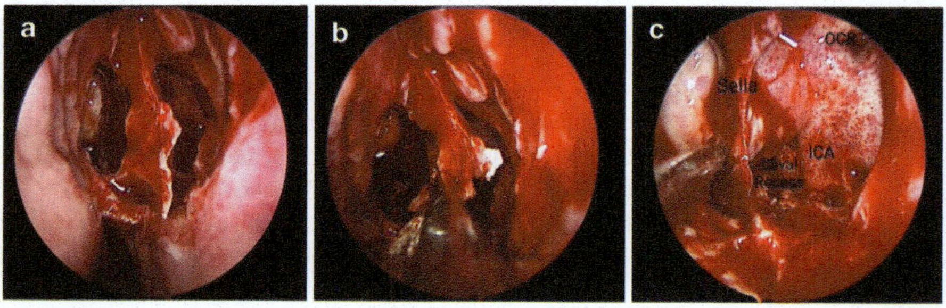


**Fig. 31.5** (**a**) "Owl eye" appearance of exposed sphenoid ostia with rostrum in-between, (**b**) Removing rostrum by Kerrison forceps, (**c**) Appearance of wide field after creating common sphenoid cavity

intra-sphenoid sinus septa can be identified inside the sphenoid sinus and removed cautiously when they are inserted in carotid or optic prominence, which can be determined by the preoperative CT scans. After wide exposure, the sellar floor, optic and carotid recesses, and clival recess are identified before opening the sellar floor [14]. In the presence of a pre-sellar or a conchal sphenoid sinus, there will be a paucity of anatomic landmarks. The neuronavigation system is very useful in these situations (Fig. 31.5).

#### 31.2.5.3 Sellar Phase

The opening of the sellar floor is performed with bone punchers or a microdrill and must be extended as required by the specific pathological process. The dura is incised in a midline position, in a linear, rectangular, or cruciate fashion (Fig. 31.6).

The superior and the inferior intercavernous sinuses are usually compressed and obliterated in patients with macroadenomas, making the dural incision bloodless; in microadenomas, and especially in Cushing disease, the entire sellar dura may be covered by one or two venous channels, which can bleed during the dural incision. To avoid this, these venous channels are sealed with bipolar coagulation forceps. The tumor is removed with ring curette. While the tumor tissue is curetted out, the shell of normal pituitary tissue is preserved along the tumor cavity [13].

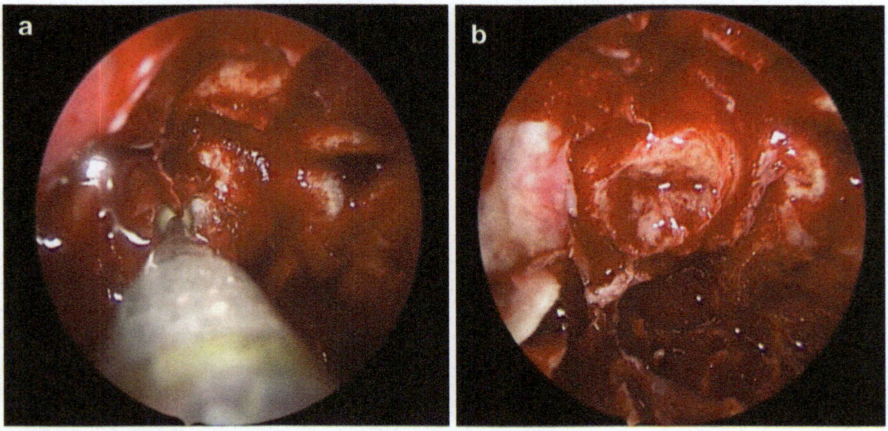


**Fig. 31.6** (**a**) Microdrill with diamond bur head used to drill sellar floor and cauterize dura, (**b**) Incised dura to reveal sellar mass

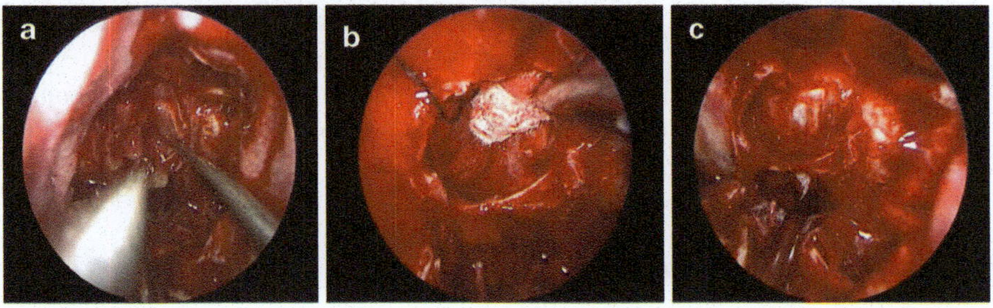


**Fig. 31.7** (**a**) Ring curette used to remove mass and biopsy taken by punch forceps, (**b**) Appearance after clearance of mass and capsule, (**c**) Arachnoid cistern protruding into sellar cavity

Tumor dissection starts from the inferior part and then the lateral part of the tumor followed by the upper part to prevent descent of the diaphragm sella, which can obscure the surgical filed. An angled endoscopes can be used to allow visualization behind the corners to remove any tumor remnants. Also, tumor extension to the cavernous sinus is sometimes difficult and venous bleeding might occur, which can be controlled by hemostatic substances and cottonoids and by gentle compressing the medial wall of cavernous sinus and irrigating for a few minutes.

After tumor removal, if the descent of the suprasellar portion of the lesion is not observed, it is useful to perform a Valsalva maneuver, which may encourage protrusion of the suprasellar cistern into the sellar cavity. After intracapsular emptying of the tumor, its pseudocapsule can be dissected from the suprasellar cistern. Attention must be taken not to rupture the arachnoid membrane that prevents cerebrospinal fluid (CSF) leak (Fig. 31.7).

At the end of the procedure, hemostasis is obtained, irrigation is performed, and the endoscope is removed gradually. Generally, the sphenoid sinus is maintained empty without any foreign materials inside it or may be filled with gel-foam and/or

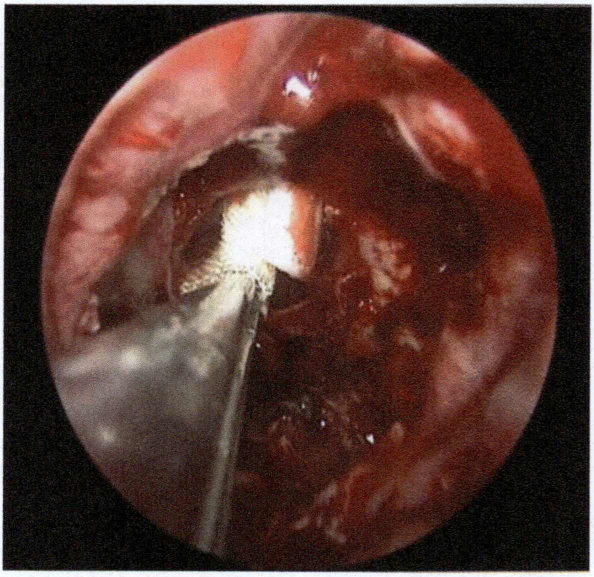

**Fig. 31.8** Gelfoam and Surgicel packing of sellar cavity to conclude surgery and hemostat

Surgicel. The middle turbinate is gently restored in a medial direction, and contact with nasal septum is avoided to prevent the formation of synechiae. Packing of the nasal cavity for a few hours is not considered necessary [11] (Fig. 31.8).

### 31.2.6 Postoperative Care

The use of the saline wash 3–4 times a day decreases nasal crusting and prevents synechiae. An antibiotic ointment is also used once daily for 1 month for local applications in the nasal cavity. Patients are kept for 2 weeks on third-generation cephalosporin (2 g/day) [13, 15].

Postoperative risk for diabetes insipidus is high, so the patients are observed in a regular hospital room for 2 days [16]. The electrolytes are measured after the operation and the next morning [15]. An endocrinological evaluation is necessary after surgery to keep postoperative hormonal balance especially that of cortisol and thyroid hormones. If patients develop CSF leak postoperatively, it should be repaired if it not stopped within 7 days. MRI is done for postoperative control after 3 months (Fig. 31.9).

**Fig. 31.9** Appearance after full healing

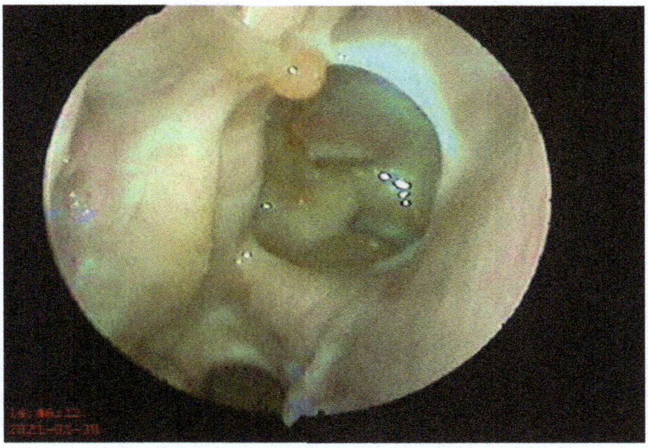

## 31.3 Surgical Complications After Endoscopic Transsphenoidal Pituitary Surgery

A. *Nasal Complications*
  (i) Nasal septum perforation (0.3–3%)
  (ii) Septal abscess and saddle nose
  (iii) Anesthesia of upper lip
  (iv) Anosmia caused by undue superior nasal septum dissection
  (v) CSF fluid leakage and meningitis
  (vi) Bleeding from the sphenopalatine artery and from the mucosal branches [17–20, 21–25].

B. *Sphenoid Sinus Complications*
  (i) Mucocele
  (ii) Sinusitis
  (iii) Fracture of the sphenoid bone with injuries of the supra or para-sellar neurovascular structures [19, 20, 23, 26, 27].

C. *Intrasellar Complications*

Subarachnoid hemorrhage, vasospasm, tension pneumocephalus, rupture of carotid artery aneurysm, and CSF leakage [17].

D. *Endocrine Complications*

Anterior pituitary and posterior pituitary insufficiency ranges between 7% and 10% [18, 28, 29, 30].

Reduction of complication rates can be achieved by:

1. Preoperative good study of the radiological imaging
2. Multidisciplinary team workup protocol before surgery
3. Better visualization of the anatomical landmarks especially when changing the endoscopic optic systems (0 °, 30 °, and 70°) for better distinction between the tumor tissue, the normal pituitary tissue, and the diaphragma.

4. Gentle usage of curved instruments and suction devices to remove tumor tissue
5. Better identification of intra-operative CSF leakages.

## References


1. Kirgis HD, Locke W. Anatomy and embryology. In: Locke W, Schally AV, editors. The hypothalamus and pituitary in health and disease. Springfield, IL: Charles C. Thomas; 1972. p. 3–65.
2. Hammer G, Radburg C. The sphenoidal sinus: an anatomical and roentgenologic study with reference to transsphenoidal hypophysectomy. Acta Radiol. 1961;56:401–22.
3. Bergland RM, Ray BS, Torack RM. Anatomical variations in the pituitary gland and adjacent-structures in 225 human autopsy cases. J Neurosurg. 1968;28:93–9.
4. Bull JWD, Schunk H. The significance of displacement of the cavernous portion of the internal carotid artery. Br J Radiol. 1962;35:801–14.
5. Goudakos JK, Markou KD, Georgalas C. Endoscopic versus microscopic trans-sphenoidal pituitary surgery: a systematic review and meta-analysis. Clin Otolaryngol. 2011;36(3):212–20.
6. Leach P, Abou-Zeid AH, Kearney T, Davis J, Trainer PJ, Gnanalingham KK. Endoscopic transsphenoidal pituitary surgery: evidence of an operative learning curve. Neurosurgery. 2010;67(5):1205–12.
7. Bansal KK, Gupta C, Varshney S, Kukreti R, Gupta A. Visual deterioration after trans-sphenoidal surgery for pituitary adenoma- a rare but severe complication: case report with review of literature (case report). Indian J Otolaryngol and Head Neck Surg (special issue). 2005:179–81.
8. Park J, Guthikonda M. The Medpor sheet as a sellar buttress after endonasal transsphenoidal surgery: technical note. Surg Neurol. 2004;61:488–93.
9. Kawamata T, Iseki H, Shibasaki T, Hori T. Endoscopic augmented reality navigation system for endonasal transsphenoidal surgery to treat pituitary tumors: technical note. Neurosurgery. 2002;50(6):1393–7.
10. Lasio G, Ferroli P, Felisati G, Broggi G. Imageguided endoscopic transnasal removal of recurrent pituitary adenomas. Neurosurgery. 2002;51(1):132–7.
11. Cappabianca P, Cavallo LM, De Divitiis E. Endoscopic endonasal transsphenoidal surgery. Neurosurgery. 2004;55(4):933–41.
12. Pell MF, Atlas MD, Biggs ND. Endoscopic pituitary tumor removal. In: Kaye AH, Black PM, editors. Operative neurosurgery. London: Churchill Livingstone; 2000. p. 715–22.
13. Jho HD, Alfieri A. Endoscopic endonasal pituitary surgery: evolution of surgical technique and equipment in 150 operations. Minim Invasive Neurosurg. 2001;44:1–12.
14. Rhoton AL, Harris FS, Renn WH. Microsurgical anatomy of the Sella region and cavernous sinus. Clin Neurosurg. 1977;24:54–85.
15. Mortini P, Losa M, Barzaghi R, Boari N, Giovanelli M. Results of transsphenoidal surgery in a large series of patients with pituitary adenoma. Neurosurgery. 2005;56:1222–33.
16. Jho HD, Carrau RL. Endoscopic endonasal transsphenoidal surgery: experience with 50 patients. J Neurosurg. 1997;87:44–51.
17. Ciric I, Ragin A, Baumgartner C, et al. Complications of transsphenoidal surgery: results of a national survey, review of the literature, and personal experience. Neurosurgery. 1997;40:225–36; discussion 236–237.
18. Frank G, Pasquini E, Farneti G, et al. The endoscopic versus the traditional approach in pituitary surgery. Neuroendocrinology. 2006;83:240–8.
19. Black PM, Zervas NT, Candia GL. Incidence and management of complications of transsphenoidal operation for pituitary adenomas. Neurosurgery. 1987;20:920–4.

20. Laws ER Jr, Kern EB. Complications of trans-sphenoidal surgery. Clin Neurosurg. 1976;23:401–16.
21. Wilson CB, Dempsey LC. Transsphenoidal microsurgical removal of 250 pituitary adenomas. J Neurosurg. 1978;48:13–22.
22. Kennedy DW, Cohn ES, Papel ID, et al. Transsphenoidal approach to the Sella: the John Hopkins experience. Laryngoscope. 1984;94:1066–74.
23. Barrow DL, Tindall GT. Loss of vision after transsphenoidal surgery. Neurosurgery. 1990;27:60–8.
24. Newmark H 3rd, Kant N, Duerksen R, et al. Orbital floor fracture: an unusual complication of trans-septal trans-sphenoidal hypophysectomy. Neurosurgery. 1983;12:555–6.
25. Cockroft KM, Carew JF, Trost D, et al. Delayed epistaxis resulting from external carotid artery injury requiring embolization: a rare complication of transsphenoidal surgery: case report. Neurosurgery. 2000;47:236–9.
26. Herman P, Lot G, Guichard JP, et al. Mucocele of the sphenoid sinus: a late complication of transsphenoidal pituitary surgery. Ann Otol Rhinol Laryngol. 1998;107:765–8.
27. Kessler L, Legaludec V, Dietemann JL, et al. Sphenoidal sinus mucocele after transsphenoidal surgery for acromegaly. Neurosurg Rev. 1999;22:222–5.
28. Semple PL, Laws ER Jr. Complications in a contemporary series of patients who underwent transsphenoidal surgery for Cushing's disease. J Neurosurg. 1999;91:175–9.
29. Laws ER Jr, Thapar K. Pituitary surgery. Endocrinol Metab Clin N Am. 1999;28:119–31.
30. Zada G, Kelly DF, Cohan P, et al. Endonasal transsphenoidal approach for pituitary adenomas and other sellar lesions: an assessment of efficacy, safety, and patient impressions. J Neurosurg. 2003;98:350–8.

# Endoscopic Approaches of Anterior Skull Base

# 32

Mostafa Ismail

**Key Points**

- Skull base forms the floor of the cranial cavity and separates the brain from other facial structures The skull base can be primarily divided into midline and lateral skull base. Midline skull base can be furtherly subdivided into three parts: the anterior, middle, and posterior parts.
- The transnasal endoscopic skull base surgery has undergone rapid advancement over the past several years. A wide range of anatomic regions and pathologies can be approached by the appropriate endoscopic approach.
- Surgical treatment of benign lesions via the endoscope has largely gained acceptance; however, its role in malignant lesions remains controversial. In this chapter, we review the transnasal endoscopic approaches to anterior part of midline skull base including the transcribriform, the transtuberculum transplanum, transellar, and transsellar transdiaphragmatic approaches.

## 32.1 Introduction

The concept of transnasal skull base surgery was credited to the ancient Egyptians, who were experts in using the sphenoethmoidal breach approach in the mummification process [1, 2]. A similar route through the sphenoid sinus has been developed and firstly proposed more than a century ago and was restricted to the treatment of tumors of the pituitary region [3, 4]. The progressive evolution in neuronavigation

**Supplementary Information** The online version contains supplementary material available at https://doi.org/10.1007/978-3-031-70077-4_32.

M. Ismail (✉)
Otolaryngology Department, Minia University, Minia, Egypt


S. Elwany (ed.), *Current Rhinology*,
https://doi.org/10.1007/978-3-031-70077-4_32

systems, the anatomical understanding, in addition to wide-angled endoscopes this approach was extended to entire midline skull base, from the crista galli to the odontoid process [5, 6]. In contrast to traditional skull base surgical approaches, the endoscopic endonasal approach offers a direct midline access to the suprasellar, retrosellar, and retroclival spaces. It avoids brain retraction and provides excellent visualization of all structure, and as a result, it offers a lower morbidity and mortality rate when compared to transcranial procedures [7].

## 32.2 Anatomy of the Anterior Skull Base

Understanding the endoscopic endonasal and endocranial anatomy of the ASB region is crucial for mastering the endoscopic endonasal approach to the area. As mentioned previously, skull base can be primarily divided into midline and lateral skull base. Midline skull base can be furtherly subdivided into three parts: the anterior, middle, and posterior parts.

From the endonasal perspective, ASB represents the part of skull base that forms the roof of ethmoids extending anteriorly to the floor and posterior border of the frontal sinus and extending posteriorly to the roof and posterior wall of the sphenoid sinus. In the center of this region is the cribriform plate on both sides, through which the olfactory tracts pass and in between the crista galli projects up centrally between the cerebral hemispheres [8]. The orbits and frontal bones form the lateral boundaries of the ASB.

From the endonasal perspective, ASB corresponds the sellar-suprasellar parachiasmatic cisterns that formed by three main cisterns; chiasmatic, suprachiasmatic, and subchiasmatic cisterns. Chiasmatic cisterns includes optic chiasm, pituitary gland, and both superior hypophyseal arteries. Suprachiasmatic cistern is formed by two cisterns; the lower one named lamina terminalis cistern that includes the A1 and A2 segments of the anterior cerebral artery, the anterior communicating artery (ACoA), and the recurrent artery of Heubner; the upper one named pericallosal cistern that includes the origin of the orbitofrontal and sometimes the frontopolar arteries. Subchiasmatic cistern has medial and lateral parts. The medial part is formed by two cisterns; interpeduncular cistern superiorly that includes the basilar artery (BA), the posterior communicating artery (PCoA), P1 and beginning of the P2 segments of the posterior cerebral artery (PCA), and the oculomotor nerve; and the prepontine cistern inferiorly that includes the superior cerebellar artery (SCA), BA, pontine perforators, and pons. The lateral part is formed by four cisterns; the carotid cistern anteromedial that includes the supraclinoid ICA, PCoA, anterior choroidal artery (AChA), and infundibular arteries; the sylvian cistern posteromedial that includes the initial part of the M1 segment and the posterior part of medial orbital gyri; the crural cistern anterolateral that includes the optic tract, the posterior segment and apex of uncus and the anterolateral surface of the cerebral peduncle, anterior choroidal artery, and origin of the P2 segment of PCA; and the ambient cistern posterolateral that includes the anterior P2 segment of the PCA and midbrain [9] (Fig. 32.1).

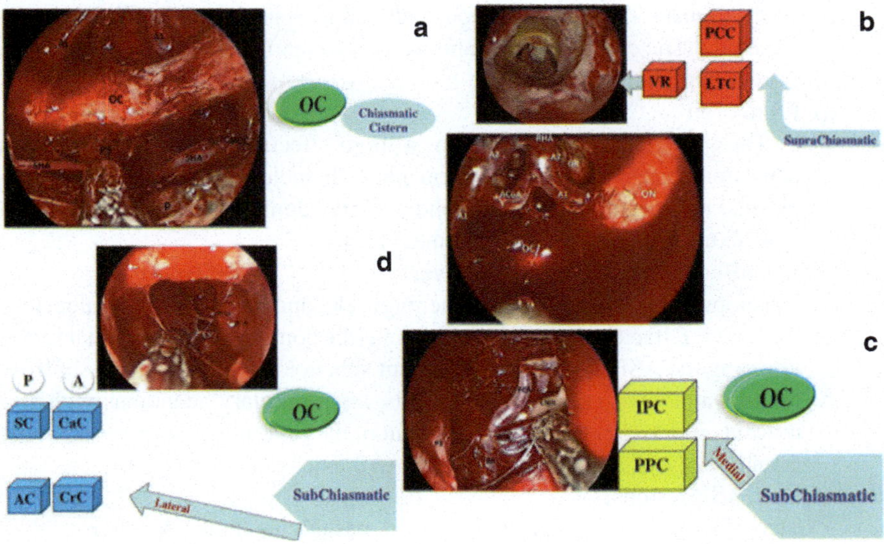


**Fig. 32.1** Endoscopic anatomy of the sellar-suprasellar parachiasmatic cisterns. (**a**) Chiasmatic cistern: OC optic chiasm, SHA superior hypophyseal artery, P pituitary gland, PS pituitary stalk. (**b**) Suprachiasmatic cisterns: LTC lamina terminalis cistern, A1, A2 segments of the anterior cerebral artery, ACoA anterior communicating artery, RHA recurrent artery of Heubner, PCC pericallosal cistern, VR third ventricle recess. (**c**) Medial part of subchiasmatic cistern: IPC interpeduncular cistern, BA basilar artery, PCA posterior cerebral artery, CNIII oculomotor nerve, PPC prepontine cistern, SCA superior cerebellar artery. (**d**) Lateral part of subchiasmatic cistern: CaC carotid cistern, SC sylvian cistern, CrC crural cistern, AC ambient cistern

## 32.3 Anterior Skull Base Pathologies

The anterior skull base (ASB) is bounded laterally by the orbital plates of the frontal bone, medially by the cribriform plate and crista galli, and anteriorly by the lesser wings of the sphenoid bone and sellar floor posteriorly. ASB may be involved by lesions arising from the nasal cavity, paranasal sinuses, orbits, and intracranial compartment. Pathology involving the ASB is subdivided into lesions intrinsic to the skull base and lesions extending from below (nasal cavity, paranasal sinuses, and orbits) or above (intracranial compartment) [10].

1. **Lesions affecting the ASB from below:**
   (i) From sinonasal cavity

   Pathological processes extending from the sinonasal region are the most common due to the thin barrier of the cribriform plate. It includes:

   A. Benign Lesions: Mucoceles, complicated rhinosinusitis, invasive fungal sinusitis, Wegener's granulomatosis, inverted papilloma, olfactory neuroblastoma, and juvenile angiofibroma.

B. Malignant Tumors: Squamous cell carcinomas, adenocarcinomas, adenoid cystic carcinoma, melanoma, undifferentiated carcinoma, sarcoma, and lymphoma.

(ii) From orbit

The thick orbital roof serves as a more effective barrier to intracranial extension than does the cribriform plate. It includes lacrimal gland neoplasms, neurogenic tumors, lymphomas, rhabdomyosarcomas, and chloromas (extramedullary myeloblastomas) [11].

2. **Lesions affecting the ASB from above:**
   (i) Developmental: Nasal gliomas, meningocele, and meningoencephaloceles.
   (ii) Acquired: Olfactory groove meningioma (the commonest intracranial lesion affecting the ASB from above), planum sphenoidale meningioma, subfrontal schwannomas, craniopharyngiomas, large pituitary adenomas with significant suprasellar and ASB extension, large Rathke cleft cysts, large arachnoid cysts, and chordomas with ASB extension.
3. **Intrinsic ASB lesions:**

   Osteomas are the commonest benign sinonasal bone tumor, and fibrous dysplasia frequently involves the ASB, aneurysmal bone cysts, primary ASB malignancies (mainly, osteosarcoma in adults and rhabdomyosarcoma in children), and metastases to the ASB are usually from breast and lung primaries [12].

## 32.4 Operative Techniques

Endoscopic endonasal transsphenoidal surgery (EETS) is not a one man show, but it needs constant collaboration between the neurosurgeon and the ENT surgeon even, for straightforward trans-sellar approaches. Endonasal structural variations have a practical significance during endoscopic endonasal approaches, so the preoperative assessment of these variations and how to precisely manage is important for minimizing the potential for perioperative surgical complications. Furthermore, the stepwise surgical approach to sphenoid sinus has demonstrated the significance of collaborative intervention into such surgical approaches of challenging anatomy [13].

In all ASB approaches, the endoscopic dissection is performed using endoscopic sinus surgery instruments with the guidance of 18-cm-long rigid endoscope with 4-mm diameter that is used for standard endoscopic sinus surgery. A light source and a digital video camera are connected to the endoscope, and images are displayed on a monitor to enable dissection.

Five waypoints should be initially followed in all ASB approaches [14]. The first waypoint is the identification of the sphenoid sinus ostium that is started with introduction of the endoscope through the right nostril. The posteroinferior part of the middle turbinate is dislocated laterally to widen the space between the middle turbinate and nasal septum. The endoscope then is angled rostrally, along the roof of the choana and the sphenoethmoidal recess, following the posteroinferior end of both middle and superior turbinates till reaching sphenoid ostium with gentile lateralization of the superior turbinate. The same procedure was repeated on the left side.

The second waypoint is the posterior septectomy that is started after identification of the sphenoid cavity, and the nasal septum is separated from the sphenoid rostrum with removal of the posterior portion of the nasal septum (about 1.5–2 cm) to allow a wide binasal approach. The nasal mucosa is detached from the vomer, anterior and inferior walls of the sphenoidal sinus, and then dissected laterally; this represents the third waypoint. A total sphenoidotomy is the fourth waypoint that means removal of the whole anterior wall of the sphenoid sinus. After removal of the inter-sphenoid sinus septum/ septa, the posterior and lateral walls of the sphenoid sinus are now visible and allowing the identification of all intrasphenoidal bony landmarks; with the sellar floor at the center, tuberculum sellae and sphenoidal planum above it, the intra-sphenoidal clival recess below, and laterally, the upper (parasellar) and lower (infrasellar) carotid prominences as well as the optic prominence can be seen with the lateral optic-carotid recess in between, this the fifth waypoint (Fig. 32.2). In cases in which a cerebrospinal fluid (CSF) leak is expected, a nasoseptal flap is elevated during the initial stage of the procedure.

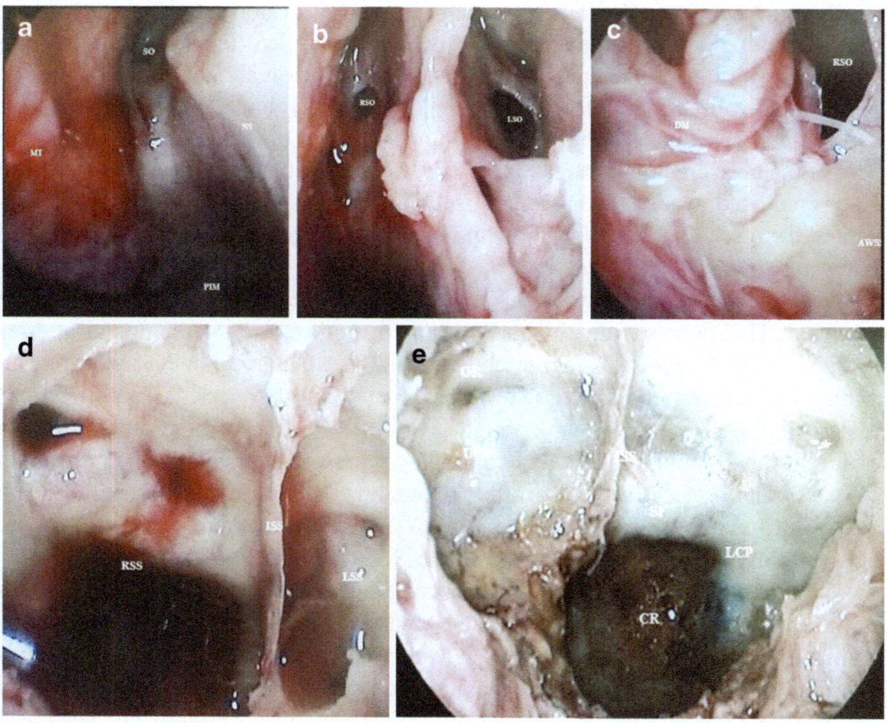


**Fig. 32.2** Five waypoints in ASB approaches. (**a**) First waypoint: Idntification of sphenoid ostium; SO, sphenoid ostium, MT middle turbinate, NS, nasal septum. (**b**) Second waypoint: Posterior septectomy: RSO right sphenoid ostium, LSO left sphenoid ostium. (**c**) Third waypoint: DM dissected mucosa, AWS anterior wall of sphenoid sinus. (**d**) Fourth waypoint: Total sphenoidotomy ISS, intersphenoid sinus septum. (**e**) Fifth waypoint: SF sellar floor, CR clival recess, OR optic recess, UCP upper carotid process, UCP lower carotid process, * Lateral opticocarotid recess (LOCR).

Four surgical approaches of the ASB will be described from anterior to posterior as following: the transcribriform approach, the transtuberculum transplanum approach, the transsellar approach, and the transsellar transdiaphragmatic approach.

1. **The Transcribriform Approach**

This approach is indicated for resection of olfactory neuroblastoma, olfactory groove meningiomas, and sinonasal tumors invading the ASB.

The transcribriform approach is defined by the approach that involves removal of the cribriform plate and ABS to access the anterior cranial fossa through a nasoethmoidal corridor. This approach extends from the posterior ethmoidal arteries and planum sphenoidale posteriorly up to the level of the crista galli and frontal sinuses anteriorly. The lamina papyracea limits this approach laterally [6, 15]. This approach can be performed unilaterally or bilaterally, according to the lesion nature. The unilateral approach is indicated for meningocele and meningoencephaloceles, whereas the bilateral approach is required for tumors.

The bilateral transcribriform approach is started by performing bilateral transnasal transethmoidal corridors involving bilateral complete anterior/posterior ethmoidectomy, bilateral sphenoidectomy, and bilateral frontal sinusotomy. This step is followed by doing submucosal resection of the cartilaginous septum and superior septectomy that it means removal of the upper third of the septal attachment to the roof of the nose creating a single, large cavity. Usually, the middle turbinate of right side is removed, while it is only lateralized on the left side [7]. For more wide exposure of the ASB, a bilateral frontal Draf III sinusotomy and the previously described five waypoints were performed.

To facilitate the drilling of this bone, all the overlying soft tissue must be removed. This consists identification of anterior and posterior ethmoidal arteries that should be coagulated and transected; then, the olfactory filaments entering and exiting the crista galli should also be coagulated and transected. The cribriform plate is removed bilaterally with a high-speed drill starting at the posterior portion of the frontoethmoidal recess and continues posteriorly to the sphenoid sinus and till the border between the cribriform plate and the lamina papyracea laterally. The crista galli is then drilled out in the midline and then fracture once it has become eggshell thin. This will create a large single cavity along the ASB [6] (Fig. 32.3).

The exposed dura mater is thoroughly coagulated and then opened on both sides of the falx keeping it intact in the midline, and this will allow exposure of the intracranial contents. If an olfactory groove meningioma is being removed, extracapsular dissection is pursued using gentle countertraction and sharp dissection and internal tumor debulking is sequentially performed on each side. For sinonasal pathologies, it is often necessary to combine this approach with other such as the transpterygoid or transorbital approaches to ensure gross total resection. For the potential intradural invasion, the coagulated dura is incised lateral to the tumor and resected with the residual tumor. Particularly for olfactory neuroblastomas, the olfactory bulbs should also be resected [16] (Fig. 32.4).

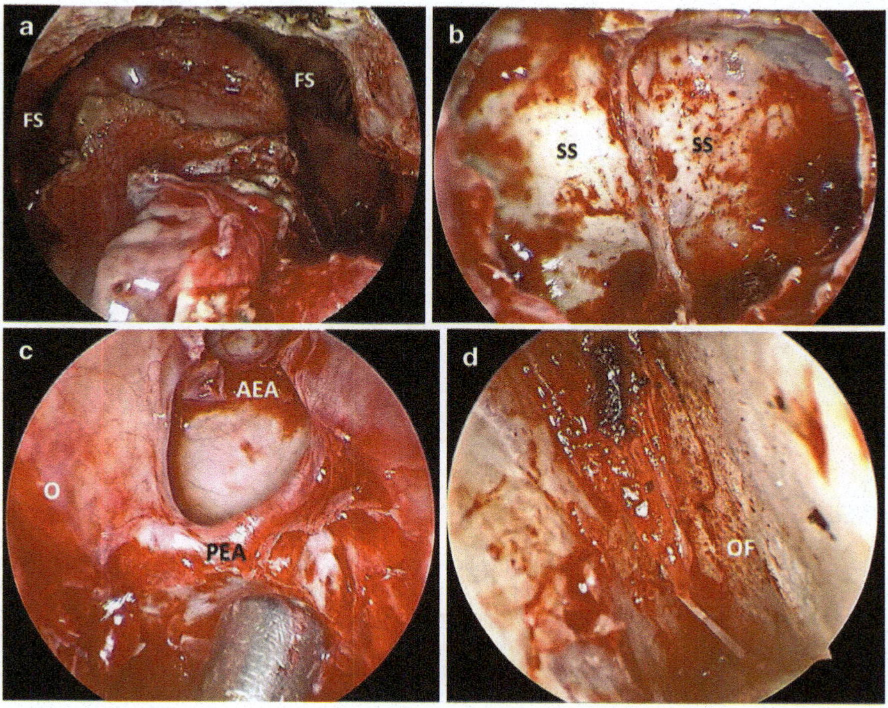


**Fig. 32.3** Endoscopic transcribriform approach started by doing (**a**) bilateral frontal Draf III sinusotomy, FS frontal sinus, followed by (**b**) bilateral sphenoidectomy, SS sphenoid sinus, followed by removal of the overlaying soft tissues in form of (**c**) coagulation of bilateral anterior ethmoidal arteries (AEA) and posterior ethmoidal arteries (PEA) then, (**d**) transection of the olfactory filaments (OF) entering and exiting the cribriform plate

The defect in the ASB may be quite large, and our preferred closure is the "gasket-seal closure" using three layers of fascia lata. First layer should be larger than the defect and placed intradural, the second layer placed extradural between dura and bone of skull base, and the last layer placed over the bony defect to cover the previous layers. A piece of bone is cut to fit the defect is placed and wedged in place over the last layer of facia lata (Fig. 32.4). Others prefer the combined gasket-seal closure with a nasoseptal vascularized flap [17].

2. **The Transtuberculum Transplanum Approach**

This approach is indicated for resection of suprasellar meningiomas, craniopharyngiomas, and pituitary macroadenomas with extensive suprasellar.

The transtuberculum transplanum approach is defined by the approach designed to access to the suprasellar region and the sphenoid planum that need a more anterior trajectory compared with the one used to reach the sellar region. This approach is started by performing the previously described five waypoints approach to sphenoid sinus [14]. This route requires a wider opening of the anterior wall of the

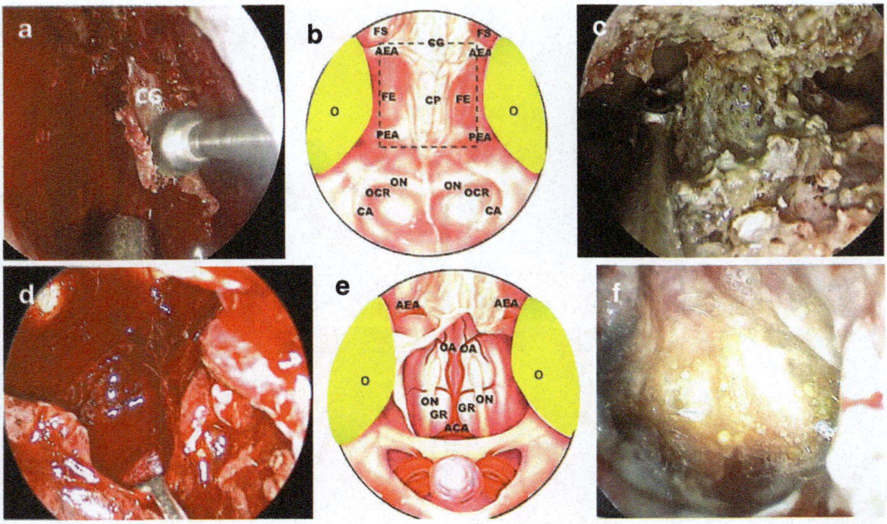


**Fig. 32.4** Endoscopic transcribriform approach (**a**–**c**) Bone drilling started by removal of both cribriform plates, drilling of crista galli (CG), and then drilling skull base bone line by dotted square stated from the lower portion of the posterior wall of frontal sinus to the sphenoid sinus and laterally till the border between the cribriform plate and the lamina papyracea. (**d**, **e**) The exposed dura mater is then opened on both sides of the falx, O orbit, ON olfactory nerve, GR gyrus rectus, ACA anterior cerebral artery. (**d**) Skull base reconstruction using three layers of fascia lata

sphenoidal sinus that is obtained by completing wide anterior and posterior ethmoidectomies [6].

Once inside the sphenoid sinus, sellar floor is removed, using a microdrill, and bony exposure is maximized by uncovering the medial borders of the cavernous sinuses. The optimal exposure usually includes bone removal of tuberculum sellae and planum sphenoidale that is firstly thinned down and is then removed carefully using a Kerrison's rongeur. Lateral limits of bone removal are the medial opticocarotid recess (MOCR) at the tuberculum sellae level, while the optic canals mark the lateral limits of bone removal at the planum sphenoidale. Removal of bone over the MOCR is important for widening the intradural exposure [7, 18].

The dura is opened with two incisions immediately superior and inferior to the SIS. The SIS was coagulated divided to obtain access to the suprasellar cistern. The upper and lower incisions were extended over the tuberculum/planum and sellar dura, respectively, in the midline (Fig. 32.5).

Extra-capsular tumor dissection is initiated by a sharp opening of the arachnoid layer of the suprasellar cistern, and the tumor dissection is proceeded. Care must be exercised to identify the pituitary stalk and the superior hypophyseal arteries as early as possible. Tumor dissection was continued on each side of the tumor laterally until the opticocarotid cistern was entered and then superiorly using a 45° endoscope with an extra care should be taken during dissection of the tumor component that in contact with the anterior part of the circle of Willis. In tumors with huge SSE

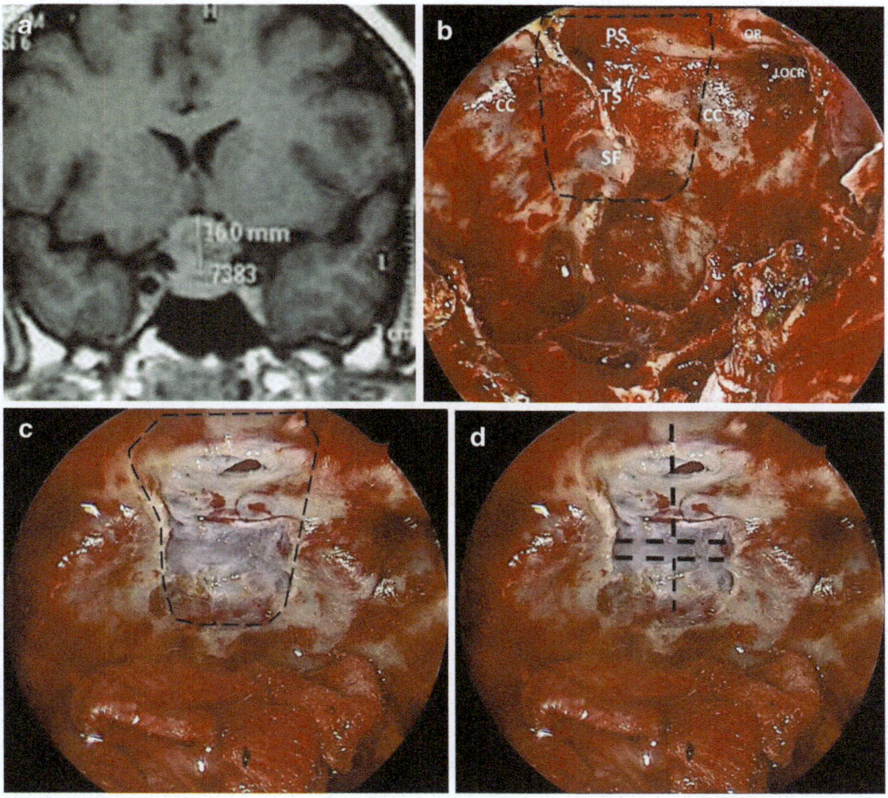


**Fig. 32.5** Endoscopic transtuberculum transplanum approach. (**a**) MRI shows suprasellar meningioma. (**b**) Bone drilling SF sellar floor, TS tuberculum sellae, PS planum sphenoidal, LOCR lateral opticocarotid recess, CC cavernous carotid, OR optic recess. (**c**) After bone drilling. (**d**) Dural opening, 2 horizontal incisions above and below coagulated SIS, 2 vertical incisions

up to the floor of the third ventricle, tumor dissection was continued posteriorly using 45° and 70° endoscopes [18, 19] (Fig. 32.6).

A multi-layered reconstruction was of critical importance to achieve a watertight closure. A piece of autologous fat was placed in the sellar cavity, followed by a layer of fascia lata placed over the bone defect and was tucked in place using a piece of bone obtained from the nasal septum. The final layer of the vascularized nasoseptal flap was then rotated to cover the entire defect with a thin layer of fibrin glue over the flap edges (Fig. 32.7.).

3. **Transsellar Approach**

This approach is indicated for resection of most of pituitary macroadenomas, Rathke's cleft cysts, and arachnoid cysts.

This approach is started by performing the previously described five waypoints approach to sphenoid sinus. Bone over the sellar face should be removed laterally

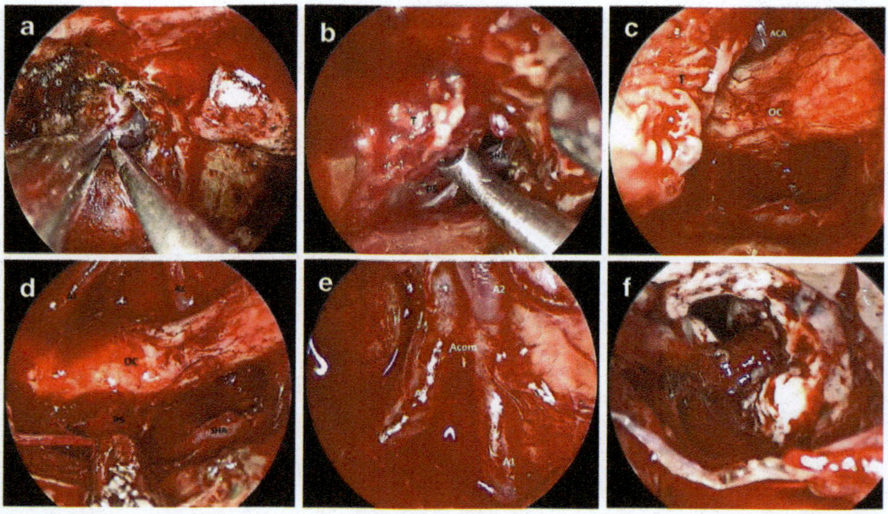


**Fig. 32.6** Extra-capsular tumor dissection in endoscopic transtuberculum transplanum approach. (**a**) Sharp opening of arachnoid layer of suprasellar cistern D dura, AR arachnoid matter, (**b**) subchiasmatic tumor dissection from pituitary stalk and the superior hypophyseal arteries T tumor, PS pituitary stalk, SHA superior hypophyseal artery, (**c**) tumor dissection continued laterally until the opticocarotid cistern OC optic chiasm, ACA anterior cerebral artery, (**d**) after complete subchiasmatic and suprachiasmatic tumor dissection A1 segment of anterior cerebral artery (**e**, **f**) angled endoscopic view showing; (**e**) superior part of circle of Willis A2 segment of anterior cerebral artery, AcoA anterior communicating artery (**f**) anterior recess of third ventricle

beyond the medial portions of the cavernous sinus and expose both the superior and inferior intercavernous sinuses creating a single large rectangular cavity within the sphenoid sinus.

After cauterization of sellar dura, it is opened widely in a cruciate fashion using a sickle knife. For resection of pituitary macroadenomas, systematic intrasellar dissection of the adenoma is mandatory using a piecemeal technique keeping the superior part of the adenoma as a last part to be removed. Resection of the suprasellar components is achieved following its spontaneous descent into the pituitary fossa in most cases that may be facilitated by enhancement of the intracranial venous pressure by Valsalva maneuver. At the end of the procedure, the integrity of the diaphragm sellae and arachnoid membrane is inspected for CSF leakage using angled endoscopes.

Sellar reconstruction at the completion of the procedure is based on CSF leakage. If there is no evident intraoperative CSF leakage, sellar reconstruction is performed by either intrasellar packing using hemostatic materials or keeping the sellar fossa empty without any packing. When an intraoperative CSF leakage is evident, intrasellar abdominal fat packing is performed [20] (Fig. 32.8.).

4. **Transsellar Transdiaphragmatic Approach**

This approach is indicated for resection of pituitary macroadenomas with extensive suprasellar.

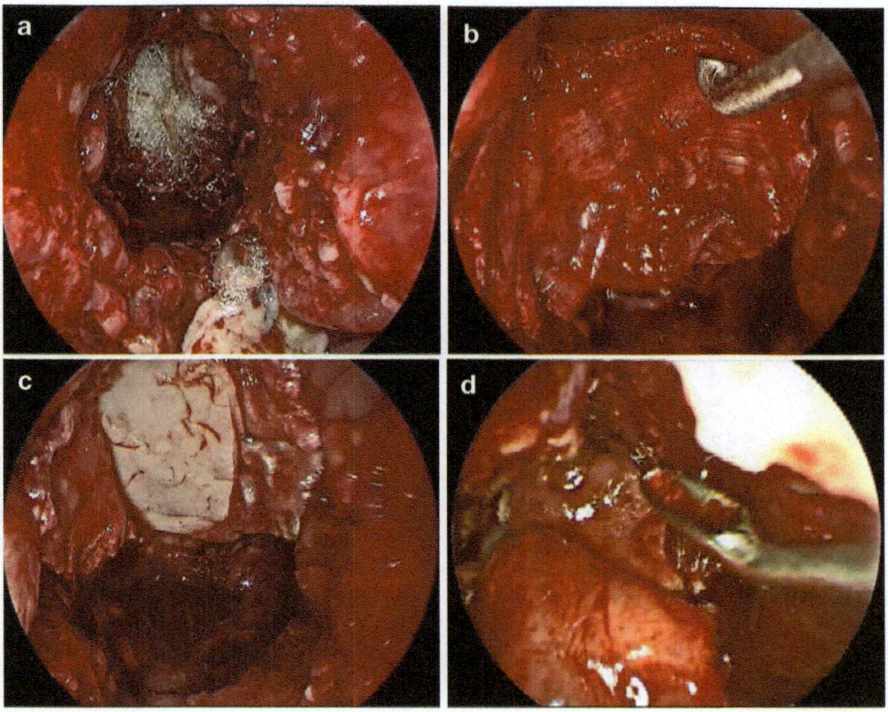


**Fig. 32.7.** Multilayer reconstruction after endoscopic transtuberculum transplanum approach. (**a**) Filling defect by a layer of fibrillar. (**b**) First layer is fascia lata. (**c**) Second layer is piece of bone from the nasal septum. (**d**) Vascularized nasoseptal flap

The transsellar transdiaphragmatic approach is defined by the approach designed to access to the suprasellar region from a posterior trajectory from inside the sellar cavity by breaching the posterior border of the diaphragma sellae. This approach was described, two decades prior; however, it was rapidly regressed in favor of the transtuberculum transplanum approach, mainly due to the inadequate angled illumination of the surgical field allowed by the microscopes and endoscopes of that time [21]. Taking advantage of the further push came from the continuous evolution of visualization and instrumentations; our, Ismail et al.'s group tried to reuse this technique, again, for extra-capsular resection of pituitary macroadenomas with extensive SSE [18].

The approach is started by performing the previously described five waypoints approach to sphenoid sinus. Then, a total sphenoidotomy is performed followed by removal of sellar floor between four blue lines. The central portion of the tuberculum sellae is thinned out and cautiously dissected from the undelaying dura so as not to injure the superior intercavernous sinus (SIS). Removal of a central 1 cm of the planum sphenoidal may be added, anteriorly, in cases with huge SSE. Then, the sellar dura is opened widely in a cruciate fashion using a sickle knife. Care should

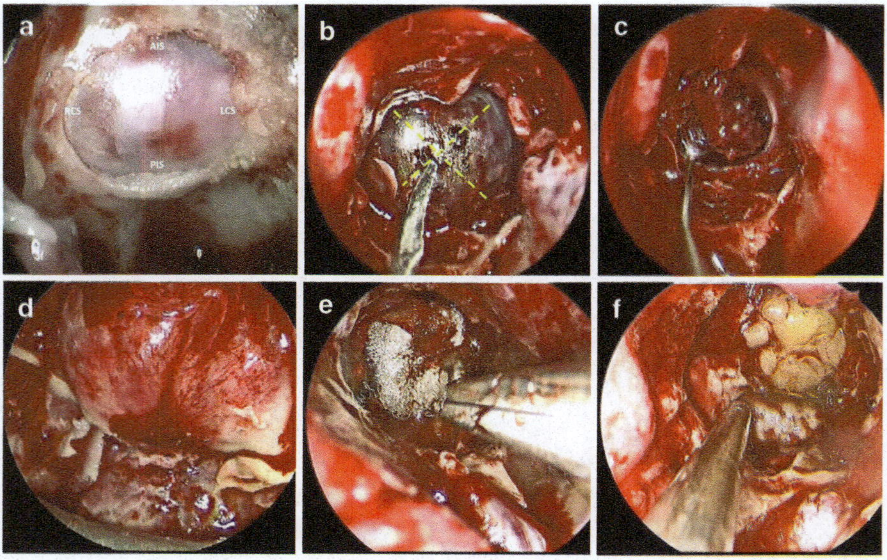


**Fig. 32.8.** Endoscopic transsellar approach. (**a**) Bone drilling, CS cavernous sinus, AIS anterior intercavernous sinus, PICS posterior intercavernous sinus, (**b**) dural opening, (**c**) resection of adenoma, (**d**) after complete resection of adenoma, (**e**) intrasellar packing using fibrillar, (**f**) intrasellar packing using abdominal fat

be taken not to extend dural opening anteriorly to avoid anterior CSF leak and SIS bleeding (Figs. 32.9 and 32.10).

Tumor dissection can be preceded through two consecutive phases. In the intra-capsular phase and after dural opening; the intrasellar tumor starts to herniate through the opening and then is removed using blunt dissectors and/or suction devices. After complete resection of the basal and lateral portions of the intrasellar tumor, the suprasellar component starts to descend partially inside the sellar cavity, and this may occur spontaneously or by applying the Valsalva maneuver. In the extra-capsular phase, angled endoscopes should be used with adding curved bendable fine blunt instruments for tumor dissection. The extra-capsular phase is initiated by sharp posterior opening of the diaphragm sellae from inside the sellar cavity; approximately 1 cm above the upper border of the dorsum sella. The posterior clinoid process is identified as the lateral limit of dural opening, on both sides.

After posterior opening of the diaphragm sellae, the posterior portion of the chiasmatic cistern is firstly encountered. Angled surgical instruments are introduced through the dural opening under direct endoscopic vision, and tumor dissection is progressed circumferentially from a caudal-to-cranial direction. The first landmarks sought should be the pituitary stalk and the posterior border of the under surface of the optic chiasm. At this point, the retrosellar region can be easily approached by advancing the angled endoscope below the optic chiasm, between the pituitary stalk medially and the paraclinoid carotid laterally exposing contents of the retrosellar

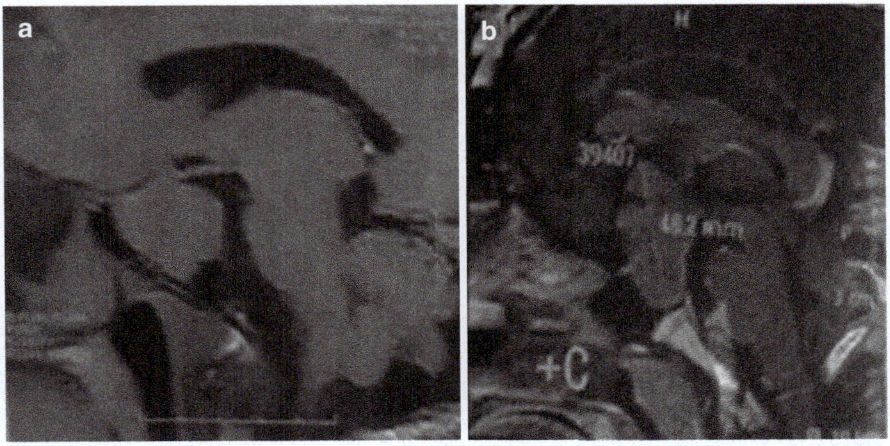


**Fig. 32.9** Contrast-enhanced T1-weighted MRI showing: preoperative sagittal views of a huge pituitary macroadenoma (**a**) grade C, Hardy's classification, and (**b**) grade D, Hardy's classification

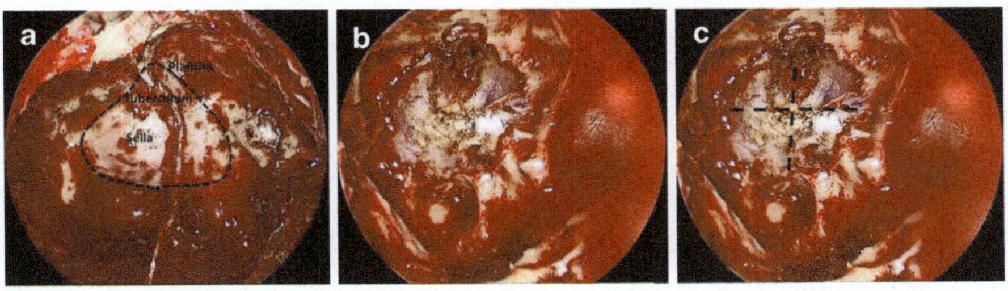


**Fig. 32.10** Endoscopic view of; (**a**) the delineated extended exposure of the sellar and suprasellar region, (**b**) the bone of sellar floor, central part of tuberculum sellae and central 1 cm of planum sphenoidal was removed, and (**c**) cruciate opening of sellar dura

region. The extra-capsular dissection is continued circumferentially till a complete clearance of the under surface of both optic nerves and optic chiasm with caution so as to adequately spare the small subchiasmatic perforators [18].

By using more long-curved surgical instruments, the suprachiasmatic cistern is entered above the optic chiasm and tumor dissection is continued under direct vision of 45° and 70° endoscopes, till identification of the anterior part of the circle of Willis. Advancing the angled endoscope below the ACoA above the chiasm may allow following tumor extension into the anterior recess of the third ventricle (Figs. 32.11 and 32.12).

After complete removal of the tumor, the surgical cavity is thoroughly irrigated with saline. Simple reconstruction is usually sufficient, and it is started by sealing the dural opening using a piece of FIBRILLAR™ and fibrin glue as a sealant. The sellar cavity is additionally packed with a piece of abdominal fat supported in place by bony fragment from the removed sphenoid rostrum (Fig. 32.13).

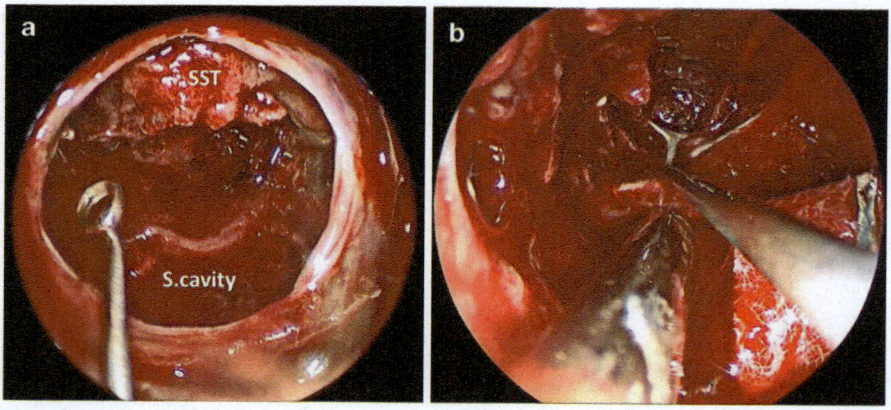


**Fig. 32.11** Endoscopic view using 0 endoscope showing; (**a**) endoscopic view after complete resection of the intrasellar tumor showing descent of the suprasellar component inside sellar cavity either, (**b**) angled endoscopic view; trying to continue the intra-capsular resection of the suprasellar component. SST suprasellar tumor

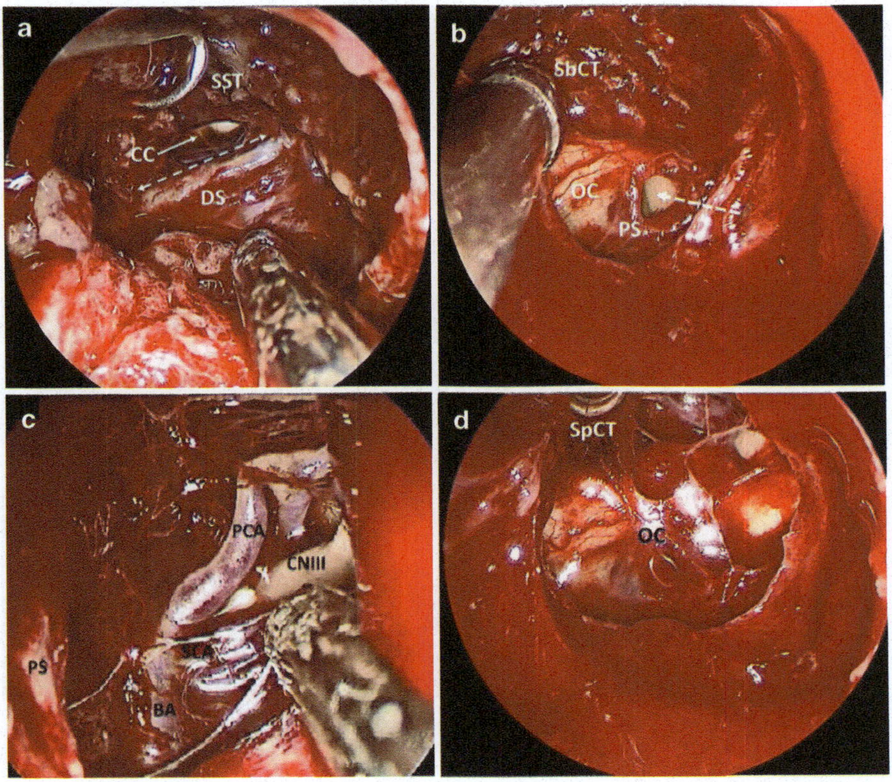


**Fig. 32.12** Angled endoscopic view showing; (**a**) posterior opening of diaphragm sellae from inside the sellar cavity (double-dotted white line) and introduction of angled instruments through the dural opening starting extra-capsular dissection from posterior portion of chiasmatic cistern. (**b**) Proceeding extra-capsular dissection from pituitary stalk and under surface of the optic chiasm, and by advancing the endoscope posteroinferiorly (single-dotted white line). (**c**) Contents of retro-sellar region were exposed. (**d**) Continuation of subchiasmatic extra-capsular dissection till complete clearance of under surface of both optic nerves and optic chiasm. SST suprasellar tumor, CC chiasmatic cistern, *DS* dorsum sellae, *SbCT* subchiasmatic tumor, *OC* optic chiasm, *PS* pituitary stalk, *BA* basilar artery, *PCA* posterior cerebral artery, *SCA* superior cerebellar artery, *CNIII* oculomotor nerve, *SpCT* suprachiasmatic tumor, *SP* subchiasmatic perforators

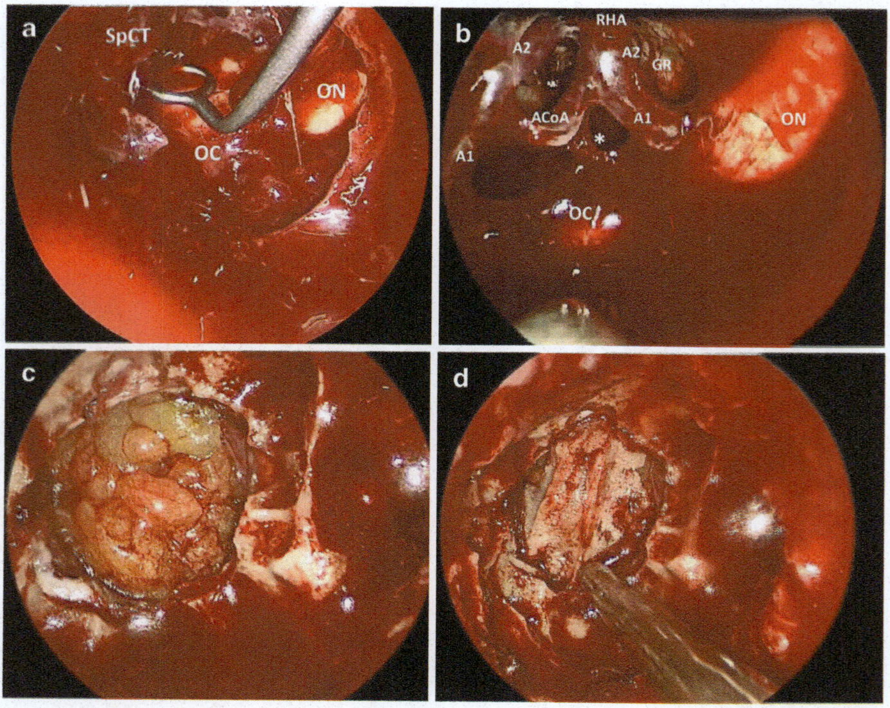


**Fig. 32.13** Angled endoscopic view showing (**a**) starting suprachiasmatic extra-capsular dissection along the anterior surface of optic nerves and chiasm, (**b**) after complete suprachiasmatic dissection, anterior part of circle of Willis was completely exposed. (**c, d**) Endoscopic view using 0 endoscope showing steps of simple skull base reconstruction. SpCT suprachiasmatic tumor, OC optic chiasm, ON optic nerve, A1 A1 segment of anterior cerebral artery, A2 A2 segment of anterior cerebral artery, AcoA anterior communicating artery, RHA recurrent artery of Heubner, GR gyrus rectus, * site of exposure of the anterior recess of third ventricle

## References

1. Lee SC, Senior BA. Endoscopic skull base surgery. Clin Exp Otorhinolaryngol. 2008;1(2):53–62.
2. Cappabianca P, de Divitiis E. Back to the Egyptians: neurosurgery via the nose: a five-thousand year history and the recent contribution of the endoscope. Neurosurg Rev. 2007;30:1–7.
3. Cappabianca P, Cavallo LM, De Divitiis E. Endoscopic endonasal transsphenoidal surgery. Neurosurgery. 2004;55(4):933–41.
4. Rosegay H. Cushing's legacy to transsphenoidal surgery. J Neurosurg. 1981;54(4):448–54.
5. Cappabianca P, Alfieri A, Colao A, Cavallo L, Fusco M, Peca C, et al. Endoscopic endonasal transsphenoidal surgery in recurrent and residual pituitary adenomas. Min-minimally invasive. Neurosurgery. 2000;43(01):38–43.
6. Kassam A, Snyderman CH, Mintz A, Gardner P, Carrau RL. Expanded endonasal approach: the rostrocaudal axis. Part I. Crista galli to the Sella turcica. Neurosurg Focus. 2005;19(1):1–12.
7. Cavallo LM, Messina A, Cappabianca P, Esposito F, de Divitiis E, Gardner P, et al. Endoscopic endonasal surgery of the midline skull base: anatomical study and clinical considerations. Neurosurg Focus. 2005;19(1):1–14.
8. Janfaza P. Surgical anatomy of the head and neck. Harvard University Press; 2011.

9. Abuzayed B, Tanriover N, Akar Z, Eraslan BS, Gazioglu N. Extended endoscopic endonasal approach to the suprasellar parachiasmatic cisterns: anatomic study. Childs Nerv Syst. 2010;26:1161–70.
10. Francies O, Makalanda L, Paraskevopolous D, Adams A. Imaging review of the anterior skull base. Acta Radiologica Open. 2018;7(5):2058460118776487.
11. Morris LGT. Chapter 60. Lesions of the anterior skull base. In: Lalwani AK, editor. Current diagnosis & treatment in otolaryngology—head & neck surgery. 3rd ed. New York: The McGraw-Hill Companies; 2012.
12. Parmar H, Gujar S, Shah G, Mukherji SK. Imaging of the anterior skull base. Neuroimaging Clin. 2009;19(3):427–39.
13. Ismail M, Abdelaziz AA, Darwish M. A comparison between collaborative and single surgeon approach in endoscopic endonasal surgery to sphenoid sinus. Eur Arch Otorhinolaryngol. 2019;276:1095–100.
14. Ismail M, Abdelhakb B, Michela O. Endoscopic sphenoid sinus anatomy in view of transsphenoidal surgery: standardized way-point cadaver dissection. Egypt J Ear Nose Throat All Sci. 2018;19(2):38–44.
15. Prevedello DM, Kassam AB, Gardner PA, Carrau RL, Snyderman CH. Expanded endoscopic endonasal approaches to the skull base. In: Cranial, craniofacial and skull base surgery. Milano: Springer; 2010. p. 239–251.
16. Greenfield JP, Anand VK, Kacker A, Seibert MJ, Singh A, Brown SM, et al. Endoscopic endonasal transethmoidal transcribriform transfovea ethmoidalis approach to the anterior cranial fossa and skull base. Neurosurgery. 2010;66(5):883–92.
17. Hadad G, Bassagasteguy L, Carrau RL, Mataza JC, Kassam A, Snyderman CH, et al. A novel reconstructive technique after endoscopic expanded endonasal approaches: vascular pedicle nasoseptal flap. Laryngoscope. 2006;116(10):1882–6.
18. Ismail M, Zidan W, Hamead K, Abdelhak B, Darwish M. Endoscopic transsellar transdiaphragmatic approach for extensive suprasellar pituitary macroadenomas. Am J Otolaryngol. 2021;42(1):102808.
19. Gardner PA, Kassam AB, Thomas A, Snyderman CH, Carrau RL, Mintz AH, et al. Endoscopic endonasal resection of anterior cranial base meningiomas. Neurosurgery. 2008;63(1):36–54.
20. Ismail M, Abdelhak B, D'Haens J, Michel O. Sellar reconstruction without intrasellar packing after endoscopic surgery of pituitary macroadenomas is better than its reputation. GMS German Med Sci. 2016:14.
21. Hashimoto N, Handa H, Yamagami T. Transsphenoidal extracapsular approach to pituitary tumors. J Neurosurg. 1986;64(1):16–20.

# 33 Cerebrospinal Fluid (CSF) Rhinorrhea

Yasser W. Khafagy, Ahmed M. Arman,
and Ahmed Y. Khafagy

**Key Points**

- Traumatic CSF rhinorrhea constitutes most of the cases of CSF rhinorrhea.
- Iatrogenic causes are rising due to the increasing rate of endoscopic skull base surgeries.
- Spontaneous resolution of iatrogenic CSF rhinorrhea is reported to be as low as 2% unlike accidental causes in which conservative treatment leads to spontaneous resolution in 85% of cases within a week.
- Spontaneous CSF leak is strongly associated with Idiopathic Intracranial Hypertension (IIH).
- Unresolved CSF leak has a 10% annual risk of developing meningitis and 40% over the long term.
- Different graft materials can be used for reconstruction, either synthetic or autologous. They can be placed underlay or overlay. However, experimental studies show that underlay becomes incorporated within the dura after the first week.
- Management of IIH is essential to avoid recurrence after surgery and includes weight loss, medical treatment, serial lumbar puncture, and surgical CSF diversion.

**Supplementary Information** The online version contains supplementary material available at https://doi.org/10.1007/978-3-031-70077-4_33.

Y. W. Khafagy (✉) · A. M. Arman
Department of Otolaryngology, Mansoura University, Mansoura, Egypt
e-mail: ykhafagy@mans.edu.eg

A. Y. Khafagy
Faculty of Medicine, Mansoura University, Mansoura, Egypt


S. Elwany (ed.), *Current Rhinology*,
https://doi.org/10.1007/978-3-031-70077-4_33

## 33.1 Introduction

Cerebrospinal fluid (CSF) is a clear watery fluid surrounding the brain and the spinal cord. It is secreted by the choroid plexus of the ventricular system, and lesser amount is formed by capillary ultrafiltration and metabolic water production. CSF then flows in the ventricular system until reaching the subarachnoid space. CSF flows through the foramen of Monro from its production sites in lateral ventricles to the third ventricle and then moves through the aqueduct of sylvius to reach the fourth ventricle, then to the subarachnoid space through the foramina of Luschka and is resorbed by arachnoid villi [1].

There are novel findings indicating that CSF circulation is a much more complex process. In fact, it is a combination of directed bulk flow, pulsatile to and from movement, and continuous bidirectional fluid exchange at the blood–brain barrier and the cell membranes at the borders between CSF and interstitial fluid spaces. Moreover, ongoing research emphasizes the role of lymphatic pathways for the drainage of CSF [2].

CSF is under continuous turnover; it is absorbed in dural venous sinuses via arachnoid villi that act as one-way valves transmitting CSF into venous sinuses when increased intracranial pressure (ICP) is 3–6 cm $H_2O$ higher than normal values. Furthermore, cervical lymphatics that run through the perineural spaces of cranial nerves drain minor portions of CSF [3].

CSF pressure, measured in the recumbent position, ranges from 5 to 15 cm $H_2O$. Recent studies suggesting an upper limit of 25 cm $H_2O$ identifies patients with idiopathic intracranial hypertension. CSF pressure can intermittently increase up to 40 cm $H_2O$ with the Valsalva maneuver, straining, and change in position. Obesity is frequently associated with an increase in CSF pressure, a 0.3 cm $H_2O$ increase in CSF pressure for each unit increase in BMI. It also normally increases in children up to 28 cm $H_2O$ and decreases by 27% after the age of 50 [4].

## 33.2 CSF Rhinorrhea

CSF rhinorrhea is due to the presence of abnormal communication between the subarachnoid space and sinonasal tract. It involves the breakdown of layers between them including the arachnoid membrane, dura mater, skull base bone, and nasal mucosa.

### 33.2.1 Etiology

CSF can occur due to traumatic and nontraumatic causes. Traumatic causes are subdivided into surgical and nonsurgical. Surgical causes include endoscopic sinus surgery and open neurosurgical approaches. Nonsurgical causes include closed head injury and penetrating head injury. Nontraumatic causes are more diverse. It may be idiopathic, inflammatory, congenital, or neoplastic [5] (Fig. 33.1).

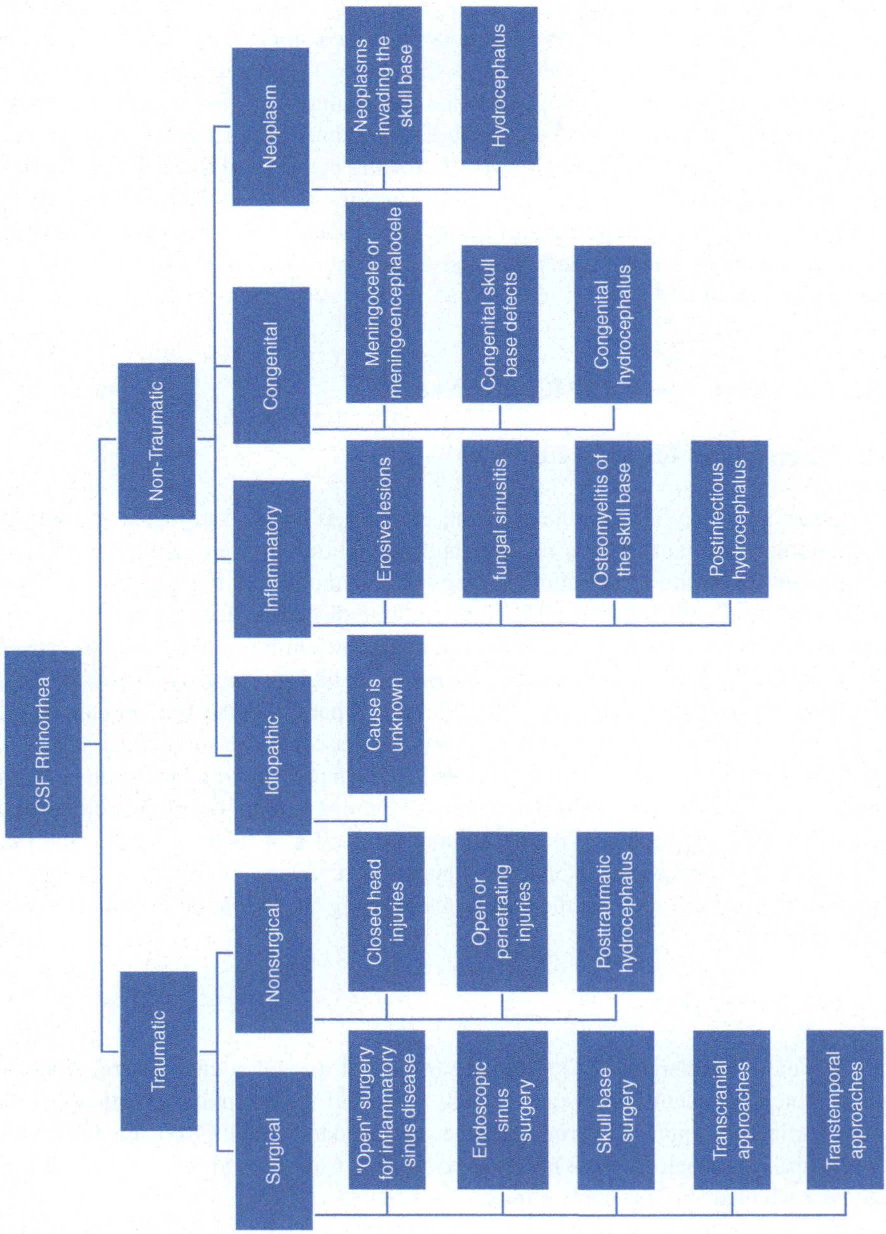


**Fig. 33.1** Different causes of CSF rhinorrhea

### 33.2.2 Complications of CSF Rhinorrhea

Ascending infection, primarily bacterial meningitis, through the communicating tract is the primary concern of CSF leakage and the major cause of comorbidity and mortality. It can lead to the spread of flora from the sinonasal cavity into the sterile subarachnoid space, which can lead to the spread of infection and subsequently causing meningitis. Patients with persistent CSF rhinorrhea have about 10% annual risk of meningitis which increases to about 40% during their overall lifetime with most episodes occurring in the first year following the onset of the leak. The mortality rate of bacterial meningitis remains 33% despite advances in antibiotic therapy with survivors having high morbidities including seizure disorder, encephalopathy, and cranial nerve defects. The actual loss of fluid is a concern in cases of rapid and extensive loss of CSF [6].

### 33.2.3 Diagnosis of CSF Rhinorrhea

A. **History and Clinical Examination**

Clear, nonsticky fluid discharge from the nose is with a salty taste (caused by high sodium content) that is copious and continuous in nontraumatic cases and scanty and intermittent in traumatic cases. It accumulates in the sinuses and leaks when the head is flexed (reservoir sign), and the discharge does not always correspond to the site of the fistula. Headache is also a presenting sign that may be caused by an increase or decrease in intracranial pressure: high-pressure types present with increasing pain that is relieved with CSF leak, whereas in the low-pressure type, pain increases in an upright position and decreases in the recumbent position. Olfactory nerve damage caused by elevated ICP can present with hyposmia or anosmia. Infection, caused by recurrent attacks of meningitis, can be the first presenting sign of fistula, especially in post-traumatic cases. If CSF is mixed with blood or nasal discharge and is placed on filtered paper, the CSF will migrate farther, leaving blood and nasal discharge in the middle and causing the formation of Halo or target sign [1].

B. **Laboratory Tests**

The nasal discharge (CSF) should be evaluated for cell count, culture, glucose, and protein concentrations, all of which should be normal in patients with IIH. Testing of sample fluid from the nose suspected to contain CSF using Glucostix test strips. Nonetheless, there is dispute over its sensitivity and specificity, and it is unclear whether it is a reliable clinical tool [7].

Beta-2 transferrin assay was found to be the gold standard when its sensitivity and specificity were compared to that of Glucostix test strips and CT (5 mm axial slice), and it is easily detectable in as little as 0.5 ml of CSF [8].

B-Trace protein is synthesized mainly in the epithelial cells of the choroid plexus and is found in CSF in concentrations 35-folds higher than in plasma. And with a specificity of 100% and a sensitivity of 91%, with immunoelectrophoresis, it is a useful marker for diagnosis of CSF leakage [9].

C. **Intrathecal Fluorescein**

Following endoscopic examination, sodium fluorescein is injected intrathecally to localize the leak. The accuracy of the test is around 96%, but its ability to identify the site of the leak precisely is limited. The effectiveness of the test depends on leakage rate, extent of defect, time of the injection, and CSF turnover rate. Some complications, such as nausea, vomiting, headache, and mild tinnitus and more severe complications such as transient pulmonary edema, seizure, coma, and even death were reported. Keerl et al. analyzed 420 administrations of the solution and found the method of administration, concentration, formulation, and idiopathic reactions to be the main reasons for complications and a 5% or lower concentration had transient side effects. They also reported that a maximum dose of 1 ml, which contains 50 mg of fluorescein, or 0.1 ml per 10 kg of body weight in Germany and a slightly lower concentration in the USA went without complications. Schlosser and Bolger reached a similar result with slow injection of 0.1 ml of 10% fluorescein diluted in 10 ml of the patient's CSF. With the lack of FDA approval, informed consent and discussion about advantages and reported risks is recommended [10, 11].

D. **Radiology**

A bone window CT of 1 mm or less intervals of the entire skull base and mastoid cavity with reformatting in all planes is very useful. At a workstation, the radiologist can carefully manipulate the data and localize the leak that may require oblique planes [12].

CT cisternography is reserved for those patients who have a negative CT scan and active leak. Gadolinium-enhanced MR cisternography is performed if there is a soft tissue opacity in the CT within an adjacent sinus to exclude a meningocele or encephalocele and to detect dural enhancement at the site of the leak. A nuclear cisternography with pledges is performed only in the most complex and difficult case. The most preferable method for evaluating CSF rhinorrhea is a combination of thin-section CT and subsequent CT cisternography. However, headache, nausea or vomiting, allergic reaction, paresthesia or seizures, and rarely, intracerebral hemorrhage are all side effects of contrast-enhanced cisternography [13].

Before diagnosis of IIH, intracranial space-occupying lesions should be ruled out, preferably by MRI. In patients with known coagulopathy, patients using oral contraceptives, or in atypical patients, cerebral venous thrombosis should be ruled out, either by magnetic resonance venography (MRV) or computed tomography venography (CTV), so using MRI with conjunction with MRV is helpful in ruling out these conditions in patients with suspected IIH [14].

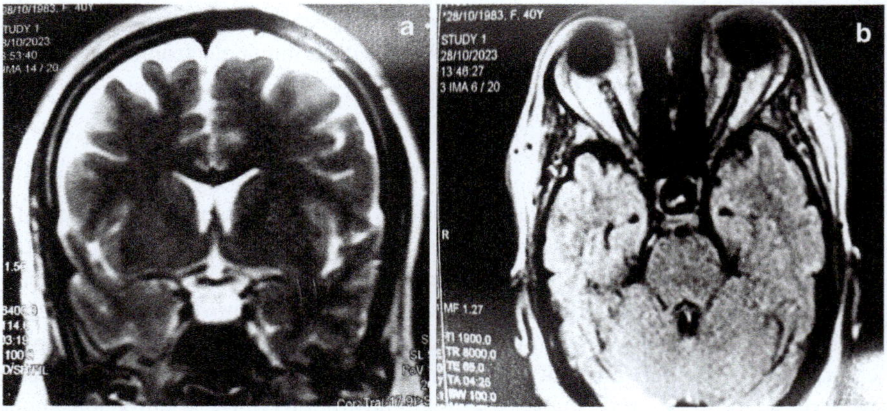


**Fig. 33.2** MRI of the brain showing an empty Sella (**a**) and thickened optic nerve (**b**) in cases of intracranial hypertension

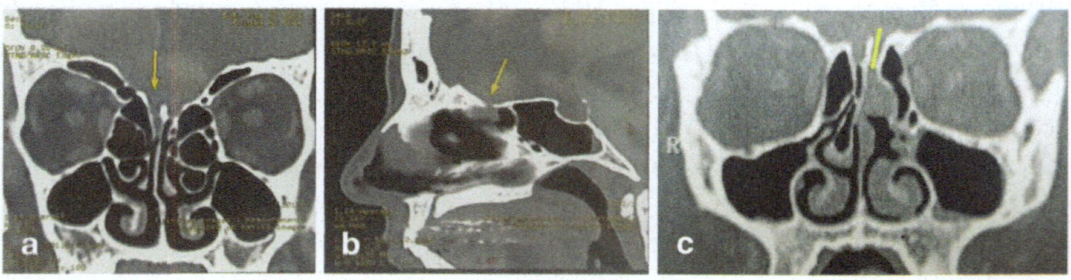


**Fig. 33.3** CT scan of PNS shows a defect in the right cribriform plate, (**a**) coronal and (**b**) sagittal views and (**c**) a left meningocele through a defect in the left cribriform plate

Although intracranial morphology in patients with IIH is usually normal under neuroimaging, long-standing raised CSF pressure causes periotic CSF distension, partial empty Sella, and changes in ventricular composition. Furthermore, 63% of patients with these findings are expected to have attenuated skull bases with arachnoid pits and thickened optic nerve sheath (Fig. 33.2) and 50–100% are found to have meningoceles (Fig. 33.3) and multiple skull defects [15].

## 33.3 Traumatic CSF Rhinorrhea

Traumatic CSF rhinorrhea is defined as the leak of CSF through the nose due to skull base trauma either accidental or iatrogenic regardless of the time of presentation.

### 33.3.1 Incidence

Traumatic CSF rhinorrhea ranges from 50% to 95% in the literature. CSF leak would appear within two days of the incident in about 50% of cases and about 75% in the 2 weeks after injury [16].

Early leaks are clearly due to a direct fracture of the skull base and concomitant dural tear. A late presentation of the leak can be due to tissue edema or a blood clot that gets resolved allowing the CSF to leak or tissue loss from wound edges [17].

### 33.3.2 Types of Traumatic CSF Rhinorrhea

Most cases of CSF rhinorrhea are traumatic, so any case with CSF rhinorrhea must be reviewed for any history of trauma or recent surgery. Traumatic CSF rhinorrhea may occur due to accidental injury or iatrogenic operative injury. Both types will have differences in the site of skull base injury, hence the development of CSF fistula and management.

A. **Accidental CSF Rhinorrhea**

Trauma can either be penetrating injury or nonpenetrating (closed) head injury. Most cases of skull base fracture do not cause CSF rhinorrhea. It will only occur in the cases when skull base fracture is associated with dural tear. The site of penetrating injury will vary according to the site of injury, and it can occur anywhere. Due to firm attachment of the dura to the skull base in the anterior cranial fossa, closed head injury may cause CSF leak. Closed head injury will mostly present with CSF fistulas at the frontal sinus and cribriform plate. Most closed head injury CSF leaks will resolve spontaneously within 7 days of injury [8, 16, 18].

B. **Iatrogenic CSF Rhinorrhea**

The rate of iatrogenic CSF rhinorrhea is reported to be increasing. This is due to the spread of endoscopic management of different rhinological and neurosurgical diseases [19].

Sinus surgery iatrogenic CSF rhinorrhea is a rare complication reported only in 0.17–0.5% of cases. However, the volume of cases of sinus surgery has highly increased in the last few decades [20–22]. Most injuries occur in the cribriform plate and ethmoid roof. The junction of the ethmoid and sphenoid skull base where the angle of the skull base slopes inferiorly is frequently found. Another common site is the thin lateral lamella especially when skull base is low in this region. New atypical injuries are emerging as a sinus balloon injury due to increase in sinus balloon use [19, 23].

The spontaneous resolution of iatrogenic CSF leaks with conservative treatment may be related to the size of the bone defect and the amount of dural injury. Iatrogenic injury can range from small skull base cracks to large defects involving dura and even brain tissue [11]. Reports of resolution with conservative treatment were as low as 2% [24].

Neurosurgical iatrogenic CSF rhinorrhea occurs after procedures involving the skull base either endoscopically or through open approaches. Iatrogenic sphenoid CSF leak after transsphenoidal pituitary surgery (0–15% occurrence) [25] is the most common site of injury after neurosurgical procedures. In these cases, conservative treatment is usually effective [26]. However, if there is no response to treatment, then reexplanation and multilayer closure may be necessary.

### 33.3.3 Presentation of Posttraumatic CSF Rhinorrhea

Cerebrospinal fluid rhinorrhea after skull base fractures is common and is present in about 40% of skull base fractures. In the acute phase following the trauma, CSF leak may be associated with event, epistaxis, nasal discharge, periorbital ecchymosis, chemosis, anosmia, cranial nerve deficits, open-head injury with CSF leakage, loss of vision, cranial nerve deficits, meningitis, and pneumocephalus. Later, patients may present with recurrent meningitis, intermittent rhinorrhea, headaches, salty taste in the throat, hyposmia, and intracranial infections. Fractures had been classified—according to the site of fractures depending on CT finding—into four types, median fracture (type I) involving the cribriform plate, medial fracture (type II) involving the roof of ethmoid and or medial frontal sinus, lateral fracture (type III) (Fig. 33.4) involving walls of the lateral frontal sinus or roof of the orbit. The last type (IV) is the complex or combinations of the three types.

Type I cribriform fractures and Type II frontoethmoidal fractures have the highest risk for intracranial infection at the rate of 60% and 43%, respectively. This may be explained by the higher incidence of larger fracture sizes and CSF rhinorrhea in these types [27]

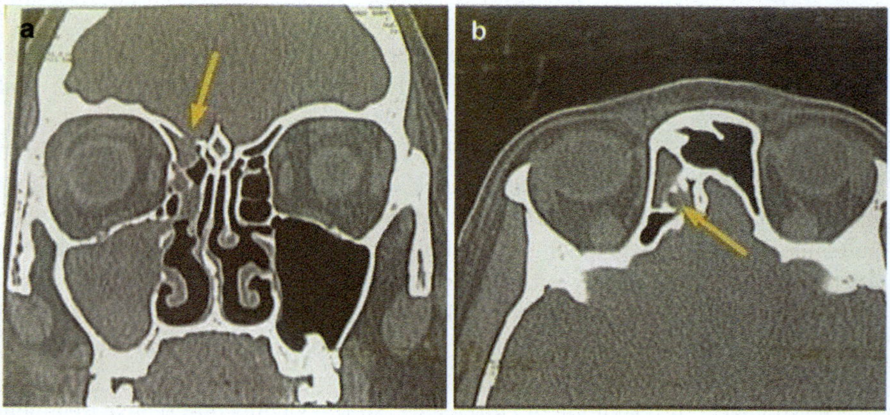


**Fig. 33.4** CT of PNS. Coronal (**a**) and sagittal (**b**) cuts showing a defect in the posterior wall of the frontal sinus with CSF leak (arrows)

**Risk of Meningitis**

The incidence of recurrent meningitis after posttraumatic CSF leaks ranges from 12.5% to 50%. The overall 30.6% risk of meningitis before surgical repair entails a risk of 18% in the first 2 weeks after injury, 7.4% per week in the first month after injury, and a cumulative risk of 85% at the ten-year follow-up [11, 28, 29].

### 33.3.4 Management

Management of traumatic CSF rhinorrhea includes conservative measures, CSF diversion, and surgical intervention.

A. **Conservative Measures:**

They are precautions designed to minimize the increase in intracranial pressure. Several measures include bed rest with elevation of head and avoidance of activities that may cause increased intracranial pressure such as nose blowing, sneezing, coughing, avoiding straining with bowel movements. Several studies have reported that spontaneous resolution with conservative management is successful in 68–85% of patients [30, 31].

As dura mater does not regenerate, the closure of the defect is usually by fibrous tissue or healing of nasal mucosa. The large defect size and the presence of an encephalocele or a meningocele would hinder the healing reducing the spontaneous cessation of the leak [11].

Spontaneous resolution occurs in 68% of posttraumatic CSF fistulas within 48 hours of injury and reaches 85% within 1 week [18].

Conservative treatment is continued for 7–10 days. If leaks persist, then additional interventional measures must be considered to prevent an intracranial infection [31, 32].

Some patients are not candidates for conservative treatment: patients with a penetrating head injury, intracranial hematoma, traumatic meningocele or encephalocele, tension pneumocephalus, and with very large defects. Those patients require prompt surgical intervention [33].

**Acetazolamide**

Less is known about its role in traumatic CSF leaks. Studies do not indicate significant benefits by adding acetazolamide in traumatic CSF leak patients [40].

Certain patients are not appropriate for conservative treatment. Those patients with a penetrating injury, intracranial hematoma, traumatic meningocele or encephalocele, significant pneumocephalus, and large defects with low potential for healing should not be treated with conservative management and require prompt surgical intervention [33].

B. **CSF Diversion**

If these precautions failed, then CSF diversion would be advocated. In most cases, lumbar draining is the method of choice for CSF diversion. External ventriculostomy draining is another method that provides CSF diversion.

(a) **Lumbar Drain**

CSF leak management has been reported to raise the success rate of nonsurgical repair to nearly 90% [34]. In contrast, there is a growing body of literature on the use of lumbar drains after skull base surgery, but many of the results are conflicting even among high-level studies. A recent meta-analysis by D'Anza et al. indicates that there is no difference in the postoperative CSF leak rate after skull base surgery with or without a lumbar drain [35].

(b) **External Ventriculostomy**

Placing an external ventriculostomy (EVD) should be considered first in patients who might benefit from an ICP monitoring device given the severity of the traumatic event and a low GCS score. In such cases, the EVD plays the dual role of ICP monitor and CSF diverter. Placement of an EVD could be preferred over a lumbar drain in patients who present with increased supratentorial pressure due to cerebral edema, intraparenchymal contusions, or other lesions not amenable to surgical evacuation [16].

C. **Surgical Management**

The indications for early surgery are penetrating injury, intracranial hematoma, meningitis, large intracranial pneumocephalus, herniation of brain tissue, and low probability of spontaneous repair.

The indications of delayed surgery are persistent CSF leakage after 10 days of conservative management, recurrence of delayed CSF leakage after 10 days of conservative management, and the presence of meningitis.

Surgical methods are classified into two groups. The first is the endoscopic approach and the second is the intracranial approach. However, nowadays, it is more popular to go for endonasal repair by endoscopic approach. Different types of grafts and flaps are used as described later on.

**Prophylactic Antibiotics**

There are conflicting reports about the usefulness of prophylactic antibiotics in patients with traumatic CSF rhinorrhea. Most review articles except few showed no significant reduction in meningitis [34, 36–38]. Prophylactic antibiotics directed toward Gram negative bacteria are used by some practitioners, may be used in patients with nasal packing or concurrent lumbar drain in place [19].

#### 33.3.4.1 Management of Iatrogenic CSF Rhinorrhea

(a) **Intraoperative**

If a CSF leak is identified during surgery, it is necessary to carefully assess the site, size and depth of the leak, signs of intracranial bleeding. It is also important to assess the integrity of the remaining skull base. If possible, the defect should be repaired during the same surgery. After identification of the defect, it should be marked, and surgery is completed, and the defect is left to be repaired at the end of the surgery. Good hemostasis is essential for proper identification of the skull base and for effective repair. Careful examination of preoperative imaging is very important for reassessment of the skull base anatomy, areas of weakness, or low skull base. If CSF leak is suspected, it is better to ask the anesthesiologist to perform a Valsalva to 40 mmHG for few minutes to evaluate the suspected area.

(b) **Postoperative:**

If the leak was not noticed during surgery, or if it is not possible to repair the injury at the time of surgery, or there is high suspicion of an injury that could not be identified, then postoperative imaging is needed. Imaging could be helpful in localizing the skull base defect, defining injury extent, and for planning of needed management. Imaging is also essential to rule out other associated intracranial complications necessitating immediate management, such as tension pneumocephalus or intracranial hemorrhage. Thin cuts of high-resolution CT scans of the skull base are obtained. In cases where intracranial incidents are suspected, MRI is also needed.

#### 33.3.4.2 Timing of Intervention

Immediate surgical intervention is indicated in cases with large skull base defects, presence of meningocele or encephalocele, tension pneumocephalus. Conservative treatment is indicated for small defects and after surgery for the skull base where repair was done during surgery and after transsphenoidal pituitary surgery. Some authors believe that iatrogenic CSF leaks that present in a delayed fashion are less likely to respond to conservative treatment alone and usually require surgical repair [39].

### 33.3.5 Positive Pressure Ventilation

The use of positive pressure ventilation in patients with obstructive sleep apnea is not uncommon. If those patients have a skull base defect or recent repair, positive pressure may be dangerous as it may lead to pneumocephalus, recurrent leaks. A recent survey among skull base surgeons showed that it is better not to use continuous positive airway pressure (CPAP) machines 2–3 weeks after surgical repair of skull base defects [36].

### 33.3.6 Paradoxical Posttraumatic CSF Rhinorrhea and CSF Rhinorrhea

Paradoxical rhinorrhea. Is rhinorrhea from the naris contralateral to the site of CSF leakage? Causes include fractures of the midline structures, the crista galli and vomer, and can also be seen when the ipsilateral naris is completely obstructed. Other causes include septal perforation and previous surgery. CSF otorhinorrhea can occur when skull base defects occur in the temporal bone, due to various causes. CSF travels from the origin of the leak, down the eustachian tube into the nasopharynx, and then into the nose [40].

## 33.4 Nontraumatic CSF Rhinorrhea

Based on ICP, nontraumatic CSF rhinorrhea is divided into two categories, elevated and normal. In the elevated category, the dural membrane breaks at its weakest point which connects the sinonasal tract to dural spaces causing the rhinorrhea, so the primary cause of elevated ICP must be addressed before restoring the continuity of the dural membrane to prevent further breakdown after repair and to prevent recurrence [40].

### 33.4.1 Neoplastic CSF Rhinorrhea

CSF flow course can be anatomically obstructed by an intracranial tumor, which causes an increase in ICP caused by elevated back pressure behind the level of obstruction that the tumor caused. Also treatment of the tumor, including chemotherapy and radiotherapy, can impair the flow of CSF by causing cerebral edema and scarring [40].

### 33.4.2 Congenital CSF Rhinorrhea

CSF leakage can be a result of a congenital defect in preexisting pathways, such as cochlear or vestibular aqueduct, oval or round window, Hyrtl's fissure, primary empty Sella syndrome, primary bony and dural defects that are free of herniation, encephaloceles, meningoceles, or meningoencephaloceles. In such cases, the case can be treated as idiopathic in nature but appears to be congenital in origin with through workup [40].

### 33.4.3 Idiopathic CSF Rhinorrhea

There is a dispute between experts around CSF rhinorrhea that is idiopathic in nature. Some experts deny its existence and believe that it always has an identifiable etiology behind it that is found after through workup. Others believe it exists but it is rare, and one of their theories involve the description of the arachnoid granulations. These granulations are found at the skull base and serve as mini herniations that herniate through the dura against the inner surface of the skull base. These herniations serve as pockets of CSF; with raised ICP it may exert pulsatile pressure on the skull base, ultimately leading to erosion of the bone and CSF leak [40].

### 33.4.4 Spontaneous CSF Leaks

**Definition**

It is CSF rhinorrhea with the absence of any inciting event. Its pathological mechanism is not clear. These leaks are associated with elevated ICP. Though spontaneous leaks are considered a variant of IIH [41], spontaneous leaks typically occur in the anterior and lateral skull base where the skull and dura are breached over a pneumatized space, over paranasal sinuses, anteriorly along the cribriform plate. An encephalocele, which is the herniation of brain through the skull base, can also occur.

#### 33.4.4.1 Pathogenesis

Elevated ICP explains the pathogenesis of spontaneous CSF leaks or encephaloceles and accounts for the demographic, clinical, and radiographic findings in this group and their similarity to the benign intracranial hypertension population [42].

Impaired CSF absorption at the arachnoid villi is the most likely theory for development of idiopathic intracranial hypertension (IIH). Arachnoid villi were shown to be obstructed in 80% to 84% of patients with empty sella syndrome (ESS) and is a common radiological finding in IIH and spontaneous CSF leaks [43].

Persistent prolonged elevations and fluctuations in CSF pressure in addition to hydrostatic pulsatile forces exerted throughout the skull causes thinning of the bony skull base, specially over sites of least resistance; this causes bony defects to form which causes spontaneous CSF leaks and encephaloceles. Sites of structural weakness include perforations in the cribriform plate, sellar diaphragm, and areas with significant pneumatization such as paranasal sinuses [44].

**Link Between CSF Rhinorrhea and Intracranial Hypertension**

Evidence has gradually accumulated that idiopathic intracranial hypertension (IIH) is associated with spontaneous leaks; such association is found in female, obese patients and patients that share specific radiographic findings, such as empty Sella, abnormalities of the optic sheath complex, globe flattening, encephaloceles, arachnoid pits, enlarged Meckel's cave, and dural ectasia. Understanding the link between IIH and spontaneous leaks is not of academic interest only: it has important management implications as this link suggests that controlling increased ICP may improve the results of spontaneous CSF leaks and reduce recurrence rates, which proves to be important before management as typical symptoms of IIH do not usually appear with spontaneous leaks which can cause the symptoms to appear with closure of the skull base defect without addressing the increased ICP [45].

**Idiopathic Intracranial Hypertension**

Idiopathic intracranial hypertension (IIH) is a neurological disorder characterized by elevated CSF pressure in the absence of any intracranial pathology or secondary causes. IIH is diagnosed by measuring lumber CSF opening pressure with normal radiological finding and normal CSF composition [42].

#### 33.4.4.2 Epidemiology and Pathogenesis

An obese woman of childbearing age is the typical patient of IIH. However, the condition can be present at any age, but obesity is more common in the childbearing age. Spontaneous prevalence also increases with the awareness of the condition and increased prevalence of obesity [45].

The pathogenesis of raised ICP is unclear with IIH disease being a disease of theories with several proposed hypotheses that have been put forward to explain it. Altered CSF dynamics, sex hormones, obesity, and an underlying prothrombotic abnormality have been suggested to play a role in the pathogenesis of this condition [46]. Also, case reports show that several drugs affect intracranial hypertension, these reports were in a few patients taking cyclosporin, tetracycline antibiotics, particularly minocycline, and oral contraceptive pills [47].

Arachnoid villi structure is changed and its function in CSF resorption is inhibited by fat-soluble vitamin retinol. Studies have shown an increase in CSF pressure in retinol-deficient animals. However, the exact mechanism is uncertain [48].

Venous hypertension has been involved as a primary mechanism for IIH and has been described as a finding in up to 90% of patients with IIH. It may arise from either intracranial source such as venous stenosis or intrathoracic sources such as obesity and central venous hypertension. The rise in CSF pressure may resolve after CSF drainage [42].

#### 33.4.4.3 Clinical Features and Disease Course

Headache is the most common presenting symptom appearing in 90% of cases, its usually generalized and worse in the morning [43]. Nonvisual manifestations that patients can present with include CSF rhinorrhea, pulsatile intracranial noises, and dizziness. Patients can also present with various types of pain, including neck pain, back or radicular pain but less common. Sixth cranial nerve palsy has been reported in 1–26% of patients where focal neurological deficits can be found but extremely uncommon in IIH patients; in addition, seventh and fourth cranial nerve palsy may be present but rarely [49].

Intracranial pulsatile noises, which the patient describes as "whooshing" or "roaring" in the ear are frequent affecting up to 60% of patients. In cases where nausea, vomiting, or photophobia occur, meningeal irritation is suspected [45].

#### 33.4.4.4 Diagnosis

Modified Dandy criteria include: (1) signs and symptoms of increased intracranial pressure (headaches, nausea, vomiting, transient obscurations of vision, papilledema). (2) No localizing neurologic signs otherwise, with the single exception being unilateral or bilateral VI nerve paresis. (3) CSF can show increased pressure, but no cytologic or chemical abnormalities otherwise. (4) Normal to small symmetric ventricles must be demonstrated (originally required ventriculography, but now demonstrated by CT) [50].

To confirm the diagnosis, a lumber puncture is done and a lumber CSF opening pressure of 150 $mmH_2O$ or more confirms the diagnosis [51].

#### 33.4.4.5 Complications of Spontaneous CSF Rhinorrhea

Complications related to CNS infections, primarily bacterial meningitis is the major cause of morbidity and mortality, followed by encephalitis and parenchymal abscess at much less rates. Some of them may resolve spontaneously, but patients with unresolved CSF leaks are at an annual risk of 10% of meningitis that increase to 40% in the long term [52].

Patients can also experience a variety of visual symptoms with transient visual obscurations being the most common and blurred or double vision and photophobia being less common. It is difficult to distinguish between IIH and chronic daily headaches in patients without papilledema, in such cases, CSF measurement should be indicated in patients with chronic daily headaches with obesity and with patients who experience pulsatile tinnitus [53].

In early stages of papilledema, indirect ophthalmoscopy with stereoscopic fundus can be of great importance as it was difficult to diagnose it with direct ophthalmoscopy earlier. Fluorescein angiography can be utilized and fluorescein leaks were observed earlier in papilledema. Visual acuity may remain earlier but deteriorate rapidly. Careful history and examination can be complemented with optical coherence tomography (OCT). The information derived from OCT can be valuable in guiding clinical decision-making in IIH [54].

With prolonged papilledema, the risk of visual acuity affection is likely to increase. An enlarged blind spot is found in virtually all patients, with visual field defects, including nasal defects, arcuate scotomas, and field constrictions, appearing in up to 90% of patients. Color vision and contrast sensitivity defects are less likely to be detected with assessment [43].

#### 33.4.4.6 Management of Spontaneous CSF Rhinorrhea

**Conservative Management**

The standard treatment of spontaneous CSF rhinorrhea is endoscopic repair. However, in patients with a BMI less than 39.15, a trial of acetazolamide 250 mg BID for 30 days is recommended as it has shown effectiveness in patients under the mentioned BMI which also highlights a relation between effectiveness of acetazolamide and BMI [55].

**Surgical Management**

The goal of reconstruction in skull base defects is to recreate the barrier and close the connection between the cranial cavity and sinonasal tract, thus decreasing the risk for brain abscess, pneumocephalus and ascending bacterial meningitis that has a rising cumulative risk that can reach up to 40% [56].

Factors that should be considered preoperatively and intraoperatively influencing the outcome include the subsequent extent of the defect and the tract connecting the sinonasal tract and cranial cavity, lateral sphenoid defect location, general health condition of the patient, high BMI, multiparity, previous intranasal or maxillofacial surgeries, and the possibility of increased CSF pressure postoperatively [57].

A. **Intracranial CSF Repair**

Bifrontal craniotomy was the first successful intracranial CSF repair reported, the approach offers direct visualization of the defect, access to the brain to manage associated injuries, and the ability to use pericranial flap in repair [58].

Complications include cerebral contusion and edema, intracranial hemorrhage, anosmia, pneumocephalus, bifrontal retraction injury, venous infarction, and bone flap infection. Up to 80% of reported cases were successful. However, others have reported recurrence rates as high as 40% [59].

B. **Endoscopic CSF Repair:**

The endonasal endoscopic repair of anterior skull base defects has become the standard in surgical management of CSF rhinorrhea. Improved illumination and magnification, enhancing exposure of the skull base defect are some advantages of this approach [60].

Current options for skull base reconstruction include avascular grafts, intranasal vascular flaps, and novel endoscopic regional flaps. Avascular graft options include autologous fascia, allogeneic collagen grafts, adipose "bath plug" grafts, bone pate, synthetic dura, Alloderm, firm grafts including bone, cartilage, Medpor, hydroxyapatite cement grafts, and free mucosal grafts [61], Leukocyte- and platelet-rich fibrin [62]. Septal grafts and middle turbinate flaps were also found to be easy to harvest and easy to place, and the overall success rate approached 93.5% [63]:

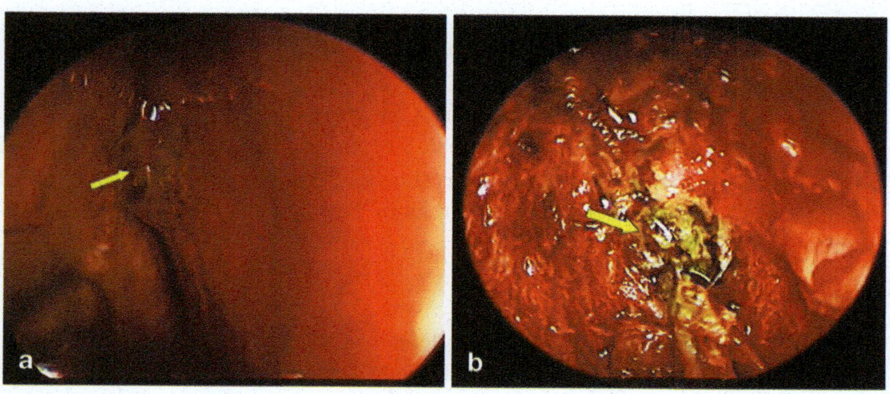


**Fig. 33.5** (**a**) A small meningocele through the upper septum (arrow) and (**b**) cribriform defect after septal dissection (arrow)

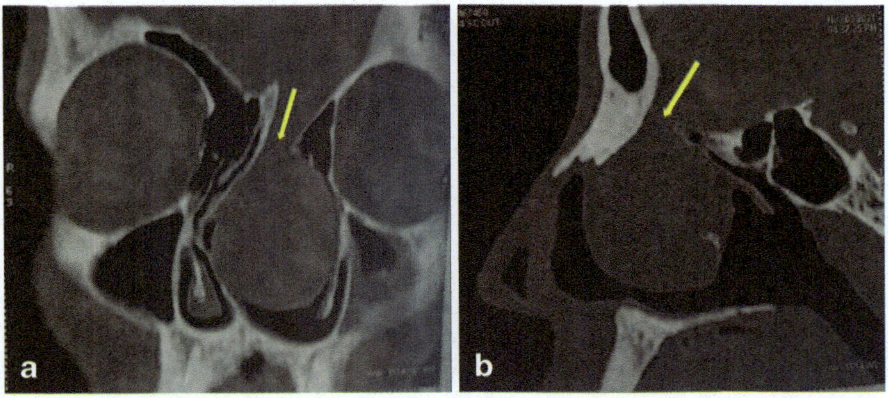

**Fig. 33.6** CT scan of PNS, coronal (**a**) and sagittal (**b**) views show a very large meningoencephalocele occupying the left nasal fossa compressing the nasal septum

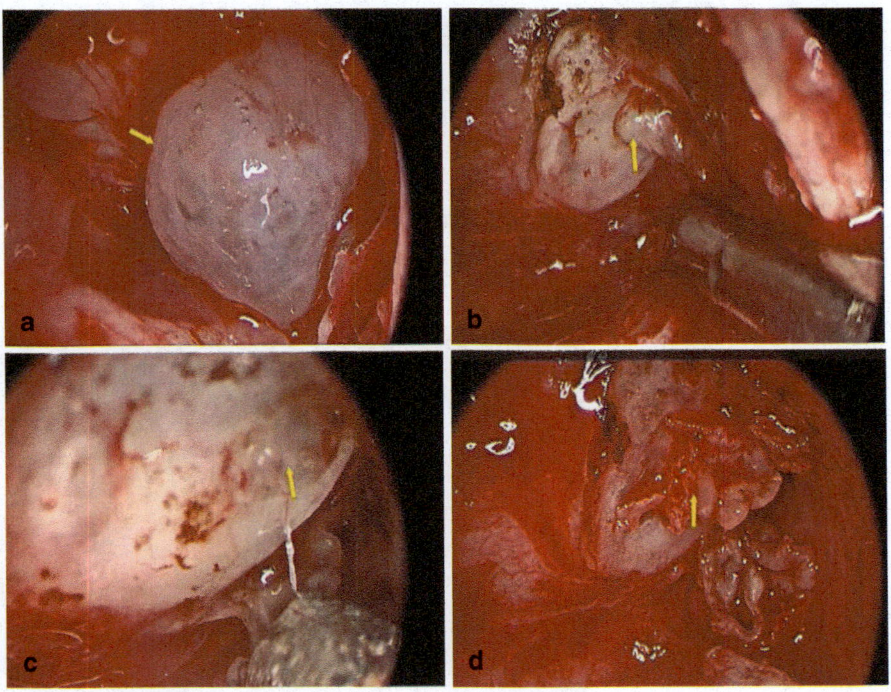

**Fig. 33.7** (**a**) Endoscopic view of the right meningocele (**b**), the meningocele coming from the skull base defect at the roof of ethmoid, (**c**) after excision of the meningocele, and (**d**) closure of the defect with a composite turbinate graft

(a) **Approach**

Using different angles and sizes of endoscopes including 4-mm 0°, 30°, and 45° endoscopes. The skull base defect is exposed according to the suspected

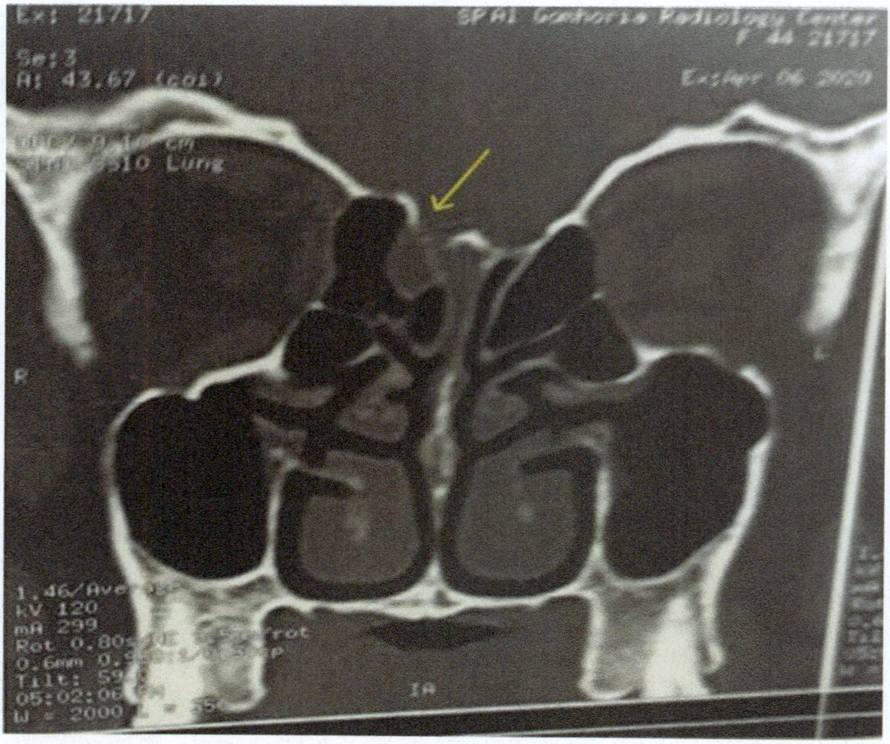


**Fig. 33.8** CNS shows the skull base defect with the meningocele at the posterior ethmoid roof

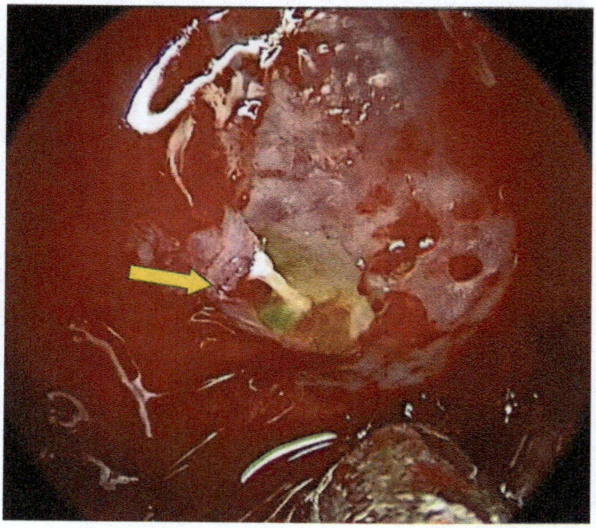

**Fig. 33.9** Endoscopic view of the CSF leak through the floor of the Sella

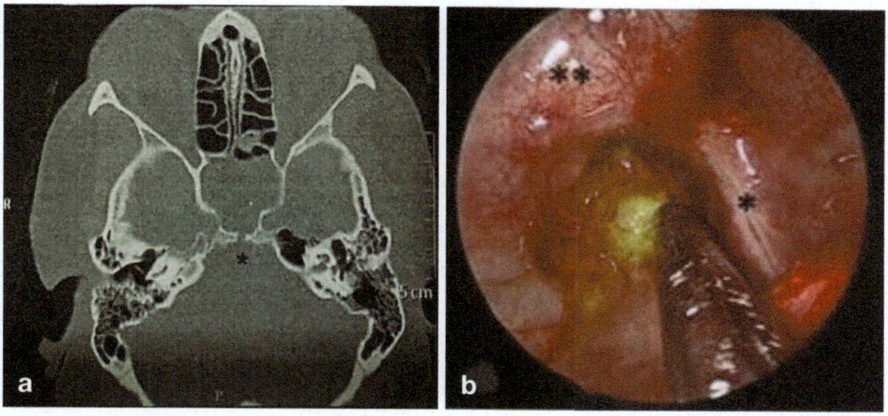


**Fig. 33.10** (**a**) CT scan of PNS. Axial view shows a small central clival defect (asterisk) with opacification of sphenoid sinus. (**b**) Endoscopic view of the same patient showing fluorescein-stained CSF from the clivus, carotid artery (asterisk), and sellar floor (double asterisk)

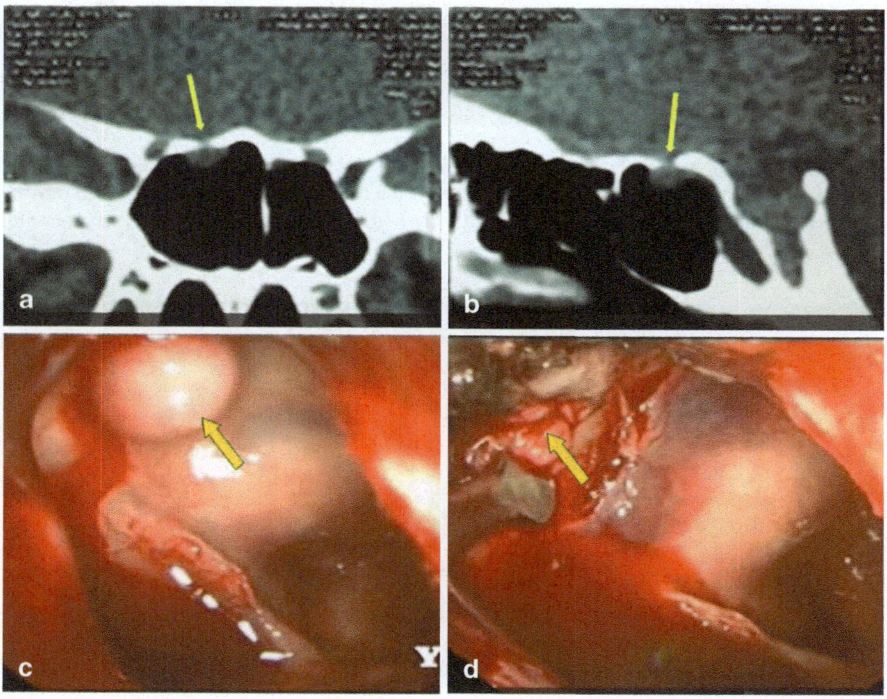


**Fig. 33.11** CT scan of PNS. Coronal (**a**) and sagittal views (**b**) showing a meningocele on the roof of sphenoid sinus, (**c**) endoscopic view of the same patient, and (**d**) repair with an inlay graft

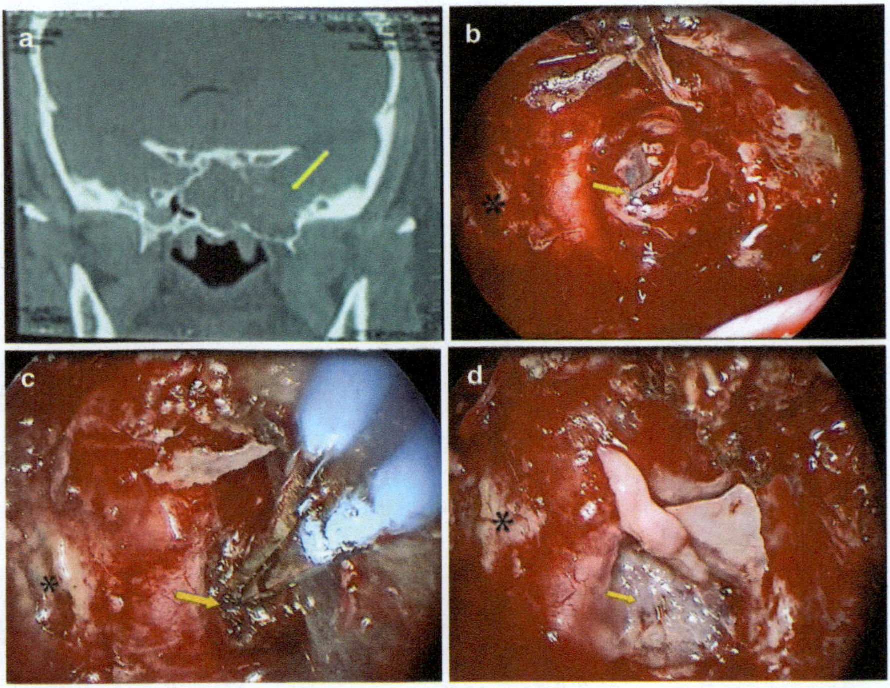


**Fig. 33.12** CT scan of PNS. (**a**) Coronal view shows a large defect at the left lateral recess of the left sphenoid sinus (arrow), (**b**) endoscopic view of the meningocele in the same patient (arrow), (**c**) the defect after cauterization of the defect (arrow), (**d**) repair of the defect in multilayer fashion (arrow), asterisk indicates the sellar floor

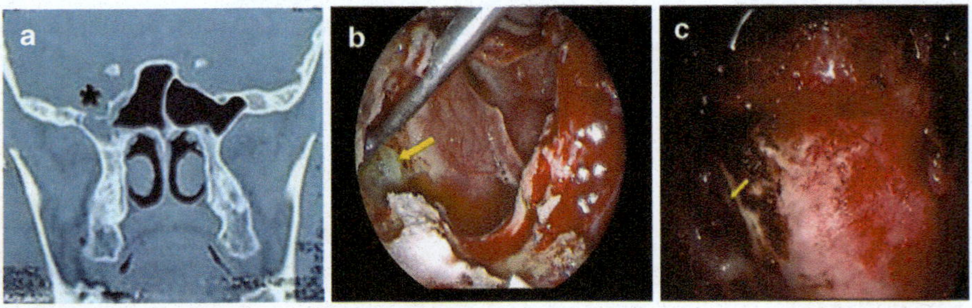


**Fig. 33.13** CT scan of PNS. (**a**) Coronal view shows a defect on the roof of the right lateral recess of the sphenoid sinus (asterisk). (**b**) Endoscopic view showing the meningocele in the right lateral recess (arrow) and (**c**) endoscopic view after complete exposure of the defect (arrow)

location of the leak depending on preoperative imaging studies. The transnasal direct approach is used for leaks in the cribriform region (Fig. 33.5) or coming through a meningocele in the midline (Fig. 33.6). The middle turbinate is medialized or partially removed to fully expose the defect in the olfactory cleft. In cases where the defect is in the lateral lamella, fovea ethmoidalis (Figs. 33.7 and 33.8), or supraorbital cell, complete ethmoidectomy is necessary for exposure and easy closure of the defect. Sphenoidotomy is done in sphenoid sinus defects and (Figs. 33.9, 33.10, and 33.11) DRAF IIb for medial frontal leaks. The transpterygoid approach was used for leaks in the lateral sphenoid sinus recess (Figs. 33.12 and 33.13) [62].

(b) **Grafts**

Grafts are either intradural or extradural. Extradural grafts are placed either with the inlay or onlay technique.

Most techniques yield similar results in experienced hands, whether underlay or onlay. Multilayer repair using different tissue materials is advocated by many authors in the literature. In experimental studies, evidence has been found that a stable underlay graft becomes incorporated with the dura after 1 week [64].

The size of the defect also has a strong impact on surgical decision for the type of grafting required. In very small defects, overlay grafts are more adequate; however, larger (>4 mm) sites can tolerate an underlay graft or multilayer closure either in underlay or overlay fashion. In cases of very large defects with elevated ICP a multilayer closure with bony underlay grafts and soft overlay grafts and local flaps are different options to use or used all together [65]:

1. **Inlay (Underlay) Graft:**

   Meningoencephaloceles at the site of the skull base defect should be cauterized and excised, and the mucosa should be separated from the surrounding bone. After identification of the skull base defect, the mucosa around the edge of the bony defect is removed for one or two millimeters. Then, the dura is dissected carefully from the inner aspect of the edge of the defect to allow for placement of the graft. The graft is then placed between the dura underneath the bony edges on all sides. The authors prefer to use a hard graft (bone or cartilage) as the first layer closing the defect. Another layer of soft tissue or composite graft is then laid down. The grafts are then supported with Surgicel pushed against these layers for insuring air tight seal of the defect. This would not be suitable for skull base cracks or very minute defects with firm adhesion of the dura to the defect. If there is a meningocele or meningoencephalocele, they are reduced carefully using bipolar cautery reaching the site of the defect. The size of the meningocele does not match the size of the defect. A large meningocele may herniate through a small defect. Also, a small meningocele may undercover a large skull base defect especially in the cribriform plate. For large skull base defects, in addition to the bony, cartilage, or composite graft, the use of a septal, turbinate flap is advised to allow for rapid healing of the defect. Inlay grafting is suited to repair skull base defects where the dura is not firmly attached to the inner surface such as defects of the posterior wall of the frontal sinus, the ethmoid roof, and, sometimes, the sphenoid sinus ( roof and lateral recess defects) [12, 66].

2. **Onlay Graft:**

   The onlay technique is recommended if there is a risk of damaging the dura, blood vessels, or nerves during dissection of the dura from the inner surface of the skull base. Also, it should be used in cases where inserting a graft in underlay fashion is impossible when the defect is only a crack or very minute. The graft is placed generally over the dural lesion and over the exposed bony margins, which have been denuded of the mucosa. The graft may be fashioned and applied as a gasket where the part of the graft is deep covering the dura and the edges are covering the bony edge. The center may be enforced with cartilage or bone chips. The graft is supported in place with layers of Surgicel, followed by a vascularized tissue flap which may be designed transnasally, using middle turbinate flap or mucoperichondrial septal flaps for fixation [67].

3. **Flaps:**

   Different local flaps have been described for reconstruction of skull base defects. A nasoseptal pedicled flap based on the nasoseptal artery, Hadad Bassagasteguy flap (HBF) had gained large popularity and had been used extensively for medium and large-sized skull base defects and after skull base surgery. Among the different vascularized flaps are the middle turbinate flap and the posterior pedicle inferior turbinate flap based on the inferior turbinate artery. Other regional vascularized flaps include the pericranial flap, palatal flap, and the transpterygoid temporoparietal fascia flap had also been described especially after surgeries involving resection of a large part of the skull base [68].

**Postoperative Measures**

During the initial healing period, a variety of sealants and packing materials, such as Gelfoam, Surgicel and Merocel, are used to stabilize the graft and help adherence to the defect site.

And in a meta-analysis published by Hegazy et al. grafts were supported in place in 61% of cases (125/204) analyzed in the study by nasal packing. The graft and nasal packing were frequently separated, using Gelfoam or Gelfilm, to prevent graft or flap avulsion during removal of nasal packing. The duration that the surgeon leaves the nasal packing is based on experience, most authors recommended packing to be left 3–5 days after surgery before removal. In addition, Fibrin glue was utilized in 52% of cases (1199/227) with high success rates but outcome analysis showed no significant improvement over each other [67].

**Success Rate**

In 2000, an analysis done by Hegazy et al. that summarized 14 studies, published between 1990 and 1999 that examined the initial experience with endoscopic CSF leak repair, found that the primary success rates in those studies ranged from 60% to 100% with an average of 90%. Many larger case series have been published later and with very high success rates of the endoscopic approach in repairing CSF fistulae after the first attempt that reached 90% and the rest were closed by the second attempt, resulting in 96% after the second attempt, that popularity of CSF leak repair using an endoscopic approach has continued to rise ever since [19].

Endoscopic repair of sinonasal CSF leaks in 48 patients (35.3% spontaneous) was reviewed and cause, site of leak, presence of a meningocele or encephalocele, inability to localize the defect, graft material, displacement, insufficient graft size, and incomplete apposition of graft to the skull base were cited as some of the variables contributing to the failure of endoscopic repair [5].

**Predictors for Failure**

Failure of repair is found to be associated with some factors, including multiparity, high BMI, symptoms and signs of visual affection as blurred vision and radiological signs of raised ICP as empty Sella, site and size of defect also affect the success rate of the repair as large defects and defects in the lateral recess of sphenoid tend to have a high rate of failure [44, 69].

Incisional pain, infection, seroma, hematoma, and scar formation are among the complications that may affect the donor site of the autograft, in addition to requiring separate operative site and additional operative time. However, the exact rates of complications are not yet outlined in the literature. These complications are not opposed when an allograft is obtained [70].

#### 33.4.4.7 Management of Associated IIH

As mentioned before, elevated ICP should be addressed before repairing the dural defect to prevent recurrence and further breakdown of the dural membrane. Hence, recurrence and failure of management is primarily attributed to failure of management of ICP elevation [71].

In 2018, a collaboration between specialists in different specialties and with various patient representatives, a guideline was developed to investigate and manage patients with IIH and associated signs and symptoms. These guidelines include management of weight, using medical and surgical lines of treatment [72]:

(a) **Weight Loss:**

As little as 6% weight reduction, whether surgically induced, as in gastric bypass, or by diet, has shown to reduce ICP and is accompanied by resolution of papilledema. Hence weight loss is heavily encouraged in all patients who are overweight [73, 74].

(b) **Medical Treatment:**

Acetazolamide is the standard treatment of IIH. Patients are usually started on a dose of 250 mg BID to ensure tolerance and the dose is increased slowly aiming for 1000–4000 mg daily as a maintenance dose. Another diuretic, like frusemide, may be tried in patients with intolerance to acetazolamide but is seldom effective [43].

Topiramate is another treatment option. It is an antiepileptic drug that can possibly reduce CSF production and could also help patients lose weight [42].

Corticosteroids are no longer used routinely in the treatment of IIH. However, it can be used initially to stabilize severe acute deterioration of vision that is not responding to standard medical treatment. However, surgical treatment must be urgently considered in such situations [45].

(c) **Serial Lumbar Punctures:**

Although little evidence in the literature of the efficacy of this procedure exists, it is advocated as a mean of ICP reduction, it is inconvenient and difficult in obese patients and is not desirable as a chronic treatment plan by most patients as well as clinicians [45].

(d) **Surgical Management:**

Surgical treatment becomes necessary when adequate medical management fails to halt visual loss progression or occasionally when patients present with severe optic neuropathy [47]. Surgical reduction of CSF is achieved by CSF diversion, which is done mostly by lumbo peritoneal shunt (LPS) (87%) which is minimally invasive in nature; it has shown rapid resolution of symptoms of high ICP and recent studies showed its effectiveness. Ventricular shunts are used but less frequently; it includes ventriculoperitoneal shunts (VPSs), ventriculoatrial shunts, and ventriculojugular shunts but are less frequently utilized (9%, 2%, and 2%, respectively) but are equally effective. They are less utilized due to proximal catheter placement difficulties [43] but recent use of the stereotactic technique has led to effective placement with good results [45]; however, most neurosurgeons prefer LP shunts.

Shunt failure is reported in up to 77% of patients due to either shunt obstruction (in 65% of cases) or over drainage, causing low-pressure headaches (in 15% of cases). Less commonly shunt migration, disconnection, and abdominal discomfort that necessitate shunt revision and lumbar radiculopathy [42].

Optic nerve sheath fenestration (ONSF) is another surgical method that has been used and has shown improvements in papilledema and visual function, also a degree of improvement in the nonoperated eye has been observed occasionally. Identified risks of failure of ONSF include lack of papilledema and long-standing symptoms. There is a lack of evidence comparing ONSF with LFS and VPS in efficacy, so the choice is based on neurosurgeons' preference and expertise [75].

Postoperative complications rate has reached as high as 40% and include pupillary dysfunction, retinal vascular complications, and transient ocular motility disturbance [76].

Recently, trials to treat venous sinus stenosis, that is thought to be playing a role in the primary mechanism of IIH, with stenting seems to be an interesting alternative in patients with demonstrable venous sinus stenosis [77]. It has shown over the past years to relieve ICP gradients, with high safety, efficacy, and with durable results and with cost analysis in its favor. However, juxta-stent narrowing and subsequent intervention with CSF diversion or additional stents is reported with recurrent headaches [78].

## Follow-Up

With no identifiable predicting factors, elevated ICP can recur months or years following the primary attack. Loss of sight might occur over different courses and throughout different time periods. Sometimes visual loss is most severe at presentation. For many its symptoms go undetected until it is severe which draws attention to the need for watchful monitoring of those patients [45].

Current practice should now include assessment of symptoms, examination of optic discs, measurement of visual acuity, and formal documentation of visual fields. Formal perimetry seems the most precise method of identifying visual loss [43].

The administration of acetazolamide caused significant reduction to ICP but to a level that is still higher than that found in most patients [79]. Permeant diversion should be considered in patients with preoperative and postoperative elevated ICP [71].

## References


1. Sakka L, Coll G, Chazal J. Anatomy and physiology of cerebrospinal fluid. Eur Ann Otorhinolaryngol Head Neck Dis. 2011;128(6):309–16.
2. Brinker T, Stopa E, Morrison J, Klinge P. A new look at cerebrospinal fluid circulation. Fluids Barriers CNS. 2014;11(1):1–16.
3. Darakchiev BJ, Pensak ML. Cerebrospinal fluid dynamics in skull base surgery. Curr Opin Otolaryngol Head Neck Surg. 2004;12(5):404–7.
4. Lee SC, Lueck CJ. Cerebrospinal fluid pressure in adults. J Neuroophthalmol. 2014;34(3):278–83.
5. Zweig JL, Carrau RL, Celin SE, Schaitkin BM, Pollice PA, Snyderman CH, Kassam A, Hegazy H. Endoscopic repair of cerebrospinal fluid leaks to the sinonasal tract: predictors of success. Otolaryngol Head Neck Surg. 2000;123(3):195–201.
6. Daudia A, Biswas D, Jones NS. Risk of meningitis with cerebrospinal fluid rhinorrhea. Ann Otol Rhinol Laryngol. 2007;116(12):902–5.
7. Chan DT, Poon WS, Ip CP, Chiu PW, Goh KY. How useful is glucose detection in diagnosing cerebrospinal fluid leak? The rational use of CT and Beta-2 transferrin assay in detection of cerebrospinal fluid fistula. Asian J Surg. 2004;27(1):39–42.
8. Abuabara A. Cerebrospinal fluid rhinorrhoea: diagnosis and management. Medicina Oral Patología Oral y Cirugía Bucal (Internet). 2007;12:397–400.
9. Schnabel C, Di Martino E, Gilsbach JM, Riediger D, Gressner AM, Kunz D. Comparison of β2-transferrin and β-trace protein for detection of cerebrospinal fluid in nasal and ear fluids. Clin Chem. 2004;50(3):661–3.
10. Keerl R, Weber RK, Draf W, Wienke A, Schaefer SD. Use of sodium fluorescein solution for detection of cerebrospinal fluid fistulas: an analysis of 420 administrations and reported complications in Europe and the United States. Laryngoscope. 2004;114(2):266–72.
11. Schlosser RJ, Bolger WE. Nasal cerebrospinal fluid leaks: critical review and surgical considerations. Laryngoscope. 2004;114(2):255–65.
12. Yadav Y, Parihar V, Janakiram N, Pande S, Bajaj J, Namdev H. Endoscopic management of cerebrospinal fluid rhinorrhea. Asian J Neurosurg. 2016;11(03):183–93.
13. Lloyd KM, DelGaudio JM, Hudgins PA. Imaging of skull base cerebrospinal fluid leaks in adults. Radiology. 2008;248(3):725–36.
14. Jinkins JR, Rudwan M, Krumina G, Tali ET. Intrathecal gadolinium-enhanced MR cisternography in the evaluation of clinically suspected cerebrospinal fluid rhinorrhea in humans: early experience. Radiology. 2002;222(2):555–9.
15. Van Zele T, Kitice A, Vellutini E, Balsalobre L, Stamm A. Primary spontaneous cerebrospinal fluid leaks located at the clivus. Allergy Rhinol. 2013;4(2).: pp.ar-2013
16. Yilmazlar S, Arslan E, Kocaeli H, Dogan S, Aksoy K, Korfali E, Doygun M. Cerebrospinal fluid leakage complicating skull base fractures: analysis of 81 cases. Neurosurg Rev. 2006;29:64–71.
17. Mccormack B, Cooper PR, Persky M, Rothstein S. Extracranial repair of cerebrospinal fluid fistulas: technique and results in 37 patients. Neurosurgery. 1990;27:412–7.
18. Bell RB, Dierks EJ, Homer L, Potter BE. Management of cerebrospinal fluid leak associated with craniomaxillofacial trauma. J Oral Maxillofac Surg. 2004;62:676–84.
19. Psaltis AJ, Schlosser RJ, Banks CA, Yawn J, Soler ZM. A systematic review of the endoscopic repair of cerebrospinal fluid leaks. Otolaryngol Head Neck Surg. 2012;147:196–203.

20. Kennedy DW, Shaman P, Han W, Selman H, Deems DA, Lanza DC. Complications of ethmoidectomy: a survey of fellows of the american academy of otolaryngology—head and neck surgery. Otolaryngol Head Neck Surg. 1994;111:589–99.
21. Ramakrishnan VR, Kingdom TT, Nayak JV, Hwang PH, Orlandi RR. Nationwide incidence of major complications in endoscopic sinus surgery. Int Forum Allergy Rhinol. 2012;2(1):34–9.
22. Bumm K, Heupel J, Bozzato A, Iro H, Hornung J. Localization and infliction pattern of iatrogenic skull base defects following endoscopic sinus surgery at a teaching hospital. Auris Nasus Larynx. 2009;36:671–6.
23. Alam ES, Hadley JA, Justice JM, Casiano RR. Significant orbital and intracranial complications from balloon sinus dilation as a stand-alone and powered dissector-assisted procedure. Laryngoscope. 2018;128:2455–9.
24. Savva A, Taylor MJ, Beatty CW. Management of cerebrospinal fluid leaks involving the temporal bone: report on 92 patients. Laryngoscope. 2003;113:50–6.
25. Kerr JT, Chu FW, Bayles SW. Cerebrospinal fluid rhinorrhea: diagnosis and management. Otolaryngol Clin North Am. 2005;38(4):597–611.
26. Lobo B, Heng A, Barkhoudarian G, Griffiths CF, Kelly DF. The expanding role of the endonasal endoscopic approach in pituitary and skull base surgery: a 2014 perspective. Surg Neurol Int. 2015;6:*82*.
27. Sakas DE, Beale DJ, Ameen AA, Whitwell HL, Whittaker KW, Krebs AJ, Abbasi KH, Dias PS. Compound anterior cranial base fractures: classification using computerized tomography scanning as a basis for selection of patients for dural repair. J Neurosurg. 1998;88:471–7.
28. Scholsem M, Scholtes F, Collignon F, Robe P, Dubuisson A, Kaschten B, Lenelle J, Martin D. Surgical management of anterior cranial base fractures with cerebrospinal fluid fistulae: a single-institution experience. Neurosurgery. 2008;62:463–71.
29. Eljamel MS, Foy PM. Acute traumatic CSF fistulae: the risk of intracranial infection. Br J Neurosurg. 1990;4:381–5.
30. Mincy JE. Posttraumatic cerebrospinal fluid fistula of the frontal fossa. J Trauma Acute Care Surg. 1966;6:618–22.
31. Brodie HA. Prophylactic antibiotics for posttraumatic cerebrospinal fluid fistulae: a meta-analysis. Arch Otolaryngol Head Neck Surg. 1997;123:749–52.
32. Leech P, Paterson A. Conservative and operative management for cerebrospinal-fluid leakage after closed head injury. Lancet. 1973;301:1013–6.
33. Oh J-W, Kim S-H, Whang K. Traumatic cerebrospinal fluid leak: diagnosis and management. Korean J Neurotrauma. 2017;13:63.
34. Friedman JA, Ebersold MJ, Quast LM. Persistent posttraumatic cerebrospinal fluid leakage. Neurosurg Focus. 2000;9:1–5.
35. D'Anza B, Tien D, Stokken JK, Recinos PF, Woodard TR, Sindwani R. Role of lumbar drains in contemporary endonasal skull base surgery: meta-analysis and systematic review. Am J Rhinol Allergy. 2016;30:430–5.
36. Ratilal BO, Costa J, Pappamikail L, Sampaio C. Antibiotic prophylaxis for preventing meningitis in patients with basilar skull fractures. Cochrane Database Syst Rev. 2015;2015:CD004884.
37. Bernal-Sprekelsen M, Bleda-Vazquez C, Carrau RL. Ascending meningitis secondary to traumatic cerebrospinal fluid leaks. Am J Rhinol. 2000;14:257–60.
38. Brodie HA, Thompson TC. Management of complications from 820 temporal bone fractures. Otol Neurotol. 1997;18:188–97.
39. Sanders-Taylor C, Anaizi A, Kosty J, Zimmer LA, Theodosopoulos PV. Sellar reconstruction and rates of delayed cerebrospinal fluid leak after endoscopic pituitary surgery. J Neurolog Surg B Skull Base. 2015;76:281–5.
40. Hoffer A, Onwuzulike K. Cerebrospinal fluid rhinorrhea. 2014. Journal: Encyclopedia of the Neurological Sciences, 2014, p. 718–721.
41. Martínez-Capoccioni G, Serramito-García R, Martín-Bailón M, García-Allut A, Martín-Martín C. Spontaneous cerebrospinal fluid leaks in the anterior skull base secondary to idiopathic intracranial hypertension. Eur Arch Otorhinolaryngol. 2017;274:2175–81.

42. Dhungana S, Sharrack B, Woodroofe N. Idiopathic intracranial hypertension. Acta Neurol Scand. 2010;121(2):71–82.
43. Ball AK, Clarke CE. Idiopathic intracranial hypertension. Lancet Neurol. 2006;5(5):433–42.
44. Pérez MA, Bialer OY, Bruce BB, Newman NJ, Biousse V. Primary spontaneous cerebrospinal fluid leaks and idiopathic intracranial hypertension. J Neuroophthalmol. 2013;33(4):330.
45. Wall M. Idiopathic intracranial hypertension. Neurol Clin. 2010;28(3):593–617.
46. Glueck CJ, Aregawi D, Goldenberg N, Golnik KC, Sieve L, Wang P. Idiopathic intracranial hypertension, polycystic-ovary syndrome, and thrombophilia. J Lab Clin Med. 2005;145(2):72–82.
47. Biousse V, Bruce BB, Newman NJ. Update on the pathophysiology and management of idiopathic intracranial hypertension. J Neurol Neurosurg Psychiatry. 2012;83(5):488–94.
48. Warner JE, Larson AJ, Bhosale P, Digre KB, Henley C, Alder SC, Katz BJ, Bernstein PS. Retinol-binding protein and retinol analysis in cerebrospinal fluid and serum of patients with and without idiopathic intracranial hypertension. J Neuroophthalmol. 2007;27(4):258–62.
49. Chen BS, Newman NJ, Biousse V. Atypical presentations of idiopathic intracranial hypertension. Taiwan J Ophthalmol. 2021;11(1):25.
50. Friedman DI, Jacobson DM. Diagnostic criteria for idiopathic intracranial hypertension. Neurology. 2002;59(10):1492–5.
51. Binder DK, Horton JC, Lawton MT, McDermott MW. Idiopathic intracranial hypertension. Neurosurgery. 2004;54(3):538–52.
52. La Fata V, McLean N, Wise SK, DelGaudio JM, Hudgins PA. CSF leaks: correlation of high-resolution CT and multiplanar reformations with intraoperative endoscopic findings. Am J Neuroradiol. 2008;29(3):536–41.
53. Aaron G, Doyle J, Vaphiades MS, Riley KO, Woodworth BA. Increased intracranial pressure in spontaneous CSF leak patients is not associated with papilledema. Otolaryngol Head Neck Surg. 2014;151(6):1061–6.
54. Chen JJ, Trobe JD. Optical coherence tomography should be used routinely to monitor patients with idiopathic intracranial hypertension. J Neuroophthalmol. 2016;36(4):453–9.
55. Tilak AM, Koehn H, Mattos J, Payne SC. Preoperative management of spontaneous cerebrospinal fluid rhinorrhea with acetazolamide. Int Forum Allergy Rhinol. 2019;9(3):265–9.
56. Alonso RC, de la Peña MJ, Caicoya AG, Rodriguez MR, Moreno EA, de Vega Fernandez VM. Spontaneous skull base meningoencephaloceles and cerebrospinal fluid fistulas. Radiographics. 2013;33(2):553–70.
57. Hadad G, Bassagasteguy L, Carrau RL, Mataza JC, Kassam A, Snyderman CH, Mintz A. A novel reconstructive technique after endoscopic expanded endonasal approaches: vascular pedicle nasoseptal flap. Laryngoscope. 2006;116(10):1882–6.
58. Lindstrom DR, Toohill RJ, Loehrl TA, Smith TL. Management of cerebrospinal fluid rhinorrhea: the Medical College of Wisconsin experience. Laryngoscope. 2004;114(6):969–74.
59. Zapalac JS, Marple BF, Schwade ND. Skull base cerebrospinal fluid fistulas: a comprehensive diagnostic algorithm. Otolaryngol Head Neck Surg. 2002;126(6):669–76.
60. Adams AS, Russell PT, Duncavage JA, Chandra RK, Turner JH. Outcomes of endoscopic repair of cerebrospinal fluid rhinorrhea without lumbar drains. Am J Rhinol Allergy. 2016;30(6):424–9.
61. Choby GW, Mattos JL, Hughes MA, Fernandez-Miranda JC, Gardner PA, Snyderman CH, Wang EW. Delayed nasoseptal flaps for endoscopic skull base reconstruction: proof of concept and evaluation of outcomes. Otolaryngol Head Neck Surg. 2015;152(2):255–9.
62. Khafagy YW, Abd Elfattah AM, Moneir W, Salem EH. Leukocyte-and platelet-rich fibrin: a new graft material in endoscopic repair of spontaneous CSF leaks. Eur Arch Otorhinolaryngol. 2018;275:2245–52.
63. Elmorsy SM, Khafagy YW. Endoscopic management of spontaneous CSF rhinorrhea with septal graft and middle turbinate rotational flap technique: a review of 31 cases. Ear Nose Throat J. 2014;93(6):E14–9.
64. Ibrahim AA, Okasha M, Elwany S. Endoscopic endonasal multilayer repair of traumatic CSF rhinorrhea. Eur Arch Otorhinolaryngol. 2016;273:921–6.

65. Prickett KK, Wise SK, DelGaudio JM. Choice of graft material and postoperative healing in endoscopic repair of cerebrospinal fluid leak. Arch Otolaryngol Head Neck Surg. 2011;137(5):457–61.
66. Roehm CE, Brown SM. Unilateral endoscopic approach for repair of frontal sinus cerebrospinal fluid leak. Skull Base. 2011;21:139–46.
67. Hegazy HM, Carrau RL, Snyderman CH, Kassam A, Zweig J. Transnasal endoscopic repair of cerebrospinal fluid rhinorrhea: a meta-analysis. Laryngoscope. 2000;110(7):1166–72.
68. Fortes FS, Carrau RL, Snyderman CH, Prevedello D, Vescan A, Mintz A, Gardner P, Kassam AB. The posterior pedicle inferior turbinate flap: a new vascularized flap for skull base reconstruction. Laryngoscope. 2007;117(8):1329–32.
69. Maltan TA, Salem EH, Eldeeb AH, Moneir W, Khafagy YW. Predictors of failure of recurrent spontaneous CSF rhinorrhea repair: a prospective cohort study. Egyptian J Otolaryngol. 2023;39(1):133.
70. Lorenz RR, Dean RL, Hurley DB, Chuang J, Citardi MJ. Endoscopic reconstruction of anterior and middle cranial fossa defects using acellular dermal allograft. Laryngoscope. 2003;113(3):496–501.
71. El Fiky L, Kotb A, Mostafa BE. A unified management for spontaneous CSF leak. Int J Otolaryngol Head Neck Surg. 2015;4(02):141.
72. Mollan SP, Davies B, Silver NC, Shaw S, Mallucci CL, Wakerley BR, Krishnan A, Chavda SV, Ramalingam S, Edwards J, Hemmings K. Idiopathic intracranial hypertension: consensus guidelines on management. J Neurol Neurosurg Psychiatry. 2018;89(10):1088–100.
73. Manfield JH, Yu KK, Efthimiou E, Darzi A, Athanasiou T, Ashrafian H. Bariatric surgery or non-surgical weight loss for idiopathic intracranial hypertension? A systematic review and comparison of meta-analyses. Obes Surg. 2017;27:513–21.
74. Fridley J, Foroozan R, Sherman V, Brandt ML, Yoshor D. Bariatric surgery for the treatment of idiopathic intracranial hypertension: a review. J Neurosurg. 2011;114(1):34–9.
75. Sinclair AJ, Kuruvath S, Sen D, Nightingale PG, Burdon MA, Flint G. Is cerebrospinal fluid shunting in idiopathic intracranial hypertension worthwhile? A 10-year review. Cephalalgia. 2011;31(16):1627–33.
76. Alsuhaibani AH, Carter KD, Nerad JA, Lee AG. Effect of optic nerve sheath fenestration on papilledema of the operated and the contralateral nonoperated eyes in idiopathic intracranial hypertension. Ophthalmology. 2011;118(2):412–4.
77. El Mekabaty A, Obuchowski NA, Luciano MG, John S, Chung CY, Moghekar A, Jones S, Hui FK. Predictors for venous sinus stent retreatment in patients with idiopathic intracranial hypertension. J Neurointervent Surg. 2017;9(12):1228–32.
78. Higgins JNP, Cousins C, Owler BK, Sarkies N, Pickard JD. Idiopathic intracranial hypertension: 12 cases treated by venous sinus stenting. J Neurol Neurosurg Psychiatry. 2003;74(12):1662–6.
79. Chaaban MR, Illing E, Riley KO, Woodworth BA. Acetazolamide for high intracranial pressure cerebrospinal fluid leaks. Int Forum Allergy Rhinol. 2013;3(9):718–21.

# Sinonasal Mucoceles

# 34

Samy Elwany

**Key Points**
- Mucoceles are expansile cystic lesions containing mucus and lined with respiratory epithelium.
- They may be unilocular or multilocular, primary or secondary.
- Secondary mucoceles may be post-traumatic, postsurgical, or in association with other diseases.
- Ethmoid and frontoethmoid mucoceles are the more common variety.
- Endoscopic marsupialization is the treatment of choice in most cases.

Sinonasal mucoceles are expansile cystic lesions containing mucus and lined with respiratory epithelium. They constitute 3% of all sinus swellings and 2.7% of non-endocrine causes of proptosis. They may be secondarily infected, resulting in a mucopyocele [1–5].

## 34.1 Types

A. According to pathogenesis:
   (a) Primary mucoceles result from retention of secretions due to obstruction of the normal outflow tract.
   (b) Secondary mucoceles occur due to trauma, surgery, or another pathology [6–8] (Figs. 34.1, 34.2, and 34.3).

S. Elwany (✉)
Department of Otolaryngology, Alexandria University, Alexandria, Egypt
e-mail: samy.elwany@alexmed.edu.eg


S. Elwany (ed.), *Current Rhinology*,
https://doi.org/10.1007/978-3-031-70077-4_34

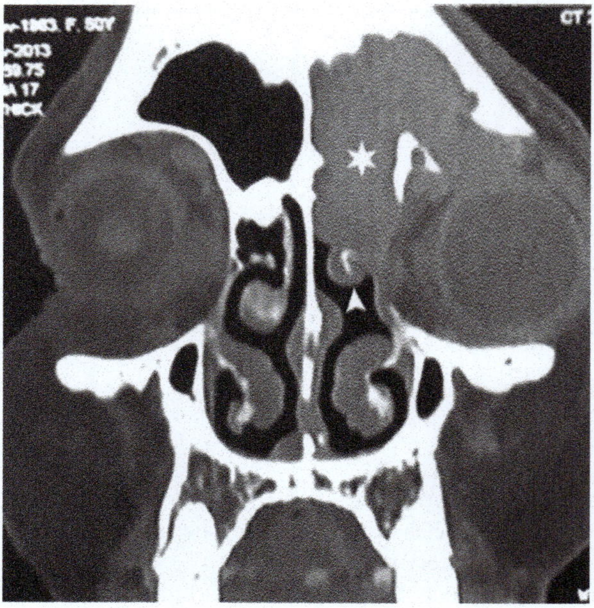

**Fig. 34.1** CT scan showing a secondary frontoethmoid mucocele (*) due to blockage of the frontal recess by a nasoseptal flap (arrowhead)

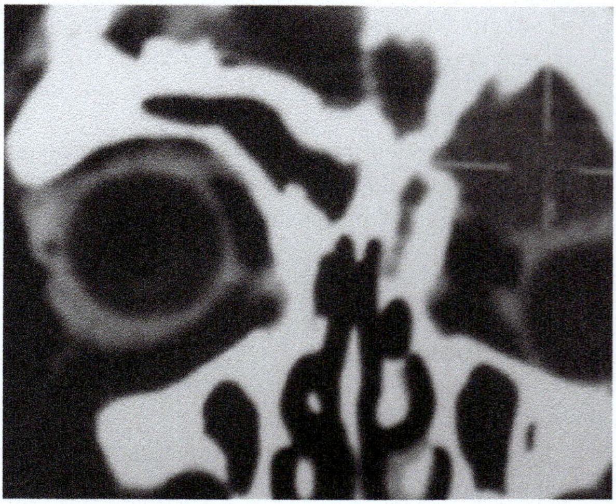

**Fig. 34.2** Left post-traumatic frontal mucocele following a car accident

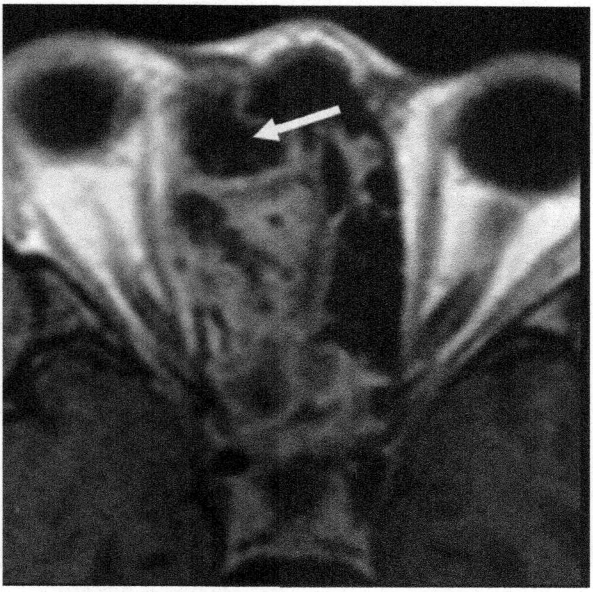

**Fig. 34.3** Secondary mucocele associated with fungal sinusitis

B. According to the number of loculi:
   (a) Unilocular
   (b) Multilocular (Fig. 34.4)

Mucocele formation and expansion leads to bony remodeling and resorption secondary to the protracted chronic inflammatory reaction.

Mucoceles develop most commonly in the frontal and ethmoid sinuses but may involve other sinuses or even an aerated turbinate [5, 9–12].

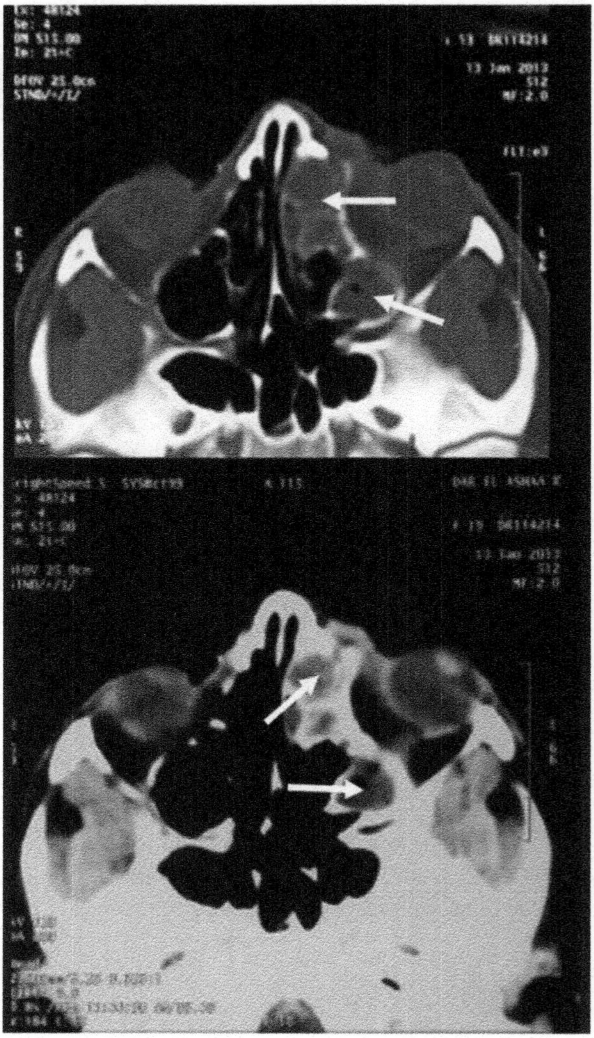

**Fig. 34.4** CT scan showing a multilocular mucocele (arrows). All loculi should be drained during surgery to avoid recurrence of symptoms

## 34.2 Clinical Picture

1. Nasal blockage (maybe predominantly unilateral) and nasal discharge [2]
2. Headache and pain behind the eyes, especially with sphenoid sinus mucoceles [13–16]
3. Cystic swelling above the medial canthus (ethmoid mucocele). It may be misinterpreted as a mucocele of the lacrimal sac (Fig. 34.5).
4. Proptosis, diplopia, and eye pain. The direction of proptosis depends on the location of the mucocele [17, 18]
5. Large frontal sinus mucoceles may erode the anterior table of the sinus and cause fluctuant external swelling [19]

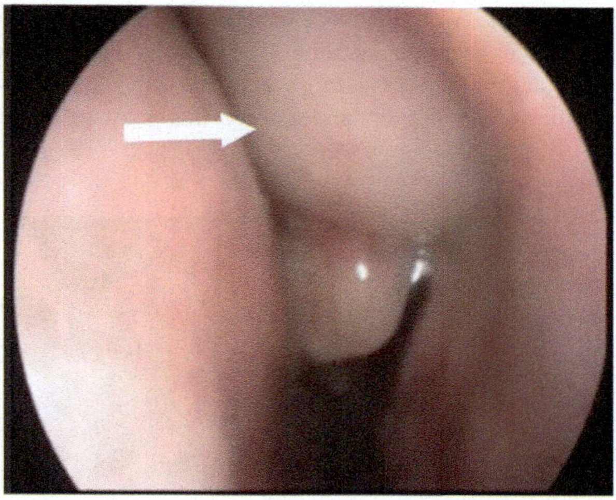

**Fig. 34.5** Typical endoscopic appearance of an ethmoid mucocele (arrow)

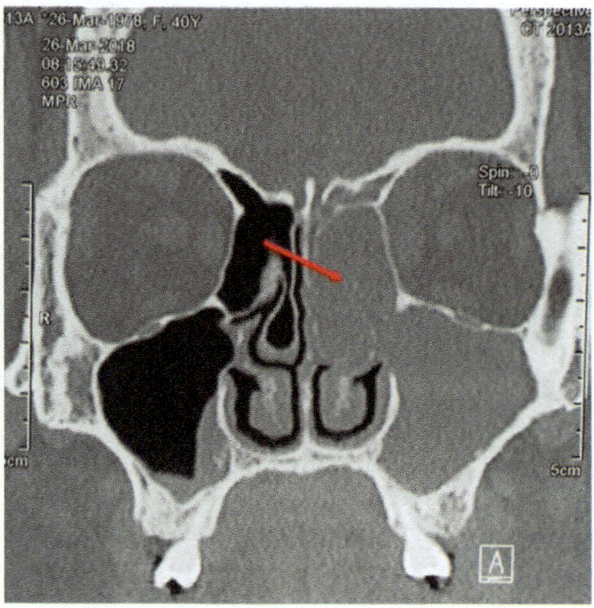


**Fig. 34.6** CT scan showing a typical ethmoid sinus mucocele

## 34.3 Radiologic Diagnosis

A. Computed tomography: Mucoceles appear in CT scan images as well-circumscribed cystic lesions with homogeneous attenuation, expanding the bony walls of the affected sinus. Bony dehiscence may be seen later (Fig. 34.6).

B. Magnetic resonance imaging (MRI): The appearance of the mucocele depends on the protein concentration of the retained mucus. Mucoceles typically appear with low intensity on T1-weighted and with high intensity on T2-weighted images. As the mucocele gets older, the protein concentration of the retained mucus increases and the MRI characteristics of the mucocele change. A long-standing mucocele will eventually show an increased T1 signal intensity and a decreased T2 signal intensity that may totally drop out (signal void) [20] (Figs. 34.7 and 34.8).

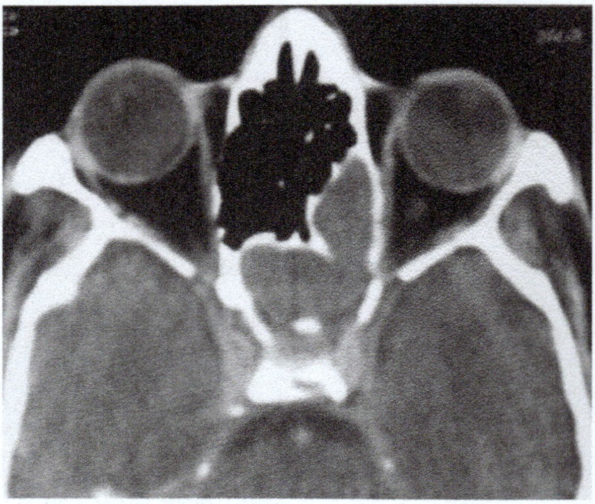

**Fig. 34.7** CT scan showing left spheno-ethmoid mucocele

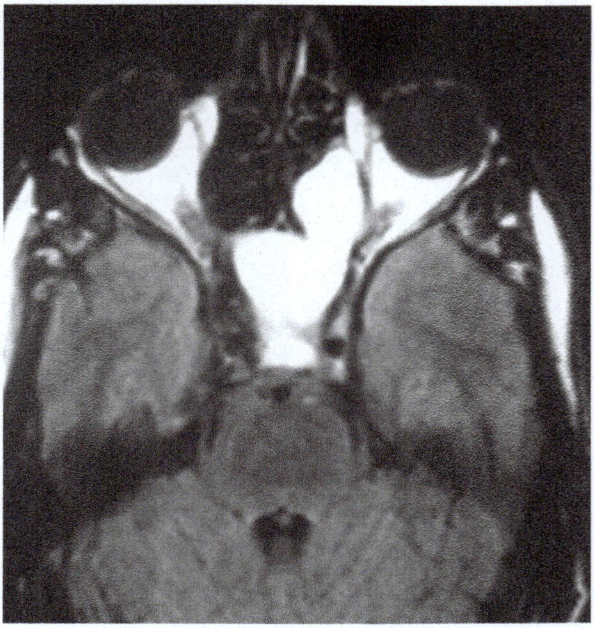

**Fig. 34.8** T1 MRI with contrast showing the enhanced contents of the mucocele

## 34.4 Treatment

Endoscopic marsupialization is the standard treatment in most cases. Marsupialization should ensure free gravitational drainage of the mucocele. All loculi of the mucocele should be widely opened. The mucosal lining of the mucocele should be left intact for faster healing (Fig. 34.9).

External and transorbital approaches such as Lynch-Howarth frontoethmoidectomy may be needed for a few selected cases when the anatomy is markedly distorted or when there is a big defect in the anterior table of the frontal sinus [21].

Causes of recurrence of mucocele formation:

1. Missed loculi, especially in the frontal sinus
2. Failure to maintain a wide communication with the nasal cavity

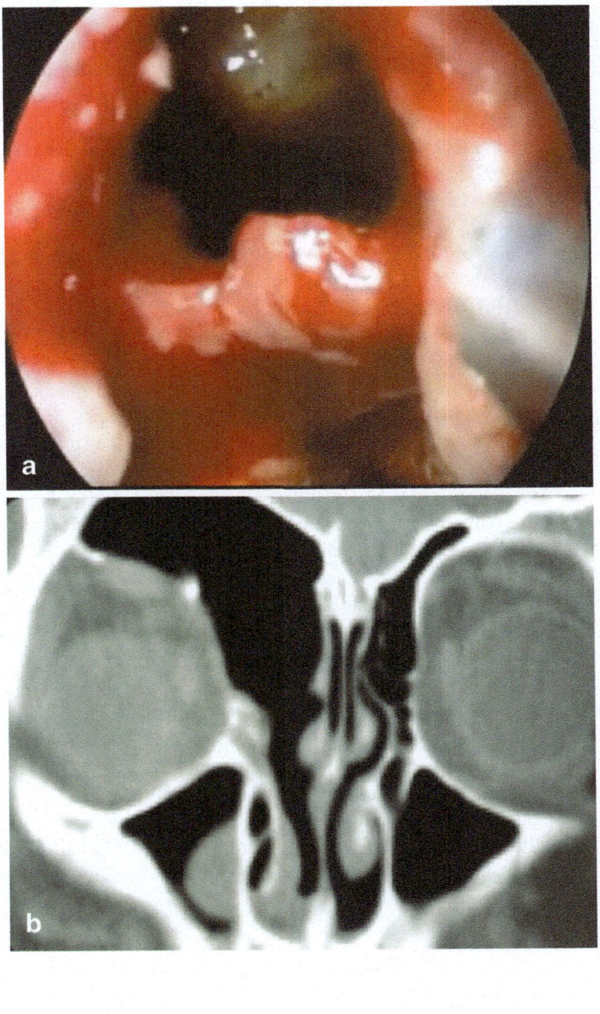


**Fig. 34.9** Endoscopic (**a**) and radiologic (**b**) procedures of a successfully marsupialized mucocele

## References


1. Madani G, Beale TJ. Sinonasal inflammatory disease. Semin Ultrasound CT MR. 2009;30:17–24. https://doi.org/10.1053/j.sult.2008.10.012.
2. Habesoglu TE, Habesoglu M, Surmeli M, Uresin T, Egeli E. Unilateral sinonasal symptoms. J Craniofac Surg. 2010;21:2019–22. https://doi.org/10.1097/SCS.0b013e3181f5389a.
3. Thompson LDR. Paranasal sinus mucocele. Ear Nose Throat J. 2012;91:276–8.
4. Olze H, Matthias C, Degenhardt P. Paediatric paranasal sinus mucoceles. Eur J Pediatr Surg. 2006;16:192–6. https://doi.org/10.1055/s-2006-924000.
5. Scangas GA, Gudis DA, Kennedy DW. The natural history and clinical characteristics of paranasal sinus mucoceles: a clinical review. Int Forum Allergy Rhinol. 2013;3:712–7. https://doi.org/10.1002/alr.21178.
6. Awad AJ, Mohyeldin A, El-Sayed IH, Aghi MK. Sinonasal morbidity following endoscopic endonasal skull base surgery. Clin Neurol Neurosurg. 2015;130:162–7. https://doi.org/10.1016/j.clineuro.2015.01.004.
7. Abou Chaaya J, Fleifel M, Arabi A. A rare presentation of intrasellar mucocele post-transsphenoidal resection of a non-secreting pituitary macroadenoma. Cureus. 2023;15:e44471. https://doi.org/10.7759/cureus.44471.
8. Hansen FS, van der Poel NA, Freling NJM, Fokkens WJ. Mucocele formation after frontal sinus obliteration. Rhinology. 2018;56:106–10. https://doi.org/10.4193/Rhin17.187.
9. Maisel RH, Deeb ME, Bone RC. Sphenoid sinus mucoceles. Laryngoscope. 1973;83:930–9. https://doi.org/10.1288/00005537-197306000-00011.
10. Gardner DG, Gullane PJ. Mucoceles of the maxillary sinus. Oral Surg Oral Med Oral Pathol. 1986;62:538–43. https://doi.org/10.1016/0030-4220(86)90317-8.
11. Suri A, Mahapatra AK, Gaikwad S, Sarkar C. Giant mucoceles of the frontal sinus: a series and review. J Clin Neurosci. 2004;11:214–8. https://doi.org/10.1016/j.jocn.2003.02.011.
12. Hssaine K, Belhoucha B, Rochdi Y, Nouri H, Aderdour L, Raji A. Paranasal sinus mucoceles: about 32 cases. Rev Stomatol Chir Maxillofac Chir Orale. 2016;117:11–4. https://doi.org/10.1016/j.revsto.2015.11.006.
13. Kösling S, Hintner M, Brandt S, Schulz T, Bloching M. Mucoceles of the sphenoid sinus. Eur J Radiol. 2004;51:1–5. https://doi.org/10.1016/j.ejrad.2003.09.002.
14. Close LG, O'Conner WE. Sphenoethmoidal mucoceles with intracranial extension. Otolaryngol Head Neck Surg. 1983;91:350–7. https://doi.org/10.1177/019459988309100402.
15. Darouassi Y, Righini CA, Reyt E. Mucoceles of the sphenoidal sinus: a report of four cases and review of the literature. B-ENT. 2005;1:181–5.
16. Yokoyama T, Inoue S, Imamura J, Nagamitsu T, Jimi Y, Katoh S, et al. Sphenoethmoidal mucoceles with intracranial extension--three case reports. Neurol Med Chir (Tokyo). 1996;36:822–8. https://doi.org/10.2176/nmc.36.822.
17. Malik M, Vahdani K, Rose GE. Ophthalmic presentation and outcome for sinonasal mucoceles. Ophthal Plast Reconstr Surg. 2023;39:44–8. https://doi.org/10.1097/IOP.0000000000002234.
18. Kim Y-S, Kim K, Lee J-G, Yoon J-H, Kim C-H. Paranasal sinus mucoceles with ophthalmologic manifestations: a 17-year review of 96 cases. Am J Rhinol Allergy. 2011;25:272–5. https://doi.org/10.2500/ajra.2011.25.3624.
19. Gavioli C, Grasso DL, Carinci F, Amoroso C, Pastore A. Mucoceles of the frontal sinus. Clinical and therapeutical considerations. Minerva Stomatol. 2002;51:385–90.
20. Bouatay R, Aouf L, Hmida B, El Korbi A, Kolsi N, Harrathi K, et al. The role of imaging in the management of sinonasal mucoceles. Pan Afr Med J. 2019;34:3. https://doi.org/10.11604/pamj.2019.34.3.18677.
21. Miller C, Berens A, Patel SA, Humphreys IM, Moe KS. Transorbital approach for improved access in the management of paranasal sinus Mucoceles. Neurol Surg B. 2019;80:593–8.

# Dacryocystorhinostomy

# 35

Yasser W. Khafagy and Noha Ahmed El-Kholy

**Key Points**

- True epiphora refers to excessive watering of the eye due to the obstruction of lacrimal passages.
- It can be due to primary "idiopathic" or secondary to inflammatory, traumatic, or neoplastic causes.
- It can be divided into four clinical grades according to the amount and type of the fluid.
- Main diagnostic tests include diagnostic probing, Schirmer's test, fluorescein dye disappearance test, syringing, dacryocystography, computed tomography, and magnetic resonance imaging.
- Conservative treatment of nasolacrimal duct obstruction may include measures to reestablish the natural flow such as topical or oral antibiotics and anti-inflammatory medications along with office-based canalicular probing and lacrimal irrigation.
- There are two approaches for dacryocystorhinostomy: external and endoscopic endonasal approaches.
- The endoscopic approach has gained more acceptance nowadays due to many reasons. These include the absence of an external scar, less periorbital ecchymosis, and less incidence of injury to the medial canthal tendon.

Y. W. Khafagy (✉) · N. A. El-Kholy
Department of Otolaryngology, Mansoura University, Mansoura, Egypt
e-mail: ykhafagy@mans.edu.eg


S. Elwany (ed.), *Current Rhinology*,
https://doi.org/10.1007/978-3-031-70077-4_35

## 35.1 Embryological Background

The lacrimal sac and nasolacrimal duct (NLD) develop as a solid epithelial cord at 5 weeks of gestation. This is followed by canalization of the cord to form the NLD at 12 weeks of gestation with the dilatation of its superior end to form the lacrimal sac. The membrane at the superior punctum is usually completely canalized at 7 months of gestation when eyelids separate and is normally patent at birth. In contrast, the inferior membrane frequently persists in the new-born. Developmental abnormalities in this region occurring typically after 4 months of gestation can result in congenital agenesis of any segment of the NLD, supernumerary puncta, canaliculi, and lacrimal fistula. The distal end of the NLD often has a membrane, and in about two-thirds of the new-borns, this remains imperforate at birth which accounts for the most common cause of congenital NLD obstruction (CNLDO) in children [1].

## 35.2 Anatomical Background

The lacrimal apparatus comprises structures involved in production (the main and accessory lacrimal glands) and transport of tears (puncta, canaliculi, lacrimal sac, nasolacrimal duct, and valves) (Fig. 35.1).

A. Lacrimal Glands

The main lacrimal gland is located in the lacrimal gland fossa, formed by the orbital plate of the frontal bone in the anterolateral part of the roof of the orbit. It is divided into two parts; orbital part and palpebral part divided by the lateral horn of

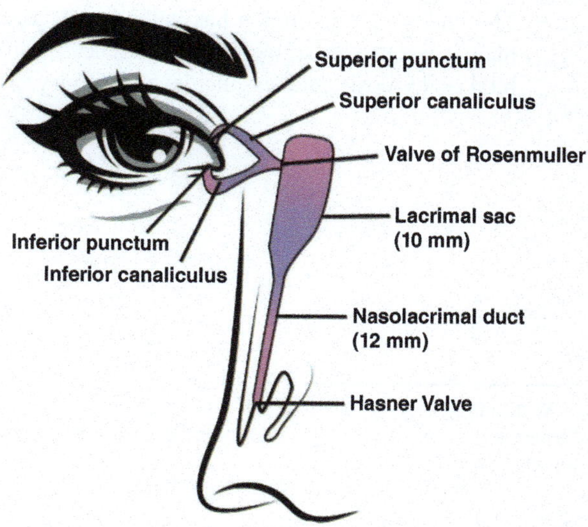


**Fig. 35.1** Diagrammatic illustration of the main anatomical landmarks of the lacrimal system

aponeurosis of the levator muscle. The orbital part is larger—nearly two-thirds of the total lacrimal gland. The palpebral part can be seen on eversion of the lids.

It has 10–12 ducts passing from the lacrimal gland and open into the lateral part of the superior fornix. One to two ducts also open into the lateral part of the inferior fornix. All the ducts pass through the palpebral part of the gland. The main blood supply is through the lacrimal artery, a branch of the ophthalmic artery. The lacrimal veins draining the gland join the ophthalmic vein, and its lymphatic drainage goes to the pre-auricular lymph nodes. Sensory nerve supply is through the lacrimal nerve, which is a branch of the ophthalmic division of the trigeminal nerve. Sympathetic innervation reaches the gland around the carotid cervical plexus and secretomotor innervation is supplied from the superior salivary nucleus [2].

B. Lacrimal Passages

Lacrimal puncta are located at the junction of the ciliary and the lacrimal portion of the lid margin upon a slight elevation called lacrimal papilla. The upper and lower puncta lie about 6 and 6.5 mm lateral to the inner canthus. The puncta are directed backward toward the eye and surrounded by a ring of dense fibrous tissue which keeps them patent. With each blink, the puncta slide in the groove between the plica semilunaris and the eyeball.

Lacrimal canaliculus has two parts, which measures 2 mm vertically and 8 mm horizontally. It lies at right angles to each other with a slight dilatation at their junction called the ampulla. The canaliculus pierces the lacrimal fascia separately and then unites to form a common canaliculus, which opens in a small diverticulum of the sac called the lacrimal sinus of Maier. The opening lies about 2.5 mm from the apex. The valve of Rosenmuller prevents the reflux from the sac to the canaliculus [3].

Lacrimal sac is located in a fossa formed by the lacrimal bone and the frontal process of the maxilla, bounded by the anterior and posterior lacrimal crests. Periorbita splits at the posterior lacrimal crest forming lacrimal fascia enclosing the sac and unites at the anterior lacrimal crest. Between the sac and the fascia lie the alveolar tissue and venous plexus, which continues around the nasolacrimal duct. It is about 15 mm long and 5 mm broad with a capacity of 20 cc. It is bounded medially by anterior ethmoidal sinus superiorly and middle meatus inferiorly. Posteriorly, it is surrounded by lacrimal fascia, lacrimal fibres of orbicularis, and orbital septum. Anterolaterally, from anterior to posterior; skin, angular vein, palpebral fibres of orbicularis muscle, medial palpebral ligament, lacrimal fibres of orbicularis muscle, and lacrimal fascia.

Nasolacrimal Duct (NLD) opens in the inferior meatus of the nose. It is about 18 mm (12–24) in length and 3 mm in diameter. The direction of the NLD is downward, backward and lateral. It has two parts: an intraosseous part (12.5 mm) and an intrameatal part (5.5 mm). The intraosseous part lies in the nasolacrimal canal formed by the maxilla and the nasal concha. The nasolacrimal canal lies lateral to the middle meatus. The intrameatal part of the NLD lies in the mucous membrane of the lateral wall of the nose. The nasolacrimal duct opens into the ostium lacrimalis which lie 30 to 35 mm from the external nares and 15 mm from the tip of the inferior turbinate. This ostium is variable in shape and location, may be multiple, and sometimes difficult to locate [2]. The lower nasolacrimal fossa and the nasolacrimal duct are narrower in females, which may account for the female predominance of nasolacrimal obstruction.

The bony canal is formed mainly by the maxilla and completed by the lacrimal bone and lacrimal process of the inferior concha. The average bony canal is slightly oval in the parasagittal plane with a width of 3.5–4.5 mm, being the widest at both ends and narrowest in the middle [4].

The NLD has numerous valves; the most important one is the valve of Hasner which is located at the distal opening of lacrimal duct at the inferior meatus and allows unidirectional tear flow. The other two valves include valve of Rosenmuller: situated at the internal opening of the common canaliculus within the lacrimal sac and valve of Krause between the sac and duct.

**Endoscopic Anatomy of the Lacrimal Sac**

The lacrimal bone extends between the frontal process of the maxilla anteriorly, to the attachment of the uncinate posteriorly. It is important to note that the lacrimal bone and sac are located just anterior to the orbit. The retrolacrimal region of the lamina papyracea is thin and trauma to the uncinate at this point may lead to penetration of the orbit. The lacrimal sac extends 9 mm above the axilla of the middle turbinate. The common canaliculus opens high on the lateral wall of the sac; this area should be exposed, and all bones should be removed during surgery for a better result [5].

The lacrimal process of the inferior turbinate represents the lower posterior part of the medial wall of the bony nasolacrimal canal. The anterior end of the middle turbinate is a constant anatomical landmark for lacrimal surgeons, since it relates closely to the position of lacrimal sac. Maxillary Line, also called lacrimal crest or ridge, is a mucosal projection along the lateral nasal wall that extends from the anterior attachment of the middle turbinate to the lateral nasal wall downward and backward toward the root of the inferior turbinate from the nasal side. It corresponds to the junction of the frontal process of maxilla anteriorly and the lacrimal bone and uncinate process posteriorly while externally it corresponds to the lacrimomaxillary suture at the junction of the frontal process of maxilla and lacrimal bone. The mid portion of the line is called "M point" and its identification is critically important during endoscopic sinus and orbital procedures [6].

## 35.3 Radiological Background

CT is a very useful diagnostic modality in the assessment of the lacrimal anatomy in relation to the surrounding bones specially in facial trauma and suspected malignancies. The anatomic relationship of the anterior ethmoid air cells to the lacrimal sac fossa is important to understand before performing dacryocystorhinostomy, in order to avoid confusion between the ethmoid and nasal cavities during creation of the ostium. A close anatomic relationship between agger nasi cells and the lacrimal sac fossa has been demonstrated in several past studies. These agger nasi cells may pneumatize the lacrimal bone, and rarely extend into the frontal process of the maxillary bone [7].

The relation of the lacrimal sac to the anterior tip of middle turbinate is variable. The sac may lie anterior, opposite, or posterior to the anterior end of middle turbinate. Anterior ethmoid air cells are present between the upper part of lacrimal fossa and nasal cavity and in more than 50% of cases agger nasi air cells extend into the frontal process of the maxilla as far as the anterior lacrimal crest [8].

## 35.4 Physiological Background

The main lacrimal gland along with the accessory glands of Krause and Wolfring are responsible for the secretion of the aqueous layer of the tear film. The tear film also comprises two other components, the lipid layer and the mucin layer, and functions to protect the ocular surface from desiccation. Periodic blinking helps in an even distribution of the tears in the conjunctival cul-de-sac (lacus lacrimalis), as also in propelling them toward the final excretory pathway [9].

The average tear flow rate is 30 microL/min and a complete recycling of the tear volume of 230 microL occurs over 7 min. The lacrimal excretory system is a mucus-lined passage with several components and the normal drainage of tears is dependent on a coordinated interaction between the anatomical and physiological well-being of these structures. Conditions that cause disruption of this normal mechanism may result in a "watering eye," also known as epiphora [10].

## 35.5 Epiphora

Epiphora is the excessive watering of eyes due to the obstruction of the lacrimal drainage system or excessive production of tears. True epiphora refers to watering due to obstruction in the tear drainage pathway "anatomical or obstructive epiphora" and must be differentiated from pseudo epiphora, which is excessive watering due to hyperlacrimation "physiological or non-obstructive epiphora" [11].

Nasolacrimal duct obstruction may be congenital or acquired:

- *Congenital Nasolacrimal Duct Obstruction* (CNLDO)

About 2–4% of infants are born with congenital obstruction of the nasolacrimal duct, which resolves spontaneously in 80–90% of cases within a few months. The most common type of CNLDO is a simple membrane at the valve of Hasner, where the nasolacrimal duct enters the nose. This membrane is generally imperforated at birth and will open spontaneously within the first few days of life. Spontaneous resolution beyond 1 year of age is possible, and in over 65% of infants aged 6–10 months it resolved with non-surgical management within 6 months [12].

- *Acquired Nasolacrimal Duct Obstruction*

In the majority of cases, the aetiology of an acquired obstruction in the lacrimal drainage apparatus remains obscure. Infection is a common associate, especially with obstructions involving the nasolacrimal duct. It is still not clear whether the infection is causal or sequential to the obstruction, or whether these two factors are simply part of a wider diathesis.

In particular, distal drainage system obstructions are idiopathic in 80% of cases, and they are referred to as "PANDO" (primary acquired nasolacrimal duct obstruction) as avascular specific inflammation, more frequent in females; this determines venous alterations with progressive atrophy or fibrosis of the lacrimal sac. Obstructions of the upper portion of the nasolacrimal duct, where the lacrimal sac goes through the bony canal, are generally related to a specific inflammation of the lacrimal sac "dacryocystitis" [13]. Secondary acquired lacrimal drainage obstruction or SALDO occurs secondary to underlying etiology as trauma, inflammation, infection, neoplasms, or other causes [14].

**Dacryocystitis**

Inflammation of the lacrimal sac (i.e., dacryocystitis) can present as an acute or chronic process. Generally, dacryocystitis occurs in association with partial or complete nasolacrimal duct obstruction [15]. Acute dacryocystitis is an aggressive infection of the lacrimal sac and is usually bacterial in origin. In the presence of tear stasis, conditions become favorable for bacterial growth in the lacrimal sac. Marked distention of the lacrimal sac occurs with accompanying erythema and pain. If the infection is left untreated, the lacrimal sac may rupture and permanent external fistula may occasionally develop. Infection may also spread to the face and eyelids forming preseptal or orbital cellulitis. Exudate accumulates within the sac causing distention and formation of a thin-walled pyocele or frank abscess [16].

Chronic dacryocystitis represents a more indolent form of lacrimal sac inflammation and infection. A reflux of mucoid or mucopurulent discharge from the lacrimal sac via the canaliculi is usually present. The walls of the lacrimal sac are usually thickened, and the lacrimal sac lumen is dilated [17].

## 35.6 Evaluation of a Case of Epiphora

### 35.6.1 History

The time of onset of epiphora, laterality, and type of discharge should be noted. It is important to ask about the intermittency of epiphora and the severity of the symptoms to get a true picture of the patient's functional problem. Epiphora in a child with a history of tearing beginning shortly after birth is indicative of an imperforate Hasner's membrane or less commonly, a bony obstruction. Epiphora due to complete nasolacrimal duct obstruction (NLDO) is usually continuous and associated with intermittent mucoid or purulent discharge. Watery discharge may be due to allergic conjunctivitis, glaucoma, reflex tearing, non-obstructive epiphora, or chronic NLDO with fibrosed sac [18].

A rapidly growing mass or bleeding from the puncta points to the diagnosis of malignancy or an ongoing granulomatous process. Unilateral epiphora is most likely due to anatomical obstruction in the lacrimal system while bilateral tearing may point to conditions like allergic conjunctivitis. History of prior facial trauma, orbital radiation, use of ophthalmic medications, any nasal allergies, and previous treatment should be elicited. Any prior intranasal surgeries undertaken should also be noted [19].

Clinical grading of Epiphora

Grade 1: Intermittent clear discharge, not causing functional problem to the patient.
Grade 2: Continuous clear discharge, not causing functional problem to the patient.
Grade 3: Continuous and copious clear discharge, causing blurred vision and/or skin excoriation and/or requiring constant wiping.
Grade 4: Mucoid or mucopurulent discharge [20].

### 35.6.2 External Examination

An examination of the lower eyelid for any laxity, ectropion, entropion, punctum eversion, or blepharitis is important. Also, examination of the medial canthus for any lacrimal sac enlargement below the medial canthal tendon and palpation of lacrimal sac is of crucial importance especially in acute dacryocystitis.

Certain facial features offer a clue to the cause of tearing. Epiphora due to an abnormal lacrimal drainage system in facial-cleft syndromes, congenital ectropion in Treacher Collin syndrome, and cicatricial ectropion in congenital ichthyosis are certain examples. Any mass lesion in the caruncle or medial eyelid can block the punctum leading to epiphora. An enlarged caruncle in thyroid eye disease (TED) can also cause epiphora due to the same reason.

Mass in the lacrimal sac region below the level of the medial canthal tendon is indicative of a lacrimal sac mucocele due to an obstruction in the distal lacrimal drainage apparatus. A mass lesion above the level of medial canthal tendon indicates malignancy or a granulomatous condition like tuberculosis, Wegener's granulomatosis (WG), or sarcoidosis. WG is also known to cause bilateral NLDO. A swelling that is hard on palpation is suggestive of a dacryolith. The presence of unilateral telecanthus may point to a swelling arising from ethmoid sinus [21].

### 35.6.3 Different Methods to Evaluate the Exact Site of Blockage in the Nasolacrimal System

1. *Slit Lamp Evaluation*

   Slit lamp evaluation should follow the external examination in every patient for a detailed assessment of the ocular adnexa and external ocular surface.

2. *Special Investigations*: Diagnostic tests are used to identify the cause of an obstruction and to choose appropriate treatment. Diagnostic tests can be classified as follows [20]:
   - Anatomical: Localize site of obstruction
     - Diagnostic probing
     - Syringing (irrigation)
     - Dacryocystography
     - CT and MRI
   - Physiological: Assess the function
     - Fluorescein dye disappearance
     - Scintigraphy
     - Saccharine test
   - Secretion: Assess secretory function
     - Schirmer's test
     - Bengal rose test
     - Tear film break-up
     - Tear lysozyme

**Schirmer's Test**

Schirmer's test is a simple clinical diagnostic procedure to rule out dry eye and hypersecretion syndromes. It consists of two parts: Schirmer's I test evaluates gross tear production and Schirmer II evaluates reflex tear production [22].

**Tear Break-up Time**

The tear break-up time is an important test to assess the mucin component of the tear function.

**ROPLAS (Regurgitation On Pressure over the Lacrimal Sac Area)**

Firm pressure is applied over the sac area and noted for any regurgitation. This must be performed before and after sac syringing to correlate with the findings of sac syringing and reach a diagnosis [23].

**FDDT**

Fluorescein dye disappearance test gives an approximate measurement of the rate of tear flow out of the conjunctival sac. The test cannot distinguish anatomical obstruction in the drainage pathway from pump failure, nor can it localize the site of blockage. It is a useful adjunct in the diagnostic evaluation of the lacrimal system, especially in children with congenital NLDO, who are uncooperative for sac syringing in the office [24].

**Sac Syringing**

Lacrimal sac syringing is the most important procedure in the evaluation of epiphora and it is generally done by ophthalmologists in an outpatient clinic under local anesthesia.

**Diagnostic Probing**

Probing is indicated when an obstruction is encountered in the lacrimal drainage apparatus at the time of sac syringing. It is useful in the identification of the exact site of blockage. A well-lubricated "0" size Bowman's probe is used for this purpose. The probe is passed along the canaliculus in which the obstruction was identified at the time of syringing or when any canaliculus when the obstruction was noted beyond the common canaliculus [25].

How to interpret a diagnostic probing test:

- A *hard stop* is when the probe is advanced along the canaliculus and encounters the lacrimal bone. This means that the probe has passed into the sac and touched its bony medial wall, and that the common canaliculus is patent.
- A *soft stop* is a spongy feeling encountered when there is an obstruction proximal to the lacrimal sac and the probe cannot be passed into the sac. In such cases the obstruction is at the common canaliculus and the lacrimal probe presses the common canaliculus and the lateral wall against the medial wall of the sac. There will also be a medial shift of the inner canthus when advancing the probe toward the lacrimal bone due to the probe displacing the common canaliculus medially.
- Reflux through the opposite punctum when syringing a hard stop suggests an obstruction of the sac or the nasolacrimal duct.

### 35.6.4 Endoscopic Nasal Examination

A precise nasal examination is essential to rule out the common nasal conditions which cause epiphora using a 4-mm, 0°, and 30° endoscope. This provides a good view of the lateral nasal wall. The health of the mucosa is assessed as significantly hypertrophied mucosa can cause blockage of the lower end of the NLD. The presence of any nasal pathology including nasal polyps and nasal anatomical variation such as deviated septum and concha Bullosa is important and should be documented in the surgical plan [26].

### 35.6.5 Dacyocystography (DCG)

Dacryocystography is an anatomical investigation and is indicated in complex cases to localize the exact site of blockage in the lacrimal apparatus. It is indicated in multiple failed surgeries, post-traumatic epiphora, and suspicious lacrimal sac tumors. It is done using a radio-opaque water-soluble fluid [27].

### 35.6.6 Dacryoscintigraphy

Nuclear lacrimal scintigraphy is a non-invasive physiological test for the evaluation of the lacrimal system. This is performed using a radiotracer, which can be detected

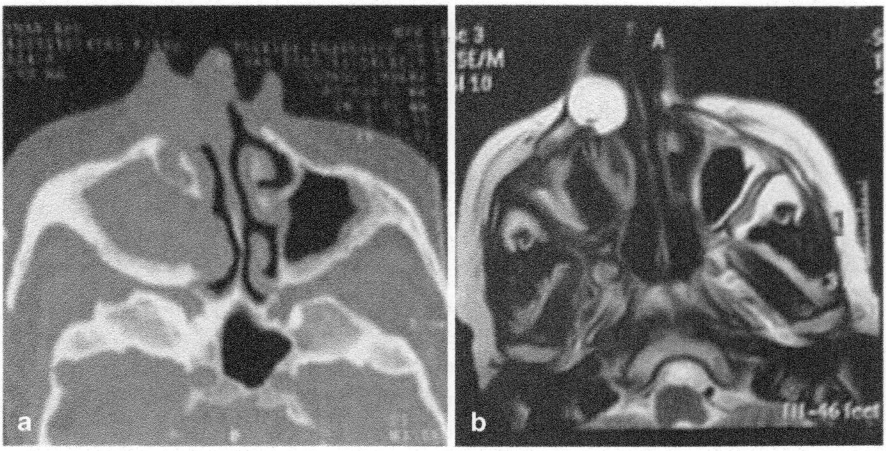

**Fig. 35.2** Radiological evaluation of a case of dacryocystocele. (**a**) Computed tomography scan of nose and paranasal sinuses, axial cuts, showing soft tissue opacity filling the right maxillary sinus with widening and expansion of the right nasolacrimal duct and external soft tissue opacity related to it. (**b**) Magnetic resonance imaging of the same patient, axial T2 weighted images, showing a cystic lesion in relation to the right nasolacrimal duct

with a gamma camera. Scintigraphy is useful in studying tear dynamics, and its main use is in the evaluation and confirmation of lacrimal pump dysfunction [28].

### 35.6.7 Computed Tomography (CT) and CT-DCG

CT-DCG is a relatively new technique which uses a water-soluble radio-opaque dye. This is indicated in cases of suspected malignancy of the lacrimal sac, facial trauma, encysted mucocele, dacryocystocele [29].

### 35.6.8 Magnetic Resonance Imaging (MRI) and MR-DCG

MRI and MR-DCG are not routinely used for lacrimal diagnostics and maybe indicated in certain cases requiring very fine resolution of the soft tissue structures [30] (Fig. 35.2).

## 35.7 Different Lines of Treatment

The treatment of nasolacrimal duct obstruction may include measures to reestablish the natural flow such as topical or oral antibiotics and anti-inflammatory medications along with office-based canalicular probing and lacrimal irrigation. The choice of antibiotic depends on initial culture and sensitivity results. Of note, unlike congenital NLDO, primary acquired NLDO in an adult generally exhibits less response to probing. Although probing with silicone tubing intubation or balloon dacryoplasty has been reported to successfully treat a subset of acquired NLDO in adults, the treatment of choice for primary acquired NLDO is DCR, which bypasses the usual site of obstruction in the distal nasolacrimal duct [31].

Dacryocystorhinostomy is the standard surgical procedure for nasolacrimal outflow tract obstruction. In dacryocystorhinostomy, the lacrimal sac is connected directly to the nose by removing the part of lacrimal bone and mucosa that separate these two structures. The earliest dacryocystorhinostomy was done by an external approach by Toti in 1904. Due to the drawbacks of the external procedure (such as external scar formation, injury to the medial canthal ligament, and periorbital ecchymosis), the endoscopic approach is considered now as the golden standard technique for management of nasolacrimal duct obstruction. The first endoscopic procedure was done by McDonough and Miring in 1989.

Endoscopic Dacryocystorhinostomy has distinct advantages such as less trauma, better cosmetic acceptability, provides a wide surgical field, minimal intraoperative bleeding, avoidance of scarring, preservation of the pumping action of the orbicularis oculi muscle, and shorter hospital stay. A transcanalicular silicone stent may be placed at the time of surgery to maintain patency of the ostium [32].

There are two clear goals of the DCR procedure. One is to make a large bony ostium into the nose and that remains so. The second is to have a mucosal lined anastomosis. Since both these purposes are well served by an external route, it is the preferred approach by many oculoplastic surgeons with high success rates. Indications of DCR include (a) persistent congenital lacrimal duct obstructions unresponsive to previous therapies, (b) primary acquired nasolacrimal duct obstructions (PANDO), and (c) secondary acquired nasolacrimal duct obstructions (SALDO).

Success rates of external DCR have long been known to be high at 90–95% [33, 34], but the effectiveness of endoscopic approaches have been more varied through the development of the technique. An early randomized study comparing endoscopic DCR to external DCR described the success rates (75% versus 91%) [35], although not achieving statistical difference. When the authors compared a third arm of endoscopic laser DCR to the same external DCR cohort, published in a separate article [36], the difference in success rates was statistically significant at 62.5% compared to the 91% [37].

It was noted that the failure of the endoscopic techniques seemed in large part due to a poor understanding of endoscopic anatomy, which led to poorly placed rhinostomies, and inadequate bone removal, which led to fibrosis and scarring of the intranasal ostium [38], unexposed common canaliculus or subsequent sump syndrome. This was addressed by ensuring wider bony ostia, extending the opening up to 8 mm superior to the uncinate and by marsupializing the lacrimal sac mucosa to expose both the common canaliculus and lower duct during surgery [39].

There is an overall result favoring external DCR, with a success rate of 84% (897/1068) for endoscopic DCR and 87% (863/993) for external DCR, but when endoscopic drilling DCR and endoscopic laser DCR are separately compared to external DCR, the success rates of endoscopic drilling DCR are comparable to external DCR (87%; 624/714), while the results of endoscopic laser DCR (77%; 273/354) clearly favor external DCR [33].

Comparison of the complications reveal that infection rates appear to be lower in endoscopic DCR. Of the studies that reported infection rates, postoperative care varied, with some using systemic and topical antibiotics [40, 41] in both groups, while some only used topical antibiotics and steroids [42].

As for cutaneous scarring, which only occurs with external DCR, it has been demonstrated that 10.8% of patients reported a scar that they had deemed cosmetically unacceptable. The reported rates of revision surgery required in the included studies are similar between endoscopic DCR and external DCR.

### 35.7.1 External DCR

Toti (1904) proposed that after creating an external approach to the lacrimal sac, its portion near the canaliculi should be preserved and absorbed into the nose, by creating a window in the lateral nasal wall. Due to late failures, Toti's technique was modified by other surgeons. Dupuy-Dutemps and Bourguet introduced mucosal anastomosis with suturing of the mucosal flaps. Fashioning the nasal mucosa and the medial wall of lacrimal sac into anterior and posterior flaps and suturing of these flaps was suggested by Ohm (1926).

The last technique is still considered the standard technique for modern external DCR and modifications are usually compared with it. Baldeschi et al. fashioned one large flap in the sac and nasal mucosa and sutured them together into the overlying orbicularis oculi to suspend the flaps away from, and prevent adhesions with, the underlying tissues with non-placement of a stent [41, 43, 44].

### 35.7.2 Endonasal Endoscopic DCR

The need for non-incisional approaches is the motivation to drain the lacrimal sac into the nose and dates back to the late nineteenth century. Caldwell in 1893 was the first to describe the endonasal approach. This technique meant an excision of the nasal mucosa anterior to the middle turbinate, drilling osteotomy through the bone, opening the lacrimal sac, and silicon stenting. The success rates for this technique range from 80% to 85% [45].

#### Operative Procedure of Endoscopic DCR (Figs. 35.3, 35.4, 35.5, 35.6, 35.7, 35.8, 35.9, and 35.10)

Under general anesthesia, decongestion of the nasal mucosa is achieved by placement of nasal pledgets that contain oxymetazoline 0.05% in the middle meatus, followed by endoscopic injection of 1% xylocaine containing 1:200,000 epinephrine into the lateral nasal wall and middle turbinate.

Lacrimal sac localization is done by determining the point of insertion of the root of the middle turbinate on the lateral nasal wall and the maxillary line as a key intranasal landmark. For surgeons who are becoming familiar with intranasal anatomy

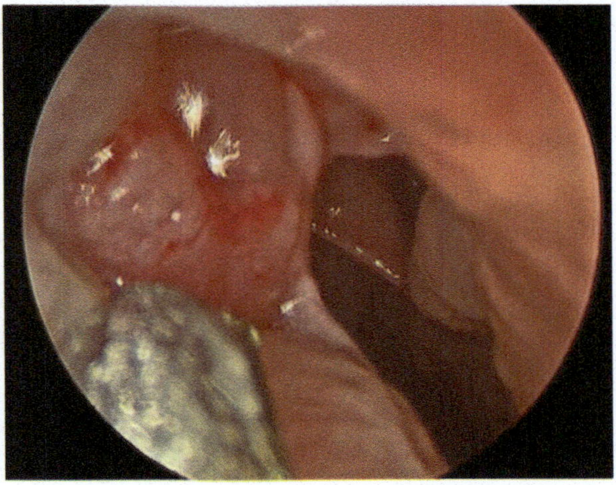

**Fig. 35.3** Intraoperative photo of the first step in endoscopic endonasal dacryocystorhinostomy showing swollen nasal mucosa over the site of the dacryocystocele

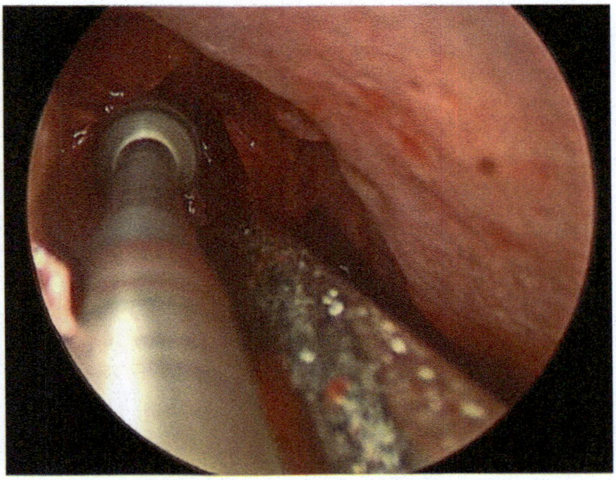

**Fig. 35.4** Drilling over the lacrimal bone to expose the lacrimal sac using a diamond burr

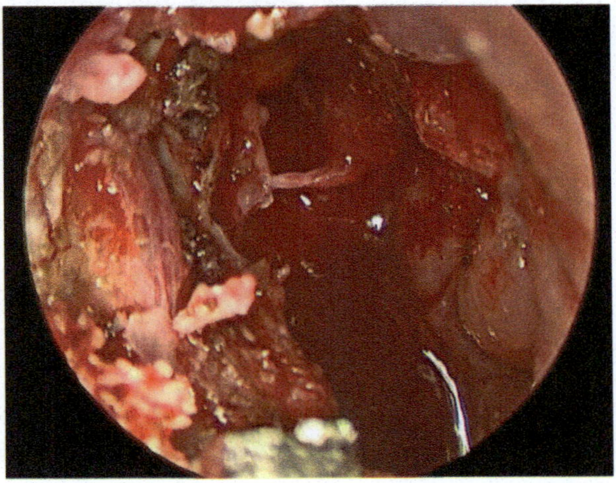

**Fig. 35.5** All the bones over lacrimal sac have been remove allowing for its complete exposure

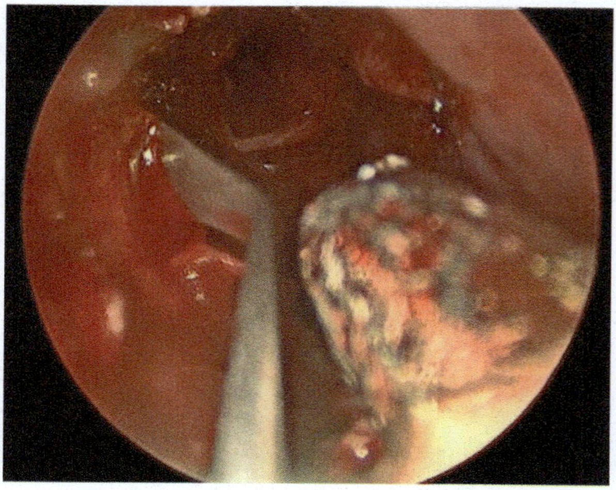

**Fig. 35.6** Incision of the lacrimal sac to evacuate the dacryocystocele

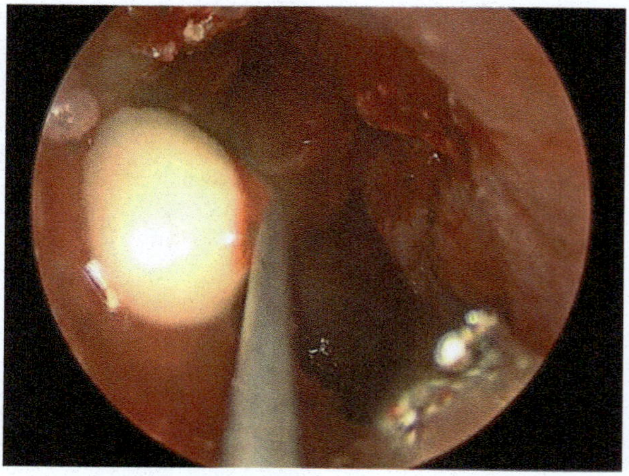

**Fig. 35.7** Endoscopic photo showing pus coming out of the lacrimal sac following its incision

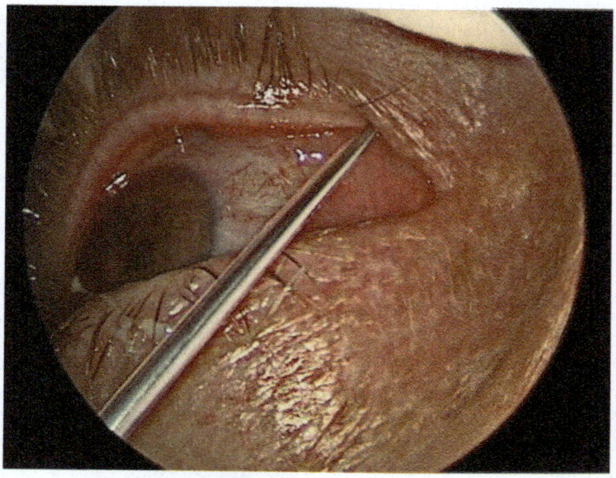

**Fig. 35.8** Probing of the superior punctum. The direction of probing starts upward then medially toward the lacrimal sac

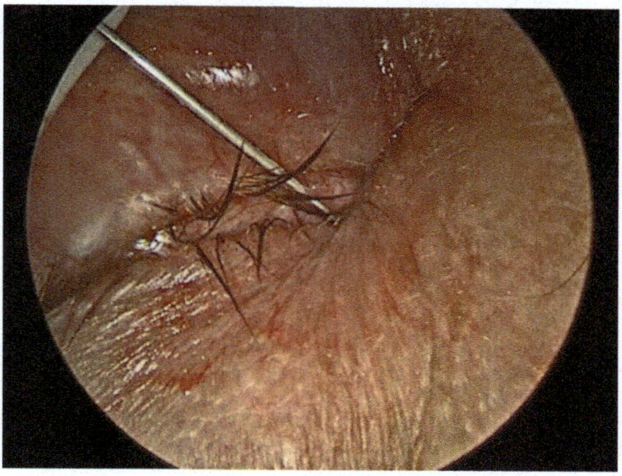

**Fig. 35.9** Probing of the inferior punctum. The direction here starts downward and then medially toward the lacrimal sac

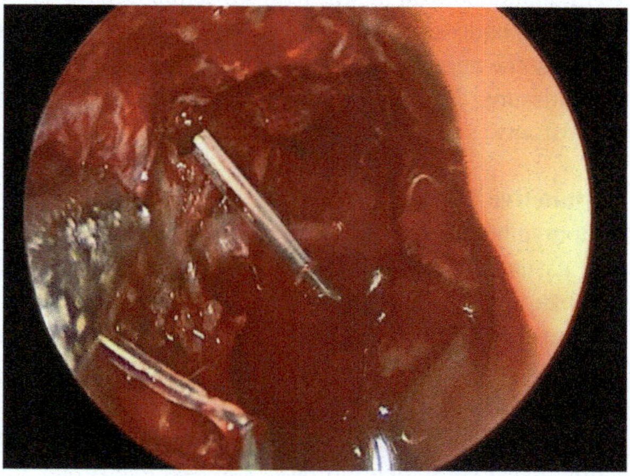

**Fig. 35.10** Endoscopic photo showing lacrimal stent passing through both superior and inferior lacrimal puncti into the nasal cavity

and surgery in patients who have atypical anatomy or a history of sinonasal procedures, it may be helpful to place a fiber optic illuminator over the lacrimal sac area at the medial canthus. The location of the lacrimal sac then may be visualized endoscopically by transillumination.

After lacrimal sac localization, the mucosa on the lateral wall is incised using a sickle knife, or electrocautery, and is elevated using a Freer elevator. It is helpful to place this incision well anterior to the location of the lacrimal sac to allow full exposure of the overlying bone. The incision is oriented vertically, extending from inferior to superior to minimize interference from bleeding. After the mucosa is elevated widely from the underlying bone, it is removed with Blakesley forceps.

To expose the lacrimal sac, the bony lacrimal fossa must be uncovered. Bone removal may be achieved by using a variety of instruments, and it should commence at the maxillary line and proceed anteriorly. Although the lacrimal bone, located posterior to the maxillary line, may be taken down with minimal force, the authors recommend the use of a high-speed drill with a diamond burr for removal of the dense frontal process of the maxilla, which is situated anteriorly creating a bony rhinostomy of adequate size and location facilitates a successful outcome. It is particularly important that the bone overlying the common canaliculus is resected completely. Generally, a rhinostomy with a vertical dimension of at least 6–8 mm is achieved in adult patients. It is common for an anterior ethmoidectomy to be required to allow satisfactory access to the lacrimal fossa by removing prominent agger nasi cells.

After removal of the overlying bone, the lacrimal sac is incised using a sickle knife. Often, it is helpful for the assistant to "tent out" the medial wall of the lacrimal sac with lacrimal probes that are introduced through the canaliculi. The medial wall of the lacrimal sac and NLD then may be removed with Blakesley forceps. An adequate rhinostomy should permit easy passage of lacrimal probes. Removal of the medial wall of the lacrimal sac in the area of the common canaliculus also may be confirmed by direct visualization of the internal common punctum with a 0° or 30° endoscope.

After the medial sac wall has been resected, a bicanalicular intubation set is used to intubate both canaliculi, with subsequent retrieval of the probes from the rhinostomy site endoscopically. The tubing is tied in the nasal vestibule in such a way as to allow the appropriate length and tension of the silicone tubing loop in the medial commissure. Thus, the closed loop formed acts as stent for the newly created rhinostomy.

**Adjunctive Measures (Use of Mitomycin C)**

Mitomycin C in a concentration of 0.02% is used if there are intra-sac synechiae, soft tissue scarring like in failed DCRs, and in the presence of complicated surgery. Intubation is also advisable for similar indications but in addition it is also used in the presence of canalicular problems and inadequate flaps [46].

**Postoperative Care**

Postoperative care usually involves local irrigation of the rhinostomy site with saline nasal spray and antibiotic–steroid eye drops are very important for the prevention of the adhesions and obstruction of rhinostomy opening. Patients are again seen after 2 weeks to clean the nose, remove crusts, and to remove early adhesions. Silastic tubes are removed in the office after 4–6 weeks.

**Complications**

Early complications include adhesions, granulations, if the tubes are tied too tightly in the nasal cavity, and epistaxis, while late complications include restenosis and failed surgery with the need for a revision surgery.

Revision surgery is occasionally indicated. It is imperative that the reason for failure is ascertained, which may include that not enough bone has been removed superiorly or inferiorly causing a sump effect with tears collecting in the sac, no wide marsupialization of the sac, missed foreign body or stones within the sac, stenosis of the superior or inferior canaliculi, and stenting that caused excessive granulations [45].

**Acknowledgement** We acknowledge Ms. Hiba Said for drawing the medical illustration.

## References


1. Hamed Azzam S, Hartstein M, Dolmetsch A, Mukari A. Assessment of Lacrijet monocanalicular intubation for congenital nasolacrimal duct obstruction. Eur J Ophthalmol. 2022;32(6):3340–5.
2. Moscato EE, Kelly JP, Weiss A. Developmental anatomy of the nasolacrimal duct: implications for congenital obstruction. Ophthalmology. 2010;117(12):2430–4.
3. Savar L, Seiff SR, Dolmetsch AM. Management of epiphora and lacrimal obstruction in adults. Pan-Am J Ophthalmol. 2014;13(2):37–43.
4. Kakizaki H, Ali MJ. The sinonasal anatomy: endoscopic lacrimal and orbital perspectives. In: Principles and practice of lacrimal surgery. Singapore: Springer; 2018. p. 49–67.
5. Vinciguerra A, Nonis A, Resti AG, Barbieri D, Bussi M, Trimarchi M. Influence of surgical techniques on endoscopic dacryocystorhinostomy: a systematic review and meta-analysis. Otolaryngol Head Neck Surg. 2021;165(1):14–22.
6. Rajak SN, Psaltis AJ. Anatomical considerations in endoscopic lacrimal surgery. Ann Anat. 2019;224:28–32.
7. Singh S, Ali MJ, Paulsen F. Dacryocystography: from theory to current practice. Ann Anat. 2019;224:33–40.
8. Gökçek A, Argin M, Altintas A. Comparison of failed and successful dacryocystorhinostomy by using computed tomographic dacryocystography findings. Eur J Ophthalmol. 2005;15(5):523–9.
9. Kopacz D, Niezgoda Ł, Fudalej E, Nowak A, Maciejewicz P. Tear film–physiology and disturbances in various diseases and disorders. In: Ocular surface diseases: some current date on tear film problem and keratoconic diagnosis. London: IntechOpen; 2021. p. 1.
10. Schaefer DP. Acquired etiologies of lacrimal system obstructions. In: The lacrimal system: diagnosis, management, and surgery. 2nd ed. Cham: Springer; 2015. p. 43–68.
11. Marcet MM, Kuk AK, Phelps PO. Evidence-based review of surgical practices in endoscopic endonasal dacryocystorhinostomy for primary acquired nasolacrimal duct obstruction and other new indications. Curr Opin Ophthalmol. 2014;25(5):443–8.
12. Takahashi Y, Kakizaki H, Chan WO, Selva D. Management of congenital nasolacrimal duct obstruction. Acta Ophthalmol. 2010;88(5):506–13.
13. Kashkouli MB, Sadeghipour A, Kaghazkanani R, Bayat A, Pakdel F, Aghai GH. Pathogenesis of primary acquired nasolacrimal duct obstruction. Orbit. 2010;29(1):11–5.
14. Karim R, Ghabrial R, Lynch T, Tang B. A comparison of external and endoscopic endonasal dacryocystorhinostomy for acquired nasolacrimal duct obstruction. Clin Ophthalmol. 2011;5:979–89.
15. Pinar-Sueiro S, Sota M, Lerchundi T-X, Gibelalde A, Berasategui B, Vilar B, et al. Dacryocystitis: systematic approach to diagnosis and therapy. Curr Infect Dis Rep. 2012;14:137–46.
16. Prat D, Magoon K, Revere KE, Katowitz JA, Katowitz WR. Management of pediatric acute dacryocystitis. Ophthalmic Plast Reconstr Surg. 2021;37(5):482–7.
17. Chakrabarti S, Dasgupta S, Banerjee M, Pal D. Role of histomorphology and chronic inflammation score in chronic dacryocystitis. J Clin Diagn Res. 2016;10(7):EC01.
18. Blackmore K, Ainsworth G, Robson A. Epiphora: an evidence based approach to the 12 minute consultation. Clin Otolaryngol. 2010;35(3):210–4.
19. Nemet AY. The etiology of epiphora: a multifactorial issue. Semin Ophthalmol. 2016;31:275–9. Taylor & Francis
20. Rao R, Kadam MY, Zaman A, Honavar SG. Evaluation of a patient with Epiphora. DCR. 2017;6
21. Avdagic E, Phelps PO. Nasolacrimal duct obstruction as an important cause of epiphora. Dis Mon. 2020;66(10):101043.
22. Mainville N, Jordan DR. Etiology of tearing: a retrospective analysis of referrals to a tertiary care oculoplastics practice. Ophthalmic Plast Reconstr Surg. 2011;27(3):155–7.

23. Alam MS, Singh P, Amitava AK, Ali MJ. Self-regurgitation on pressure over lacrimal sac in cases of primary-acquired nasolacrimal duct obstruction: correlation with physician examination and patients' perceptions. Saudi J Ophthalmol. 2021;35(3):217–9.
24. Kashkouli MB, Mirzajani H, Jamshidian-Tehrani M, Shahrzad S, Sanjari MS. Fluorescein dye disappearance test: a reliable test in assessment of success after dacryocystorhinostomy procedure. Ophthalmic Plast Reconstr Surg. 2015;31(4):296–9.
25. Kavitha C, Manipur SR, Acharya P, Lakshmi B. Clinical study of efficacy of probing as a treatment for epiphora in adults. J Clin Ophthalmol Res. 2019;7(1):5–7.
26. MacEwen C, Young J, Barras C, Ram B, White P. Value of nasal endoscopy and probing in the diagnosis and management of children with congenital epiphora. Br J Ophthalmol. 2001;85(3):314–8.
27. Bae SH, Park J, Lee JK. Comparison of digital subtraction dacryocystography and dacryoendoscopy in patients with epiphora. Eye. 2021;35(3):877–82.
28. Gholamrezanezhad A, Fard-Esfahani A, Sadeghi-Tari A, Mirpour S, Saghari M, Eftekhari M, et al. Quantitative assessment of dacryoscintigraphic images in the evaluation of epiphora. Orbit. 2007;26(4):229–35.
29. Papathanassiou S, Koch T, Suhling MC, Lenarz T, Durisin M, Stolle SR, et al. Computed tomography versus dacryocystography for the evaluation of the nasolacrimal duct—a study with 72 patients. Laryngoscope Investig Otolaryngol. 2019;4(4):393–8.
30. Cubuk R, Tasali N, Aydin S, Saydam B, Sengor T. Dynamic MR dacryocystography in patients with epiphora. Eur J Radiol. 2010;73(2):230–3.
31. Ali MJ, Naik MN. Efficacy of endoscopic guided anterograde 3 mm balloon dacryoplasty with silicone intubation in treatment of acquired partial nasolacrimal duct obstruction in adults. Saudi J Ophthalmol. 2014;28(1):40–3.
32. Smirnov G, Tuomilehto H, Teräsvirta M, Nuutinen J, Seppä J. Silicone tubing is not necessary after primary endoscopic dacryocystorhinostomy: a prospective randomized study. Am J Rhinol. 2008;22(2):214–7.
33. Welham R, Wulc AE. Management of unsuccessful lacrimal surgery. Br J Ophthalmol. 1987;71(2):152–7.
34. Walland MJ, Rose GE. Factors affecting the success rate of open lacrimal surgery. Br J Ophthalmol. 1994;78(12):888–91.
35. Hartikainen J, Antila J, Varpula M, Puukka P, Seppä H, Grénman R. Prospective randomized comparison of endonasal endoscopic dacryocystorhinostomy and external dacryocystorhinostomy. Laryngoscope. 1998;108(12):1861–6.
36. Hartikainen J, Grenman R, Puukka P, Seppä H. Prospective randomized comparison of external dacryocystorhinostomy and endonasal laser dacryocystorhinostomy. Ophthalmology. 1998;105(6):1106–13.
37. Sprekelsen MB, Barberán MT. Endoscopic dacryocystorhinostomy: surgical technique and results. Laryngoscope. 1996;106(2):187–9.
38. Tsirbas A, Davis G, Wormald PJ. Mechanical endonasal dacryocystorhinostomy versus external dacryocystorhinostomy. Ophthalmic Plast Reconstr Surg. 2004;20(1):50–6.
39. Tsirbas A, Wormald PJ. Endonasal dacryocystorhinostomy with mucosal flaps. Am J Ophthalmol. 2003;135(1):76–83.
40. Cokkeser Y, Evereklioglu C, Er H. Comparative external versus endoscopic dacryocystorhinostomy: results in 115 patients (130 eyes). Otolaryngol Head Neck Surg. 2000;123(4):488–91.
41. Dolman PJ. Comparison of external dacryocystorhinostomy with nonlaser endonasal dacryocystorhinostomy. Ophthalmology. 2003;110(1):78–84.
42. Leong SC, Karkos PD, Burgess P, Halliwell M, Hampal S. A comparison of outcomes between nonlaser endoscopic endonasal and external dacryocystorhinostomy: single-center experience and a review of British trends. Am J Otolaryngol. 2010;31(1):32–7.
43. Baldeschi L, Nardi M, Hintschich CR, Koornneef L. Anterior suspended flaps: a modified approach for external dacryocystorhinostomy. Br J Ophthalmol. 1998;82(7):790–2.

44. Mohan N, Bhaskar G, Sinha BP, AnkitaKumari A. Flapless modified Toti's procedure with use of circumostealMitomycin C as an adjunctive therapy in management of failed Dacryocystorhinostomy (DCR). J Med Sci Clin Res. 2019;7(7):956–61.
45. Mathew M, McGuiness R, Webb L, Murray S, Esakowitz L. Patient satisfaction in our initial experience with endonasal endoscopic non-laser dacryocystorhinostomy. Orbit. 2004;23(2):77–85.
46. Cheng S-m, Feng Y-f, Xu L, Li Y, Huang J-h. Efficacy of mitomycin C in endoscopic dacryocystorhinostomy: a systematic review and meta-analysis. PLoS One. 2013;8(5):e62737.

# Transorbital Endoscopic Surgery (TOES) 36

Ahmed A. Ibrahim and Sundus A. Alsedra

**Key Points**

- Endoscopic-assisted surgical approaches to the orbit are mainly performed via transnasal routes while nontransnasal endoscopic approaches inside and around the orbit are still rarely adopted in practice.
- The orbit should not only be considered the site of a pathologic finding, but also seen as a corridor for access to deeper areas.
- It requires great precision and care to save the structural integrity of the vital intraorbital content and functions as well as to preserve the aesthetics of the face.
- It should be performed on a case-to-case basis providing the most possible direct access to the lesion while minimizing any trauma to adjacent structures.
- The anatomy of the orbit and orbital apex is complex owing to the close relation between the carotid arteries, optic nerves, pituitary gland, and cavernous sinus.

## 36.1 Background

The end of the nineteenth century was the starting point of orbital surgery in the management of retrobulbar, intraorbital lesions, and orbital decompression mainly in Grave's diseases. Later in the beginning of 1950, they used lateral orbitotomy as an approach for

**Supplementary Information** The online version contains supplementary material available at https://doi.org/10.1007/978-3-031-70077-4_36.

A. A. Ibrahim (✉)
Alexandria University, Alexandria, Egypt

S. A. Alsedra
Al Yarmouk Teaching Hospital, Baghdad, Iraq


S. Elwany (ed.), *Current Rhinology*,
https://doi.org/10.1007/978-3-031-70077-4_36

certain intracranial pathologies. With progression of endoscopic surgery, advanced approaches have been innovated in dealing with skull base, sinonasal, and lastly transorbital surgery. These endoscopic transnasal and transorbital approaches provide an excellent corridor for what is called the sino-orbito-cranial interface. This corridor for inside and around the orbit is evolving in limited practice with widening surgical indications and with the need for good collaboration between multiple correlated specialties [1].

## 36.2 Anatomy

The orbit is a cone-shaped bony cavity with openings into the cranium that include the optic canal and superior orbital fissure together forming the orbital apex. The optic canal contains both the optic nerve and ophthalmic artery. The superior orbital fissure contains the oculomotor nerve, ophthalmic division of the trigeminal nerve, superior ophthalmic vein, and sympathetic fibers from the cavernous sinus. Endoscopic endonasal anatomy of the superior orbital fissure and orbital apex regions are critical considerations for clinical applications [2].

## 36.3 The Main Differential Diagnoses of Orbital Lesions

- Inflammatory/infectious lesion
- Dermoid cyst
- Grave's disease
- Vascular malformation (capillary hemangioma, cavernous hemangioma, and hemangiopericytoma)
- Lymphoproliferative disease
- Neurogenic tumors (meningioma and schwannoma)
- Mesenchymal and metastatic tumors

## 36.4 Preparation for Surgery

**Surgical Planning**

- The patient should be evaluated by a multidisciplinary team.
- A full radiologic study for preoperative planning of our approach.

**Operative Settings**

- Patient position like any standard nasal endoscopic surgical procedures.
- It is preferred to have a two-screen monitor for more than two surgeons.
- Usually, the head of the patient is not fixed unless an intracranial dissection will be carried out.
- A navigation system is of great importance especially in intraconal and intracranial dissection.
- Our setting let us work using four to six hands in the surgical field during the procedure (Fig. 36.1).

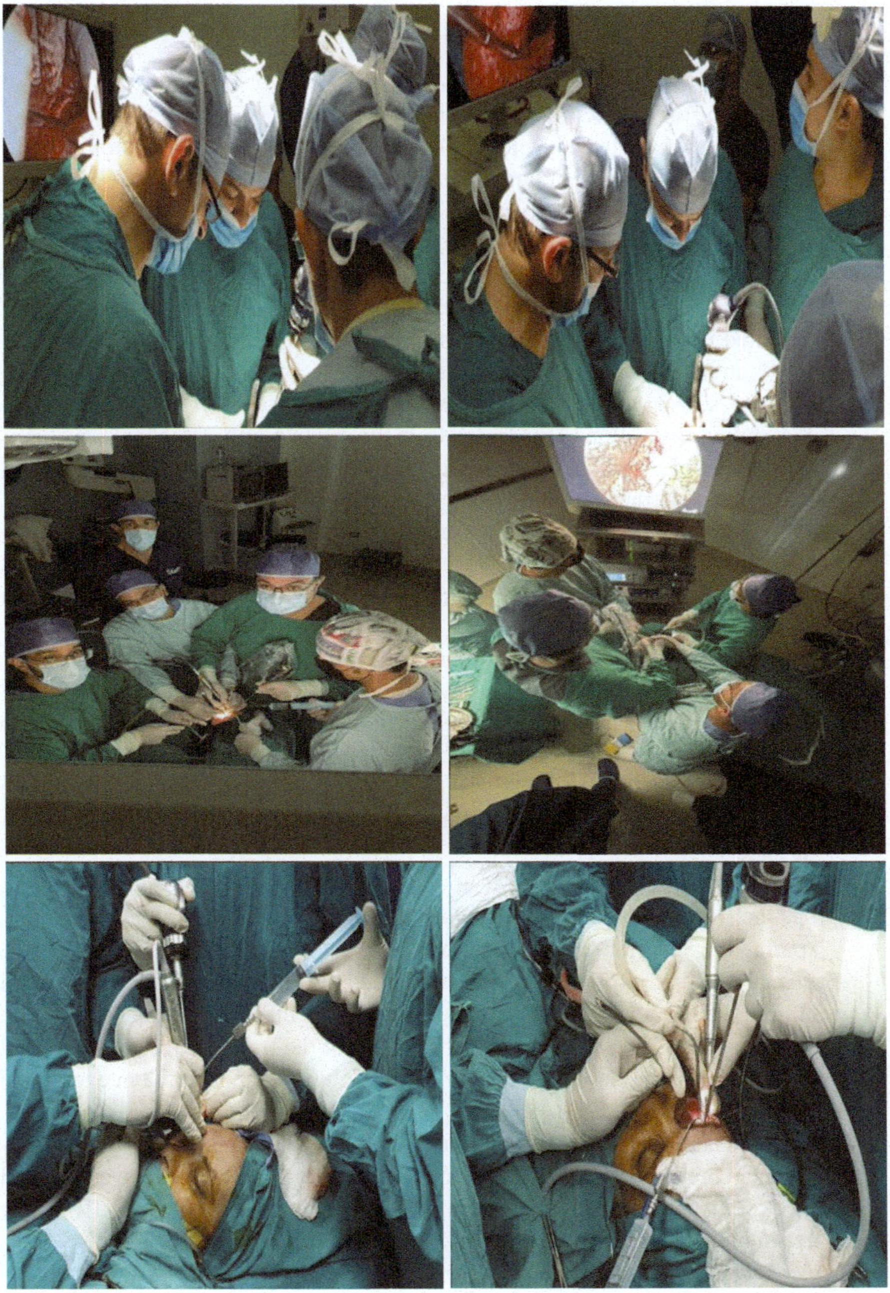

**Fig. 36.1** Operative setting using four to six hands technique for TONES

## 36.5 Surgical Approaches

- *Transnasal for intraconal or extraconal lesions*
  - Subtotal or total resection of the middle turbinate.
  - Complete sphenoethmoidectomy and mega middle meatus antrostomy.
  - Exposure and removal of lamina papyracea.
  - Periorbital exposure and opening.
  - Extraconal and intraconal fat management as needed.
  - Medial collateral veins are identified and managed.
  - Medial, inferior rectus, and superior oblique muscles are identified and retracted using slings or curved instruments for dealing with lesions according to an intraconal extension of dissection.
  - Anterior septal window for contralateral instrumentation if needed.
  - Meticulous dissection of the lesion from the surrounding intraconal structures.
  - Caretaking of the anterior ethmoidal and the central retinal arteries.
  - Finally, reconstruction if needed.
- *Blepharoplasty endoscopic-assisted approach (superior eyelid approach)*
  - A skin incision is made on a lid crease in the superior eyelid.
  - The orbicularis oculi muscle should be identified and a suborbicularis flap is raised.
  - Dissection is carried out in a supero-lateral direction until the orbital rim is reached.
  - The decision on whether the orbital septum should be spared or opened is subject to the target site of surgery.
  - If an opening in the periorbita is created, orbital fat will protrude into the operative field and should be managed with malleable retractors or silastic sheets.
  - If needed, the levator palpebrae aponeurosis and Müller's muscle can be cut, but they should be carefully re-approximated at the end of the procedure, sparing the superior oblique tendon.
  - In an extraconal approach, careful dissection of the periorbita from the orbital bones is carried out as far as the superior and inferior orbital fissure. The greater wing of the sphenoid and orbital part of the frontal bone can be drilled out to expose the dura of the anterior and middle cranial fossa according to requirements.
  - Multiple landmarks can be used like the lateral rectus muscle; lacrimal neurovascular bundles; and more posteriorly and laterally, the ciliary artery and short ciliary nerves that arise from the ciliary ganglion; branch of III nerve; and superior ophthalmic vein.
- *Transorbital neuroendoscopic surgery (TONES—combined direct and endoscopic approach) Six Hands participants*
  - The approach is similar to the superior eye lid approach in the beginning and the periorbital is carefully dissected from the orbital bones as far as the superior and inferior orbital fissures, during which several communication vessels were coagulated for hemostasis.

- In a middle cranial fossa approach, the greater wing of the sphenoid should be removed as far as the dura mater. In this case, the supero-medial boundary of the approach is defined by the superior orbital fissure, while the lateral boundary is delineated by the temporalis muscle. Superiorly, the approach can be partially extended to the lesser wing of the sphenoid toward the anterior clinoid process. If necessary, the frontal bone can be partially resected, and the spheno-orbital sinus can be coagulated.
- Removal of the bony walls of the orbit depends on the lesion site and extension, which is performed by using coarse diamond burr to achieve more hemostasis.
- In case of an intracranial approach, the dura is opened and the anterior part of the temporal lobe of the brain is reached.
- In an anterior cranial fossa approach, craniotomy is performed by removing the orbital part of the frontal bone, along with partial removal of the lesser sphenoid wing. The greater wing of the sphenoid is left intact. The dura is exposed and opened according to individual requirements.
- The greater wing of the sphenoid and orbital part of the frontal bone can be drilled out to expose the dura of the anterior and middle cranial fossa. Specific work is done according to individual requirements.

• *Biportal approach for intraconal or extraconal lesions*
• This is a combination of the superior or inferior eyelid approach with the transnasal approach. This is used for certain orbital tumors which need wide access to be removed by a multi-portal gateway.

## 36.6 Advantages

Skull base approaches through the orbit have become an alternative for open or endoscopic aggressive craniofacial approaches:

1. Hospitalization and the need for a high dependency unit had markedly decreased.
2. No intracranial affection like brain edema from excessive traction was observed.
3. Also the best cosmetic outcome is achieved when compared to external approaches.
4. The approach provides a coplanar visualization without crossing the field of endoscopy.
5. In addition to dealing with the skull base, a multiportal approach combining the transorbital with a transnasal or transmaxillary approach has gained a wide scope of working distance between endoscopy with further use of other instruments.
6. A multiportal use of endoscopy can be attempted with increasing access to multiple targets without affecting the visual function or extraocular muscle movements [3, 4].

## 36.7 Complications

1. Neuro-Vascular injury.
2. Diplopia.
3. Visual impairment.
4. Enophthalmos.

**Cases (Figs. 36.2, 36.3, and 36.4)**

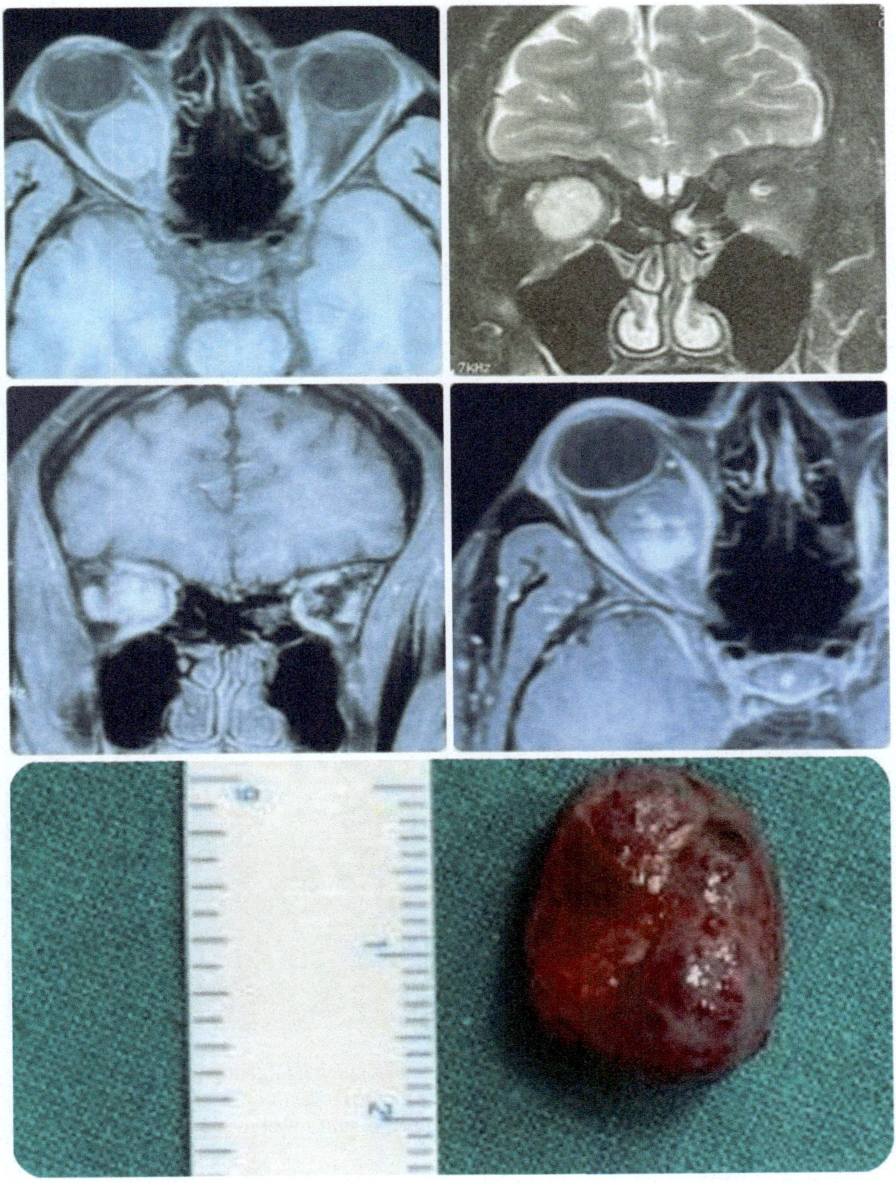

**Fig. 36.2** A case with right side intraconal orbital hemangioma with a smooth surface 2×2×3 cm, ovoid in shape, heterogeneous matrix, matted post-contrast enhancement, occupying the postero-medial surface of the globe and exerts a mass effect with smooth bowing of the optic nerve and displacement of the medial rectus muscle. The case was managed by an endonasal transorbital intraconal approach

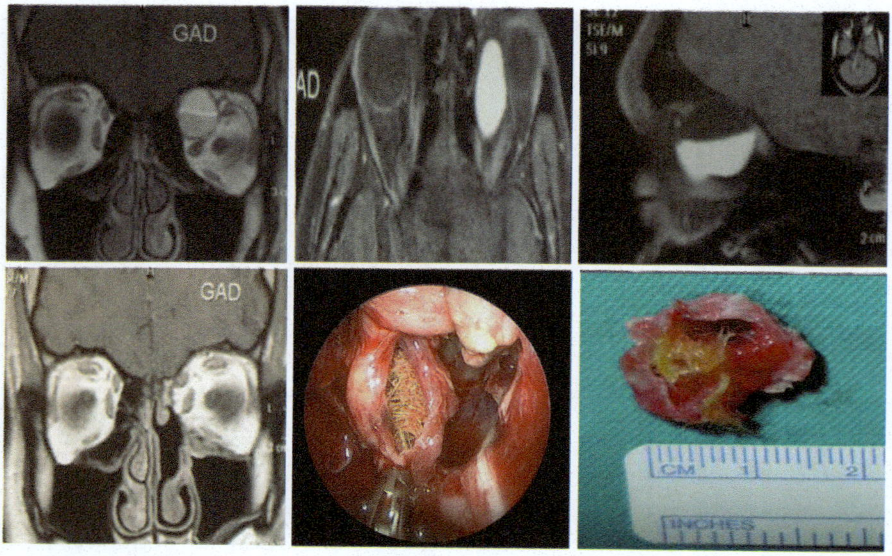


**Fig. 36.3** A case of intranasal dermoid 1×2×2 cm, with a smooth surface and a fluid level inside, occupying the superior medial aspect of the left orbit, managed by an endonasal transorbital intraconal approach

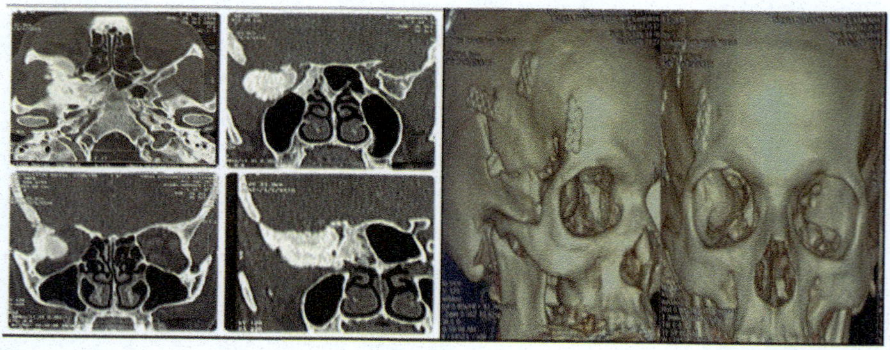

**Fig. 36.4** A case of recurrent orbital intra-osseous meningioma targeting the lateral right orbit, involving the greater wing and adjacent body of the sphenoid bone (3×3×2 cm). Encroaching upon the orbital apex, optic canal, foremen rotundum, vidian canal as well as the superior and inferior orbital fissures

## References


1. Dallan I, Castelnuovo P, Locatelli D, Turri-Zanoni M, AlQahtani A, Battaglia P, Hirt B, Sellari-Franceschini S. Multiportal combined transorbital transnasal endoscopic approach for the management of selected skull base lesions: preliminary experience. World Neurosurg. 2015;84(1):97–107.
2. Dallan I, Castelnuovo P, de Notaris M, Sellari-Franceschini S, Lenzi R, Turri-Zanoni M, Battaglia P, Prats-Galino A. Endoscopic endonasal anatomy of superior orbital fissure and

orbital apex regions: critical considerations for clinical applications. Eur Arch Otorrinolaringol. 2013;270:1643–9.
3. Bernal-Sprekelsen M, Alobid I, Enseñat J, Prats-Galino A. Endoscopic approaches to the paranasal sinuses and skull base: a step-by-step anatomic dissection guide. Stuttgart: Thieme; 2017.
4. Moe KS, Bergeron CM, Ellenbogen RG. Transorbital neuroendoscopic surgery. Neurosurgery. 2010;67(3):ons16–28.

# 3D Endoscopic Sinonasal Surgery

37

Amr Kholief

**Key Points**

- Three-dimensional (3D) endoscopes were available to be used in endoscopic sinus procedures.
- 3D endoscopy gives a real-time depth perception that could, in theory, address visual misperceptions.
- There are several current designs to mimic binocular vision in 3D visualization technology. These include dual-channel technology, shutter mechanism technology, and the insect eye technology.
- Stereoscopic vision allows for a better visualization of textures and curvatures of the surfaces. Some centers have found that 3D endoscopic procedures result in shorter operative times.
- Some surgeons reported discomforts such as eye strain, headache, fatigue, or dizziness during 3D surgery. Also, soiling of one lens interferes with visualization.

## 37.1 Introduction

Despite the recent development of new surgical procedures, including endoscopes, three-dimensional (3D) endoscopes were available to be used in endoscopic sinus procedures, and many studies have explained the role and restrictions of the 3D endoscopic system in sinus or skull base surgical approaches [1]. In these studies, 3D images were reconstructed from many two dimensional (2D) images captured by using special lenses that simulate the compound eye of bees from different angles [2].

A. Kholief (✉)
Department of Otolaryngology, Alexandria University, Alexandria, Egypt


S. Elwany (ed.), *Current Rhinology*,
https://doi.org/10.1007/978-3-031-70077-4_37

The availability of endoscopy transformed the viewing of the field during surgery, that allowed a lot of minimally invasive surgeries and major procedures to be carried out. Lowered postoperative morbidity and quicker recovery periods were seen thereafter. With endoscopy there is a loss of stereopsis, which can limit depth perception and consequently the ability to identify and manage anatomical and surgical structures [3].

3D endoscopy gives a real-time depth perception that could, in theory, address visual misperceptions. A new study concluded complications or hazards in 2D endoscopic sinonasal surgery that did not improve since the late 1990s. The introduction of 3D endoscopy will allow the way for change [4].

The application of endoscopy to surgery is a primary example of how technical innovations influence medicine and surgical outcomes in 1806. Phillip Bozzini invented the endoscope. It was formed of an eyepiece and container and used as a candle for light [5].

The original endoscopes were used as cystoscopes (used to visualize the urinary bladder) and allowed visualization of structures beyond the reach of the microscope. Hirschmann was the first to report the use of a modified type of this scope to visualize the maxillary sinus in 1901. During this period of time, he became a pioneer of ENT surgery [6].

## 37.2 The Evolution of Skull Base Surgery

Extended endoscopic endonasal approaches are increasingly carried out in dealing with various intracranial and cranial base lesions. Among that huge spectrum, a lot of lesions like pituitary adenomas and encephaloceles of the cribriform plate are involved and easily reached through the endonasal access [7].

On the other end, many challenging pathological lesions like meningiomas, esthesioneuroblastomas, suprasellar craniopharyngiomas, and chordomas are in need of the endoscopic approaches, as they often require massive drilling of the skull base and can surround or invade neurovascular structures. However, these same challenges face the surgeon while using open transcranial approaches to treat the same lesions [8].

During 1960s, around the same time as Basil Hirschowitz upgraded a fiberoptic system for endoscopy, Harold Hopkins also made a lot of modifications to improve the optical efficiency nine-fold by using glass rods which were placed between lenses. Karl Storz compounded these two innovations to get the modern rigid endoscope which saw a rapid uptake in hospitals in various surgical disciplines, including ENT specialty [4].

In 1932, Walter Dandy, widely described as the pioneer of neuroendoscopy at that time, reported his use of endoscopic ventriculostomy to remove the choroid plexus in a case of hydrocephaly [9].

Skull base endoscopic surgery is primarily concerned with the transsphenoidal surgical pathway to the pituitary, which has seen variable use over the last 100 years. Sir Victor Horsley likely performed the initial pituitary surgery in 1889, and unfortunately this went undocumented at this time [10]. After 4 years, Caton and Paul published a study outlining their excision of the pituitary gland using a lateral sub-temporal approach [11]. The transsphenoidal pathway to the pituitary was described and introduced by Schloffer in 1907 [12]. Then Harvey Cushing and Oscar Hirsch pioneered the transsphenoidal route, coincidentally both using the same submucosal septal resection method for the first time independently on the same day in 1910 [13].

Hirsch used the endonasal approach, essentially that which is used today, whereas Cushing favored a sublabial approach. Harvey Cushing first used the transsphenoidal approach in 1909 on a patient with acromegaly and continued to use this approach for 20 years [14].

Many complications like cerebrospinal fluid (CSF) rhinorrhea, difficulty in controlling bleeding and postoperative cerebral edema directed him to abandon it in 1929 and opt the transfrontal route through the frontal bone with retraction of the frontal lobe of the brain [15].

The landmark 1997 paper from Jho and Carrau introduced the recent and updated endoscopic pituitary surgery through the transsphenoidal approach, observing safety and efficacy of endoscopy alongside decreased morbidity in a series of 50 patients. At the time, many surgeons criticized the defect in stereoscopic vision, difficulty in controlling bleeding, and increasing incidence of CSF leaks [16].

A recent systematic review reported that the endoscopic transsphenoidal route of pituitary surgery is associated with decreased complication rates and shorter lengths of stay in hospital [17], which is likely due to the expanded view and reduced surgical injury rates. While these authors found that tumor resection rates are not improved with the use of the endoscope, two more recent meta-analyses found higher rates of total gross removal and remission for functioning pituitary tumors. [18]

The essential advantage of the transsphenoidal approach is that it provides a direct anatomical pathway to the pituitary gland without requiring the avoidance of major neurovascular structures [19]. This is not the case where brain retraction is used [20].

## 37.3 Advances in Skull Base Endoscopy

Presentation of endoscopy was a step back in terms of depth perception. The image produced by traditional endoscopes is two dimensional, resulting in a loss of stereopsis [21].

Although the endoscope offered a lot of advantages, unfortunately it did not give the ability to display a binocular vision. A 2D image of the surgical field was obtained by monocular endoscope and displays, but this was associated with impairment of depth perception, size estimation, and hand–eye coordination. Many studies related to human kinetics have explained that the important requirement for monocular cues are longer times of movements and the tendency to underestimate spaces between surgical landmarks [22].

Experienced surgeons use intuitive clues to perceive depth, using tactile and visual clues to understand spatial relationships of relevant structures. These may not be sufficient to avoid visual misperceptions, which have been shown to be the cause of 97% of laparoscopic bile duct injuries [23].

Despite many limitations during the use of 2D endoscope, the endoscopic surgeons have gained experience to create 3D construction from monocular cues. These cues are relative color/texture gradients, structure/size, and motion parallax; surgeons also were depending on haptic cues and many surgical movements to deduce the spatial relationships [24].

3D endoscopy has been introduced in ENT surgery with the purpose of addressing these misperceptions and the loss of depth perception.

Although many technical updates have been used for upgrading monocular cues of endoscope, 2D visualization was unable to gain the same depth perception obtained from binocular cues such as convergence, stereopsis, and vertical disparities. The visual centers of the human cortex of the brain superimposes two subtly different retinal images obtained from different viewing angles to achieve stereopsis. Similarly, the majority of the stereoscopic systems offer two little different images, which are displayed separately afterward to each eye, thereby giving the 3D view of a surgical field. Until recently, there are two main image generation strategies that have been used for stereopsis which are called the dual-channel and shutter mechanism technologies [25].

There are several current designs to mimic binocular vision in 3D visualization technology:

1. *Dual-channel technology*: This utilizes two distinct images generated from either a camera or video chip to render 3D images; so the changes in color, brightness, and sharpness gained from two cameras are obtained using two scopes, and the dual image is projected on to a screen. This might result in surgeon discomfort or side effects like ocular fatigue, headache, nausea, or migraine; in addition, the narrow inter-pupillary distance between the endoscopes or chips produces a weak 3D effect [26] Figs. 37.1 and 37.2.
2. *Shutter mechanism technology*: This technology depends on temporal shifts produced by a single camera which then generates rapidly alternating, slightly different images to render stereopsis. This design was applied by first generation Karl Storz 3D scopes, relies on the principle that the camera is always slightly moving. It analyzes minor angle changes between frames and uses a shutter mechanism to create a stereoscopic image. This gives a improper 3D effect due to the unpredictable movement and instability of the endoscope. It can be generated using a single optical endoscope, so only the camera and image processing unit are required to be replaced which makes it easier to incorporate into hospitals [27].
3. *The insect-eye technology*: This technology used by VisionSense Ltd. employs a collection of many microscopic lenses on a single video chip at the distal end of the endoscope. These lenses provide multiple images of the target, which are divided into "right" or "left" images and displayed into each eye of the surgeon, who wears polarized glasses. This technology only uses one video chip, thus avoiding side effects associated with the dual camera technologies [8].

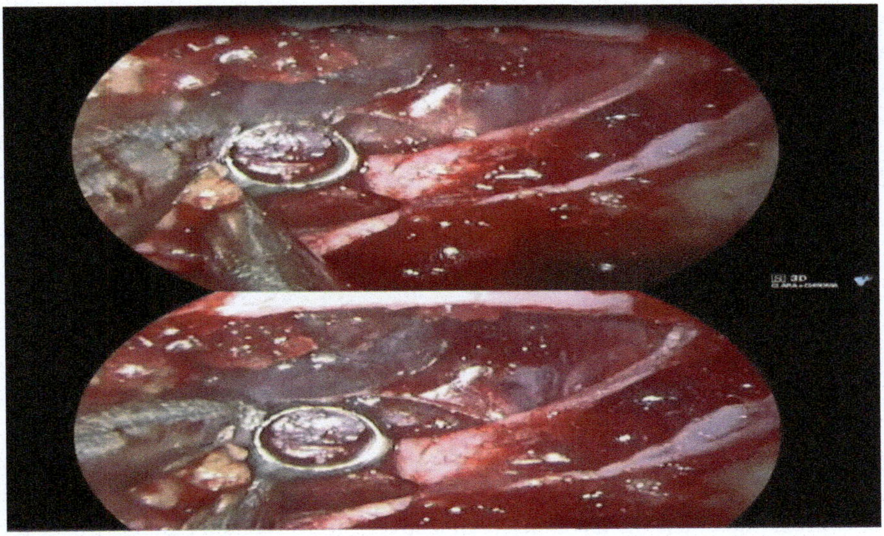

**Fig. 37.1** 3D view of the transsphenoidal approach of pituitary macroadenoma surgery. Note the double image of the view created by 3D Storz endoscope "dual-channel technology"

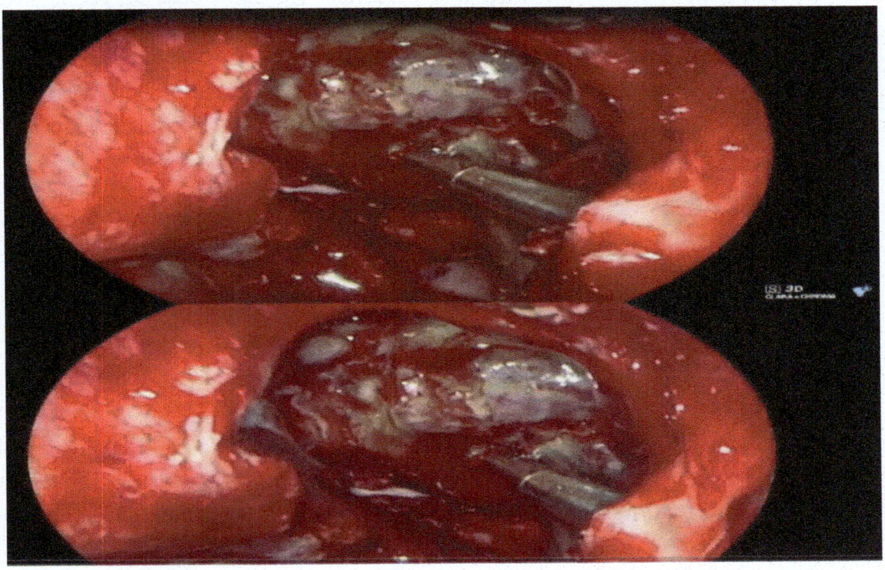

**Fig. 37.2** 3D view of the transsphenoidal approach of pituitary macroadenoma surgery after complete tumor resection created by 3D Storz endoscope "dual-channel technology"

## 37.4 Field of View (FOV) Evaluation

Van Gompel et al. stated that the FOV of the 2D endoscope was 8.3 cm and that of the 3D VisionSense endoscope was calculated as 4.0 cm at a specific distance of 6 cm which equates to 52% reduction in FOV. These results were calculated using a

VisionSense (VSII) 3D endoscope, which is considered an older version of VisionSense 3D endoscope used [28].

During calculation of the FOV, Van Gompel did not use a conventional method as previously stated, so the endoscopic FOV was measured and called an angular field of view (FOVA). Other studies, including our own, have demonstrated a lesser reduction in the field of view [29].

## 37.5 Advantages of the 3D Endoscope

It has been proposed that 3D endoscopy will decrease the barrier in using endoscopy experienced as a result of lack of stereoscopic vision, so the learning curve of novices will be reduced. Other studies have advocated the role of 3D visualization in surgical training [30].

Many simulated papers have found that participants prefer 3D technology, especially novices, owing to a subjectively greater degree of depth perception and less effort required to use the technology. Objectively, trials found a reduced frequency of past pointing, lower error rates, and increased accuracy of movement [31].

Stereoscopic vision allows for a better visualization of textures and curvatures of the surfaces which is very essential and beneficial for skull base surgeons who depend on many subtleties of the ventral skull base surgical field for safe entry into the cranial vault [32].

Some centers have found that 3D endoscopic procedures result in shorter operative times, particularly in pituitary adenoma resection where a 30-min reduction in operating time was observed [32].

## 37.6 Disadvantages of the 3D Endoscope

It is widely reported that soiling of one lens results in poor visualization. This can be improved with proper irrigation. One study reported that the high definition system (3DHD) system responds better to blood soiling than the standard definition (3DSD) version [33].

Interestingly, up to 2% of the population are unable to perceive 3D images and so will not see the benefits of 3D technology. This condition is known as amblyopia [34]. It was also reported that i2D endoscopes provide better image quality (brilliance and color) than 3D endoscopes [32].

Many authors in nonclinical and clinical approaches reported similar results. Furthermore, some surgeon discomforts like eye strain, headache, fatigue, or dizziness were reported by few surgeons in many studies while using the 3D endoscope [35].

A study was done in 1995 which was performed using a 3D dual camera endoscope and the result was that 20 of 32 surgeons with variable surgical experiences while doing laparoscopic surgeries reported superior depth perception but 15 of 32 noted no betterment of surgical maneuvers. About 40% of surgeons described worse image resolution and illumination of the surgical field compared to 2D endoscope [36].

**Fig. 37.3** Comparison between 3D and 2D endoscopes

| | 3D | 2D |
|---|---|---|
| Depth perception | +++ | +/– |
| Anatomical Details | ++ | + |
| Field of view | ++ | ++ |
| Color | + | ++ |
| Brilliance | + | ++ |
| Image distortion | + | No |
| Time for preops | ++ | + |
| Fogging | ++ | + |
| Angled endoscopes | +/– | ++ |
| Ease of use | + | ++ |
| Headache, Nausea..... | + | – |

Figure 37.3 compares 3D and 2D endoscopes.

**Future**

In the future, 3D technology would apply an integration of scans and navigation system to render an augmented reality display, so surgeons would see what is beyond that which is visible. For example, the pathway of the internal carotid artery would be demonstrated below the superior/posterior wall of the sphenoid sinus [27].

The idea of integration of a digital image (which contains the volumetric position of each pixel) with CT or MRI scans to construct a hybrid image. Incorporation of this technology to advanced surgery like robotic surgery would offer pre-programed tasks [37].

Several publications have mentioned that the use of 3D technology will impact the art of surgical training like simulators where there is no harm on patient safety [38].

**Acknowledgments** I would like to express my deep thanks to Mr. Shahzada Ahmed, consultant and clinical lead of ENT department at Queen Elizabeth Hospital, Birmingham, United Kingdom for his continued support. Also, many thanks to the team at Karl Storz GmbH & Co. (Tuttlingen, Germany) who provided The Karl Storz 3D endoscope tools.

## References

1. Shah RN, Leight WD, Patel MR, Surowitz JB, Wong YT, Wheless SA, et al. A controlled laboratory and clinical evaluation of a three-dimensional endoscope for endonasal sinus and skull base surgery. Am J Rhinol Allergy. 2011;25(3):141–4.
2. Szold A. Seeing is believing: visualization systems in endoscopic surgery (video, HDTV, stereoscopy, and beyond). Surg Endosc Other Interv Tech. 2005;19:730–3.
3. Dehdashti AR, Ganna A, Karabatsou K, Gentili F. Pure endoscopic endonasal approach for pituitary adenomas: early surgical results in 200 patients and comparison with previous microsurgical series. Neurosurgery. 2008;62(5):1006–17.

4. Lee SC, Senior BA. Endoscopic skull base surgery. Clin Exp Otorhinolaryngol. 2008;1(2):53–62.
5. Dehdashti AR, Karabatsou K, Ganna A, Witterick I, Gentili F. Expanded endoscopic endonasal approach for treatment of clival chordomas: early results in 12 patients. Neurosurgery. 2008;63(2):299–309.
6. Grosvenor AE, Laws ER. The evolution of extracranial approaches to the pituitary and anterior skull base. Pituitary. 2008;11:337–45.
7. Byrn JC, Schluender S, Divino CM, Conrad J, Gurland B, Shlasko E, Szold A. Three-dimensional imaging improves surgical performance for both novice and experienced operators using the da Vinci Robot System. Am J Surg. 2007;193(4):519–22.
8. Di Ieva A, Tam M, Tschabitscher M, Cusimano MD. A journey into the technical evolution of neuroendoscopy. World Neurosurg. 2014;82(6):e777–89.
9. Doglietto F, Prevedello DM, Jane JA, Han J, Laws ER. A brief history of endoscopic transsphenoidal surgery—from Philipp Bozzini to the First World Congress of Endoscopic Skull Base Surgery. Neurosurg Focus. 2005;19(6):1–6.
10. Laws ER, Dunn IF. The evolution of surgeryethe soul of neurosurgery. In: Meningiomas of the Skull Base. Stuttgart: Thieme; 2019.
11. Linder TE, Simmen D, Stool SE. Revolutionary inventions in the 20th century: the history of endoscopy. Arch Otolaryngol Head Neck Surg. 1997;123(11):1161–3.
12. Govindaraj S, Adappa ND, Kennedy DW. Endoscopic sinus surgery: evolution and technical innovations. J Laryngol Otol. 2010;124(3):242–50.
13. Kennedy DW. Functional endoscopic sinus surgery. Tech Arch Otolaryngol. 1985;111(10):643–9.
14. Caton R. Notes of a case of acromegaly treated by operation. Br Med J. 1893;2(1722):1421.
15. Cohen-Gadol AA, Liu JK, Laws ER. Cushing's first case of transsphenoidal surgery: the launch of the pituitary surgery era. J Neurosurg. 2005;103(3):570–4.
16. Cohen-Gadol AA, Laws ER, Cole CD, Kan P, Couldwell WT. Harvey Cushing and Oskar Hirsch: early forefathers of modern transsphenoidal surgery. J Neurosurg. 2005;103(6):1096–104.
17. Goudakos JK, Markou KD, Georgalas C. Endoscopic versus microscopic trans-sphenoidal pituitary surgery: a systematic review and meta-analysis. Clin Otolaryngol. 2011;36(3):212–20.
18. Gao Y, Zhong C, Wang Y, Xu S, Guo Y, Dai C, et al. Endoscopic versus microscopic transsphenoidal pituitary adenoma surgery: a meta-analysis. World J Surg Oncol. 2014;12:1–12.
19. García-Garrigós E, Arenas-Jiménez JJ, Monjas-Cánovas I, Abarca-Olivas J, Cortés-Vela JJ, De La Hoz-Rosa J, Guirau-Rubio MD. Transsphenoidal approach in endoscopic endonasal surgery for skull base lesions: what radiologists and surgeons need to know. Radiographics. 2015;35(4):1170–85.
20. Hamid O, El Fiky L, Hassan O, Kotb A, El Fiky S. Anatomic variations of the sphenoid sinus and their impact on trans-sphenoid pituitary surgery. Skull Base. 2007;18:9–15.
21. Cote M, Kalra R, Wilson T, Orlandi RR, Couldwell WT. Surgical fidelity: comparing the microscope and the endoscope. Acta Neurochir. 2013;155:2299–303.
22. Stammberger HR, Kennedy DW. Paranasal sinuses: anatomic terminology and nomenclature. Ann Otol Rhinol Laryngol. 1995;104(10_suppl):7–16.
23. Way LW, Stewart L, Gantert W, Liu K, Lee CM, Whang K, Hunter JG. Causes and prevention of laparoscopic bile duct injuries: analysis of 252 cases from a human factors and cognitive psychology perspective. Ann Surg. 2003;237(4):460.
24. Banna M, Olutola PS. Patterns of pneumatization and septation of the sphenoidal sinus. J Can Assoc Radiol. 1983;34(4):291–3.
25. Reichelt S, Häussler R, Fütterer G, Leister N. Depth cues in human visual perception and their realization in 3D displays. In: Three-dimensional imaging, visualization, and display 2010 and display technologies and applications for defense, security, and avionics IV, vol. 7690. SpIE; 2010. p. 92–103.
26. Radermacher K, Pichler CV, Fischer S, Rau G. 3D-visualisation in surgery. Helmholtz-Institute Aachen; 1998.

27. Brown SM, Tabaee A, Singh A, Schwartz TH, Anand VK. Three-dimensional endoscopic sinus surgery: feasibility and technical aspects. Otolaryngol Head Neck Surg. 2008;138(3):400–2.
28. Van Gompel JJ, Tabor MH, Youssef AS, Lau T, Carlson AP, Van Loveren HR, Agazzi S. Field of view comparison between two-dimensional and three-dimensional endoscopy. Laryngoscope. 2014;124(2):387–90.
29. Zaidi HA, Zehri A, Smith TR, Nakaji P, Laws ER Jr. Efficacy of three-dimensional endoscopy for ventral skull base pathology: a systematic review of the literature. World Neurosurg. 2016;86:419–31.
30. Verdaasdonk EGG, Stassen LPS, Monteny LJ, Dankelman J. Validation of a new basic virtual reality simulator for training of basic endoscopic skills: the SIMENDO. Surg Endosc Other Interv Tech. 2006;20:511–8.
31. Egi H, Hattori M, Suzuki T, Sawada H, Kurita Y, Ohdan H. The usefulness of 3-dimensional endoscope systems in endoscopic surgery. Surg Endosc. 2016;30:4562–8.
32. Kholief A, Ali A, Elwany S, Ahmed S, Youssef A, Zahran M. Evaluation of the three-dimensional endoscopy in basic and extended nasal procedures: a clinical and cadaveric study. Int Arch Otorhinolaryngol. 2023;27(4):e620–4.
33. Nassimizadeh A, Muzaffar SJ, Nassimizadeh M, Beech T, Ahmed SK. Three-dimensional hand-to-gland combat: the future of endoscopic surgery? J Neurol Surg Rep. 2015;76(02):e200–4.
34. Webber AL, Wood J. Amblyopia: prevalence, natural history, functional effects and treatment. Clin Exp Optom. 2005;88(6):365–75.
35. Botanov Y, Ilardi SS. The acute side effects of bright light therapy: a placebo-controlled investigation. PLoS One. 2013;8(9):e75893.
36. Cappabianca P, Cavallo LM, Esposito F, De Divitiis O, Messina A, De Divitiis E. Extended endoscopic endonasal approach to the midline skull base: the evolving role of transsphenoidal surgery. Adv Tech Stand Neurosurg. 2008;33:151–99.
37. Teistler M, Breiman RS, Lison T, Bott OJ, Pretschner DP, Aziz A, Nowinski WL. Simplifying the exploration of volumetric images: development of a 3D user interface for the radiologist's workplace. J Digit Imaging. 2008;21:2–12.
38. van Dongen KW, Ahlberg G, Bonavina L, Carter FJ, Grantcharov TP, Hyltander A, et al. European consensus on a competency-based virtual reality training program for basic endoscopic surgical psychomotor skills. Surg Endosc. 2011 Jan;25(1):166–71.

# Fibro-Osseous Lesions of the Nose and Paranasal Sinuses

# 38

Ahmed A. Ibrahim, Haitham Morsi, and Sundus A. Alsedra

**Key Points**

- Benign tumors are characterized by the replacement of the normal bone by a fibrous cellular stroma containing various amounts of foci of mineralization or ossification.
- They are usually divided into three different entities: osteoma, fibrous dysplasia (FD), and ossifying fibroma (OF).
- They can have overlapping histologic features. Hence, definitive diagnosis incorporates clinical history (e.g., the age of the patient, the location, and progression of growth), radiologic appearance, and histopathology.
- Surgical resection of these lesions can be challenging due to their complex anatomic relationships in the skull base and orbit and their tendency to surround neurovascular structures.

**Supplementary Information** The online version contains supplementary material available at https://doi.org/10.1007/978-3-031-70077-4_38.

A. A. Ibrahim (✉)
Alexandria University, Alexandria, Egypt

H. Morsi
Alexandria University Hospital/Canadian Hospital, Dubai, UAE

S. A. Alsedra
Al Yarmouk Teaching Hospital, Baghdad, Iraq


S. Elwany (ed.), *Current Rhinology*,
https://doi.org/10.1007/978-3-031-70077-4_38

## 38.1 Background

The nose and paranasal sinuses can be affected by a wide range of disorders including inflammatory, infectious, and neoplastic disorders, among which is a class of benign bony neoplasm known as fibro-osseous lesions. They are benign and a slowly progressive disorder of the bone which is characterized by the replacement of the normal bone by fibroblasts and a variably mineralized collagen matrix leading to fibrous stroma mixed with ossifying or cement-like tissue [1].

Fibrous dysplasia (FD), ossifying fibroma (OF), and osteoma all fall under this category along a continuum from the least to the most bony content. They are frequently asymptomatic, where they are incidentally found on imaging taken for another reason. Over time if extended, symptoms may arise from the space-occupying compression of surrounding structures causing chronic rhinosinusitis and mucoceles, facial deformity, orbital, or neurological complications [2–3].

The surgical removal and pathologic evaluation of these lesions is often challenging due to their complex anatomic locations in the skull base and orbit, and their tendency to surround the adjacent neurovascular structures, so conventional wisdom advocates intervention when these lesions are symptomatic, or when they show rapid growth [4].

## 38.2 Osteomas

These are the most common benign lesions of the paranasal sinuses with a prevalence of 3% and arising from the frontoethmoid region. Osteomas are the most frequent bone tumors of the facial region. They arise mainly in the frontal and ethmoid sinuses in the close vicinity of the nasofrontal duct. Involvement of the sphenoid sinus region is extremely rare. Lesions larger than 3 cm in diameter are considered giant tumors.

Most sinonasal osteomas are solitary. Multiple osteomas raise the possibility of Gardner syndrome (colorectal polyps prone to malignant degeneration, skeletal abnormalities, and supernumerary teeth).

Osteomas are typically smooth and lobulated in appearance and covered by the sinus mucosa. Histologically, there are three types of osteomas.

- The eburnated type (the ivory or compact type). The osteoma is very dense and lacks haversian canals. It arises from membranous elements.
- The mature type (spongy type) is composed of a softer cancellous bone. It arises from cartilaginous elements.
- The mixed type of osteoma which contains elements of both the eburnated and mature forms [5].

There are three main theories regarding the etiology of osteomas: developmental, traumatic, and infectious. The developmental theory proposes that reactivation of embryonic stem cells leads to uncontrolled bone formation. The traumatic and infectious theories propose an inflammatory process as the initiating factor for bony tumor formation [6].

Clinical presentation

- Osteomas are frequently asymptomatic and discovered incidentally.
- Symptoms arise from mass effect as the lesion impinges on normal structures.
- Extra sinus complications may occur.
- Orbital complications include: diplopia, epiphora, facial distortion, and even blindness.
- Intracranial complications include: mucoceles, meningitis, frontal abscess, cerebrospinal fluid (CSF) leak, or pneumatocele.

Radiologically: osteomas are best demonstrated by plain films or computed tomography (CT). On CT, an osteoma appears as very dense, homogeneous, well-circumscribed mass attached with an apparent range of broad to narrow pedicle to an adjacent bone. The surrounding bone is normal and does not have a lytic or moth-eaten appearance (Fig. 38.1). An MRI may be needed in the presence of a complication such as mucocele formation. (Fig. 38.2).

Surgical approaches can be classified as external, endoscopic, or a combination of both (above and below [7]) (Figs. 38.3 and 38.4).

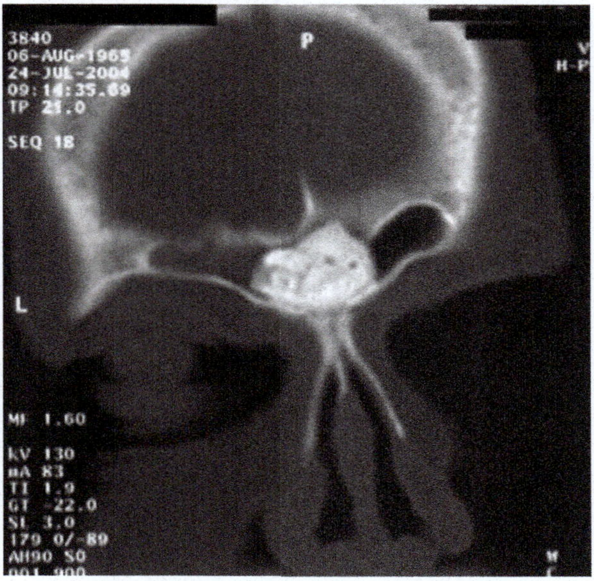


**Fig. 38.1** Large frontoethmoid osteoma

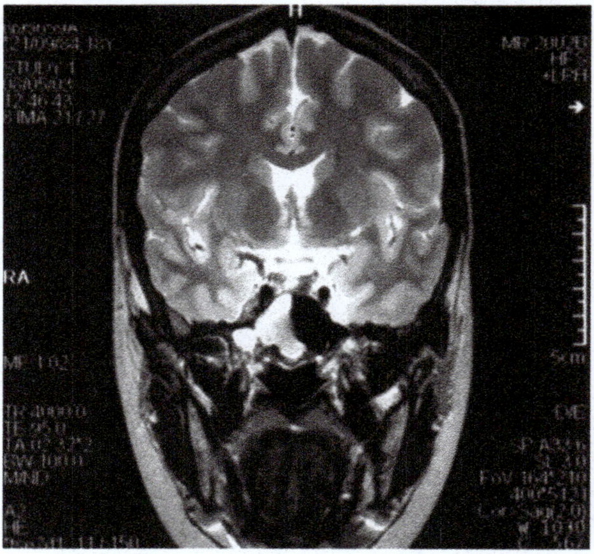

**Fig. 38.2** Preoperative coronal T1-weighted unenhanced MRI view, localizing a large osteoma with an adjacent mucocele in the right half of the sphenoid sinus

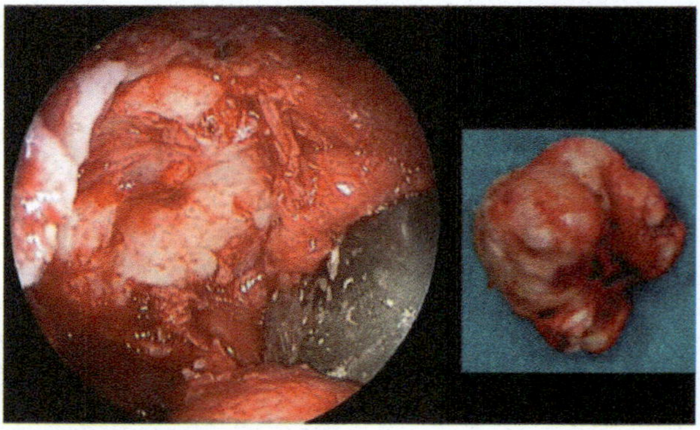

**Fig. 38.3** Endoscopic resection of bug frontoethmoid osteoma

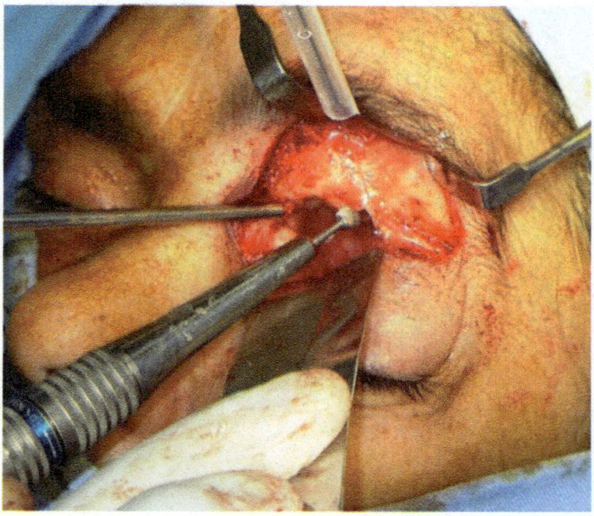

**Fig. 38.4** Excision of frontoethmoid osteoma through a blephroplasty incision

## 38.3 Fibrous Dysplasia (FD)

Fibrous dysplasia is a developmental anomaly of the facial bones, in which normally a mineralized bone is replaced by proliferating fibrous tissue and immature woven bone, which is benign. It is related to a set of mutations in the GNAS1 gene, located on chromosome 20q2.

The incidence of FD involving the sinonasal system is unknown. Men and women are equally affected. The frontoethmoid and sphenoid sinus are the most commonly affected sinuses.

FD usually presents in adolescent and young women. It is slowly growing and tends to stabilize at the age of sexual maturity. Two forms are present:

- *Monostotic*: unique or multiple lesions in a single bone.
- *Polyostotic*: multiple lesions involving different bones.
- Dissemination of pathological bone changes connected to other disturbances such as McCune–Albright syndrome, which is accompanied by endocrine dysfunction as precocious puberty and/or hyperthyroidism and café-au-lait patches.

Clinical Picture

- Symptoms and signs of narrowing of neural foramina, fissures, and canals (e.g., optic nerve),
- Cosmetic deformities.

**Radiology**

On CT scan:

- CT appearance of fibrous dysplasia varies, but the typical ground glass appearance is the most common and highly suggestive of FD [8].
- A mixed density pattern prevails in 50% cases.
- Lucent "pseudo"-cystic appearance is seen in 25% of tumors.

On MRI:

- Most useful in assessing the impact of the fibrosseous lesion on adjacent cranial nerves, vessels, orbital contents, and brain parenchyma.
- FD lesion appears intermediately in T1 and is hypo intense in T2.

CT appearance of fibrous dysplasia varies, but the typical ground glass appearance is the most common and highly suggestive of FD [8].

Asymptomatic fibrous dysplasia does not require treatment. Surgical drilling is indicated for lesions compressing adjacent structures or causing cosmetic deformities (Fig. 38.5).

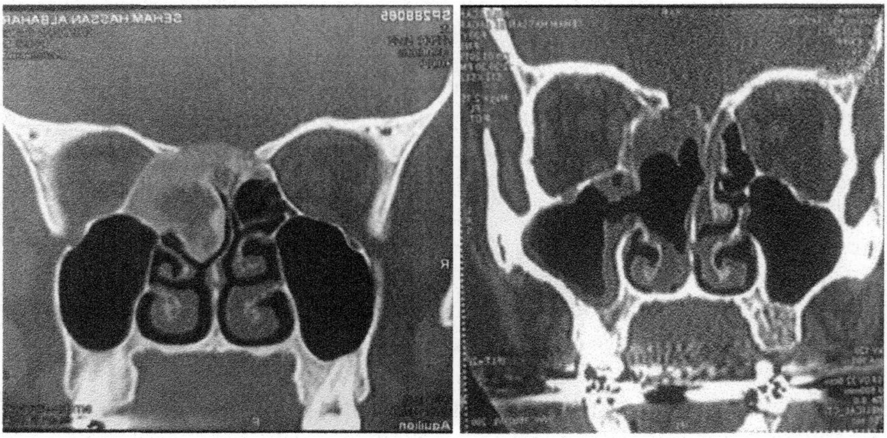

**Fig. 38.5** Preoperative (right) and postoperative (left) CT of fibrous dysplasia involving the frontoethmoid region and displacing the skull base and lamina papyracea

## 38.4 Ossifying Fibroma (OF)

This is also known as cemento-ossifying fibroma, psammomatoid ossifying fibroma, and juvenile ossifying fibroma. It is the most concerning of the fibro-osseous lesions. OF occurs more frequently in the third and fourth decades of life. It has a higher incidence in the black population.

It involves more commonly the mandible (molar and premolar periapical regions) and when arising outside the mandible, it appears to affect the ethmoid and maxillary sinuses most frequently.

OF appears as a smooth masse covered with mucosa. Histologically, it shows trabeculae of the lamellar bone, a variable amount of vascularized stroma and osteoblastic rimming of the trabeculae leading to cortical expansion of the affected bone.

On CT imaging, it appears as a sharply circumscribed round or oval lesion with an eggshell rim and a central radiolucency.

Ossifying fibromas are typically painless, but because of their aggressive and locally destructive nature, complete removal is advised when causing symptoms [3] (Fig. 38.6).

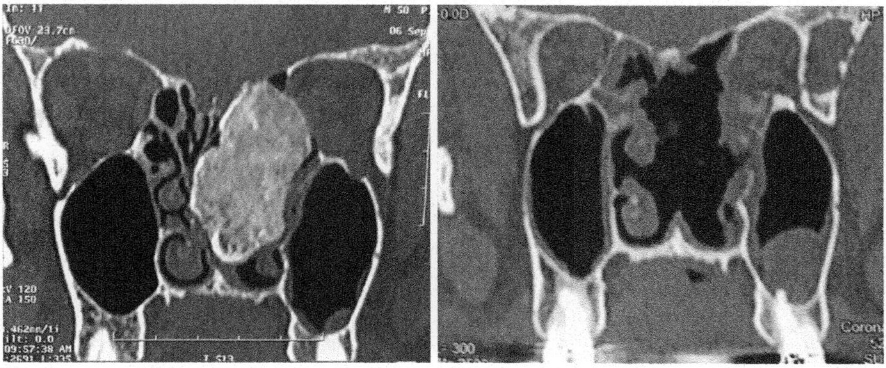

**Fig. 38.6** Preoperative (right) and postoperative (left) ossifying fibroma in the left frontoethmoid region and extending to the nasal cavity

## References


1. Stapleton AL, Tyler-Kabara EC, Gardner PA, Snyderman CH. Endoscopic endonasal surgery for benign fibro-osseous lesions of the pediatric skull base. Laryngoscope. 2015;125:2199–203. https://doi.org/10.1002/lary.25070.
2. Mehta D, Clifton N, McClelland L, Jones NS. Pediatric fibro-osseous lesions of the nose and paranasal sinuses. Int J Pediatric Otorhinolaryngol. 2006;70(2):193–9. https://doi.org/10.1016/j.ijporl.2005.09.031.
3. Eller R, Sillers M. Common fibro-osseous lesions of the paranasal sinuses. Otolaryngol Clin N Am. 2006 Jun;39(3):585–600, x. https://doi.org/10.1016/j.otc.2006.01.013.
4. Brodish BN, Morgan CE, Sillers MJ. Endoscopic resection of fibro-osseous lesions of the paranasal sinuses. Am J Rhinol. 1999;13(1):11–6. https://doi.org/10.2500/105065899781389830.
5. Chen C, Selva D, Wormald PJ. Endoscopic modified lothrop procedure: an alternative for frontal osteoma excision. Rhinology. 2004;42(4):239–43.
6. Lund VJ, Stammberger H, Nicolai P, et al. European position paper on endoscopic management of tumours of the nose, paranasal sinuses and skull base. Rhinol Suppl. 2010;22:1–143.
7. Phillips J, Woodworth BA. Fibro-osseous lesions of the paranasal sinuses. In: Sataloff RT, editor. Sataloff's comprehensive textbook of otolaryngology: rhinology/allergy and immunology, vol. 2. 1st ed. New Delhi: Jaypee Brothers Medical Publisher; 2016. p. 263–72.
8. Nair S. The frontal sinus. In: Watkinson JC, Clarke RW, editors. Scott-Brown's otorhinolaryngology head and neck surgery: basic sciences, head and neck endocrine surgery, rhinology, vol. 1. 8th ed. Boca Raton: Taylor & Francis Group Publisher; 2018. p. 1081–106.

# Inverted Papilloma

# 39

Ibrahim Rezk Mohamed and Khaled Gamal Dahy Ahmed

**Key Points**

- Inverted papilloma is the second most frequent benign tumor of the sinonasal tract.
- Inverted papilloma is the most common surgical indication for benign tumors of the sinonasal tract.
- Inverted papilloma predominantly arises from the lateral nasal wall and medial wall of maxillary sinus.
- Unilateral nasal obstruction is the most common symptom in patients with inverted papilloma.
- The vast majority of malignant tumors arising from inverted papillomas are squamous cell carcinomas.
- The so-called cerebriform-columnar pattern, which is highly predictive of inverted papilloma, can be easily detected by MRI.
- The site of origin of the lesion can be reliably identified when associated with a bony strut, focal hyperostosis, and osteitic changes on a CT image but may also be identified on an MRI image.
- Endoscopic transnasal surgery is the gold standard of treatment for inverted papilloma.
- Endoscopic resection of inverted papilloma has shifted toward a pedicle-oriented technique.
- Incomplete resection, high-stage disease, dysplasia, high-risk human papilloma (HPV), and smoking are the most relevant risk factors for recurrence.

I. R. Mohamed (✉) · K. G. D. Ahmed
Department of Otolaryngology, Sohag University, Sohag, Egypt


S. Elwany (ed.), *Current Rhinology*,
https://doi.org/10.1007/978-3-031-70077-4_39

## 39.1 Background

Schneiderian papillomas (SPs) of the nose, also known as sinonasal papillomas, were first identified by Ward in 1854. These benign lesions have the name C. Victor Schneider in recognition of the man who first established that the ectoderm is the source of catarrh and not the cerebrospinal fluid (CSF) in the 1600s. Kramer and Som distinguished SPs from inflammatory nasal polyps by classifying SPs as actual nasal neoplasms and referring to them as true papillomas. Ringertz was the first to notice how SPs vary from other kinds of papillomas in that they have a propensity to invert into the connective tissue stroma.

SPs are a distinct class of benign lesions that develop on the sinonasal tract's mucosal surfaces. The histopathologic characteristics of these neoplastic lesions allow for easy identification. SPs, also known as inverting papillomas, have many synonyms (e.g., epithelial papilloma, transitional cell papilloma, squamous cell papilloma). The sinonasal mucosa, in contrast to the remainder of the upper respiratory tract mucosa, is ectodermal in origin and first develops in the fourth week of pregnancy from the stomodeum (a primitive mouth). The mucosal lining of the nasopharynx, which is of endodermal origin but has a similar histology, is continuous with the sinonasal mucosa.

Rarely do lesions with similar histologic and biologic characteristics develop beyond the nasal cavity. These show the Schneiderian membrane migrating ectopically during development. The lacrimal sac, the middle ear region, and the pharynx are examples of extrasinonasal places where SPs may manifest. These extranasal papillomas may come back after insufficient excision, just like SPs.

## 39.2 Epidemiology

Nasal cavity papillomas (Schneiderian papillomas) include three types: inverted (endophytic), fungiform (exophytic), and cylindrical (oncocytic). The inverted and cylindrical types usually originate from the lateral nasal wall. The fungiform type usually originates from the nasal septum.

Inverted papilloma (IP) is a benign neoplasm characterized by invagination of the neoplastic epithelium into the underlying stroma, without transgression of the basement membrane.

Inverted papilloma is the second most frequent benign tumor of the sinonasal tract after osteoma and is the most frequent papilloma of the sinonasal region, arising from the sinonasal epithelial lining. An estimated 0.74–2.3 new cases may be expected per 100,000 population annually. It comprises 0.5–5% of primary nasal tumors.

Males are more commonly affected than females (2.5 to 3: 1 male to female ratio), and the tumor is the most frequent in the fifth and sixth decades of life.

Although the tumor is benign, it may be locally destructive and they have a tendency for recurrence, with a recurrence rate of 5–25%.

The incidence of being associated with malignancy (squamous cell carcinoma) or develop secondary malignancy is 5–15%. The rates of synchronous and metachronous malignancy are reported to be about 10.1% and 1.1%, respectively [1].

The lateral nasal wall and maxillary sinus: maxillary medial wall is the most common site of origin. Frontal and sphenoid sinuses are rarely involved primarily.

About 30% of cases originate from multiple sites (multicentric) with increased risk of leaving residual tumor tissue after surgery. Inverted papilloma may rarely be bilateral [1].

## 39.3 Aetiology and Genetic Profile

Exposure to an organic solvent seems to be related to a higher risk of developing inverted papilloma, while no association has been demonstrated with smoking or alcohol consumption.

Cigarette smoking increases the risk of recurrence for sinonasal inverted papilloma, and also increases the risk of malignant transformation [2, 3].

The presence of human papillomavirus (HPV) in inverted papilloma has been extensively investigated, but its role is still a matter of debate. Low-risk HPV (HPV 6 and 11) is 2.8 times as frequent as high-risk HPV (HPV 16 and 18) in inverted papilloma. However, high-risk HPV is more frequent in cases with high-grade dysplasia and carcinoma (55%). HPV detection rates increase in dysplastic inverted papilloma and SCC-ex-inverted papilloma with an increasing ratio of HR to LR HPV types, compared to nondysplastic inverted papilloma [4].

From a small number of cases studied, it appears that activating mutations in the epidermal growth factor receptor (EGFR) gene have a high prevalence in inverted papilloma and in concurrent squamous cell carcinomas arising from inverted papilloma [5].

## 39.4 Pathology

**Site**

Inverted papilloma originates most commonly from the lateral nasal wall around the middle meatus (89%) and involves the medial wall of the maxillary sinus. The tumor, however, may involve other walls of the maxillary sinus and extend to other sinuses. Orbital and intracranial spread of the tumor has been reported.

The lateral nasal wall and maxillary sinus: maxillary medial wall is the most common site of origin. Frontal and sphenoid sinuses are rarely involved primarily.

About 30% of cases originate from multiple sites (multicentric) with increased risk of leaving residual tumor tissue after surgery. Inverted papilloma may rarely be bilateral [1].

**Macroscopic Appearance**

Grossly, nasal endoscopy typically shows a pale, polypoidal mass with a papillary appearance protruding from the middle meatus. In any case, a biopsy performed under endoscopic guidance is indicated to establish definitive histology.

**Microscopic Appearance**

Histologically, inverted papilloma has an endophytic or inverted growth pattern consisting of thickened epithelium growing inward into the underlying connective tissue stroma to form large clefts, ribbons, and islands. The epithelium varies in cellularity and is composed of squamous, transitional, and columnar cells.

Multiple inversions of the surface epithelium into the underlying stroma, composed of squamous and/or columnar cells and lined by a distinct and intact continuous basement membrane, is the typical morphology of inverted papilloma. Non-keratinizing squamous or transitional epithelium, 5–30 cells thick, frequently predominates, and is covered by a layer of ciliated columnar cells (Fig. 39.1).

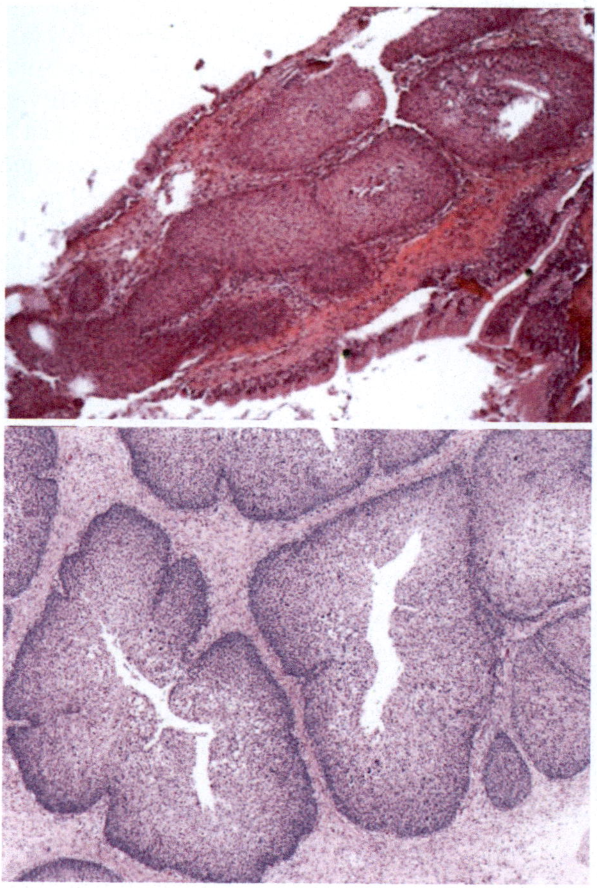

**Fig. 39.1** Histologic cross-section of sinonasal inverted papilloma. Invagination of superficial epithelium into underlying stroma (black asterisks)

Infiltration of the epithelium by neutrophils (so-called transmigrating neutrophils) is frequently seen. There is usually a loss of underlying seromucinous glands. The stroma may be either loose or dense and may be inflamed. Premalignant and malignant features, dysplasia, carcinoma in situ, and invasive carcinoma can be seen arising in inverted papilloma [1].

## 39.5 Clinical Behavior

Almost always, sinonasal SPs are unilateral. The three basic clinical characteristics of tumors are their propensity to recur, their ability to destroy nearby structures, and their propensity to be malignant.

The rate of recurrence of these neoplastic tumors varies greatly (0–78%), primarily dependent on the surgical method and degree of resection. Another explanation for the high recurrence rate has been theorized to be the multicentric origin of SPs; however, this has only sometimes been supported by evidence.

Malignant transformation is observed in 5–15% of cases; synchronous occurrence is more frequent than metachronous. The vast majority of malignant tumors arising from inverted papilloma are squamous cell carcinomas, but other tumors such as sinonasal undifferentiated carcinomas, mucoepidermoid carcinoma, and verrucous carcinoma may rarely occur.

## 39.6 Clinical Features

**History**

Patients may present with non-specific symptoms such as nasal obstruction, epistaxis, rhinorrhoea, hyposmia, and headaches of long duration.

Unilateral nasal obstruction is the most common symptom prompting the patient to seek an otorhinolaryngologic consultation.

Unilateral rhinosinusitis with related symptoms, such as headache and facial pain, may be caused by mechanic obstruction of sinus drainage.

Epiphora, proptosis, and diplopia may be associated with advanced lesions involving the orbit and should raise the suspicion of malignant transformation.

**Nasal Examination**

Nasal endoscopy typically shows a pale, polypoidal mass with a papillary appearance protruding from the middle meatus. It has an irregular, friable appearance, and they often bleed when touched (Fig. 39.2). They are reddish gray and may completely fill the nasal cavity, extending from the vestibule to the nasopharynx. The nasal septum is often bowed to the contralateral side. Proptosis and facial swelling sometimes develop secondary to expansion of the papillomatous lesion. In any case, a biopsy performed under endoscopic guidance is indicated to establish definitive histology.

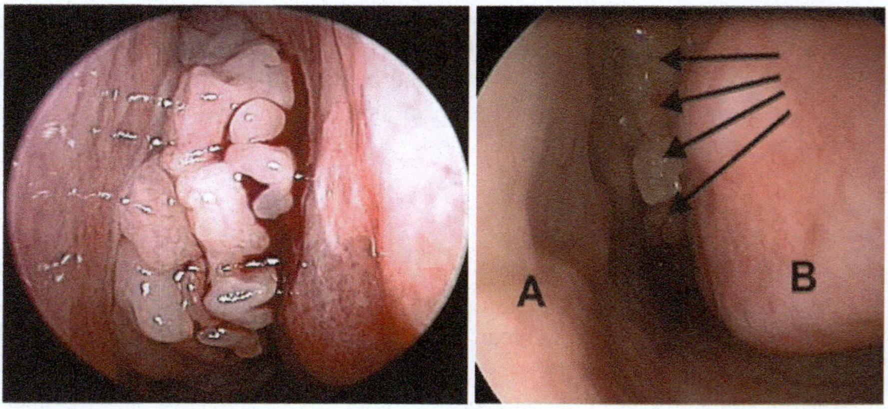


**Fig. 39.2** Nasal endoscopy of IP reveal papillary appearance of the lesion protruding from the middle meatus (black arrows) with irregular, friable appearance, and bleed on touch. (**a**) nasal septum and (**b**) inferior turbinate

## 39.7 Differential Diagnosis

General imaging differential considerations include:

- Sinonasal carcinoma: Unfortunately imaging is unable to confidently distinguish between inverted papillomas, inverted papilloma with malignancy, and pure malignancy.
- Antrochoanal polyp: Non-enhancing, peripheral mucosal enhancement may be present.
- Juvenile nasopharyngeal angiofibroma (JNA).
- Olfactory neuroblastoma.
- Paranasal sinus mucocele.
- Respiratory epithelial adenomatoid hamartoma (REAH): Significant widening of the olfactory cleft (OC) with the characteristic location (in the anterior half of the OC).

## 39.8 Radiologic Features

Imaging studies are required to assess the extent, site of origin of the tumor, and its relationship with surrounding structures (i.e., orbit, skull base, optic nerve, and internal carotid artery), and assess possible malignancy.

**On CT Scans**

Inverted papilloma appears as soft tissue density. With contrast, the tumor enhances heterogeneously. Hyperdense areas may be observed within the tumor. Remodeling of the bony sinus walls is frequent. Islands of tumor cells have been reported to exist

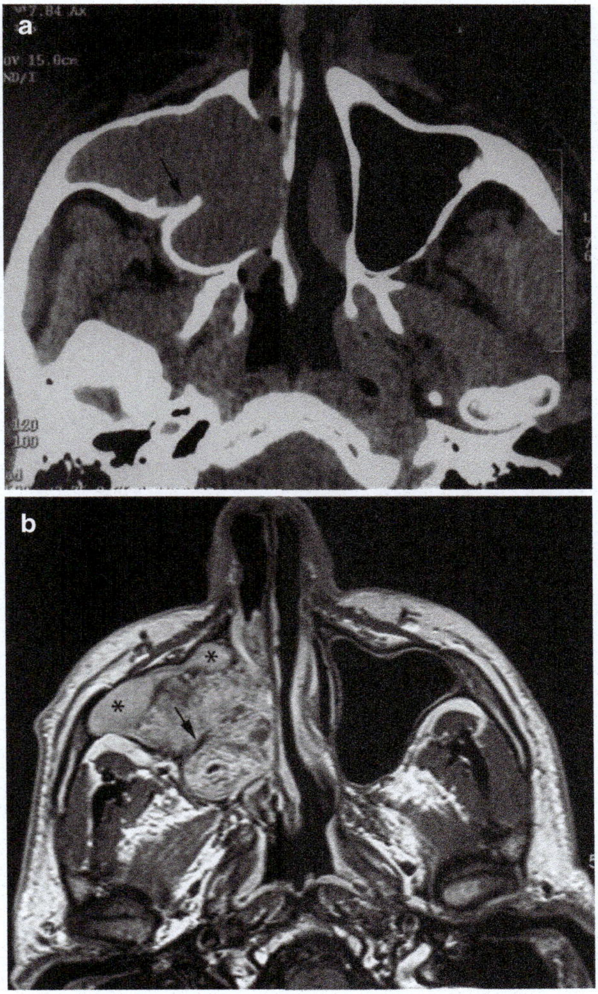


**Fig. 39.3** (**a**) CT scan axial plane reveals right maxillary sinus inverted papilloma; sinus walls are expanded and remodeled, with focal strut along the posterior wall of the maxillary sinus, representing the site of origin of the lesion (arrows). (**b**) Contrast-enhanced T1-weighted spin-echo MR image, axial plane. It displays the typical cerebriform-columnar pattern and better discrimination between neoplasm and retained secretions (asterisks)

within the bone at the site of origin of the tumor. The presence of a focal, often cone-shaped, hyperostosis has been reported to correlate with the point of origin of the lesions. This is useful not only in suggesting the diagnosis, but also in aiding surgical planning, as the location of tumor origin determines the extent of surgery required (Figs. 39.3a and 39.4a).

## On MRI

T1: isointense to muscle.

T2: Generally hyperintense to muscle. Alternating hypointense lines.

T1 C+ (Gd): Heterogeneous enhancement. Alternating hypointense lines.

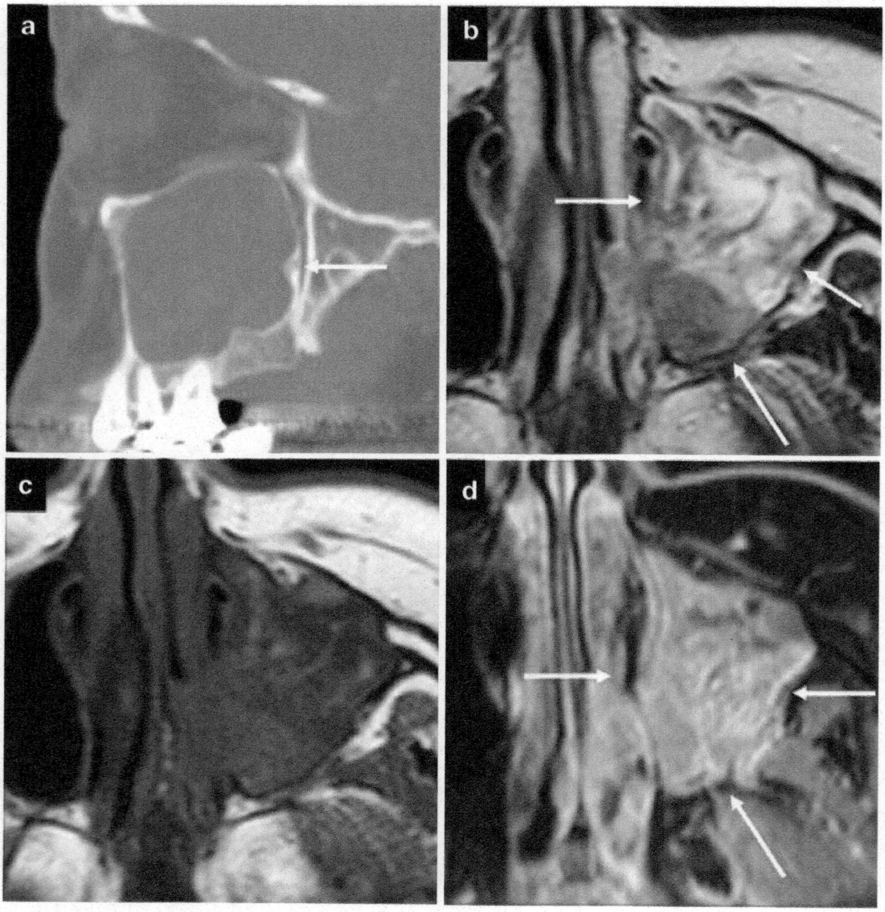


**Fig. 39.4** CT scan sagittal plane shows a mass lesion in the left maxillary sinus and localized hyperostosis of the posterior wall of the maxillary sinus on the bone window (arrow) (**a**), which indicates the origin of the inverted papilloma. T2-weighted image shows a lobulated shape mass with a CCP (arrows) (**b**). T1-weighted image shows hypointensity (**c**) with heterogeneous contrast enhancement after contrast administration (arrows) (**d**)

On postcontrast, T1W MRI inverted papilloma shows a convoluted cerebriform enhancing pattern that can be easily detected by MR as alternating roughly parallel lines of high and low signal, that is present in 50–80% of cases. MRI also differentiates the tumor from secretions. The so-called cerebriform-columnar pattern, which is highly predictive of inverted papilloma and differentiates it from other tumors (Figs. 39.3 and 39.4).

The site of origin of the lesion can be reliably identified when associated with a bony strut, focal hyperostosis, and osteitic changes on CT but may also be identified on MRI.

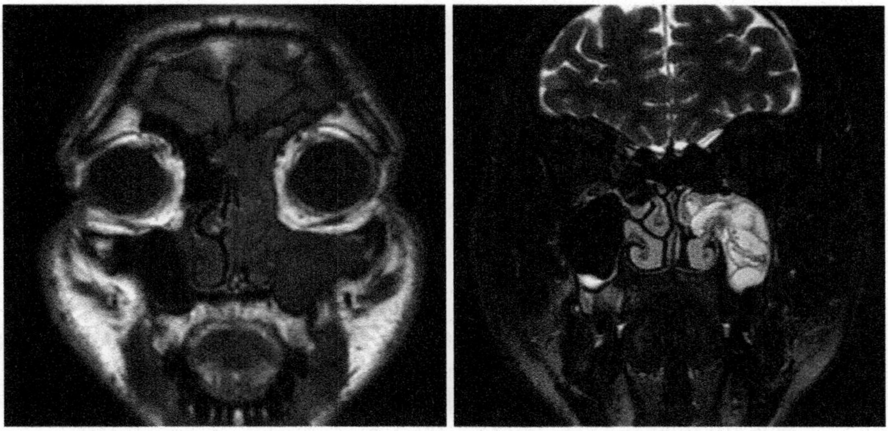

**Fig. 39.5** T1-weighted MR image shows hypointensity with heterogeneous contrast enhancement after contrast administration with the typical cerebriform-columnar pattern

Finally, MRI may also suggest a malignant transformation of the lesion on the basis of the loss of the typical cerebriform-columnar pattern and the evidence of aggressive and infiltrative tumor growth (Fig. 39.5) [6].

## 39.9 Biopsy

In any case, a biopsy performed under endoscopic guidance is indicated to establish definitive histology. Imaging should be done before biopsy to avoid possible vascular or brain injury.

## 39.10 Staging Systems

There is no standard staging system. A staging system is essential for determining the optimal surgical approach and predicting postoperative outcomes for inverted papilloma (IP). The Krouse, Oikawa, Cannady, and Han staging systems, which are based on the extent of IP, and the Meng system, which is based on the site of origin.

*Krouse staging system*

- Stage T1: limited to one area of the nasal cavity.
- Stage T2: involvement of the medial wall of the maxillary or ethmoid sinuses and/or the ostiomeatal unit.
- Stage T3: involvement of the superior, inferior, posterior, anterior, or lateral walls of the maxillary sinus, sphenoid sinus, and/or frontal sinus.
- Stage T4: tumors with extra-sinonasal spread or malignancy.

*Oikawa staging system*

- T3A: No extension to frontal sinus or supraorbital recess
- T3B: Involving frontal sinus or supraorbital recess

*Cannady staging system*

- Group A: confined to the nasal cavity, medial maxillary sinus, and ethmoid sinus (recurrence rate = 3%).
- Group B: involving the lateral maxillary sinus, sphenoid sinus, or frontal sinus (recurrence rate = 19%).
- Group C: extra-sinus extension (recurrence rate = 35%).

*Han staging system*

- Group I: It is confined to the nasal cavity, lateral nasal wall, medial wall of the maxillary sinus, ethmoid sinus, and sphenoid sinus.
- Group II: It involves lateral to medial wall of the maxillary sinus.
- Group III: It involves the frontal sinus.
- Group IV: It involves regions beyond the sinonasal cavities.

*Meng staging system*

- Stage 1: Site of origin of IP is confined to the nasal cavity.
- Stage 2: Site of origin of IP involves ethmoid sinus except for the supraorbital region, posterior, lateral, or superior wall of the maxillary sinus, medial to Sternberg's canal of the sphenoid sinus, facial midline to lamina papyracea of the frontal sinus.
- Stage 3: Site of origin of IP involves the supraorbital region, inferior, anterior, or medial wall of the maxillary sinus, lateral to Sternberg's canal of the sphenoid sinus, lamina papyracea to central pupil line or invades both of the frontal sinuses.
- Stage 4: Site of origin of IP involves the region of the frontal sinus lateral to the central pupil line.

The staging systems proposed by Han and Meng were found to be accurate in terms of tumor recurrence. We recommend the use of the Han staging system before surgery and the Meng system after intraoperative identification of the origin of the tumor [7–9].

## 39.11 Management

### 39.11.1 Endoscopic Approach

*Endoscopic transnasal surgery* is the gold standard of treatment for inverted papilloma.

Endoscopic medial maxillectomy and complete resection of the tumor is the classic treatment of inverted papilloma.

**The Goals of Endoscopic Surgery**

- Dissecting of all diseased mucosa and sending it for histologic examination to exclude the presence of malignancy.
- Drilling the bone at the site origin to decrease the chances of recurrence.
- Creation of a large marsupialized cavity for post-operative endoscopic inspection.

**Types of Endoscopic Resection**

- *Type 1: Simple ESS*: It is indicated for diseases involving middle meatus, ethmoid, superior meatus, sphenoid, or combination of these structures.
- *Type 2: Medial Maxillectomy*: It is indicated for diseases involving maxillary sinus mucosa (but not the lateral or the anterior walls).
- *Type 3: Sturman-Canfield operation/Endoscopic Denker operation*: It includes the removal of medial portion of anterior maxillary wall to enable access to all the antrum walls. It is indicated for diseases involving anterior or lateral walls of maxillary sinus mucosa.

**Advantages of Endoscopic Approach**

An endoscopic approach has a lower recurrence rate compared to external approaches. Three recent meta-analyses comparing endoscopic and external approaches clearly showed that endoscopic resection is associated with a reduction of the risk of recurrence by between one-third and one-half [10–13].

Moreover, unquestionable advantages of endoscopic surgery over external approaches are the absence of facial incision, facial swelling, and a reduction in postoperative pain and paresthesia. Therefore, endoscopic surgery is preferred whenever possible.

**Contraindications of Endoscopic Approach**

However, an exclusive endoscopic approach may be contraindicated in the following situations:

1. Synchronous malignancy involving critical areas.
2. Site of origin on the anterior wall or lateral recess of the frontal sinus, or massive involvement of the mucosa of the frontal sinus.
3. Orbital involvement, which is a very uncommon situation.
4. Significant scarring and anatomic distortion that are usually found in patients who have already undergone one or more surgical procedures.

**Modifications of the Endoscopic Medial Maxillectomy (EMM) Procedure**

The aim is to gain adequate antero-inferior access to the maxillary sinus based on the supposed origin and extent of the IP.

1. *Pedicle-oriented endoscopic surgery (POES)*:

Recently, a more conservative approach, pedicle-oriented endoscopic surgery (POES), offers good control of the disease, shorter operating times, avoidance of unnecessary surgery with respect to uninvolved structures, and permits a follow-up aimed at the site of the pedicle attachment.

Briefly, the procedure starts with debulking of the intranasal part of the tumor with the aim of detecting the site of origin of the lesion. Subsequently, both the subperiosteal dissection of the mucosa and drilling of the underlying bone are limited to the point of insertion of the tumor.

No difference in terms of recurrence rate was observed, while a decrease in postoperative complications was experienced with the new technique [14–16].

2. *Modular classification of endoscopic medial maxillectomies (EMMs)*:

Recently, a modular classification of endoscopic medial maxillectomies (EMMs) has been proposed, which progressively widens the size of the targeted area exposed.

There are four types of EMMs (A–D), with a transseptal variant for each, identified. In the axial plane, type A exposed the vidian canal and foramen rotundum, type B exposed the foramen ovale and foramen spinosum, and transseptal type C or type D exposed the coronoid process. In the sagittal plane, type A exposed the vidian canal, and type B exposed the foramen ovale and styloid process. Transseptal type C exposed the pterygomaxillary fissure, and type D exposed the inferior border of the lateral pterygoid plate. The nasal floor limits the downward angle in transseptal approaches. The width of the piriform aperture independently influenced surgical volume of types B and C.

The clear advantage is the possibility of minimizing the corridor on the basis of the surgical need, with the option of intraoperative shift to a larger approach if there is inadequate exposure [17].

It can provide access to almost the whole maxillary sinus and is indicated in cases of inverted papillomas originating from the inferior portion of the lateral and/or anterior walls of the maxillary sinus. Preliminary results have shown good oncologic control and a significant decrease in epiphora and dacryocystitis compared with classical extended medial maxillectomies.

3. *"TuNa-saving" technique*

A new surgical approach, the "TuNa-saving" technique, is a modified medial maxillectomy for selected cases of maxillary sinus inverted papilloma.

In this technique, the endoscopic medial maxillectomy was performed while preserving the head of the inferior turbinate and the nasolacrimal duct ("Tu" for "Turbinate" and "Na" for "Nasolacrimal duct," "TuNa-saving"). This technique allowed for good oncological control and a reduction in the rate of complications [18].

4. *Prelacrimal approach*

The prelacrimal approach provides direct access inside the maxillary sinus by removing the bone between the lacrimal pathway and the piriform aperture (with a possible extension to the medial part of the anterior maxillary wall). The lateral nasal wall is completely preserved. Results are promising with good oncologic control, no epiphora or dry nose. However, a possible drawback may be the impossibility to have full visualization of the maxillary sinus during nasal endoscopy at follow-up [19].

### 39.11.2 External Approach

Open En bloc resection with medial maxillectomy through lateral rhinotomy or midfacial degloving approaches.

Whatever the approach, the key concept for a radical resection is to dissect the involved mucosa in the subperiosteal plane and drill the underlying bone. Histopathological evidence of bone involvement indicates the importance of removal of the underlying bone at the time of endoscopic tumor resection. Thus, the extent of the operation is determined by the site of origin and area of mucosa involved by the lesion [20].

**Lateral Rhinotom Approach**

The lateral rhinotomy approach involves a curvilinear incision between the medial canthus and the dorsum of the nose. For this procedure, start the incision under the medial end of the eyebrow, extend the incision inferiorly between the medial canthus and the nasal dorsum and along the deep nasal-cheek groove adjacent to the ala of the nose. Then, swing the incision up onto the floor of the nose. The incision includes the full thickness of the skin down to the periosteum. A gentle W- or Z-plasty incision can be incorporated into the medial canthus region to help prevent postoperative webbing of the soft tissue.

After the skin incision is made, elevate the periosteum to expose the medial orbital wall, the anterior maxillary wall up to the infraorbital foramen, and the piriform aperture. The nasal bones can be retracted medially after medial and lateral osteotomies are performed. To achieve en bloc resection, perform osteotomies through the inferior and anterior aspects of the medial wall of the maxilla, through the medial wall of the orbit just inferior to the frontoethmoid suture line, and through the inferior orbital rim and orbital floor. By connecting these osteotomies, the specimen can be mobilized by using a heavy, curved Mayo scissors, which can be used to separate the specimen from the posterior wall of the maxillary sinus.

For medial maxillectomy, include the region of the lacrimal fossa, the infraorbital rim, and the prelacrimal recess of the maxillary sinus. Divide the lateral nasal wall along the floor of the nose. Amputate the middle turbinate below its superior attachment and remove the entire lateral wall intact after its detachment from the rest of the infraorbital rim.

To avoid epiphora, which is a common postoperative complication of this procedure, always incorporate dacryocystorhinostomy. Dacryocystorhinostomy can be accomplished by catheterization of the lacrimal duct by using an indwelling silicone tube (Guibor tube) or by incising the lacrimal sac vertically and sewing the edges to the adjacent tissues.

The medial canthus is usually displaced from its insertion and should be fixed to prevent unsightly telecanthus. If the tendon elevated is attached to the periosteum, it resumes its normal position after careful closure of the periosteum. Sometimes, the tendon is transected and should be tagged and approximated at the end of the procedure. Transnasal wiring is required if the lacrimal crest and adjacent bone are included in the resection.

**Midfacial Degloving Approach**

An alternative, versatile, and recommended approach is midfacial degloving for total excision of the SP. This approach consists of lifting the soft tissue from the mid portion of the face by means of a sublabial incision.

Four types of incisions are required in the midfacial degloving approach: (1) bilateral intercartilaginous incisions, (2) a complete septocolumellar transfixion incision, (3) bilateral sublabial incisions from the maxillary tuberosity to the tuberosity, and (4) bilateral pyriform aperture incisions extending to the vestibule. These incisions facilitate exposure of the pyriform aperture and the lateral nasal wall. En bloc resection of the lateral nasal wall is easy to perform, and it affords the possibility of extending the procedure to include the sphenoethmoidectomy and the medial orbital wall as dictated by the extent of the lesion.

Advantages of this approach include no external scarring, good visibility of the operative field, and simultaneous bilateral exposure. In addition, the recurrence rate of SP excised by using the midfacial degloving procedure is similar to those of lateral rhinotomy and medial maxillectomy. As with the lateral rhinotomy, the midfacial degloving approach can be combined with the craniofacial approach to treat lesions involving the base of the skull or anterior cranial fossa.

The primary limitation of the midfacial degloving approach is when surgery is required for more extensive tumors that invade the supraorbital ethmoid cells or the frontal sinus, which require a separate incision. Septal translocation through a sublabial incision is another approach that shares the same advantages of the midfacial degloving approach. It provides wide exposure with no external scarring.

## 39.12 Frontal Sinus Inverted Papilloma

Frontal sinus inverted papilloma is more difficult to treat. It is important to differentiate between papillomas arising from the lateral nasal wall and extending into the frontal sinus and the more difficult-to-treat papillomas whose site of origin is within the frontal sinus (Fig. 39.6).

Different degrees of frontal sinus involvement can be observed. The surgical choice may involve a Draf IIB or Draf III endoscopic sinusotomy or a combination of an endoscopic approach with external sinusotomy through an osteoplastic flap depending on the extent of frontal sinus mucosa involvement, a finding that can only be assessed at the time of surgery.

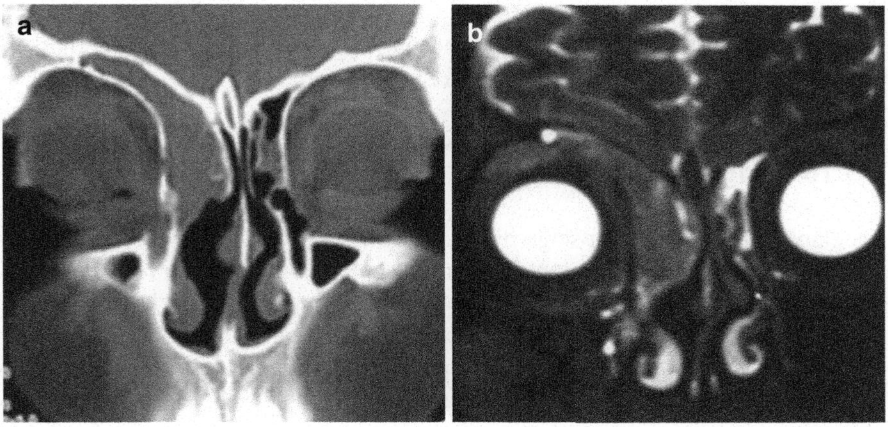


**Fig. 39.6** (**a**) CT scan showing inverted papilloma extending to the right frontal sinus. (**b**) T2-weighted MRI shows the heterogenous enhancement of the papilloma

An external approach through osteoblastic or eyebrow incisions may be needed for papilloma involving the extreme lateral frontal sinus.

## 39.13 Inverted Papilloma with Orbital or Intracranial Extension

For papilloma with orbital or intracranial extensions, it is important to preserve the periorbita and the dura to prevent extension of the tumor into the orbit or beyond the dura.

## 39.14 Radiation

Indications:

- Patients with SCC.
- Multiple recurrent disease (controversial).
- Incompletely resectable disease (controversial).

## 39.15 Postoperative Follow-Up

**Endoscopic Inspection**
Postoperative surveillance is almost exclusively clinical. Regardless of the access selected, resection of inverted papilloma should lead to the creation of a large cavity that will allow wide access for endoscopic inspection during follow-up. This is performed every 4 months during the first 2 years, every 6 months until the fifth, and then yearly until the tenth year.

**Imaging**
Postoperatively, MRI or CT is indicated only when a sinus that was originally involved by the lesion is not accessible for exploration.

## 39.16 Prognosis

Incomplete resection, high-stage disease, high-risk HPV, dysplasia, and smoking are the most relevant risk factors for recurrence. Smoking has been recently recognized as a risk factor for recurrence and malignant transformation. High-risk HPV (HPV 16 and 18) is considered a risk factor for malignant transformation [1–3].

Recurrence rates after transnasal resection of inverted papilloma dramatically decreased after the introduction of microscopic and endoscopic techniques. In a recent meta-analysis, the recurrence rates after endoscopic resection and external and combined approaches were 13.8%, 18.7%, and 12.9%, respectively [11].

In a recent meta-analysis, Krouse stage 3 (involvement of any wall of the maxillary sinus except the medial, frontal sinus, or sphenoid sinus) yielded a significant increase in the risk of recurrence (51%) when compared with stage 2 (involvement of ostiomeatal complex region, ethmoid, or medial wall of the maxillary sinus) [21].

Finally, dysplasia is emerging as an effective predictor of recurrence. In a recent study, the presence of dysplasia conferred a ten-fold higher risk of recurrence [22].

## References


1. El-Naggar AK, et al. WHO classification of head and neck tumours. Lyon: IARC; 2017.
2. Hong SL, et al. Smoking and malignancy in sinonasal inverted papilloma. Laryngoscope. 2013;123(5):1087–91.
3. Moon IJ, et al. Cigarette smoking increases risk of recurrence for sinonasal inverted papilloma. Am J Rhinol Allergy. 2010;24(5):325–9.
4. Lawson W, Schlecht NF, Brandwein-Gensler M. The role of the human papillomavirus in the pathogenesis of Schneiderian inverted papillomas: an analytic overview of the evidence. Head Neck Pathol. 2008;2:49–59.
5. Udager AM, et al. High-frequency targetable EGFR mutations in sinonasal squamous cell carcinomas arising from inverted sinonasal papilloma. Cancer Res. 2015;75(13):2600–6.
6. Lee DK, et al. Focal hyperostosis on CT of sinonasal inverted papilloma as a predictor of tumor origin. Am J Neuroradiol. 2007;28(4):618–21.
7. Krouse JH. Development of a staging system for inverted papilloma. Laryngoscope. 2000;110(6):965–8.
8. Meng Y, et al. Origin site-based staging system of sinonasal inverted papilloma for application to endoscopic sinus surgery. Head Neck. 2019;41(2):440–7.
9. Nakayama T, et al. Comparison of current staging systems for sinonasal inverted papilloma. Am J Rhinol Allergy. 2021;35(1):64–71.
10. Busquets JM, Hwang PH. Endoscopic resection of sinonasal inverted papilloma: a meta-analysis. Otolaryngol Head Neck Surg. 2006;134(3):476–82.
11. Goudakos JK, et al. Endoscopic resection of sinonasal inverted papilloma: systematic review and metaanalysis. Am J Rhinol Allergy. 2018;32(3):167–74.
12. Kim JS, Kwon SH. Recurrence of sinonasal inverted papilloma following surgical approach: a meta-analysis. Laryngoscope. 2017;127(1):52–8.

13. Peng R, et al. Outcomes of sinonasal inverted papilloma resection by surgical approach: an updated systematic review and meta-analysis. In: International forum of allergy & rhinology. Wiley Online Library; 2019.
14. Kamel RH, Abdel Fattah AF, Awad AG. Origin oriented management of inverted papilloma of the frontal sinus. Rhinology. 2012;50(3):262–8.
15. Landsberg R, et al. Attachment-oriented endoscopic surgical strategy for sinonasal inverted papilloma. Am J Rhinol. 2008;22(6):629–34.
16. Pagella F, et al. Evolution in the treatment of sinonasal inverted papilloma: pedicle-oriented endoscopic surgery. Am J Rhinol Allergy. 2014;28(1):75–81.
17. Schreiber A, et al. Modular endoscopic medial maxillectomies: quantitative analysis of surgical exposure in a preclinical setting. World Neurosurg. 2017;100:44–55.
18. Pagella F, et al. "TuNa-saving" endoscopic medial maxillectomy: a surgical technique for maxillary inverted papilloma. Eur Arch Otorhinolaryngol. 2017;274:2785–91.
19. Suzuki M, et al. Modified transnasal endoscopic medial maxillectomy through prelacrimal duct approach. Laryngoscope. 2017;127(10):2205–9.
20. Liang N, et al. Bone involvement: histopathological evidence for endoscopic management of sinonasal inverted papilloma. Laryngoscope. 2017;127(12):2703–8.
21. Lisan Q, Moya-Plana A, Bonfils P. Association of Krouse classification for sinonasal inverted papilloma with recurrence: a systematic review and meta-analysis. JAMA Otolaryngol Head Neck Surg. 2017;143(11):1104–10.
22. Safadi A, et al. The clinical behavior of sinonasal inverted papilloma with cellular dysplasia: case series and review of the literature. Eur Arch Otorhinolaryngol. 2017;274:3375–82.

# Juvenile Angiofibroma (JNA)

# 40

Hussam Elbosraty

**Key Points**

- JNA is a benign, nonencapsulated, highly vascular tumor, occurring almost exclusively in adolescent males. The tumor usually presents with recurrent epistaxis and nasal obstruction.
- The typical age range of JNA is 9 to 25 years.
- The tumor usually arises from the sphenopalatine foramen, vidian canal, and pterygoid wedge.
- The tumor spreads along the path of least resistance, virtually in all directions, to involve many vital structures.
- Radiology is usually diagnostic. Biopsies are prohibited.
- Treatment of choice is the surgical resection of the tumor.

## 40.1 Introduction

JNA is a benign, nonencapsulated, highly vascular tumor, occurring almost exclusively in adolescent males. It occupies approximately 0.05% to 0.5% of all head and neck masses [1, 2]. Individuals from India and the Middle East appear to have an increased incidence when compared to those of European descent [3].

The typical age range of JNA is 9 to 25 years, and though there have been case reports of NA diagnoses in older males, this is still considered a rare occurrence [4]. Though histologically benign, it often demonstrates aggressive features with local destruction and invasion into the surrounding structures [5].

**Supplementary Information** The online version contains supplementary material available at https://doi.org/10.1007/978-3-031-70077-4_40.

H. Elbosraty (✉)
Department of Otolaryngology, Cairo University, Cairo, Egypt


S. Elwany (ed.), *Current Rhinology*,
https://doi.org/10.1007/978-3-031-70077-4_40

Hippocrates first described this tumor in the fourth century B.C [6]. The term "juvenile nasopharyngeal angiofibroma" was coined by Chaveau in 1906 and his works resparked the interest in JNA [7].

The prevalence in males may be explained by high androgen receptor (AR) expression suggesting that JNA is androgen-dependent [8].

Many theories had been postulated to explain the etiology and the pathogenesis of JNA like the proliferation of fibrocartilage or the periosteum of the skull base between the basisphenoid and basiocciput or fetal erectile tissue, which proliferates under hormonal influence (pseudo-tumor theory), a hamartoma, hemangioma, paraganglioma [9–12]

## 40.2 Site of Origin

Juvenile nasopharyngeal angiofibroma can arise from any one of the following sites:

1. Sphenopalatine foramen: The upper margin of the sphenopalatine is considered as the most common site of origin of JNA. The sphenopalatine foramen is the point of trifurcation of three bones: palatine (perpendicular plate, orbital process, and sphenoidal process), vomer (horizontal ala), and sphenoid (specifically the root of the pterygoid process).
2. Vidian canal: The vidian canal/pterygoid canal arises from the anterior wall of the foramen lacerum and opens into the posterior wall of the pterygopalatine fossa. Literature states this as the potential site of origin in cases with laterally extended JNAs having little/no involvement of the sphenopalatine foramen/nasopharynx.
3. Pterygoid wedge: The pterygoid wedge is found to be the most common site of recurrence [13]. Drilling of the pterygoid wedge during primary surgery significantly reduces the risk of recurrence. First branchial arch artery theory for the origin of JNA supports this, as the first branchial arch artery is connected to the C4 segment of the internal carotid artery (ICA), its incomplete regression also explains how JNAs acquire blood supply from ICA despite no anatomical proximity [14].

## 40.3 Extensions of JNA

The tumor grows in the submucosal plane along the superior border of the choana and the roof of the nasopharynx to reach the nasal septum. It impinges on adjacent structures and causes pressure erosion of the bone. This invasiveness and extensiveness lead to high recurrence rates of 0–57% [15]. The tumor spreads along the path of least resistance to involve many vital structures.

*Medially*, it extends into the nasopharynx and grows submucosally. It can occupy the entire nasopharynx to cause bilateral nasal obstruction and nasal intonation of voice (rhinolalia clausa). The tumor mass may depress the soft palate and hang in the oropharynx. The blockage of Eustachian tube(s) may result in conductive hearing loss (otitis media with effusion).

*Anteriorly*, it enters the nasal cavity first causing unilateral nasal obstruction, epistaxis, and then it pushes the nasal septum toward the opposite side to produce contralateral nasal obstruction as well. Further tumor growth allows it to involve ethmoidal sinuses with flattening of the nasal bridge and an increase in the intercanthal distance. An associated proptosis gives a classical "frog-face deformity." The tumor may encroach upon and erode the anterior wall of sphenoid sinus.

*Laterally*, it extends to the pterygopalatine fossa causing an anterior bowing of the posterior wall of maxillary sinus (Holman-Miller sign), and then into the orbit via the inferior orbital fissure. This produces proptosis. Further involvement of an orbital apex results in loss of vision. An involvement of extraocular muscles produces diplopia. From the pterygopalatine fossa, the tumor grows laterally to invade the infratemporal fossa via the pterygomaxillary fissure. This causes facial swelling and fullness in the cheek, along the vidian canal to reach the foramen lacerum. Which opens in the middle cranial fossa. An erosion of the anterior face of the greater wing of the sphenoid causes the entry of the tumor into the middle cranial fossa (Figs. 40.1 and 40.2).

*Posteriorly*, the tumor can erode the pterygoid process and spread downward into the pterygoid fossa. It can reach as far as the parapharyngeal space. Posterolateral extension from the nasopharynx can cause extension into the fossa of Rosenmuller and extension from the apex of this fossa results in intracranial extension by eroding the carotid canal and petrous apex.

*Intracranial extension of the tumor* **may occur through one of the following routes:**

(i) From the infratemporal fossa, it erodes the anterior face of the greater wing of the sphenoid and/or through foramen ovale causing its widening into the middle cranial fossa. In such cases, the tumor lies lateral to the Internal Carotid Artery (ICA) and Cavernous Sinus (CS).

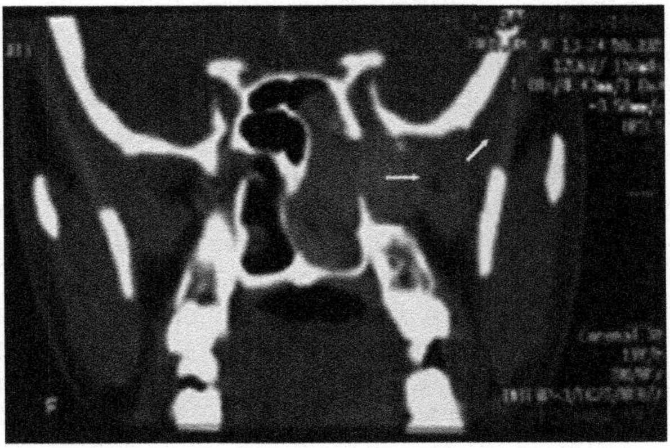

**Fig. 40.1** Lateral extension of JNA into the pterygopalatine fossa and infratemporal fossa. (Note the widening of the sphenopalatine foramen, bowing of the nasal septum, and extension onto the sphenoid sinus)

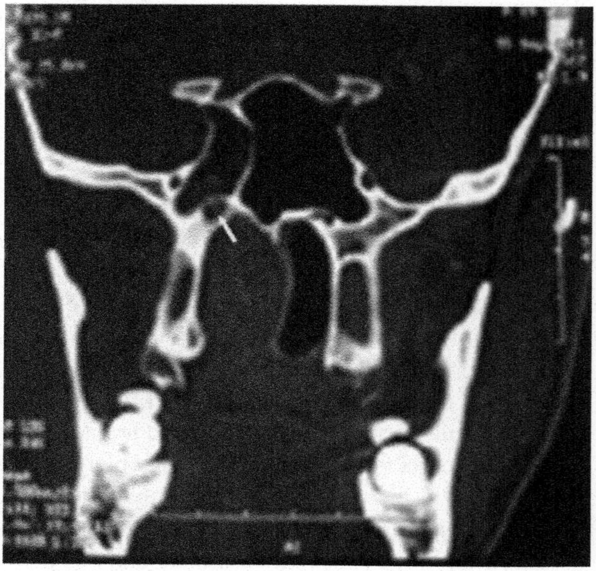

**Fig. 40.2** Tumor invasion of the vidian canal

(ii) From the pterygopalatine fossa through the inferior orbital fissure to the orbit toward orbital apex and superior orbital fissure to the middle cranial fossa. In this case, the tumor lies anterolateral to ICA and lateral to CS.

(iii) From the sphenoid sinus ➔ erosion of the roof of sphenoid sinus ➔ intracranial spread. The tumor lies medial to the ICA and lateral to the pituitary gland.

(iv) From the pterygopalatine fossa through the pterygoid (vidian) canal to the foramen lacerum to the middle cranial fossa. Encasement of ICA is seen early.

(v) Through the fossa of Rosenmuller ➔ erodes carotid canal and petrous apex ➔ intracranial spread.

(vi) From the nasal cavity ➔ through cribriform plate ➔ anterior cranial fossa (Rare).

## 40.4 Pathology of JNA

JNA classically presents as a painless, progressive unilateral nasal obstruction. Epistaxis, rhinorrhea, and pain may also be seen. Clinical examination reveals a firm vascular reddish, or reddish-purple mass in the nasopharynx and nose. As this tumor is aggressive and expansile, it invades adjacent structures causing further symptoms. Impaired Eustachian tube function, facial deformity, proptosis, and changes in visual acuity may be seen. Invasion of the intracranial region may lead to cranial nerve palsy.

Macroscopically this tumor appears as a rounded, circumscribed, nonencapsulated mucosa covered mass. The color depends on the vascular component and may vary from pale white in less vascular lesions to a pink and wine-colored mass in highly vascularized ones. Histopathologically, JNA shows a fibrocellular stroma with spindle cells and haphazardly arranged collagen interspersed with an irregular vascular pattern. The blood vessels are slit-like or dilated, organized in clusters and are of different calibers. A higher density toward the periphery is noted, which was seen in the present case too. The muscular lining of the blood vessel is absent in small and incomplete in larger vessels. A typical staghorn type of appearance is seen. Finally, numerous inflammatory cells such as mast cells and T-lymphocytes are seen [16]. Immunohistochemistry (IHC) tests act as ancillary tests for juvenile nasopharyngeal angiofibroma. Various IHC tests are available like vimentin, Androgen receptor, CD 31, CD 34, β Catenin.

## 40.5 Radiology

CT images show a heterodense mass that is centered in the sphenopalatine foramen. Avid enhancement is noted on contrast-enhanced CT (CECT) [17].

Lloyd's criteria for the diagnosis of JNA on CECT: [18]

(i) Mass lesion in the nasopharynx/nasal cavity and pterygopalatine fossa
(ii) Erosion of the posterior bony margin of the sphenopalatine foramen with an extension into the upper medial pterygoid plate.
(iii) Ram Haran sign: In JNA patients, coronal cuts of CT Nose-PNS show widening of the pterygoid wedge. It appears as a quadrilateral area rather than a normal triangular area. (Fig. 40.3)
(iv) Holman-Miller sign/Antral sign: Anterior bowing of the posterior wall of the maxillary antrum. This is due to the tumor mass completely filling the pterygopalatine fossa (Fig. 40.4)
(v) Hondousa sign: Widening of the gap between the maxillary body and ramus of the mandible. This occurs when the tumor mass involves infratemporal fossa.

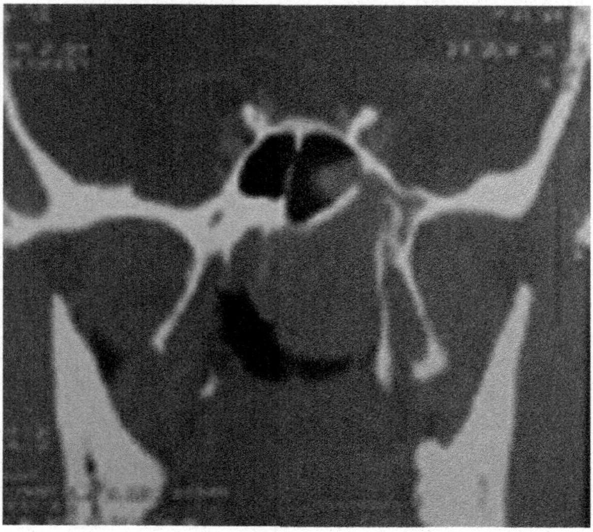

**Fig. 40.3** Invasion of the left (Lt.) pterygoid wedge (Ram Haran sign)

Chopstick sign: When contrast-enhanced CT (CECT) is used for post-operative surveillance to detect a residual/recurrent tumor, it shows "floating" medial and lateral pterygoid plates in cases where the root of the pterygoid base is drilled. These pterygoid plates are visualized separately to appear like a pair of chopsticks [19].

Contrast-enhanced MRI (CE-MRI) is the investigation of choice for advanced JNA tumors, particularly those with intracranial involvement) (Fig. 40.5), intraorbital, or parapharyngeal space involvement. It can accurately determine the extent of the tumor. The lesion shows low signal intensity in T1-weighted images but heterogeneous intermediate signal intensity in T2-weighted images. "Salt and pepper" appearance on contrast MRI is characteristic due to flow-void areas (T2WI and contrast-enhanced T1WI) [13].

Fat suppression MRI: This has been useful in detecting bone invasion by the tumor. The normal pterygoid wedge should be hypointense owing to fat-rich marrow. Any iso/hyper-intensity in that area indicates invasion by the tumor, therefore mandating bone drilling to avoid recurrence. MRI is also the preferred modality for post-operative long-term surveillance because of its superior soft tissue differentiation quality without any radiation exposure.

Angiography is a useful adjunct in the diagnosis of vascular tumors. The location and size of the tumor and feeding vessels are clearly demonstrated by this technique. The vascular supply to JNAs is primarily from distal internal maxillary artery branches, particularly the sphenopalatine, descending palatine, and posterior superior alveolar branches. JNAs may also be supplied by the ascending pharyngeal artery [20]. Given the extensive vascularity of the tumor, a biopsy should not be a consideration in the diagnostic evaluation of JNA especially in a clinical setting.

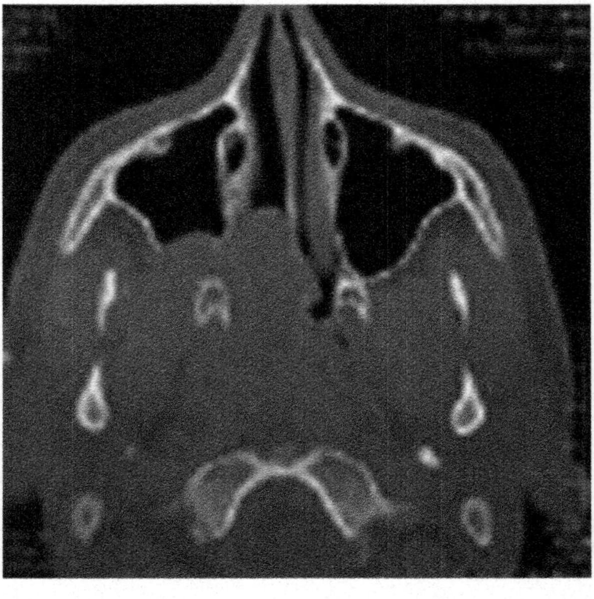

**Fig. 40.4** Bowing of the posterior maxillary sinus wall (Holman-Miller sign)

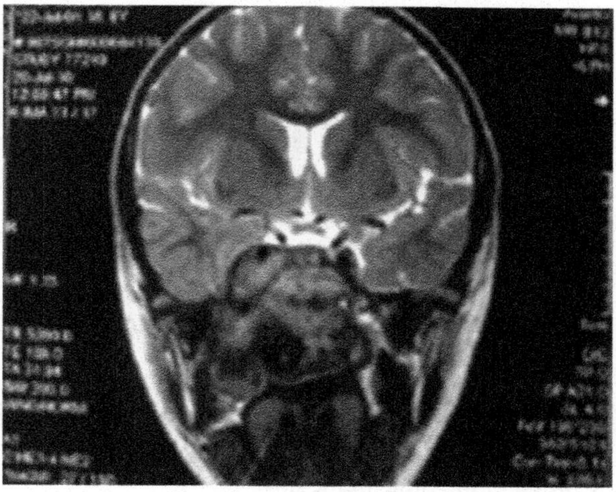

**Fig. 40.5** JNA encasing internal carotid artery

## 40.6 Staging Systems

Many staging systems have been proposed over the years, each has its own merits and demerits:

*Andrews-Fisch's staging system* [21]
- I Confined to the nose or nasopharyngeal vault
- II Invasion of the pterygopalatine fossa or maxillary/ethmoid/sphenoid sinuses with bone destruction
- IIIA Extension into the infra-temporal fossa or orbit
- IIIB Intracranial but extradural extension (parasellar area)
- IVA Intracranial intradural extension without involving cavernous sinus/optic chiasma/pituitary fossa (mnemonic C-O-P)
- IVB Intracranial intradural extension involving cavernous sinus/optic chiasma/pituitary fossa

*Radkowski's staging system* [22]
- IA Involvement of the nose or nasopharyngeal vault
- IB Extension into one or more sinuses
- IIA Minimal extension into the pterygopalatine fossa
- IIB Complete extension into the pterygopalatine fossa
- IIC Extension into infratemporal fossa/posterior to pterygoid plates
- IIIA Minimal skull base involvement (middle cranial fossa/base of pterygoid plates)
- IIIB Extensive intracranial involvement with or without involvement of the cavernous sinus.

*UPMC (University of Pittsburgh Medical Center)/Snyderman* **(only valid for tumors which are preoperatively embolized)** [23]

- I Nasal cavity, medial pterygopalatine fossa
- II Paranasal sinuses and lateral pterygopalatine fossa, no residual vascularity
- III Skull base erosion, orbit, infratemporal fossa, no residual vascularity
- IV Skull base erosion, orbit, infratemporal fossa, with residual vascularity from ICA
- V Intracranial extension with residual vascularity from ICA
- VM Medial cavernous sinus
- VL Middle cranial fossa

## 40.7 Treatment

Treatment of choice is the surgical resection of the tumor. Attribution of the oldest reported surgical treatment of JNA is to Hippocrates, recorded as a "longitudinal splitting of the ridge of the nose." [24]

Many surgical approaches are performed and, in some instances, combined approaches need to be used as lateral rhinotomy, transpalatal, transfacial, transnasal, sublabial/Le Fort I, transmaxillary, and infratemporal surgical corridors [25]. When possible, many cases now are treated endoscopically with an endonasal approach and may be augmented with an anterior maxillotomy or other craniotomy approaches, as needed [26].

Controlled hypotension while under general anesthesia is typically employed, with epinephrine to contract the nasal mucosa and improve the operative view. During the endonasal approach, parts of the inferior and middle turbinates may need to be resected to improve visualization. Also, depending on tumor size, the ethmoid air cells and maxillary ostium may need to be opened.for further access to tumor boundaries, especially when removal of the posterior wall of the maxillary sinus is needed to access the pterygopalatine or infratemporal fossae [27].

The strategy regarding these masses is to determine the periphery and extent of the tumor by dissecting around the margins, with as little manipulation as possible of the tumor itself. This approach allows the identification of key anatomic landmarks while keeping the tumor en bloc.

### 40.7.1 Surgical Considerations for Endoscopic JNA Surgery

The tumor size and extent decide the exact endoscopic approach required. While smaller tumors are managed via an endonasal approach, medium to large-sized tumors require an endoscopic Denker's or a more extensive transpterygoid approach [28]. Extended anterior skull base approaches are recommended for intracranial lesions [29].

### 40.7.2 Tricks in Endoscopic Resection of JNA

1. Exposure is the key to a successful surgery. Adequate exposure allows an identification of tumor limits, delineation of feeder vessels, and assessment of tumor's relation with vital structures.
2. Try to identify and control the feeding artery first (sphenopalatine and internal maxillary artery), before starting with tumor dissection (Fig. 40.6).
3. Posterior septectomy greatly increases the access to the tumor (Fig. 40.7)

4. Dissection is carried along the tumor pseudocapsule from the lateral to the medial direction. Injury to the tumor surface can provoke massive bleeding.
5. For larger tumors, a four-handed technique is recommended. For large tumors with extensive lateral extension into the infratemporal fossa/parapharyngeal space, the four-port Bradoo's technique is a worthy option [30]. Large tumors may be removed through the oral cavity (Fig. 40.8).
6. Drilling of the pterygoid base at the end of the procedure should be a routine practice to minimize tumor recurrence rates.
7. Hemostatic materials like Surgicel, Floseal, Tissel, bipolar cautery, and readily available fresh blood units should be available.
8. The possibility to convert an endoscopic approach into an open approach at any given time during the surgery should be a choice if needed.

Although surgical resection is the primary treatment of choice, radiation therapy can be an adjuvant therapy for residual or recurrent disease; this primarily takes

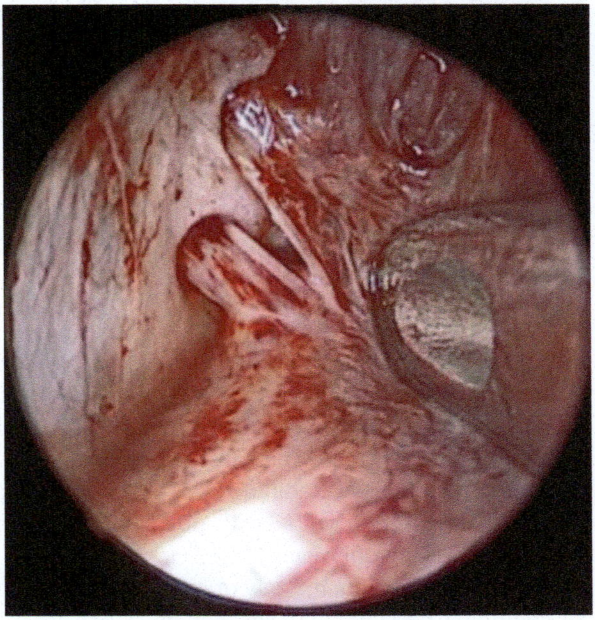

**Fig. 40.6** Exposure of sphenopalatine artery

**Fig. 40.7** Posterior septectomy

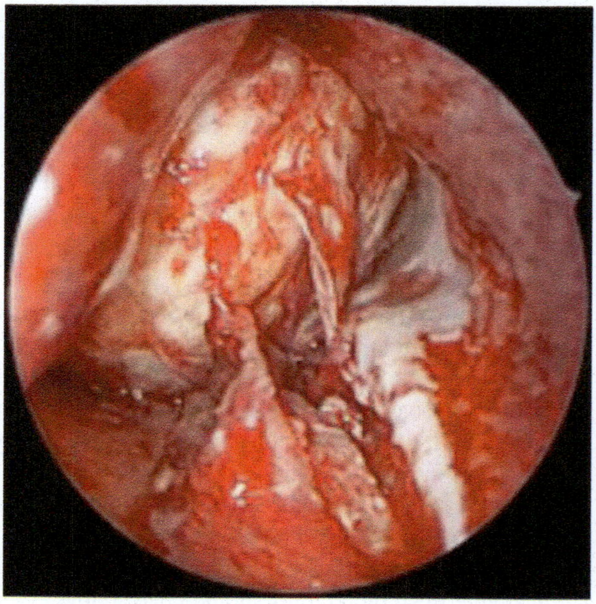

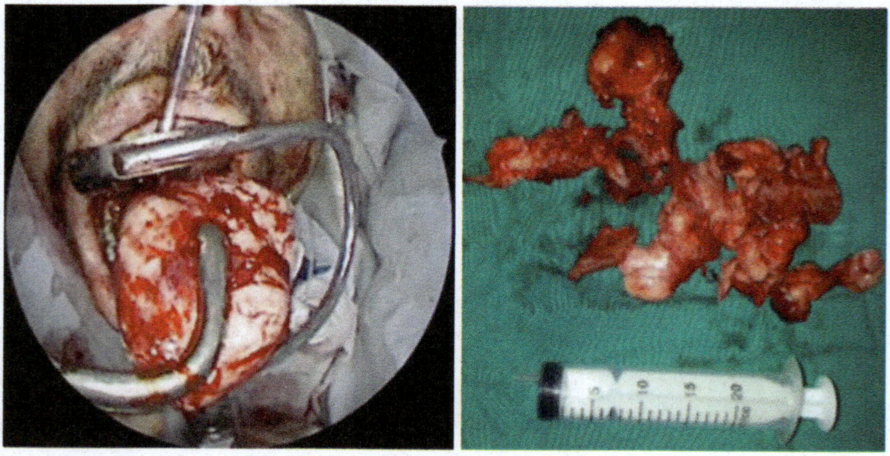

**Fig. 40.8** Removal of the tumor through the oral cavity

place in the setting of advanced tumors that involve critical areas, or those with an intracranial extension that may not be completely resectable. To some this remains controversial owing to concerns over long-term morbidity or the possibility of secondary neoplasm from the high doses of radiation [31].

Intensity Modulated Radiotherapy (IMRT), Gamma knife, and cyber knife are being applied in association with other treatment modalities to achieve desired results in large angiofibromas [32].

Hormonal therapy in the way of androgen receptor blockers such as flutamide is an additional possible adjuvant therapy. These have been shown to help reduce tumor size prior to surgical resection or in the setting of recurrence, but do not have curative results on their own [33].

### 40.7.3 Complications During Management

The most significant complication of JNA is blood loss, primarily in the operative/procedural setting and can be fatal in the absence of proper precautions. Exophthalmos, facial/orbital deformity, vision loss, and loss of extraocular movements can occur from orbital invasion by the tumor. Vision loss can also be a potential complication of nontarget embolization if there is an internal carotid artery branch involvement. Other severe complications of preoperative embolization include arterial vasospasm, facial palsy, infarction, or cranial nerve injury. More self-limiting, less severe complications include facial swelling, pain or abnormal sensation, headache, or nausea/vomiting. Surgical complications can include much of the same, with the addition of scarring and facial deformity. Hormonal therapy, if employed, can lead to feminization as a complication or at least an undesirable side effect in adolescent boys.

## References

1. Alshaikh NA, Eleftheriadou A. Juvenile nasopharyngeal angiofibroma staging: an overview. Ear Nose Throat J. 2015;94(6):E12–22.
2. Allensworth JJ, Troob SH, Lanciault C, Andersen PE. High-grade malignant transformation of a radiation-naïve nasopharyngeal angiofibroma. Head Neck. 2016;38(Suppl 1):E2425–7.
3. López F, Triantafyllou A, Snyderman CH, Hunt JL, Suárez C, Lund VJ, Strojan P, Saba NF, Nixon IJ, Devaney KO, Alobid I, Bernal-Sprekelsen M, Hanna EY, Rinaldo A, Ferlito A. Nasal juvenile angiofibroma: current perspectives with emphasis on management. Head Neck. 2017;39(5):1033–45.
4. McGarey PO, David AP, Payne SC. Nasopharyngeal angiofibroma in a 32-year-old man. BMJ Case Rep. 2018;2018:2018.
5. Szymańska A, Szymański M, Czekajska-Chehab E, Szczerbo-Trojanowska M. Invasive growth patterns of juvenile nasopharyngeal angiofibroma: radiological imaging and clinical implications. Acta Radiol. 2014;55(6):725–31.
6. Martin H, Ehrlich HE, Abels JC. Juvenile nasopharyngeal angiofibroma. Ann Surg. 1948;127(3):513–36.
7. Chaveau C. Histoire de maladies du pharynx. Vol 5. Paris: J.B. Bailliere et fils; 1906 (as in Janakiram, N., Wormald, P. and Sharma, S. Juvenile Nasopharyngeal Angiofibroma. Noida, India: Thieme; 2017:3).
8. Schick B, Rippel C, Brunner C, Jung V, Plinkert PK, Urbschat S. Numerical sex chromosome aberrations in juvenile angiofibromas: genetic evidence for an androgen-dependent tumor? Oncol Rep. 2003;10:1251–5.
9. Bensch H, Ewing J. Neoplastic disease. 4th ed. Philadelphia: Saunders and Co.; 1941.
10. Ringertz N. Pathology of malignant tumors arising in nasal and paranasal cavities and maxilla. Acta Otolaryngol Suppl (Stockh). 1938;27:158–61.
11. Sternberg SS. Pathology of juvenile nasopharyngeal angiofibroma: a lesion of adolescent males. Cancer. 1954;7:15–28.
12. Osborn DA. The so-called juvenile angio-fibroma of the nasopharynx. J Laryngol Otol. 1959;73(5):295–316.

13. Janakiram, N., Wormald, P. and Sharma, S. Juvenile nasopharyngeal angiofibroma. Noida: Thieme; 2017:45, 54, 222.
14. Schick B. Juvenile nasopharyngeal angiofibroma. In: Watkinson JC, Clarke RW, editors. 8. Scott-Brown's Otorhinolaryngology Head & Neck Surgery: Volume 1. Boca Raton: CRC Press; 2019. p. 1265–8.
15. Bremer JW, Neel HB 3rd, DeSanto LW, Jones GC. Angiofibroma: treatment trends in 150 patients during 40 years. Laryngoscope. 1986;96:1321–9.
16. Wendler O, Schäfer R, Schick B. Mast cells and T-lymphocytes in juvenile angiofibromas. Eur Arch Otorrinolaringol. 2007;264:769–75.
17. Garça MF, Yuca SA, Yuca K. Juvenile nasopharyngeal angiofibroma. Eur J Gen Med. 2010;7:419–25.
18. Lloyd G, Howard D, Lund VJ, Savy L. Imaging for juvenile angiofibroma. J Laryngol Otol. 2000;114(9):727–30.
19. Janakiram TN, Sharma SB, Samavedam UC, Deshmukh O, Rajalingam B. Imaging in juvenile nasopharyngeal Angiofibroma: clinical significance of Ramharan and chopstick sign. Indian J Otolaryngol Head Neck Surg. 2017;69(1):81–7.
20. Wu AW, Mowry SE, Vinuela F, Abemayor E, Wang MB. Bilateral vascular supply in juvenile nasopharyngeal angiofibromas. Laryngoscope. 2011;121:639–43.
21. Andrews JC, Fisch U, Valavanis A, et al. The surgical management of extensive nasopharyngeal angiofibromas with the infratemporal fossa approach. Laryngoscope. 1989;99(4):429–37.
22. Radkowski D, McGill T, Healy GB, et al. Angiofibroma. Changes in staging and treatment. Arch Otolaryngol Head Neck Surg. 1996;122(2):122–9.
23. Snyderman CH, Pant H, Carrau RL, Gardner P. A new endoscopic staging system for angiofibromas. Arch Otolaryngol Head Neck Surg. 2010;136(6):588–94. https://doi.org/10.1001/archoto.2010.83.
24. Mair EA, Battiata A, Casler JD. Endoscopic laser-assisted excision of juvenile nasopharyngeal angiofibromas. Arch Otolaryngol Head Neck Surg. 2003;129(4):454–9.
25. Park CK, Kim DG, Paek SH, Chung HT, Jung HW. Recurrent juvenile nasopharyngeal angiofibroma treated with gamma knife surgery. J Korean Med Sci. 2006;21(4):773–7.
26. Snyderman CH, Pant H. Endoscopic management of vascular sinonasal tumors, including angiofibroma. Otolaryngol Clin North Am. 2016;49(3):791–807.
27. Ye D, Shen Z, Wang G, Deng H, Qiu S, Zhang Y. Analysis of factors in successful nasal endoscopic resection of nasopharyngeal angiofibroma. Acta Otolaryngol. 2016;136(2):205–13.
28. Ahmed Y, Carrau RL, Ahmed T, Ahmed AI. Endoscopic approach to the infratemporal fossa. Alex J Med. 2014;50(2):127–30. https://doi.org/10.1016/j.ajme.2013.12.001.
29. Snyderman CH, Gardner PA, Fernandez-Miranda JC, Wang EW. Extended anterior skull base approaches. In: Watkinson JC, Clarke RW, editors. 8. Scott-Brown's otorhinolaryngology head & neck surgery: Volume 1. Boca Raton: CRC Press; 2019. p. 1289–303.
30. Bradoo R, Joshi A, Shah K, Patel T, Lohiya T. The four-port Bradoo technique: an alternative to the modified endoscopic Denker's approach for Giant JNA. Indian J Otolaryngol Head Neck Surg. 2017;69(3):277–81. https://doi.org/10.1007/s12070-017-1150-1.
31. Lee JT, Chen P, Safa A, Juillard G, Calcaterra TC. The role of radiation in the treatment of advanced juvenile angiofibroma. Laryngoscope. 2002;112(7 Pt 1):1213–20.
32. Dare AO, Gibbons KJ, Proulx GM, Fenstermaker RA. Resection followed by radiosurgery for advanced juvenile nasopharyngeal angiofibroma: report of two cases. Neurosurgery. 2003;52(5):1207–11.
33. Scholfield DW, Brundler MA, McDermott AL, Mussai F, Kearns P. Adjunctive treatment in juvenile nasopharyngeal angiofibroma: how should we approach recurrence? J Pediatr Hematol Oncol. 2016;38(3):235–9.

# Sino-nasal Cancers

# 41

Hisham Khalil, Mostafa Mehana, and Yazan Kanaan

**Key Points**

- Sino-nasal tumours include benign and malignant lesions of the sino-nasal tract. Tumours are either of epithelial or non-epithelial origin.
- Sino-nasal cancers (SNCs) are rare and represent around 1% of all body tumours.
- Patients with SNC often present late as symptoms often mimic those of rhinitis or rhinosinusitis.
- There is a paucity of level I and II evidence in the literature to support treatment decisions. The management is best overseen in specialised centres through a multi-disciplinary team (MDT). The treatment will depend on patient factors and choice, histology stage of the disease and the expertise of the MDT.

## 41.1 Introduction

Sino-nasal tumours are a group of diverse disorders that include benign and malignant lesions of the sino-nasal tract. The tissue of origin is either epithelial, bone or cartilage, glandular structures, lymphoid and connective tissue, and specialised neuronal cells. Some of these lesions predominantly affect the anterior skull base and it will be dealt with in a separate chapter.

H. Khalil (✉)
University Hospitals Plymouth NHS Trust, Plymouth, UK

Peninsula Medical School, University of Plymouth, Plymouth, UK
e-mail: hisham.khalil@plymouth.ac.uk

M. Mehana · Y. Kanaan
University Hospitals Plymouth NHS Trust, Plymouth, UK


S. Elwany (ed.), *Current Rhinology*,
https://doi.org/10.1007/978-3-031-70077-4_41

Sino-nasal cancers (SNCs) are rare tumours of the nasal cavity and paranasal sinuses, accounting for less than 1% of all malignancies [1] and about 3–5% of head and neck malignancies [2]. Most sino-nasal cancers are histologically squamous cell carcinomas, with adenocarcinomas being the second most common histology subtype [3]. The primary risk factor for SNC is smoking. Other risk factors include exposure to hard wood dust for adenocarcinoma of the maxillary sinust [4], with other occupational risk factors including leather dust, nickel, and radium [5]. Within the United Kingdom, SNC is the second most common cancer site for occupational attribution [6]. There has been a correlation between EBV [7] and nasal lymphoma. There is also an association between HPV and sinonasal squamous cell carcinoma (SCC) [8].

Mahalingappa and Khalil reported five-year results of treating 30 patients with SNC. The nasal cavity was the most common site for presentation, followed by the maxillary sinuses. Fifty per cent of patients had a squamous cell carcinoma and 27 per cent had a malignant melanoma. Half of the patients presented at stage IV of the cancer and 20 per cent at stage III. Thirty-seven per cent of patients underwent surgical management and only 20 per cent of the total patient group underwent endoscopic surgery. The mortality was 30 per cent over the studied period. They concluded that late-stage presentation SNC has resulted in increased patient mortality in their case series. They also found a high incidence of malignant melanoma with high recurrence but also high survival rates [9].

## 41.2 Classification of Sino-Nasal Cancer

The WHO classification of SNC includes the following [10]:

- Malignant epithelial tumours
- Neuroendocrine tumours
- Benign epithelial tumours
- Soft tissue tumours
- Tumours of bone and cartilage
- Haematolymphoid tumours
- Neuroectodermal tumours
- Germ cell tumours
- Secondary tumours

### 41.2.1 Epithelial Cancers

- Squamous cell carcinoma
- Adenoid cystic carcinoma
- Adenocarcinoma
- Malignant melanomas
- Olfactory neuroblastomas
- Sino-nasal undifferentiated carcinoma

### 41.2.2 Non-epithelial Cancer

- Malignant lymphoma
- Sarcomas

### 41.2.3 Squamous Cell Carcinoma

Histological subtypes of SCC include keratinising SCC, non-keratinising SCC, basiloid, papillary, adenosquamous and spindle cell varieties. Given the rarity of these tumours, pathologists may experience difficulty in differentiating these tumours from other histological types of sino-nasal cancer.

### 41.2.4 Adenocarcinoma

Sino-nasal adenocarcinoma arises from the epithelial lining of the sino-nasal tract including the goblet cells or minor salivary glands. The sub-types of sino-nasal adenocarcinoma therefore include salivary-gland and non-salivary glands sub-types. Adenoid cystic carcinoma (AdCC) is the most common salivary-type carcinoma. This malignancy is known for its peri-neural spread.

### 41.2.5 Sino-nasal Malignant Melanoma

Sino-nasal malignant melanomas are rare tumours that account for between 0.5 and 2% malignant melanomas. They have a relatively poor prognosis due to late presentation. Risk factors and aetiology remain unclear. The incidence is slightly higher in white men over the age of sixty. Most patients present with unilateral epistaxis and nasal obstruction. The histology usually reveals an undifferentiated tumour with the diagnosis clinched with immunohistochemistry, e.g. demonstrating positivity for vimentin, S100, and HMB45 (human melanoma black 45).

### 41.2.6 Sino-nasal Undifferentiated Carcinoma (SNUC)

SNUCs are a very rare group of sino-nasal tumours of unknown aetiology. It has an estimated incidence of 0.02 per 100,000. Most patients with SNUC are diagnosed at a late stage in their disease, with a poor prognosis. Pathological examination of SNUC typically reveals large tumours with fungating and poorly defined margins that invade adjacent structures. The histologic appearance is characterised by sheets, trabecular, and ribbon-like arrangements of small to medium-size undifferentiated cells. These cells often have high nuclear to cytoplasmic ratio, high mitotic rate, and prominent tumour necrosis. Lymphovascular and neural invasion are often also identified. It is immunohistochemically distinct from other sino-nasal malignancies such as lymphoma, neuroendocrine carcinoma, mucosal melanoma, nasopharyngeal carcinoma, and olfactory neuroblastoma. Cytokeratin staining is positive while staining for leucocyte common antigen.

### 41.2.7 Olfactory Neuroblastoma (Esthesioneuroblastoma)

Olfactory neuroblastoma is a rare type of cancer, making up to only 3% of nasal cavity tumour cases. Olfactory neuroblastoma affects only about one person per 2.5 million each year. Olfactory neuroblastoma can form at any age but is most commonly seen in people aged 50 to 70 years old. The tumour arises from the olfactory bipolar cells of the olfactory cleft area of the nasal cavity.

### 41.2.8 Sino-nasal Lymphomas

Sino-nasal lymphomas are of the non-Hodgkin type. Sino-nasal Non-Hodgkin's lymphoma (NHL) These could be B cell or T cell lymphomas. The NK T cell lymphomas are some of the most malignant of SNCs.

### 41.2.9 Rare Miscellaneous Types of SNC

Rare histological types of SNC include carcinosarcomas and hemangiopericytoma.

## 41.3 Staging of Sino-nasal Cancers

The staging of SNC will depend on whether it is epithelial, or non-epithelial, e.g. a malignant lymphoma. The Tumour Nodal metastasis Distant Metastasis (TNM) staging system is usually employed for staging nasal andsinus cancer except for sino-nasal lymphoma. There are variations depending on the site of origin of the nasal and paranasal sinus cancer. This is sometimes difficult to ascertain in advanced stages of the disease.

An example for the T Staging of the TNM staging for maxillary sinus cancer is included [11] (Table 41.1)

**Table 41.1** Tumour staging of cancer of the maxillary sinus

| Tumour size (T) | |
|---|---|
| Tx | Cancer can't be assessed |
| Tis | Carcinoma in situ |
| T1 | Tumour limited to maxillary sinus mucosa without erosion or destruction of the bone |
| T2 | Tumour causing erosion or destruction of the bone including extension to the hard palate and / or middle meatus but excluding extension to the posterior wall of the maxillary sinus and the pterygopalatine fossa |
| T3 | Tumour involves any of the following structures: bone of the posterior wall of the maxillary sinus, pterygopalatine fossa, subcutaneous tissues, medial or inferior wall of the orbit, ethmoid sinuses |
| T4a | Moderately advanced local disease. Cancer involves anterior orbital contents, skin of the cheek, pterygoid plates, cribriform plate, sphenoid sinus, frontal sinus |
| T4b | Very advanced local disease<br>Tumour involves any of the following: orbital apex, dura, brain, middle cranial fossa, cranial nerves except the maxillary division of the trigeminal nerve, nasopharynx or clivus |

## 41.4 The Diagnostic Approach to Patients with Sino-nasal Cancer

The vague presentations of sino-nasal cancer often lead to a late diagnosis. Patients often experience symptoms that are not dissimilar to those of rhinitis and rhinosinusitis including nasal congestion and facial discomfort with or without a change in the sense of smell.

**Symptoms and Signs**

The early symptoms that should raise a suspicion of a sino-nasal cancer include:

- Unilateral nasal obstruction with epistaxis more than 3 weeks
- Unilateral purulent nasal discharge which may or may not be blood-stained, for more than 3 weeks
- A health professional or the patient noticing a unilateral nasal mass.

Late symptoms include facial swellings and pain, headaches, visual disturbance, unexplained loose dentition or ill-fitting dentures, unilateral proptosis, and unilateral cranial nerve palsy.

The examination of a patient with suspected SNC should include inspection and palpation of the face and neck, cranial nerves assessment, and a comprehensive ENT examination including a nasal endoscopy. Nasal endoscopy whether flexible or rigid should ascertain the presence of nasal lesions, morphologic appearance, site of origin if apparent as well as involvement of the olfactory cleft and post-nasal space. Further clinical assessments will depend on the patient symptoms and findings. For example, a detailed ophthalmological assessment in patients with visual symptoms.

**Investigations**
Patients with highly suspicious symptoms and in the absence of a detectable nasal mass on nasal endoscopy should have an initial CT of the sinuses and further imaging, e.g. MRI of the sinuses, and requested accordingly. In patients with a detectable nasal mass on nasal endoscopy, both CT and MRI scans of the sinuses should be requested prior to nasal endoscopy. Patients also presenting with cervical lymphadenopathy should have an ultrasound-guided Fine Needle Aspiration biopsy of a representative lymph node for cytological examination. If SNC is confirmed on histology, staging MRI scans of the neck and CT of the thorax, abdominal cavity and pelvis are requested.

Biopsies of sino-nasal masses are taken after endoscopic image documentation of the lesion, followed by targeted biopsies of abnormal tissue to ensure a representative sample. Histopathological assessment of biopsies is preferably carried out be a dedicated head and neck cancer pathologist.

### 41.4.1 Treatment of Sino-nasal Cancer

The management of SNC is through a multi-disciplinary approach and will depend on various factors including the patient profile and choice, histological type and stage of the cancer and expertise of the multi-disciplinary team (MDT) in the treatment centre. These variables impact the shared decision-making with patients and the MDT ensuring that patients are fully informed of the pros and cons of each treatment strategy as well as non-treatment.

In sino-nasal lymphoma, the role of surgery is limited to taking a biopsy for histological confirmation. The treatment is usually by radiotherapy alone or combined with chemotherapy depending on the histological sub-type and stage of the disease. For other types of SNC, the best chance of cure is achieved with complete surgical excision with clear margins. However, this is often not achievable due to the late stage at presentation. Patient choice may also dictate the treatment even if not oncologically sound. For example, preservation of the orbit even if this leaves residual disease which is then addressed with radiotherapy and chemotherapy. The available evidence does not suggest that more conservative endoscopic resections have inferior outcomes compared to more extensive traditional approaches such as a total maxillectomy or craniofacial resection. The overall prognosis of SNC remains poor with 5-year survival rates ranging from 50–60% on average. There has been an improvement of survival rates over the last decade. The use of induction chemotherapy and chemoradiotherapy as well as proton-beam therapy has resulted in prolonged periods of remission of disease and improved 5-year survival of SNCs that were deemed uncurable in the past [12].

More recently, there has been an increased attention towards HPV-related SCC with evidence of over-expression of p16 and presence of HPV DNA. There are some studies that suggest better prognosis in HPV-related SCC. There is a need for large multi-centre trials comparing different treatment modalities and outcomes in the various histological types and sub-types.

## 41.5 Case Study

A 55-year-old man presented acutely to the Emergency Department with a right periorbital swelling, headaches, and recurrent right epistaxis. An initial ENT assessment revealed a right sino-nasal mass extending into the orbit and right skull base. CT and MRI of the sinuses (Figs. 41.1 and 41.2) and further staging imaging revealed a T4bNoMo right sino-nasal tumour which a biopsy confirmed to be a Sino-nasal Undifferentiated Carcinoma. Following a MDT discussion and patient agreement, the patient underwent induction chemotherapy with Taxotere, Cisplatinum and Fluouracil (TPF) resulting in significant regression in the tumour. This was then followed by radical radiotherapy and radiotherapy.

The patient had complete regression of the tumour but developed right ocular pain and epiphora. There was evidence of mucosal thickening in the right sino-nasal tract in post-treatment scans but repeated biopsies confirmed the patient was free of disease.

The patient remained free of disease for 3 years following his treatment and undergoes 2 month outpatient follow-up with nasal endoscopic examinations. He also has 6 month MRI scans of the sinuses alternating with 6 month nasal biopsies. (Fig. 41.3)

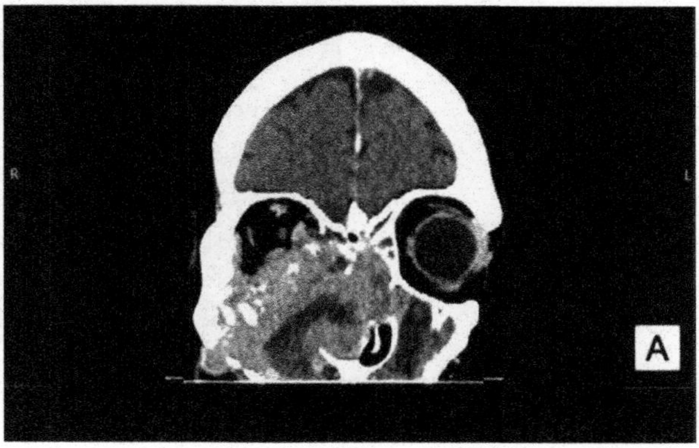


**Fig. 41.1** CT Sinuses: pre-treatment CT of the sinuses demonstrating an extensive sino-nasal tumour involving the right orbit, skull base and extending to the left nasal cavity

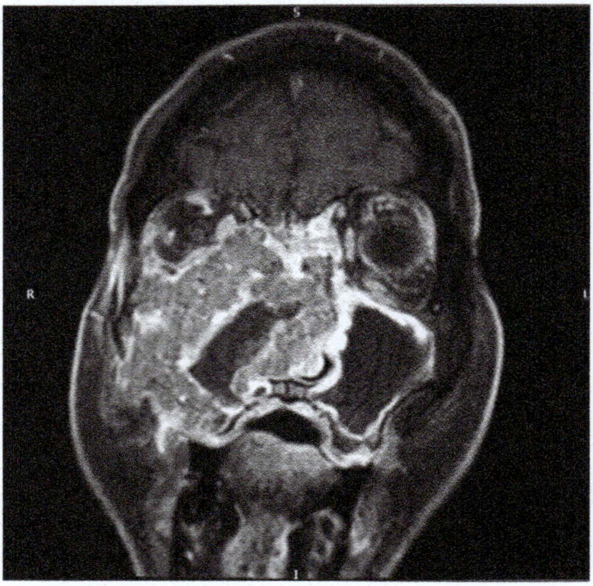


**Fig. 41.2** MRI Sinuses: pre-treatment MRI of the sinuses demonstrating an extensive sino-nasal tumour involving the right orbit, skull base and extending to the left nasal cavity

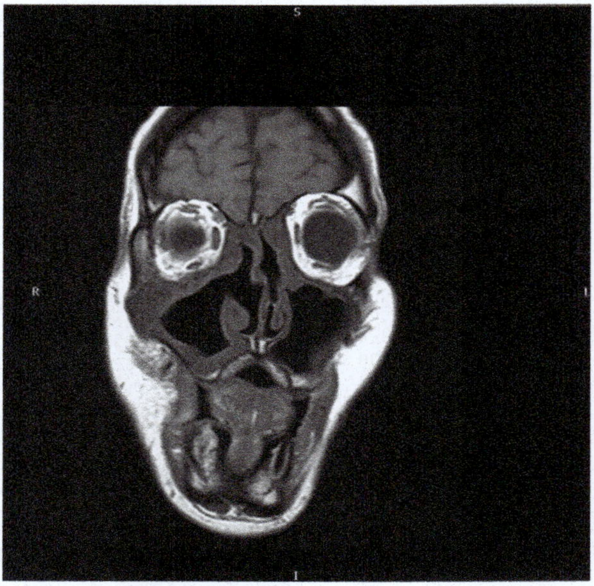


**Fig. 41.3** Post-treatment MRI, free of disease

## References


1. Tufano RP, Mokadam NA, Montone KT, Weinstein GS, Chalian AA, Wolf PF, et al. Malignanant tumours of the nose and paranasal sinuses:hospital of the University of Pennsylvania experience 1990-1997. Am J Rhinol. 1999;13:117–23.
2. Tiwari R, Hardillo JA, Mehta D, Slotman B, Tobi H, Croonenburg E, et al. Squamous cell carcinoma of maxillary sinus. Head Neck. 2000;22:164–9.
3. Franchi A, Miligi L, Palomba A, Giovannetti L, Santucci M. Sino-nasal carinomas: recent advances in molecular and phenotypic characterization and their clinical implications. Crit Rev Oncol Hematol. 2011;79(3):265–77.
4. World Health Organisation. Wood Dust. IARC Monogr Eval Carcinog Risks Hum. 1995;62:35–7.
5. El Ghissassi F, Baan R, Straif K, Grosse Y, Secretan B, Bouvard V, et al. A review of human carcinogens. Part D: Radiation. Lancet Oncol. 2009;10(8):751–2.
6. Rushton L, Hutchings SJ, Fortunato L, Young C, Evans GS, Brown T, et al. Occupational cancer burden in Great Britain. Br J Cancer. 2012;107(Suppl. 1):S3–7.
7. Feng YF, Wu QL, Zong YS. Correlation of immunophenotype of sino-nasal non-Hodgkin's lymphoma to Epstein-Barr virus infection. Ai zheng. 2007;26(11):1170–6.
8. Alos L, Moyano S, Nadal A. Alobid I et alHuman papillomaviruses are identified in a subgroup of sino-nasal squamous cell carcinomas with favorable outcome. Cancer. 2009;115(12):2701–9. https://doi.org/10.1002/cncr.24309.
9. Mahalingappa YB, Khalil HS. Sino-nasal malignancy: presentation and outcomes. J Laryngol Otol. 2014;128(7):654–7.
10. Agarwal A, Bhatt AA, Bathla G, Kanekar S, Soni N, Murray J, Vijay K, Vibhute P, Rhyner PH. Update from the 5th edition of the WHO classification of nasal, paranasal, and skull base tumors: imaging overview with histopathologic and genetic correlation. AJNR Am J Neuroradiol. 2023;44(10):1116–25. https://doi.org/10.3174/ajnr.A7960. Epub 2023 Aug 17. PMID.
11. American Joint Committee on Cancer (AJCC). AJC cancer staging manual. 8th ed. New York: Springer; 2017.
12. Liu Q, Huang X, Chen X, Zhang J, Wang J, Qu Y, Wang K, Wu R, Zhang Y, Xiao J, Yi J, Luo J. Long-term outcomes of endoscopic resection versus open surgery for locally advanced sinonasal malignancies in combination with radiotherapy. J Neurol Surg B Skull Base. 2022;85(1):28–37. https://doi.org/10.1055/a-1980-8567. PMID: 38274487; PMCID: PMC10807958.

# Anterior Skull Base Tumors

# 42

Muhammad Shahzad, Samiul Muquit, and Hisham Khalil

**Key Points**

- Anterior skull base tumors are a diverse group of lesions that may arise from the anterior skull base, the sinonasal tract, the intracranial cavity, or may be metastatic lesions.
- The histology of these lesions are variable.
- The tumors may present late as the initial symptoms may be vague and non-specific.
- Patients with anterior skull base lesions are best managed in specialized centers through a multidisciplinary team. The choice of treatment and prognosis depend on patient factors, tissue of origin, and stage of the disease.

M. Shahzad
Department of Neurosurgery, Southwest Neurosurgery Centre, University Hospitals Plymouth NHS Trust, Plymouth, UK

S. Muquit
Department of Neurosurgery, Southwest Neurosurgery Centre, University Hospitals Plymouth NHS Trust, Plymouth, UK

Peninsula Medical School, University of Plymouth, Plymouth, UK

H. Khalil (✉)
Peninsula Medical School, University of Plymouth, Plymouth, UK

University Hospitals Plymouth NHS Trust, Plymouth, UK
e-mail: hisham.khalil@plymouth.ac.uk


S. Elwany (ed.), *Current Rhinology*,
https://doi.org/10.1007/978-3-031-70077-4_42

## 42.1 Introduction

Anterior skull base tumors arise directly from the skull base; these are an extension of sinonasal or intracranial tumors or are metastatic lesions. Anterior skull base tumors are therefore a diverse group of disorders with varied histology and presentations. They are best managed by multi-disciplinary teams with expertise in neurosurgery, neurology, otolaryngology, maxillofacial surgery, ophthalmology, neuro-radiology, neuro-oncology, neuro-pathology, specialist nursing, and inputs from allied health professions.

## 42.2 Clival Chordomas

The deeply seated position of tumors at the clivus, along with their proximity to important neurovascular structures, make them a significant surgical challenge in terms of exposure and removal. Surgical approaches for treating these neoplasms have been completely transformed by recent developments in visualization technologies and endoscopic microinstrumentation. Less invasive endonasal endoscopic techniques have taken the place of traditional aggressive surgical methods. On occasion, these anterior approaches are supplemented with lateral or posterolateral techniques to ensure comprehensive removal, which is a critical factor influencing the prognosis of the patient. Because the tumors in this location tend to invade the clival bone, surgical resection may be required regardless of the particular pathology and may extend beyond the margins that are observably affected. Usually quite large at the time of diagnosis, these tumors can spread into nearby regions like the parasellar region, the anterior cranial fossa, the nasal cavity, the paranasal sinuses, the nasopharynx, or the middle fossa [1–3].

## 42.3 Anatomy

The clivus, comprising the basilar part of the occipital bone and the body of the sphenoid bone, spans from the dorsum sellae to the foramen magnum. Its superior aspect is framed by the petroclival fissure laterally and the petrous temporal bone, leading to the jugular foramen. The antero inferior aspect of the clivus bears the pharyngeal tubercle which serves as an attachment site for the pharyngeal raphe and anterior longitudinal ligament. Laterally, the supracondylar groove indicates the position of the underlying hypoglossal canal. The clival dura features a complex venous system, including the clival venous plexus and inferior petrosal sinus, which connects to the posterior cavernous sinus and jugular bulb. The abducens nerve's trajectory through this area and the adjacent anatomical landmarks, including the Eustachian tube and the internal carotid artery, are critical for surgical access. The posterior aspect of clivus is related to the brainstem and vertebrobasilar arteries.

## 42.4 Imaging

High-resolution CT scans are essential for identifying areas of bone destruction and determining the degree of bone involvement by clival tumors, particularly chordomas. They are especially helpful in assessing the optic and carotid canals. When tumoral calcification is present, it is easily detected. Cervical spine dynamic plain radiographs in flexion and extension are advised when occipitocervical stability is in doubt. Critical surrounding neurovascular structures can be identified with multiplanar magnetic resonance imaging (MRI), both with and without contrast enhancement. MRI is also excellent at mapping tumor boundaries. Tumoral contrast can be better seen in areas rich in fat when fat signal is suppressed by defining the spatial relationship between the tumor, the clival bone, and the internal carotid artery. CT angiography is an essential tool for surgical intervention planning. Intraoperative navigation systems can be designed to precisely guide surgery by integrating this imaging with volumetric MRI data. While not always required, routine cerebral angiography is useful for identifying venous drainage patterns, vascular anomalies, and narrowing when detailed vascular mapping is needed. Preoperative evaluation may include temporary balloon occlusion tests and additional cerebrovascular reserve tests, such as transcranial Doppler, to assess the patient's ability to tolerate such vascular interventions in cases where carotid artery compromise is anticipated or arterial injury risk is significant [1, 3–5].

Meningioma, chondrosarcoma (usually paramedian), pituitary adenoma, metastatic lesions, nasopharyngeal carcinoma, plasmacytoma, and sphenoid sinus cancers are among the possible diagnoses for a clival mass displaying invasive features. When compared with the high signal intensity of clival marrow fat, chordomas on T1-weighted MRI generally show an intermediate to low signal intensity. T1-weighted images might show intermittently high contrast areas inside the tumor, which could be a sign of mucin release or intratumoral bleeding. Since the tumor's vacuolated cells contain a rich amount of fluid, T2-weighted MRI frequently displays a high signal intensity. T2 hypointensity is produced by areas of calcification, hemorrhage, or dense mucus rich in proteins. A characteristic "honeycomb" pattern of contrast enhancement ranging from moderate to significant reflects the multilobulated structure of the tumor in MRI images, where low-intensity septations divide high-signal intensity lobules. While chordomas typically appear along the midline, chondrosarcomas typically appear along the lateral aspects of the petroclival fissure. However, because chondrosarcomas have recognizable calcification patterns, CT scans may help differentiate. With a dural base and a sharply defined, uniformly contrast-enhancing appearance, meningiomas in the clival region are distinguished on MRI by their potential for hyperostosis but without the bone destruction characteristic of chordomas. Since nasopharyngeal cancers like carcinoma, lymphoma, and plasmacytomas can extend anteriorly and are associated with cervical lymphadenopathy, it is crucial to consider them in the differential diagnosis when evaluating clival chordoma. These cancers can resemble the lytic destruction of the skull base observed in chordomas. Similarly, when a large mass obscures the pituitary gland, pituitary macroadenomas may present in a way that suggests clival origin. The diagnostic marker for pituitary macroadenomas is significantly elevated serum prolactin levels [6].

## 42.5 Assessment

A thorough medical history and physical examination are necessary for every patient, along with a neuro-ophthalmologic evaluation. Less than one-third have a neuro-ophthalmological exam that is normal. Patients who have upper clival tumors are evaluated thoroughly for hypothalamic or pituitary dysfunction. A thorough evaluation of the cranial nerves and hearing is performed on patients with mid-to lower-clival tumors. This usually entails direct laryngoscopy and audiometry. Clival tumor symptoms differ depending on where the tumor extends; however, they frequently manifest as headaches, diplopia from impairment of the abducens nerve, and other cranial nerve deficits. Ataxia and motor weakness can be caused by an enlargement that compresses the brainstem or cerebellum, while nasal obstruction, epistaxis, and fullness in the throat can be brought on by an extension into the retropharyngeal space or nasal cavity [7].

## 42.6 Surgical Management

Various surgical techniques have been used to access the clivus; the choice of a specific technique is based on the characteristics of the tumor, the anatomy and functional requirements of each patient, as well as the experience and preference of the surgical team. An endoscopic transsphenoidal approach is often the best option for small, centrally located upper clival tumors without lateral expansion, while a combined endoscopic and open intracranial approach may be necessary for larger tumors with lateral and intradural growth to ensure a complete removal. Open surgical techniques are no longer as necessary, thanks to advancements in high-definition imaging and specialized endoscopic surgical instruments.

### 42.6.1 Transsphenoidal

Providing good access to the sphenoid sinus, sella turcica, and the clivus, the transsphenoidal technique is useful for excising smaller tumors in the upper and middle sections of the clivus. Though lateral visibility can be improved by accessing the medial maxillary sinus and excising the pterygoid plate, it is limited in its ability to provide inferior and lateral exposure. An extensive bone removal technique is limited by a narrow and deep surgical field. The endoscopic endonasal transsphenoidal approach is the method of choice these days because it greatly improves visual clarity, makes surgical maneuvering easier, and expands the access [8, 9].

### 42.6.2 Transsphenoethmoidal Approach

The majority of tumors located within the sphenoid sinus and clivus can be adequately accessed with the use of techniques like external ethmoidectomy, which can optionally be combined with medial maxillectomy, to improve the reach of the microscopic transsphenoidal method. Better accessibility is provided by this method, especially when combined with medial maxillectomy for tumors extending inferiorly or narrow ethmoid sinuses. Though there is a chance for increased inferior exposure with a medial maxillectomy, it still requires facial incisions and has exposure limitations, particularly laterally where the reach is only about 2 cm from the midline [10].

### 42.6.3 Transoral

The posterior pharyngeal wall and soft palate can be divided exposing the clivus and upper cervical spine. This approach provides comparatively limited access and is primarily utilized for odontoidectomy procedures. This method works well for treating small lower clival tumors or performing tumor biopsies. Nevertheless, postoperative management of cerebrospinal fluid (CSF) leakage faces difficulties. It is possible to place fat or fascial grafts behind the pharyngeal wall, but doing so is challenging and frequently results in gaps and a higher risk of CSF leakage. Thus, unless other approaches are judged inappropriate, the transoral-transpalatal route is not advised as the main course of action for treating intradural lesions close to the foramen magnum [11, 12].

### 42.6.4 Transmaxillary

For clival tumors that extend into the nasopharynx or craniocervical junction, transmaxillary approaches are useful, particularly in cases where lateral growth is minimal. There are several documented variations on this strategy, including the unilateral maxillotomy and the Le Fort I osteotomy with possible palate division. Difficulties arise from the possibility of ischemic osteonecrosis resulting from multi-segment osteotomies, which can be reduced by protecting the soft palate and preserving soft tissue attachments. The main issue is still how hard it is to control CSF leakage; packing materials are needed for direct dural repair, which is frequently impractical. CSF leakage has been lessened with the use of vascularized mucosal flaps. Currently, this method is mostly used for maxillary sinus resections in cases of cancer [13, 14].

### 42.6.5 Transmandibular

The transmandibular approach provides a wide range of access to the base of the skull, particularly control over the cranial nerves IX to XII and the vasculature. This method makes it easier to expose the anterior cranial fossa to the lower clivus, anterior cervical spine up to C7 as well as the infratemporal fossa to the contralateral medial pterygoid plate. It is mainly recommended for large tumors occupying the lateral and middle compartments of the skull base, as well as lesions at the upper cervical spine and craniocervical junction that require extensive resection of soft tissue and bone. The expected morbidity of this procedure, which includes significant anatomical dissection, includes the need for a temporary tracheostomy, conductive hearing loss, otitis media from the division of the Eustachian tube, and transient swallowing difficulties. The transmandibular approach is indicated only in cases where significant symptom relief or gross total resection is feasible due to its significant associated morbidity, which makes it a decision that should be carefully considered before proceeding. Notable improvements in endoscopic techniques, potentially enhanced by posterolateral approaches, have largely replaced the necessity for such a lengthy surgical procedure, highlighting the significance of considering less invasive options when practical [15].

### 42.6.6 Transbasal

The transbasal approach lessens frontal lobe retraction and allows exposure of posteriorly and laterally related structures, such as the medial walls of the cavernous sinus and the hypoglossal canals. The procedure includes extradural clivus resection, bilateral orbital osteotomy (removal of supraorbital bar), ethmoidectomy, and sphenoidectomy. The hypoglossal canals inferolaterally and the foramen magnum inferiorly define the limits of exposure; the intracavernous carotid arteries form the superolateral limits. When utilizing the extended transbasal approach, the posterior clinoids, dorsum sella, and the area behind and above the pituitary gland are blind spots. Because endoscopic methods provide better visualization and access to the entire clivus without requiring manipulation of the frontal lobes, they have rendered this approach unnecessary [16].

### 42.6.7 Transpetrous

The need for an anterior, posterior, or total petrosectomy will depend on the location of the tumor. An anterior petrosectomy provides access to tumor extensions close to the petroclival synchondrosis, posterior cavernous sinus, and cerebellopontine areas. The petrosal or subtemporal-retrolabyrinthine approach is the best posterior transpetrous technique for large posterolateral intradural tumors, whereas the infratemporal fossa (ITF) approach is the best for both extradural and intradural growths. By removing extradural tumors, this technique may enhance neurological outcomes by precisely identifying and conserving jugular foramen structures. A total petrosectomy provides wide access over several cranial fossae but comes with a number of serious risks, such as damage to the inner ear and facial nerve [17].

### 42.6.8 Endoscopic Endonasal

Endoscopic endonasal procedures, which make use of the nasopharyngeal passage, provide a direct path to the clivus and greatly reduce the amount of neurovascular and soft tissue manipulation required. This is now generally accepted as the preferred technique, especially in the treatment of clival chordomas. For this purpose, the clivus is anatomically divided into three segments: the upper, middle, and lower thirds, respectively, with cranial nerves in the cavernous sinus representing the upper third, paraclival carotid arteries representing the middle third, and Eustachian tubes representing the lower third. With lateral disease spreading past the abducens nerve indicating its limitation, this approach allows access to the ventral aspect of the brainstem and vertebrobasilar system. MRI and CT angiography (CT-A) are required as part of preoperative planning to assess the need for access to both soft and bony structures. This includes evaluating any potential lateral extensions beyond the occipital condyles and petroclival synchondrosis. To prepare for potential carotid injury, CT-A is essential for evaluating the integrity of the bone surrounding the carotid arteries and the extent of the Willis circle. Preoperative placement of a lumbar drain, which stays clamped during surgery but is accessible for CSF management afterward, is necessary for anticipated significant CSF leaks. The patient is placed in a rigid head fixation tilted at a 30° angle. The initial step in sinonasal dissection involves creating a nasoseptal flap, based on the sphenopalatine artery, designed to cover the surgical defect. To optimize its area, this flap is extended along the nasal floor and toward the columella. Bilateral flaps could be prepared in cases of extensive clival defects. Critical anatomical landmarks are exposed by opening the paranasal sinuses, which is achieved through procedures like sphenoidotomies and ethmoidectomies. For comprehensive access, other procedures such as opening the pterygopalatine fossae and performing maxillary antrostomies might be required. In order to enable the transpterygoid approach without compromising nasal flaps, the vidian neurovascular bundle is recognized and controlled. Using a U-shaped mucosal incision, the sphenoid sinus floor, which extends to the clivus and vidian canals, is removed to allow for lower clival access. Longus coli dissection or resection may also be necessary. Based on the tumor's progression and the particular posterior fossa regions that require attention, the surgical approach for clival tumors is modified. The upper clival approach exposes the medial sides of the cavernous carotid arteries and removes the ventral surface and floor of the sella, making access to the cavernous sinuses and interpeduncular cistern easier. Either an extradural approach or a transcavernous technique involving pituitary mobilization is used to remove posterior clinoids. For lateral cavernous sinus tumor extension, endoscopic resection is performed using precise dural incisions. The abducens nerve is vulnerable during these excisions and should be monitored. Tumors that spread into the prepontine cistern and petrous apex are addressed by the midclival approach; however, adequate lateral access requires a transpterygoid approach. For thorough tumor management, this entails sinonasal access, which includes dissection within the pterygopalatine fossa and medial maxillectomy. With reference to V3, the horizontal petrous carotid segment is exposed with precision, along with the paraclival and lateral carotid artery segments. This entails excising the thin bone that covers the superior portion of the Eustachian tube and the carotid artery. Next, the fibrocartilaginous region close to the foramen lacerum is cut. Detaching the tensor veli palatini and medial pterygoid muscles improves the exposure of the Eustachian tube. The levator veli palatini muscle is further detached to provide full visibility of the cartilaginous section of the tube. The Eustachian tube can be partially resected or mobilized for access in order to effectively reach the medial jugular foramen, petrous apex, and lateral clivus, depending on the specific disease being addressed and the surgical goals. In lower clival techniques, the emphasis is on treating bone disease that has spread laterally beyond these structures and managing the occipital condyles. The occipital condyles, which are located about ten and two o'clock in relation to the ventral aspect of the foramen magnum, may require partial resection via an endonasal technique in order to improve access in the case of lateral intradural disease. Limitations occur when the disease progresses past the condyles, in which case the condition must be managed with an extensive lateral craniotomy or with an endoscopic transpterygoid approach with mobilization of the Eustachian tube [18–22].

#### 42.6.8.1 Reconstruction

A layered approach is used to perform dural reconstruction, with a focus on vascularized repair for carotid artery coverage, prevention of CSF fistulas, and promoting healing of the skull base, particularly prior to starting any adjunctive therapies. In cases of extensive defects following total clival resection, extra flaps from the pericranial, temporoparietal, and inferior turbinate fascia are combined with the standard nasal septal flap to ensure sufficient vascularized coverage [23–25].

### 42.6.9 Transcondylar

Because of its direct access and surgical benefits, the transcondylar approach is advantageous for tumors extending laterally from the lower clivus to the atlanto-occipital joint, jugular foramen, or upper cervical spine. This technique provides control over the vertebral artery, a large and easily accessible field, and a sterile surgical environment. In an event that craniocervical fixation is required, it enables prompt neural decompression and direct visualization and access to the craniocervical junction. This method works especially well for large lower clival chordomas because it allows for phased surgeries with posterior and possibly anterior interventions to remove the tumor completely. A supine position with the head turned away from the surgical site and slightly elevated, or directly on the side, is recommended for patient setup. There are different ways to make the incision; one popular method is a retroauricular C-shaped cut; another option is to trace from the upper border of the sternomastoid, across the mastoid, to the occipital crest and external occipital protuberance. The decision is made based on the extent of the tumor, whether or not more surgical access may be required, and whether or not occipitocervical fusion is also being done. After lifting the flap, the jugular vein is visible through the anterior border of the sternomastoid muscle. Next, the muscle is separated from the mastoid tip and retracted posterolaterally by moving superiorly. The accessory nerve is situated close to the jugular vein and is cautiously dissected in the direction of the base of the skull, making sure that the fatty tissue that surrounds it acts as a protective layer and that its distal end, which is near the sternomastoid, is also released for inferior mobilization. For orientation, locate the transverse process of the atlas immediately below and in front of the tip of the mastoid. With consideration for the location of the vertebral artery beneath these muscles, the rectus minor, superior and inferior oblique, and levator scapulae muscles are carefully released from the transverse process of the atlas. The vertebral artery first becomes visible between the transverse processes of C1 and C2, where the anterior branch of the C2 nerve root crosses it. Above C1, the dissection proceeds in a subperiosteal direction, moving posteriorly along its arch. In order to provide unobstructed access to the lateral aspect of the foramen magnum, the surrounding structures, such as the transverse process and anterior arch of C1, are meticulously freed, translocated, and prepared. The sigmoid sinus and jugular bulb are exposed during a complete mastoidectomy, with the jugular foramen establishing the upper limit of exposure. If tumor growth gets too big, a transpetrous procedure might be required. For improved access, a retromastoid craniotomy may be included. The extent of condylar resection depends on how far the tumor can spread, with the hypoglossal nerve being especially protected. When more than half of the condyle is excised, it is frequently necessary to perform occipitocervical stabilization, either simultaneously or as a follow-up procedure. Rigid collars are used to provide temporary stability. With the preservation of the vertebral artery and lower cranial nerves (CNs) as top priorities, the tumor is carefully removed using ultrasonic aspiration or suction in conjunction with bipolar cautery. CN monitoring further improves surgical safety. Dissection focuses moving from unaffected to affected areas, which is particularly important in fields that have been surgically altered or scarred in the past. In order to reduce the risk of CSF leakage during dural reconstruction, standard techniques such as primary closure and patch duraplasty strive for a watertight seal. The back of the operating bed is raised, and the patient is positioned laterally with the tumor side facing upward. The patient's head is first placed in a neutral position to mark the incision site, and then it is flexed laterally downward without rotating. In order to facilitate access for possible craniocervical fixation, a hockey stick-shaped incision is made from above the ear to the posterior midline of the neck. In order to expose the mastoid and digastric grooves, soft tissue dissection entails lifting the suboccipital muscles from the occipital bone in one piece and carefully dissecting beneath the groove so as to preserve the vertebral artery. For positioning, the patient is arranged on their side, with the side to be operated on facing upward, and the head positioned slightly raised and angled away without rotation. A potential craniocervical fixation involves an incision shaped like a hockey stick that extends from above the ear to the posterior midpoint of the neck. To reveal the mastoid and digastric groove, the suboccipital muscles are gently raised from the occipital bone in one piece and extended laterally. To prevent damage to the vertebral artery and to avoid using electrocautery, dissection below the digastric groove is done carefully. The vertebral artery third segment at C1's sulcus arteriosus is visible when the musculature covering the cervical arch and the spinal components of C2 are methodically separated. The C2 nerve root crosses the upper segment of the vertebral artery behind it, laterally between C1 and C2.

Near the jugular bulb is where the sigmoid sinus is visible after a suboccipital craniotomy. To gain access to the vertebral artery, the bone is carefully removed in the direction of the jugular fossa and jugular tubercle. The vertebral artery is then carefully released and repositioned to provide detailed access to the occipital condyle. In order to achieve complete exposure and subsequent tumor resection, this procedure might necessitate severing the C2 nerve root, underscoring the meticulous and exacting approach required for such intricate surgical procedures. Running from a posterior-medial to an anterior-lateral orientation and angled at about a 45° angle with respect to the sagittal plane, the hypoglossal canal crosses the intersection of the posterior and middle thirds of the occipital condyle.

The extradurally initiated tumor resection process begins with careful protection of vital structures such as the anterior jugular vein system, hypoglossal nerve, vertebral artery, and lower cranial nerves. Rectus capitus lateralis muscle helps to divide the vertebral artery from the jugular vein and jugular fossa anteriorly. The dura is sliced posterior to the vertebral artery and extended superiorly and inferiorly as necessary after the extradural tumor is removed. The upper dentate ligaments are severed to improve dissection and maneuverability. The C1 and C2 nerve roots may also be sectioned if needed. Anterior or posterior transposition is possible upon release of the spinal accessory nerve's rootlets. Dissection is guided to the vertebral artery's junction with the basilar artery by meticulous adherence to its course, which is followed methodically as one moves from normal to anomalous anatomy. Notably, the rootlets of the hypoglossal nerve may be divided by the vertebral artery, but those of the cranial nerves IX, X, and XI always lie posterior to the vertebral artery. Access anterior to the vertebral artery can be made easier if necessary by extending the dural incisions surrounding its dural entry.

In most cases, it is possible to ensure a watertight primary closure of the dura but, if necessary, a dural patch should be immediately considered. If dura resection anterior to the vertebral artery has occurred or if circumvertebral dural incisions have been made, primary dural closure is unlikely and a multilayered reconstruction strategy is required. Instead, we choose to apply an easily accessible, pliable intra- and extradurally available dural substitute. Subcutaneous fat from sources that are commercially available and tissue adhesives are added to this. Then, the suboccipital and cervical musculature are precisely approximated, and the occipital bone flap is replaced and plated in place. When it is anticipated that the patient may experience craniocervical instability, the patient is carefully repositioned into a prone position, and fluoroscopy is used to verify alignment. After that, a cervical occipital fusion is performed. An alternative interim management strategy is to place the patient in a stiff collar and postpone the occipital cervical fusion until a later stage, depending on the probability and degree of craniospinal instability [26–30].

### 42.6.10 Postoperative Care

The timely detection and aggressive treatment of lower cranial neuropathy is a critical component of postoperative care for patients having clival resection. Immediately following surgery, speech and language teams thoroughly evaluate every patient, including a thorough assessment of swallowing. Further diagnostic techniques like direct laryngoscopy or modified barium swallow might be necessary. Oral intake is only allowed when it is considered safe. CSF leakage is a possible consequence of endoscopic clival resection and can be caused by technical difficulties with reconstruction, graft displacement, or underlying hydrocephalus, including acute cases linked to posterior fossa syndrome. Of all the procedures involving the skull base, endoscopic reconstruction of transclival defects presents special difficulties because of anatomical factors like the size of the defect, the length of exposed internal carotid arteries on both sides, and the possibility of spaces inside the clival recess. Management decisions are also influenced by patient-specific factors, such as an elevated body mass index. Separating "low-flow" from "high-flow" leaks is essential for managing CSF leaks. This must be done based on imaging results and clinical assessment, including checking for pneumocephalus in CT scans. Low-flow leaks frequently respond well to CSF diversion via lumbar drainage; recurrent leaks, assuming an underlying pressure-related etiology, warrant consideration for ventriculoperitoneal shunt placement. Conversely, high-flow leaks, typically associated with significant pneumocephalus, require immediate surgical exploration of the reconstruction to determine the cause of failure. Comprehensive reconstruction is required for subsequent revision, and depending on how well the initial reconstruction worked, secondary vascularized flaps like pericranial and temporoparietal fascial flaps may be used. Extended CSF diversion strategies are also used. Reevaluating the reconstruction during surgery and placing a ventriculoperitoneal shunt may be required if leaks continue after revision. Prisms and extraocular muscle surgery performed under ophthalmological supervision are the next line of treatment for ocular movement abnormalities after patching. One of the first things done after surgery is a noncontrast CT scan of the brain to look for any subclinical problems. A baseline postoperative magnetic resonance image is obtained 48 hours after surgery. Additionally, if clinically indicated, flexion-extension radiographs are obtained along with dynamic imaging of the craniocervical junction. Adequate monitoring, encompassing clinical assessment and imaging, is essential, with a frequency determined by the tumor pathology. For chordoma or chondrosarcoma patients without visualized tumor on baseline postoperative imaging, additional imaging is scheduled at three-month intervals for the first year, followed by six-month intervals for the next two years, and yearly thereafter. Referral to a specialized radiation treatment facility is advised upon detection of residual disease; ideally, this facility will have proton beam capability and experienced radiation oncologists who are knowledgeable about treating clival disease. In addition, a referral to medical oncology might be necessary. The treatment of local disease that is residual or recurrent is complex and outside the purview of this chapter. The development of appropriate management strategies requires a thorough analysis of a number of variables, such as the patient's clinical status, the size and location of recurrences, the initial tumor histology, the extent of prior resection, and the features of previous radiation.

## 42.7 Case Study

A 50-year-old woman presented with a history of frontal headaches and fits. Imaging revealed an anterior fossa tumor. The appearances were initially suggestive of an anterior cranial fossa meningioma but the destruction of the anterior skull base and extension into the nasal cavity raised suspicion of other lesions.

An examination of the nasal cavity under anesthesia and a diagnostic nasal endoscopy and biopsy revealed a diagnosis of a non-Hodgkin's lymphoma. The patient was successfully treated with chemotherapy with complete remission. There has been no evidence of a post-treatment CSF leak, and the patient remains free of disease three years after completion of her treatment (Figs. 42.1 and 42.2).

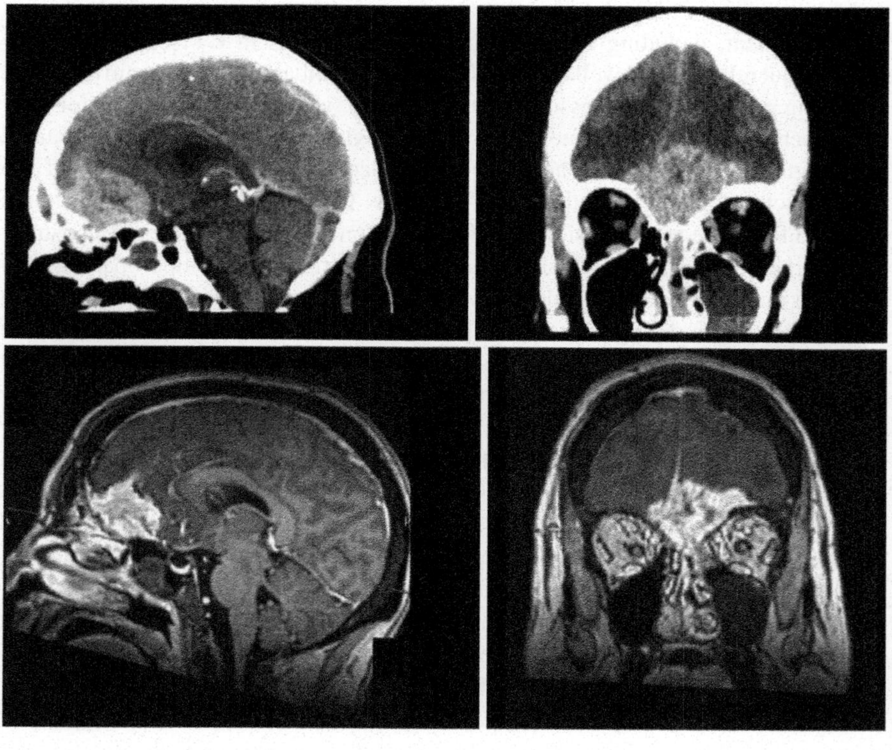

**Fig. 42.1** Pretreatment CT and MRI

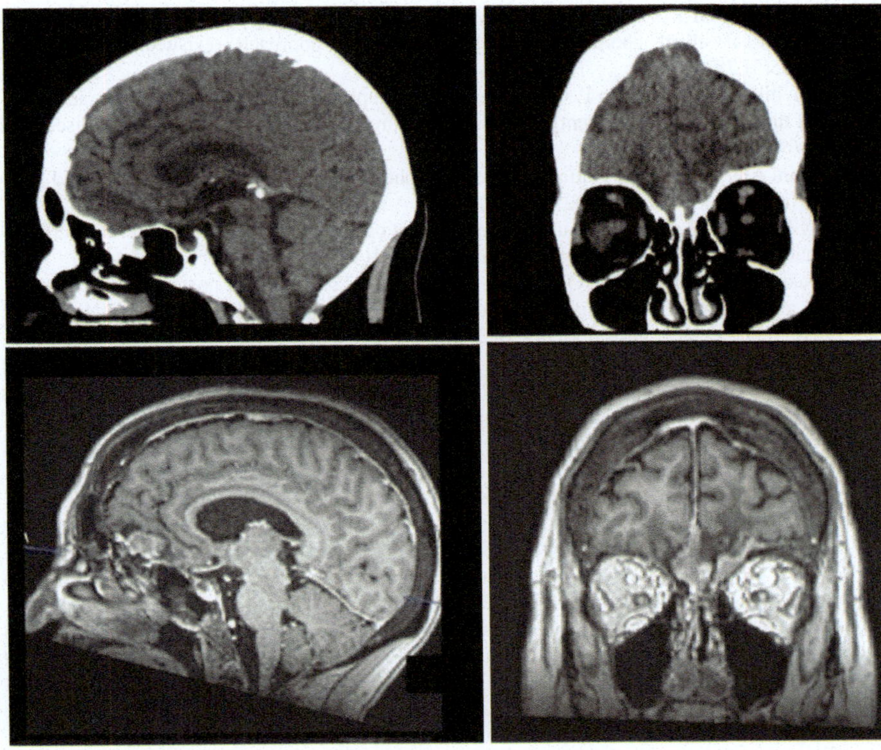

**Fig. 42.2** Post-treatment CT and MRI scans

## References


1. Colli BO, Al-Mefty O. Chordomas of the skull base: follow-up review and prognostic factors. Neurosurg Focus. 2001;10(3):E1. https://doi.org/10.3171/foc.2001.10.3.2.
2. Diaz RJ, Guduk M, Romagnuolo R, Smith CA, Northcott P, Shih D, Berisha F, Flanagan A, Munoz DG, Cusimano MD, Pamir MN, Rutka JT. High-resolution whole-genome analysis of skull base chordomas implicates FHIT loss in chordoma pathogenesis. Neoplasia. 2012;14(9):788–98.
3. Fernandez-Miranda JC, Gardner PA, Snyderman CH, Devaney KO, Mendenhall WM, Suarez C, Rinaldo A, Ferlito A. Clival chordomas: a pathological, surgical, and radiotherapeutic review. Head Neck. 2014;36(6):892–906. https://doi.org/10.1002/hed.23415.
4. Hoch BL, Nielsen GP, Liebsch NJ, Rosenberg AE. Base of skull chordomas in children and adolescents: a clinicopathologic study of 73 cases. Am J Surg Pathol. 2006;30(7):811–8. https://doi.org/10.1097/01.pas.0000209828.39477.ab.
5. Lanzino G, Dumont AS, Lopes MB, Laws ER Jr. Skull base chordomas: overview of disease, management options, and outcome. Neurosurg Focus. 2001;10(3):E12.
6. Curtin HD, Rabinov JD, Som PM. Central skull base. In: Head and neck imaging. Mosby, Saint Louis; 2003.
7. Laws E. Clivus chordomas. In: Sekhar LN, Janecka IP, editors. Surgery of cranial base tumors. New York: Raven Press; 1993. p. 679–85.

8. Maira G, Pallini R, Anile C, Fernandez E, Salvinelli F, La Rocca LM, Rossi GF. Surgical treatment of clival chordomas: the transsphenoidal approach revisited. J Neurosurg. 1996;85(5):784–92.
9. de Divitiis E, Cappabianca P, Cavallo LM. Endoscopic transsphenoidal approach: adaptability of the procedure to different sellar lesions. Neurosurgery. 2002;51(3):699–705; discussion 705–697.
10. Lalwani AK, Kaplan MJ, Gutin PH. The transsphenoethmoid approach to the sphenoid sinus and clivus. Neurosurgery. 1992;31(6):1008–14.
11. Yang SY, Gao YZ. Clinical results of the transoral operation for lesions of the craniovertebral junction and its abnormalities. Surg Neurol. 1999;51(1):16–20.
12. Hayakawa T, Kamikawa K, Ohnishi T, Yoshimine T. Prevention of postoperative complications after a transoral transclival approach to basilar aneurysms. Technical note. J Neurosurg. 1981;54(5):699–703. https://doi.org/10.3171/jns.1981.54.5.0699.
13. Kassam AB, Gardner P, Snyderman C, Mintz A, Carrau R. Expanded endonasal approach: fully endoscopic, completely transnasal approach to the middle third of the clivus, petrous bone, middle cranial fossa, and infratemporal fossa. Neurosurg Focus. 2005;19(1):E6.
14. Cavallo LM, Messina A, Gardner P, Esposito F, Kassam AB, Cappabianca P, de Divitiis E, Tschabitscher M. Extended endoscopic endonasal approach to the pterygopalatine fossa: anatomical study and clinical considerations. Neurosurg Focus. 2005;19(1):E5.
15. James D, Crockard HA. Surgical access to the base of skull and upper cervical spine by extended maxillotomy. Neurosurgery. 1991;29(3):411–6.
16. Sekhar LN, Nanda A, Sen CN, Snyderman CN, Janecka IP. The extended frontal approach to tumors of the anterior, middle, and posterior skull base. J Neurosurg. 1992;76(2):198–206.
17. Harsh GR, Sekhar LN. The subtemporal, transcavernous, anterior transpetrosal approach to the upper brain stem and clivus. J Neurosurg. 1992;77(5):709–17. https://doi.org/10.3171/jns.1992.77.5.0709.
18. Chibbaro S, Cornelius JF, Froelich S, Tigan L, Kehrli P, Debry C, Romano A, Herman P, George B, Bresson D. Endoscopic endonasal approach in the management of skull base chordomas—clinical experience on a large series, technique, outcome, and pitfalls. Neurosurg Rev. 2014;37(2):217–224; discussion 224–215. https://doi.org/10.1007/s10143-013-0503-9.
19. Fatemi N, Dusick JR, Gorgulho AA, Mattozo CA, Moftakhar P, De Salles AA, Kelly DF. Endonasal microscopic removal of clival chordomas. Surg Neurol. 2008;69(4):331–8. https://doi.org/10.1016/j.surneu.2007.08.035.
20. Fraser JF, Nyquist GG, Moore N, Anand VK, Schwartz TH. Endoscopic endonasal transclival resection of chordomas: operative technique, clinical outcome, and review of the literature. J Neurosurg. 2010;112(5):1061–9. https://doi.org/10.3171/2009.7.JNS081504.
21. Koutourousiou M, Gardner PA, Tormenti MJ, Henry SL, Stefko ST, Kassam AB, Fernandez-Miranda JC, Snyderman CH. Endoscopic endonasal approach for resection of cranial base chordomas: outcomes and learning curve. Neurosurgery. 2012;71(3):614–24; discussion 624–615. https://doi.org/10.1227/NEU.0b013e31825ea3e0.
22. Stippler M, Gardner PA, Snyderman CH, Carrau RL, Prevedello DM, Kassam AB. Endoscopic endonasal approach for clival chordomas. Neurosurgery. 2009;64(2):268–277; discussion 277–268. https://doi.org/10.1227/01.NEU.0000338071.01241.E2.00006123-200902000-00008[pii]
23. Cavallo LM, Messina A, Esposito F, de Divitiis O, Dal Fabbro M, de Divitiis E, Cappabianca P. Skull base reconstruction in the extended endoscopic transsphenoidal approach for suprasellar lesions. J Neurosurg. 2007;107(4):713–20.
24. Esposito F, Dusick JR, Fatemi N, Kelly DF. Graded repair of cranial base defects and cerebrospinal fluid leaks in transsphenoidal surgery. Neurosurgery. 2007;60(4 Suppl 2):295–303; discussion 303–304.
25. Leng LZ, Brown S, Anand VK, Schwartz TH. "Gasket-seal" watertight closure in minimal-access endoscopic cranial base surgery. Neurosurgery. 2008;62(5 Suppl 2)

26. Liu JK, Couldwell WT. Far-lateral transcondylar approach: surgical technique and its application in neurenteric cysts of the cervicomedullary junction. Report of two cases. Neurosurg Focus. 2005;19(2):E9.
27. Morera VA, Fernandez-Miranda JC, Prevedello DM, Madhok R, Barges-Coll J, Gardner P, Carrau R, Snyderman CH, Rhoton AL Jr, Kassam AB. "Far-medial" expanded endonasal approach to the inferior third of the clivus: the transcondylar and transjugular tubercle approaches. Neurosurgery. 2010;66(6):211–9; discussion 219–220. https://doi.org/10.1227/01.NEU.0000369926.01891.5D.
28. Wen HT, Rhoton AL Jr, Katsuta T, de Oliveira E. Microsurgical anatomy of the transcondylar, supracondylar, and paracondylar extensions of the far-lateral approach. J Neurosurg. 1997;87(4):555–85.
29. Bertalanffy H, Seeger W. The dorsolateral, suboccipital, transcondylar approach to the lower clivus and anterior portion of the craniocervical junction. Neurosurgery. 1991;29(6):815–21.
30. Arnold H, Sepehrnia A. Extreme lateral transcondylar approach. J Neurosurg. 1995;82(2):313.

# 43 Endoscopic Surgery for Malignant Sinonasal Tumors

Mario Turri-Zanoni, Giacomo Gravante, and Paolo Castelnuovo

**Key Points**

- Endoscopic surgery offers advantages such as reduced morbidity, avoidance of brain retraction, minimal scarring, and short hospitalization, leading to safe and effective tumor removal.
- Indications and contraindications are detailed, considering tumor characteristics and locations, with the possibility of shifting to a combined cranio-endoscopic resection in borderline cases.
- The importance of considering tumor characteristics and staging is mandatory when choosing appropriate treatment.

## 43.1 Background

Malignant tumors affecting the sinonasal tract are uncommon and display various histological compositions, impacting their biological behavior and prognosis alongside factors like size and location [1]. Treatment approaches, ranging from surgery to radiation and chemotherapy, either singularly or in combination, are tailored based on these considerations. While in the past, surgical procedures predominantly relied on open approaches like craniofacial resection (CFR) [2], recent decades have witnessed advancements in endoscopic techniques, offering safer and equally effective tumor removal strategies [3]. Endoscopic procedures boast advantages such as

M. Turri-Zanoni (✉) · G. Gravante · P. Castelnuovo
Department of Otorhinolaryngology and Skull Base Surgery, University of Insubria, Varese, Italy


S. Elwany (ed.), *Current Rhinology*,
https://doi.org/10.1007/978-3-031-70077-4_43

minimized morbidity, avoidance of brain retraction, reduced facial scarring, and shorter hospitalization time. The precision of endoscopic visualization enables surgeons to precisely discern tumor margins and affected anatomical structures, contributing to better outcomes in treatment.

## 43.2 Indications and Contraindications

Over time, endoscopic approaches have gained momentum, expanding the limits and indications, largely propelled by advancements in instrumentation and technology [1, 4]. Presently, the indications and contraindications for an endoscopic approach are updated and documented in Table 43.1 and displayed in Fig. 43.1, taking into account previous indications reported by Castelnuovo et al. in 2016, and more recent indications, as given by Lopéz et al. in 2022. However, it is important

**Table 43.1** Indications and contraindications of transnasal endoscopic surgery for malignancies of the sinus and skull base

| Tumor location | Endoscopic approach | Open approach | Unresectable |
|---|---|---|---|
| Ethmoid (nasal cavity and box) | Ethmoid cancer involving lamina papyracea, cribriform plate, or roof of the ethmoid | Infiltration in nasal bones, palate, skin, and subcutaneous tissue | Brain infiltration with vascular involvement |
| | Limited dural infiltration, olfactory bulb involvement, focal midline brain invasion | Dural infiltration extended laterally over the orbital roofs, brain infiltration[a] | |
| Maxillary sinus | Medial, posterior, and/or superior maxillary walls | Lateral, anterior, and/or inferior wall involvement. Skin or subcutaneous tissue involvement | |
| Frontal sinus | Lesion abutting into the frontal sinus or involving the medial portion or originating from the lower third | Erosion of the anterior or posterior wall, massive involvement of the frontal sinus, skin, or subcutaneous tissue involvement. Limited dural infiltration, brain infiltration[a] | Brain infiltration with vascular involvement |
| Sphenoid sinus | Anterior wall involvement. Limited lateral/posterior wall involvement | Planum sphenoidale involvement[a] | Relevant posterior/lateral wall involvement, cavernous sinus involvement, optical chiasm involvement, internal carotid artery involvement |

[a] Elegible for cranio-endoscopic approach

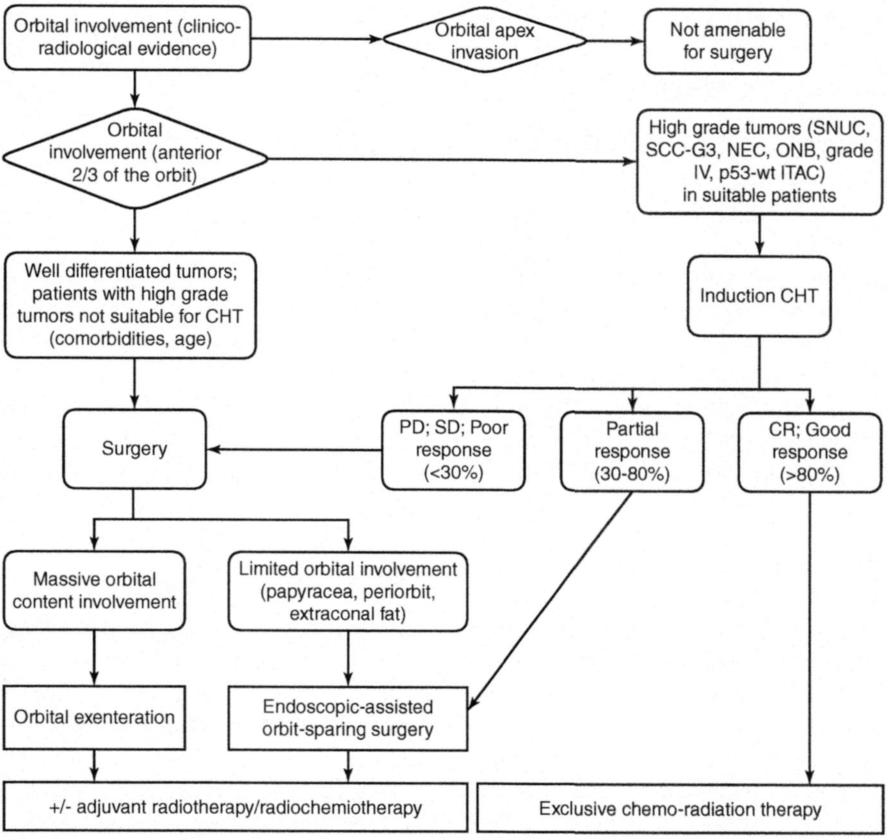


**Fig. 43.1** Indications and limits in endoscopic and open approaches. (**A**) Coronal CT scan showing sites amenable to endoscopic surgery (blue area), open surgery (purple area), and combined approaches (yellow area). (**B**) Sagittal CT scan showing sites amenable to endoscopic surgery (blue area), open surgery (purple area), combined approaches (yellow area), and unresectable (red area). (**C**) Axial CT scan showing sites amenable of endoscopic surgery (blue area), open surgery (purple area), cranio-endoscopic approach (yellow area), and unresectable regions (red area). Blue dotted line shows the limits of endoscopic nasopharyngectomy

to note that a purely endoscopic approach may not always be the optimal technique for achieving complete resection of a given tumor. In borderline cases, patients should be informed about the potential option of shifting to a combined cranio-endoscopic resection, depending on the disease's extent as assessed intraoperatively by the surgeon. Furthermore, the resection methods may differ based on the involved subsite within the sinonasal tract: ethmoid complex, frontal sinus, sphenoid sinus, or maxillary sinus. Each subsite presents unique challenges, necessitating standardized and specific endoscopic surgical techniques that are intricately tied to the anatomical complexity of the involved sinus and its specific relationship with adjacent structures. In the next sections, attention will be focused on tailored endoscopic surgical approaches, based on involved subsite.

## 43.3 Endoscopic Surgical Techniques

### 43.3.1 Instrumentation

- HD camera and monitors with a recording system.
- 0 and 45° endoscopes.
- Long-handle endoscopic bipolar forceps; curved and double-curved cutting instruments.
- Diode laser supports.
- Microdebrider and powered instruments, long stem, and curved drills.
- Long dissection instruments and dural reconstruction instruments.
- Intranasal vascular Doppler.
- Cavitron® ultrasonic surgical aspirator can be helpful in selected cases where the tumor is closely adjacent to vital structures.
- Magnetic navigation system [5].

### 43.3.2 Surgical Setup

The patient is positioned in a supine position with a 10–20° reverse-Trendelenburg tilt, and the head slightly extended. The surgeon takes position on the patient's right side, the assistant on the left, and the nurse on the right of the operating surgeon. The anesthesiologist is stationed on the patient's left, overseeing the anesthesia equipment positioned alongside the assistant at the base of the surgical bed. Hypotensive general anesthesia is administered as per protocol [6]. A preoperative antibiotic regimen, typically third-generation cephalosporin, is administered for prophylaxis. Prior to surgery, the nasal cavities are packed with cottonoids soaked in a solution comprising 2% oxymetazoline, 1% oxybuprocaine, and adrenaline (1:100,000) to minimize bleeding and optimize transnasal visualization [5].

### 43.3.3 Ethmoid Complex Involvement

Depending on the extent of the disease, the transnasal endoscopic resection may involve unilateral or bilateral approaches [7, 8]. In a unilateral resection, the procedure extends anteroposteriorly from the posterior wall of the frontal sinus to the planum sphenoidale and laterolaterally from the nasal septum to the lamina papyracea. In a bilateral resection, the procedure extends from one lamina papyracea to its opposite counterpart. The sequential steps of the endoscopic endonasal resection (EER) technique encompass six primary surgical phases (Fig. 43.2) [5].

1. Identification of Tumor Origin

   Gradual debulking of the lesion aids in pinpointing the precise origin of the tumor, ensuring meticulous respect for surrounding anatomical landmarks criti-

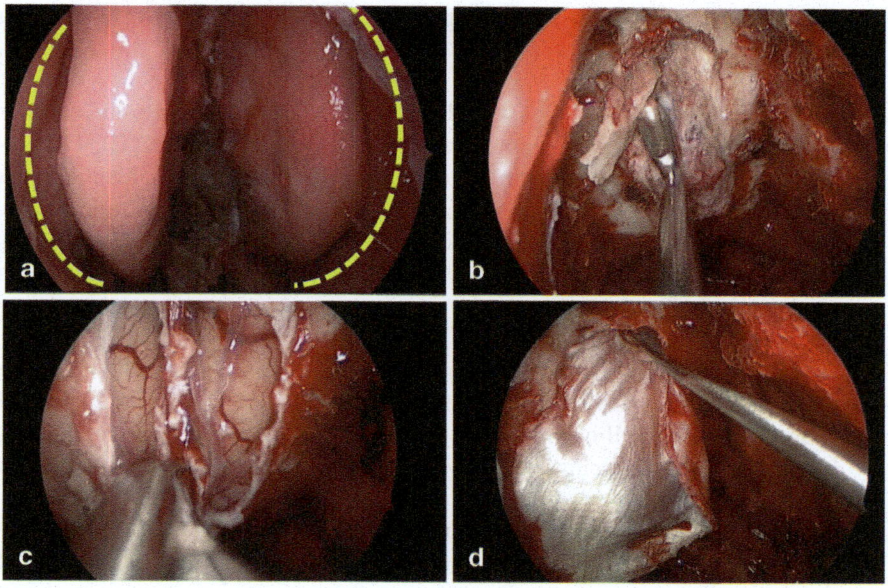


**Fig. 43.2** Surgical steps of endoscopic endonasal resection. (**A**) Subperiosteal dissection (dotted lines) to remove the ethmoidal box. (**B**) After removal of the bony ethmoidal roof and crista galli, the dura mater is exposed. (**C**) Transnasal resection of dura mater. (**D**) Endonasal skull base reconstruction using layers of autologous materials (fascia lata)

cal for subsequent surgical phases. En bloc resection is feasible solely for smaller tumors [3, 5, 6].

2. Exposure of the Surgical Field

    This phase involves removing two-thirds of the nasal septum, creating ample space for enhanced maneuverability of endoscopic instruments using the "2-nostrils 4-hands" technique. Extending removal is essential to delineate the anterosuperior margin through frontal sinusotomy (Draf IIb for unilateral EER or Draf III for bilateral EER) and the posteroinferior margin through extensive sphenoidotomy involving intersphenoidal septum and sphenoidal rostrum [3, 5, 6].

3. Centripetal Removal

    Once the posteroinferior and anterosuperior margins are visible, unilateral or bilateral subperiosteal dissection of the nasal-ethmoidal-sphenoidal complex exposes the lateral margins [6]. When the tumor is in close proximity to the lamina papyracea or involves it, this structure is integrated into the dissection. In cases where disease extension demands, an endoscopic medial maxillectomy can be executed for effective control of the entire maxillary sinus (see Sect. 43.3.4). Superiorly, the dissection proceeds anteroposteriorly by excising olfactory fibers and the basal lamella of the ethmoidal turbinate(s) to mobilize the specimen. The entire nasal–ethmoidal–sphenoidal complex is then centralized within the nasal fossa (centripetal technique) for transoral or nasal vestibule removal. Frozen sections verify surgical margins, and if necessary, resection extends until clear margins are achieved [3, 5, 6].

4. Skull Base Removal

   Based on disease extension, EER might extend to encompass the anterior skull base (endoscopic resection with transnasal craniectomy; ERTC). The ethmoid roof is exposed using a drill equipped with a diamond burr. Identification and careful cauterization of the anterior and posterior ethmoidal arteries occur, followed by their division. Delicate detachment and removal of the crista galli is conducted with blunt instruments, ensuring preservation of the dural layer's integrity [3, 5, 6].

5. Intracranial Step

   For effective subsequent skull base reconstruction, proper dissection of the epidural space over the lateral orbital roofs, posterior planum sphenoidale, and anterior posterior wall of the frontal sinus is crucial before dura resection. The dura is incised and circumferentially cut away from the suspected tumor area using angled scissors or a specialized scalpel. The falx cerebri is managed by clipping or cauterization in its anterior portion before resection to prevent sagittal sinus bleeding. The posterior portion, specifically at the sphenoethmoidal planum level, is then resected. Dissection of the arachnoid plane from the brain parenchyma over the intracranial tumor region occurs. Subsequently, the specimen, including residual tumor, anterior skull base, and overlying dura, with one or both olfactory bulbs, is transnasally removed. Dural margins undergo frozen section analysis. For small tumors, dural resection is viable [3, 5, 6].

6. Skull Base Reconstruction

   Following the tumor removal, the skull base defect is reconstructed using the endoscopic endonasal multilayer technique, preferably employing autologous materials. From our experience, we have found that fascia lata and/or the iliotibial tract possess optimal characteristics in terms of thickness, pliability, and strength for this purpose. For the initial layer of duraplasty within the dura, the graft should be approximately 30% larger than the dural defect. In bilateral resection cases, it split along the midline to accommodate the falx cerebri. The second layer, both within and outside the skull, is carefully sized and placed between the previously loosened dura and the remaining skull base bone. Fatty tissue fragments are inserted to fill the space between the second and third layers and smooth the exposed skull base. The third outer layer must cover the entire exposed anterior skull base without overlapping the frontal sinusotomies. Borders of the second and third layers are sealed with small amounts of fibrin glue. We avoid using bone or cartilage grafts to prevent complications like radionecrosis, infections, or postoperative extrusion following radiotherapy. In cases where the tumor does not involve the nasal septum and lacks multiple localized areas, the third layer of reconstruction can be harvested using mucoperiosteal/mucoperichondrial pedicled flaps. These flaps, such as the Hadad-Bassagasteguy flap [9] or the septal flip flap [10, 11] vascularized by ethmoidal arteries, aid in rapid healing of the surgical site and reduce postoperative nasal crusting, particularly beneficial for patients requiring postoperative radiation therapy. In specific instances, the frontal sinusotomies can be stented with rolled polymeric silicone sheaths to facilitate subsequent frontal sinus cleaning without risks to the duraplasty. The surgical cavity is typically packed for approximately 48 h postprocedure [3, 5, 6].

### 43.3.4 Maxillary Sinus Involvement

An endoscopic approach for maxillary sinus tumors can be considered in cases where the tumor is limited to the early stages and localized to medial, posterior, and/or superior maxillary walls. Moreover, such an approach is advisable when there is no extensive invasion into surrounding critical structures, such as the orbit, lacrimal sac, or adjacent soft tissues. For tumors involving the medial maxillary wall, a transnasal endoscopic partial maxillectomy (TEPM) type 3 or 4 is recommended, as described by Turri et al. [12]:

- *TEPM 3A:*
- This procedure involves the removal of the medial maxillary wall along with the lower turbinate, establishing a connection between the nasal floor and the floor of the maxillary sinus. The resection includes the lacrimal bone, and the nasolacrimal duct is transected a few millimeters distal to the lacrimal sac. This approach enhances surgical maneuverability within the maxillary sinus, providing increased accessibility for inspection and optimal management of retrolacrimal recess, an important area for achieving a thorough resection.
- *TEPM 3B:*
- The removal of the pyriform aperture involves the partial or complete drilling of the ascending branch of the maxillary bone through a transnasal approach. This procedure enhances control over the anterior half of the maxillary sinus, particularly addressing the alveolar recess and the zygomatic recess. Additionally, it serves to extend the surgical pivot point during expanded transnasal transmaxillary transpterygoid approaches targeting areas like the infratemporal fossa, nasopharynx, and upper parapharyngeal space.
- *TEPM 4:*
- The resection is expanded toward the anterior wall of the maxillary sinus, allowing for complete removal up to the zygomatic bone, as necessary. The dissection's upper boundary is set by a horizontal plane that passes through the infraorbital foramen to safeguard the infraorbital nerve and avoid the orbit contents. Yet, in specific situations, this method might be extended upward by removing the superior wall of the maxillary sinus (the orbital floor) while preserving the periorbital layer. This technique allows for addressing pathologies related to the anterior wall of the maxillary sinus, provided they do not involve the entire wall thickness and don't involve the soft tissues.

Tumors involving the upper wall can be managed endoscopically by removing it provided that the orbital contents are not affected by the disease (see Sect. 43.4.3).

Similarly, the posterior wall can be endoscopically removed, allowing for the management of malignancies extending into the pterygopalatine or infratemporal fossa (see Sect. 43.4.1).

### 43.3.5 Frontal Sinus Involvement

Frontal sinus malignancies could undergo exclusive endoscopic surgery in selected cases: lesion abutting into the frontal sinus or involving the medial portion or originating from the lower third. The optimal surgical procedure in such cases is Draf type III, also known as the endoscopic modified Lothrop procedure (EMLP), and consists of the bilateral removal of the frontal sinus floor anteriorly to the roots of the middle turbinates between the two medial walls of the orbit. This procedure includes superior nasal septectomy and intersinus septectomy [13, 14]. To widen access to the lateral aspect of the frontal sinus, which is often challenging in endoscopic nasal approaches, an orbital transposition is effective [15]. Orbital transposition entails removing the bony supero-medial angle of the orbit to temporarily shift the orbital contents laterally, facilitating complete access to the supraorbital recess. In specific instances, achieving access to the far lateral section of the frontal sinus can involve partial resection of the opposite pyriform aperture to further shift the pivot point for the curved instruments [16]. Whenever frontal sinus is completely obliterated by the mass and/or anterior or posterior walls are involved by disease, a combined endoscopic-external approach is advisable. External options encompass frontal osteoplastic flap (OPF), with or without cranialization of the sinus, or even more aggressive procedures, such as Riedel's operation, that consists of removing the anterior wall and floor of the frontal sinus, and its modification according to Mosher's, with removal of the frontal sinus anterior and posterior walls [17].

### 43.3.6 Sphenoid Sinus Involvement

Sphenoid sinus is a critical region within the sinonasal tract, due to its close relation with vital structures: internal carotid artery (ICA), pituitary gland, cavernous sinus, optic chiasm, maxillary division of trigeminal nerve, and vidian nerve. Thus, tumors involving sphenoid sinus have very selected indications for endoscopic surgery, that is, anterior wall involvement and limited lateral/posterior wall involvement without outreaching of the aforementioned critical structures [18, 19]. Tumors of the sphenoid sinus can directly originate within it or arise from the ethmoid or septum and extend into it. In both scenarios, the ethmoid and septum are often involved. Therefore, surgical steps should typically include posterior septectomy, centripetal removal of one or both ethmoid boxes, and resection of the rostrum and anterior wall of the sphenoid sinus. The boundaries of anterior sphenoidectomy are defined as follows: superiorly by the planum sphenoidale, inferiorly by the basisphenoid up to the junction between superior and middle clivus, and laterally by a plane passing through the medial edge of the orbital apex. Whenever the planum sphenoidale is affected, a combined cranio-endoscopic approach is preferred [18, 19].

## 43.4 Surrounding Areas Management

### 43.4.1 Pterygopalatine and Infratemporal Fossa

Pterygopalatine (PPF) and infratemporal fossa (ITF) can be involved by primary tumors originating within them or by direct spread of tumors from neighboring regions, such as the sinonasal tract. Additionally, they can serve as sites for metastasis from tumors originating in various organs. Pterygomaxillary fissure and the inferior projection of the infraorbital canal represent the boundary between PPF, which is located medially to it, and ITF, which is located lateral to it [20]. Endoscopic approach is advisable for PPF and ITF tumors, but an exclusive endoscopic procedure is contraindicated in cases of extensive involvement of the ITF, where a combined approach is preferable. The absolute contraindication for surgery arises when the ICA in the parapharyngeal space is involved [1, 4]. In order to endoscopically access such spaces, a TEPM type 3 or 4 is recommended, and the choice depends on the lateral extent of the tumor in the ITF to gain more fulcrum and maneuverability. The postero-lateral wall of the maxillary sinus is the anterior limit of PPF and ITF. After the removal of the bony wall, the PPF and ITF periosteum is exposed. Through this frontal approach and subsequent removal of fatty tissue, the foremost (frontal) structures consist of the maxillary artery and its branches, traversing the surgical area in an anterior, superior, and medial direction, while the nervous components are situated deeper within the plane. The malignant tumor involving such areas is excised from the outer edges and progressing toward the core to ensure clear surgical margins, which are confirmed through frozen sections. This process may involve sacrificing neuro-muscular structures to achieve negative surgical margins. The maxillary artery is promptly ligated or clipped upon identification during tumor removal to prevent bleeding either during or after the operation. Upon completion of the procedure, the surgical site with a graft or a mucoperiosteal flap [20–22].

### 43.4.2 Lacrimal Duct System

The lacrimal pathway constitutes a system closely associated with the sinonasal region, and its involvement can occur when dealing with malignant tumors. The indication for an exclusive endoscopic resection for sinonasal tumors invading the lacrimal pathways is determined by two potential scenarios: invasion of the nasolacrimal duct or invasion of the medial wall of the lacrimal sac. All other cases require a combined endoscopic and open approach [1]. In case of inferior half of nasolacrimal duct invasion without the involvement of the lacrimal sac, the endoscopic procedure includes a medial maxillectomy with the transection of the nasolacrimal duct at the level of the lower orbital wall, corresponding to the junction of the lacrimal sac with nasolacrimal duct. Whenever the upper third of nasolacrimal duct or the medial lacrimal sac is involved by tumor, the resection must include these structures, being aware that bony structures, except for lacrimal bone and papyracea, and orbital contents are not invaded [23]. While severing the nasolacrimal duct sharply should not encourage subsequent scarring, numerous authors propose employing supplementary methods like marsupialization, flap creation, transcanalicular stenting, distal stenting, or simultaneous dacryocystorhinostomy procedures to mitigate the likelihood of postoperative tearing [12, 24–26]. Nevertheless, this might not be imperative, given the outcome of 4.8% of patients experiencing tearing in literature [23].

### 43.4.3 Orbit

The frequency of tumors from the sinonasal region spreading into the orbit varies based on the tumor's origin, its histological type, and its aggressiveness, affecting negatively both overall and disease-free survival [27]. It's documented to occur in around 62–82% of ethmoid tumors, 55% of maxillary tumors, and 46% of tumors originating in the nasal cavity [28]. Orbital preservation or exenteration depends on the degree of orbital invasion and tumor biology. In particular, the degree of orbital involvement should be established between various levels, from bony wall erosion and periosteum involvement to deeper penetration into the soft tissues of the orbit and invasion of the orbital apex. Moreover, tumor biology and behavior affect the response to treatment, so that some histotypes benefit from multimodal treatment rather than a primary surgical approach. A comprehensive algorithm for orbital invasion management was proposed by Turri et al. in 2019, based on 163 patients, and displayed in Diagram 43.1 [29].

### 43.4.4 Nasopharynx

Malignant sinonasal tumors may abut into nasopharynx or invade it. This latter case must be carefully considered and can be suitable for specific resection, described as nasopharyngectomy type 1–3. The extent of the surgical removal is categorized into three subtypes based on the spread of the disease. Type 1 NER is restricted to the supero-posterior wall of the nasopharynx, reaching the bony floor of the sphenoid sinus above and the pharyngo-basilar/prevertebral fascia posteriorly. Type 2 NER expands superiorly to encompass the anterior wall and floor of the sphenoid sinus. Type 3 NER extends outward to include the lateral wall of the nasopharynx and the cartilaginous segment of the Eustachian tube [30]. In instances of types 1 and 2 NER, the surgical wound can be intentionally left to heal by secondary intention. However, in cases where an extensive resection exposing the ICA and/or skull base is performed (selected cases of type 3 NER), the surgical area was covered using a

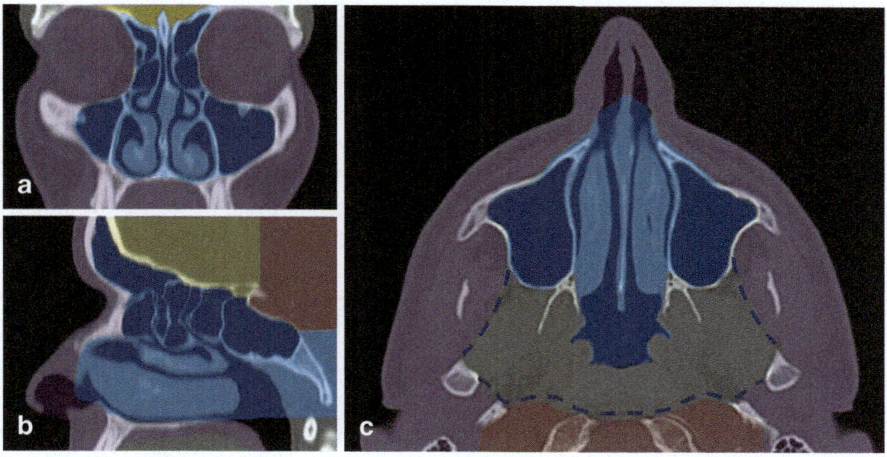


**Diagram 43.1** Management of orbital invasion. *CHT* chemotherapy, *CR* complete response, *ITAC* intestinal type adenocarcinoma, *NEC* neuroendocrine carcinoma, *ONB* olfactory neuroblastoma, *PD* progression of disease, *SCC-G3* poorly differentiated squamous cell carcinoma, *SD* stable disease, *SNUC* sinonasal undifferentiated carcinoma

pedicled flap (mainly the Hadad flap). When the tumor extends bilaterally, involving the nasal septum, or when the defects are too large to be covered, or in situations of radiation-induced nasal mucosa degeneration, a temporo-parietal fascia flap (TPFF) is harvested and inserted into the nose through a trans-pterygoid tunnel [30–32].

## 43.5 Complications and Oncological Outcomes

Both endoscopic approach and open craniofacial surgery carry potential postoperative morbidity and mortality. CFR complications range from 12% to 47%, with a 4% average mortality rate [4, 33]. Conversely, endoscopic resections were associated with lower major complication rates (6.6–25.9%) than open approaches, with a mortality rate of around 0–1% [34–37]. Moreover, the endoscopic approach significantly reduces hospital stays. Potential complications can be categorized into five primary groups:

1. Systemic (sepsis, fever)
2. Central nervous system (meningitis, brain abscess, pneumocephalus, cranial nerve injuries, etc.)
3. Orbital (orbital hematoma, pneumorbit, epiphora, etc.)
4. Vascular (intraoperative bleeding from sphenopalatine, ethmoidal, frontopolar, medial orbitofrontal, or internal carotid arteries [ICA]; nasal bleeding after nasal packing removal)
5. Skull base reconstruction failure [5]

Notably, endoscopic procedures involving the ICA require careful consideration. In this context, advances in navigational aids and acoustic doppler have drastically helped reduce complications. Some authors emphasized the specific occurrence of CSF leaks in endoscopic versus open approaches. Although this was a concern in the past, significant technological advancements in the reconstruction of skull base defects have led to a substantial reduction in postoperative CSF leak rates. The adoption of multilayer techniques involving pedicled mucosal flaps and "minimally invasive" pericranial flaps to seal endoscopic dural defects has played a significant role in diminishing the incidence of CSF leaks [4].

Multiple reviews and meta-analyses comparing outcomes between endoscopic and open craniofacial resections consistently show comparable survival data [38]. A systematic review of 226 patients revealed no significant differences in 5-year overall survival (OS), disease-specific survival (DSS), and locoregional control between endoscopic and traditional CFR for T1 and T2 sinonasal malignancies [39]. For olfactory neuroblastoma, a stage-matched analysis on 109 cases demonstrated significant improvement in the EER group for Kadish stage C. Margin clearance was greater for both Kadish stage B and C in the EER group, with margin status identified as a crucial predictor of survival [40]. Another meta-analysis of olfactory neuroblastoma confirmed better overall survival and DSS with endoscopic surgery, particularly for Kadish stage C and D patients [41]. Similar trends were observed in sinonasal adenocarcinoma, where endoscopic treatment showed improved survival outcomes. A pooled analysis indicated lower local recurrence rates in the endoscopic group, especially for T2, T3, and T4 tumors [37]. Mucosal melanoma, in contrast, continues to exhibit poor survival outcomes, with limited improvement noted compared to squamous cell carcinoma and adenocarcinoma. Open CFR for mucosal melanoma demonstrated a 3-year DSS of 29.7%, while endoscopic cohorts reported a 5-year DFS of 39% [42, 43]. The unique challenge in mucosal melanoma lies in the requirement for wider margins due to high false-negative rates of intraoperative frozen margins [44]. Overall, these findings emphasize the importance of considering tumor characteristics and staging when evaluating the outcomes of endoscopic versus open approaches in sinonasal malignancies.

## References

1. Castelnuovo P, Turri-Zanoni M, Battaglia P, Antognoni P, Bossi P, Locatelli D. Sinonasal malignancies of anterior skull base. Otolaryngol Clin North Am. 2016;49(1):183–200. https://doi.org/10.1016/j.otc.2015.09.012.
2. Ketcham AS, Wilkins RH, Van Buren JM, Smith RR. A combined intracranial facial approach to the paranasal sinuses. Am J Surg. 1963;106(5):698–703. https://doi.org/10.1016/0002-9610(63)90387-8.
3. Castelnuovo P, et al. Endoscopic endonasal surgery for malignancies of the anterior cranial base. World Neurosurg. 2014;82(6):S22–31. https://doi.org/10.1016/j.wneu.2014.07.021.
4. López F, et al. The selective role of open and endoscopic approaches for sinonasal malignant tumours. Adv Ther. 2022;39(6):2379–97. https://doi.org/10.1007/s12325-022-02080-x.

5. Battaglia P, Lambertoni A, Castelnuovo P. Transnasal endoscopic surgery: surgical techniques and complications. In: Nicolai P, Bradley PJ, editors. Advances in oto-rhino-laryngology, vol. 84. Basel: S. Karger AG; 2020. p. 46–55. https://doi.org/10.1159/000457924.
6. Castelnuovo P, Battaglia P, Locatelli D, Delù G, Sberze F, Bignami M. Endonasal micro-endoscopic treatment of malignant tumors of the paranasal sinuses and anterior skull base. Oper Tech Otolaryngol Head Neck Surg. 2006;17(3):152–67. https://doi.org/10.1016/j.otot.2006.06.002.
7. Tajudeen BA, et al. Smell preservation following endoscopic unilateral resection of esthesioneuroblastoma: a multi-institutional experience. Int Forum Allergy Rhinol. 2016;6(10):1047–50. https://doi.org/10.1002/alr.21794.
8. Schreiber A, et al. Unilateral endoscopic resection with transnasal craniectomy for sinonasal intestinal-type adenocarcinoma: a bi-institutional case-control study on 54 patients. Oral Oncol. 2018;87:89–96. https://doi.org/10.1016/j.oraloncology.2018.10.027.
9. Hadad G, et al. A novel reconstructive technique after endoscopic expanded endonasal approaches: vascular pedicle nasoseptal flap. Laryngoscope. 2006;116(10):1882–6. https://doi.org/10.1097/01.mlg.0000234933.37779.e4.
10. Battaglia P, et al. Septal flip flap for anterior skull base reconstruction after endoscopic resection of sinonasal cancers: preliminary outcomes. Acta Otorhinolaryngol Ital. 2016;36(3):194–8. https://doi.org/10.14639/0392-100X-748.
11. Villaret AB, et al. Endoscopic transnasal craniectomy in the management of selected sinonasal malignancies. Am J Rhinol Allergy. 2010;24(1):60–5. https://doi.org/10.2500/ajra.2010.24.3397.
12. Turri-Zanoni M, et al. Transnasal endoscopic partial maxillectomy: operative nuances and proposal for a comprehensive classification system based on 1378 cases. Head Neck. 2017;39(4):754–66. https://doi.org/10.1002/hed.24676.
13. Turri-Zanoni M, Battaglia P, Bignami M, Castelnuovo P, Arosio AD. Comprehensive access strategies to the frontal sinus. Curr Opin Otolaryngol Head Neck Surg. 2023;31(1):57–64. https://doi.org/10.1097/MOO.0000000000000864.
14. Sileo G, et al. Sinonasal malignancies involving the frontal sinus: a mono-institutional experience of 84 cases and systematic literature review. J Clin Med. 2023;12(9):3186. https://doi.org/10.3390/jcm12093186.
15. Karligkiotis A, et al. Endoscopic endonasal orbital transposition to expand the frontal sinus approaches. Am J Rhinol Allergy. 2015;29(6):449–56. https://doi.org/10.2500/ajra.2015.29.4230.
16. Papatsoutsos E, et al. Defining the limits and indications of the Draf III endoscopic approach to the lateral frontal sinus and maximizing visualization and maneuverability: a cadaveric and radiological study. Eur Arch Otorhinolaryngol. 2022;279(10):4969–76. https://doi.org/10.1007/s00405-022-07323-9.
17. Pietrobon G, et al. Frontal sinus ablation (Riedel-Mosherâ€™s procedure): indications and role in the endonasal endoscopic era. Rhinology. 2019;57(4):293–302. https://doi.org/10.4193/Rhin18.197.
18. Martin TJ, Smith TL, Smith MM, Loehrl TA. Evaluation and surgical management of isolated sphenoid sinus disease. Arch Otolaryngol Head Neck Surg. 2002;128(12):1413–9. https://doi.org/10.1001/archotol.128.12.1413.
19. Ghosh R, et al. Sphenoid sinus malignancies: a population-based comprehensive analysis. Int Forum Allergy Rhinol. 2016;6(7):752–9. https://doi.org/10.1002/alr.21733.
20. Zoli M, et al. Infra-temporal and pterygo-palatine fossae tumors: a frontier in endoscopic endonasal surgery—description of the surgical anatomy of the approach and report of illustrative cases. Int J Environ Res Public Health. 2022;19(11):6413. https://doi.org/10.3390/ijerph19116413.
21. Karkas A, Zimmer LA, Theodosopoulos PV, Keller JT, Prades J-M. Endonasal endoscopic approach to the pterygopalatine and infratemporal fossae. Eur Ann Otorhinolaryngol Head Neck Dis. 2021;138(5):391–5. https://doi.org/10.1016/j.anorl.2020.12.009.

22. Oakley GM, Harvey RJ. Endoscopic resection of pterygopalatine fossa and infratemporal fossa malignancies. Otolaryngol Clin North Am. 2017;50(2):301–13. https://doi.org/10.1016/j.otc.2016.12.007.
23. Sieśkiewicz A, et al. Assessment of lacrimal duct patency in patients undergoing endoscopic medial maxillectomy. J Clin Med. 2021;10(2):245. https://doi.org/10.3390/jcm10020245.
24. Yeo N-K, Wang JH, Chung Y-S, Jang YJ, Lee B-J. Contributing factors to prevent prolonged epiphora after maxillectomy. Arch Otolaryngol Head Neck Surg. 2010;136(3):229–33. https://doi.org/10.1001/archoto.2010.18.
25. Imre A, et al. Transection of nasolacrimal duct in endoscopic medial maxillectomy: implication on epiphora. J Craniofac Surg. 2015;26(7):e616–9. https://doi.org/10.1097/SCS.0000000000002115.
26. Sadeghi N, Al-Dhahri S, Manoukian JJ. Transnasal endoscopic medial maxillectomy for inverting papilloma. Laryngoscope. 2003;113(4):749–53. https://doi.org/10.1097/00005537-200304000-00031.
27. Muscatello L, Fortunato S, Seccia V, Marchetti M, Lenzi R. The implications of orbital invasion in sinonasal tract malignancies. Orbit. 2016;35(5):278–84. https://doi.org/10.1080/01676830.2016.1193532.
28. Neel GS, Nagel TH, Hoxworth JM, Lal D. Management of orbital involvement in sinonasal and ventral skull base malignancies. Otolaryngol Clin North Am. 2017;50(2):347–64. https://doi.org/10.1016/j.otc.2016.12.010.
29. Turri-Zanoni M, et al. Multidisciplinary treatment algorithm for the management of sinonasal cancers with orbital invasion: a retrospective study. Head Neck. 2019;41(8):2777–88. https://doi.org/10.1002/hed.25759.
30. Castelnuovo P, et al. Endoscopic endonasal nasopharyngectomy in selected cancers. Otolaryngol Head Neck Surg. 2013;149(3):424–30. https://doi.org/10.1177/0194599813493073.
31. Chen M-Y, et al. Use of a posterior pedicle nasal septum and floor mucoperiosteum flap to resurface the nasopharynx after endoscopic nasopharyngectomy for recurrent nasopharyngeal carcinoma. Head Neck. 2012;34(10):1383–8. https://doi.org/10.1002/hed.21928.
32. Ong YK, Solares CA, Lee S, Snyderman CH, Fernandez-Miranda J, Gardner PA. Endoscopic nasopharyngectomy and its role in managing locally recurrent nasopharyngeal carcinoma. Otolaryngol Clin North Am. 2011;44(5):1141–54. https://doi.org/10.1016/j.otc.2011.07.002.
33. König M, Osnes T, Jebsen P, Meling TR. Craniofacial resection of malignant tumors of the anterior skull base: a case series and a systematic review. Acta Neurochir (Wien). 2018;160(12):2339–48. https://doi.org/10.1007/s00701-018-3716-4.
34. Ganly I, et al. Complications of craniofacial resection for malignant tumors of the skull base: report of an International Collaborative Study. Head Neck. 2005;27(6):445–51. https://doi.org/10.1002/hed.20166.
35. Zhang Y, et al. A modified endovascular treatment protocol for iatrogenic internal carotid artery injuries following endoscopic endonasal surgery. J Neurosurg. 2019;132(2):343–50. https://doi.org/10.3171/2018.8.JNS181048.
36. Snyderman CH, Kassam AB, Carrau R, Mintz A. Endoscopic reconstruction of cranial base defects following endonasal skull base surgery. Skull Base. 2007;17(1):73–8. https://doi.org/10.1055/s-2006-959337.
37. Meccariello G, et al. Endoscopic nasal versus open approach for the management of sinonasal adenocarcinoma: a pooled-analysis of 1826 patients. Head Neck. 2016;38(1):E2267–74. https://doi.org/10.1002/hed.24182.
38. Carlton DA, David Beahm D, Chiu AG. Sinonasal malignancies: endoscopic treatment outcomes. Laryngoscope Investig Otolaryngol. 2019;4(2):259–63. https://doi.org/10.1002/lio2.249.
39. Higgins TS, Thorp B, Rawlings BA, Han JK. Outcome results of endoscopic vs craniofacial resection of sinonasal malignancies: a systematic review and pooled-data analysis. Int Forum Allergy Rhinol. 2011;1(4):255–61. https://doi.org/10.1002/alr.20051.
40. Harvey RJ, et al. Survival outcomes for stage-matched endoscopic and open resection of olfactory neuroblastoma. Head Neck. 2017;39(12):2425–32. https://doi.org/10.1002/hed.24912.

41. Fu TS, Monteiro E, Muhanna N, Goldstein DP, de Almeida JR. Comparison of outcomes for open versus endoscopic approaches for olfactory neuroblastoma: a systematic review and individual participant data meta-analysis. Head Neck. 2016;38(1):E2306–16. https://doi.org/10.1002/hed.24233.
42. Ganly I, et al. Craniofacial resection for malignant melanoma of the skull base: report of an international collaborative study. Arch Otolaryngol Head Neck Surg. 2006;132(1):73–8. https://doi.org/10.1001/archotol.132.1.73.
43. Lund VJ, Wei WI. Endoscopic surgery for malignant sinonasal tumours: an eighteen year experience. Rhinology. 2015;53(3):204–11. https://doi.org/10.4193/Rhino14.318.
44. Chiu AG, Ma Y. Accuracy of intraoperative frozen margins for sinonasal malignancies and its implications for endoscopic resection of sinonasal melanomas. Int Forum Allergy Rhinol. 2013;3(2):157–60. https://doi.org/10.1002/alr.21075.

# Benign Swellings of the Nasopharynx 44

Hisham Khalil and Ra'ed Al-Ashqar

**Key Points**

- The nasopharynx or postnasal space can be affected by several benign lesions including cysts and benign tumours.
- The ones commonly encountered in clinical practice include hypertrophy of the lymphoid tissue of the postnasal space, Thornwaldt cysts, and juvenile nasopharyngeal angiofibroma.
- The diagnostic approach includes a focused history, ENT examination including a nasal endoscopy, neck palpation, and where required imaging including CT, MRI, and biopsy where indicated.

## 44.1 Thornwaldt Cysts

Thornwaldt cysts are relatively rare cystic swellings encountered in the postero-superior aspect of the nasopharynx. They are usually asymptomatic but if large enough can cause nasal obstruction, postnasal drip, headaches, and manifestations of Eustachian tube occlusion such as ear fullness, conductive hearing loss, and a middle ear effusion.

H. Khalil (✉)
University Hospitals Plymouth NHS Trust, Plymouth, UK

Peninsula Medical School, University of Plymouth, Plymouth, UK
e-mail: Hisham.khalil@plymouth.ac.uk

R. Al-Ashqar
Peninsula Medical School, University of Plymouth, Plymouth, UK


S. Elwany (ed.), *Current Rhinology*,
https://doi.org/10.1007/978-3-031-70077-4_44

The treatment of symptomatic cysts is usually by endoscopic marsupialization through 'uncapping' of the cyst. There is a need to use a combination of imaging, usually MRI and a biopsy, to exclude other more sinister lesions [1].

## 44.2 Juvenile Nasopharyngeal Angiofibroma

### 44.2.1 Introduction

Juvenile nasopharyngeal angiofibroma (JNA) is a rare, benign tumour of vascular tissue that has locally destructive properties. The lesion accounts for less than 0.5% of head and neck tumour and occurs almost exclusively in young adult male patients. The presumed site of origin is near the superior border of the periosteum of the sphenopalatine foramen. From there, it tends to spread towards the nasopharynx, nasal cavity, paranasal sinuses, and orbits. It can also invade the skull base with intracranial extension.

### 44.2.2 Pathogenesis and Risk Factors

The exact aetiology and pathogenesis of JNA remain unknown. The almost exclusive occurrence in young adult males suggested a hormonal or genetic influence. A recent study by Safhi et al. demonstrated significant upregulation of the fibroblast growth factor receptor 3/4 genes in JNA patients with a stronger association in smokers. There are also reports of a higher incidence of recurrence after excision and more severe bleeding amongst smokers [2, 3].

### 44.2.3 Staging of JNA

There are several staging systems for JNA in use. The Andrews–Fisch classification was introduced in 1989 as a modification of the original Fisch classification. (Table 44.1) The staging system provides the surgeon with a guide to surgical routes for excision [4].

**Table 44.1** The Andrews–Fisch staging of JNA

| | | |
|---|---|---|
| Stage I | Tumour confined to the site of origin at the sphenopalatine foramen may extend unimpeded into the nasopharynx and nasal cavity | |
| Stage II | Involvement of the pterygopalatine fossa or the regional paranasal sinuses (the next major sequence of invasion) | |
| Stage III | Involvement of the infratemporal fossa or orbital region | |
| | Stage IIIa | Without intracranial extension |
| | Stage IIIb | With extradural intracranial (parasellar) extension |
| Stage IV | Intracranial intradural extension | |
| | Stage IVa | Without cavernous sinus, pituitary or optic chiasma infiltration |
| | Stage IVb | With the involvement of cavernous sinus/ pituitary fossa/or optic chiasma |

### 44.2.4 Diagnosis

The diagnostic approach to nasopharyngeal angiofibroma depends on a history of nasal obstruction and recurrent severe epistaxis in a young adult male with a vascular lesion in the posterior nasal cavity and nasopharynx demonstrated on nasal endoscopy. The diagnosis is clinched with a combination of CT angiography and MRI, which are also required for staging. There should be no attempt at biopsy except as part of a definitive exciton and usually after embolization.

### 44.2.5 Surgical Excision

The planning of a surgical excision depends on the stage of the JNA, whether the procedure is a primary or revision surgery. The choice of endoscopic versus external or combined external and endoscopic procedures is also influenced by the expertise of the surgical team.

Pre-operative embolization is usually feasible in primary excision,which is a primary or revision procedure. This is best carried out 24–48 h before the procedure to minimize the impact of re-opening of collateral circulation. The surgical approaches include endoscopic transnasal, transpalatal, Denker approach, facial translocation, medial maxillectomy, and infratemporal fossa with or without craniotomy. Segmental endoscopic resections are very effective for early stage disease. External or combined approaches may be necessary for access to more extensive and recurrent diseases [5].

### 44.2.6 Adjunct Treatment

Radiotherapy is reserved for advanced stage and some recurrent diseases where total resection is not feasible. This should be balanced with the risk of delayed-onset radiation-induced malignancy. More recently proton-beam therapy has been used over traditional radiotherapy techniques for the treatment of advanced JNA [6].

**Case Study**

A 27-year-old man was referred to the ENT outpatients with nasal obstruction and recurrent epistaxis (bilateral) and smooth soft tissue mass in the nasopharynx (Fig. 44.1). An MRI with contrast demonstrated an enhancing lesion in the nasopharynx with an extension into the left nasal cavity (Fig. 44.2).

An MRI scan with contrast demonstrated an enhancing lesion in the nasopharynx with an extension into the left nasal cavity (Figs. 44.2 and 44.3).

The patient had embolization 36 h prior to surgery. Complete excision was achieved through a trans-nasal endoscopic excision using a microdebrider and bipolar diathermy to the left sphenopalatine foramen. The patient made a complete recovery without complications or recurrence of the lesion.

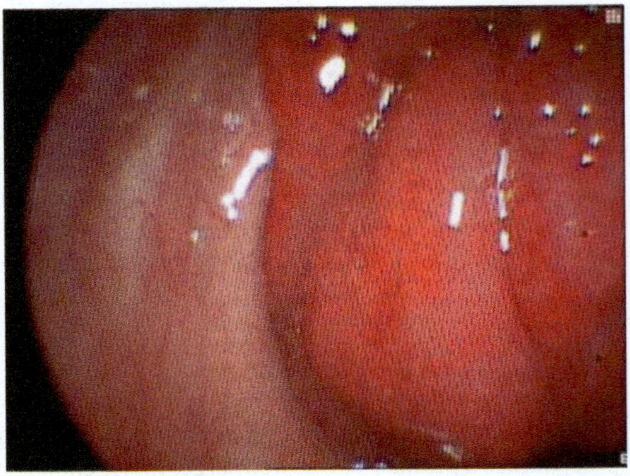

**Fig. 44.1** Endoscopic view of the left posterior nasal cavity and nasopharynx

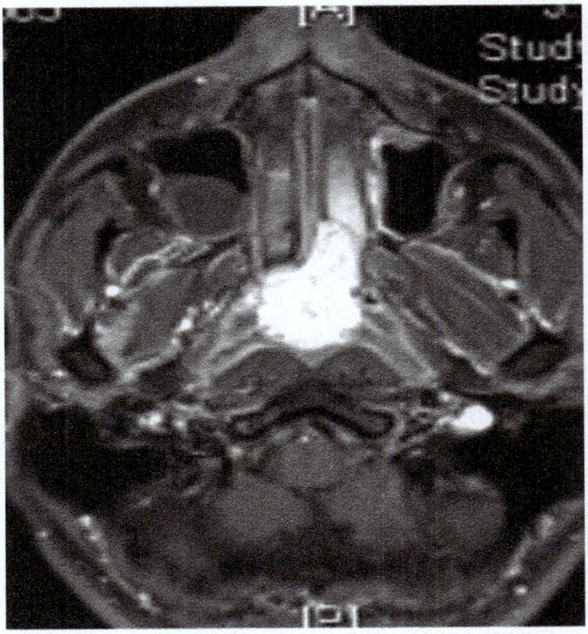

**Fig. 44.2** Coronal MRI scan with contrast demonstrated an enhancing lesion in the nasopharynx with an extension into the left nasal cavity

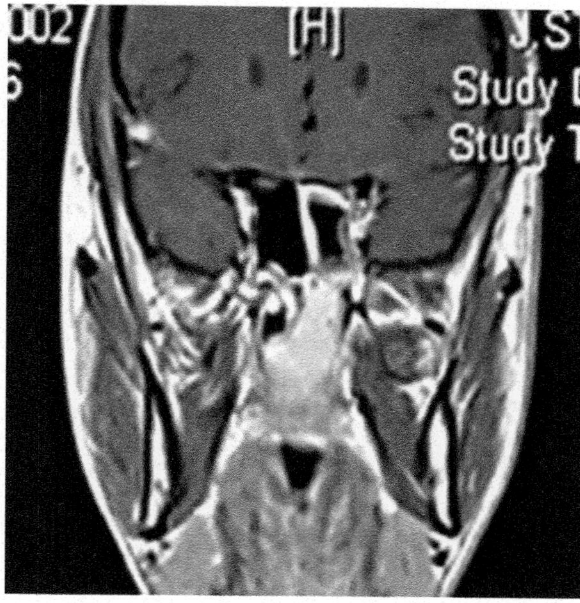


**Fig. 44.3** Axial and coronal MRI scan demonstrating an enhancing lesion in the nasopharynx with an extension into the left nasal cavity

## References


1. Jyotirmay H, Arun Kumar SJ, Preetam P, et al. Recent trends in the management of Thornwaldts cyst: a case report. J Clin Diagn Res. 2014;8(8):KD03–4.
2. Ferouz AS, Mohr RM, Paul P. Juvenile nasopharyngeal angiofibroma and familial adenomatous polyposis: an association? Otolaryngol Head Neck Surg. 1995;113(4):435–9. https://doi.org/10.1016/S0194-59989570081-1.
3. Safhi FA, Al-Hazani TMI, Jalal AS, Alduwish MA, Alshaya DS, Almufareh NA, Domiaty DM, Alshehri E, Al-Shamrani SM, Abboosh TS, Alotaibi MA, Alwaili MA, Al-Qahtani WS. FGFR3 and FGFR4 overexpression in juvenile nasopharyngeal angiofibroma: impact of smoking history and implications for personalized management. J Appl Genet. 2023;64(4):749–58. https://doi.org/10.1007/s13353-023-00780-w. Epub 2023 Sep 1.
4. Alshaikh NA, Eleftheriadou A. Juvenile nasopharyngeal angiofibroma staging: an overview. Ear Nose Throat J. 2015;94(6):E12–22. https://doi.org/10.1177/014556131509400615.
5. Cohen-Cohen S, Scheitler KM, Choby G, Janus J, Moore EJ, Kasperbauer JL, Cloft HJ, Link M, Gompel JJV. Contemporary surgical management of juvenile nasopharyngeal angiofibroma. J Neurol Surg B Skull Base. 2021;83(Suppl 2):e266–73. https://doi.org/10.1055/s-0041-1725031. PMID: 35832970; PMCID: PMC9272285.
6. Hoeltgen L, Tessonnier T, Meixner E, Hoeen P, et al. Proton therapy for advanced juvenile nasopharyngeal angiofibroma. Cancers. 2023;15(20):5022.

# Nasopharyngeal Carcinoma

45

Ra'ed Al-Ashqar and Hisham Khalil

**Key Points**

- The differential diagnosis of lesions of the nasopharynx includes Thornwaldt's cyst, juvenile nasopharyngeal angiofibroma (JNA) and nasopharyngeal cancer (NPC).
- A focused history, nasal endoscopy, contrast CT and MRI are part of the diagnostic workup in patients with nasopharyngeal lesions.
- Pre-operative embolization is beneficial for patients undergoing primary excision of JNA.
- Endoscopic and/or external approaches are employed for excision depending on the stage of the JNA.
- The primary treatment for NPC is radiotherapy ± chemotherapy with surgery reserved for recurrences.

## 45.1 Introduction

Nasopharyngeal carcinoma (NPC) is a rare malignancy arising from the epithelium of the nasopharynx. It is unique within the context of head and neck tumours as its deep location of origin gives rise to a wide range of possible clinical presentations, making early diagnosis a distinct challenge. It is, by definition, a squamous cell carcinoma (SCC) of the nasopharynx, further classified as keratinizing, non-keratinizing and basaloid types. However, its unique biology, as well as its complex association with a variety of environmental, viral and genetic factors, makes the

R. Al-Ashqar · H. Khalil (✉)
University Hospitals Plymouth NHS Trust, Plymouth, UK
e-mail: hisham.khalil@plymouth.ac.uk





S. Elwany (ed.), *Current Rhinology*,
https://doi.org/10.1007/978-3-031-70077-4_45

diagnosis and management of this cancer different to all other head and neck tumours. In this chapter, we aim to outline these features of nasopharyngeal carcinoma, as well as go in-depth on the typical and atypical presentations of this condition, its epidemiology, as well as a look into a challenging presentation of NPC.

## 45.2 Classification

The most commonly used classification system for nasopharyngeal carcinoma is the World Health Organization (WHO) classification. According to the most recent updates from the WHO, NPC is classified into three subtypes: keratinizing (WHO type 1), non-keratinizing and basaloid SCC. Non-keratinizing carcinoma is further divided into differentiated (WHO type 2) and undifferentiated (WHO type 3) types [1, 2]. Keratinizing SCC appears to have a closer pathogenesis than other aerodigestive tract squamous cell carcinomas, and smoking is a recognized risk factor for this type of NPC, as it is with other head and neck SCCs [2]. However, the most common type of NPC is the non-keratinizing type, which almost invariably displays an association with the Epstein Barr Virus (EBV). This association has given rise to the endemic nature of this carcinoma, with the vast majority (>95%) of NPC cases in these regions being associated with the presence of EBV [1–3]. Basaloid NPC represents the rarest subtype of NPC worldwide.

## 45.3 Staging

As with the majority of head and neck tumours, the staging of nasopharyngeal carcinomas is through the tumour, nodes and metastasis (TNM) system based on the International Union Against Cancer and American Joint Committee on Cancer (AJCC) system. Although the different subtypes of NPC may differ in their pathogenesis, the staging system remains the same for all, and prognosis for all types primarily depends on the stage at presentation [2, 4]. Figure 45.1 outlines the most recent TNM staging system applicable to all types of nasopharyngeal carcinomas.

## 45.4 Pathogenesis and Risk Factors

The aetiology of nasopharyngeal involves a complex interaction between viral, genetic and environmental factors. While keratinizing NPC risk seems to be increased by smoking in a similar process to other head and neck squamous cell carcinomas [2], the more common non-keratinizing NPC appears closely related to the presence of EBV. The mechanism of development of NPC from EBV is unclear to date although many theories exist. What is clear, however, is that almost all tumour cells in these cases express EBV, which can be shown through a variety of methods, most commonly through in situ hybridization for EBV RNA [1, 2, 5]. In

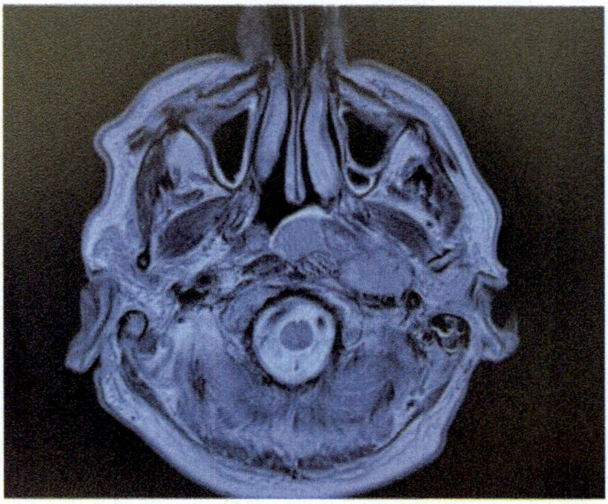

**Fig. 45.1** Axial RI scan demonstrating a left nasopharyngeal mass

the case of non-keratinizing NPC, the virus exists in almost all cases and in a latent state exclusively within the tumour cells, absent from the surrounding stroma [5]. Another feature that differentiates non-keratinizing from keratinizing NPC is the infiltration of malignant cells with lymphocytes (predominantly T-cells) and plasma cells, which may propagate the growth of EBV-infected NPC cells in these patients [6].

Genetic susceptibility to the development of NPC has also been demonstrated, primarily through a number of human leukocyte antigens (HLA) haplotypes, such as HLA-A2, AW19 and BW46 [6, 7]. Some studies have found that the familial risk of developing NPC is among the highest of any malignancy [8].

Other environmental risk factors have been identified for the development of NPC. As mentioned previously, smoking appears to increase the incidence of NPC in both low and high-incidence populations although more markedly affects the incidence of well-differentiated keratinizing NPC [2]. Furthermore, consumption of alcohol, salted fish and preserved foods (possibly due to their high nitrosamine content) has been shown to increase the risk of NPC [2, 5, 6, 9, 10].

## 45.5 Epidemiology

The epidemiology of NPC has long been a source of interest due to its unique geographic distribution as well as its association with EBV. The global incidence of NPC is around less than 1 in 100,000 people yearly, with around 129,000 new cases reported worldwide in 2018 and 133,000 cases in 2020 [9, 11–13]. However, the geographic distribution of these cases varies greatly, with over 70% of all cases presenting in the 'endemic' regions, mostly in East and Southeast Asia [13]. In these endemic regions, over 95% of NPC cases are of the non-keratinizing variety (mostly undifferentiated) [2, 7], and while keratinizing NPC makes up a more significant proportion of cases in non-endemic countries, non-keratinizing NPC remains more prevalent worldwide [1].

NPC incidence is from two to three times more common in males than in females globally [11, 13]. In non-endemic populations, it shows a bimodal distribution by age, with a small peak in incidence in young adulthood (ages 15–25) and a second larger peak from 65 to 80 years of age. Comparatively, in endemic areas, there appears to be only one peak for NPC incidence from 45 to 59 years of age, followed by a decline in incidence [11].

Adding to the credibility of the genetic element of risk for the development of NPC, many studies have found that NPC incidence varies greatly between different races and ethnic backgrounds, even within endemic areas. For example, in southern China, the Cantonese-speaking population were found to have almost double the risk of developing NPC compared to groups of other dialects within the region [11].

## 45.6 Patient Profiling

As with any other disease, it is important to be aware of the typical presentations of a condition in order to ease the process of diagnosis in a clinical setting. While not all patients will present in a similar fashion, having a typical patient profile in mind is a useful tool to enable clinicians to suspect NPC in most cases. Unfortunately, early lesions within the nasopharynx, due to its location, may produce trivial nasal symptoms, which are often ignored by both the patient and the physician. As such, NPC is often detected at a later stage [14]. Furthermore, the anatomic location of the nasopharynx makes NPC amenable to spread in multiple directions and affecting adjacent structures, causing symptoms that may not be immediately attributable to a nasal tumour, making it vital that we are knowledgeable about the symptomatology of nasopharyngeal tumours.

First and foremost, in the case of NPC, one should be wary of the patient's ethnic background, age group, family history of NPC and smoking status, and physicians residing in what are considered endemic areas certainly should have a high index of suspicion for NPC in any patient presenting with the typical symptoms.

While NPC originates within the nasopharynx, what is often seen as the most common presentation of NPC is the presence of a lump in the neck, which may be both unilateral or bilateral, most commonly found to be involved level II, level III and level V lymph nodes. Up to 75% of NPC patients present with involvement of their cervical lymph nodes, making this a significant finding that should indicate a high level of suspicion for NPC [9, 15, 16].

As NPC most commonly originates in the fossa of Rosenmuller, in close relation to the eustachian tube opening, invasion into the eustachian tube or mass effect from the tumour bulk encroaching on the eustachian tube may lead to otological symptoms in NPC patients [9, 17]. Often, these present as unilateral hearing loss, aural fullness and occasionally tinnitus. These symptoms are easy to write off as secondary eustachian tube dysfunction. It is therefore vital that in any patient found to have unilateral middle ear effusion, be it symptomatic or not, a nasopharyngeal examination must be performed [17].

While nasal symptoms are often mild or delayed in nasopharyngeal carcinoma, they remain one of the most common presentations of NPC. The most common of these symptoms is bloody nasal discharge (often unilateral) with nasal obstruction often presenting late when the tumour bulk has reached a size where it can obstruct the posterior choana [9]. Other possible nasal symptoms to consider are cacosmia and blood-stained postnasal drip.

Invasion of NPC into the clivus or pterygopalatine fossa may lead to the development of occipital headaches or facial pain/numbness, respectively. Headaches are likely the most common neurological presentation in NPC and in some cases the sole presenting symptom [18, 19].

## 45.7 Atypical Presentations

Nasopharyngeal carcinomas present with a very wide array of symptoms, generally classified as nasal, otological, neck symptoms and neurological, making it quite a complex carcinoma to suspect clinically. While most otolaryngologists are aware of the common presentations of NPC, it is useful to also be wary of the more atypical presentations of this carcinoma. At the outset, while NPC is relatively rare in non-endemic populations, one must not ignore the common symptoms in any patient regardless of age or background.

Of the uncommon presentations in NPC, due to its presentation mainly in the later stages of the disease, is the presentation with cranial nerve palsies. Most commonly, cranial nerves V1, V2 and V3 may be involved in presentation due to direct invasion by the tumour [20]. Furthermore, invasion into the cavernous sinus, and rarely, the orbital apex, may present with oculomotor trochlear, and most commonly abducens nerve palsies, with patients presenting with opthalmoplegia or diplopia [9, 20]. Some studies report significant intracranial extension of NPC presenting with neurological sequelae without clear nasopharyngeal disease, making it vital that we are aware of the invasive capability of NPC, maintaining a high index of suspicion [21].

Another recognized rare phenomenon associated with nasopharyngeal carcinoma, as well as other malignancies arising from the lateral wall of the nasopharynx, is the development of ipsilateral conductive hearing loss, trigeminal neuralgia and palatal asymmetry. This is a triad of symptoms known as Trotter's Triad, the presence of which should illicit high suspicion of occult nasopharyngeal malignancy [22].

Direct invasion or metastatic spread of the tumour towards or around the carotid sheath may present as Horner syndrome, which is a very rare presentation of NPC [23, 24]. Similarly, there has been a reported case of NPC presenting as Lemierre Syndrome, with the patient presenting with fever, neck pain and swelling and trismus [25]. This is a wholly atypical presentation for a nasopharyngeal carcinoma. Furthermore, on rare occasions, patients may present with trismus due to NPC invasion through the masticator space [26]. In all cases, nasopharyngeal disease may be unclear at the time of presentation.

Paraneoplastic syndrome is a rare entity, representing the indirect effects of tumour metabolites or autoimmune responses to them rather than by direct invasion by the tumour. While extremely rare, paraneoplastic syndromes have been found to be associated with some cases of NPC. The most common of these is dermatomyositis (believed to be involved in 1 in 1000 NPC cases), but others have been reported such as Syndrome of Inappropriate Antidiuretic Hormone Release (SIADH), immune thrombocytopenia, Cushing syndrome and demyelinating motor neuropathy [27]. Dermatomyositis may present with a constellation of symptoms, most commonly starting with a purple-red skin rash, discolouration of the eyelids, dysphagia and developing into muscle weakness [28]. One study found that the prevalence of NPC in patients with dermatomyositis was 3.3% [29].

While the symptoms of NPC are most commonly due to local invasion, an uncommon presentation is due to symptoms caused by distant metastasis. The most common sites of distant metastasis for NPC are the bone, lung and liver [9, 30]. It is often difficult to differentiate a primary lymphoepithelial tumour in the lung from a metastatic tumour originating from an NPC, and this may result in a delay in appropriate management. It is therefore important to utilize all tools available to localize the origin [9, 31]. Positron Emission Tomography (PET) scan is a useful tool in this scenario. Additionally, identifying EBV RNA within tumour cells is an exceptionally useful way to identify lesions originating from an NPC.

It is clear at this point that nasopharyngeal carcinomas have an extraordinarily broad range of possible presentations, often presenting in ways unrelated to the site of tumour origin. It is therefore prudent to educate ourselves on these rare but possible presentations, along with knowledge of high-risk features and populations, in order to avoid missing this challenging diagnosis (Table 45.1).

**Table 45.1** Based on the seventh edition AJCC TNM classification system for nasopharyngeal carcinomas

| AJCC stage | Grouping | Description |
|---|---|---|
| 0 | Tis | Tis: Tumour only involving the superficial lining of the nasopharynx with no deep growth |
| | N0 | N0: No regional lymph node spread |
| | M0 | M0: No distant spread |
| I | T1 | T1: Tumour within the nasopharynx. There may be growth into the oropharynx or the nasal cavity, but no further |
| | N0 | N0: No regional lymph node spread |
| | M0 | M0: No distant spread |
| II | T1 (or T0) | T1: Tumour within the nasopharynx. There may be growth into the oropharynx or the nasal cavity, but no further (OR T0) |
| | N1 | N1: The tumour has spread to 1 or more lymph nodes on one side of the neck (unilateral cervical) or spread to lymph nodes behind the throat (retropharyngeal). No lymph nodes are greater than 6 cm across and all above the supraclavicular fossa |
| | M0 | M0: No distant spread |
| | T2 | T2: The tumour has grown into the parapharyngeal space on either side but without bony invasion |
| | N0 (or N1) | N0: No regional lymph node spread (OR N1) |
| | M0 | M0: No distant spread |

(continued)

**Table 45.1** (continued)

| AJCC stage | Grouping | Description |
|---|---|---|
| III | T1 (or T0) | T1: Tumour within the nasopharynx. There may be growth into the oropharynx or the nasal cavity, but no further (OR T0) |
| | N2 | N2: Bilateral cervical lymph node involvement, with none larger than 6 cm, and all above the supraclavicular fossa |
| | M0 | M0: No distant spread |
| | T2 | T2: The tumour has grown into the parapharyngeal space on either side but without bony invasion |
| | N2 | N2: Bilateral cervical lymph node involvement, with none larger than 6 cm, and all above the supraclavicular fossa |
| | M0 | M0: No distant spread |
| | T3 | T3: The tumour has grown into nearby bony structures or the paranasal sinuses |
| | N0/1/2 | N0: No regional lymph node spread (OR N1, N2) |
| | M0 | M0: No distant spread |
| IVA | T4 | T4: Tumour extends into the intracranial space or involves the cranial nerves, hypopharynx, orbit or infratemporal fossa/masticator space |
| | N0/1/2 | N0: No regional lymph node spread (OR N1, N2) |
| | M0 | M0: No distant spread |
| | Any T | T: Any T stage |
| | N3 | N3: Tumour involves regional lymph nodes, with a size greater than 6 cm, or involving the supraclavicular fossa |
| | M0 | M0: No distant spread |
| IVB | Any T | T: Any T stage |
| | Any N | N: Any N stage |
| | M1 | M1: There is distant spread of the tumour |

## 45.8 Diagnosis

The diagnosis of nasopharyngeal carcinoma requires clinicians to be vigilant and thorough in all steps of the process. As with any diagnosis, detailed history taking must be done for every patient, and NPC should be considered a differential diagnosis for any patient with symptoms within the classes of symptoms outlined above, be it nasal symptoms, otological symptoms, neck symptoms or neurological symptoms. Focus should also be placed on family history, as well as the patient's ethnic background, with a high index of suspicion for patients from endemic regions.

When NPC is suspected, a full head and neck examination must be performed, with a focus on neck examination looking for cervical lymphadenopathy, as well as close inspection of the ears in search of otitis media with effusion. The most important aspect of the examination, however, is the inspection of the nasopharynx. The current wide availability of rigid and flexible scopes has made nasopharyngoscopy much more accessible and efficient, making this the mainstay of examination [9, 32]. Close inspection of the nasopharynx must be done, with a focus on the posterior edge of the eustachian tube opening and the lateral recess of the nasopharynx (fossa of Rosenmuller). As clarified before, not all NPC presents as a clear nasopharyngeal mass, and as such, any suspicious swelling or lesion within the region should be considered significant. Most commonly, NPC visualized in the nasopharynx will appear as a mass or swelling with overlying abnormal capillaries that bleed easily on contact [33].

When visualized or suspected, the most useful tool to finalize a diagnosis of NPC is a nasopharyngeal biopsy. Often, a biopsy can easily be taken from the nasopharynx under local anaesthesia, even in the outpatient clinic setting, making it a fast and efficient method of diagnosis. If there is a significant risk of bleeding or multiple deep biopsies are required, with further closer inspection of the nasopharynx, it may be done under general anaesthesia [9].

While a biopsy positive for NPC finalizes the diagnosis, further testing is also required for staging and may also be a useful tool in the case of an unclear pathology. The most important of these is the role of imaging. The primary imaging tool in the case of NPC is MRI scanning due to its excellent soft tissue delineation, making it accurate at identifying tumour extent, invasion and infiltration [34]. In the absence of MRI, CT scanning is an inferior yet useful alternative. Other useful tools are PET-CT scans, with a growing role in localizing tumours and identifying distant metastasis, and ultrasound scanning, which is a very cheap and widely available method of investigating involved neck lymph nodes, with the added benefit of being able to take fine needle aspiration cytology [9, 35].

As mentioned before, another potentially useful tool in the diagnosis of NPC is testing for EBV antibodies in the serum. The most used antibody markers for NPC screening are anti-viral capsid, anti-early antigen and EBV nuclear antigen 1 IgA antibodies. However, these tests are not specific to only NPC and can be positive in the presence of any other EBV-related disease and as such, are a more useful tool for screening in high-risk areas [36]. Another new method for the detection of EBV in NPC is the detection of EBV DNA in nasopharyngeal brush cytology by PCR. While this method is still novel and under review, initial results show promising sensitivity and specificity [37].

## 45.9 Management

Nasopharyngeal carcinoma, specifically the most common non-keratinizing subtype, is a radiosensitive tumour. As such, radiotherapy, namely intensity-modulated radiotherapy (IMRT), is the mainstay of treatment for primary NPC in all its stages given there is no distant metastasis. In the early stages of NPC (stages I and II), radiotherapy alone is often all that is needed for treatment [9]. At later stages, however, concurrent chemoradiotherapy offers high local control rates. Platinum-based chemotherapeutic agents, most commonly cisplatin, are used concurrently with IMRT in order to control advanced disease. Some advocate the use of additional adjuvant chemotherapy with cisplatin and fluorouracil in order to further control disease and reduce recurrence rates, but data on its efficacy is less clear [9, 38].

IMRT involves differential radiation doses to different regions of the head and neck, with concentrated doses of radiation (usually 70 Gy) given to the tumour itself and directly involved sites, a slightly lower dose (60 Gy) given to involved neck lymph nodes and an even lower dose to uninvolved nodes [9, 38]. This is now the mainstay of radiotherapy treatment in NPC.

Post-treatment, patients should undergo regular follow-up long-term, as disease recurrence may occur many years after treatment. As such, it is pertinent to perform regular nasal endoscopies every few months post-treatment to rule out recurrence, with a biopsy of any suspicious lesions visualized in the nasopharynx [39].

With the advent of IMRT and concurrent chemoradiation in the treatment of NPC, control rates for the disease have shown a significant improvement in recent years, with mortality rates from NPC decreasing significantly worldwide and local control rates for the disease 5 years after treatment improving significantly [40].

Treatment failure most commonly occurs due to distant disease. In the case of advanced disease with distant metastasis, to date, the only option for treatment remains chemotherapy, and while response rates are not poor, the mortality rate remains high in patients presenting at this late stage [9].

Surgical management in cases of NPC is generally reserved for recurrent disease or local failure. Radiotherapy may also be used in cases of local or nodal recurrence [9]. In the case of surgical salvage therapy, it is limited due to the excessively difficult access to the nasopharynx surgically. As such, treatment involves significant morbidity to the patient. Surgical approaches for salvage treatment vary according to the stage and local extent of disease, from an endoscopic approach, lateral skull base approach, midface degloving, maxillary swing and transpalatal approaches [41].

### 45.9.1 Complications of Treatment

As the main treatment in NPC is radiotherapy, it is expected that there are often significant morbidities associated with the management. Most commonly, local nasal complications occur, with nasal dryness, crusting, hyposmia, adhesions and sinusitis being the most common, treated accordingly. Other common issues are mucositis of the oral cavity and oropharynx and development of xerostomia, as well as development of otologic complications such as otitis externa or persistent otitis media. Dysphagia, neck stiffness and trismus may also develop after neck irradiation, significantly affecting quality of life when present [42, 43].

Most importantly, irradiation of the head and neck may increase the risk of future malignancy developing in any of the involved areas, commonly mucosal squamous cell carcinomas or sarcomas, and physicians should remain vigilant long-term in these patients in order to diagnose such conditions early [44].

As such, treatment of NPC in itself involves significant morbidity for the patient, requiring care and attention long term post-treatment in order to maintain a stable quality of life and avoid further progression of the disease. Clinicians must be cautious and aware of the array of issues faced by these complex patients in order to be able to manage them accordingly.

## 45.10 Conclusion

Nasopharyngeal carcinoma is a complex disease, with a wide array of presenting symptoms and a unique geographical distribution and pathogenesis, posing a challenge to healthcare workers and patients alike in the diagnosis. Recent advances in diagnostic tools and knowledge of disease aetiology have led to earlier diagnosis of disease, and the advent of IMRT and concurrent chemoradiation have significantly improved control rates for NPC patients. However, we must still remain vigilant in order to appropriately manage this complex condition and the morbidity associated with its treatment, and knowledge is the first and most important tool in order to achieve the best long-term outcomes.

**Case Study**

We present the case of a 78-year-old Caucasian patient, whose only relevant history was that of chronic rhinosinusitis with nasal polyps, operated multiple times over 10 years previously. This patient presented to the Emergency Department complaining primarily of severe hiccups and persistent headaches. The only other relevant symptoms, only revealed after detailed questioning, were a mild salty taste in the mouth and a sense of pressure in his left ear. An MRI of his paranasal sinuses and brain revealed a large left parapharyngeal mass with retropharyngeal extension, not impinging on his airway. He was therefore referred to our clinic, where a flexible nasal endoscopy revealed a mild fullness of the lateral postnasal space on the left. Accordingly, he was scheduled for a postnasal space biopsy, the results of which revealed a nasopharyngeal carcinoma. He went on to be treated with radiotherapy and remains to this day recurrence-free.

This case highlights the often-unclear presentation of NPC, with the non-specific symptoms of hiccups and headaches in this situation leading to an incidental finding of a parapharyngeal mass on MRI. The endoscopic findings in the nasopharynx were mild with no clear disease visualized. As such, it would be very easy to miss a diagnosis of nasopharyngeal carcinoma where a biopsy was not taken from the patient, making it prudent to be aware of all the possible constellations of presentations this unique carcinoma may present.

## References

1. Badoual C. Update from the 5th Edition of the World Health Organization Classification of Head and Neck Tumors: oropharynx and nasopharynx. Head Neck Pathol. 2022;16(1):19–30. https://doi.org/10.1007/s12105-022-01449-2. Epub 2022 Mar 21. PMID: 35312986; PMCID: PMC9019010.
2. Stelow EB, Wenig BM. Update from the 4th edition of the World Health Organization Classification of Head and Neck Tumours: nasopharynx. Head Neck Pathol. 2017;11(1):16–22. https://doi.org/10.1007/s12105-017-0787-0. Epub 2017 Feb 28. PMID: 28247232; PMCID: PMC5340728.
3. Brennan B. Nasopharyngeal carcinoma. Orphanet J Rare Dis. 2006;1:23. https://doi.org/10.1186/1750-1172-1-23. PMID: 16800883; PMCID: PMC1559589.

4. Guo R, Mao YP, Tang LL, Chen L, Sun Y, Ma J. The evolution of nasopharyngeal carcinoma staging. Br J Radiol. 2019;92(1102):20190244. https://doi.org/10.1259/bjr.20190244. Epub 2019 Jul 12. PMID: 31298937; PMCID: PMC6774596.
5. Young LS, Dawson CW. Epstein-Barr virus and nasopharyngeal carcinoma. Chin J Cancer. 2014;33(12):581–90. https://doi.org/10.5732/cjc.014.10197. Epub 2014 Nov 21. PMID: 25418193; PMCID: PMC4308653.
6. Tsao SW, Tsang CM, Lo KW. Epstein-Barr virus infection and nasopharyngeal carcinoma. Philos Trans R Soc Lond Ser B Biol Sci. 2017;372(1732):20160270. https://doi.org/10.1098/rstb.2016.0270. PMID: 28893937; PMCID: PMC5597737.
7. Zhou X, Cui J, Macias V, Kajdacsy-Balla AA, Ye H, Wang J, Rao PN. The progress on genetic analysis of nasopharyngeal carcinoma. Comp Funct Genomics. 2007;2007:57513. https://doi.org/10.1155/2007/57513. PMID: 18288251; PMCID: PMC2233780.
8. Liu Z, Chang ET, Liu Q, Cai Y, Zhang Z, Chen G, Huang QH, Xie SH, Cao SM, Shao JY, Jia WH, Zheng Y, Liao J, Chen Y, Lin L, Liang L, Ernberg I, Vaughan TL, Adami HO, Huang G, Zeng Y, Zeng YX, Ye W. Quantification of familial risk of nasopharyngeal carcinoma in a high-incidence area. Cancer. 2017;123(14):2716–25. https://doi.org/10.1002/cncr.30643. Epub 2017 Feb 27. PMID: 28241094; PMCID: PMC5498222.
9. Shah AB, Nagalli S. Nasopharyngeal carcinoma [Updated 2022 Oct 1]. In: StatPearls [Internet]. Treasure Island: StatPearls Publishing; 2024. https://www.ncbi.nlm.nih.gov/books/NBK554588/.
10. Okekpa SI, Mydin RBSMN, Mangantig E, NSA A, SNS Z, Kaur G, Musa Y. Nasopharyngeal carcinoma (NPC) risk factors: a systematic review and meta-analysis of the association with lifestyle, diets, socioeconomic and sociodemographic in Asian region. Asian Pac J Cancer Prev. 2019;20(11):3505–14. https://doi.org/10.31557/APJCP.2019.20.11.3505. PMID: 31759378; PMCID: PMC7063023.
11. Chang ET, Ye W, Zeng Y-X, Adami H-O. The evolving epidemiology of nasopharyngeal carcinoma. Cancer Epidemiol Biomarkers Prev. 2021;30(6):1035–47. https://doi.org/10.1158/1055-9965.EPI-20-1702.
12. Zhang Y, Rumgay H, Li M, Cao S, Chen W. Nasopharyngeal cancer incidence and mortality in 185 countries in 2020 and the projected burden in 2040: population-based global epidemiological profiling. JMIR Public Health Surveill. 2023;9:e49968. https://doi.org/10.2196/49968. https://publichealth.jmir.org/2023/1/e49968.
13. Yu H, Yin X, Mao Y, Chen M, Tang Q, Yan S. The global burden of nasopharyngeal carcinoma from 2009 to 2019: an observational study based on the Global Burden of Disease Study 2019. Eur Arch Otorhinolaryngol. 2022;279(3):1519–33. https://doi.org/10.1007/s00405-021-06922-2. Epub 2021 Jun 19. PMID: 34146150; PMCID: PMC8897385.
14. Song Y, Cheng W, Li H, Liu X. The global, regional, national burden of nasopharyngeal cancer and its attributable risk factors (1990–2019) and predictions to 2035. Cancer Med. 2022;11(22):4310–20. https://doi.org/10.1002/cam4.4783. Epub 2022 Apr 27. PMID: 35475595; PMCID: PMC9678109.
15. Ho FC, Tham IW, Earnest A, Lee KM, Lu JJ. Patterns of regional lymph node metastasis of nasopharyngeal carcinoma: a meta-analysis of clinical evidence. BMC Cancer. 2012;12:98. https://doi.org/10.1186/1471-2407-12-98. PMID: 22433671; PMCID: PMC3353248.
16. Tiong TS, Selva KS. Clinical presentation of nasopharyngeal carcinoma in Sarawak Malaysia. Med J Malaysia. 2005;60(5):624–8. PMID: 16515114.
17. Woollons AC, Morton RP. When does middle ear effusion signify nasopharyngeal cancer? N Z Med J. 1994;107(991):507–9. PMID: 7830981.
18. Alshahrani EH, Ismail A. Nasopharyngeal carcinoma presenting with occipital headache as a sole symptom in a young adult male: a case report. Cureus. 2023;15(4):e37801. https://doi.org/10.7759/cureus.37801. PMID: 37214037; PMCID: PMC10198749.
19. Wu Z-X, Xiang L, Rong J-F, He H-L, Li D. Nasopharyngeal carcinoma with headaches as the main symptom: a potential diagnostic pitfall. J Cancer Res Ther. 2016;12(1):209–14. https://doi.org/10.4103/0973-1482.157334.

20. Chow JCH, Lee A, Bao KKH, Cheung KM, Chan JCH, Tam AHP, Sung WWY, Tsui TYM, Chuk EYH, Chung DHS, Wong KH, Prayongrat A, Lertbutsayanukul C, Kannarunimit D, Chakkabat C, Kitpanit S. Cranial neuropathies in advanced nasopharyngeal carcinoma: neurological recovery after modern radiotherapy and systemic chemotherapy. Radiother Oncol. 2021;163:221–8. https://doi.org/10.1016/j.radonc.2021.08.022. Epub 2021 Sep 8. PMID: 34506830.
21. Pollard C III, Mesko SM, Ginsberg LE, Kies MS, Raza SM, Su SY, Tung S, Phan J. Nasopharyngeal carcinoma presenting as an inconspicuous primary lesion with extensive cavernous sinus involvement and temporal lobe extension: a case report and review of literature. Clin Case Rep. 2017;5(10):1682–8. https://doi.org/10.1002/ccr3.1166. PMID: 29026572; PMCID: PMC5628216.
22. Sakthivel P, Mohamed A, Guwariya M, Chirom AS. Trotter's triad. BMJ Case Rep. 2020;13(9):e237392. https://doi.org/10.1136/bcr-2020-237392. PMID: 32907871; PMCID: PMC7481091.
23. Jiménez-Caballero PE, Marsal-Alonso C, Alvarez-Tejerina A. Sindrome de Horner como primera manifestación del cáncer de cavum. A propósito de dos casos [Horner syndrome as the first symptom of nasopharyngeal cancer. Two case reports]. Rev Neurol. 2005;40(9):541–3. Spanish. PMID: 15898015.
24. Padungkiatsagul T, Poonyathalang A, Jindahra P, Cheecharoen P, Vanikieti K. Isolated Horner syndrome as a rare initial presentation of nasopharyngeal carcinoma: a case report. Int Med Case Rep J. 2018;11:271–6. https://doi.org/10.2147/IMCRJ.S177337. PMID: 30425588; PMCID: PMC6202048.
25. Ito T, Majima H, Ozawa T, Maeda M, Iwamoto S, Hirayama M, Azuma E. An unusual presentation of nasopharyngeal carcinoma as Lemierre syndrome. Am J Case Rep. 2019;20:263–7. https://doi.org/10.12659/AJCR.913755. PMID: 30814483; PMCID: PMC6441307.
26. Ozyar E, Cengiz M, Gurkaynak M, Atahan IL. Trismus as a presenting symptom in nasopharyngeal carcinoma. Radiother Oncol. 2005;77(1):73–6. https://doi.org/10.1016/j.radonc.2005.07.006. Epub 2005 Sep 12. PMID: 16154654.
27. Ng SY, Kongg MH, Yunus MR. Paraneoplastic neurological disorder in nasopharyngeal carcinoma. Malays J Med Sci. 2017;24(1):113–6. https://doi.org/10.21315/mjms2017.24.1.12. Epub 2017 Feb 24. PMID: 28381934; PMCID: PMC5346009.
28. Qudsiya Z, Waseem M. Dermatomyositis [Updated 2023 Aug 7]. In: StatPearls [Internet]. Treasure Island: StatPearls Publishing; 2024. https://www.ncbi.nlm.nih.gov/books/NBK558917/.
29. Irekeola AA, Shueb RH, Engku Nur Syafirah EAR, Wada Y, Abdul Rahman Z, Ahmad S, Mohamud R, Mat Lazim N, Yean CY. Prevalence of nasopharyngeal carcinoma in patients with dermatomyositis: a systematic review and meta-analysis. Cancers. 2021;13(8):1886. https://doi.org/10.3390/cancers13081886.
30. Qu W, Li S, Zhang M, Qiao Q. Pattern and prognosis of distant metastases in nasopharyngeal carcinoma: a large-population retrospective analysis. Cancer Med. 2020;9(17):6147–58. https://doi.org/10.1002/cam4.3301. Epub 2020 Jul 10. PMID: 32649056; PMCID: PMC7476823.
31. Chuang M-K, Hong R-L. Nasopharyngeal carcinoma and pulmonary lymphoepithelioma-like carcinoma—metastases or synchronous second primary cancer. J Cancer Res Pract. 2015;2(3):248–54. https://doi.org/10.6323/JCRP.2015.2.3.08. ISSN 2311-3006.
32. Jicman Stan D, Niculet E, Lungu M, Onisor C, Rebegea L, Vesa D, Bezman L, Bujoreanu FC, Sarbu MI, Mihailov R, Fotea S, Tatu AL. Nasopharyngeal carcinoma: a new synthesis of literature data (review). Exp Ther Med. 2022;23(2):136. https://doi.org/10.3892/etm.2021.11059. Epub 2021 Dec 13. PMID: 35069817; PMCID: PMC8756428.
33. Low WK. The contact bleeding sign of nasopharyngeal carcinoma. Head Neck. 1997;19(7):617–9. https://doi.org/10.1002/(sici)1097-0347(199710)19:7<617::aid-hed9>3.0.co;2-a. PMID: 9323151.
34. Goh J, Lim K. Imaging of nasopharyngeal carcinoma. Ann Acad Med Singap. 2009;38(9):809–16. PMID: 19816641.

35. King AD, Bhatia KS. Magnetic resonance imaging staging of nasopharyngeal carcinoma in the head and neck. World J Radiol. 2010;2(5):159–65. https://doi.org/10.4329/wjr.v2.i5.159. PMID: 21161030; PMCID: PMC2999022.
36. Liu W, Chen G, Gong X, et al. The diagnostic value of EBV-DNA and EBV-related antibodies detection for nasopharyngeal carcinoma: a meta-analysis. Cancer Cell Int. 2021;21:164. https://doi.org/10.1186/s12935-021-01862-7.
37. Tune CE, Liavaag P-G, Freeman JL, van den Brekel MWM, Shpitzer T, Kerrebijn JDF, Payne D, Irish JC, Ng R, Cheung RK, Dosch H-M. Nasopharyngeal brush biopsies and detection of nasopharyngeal cancer in a high-risk population. JNCI J Natl Cancer Inst. 1999;91(9):796–800. https://doi.org/10.1093/jnci/91.9.796.
38. Jiromaru R, Nakagawa T, Yasumatsu R. Advanced nasopharyngeal carcinoma: current and emerging treatment options. Cancer Manag Res. 2022;14:2681–9. https://doi.org/10.2147/CMAR.S341472. PMID: 36117730; PMCID: PMC9480178.
39. Zhou GQ, Wu CF, Deng B, et al. An optimal posttreatment surveillance strategy for cancer survivors based on an individualized risk-based approach. Nat Commun. 2020;11:3872. https://doi.org/10.1038/s41467-020-17672-w.
40. Bai R, Sun J, Xu Y, Sun Z, Zhao X. Incidence and mortality trends of nasopharynx cancer from 1990 to 2019 in China: an age-period-cohort analysis. BMC Public Health. 2022;22(1):1351. https://doi.org/10.1186/s12889-022-13688-7. PMID: 35840964; PMCID: PMC9284805.
41. Tsang RK, Wei WI. Salvage surgery for nasopharyngeal cancer. World J Otorhinolaryngol Head Neck Surg. 2015;1(1):34–43. https://doi.org/10.1016/j.wjorl.2015.09.006. PMID: 29204538; PMCID: PMC5698510.
42. Fang C, Zhong Y, Chen T, Li D, Li C, Qi X, Zhu J, Wang R, Zhu J, Wang S, Ruan Y, Zhou M. Impairment mechanism of nasal mucosa after radiotherapy for nasopharyngeal carcinoma. Front Oncol. 2022;12:1010131. https://doi.org/10.3389/fonc.2022.1010131. PMID: 36591522; PMCID: PMC9797686.
43. Wang C, Wang F, Min X, Zhang Q, Shen LJ, Jiang Y, Yan J. Toxicities of chemoradiotherapy and radiotherapy in nasopharyngeal carcinoma: an updated meta-analysis. J Int Med Res. 2019;47(7):2832–47. https://doi.org/10.1177/0300060519858031. Epub 2019 Jul 5. PMID: 31272262; PMCID: PMC6683919.
44. Wang WJ, Li M, Pan XB. Risk factors of secondary cancer in nasopharyngeal carcinoma patients after radiotherapy. J Cancer. 2022;13(13):3452–62. https://doi.org/10.7150/jca.77768. PMID: 36313032; PMCID: PMC9608213.

# External Approaches to the Nose and Paranasal Sinuses

# 46

Alaa Eldin Elfeky

**Key Points**

- External approaches to the nasal cavity and paranasal sinuses are procedures performed directly on the skin or mucous membrane to expose the facial skeleton and provide adequate space for osteotomies.
- Although endoscopic endonasal techniques in sinus surgery have reduced the indications for external approaches, it is not technically possible to use this in all cases and external approaches may be needed.
- The sinonasal surgeon should be familiar with external approaches.

**Principal Goals of Using External Approach**

1. To remove the lesion completely.
2. To protect the intracranial structures.
3. To control CSF leakage.
4. To prevent posttraumatic inflammatory complications.
5. To restore facial bone contour and symmetry.

## 46.1 Classifications

According to anatomical sites and indications, external approaches can be indicated alone or can be combined with another approach for the following.

A. E. Elfeky (✉)
Faculty of Medicine, Zagazig University, Zagazig, Egypt
e-mail: AMElfeky@medicine.zu.edu.eg


S. Elwany (ed.), *Current Rhinology*,
https://doi.org/10.1007/978-3-031-70077-4_46

1. Nasal fossa and paranasal sinuses
   (a) Lateral rhinotomy
   (b) Mid-facial degloving
2. Frontal sinus
   (a) Trephination
   (b) Lynch procedure
   (c) Osteoplastic approach (bicoronal)
   (d) Open sky
   (e) Gullwing
   (f) Butterfly
3. Maxillary sinus
   (a) Caldwell-Luc
   (b) Swing maxillotomy
   (c) Weber-Ferguson
4. Ethmoid sinus
   (a) External ethmoidectomy
   (b) Transorbital ethmoidectomy
5. Sphenoid sinus
   (a) Sublabial transseptal approach
   (b) External sphenoethmoidectomy
6. Ligation of ethmoidal arteries.
7. Ligation of the internal maxillary artery

## 46.2 Relevant Anatomy

*The lateral wall of the nose* comprises the ethmoid labyrinth and middle turbinate, the medial wall of the maxilla, and the separate inferior turbinate. The nasal septum is medial, the orbital periosteum is lateral, the anterior skull base is superior, the hard palate is inferior and the nasopharynx and the sphenoid sinus are posterior.

*The lacrimal sac* lies posterior to the anterior lacrimal crest, and the bony naso-lacrimal duct passes inferiorly to open into the inferior meatus.

*The cribriform plates* of the ethmoid lie at approximately pupillary level, and the ethmoidal vessels provide an indication of the level of the cribriform plate.

*The anterior and posterior ethmoidal arteries* pass medially from the ophthalmic artery across the roof of the ethmoid into the nose. Mean distances of 24, 12 and 6 mm are important. A mean distance of 24 mm separates the anterior lacrimal crest from the anterior ethmoid artery, 12 mm separates the anterior ethmoidal artery from the posterior ethmoidal artery and 6 mm separates the posterior ethmoidal artery from the optic canal.

*The infraorbital nerve* exits its foramen on the anterior surface of the maxilla, just below the midpoint of the inferior orbital rim. It gives sensation to the skin of the cheek, upper lip, lateral nose and gingivae.

*The supratrochlear nerve* passes superiorly through the supratrochlear notch giving sensation to the forehead and anterior scalp.

## 46.3 Preoperative Assessment

The patient should undergo adequate clinical and radiological assessment. *CT* accurately identifies the extent of the lesion, bone destruction and cribriform plate invasion. *MRI* further demonstrates intracranial extension and dural penetration and differentiates tumours from mucous or mucosal swelling within the sinuses.

*Endoscopic examination* of the nose, nasopharynx and related areas should be carried out. *Histopathology* of the lesion should be confirmed by biopsy under local anaesthesia or by formal examination under general anaesthesia. *Distant metastasis* should be excluded by imaging of the neck, chest and abdomen or a bone scan.

*Eye assessment* of the visual field, visual acuity or proptosis by an ophthalmologist is mandatory.

### 46.3.1 Preoperative Counselling

The patient should be fully informed about the risks, surgical complications and the expected outcome. The surgeon usually explained some postoperative significant conditions such as bruising and swelling, that take several weeks to resolve, or temporary paraesthesia in the distribution of the infraorbital nerve. *Preoperative consent* includes discussing the facial incision, injury to the optic, supraorbital and supratrochlear nerves and CSF leak.

### 46.3.2 Preoperative Preparation

The operations are usually performed under general anaesthesia with an endotracheal tube placed centrally in the mouth and a pharyngeal pack. A ribbon gauze soaked with 1:1000 adrenaline is placed intranasally, and 1:200,000 adrenaline is injected into the incision sites. Perioperative antibiotics and metronidazole injections are advisable. The patient lies in the reversed Trendelenburg position with 15° of head-up tilt. The eyes should be taped or a temporary tarsorrhaphy performed on the side of the procedure.

## 46.4 Nasal Fossa and Paranasal Sinuses

### 46.4.1 Lateral Rhinotomy [1, 2]

#### 46.4.1.1 Indications

1. To allow resecting of a nasal tumour involving the lateral nasal wall, e.g., inverted papilloma.
2. To allow resecting of a limited tumour of the ethmoid sinuses.
3. To allow resecting of a lacrimal sac tumour.
4. To allow accessing a septal lesion or tumour.

5. To allow accessing a posterior nasal tumour, e.g., juvenile angiofibroma.
6. To allow debulking of an extensive nasal tumour before palliative radiotherapy or chemotherapy.
7. To remove a quite large and impacted foreign body in the nose, e.g., rhinoliths.
8. To be used as a part with other incisions in a major operation, e.g., maxillectomy.

#### 46.4.1.2 Contraindications

1. If the tumour is too extensive to be adequately removed, e.g., orbital involvement or intracranial spread.
2. If the tumour extends too far laterally or posteriorly.

#### 46.4.1.3 Incision

The incision for lateral rhinotomy extends from just above the medial canthus along the lateral aspect of the nose into the alar crease. If necessary, a wider exposure may be gained by splitting the upper lip (Fig. 46.1).

#### 46.4.1.4 Procedure

The incision is made by a scalpel, and the underlying soft tissues are dissected with electrocautery. The periosteum, together with the soft tissue, is elevated off the anterior wall of the maxilla as far lateral as the lateral aspect of the maxillary antrum and as far superior as the orbital rim to expose and preserve the infraorbital nerve.

The periorbita is then undermined off the lamina papyracea. Staying below the fronto-ethmoid suture line is a safety feature to avoid entrance into the anterior cranial fossa. The nasal cavity is then entered by incising the mucosa along the piriform aperture.

#### 46.4.1.5 Closure

The subcutaneous tissue is closed with 4-0 vicryl sutures placed close together.

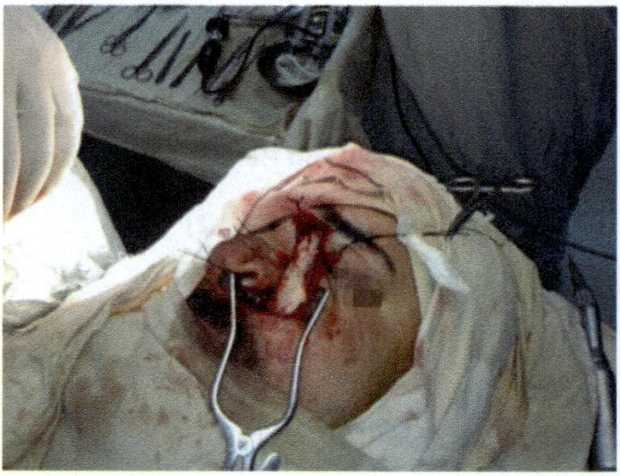

**Fig. 46.1** Lateral rhinotomy incision

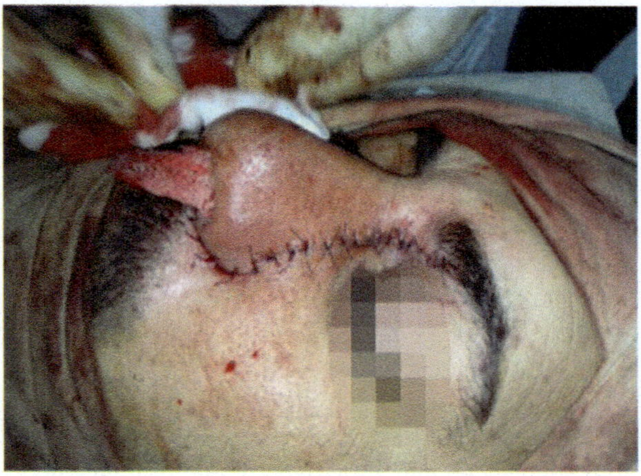

**Fig. 46.2** Closure of lateral rhinotomy incision

A 6-0 silk suture is used for the skin closure. If the lip has been split, the incision should be closed in four layers (mucosa, muscle, subcutaneous tissue and skin). A gentle pressure dressing may be used to prevent oedema of the face and upper lip (Fig. 46.2).

#### 46.4.1.6 Complications

1. Optic
   (a) Diplopia: Occurs due to trochlear trauma or displacement and is usually transient.
   (b) Epiphora: Occurs due to nasolacrimal duct trauma or stenosis and usually corrected by stenting the duct.
2. Nasal
   (a) CSF rhinorrhoea: If osteotomy during operation is performed superior to the frontoethmoid suture and should be repaired immediately.
   (b) Frontoethmoidal mucocele: This may occur later due to frontonasal duct stenosis or obstruction. This may be avoided by recognizing and stenting the duct during operation.
3. Neurological
   (a) Facial paraesthesia: Due to injury of the infraorbital nerve and may be avoided by limiting the dissection medial to the infraorbital nerve.
   (b) Dental paraesthesia: Due to injury of the superior alveolar nerve.
4. Cosmetic
   (a) Medial canthal webbing: Due to malalignment during skin closure. This may be avoided by accurate repositioning of the medial canthal ligament.
   (b) Unacceptable scar: Due to placement of the incision after distortion with infiltration anaesthesia. This may be avoided by ensuring precise realignment during skin closure.

## 46.4.2 Midfacial Degloving [3, 4]

### 46.4.2.1 Indications

1. Resection of sinonasal disease, e.g., dermoid cyst or hereditary haemorrhagic telangiectasia.
2. Resection of a benign tumour, e.g., inverted papilloma, angiofibroma and fibro-osseous dysplasia.
3. Resection of a selected low-grade malignant tumour of the maxillary, ethmoid or sphenoid sinus.
4. Resection of a limited malignant tumour of the inferior aspect of the nasal cavity or nasal septum.
5. Repair of a large septal perforation.
6. Repair of a midfacial fracture.
7. Patients who may have hyperplastic or pigmented scar.

### 46.4.2.2 Contraindications

1. Tumours extending to orbit, frontal sinus or cribriform plate.
2. It gives limited exposure to lesions of the superior ethmoid and frontoethmoidal recess.

### 46.4.2.3 Incision

A bilateral sublabial incision is made straight down to the bone from one maxillary tubercle to the other.

Bilateral septo-columellar and intercartilaginous incisions are made. A transfixion incision is made and connected to the intercartilaginous incision. An incision is carried laterally across the floor of the nose to join the transfixion incision and the intercartilaginous incision.

### 46.4.2.4 Procedure

The soft tissue attachments to the bone are sharply divided to release the nasal tip and expose the gingivobuccal sulcus. The upper lip is retracted, and the soft tissues are undermined as high as the orbital rim and infraorbital nerve. Superior and lateral dissection can deglove completely the mid-third of the face giving access to the nasal cavity and maxillae (Fig. 46.3).

### 46.4.2.5 Closure

After meticulous haemostasis, the frenulum must be correctly repositioned in the midline, and the sublabial and vestibular incisions can be sutured with 4-0 vicryl.

### 46.4.2.6 Complications

1. Stenosis of the vestibule: This may be avoided by proper repositioning and suturing of the nasal sutures.
2. Epiphora: This may be avoided by opening the lacrimal sac and suturing it to the surrounding soft tissue.

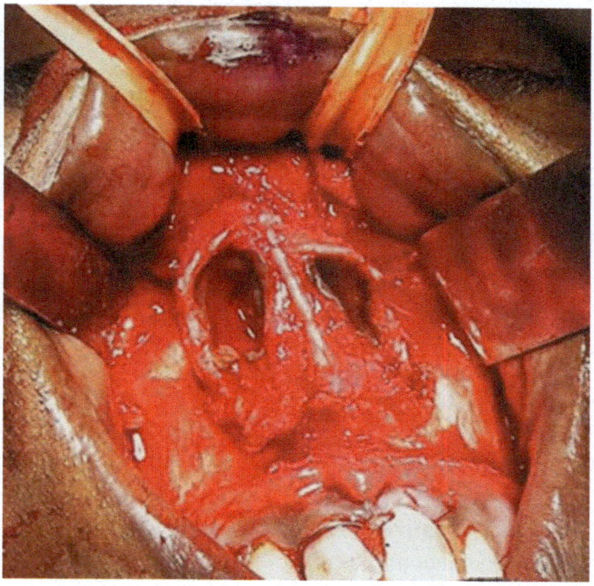

**Fig. 46.3** Mid-facial degloving

## 46.5 Frontal Sinus

### 46.5.1 Trephination [5, 6]

#### 46.5.1.1 Indication

1. Acute frontal sinusitis if symptoms fail to improve within 48 h of medical treatment.
2. If there is progression of the disease as characterized by symptoms and signs despite treatment.
3. Acute frontal sinusitis with orbital or intracranial complications.
4. Excision of small osteoma of the frontal sinus.

#### 46.5.1.2 Contraindications

1. The presence of anaplastic frontal sinus.
2. A history of keloid development.

#### 46.5.1.3 Incision

A 1-cm brow incision is made medial to the supraorbital nerve.

#### 46.5.1.4 Procedure

The periosteum is elevated to expose the anterior wall of the frontal sinus. A cutting burr is used to drill through the sinus. Commercial trephination sets are available to perform limited trephination through a very small incision (Fig. 46.4).

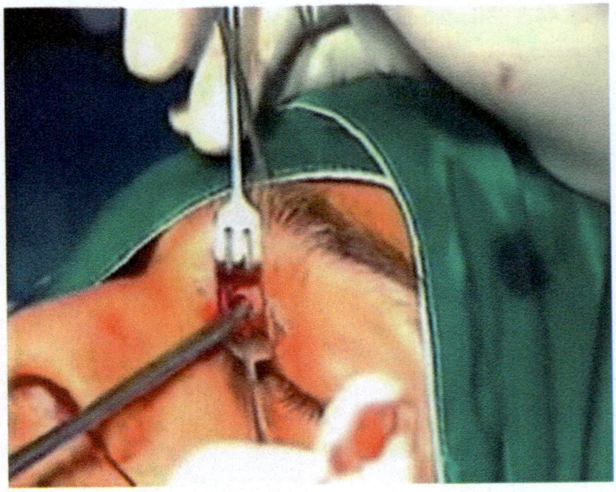

**Fig. 46.4** Trephination of the frontal sinus

#### 46.5.1.5 Closure

The subcutaneous tissue is closed with 3-0 vicryl, and the skin is closed with 4-0 silk.

#### 46.5.1.6 Complications

1. Injury of the orbit or anterior cranial fossa: This may be avoided by preoperatively reviewing the CT to estimate the depth and relations of the frontal sinus.
2. Recurrence: This can be avoided by removing the lateral wall of the frontonasal recess to provide communication between the frontal sinus and the middle meatus.

### 46.5.2 Lynch Procedure [7, 8]

#### 46.5.2.1 Indications

Patients who are not candidates for an endoscopic approach because of anatomic limitations have the following:

1. Chronic frontoethmoiditis unresponsive to medical treatment
2. Frontoehmoiditis with orbital complications
3. Frontoethmoidal mucocele
4. Frontoethmoidal recurrent polyposis
5. Dacryocystorhinostomy
6. Repair of CSF leak
7. Transethmoidal hypophysectomy

#### 46.5.2.2 Contraindications

1. The presence of anaplastic frontal sinus
2. A history of keloid development

#### 46.5.2.3 Incision

A curved incision is made midway between the nasal bridge and the medial canthus. Starting above the medial aspect of the upper eyelid and then carried inferiorly down to the level of the medial canthus.

#### 46.5.2.4 Procedure

The periosteum is elevated to expose the nasal process of the maxilla, the medial wall of the orbit and the frontal bone.

The lacrimal sac is elevated from its groove and displaced laterally. As dissection proceeds posteriorly, the lamina papyracea can be encountered and penetrated. Further dissection displays the anterior ethmoidal artery and then the posterior ethmoidal artery. A cutting burr is used to trephine the floor of the frontal sinus to communicate it with the anterior ethmoid air cells, which are usually removed until free communication with the middle meatus is obtained (Fig. 46.5).

#### 46.5.2.5 Closure

The periosteum of the trochlear region is reattached to that of the frontal region by non-absorbable vicryl, and the skin is closed with 4-0 silk. The frontal sinus may be drained with a temporary silastic tube into the middle meatus.

#### 46.5.2.6 Complications

1. Recurrence of the original pathology. This is usually due to frontonasal duct obstruction, which may be avoided by inserting a 1-cm diameter silastic tube running from the frontal sinus into the middle meatus.
2. Paraesthesia of the frontal region: This is due to injury of the supratrochlear nerve and may be avoided by placing the incision medial to the supratrochlear notch.

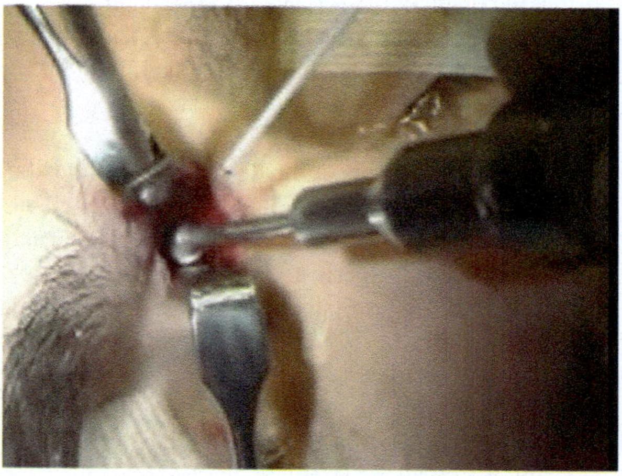

**Fig. 46.5** Lynch procedure

3. CSF leakage: This is due to penetration of the regions of the cribriform plate or superior attachment of the middle turbinate and can be avoided by careful reviewing of the CT preoperatively.
4. Diplopia: This is due to under-action of the superior oblique and is usually temporary and improves with time.

### 46.5.3 Osteoplastic Approach (Bicoronal) [9, 10]

#### 46.5.3.1 Indications

1. Trauma to the frontal sinus.
   (a) The anterior table is comminuted or displaced.
   (b) The posterior table displaced or the presence of bone fragments.
   (c) Sinus floor fractures involving the nasofrontal duct.
2. Chronic suppuration of the frontal sinus which has failed to respond to all other means of treatment.
3. Frontal mucocele.
4. Tumours of the frontal sinus, e.g., osteoma and fibrous dysplasia.

#### 46.5.3.2 Contraindications

1. Baldness
2. Strong family history of male pattern baldness

#### 46.5.3.3 Special Preoperative Preparation

1. A template of the frontal sinus is designed from an anteroposterior radiograph taken at 6 ft. of distance (Caldwell's view).
2. The hair is shaved 2–3 cm behind the hairline.
3. The patient lies in the reversed Trendelenburg position, with the head placed so that the plane of the forehead is horizontal.
4. Bilateral temporary tarsorrhaphies are performed.
5. The line of incision is infiltrated with 1:200,000 adrenaline.

#### 46.5.3.4 Incision

1. A bicoronal incision is made 2–3 cm behind the hairline, in a strip that has been shaved.
2. It is made through the skin, subcutaneous tissue and frontalis muscle, taking care not to damage the periosteum.
3. It is extended infero-laterally to just anterior to the root of the helix (Fig. 46.6).

#### 46.5.3.5 Procedure

1. The flap is raised in the plane between the frontalis muscle and the periosteum, as far as the supraorbital rims and glabella (Fig. 46.7).
2. Using the sterilized template, the frontal sinus is outlined using a marking pen.
3. The periosteum is incised around the outline and elevated 2–3 mm on either side.

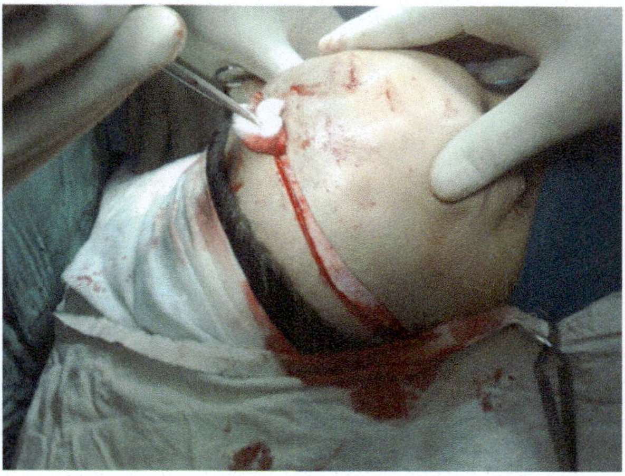

**Fig. 46.6** Bicoronal incision

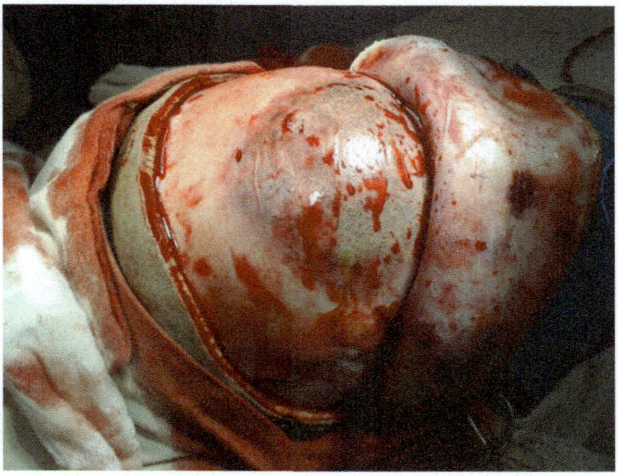

**Fig. 46.7** Elevation of the flap

4. The bone is cut with a fissure burr just within the outline and is bevelled to provide a supportive rim on closure (Fig. 46.8).
5. Care is taken to preserve the supraorbital and supratrochlear nerves.
6. The intersinus septum is broken with an osteotome allowing the flap to be moved down and forward, hinged inferiorly (Fig. 46.9).
7. The diseased mucosa or tumour can be removed.
8. If the nasofrontal duct is patent, it is better to preserve the mucous membrane and leave the duct intact.
9. If the duct is obstructed anywhere along its course from the frontal sinus to the infundibulum, either strip the mucosa very carefully and completely obliterate the duct or remove the obstruction and stent the duct.

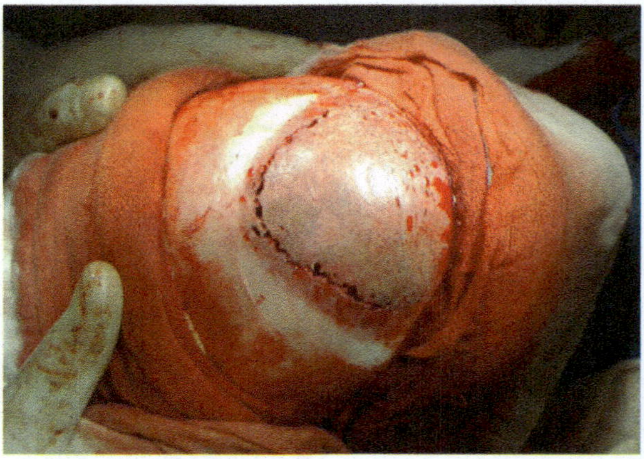

**Fig. 46.8** Outlining of the bony flap

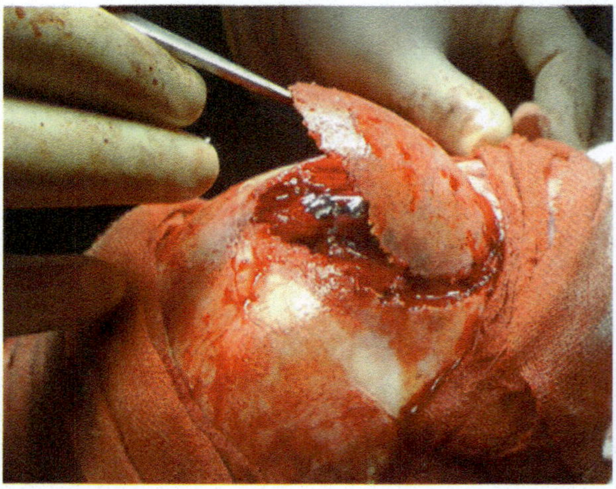

**Fig. 46.9** Elevation of the bony flap

#### 46.5.3.6 Closure

1. The bone flap is returned to its anatomic site.
2. Drill holes are placed in the bone flap and the surrounding bone to allow fixation of the flap with silk (Fig. 46.10).
3. The periosteal layer is sutured with vicryl.
4. Stables are used to close the skin (Fig. 46.11).
5. Drains may be inserted laterally.
6. A pressure dressing is applied for 48 h.

#### 46.5.3.7 Pitfalls, Complications and Instructions

1. Postoperative wound infection is relatively uncommon.
   (a) Perioperative and postoperative antibiotics contribute to the low incidence.
2. Haematoma under the flap.
   (a) This can be prevented by careful hemostasis, drains and a pressure dressing.

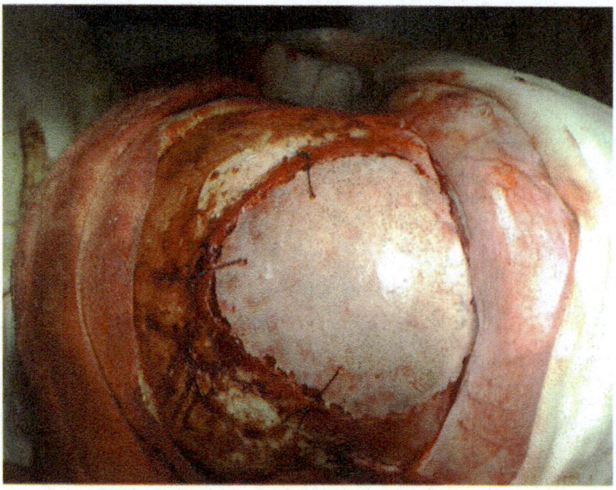

**Fig. 46.10** Fixation of the bony flap into place

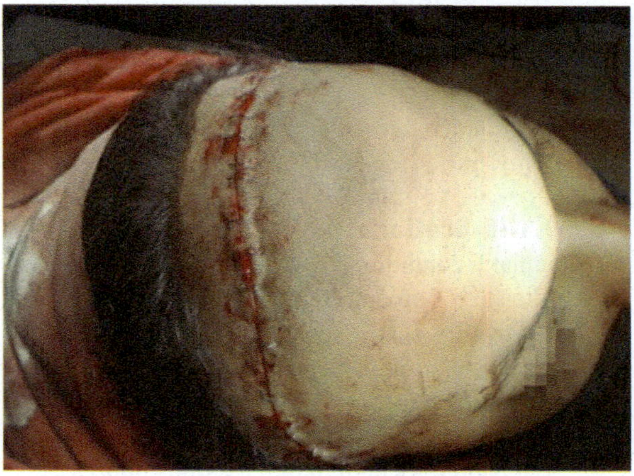

**Fig. 46.11** Closure of skin incision

3. Necrosis of the flap.
   (a) Preservation of the periosteum along the inferior edge of the anterior frontal sinus bone flap, forming a hinge, is most important because this is the source of blood supply to the periosteal bone flap.
4. Injury to the inner table during the initial cut through the outer table.
   (a) Bevel bone cuts inwards towards the sinus and makes it slightly smaller than the X-ray template.
5. Cerebrospinal fluid leak.
   (a) This is usually due to injury or trauma to the posterior table with a dural tear.
   (b) Preoperatively, the status of the posterior table should be carefully evaluated in every patient.
   (c) When compromise either due to infection or trauma is encountered, explore and repair dural defects at the time of the surgical procedure.

#### 46.5.3.8 Other Incisions

1. Open sky [11]
   (a) Two incisions in the medial orbital region connect over the nasal bridge.
   (b) It leaves a deforming scar over the nasion region.
2. Gullwing (eyeglass or spectacle) [11]
   (a) Two curved incisions at or inferior to the brow, ending at the nasion.
   (b) It leaves unattractive scars, which are highly visible because of their presence in the prominence on the brow and the resultant reflection of the light.
   (c) It usually divides the supraorbital nerve which results in paresthesia and numbness of the forehead.
3. Butterfly [11]
   (a) A combination of gullwing and the open sky incisions.
   (b) It leaves a deforming H-shaped scar over the brows and the nasion region.

## 46.6 Maxillary Sinus

### 46.6.1 Caldwell-Luc Operation [12, 13]

The technique of creating an opening in the canine fossa with an intranasal antrostomy.

#### 46.6.1.1 Indications

1. Traumatic conditions:
   Closure of oroantral fistula
2. Inflammatory conditions:
   This operation has been replaced by endoscopic techniques in most inflammatory conditions.
3. Neoplastic conditions:
   Excision of benign maxillary sinus tumour
   Biopsy and staging of palatal carcinoma
4. Access to other spaces:
   Access to pterygopalatine fossa
   Access to orbital floor
   Access to the medial wall of the maxilla

#### 46.6.1.2 Contraindications

Children less than 7 years of age
When a malignant lesion of the maxillary sinus is suspected

#### 46.6.1.3 Incision

A sublabial incision is carried from the canine tooth to the first molar. It is important to leave a 5-mm cuff of mucosa above the gingiva to facilitate closure of the mucosa at the end of the procedure.

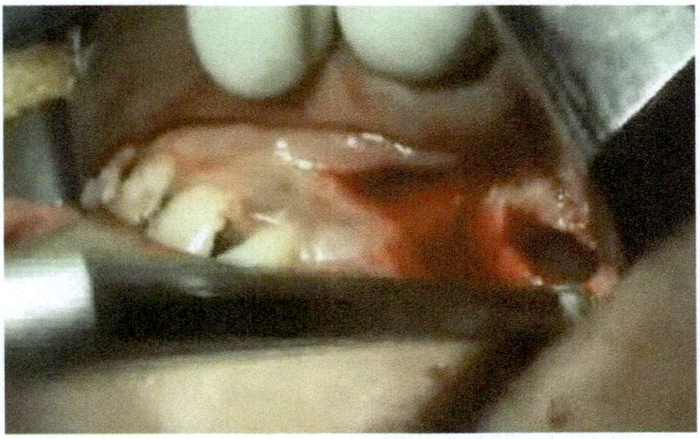

**Fig. 46.12** Caldwell-Luc operation

#### 46.6.1.4 Procedure

Dissecting in the subperiosteal plane, the soft tissue of the cheek is elevated to the level of the infraorbital nerve. The ideal place to open the maxillary sinus is the canine fossa, which is an area of thin bone just superior to the root of the canine tooth. A small hole is made with a drill or osteotome and enlarged with a bone rongeur to the margins of the sinus (pyriform sinus, orbital rim and maxillary alveolus) (Fig. 46.12).

#### 46.6.1.5 Closure

The mucosal flap of the incision is approximated with interrupted or continuous vicryl sutures.

#### 46.6.1.6 Complications

1. Facial oedema
2. Injure the infraorbital nerve
3. In paediatric patients, asymmetry of the facial skeleton and delayed eruption of secondary teeth

### 46.6.2 Swing Maxillotomy [14, 15]

It is an approach designed to facilitate access to the nasopharynx and middle cranial fossa skull base.

#### 46.6.2.1 Indications

1. Resection of tumours of the nasopharynx
2. Resection of tumours of the pterygopalatine fossa and pterygomaxillary fissure
3. Resection of palatal tumours
4. Resection of chordoma extending to the nasopharynx

#### 46.6.2.2 Contraindications

1. Tumours extending intracranially.

2. Severe trismus: Difficult to use osteotomes intraorally.
3. Children: The procedure may affect the development of the maxilla.

#### 46.6.2.3 Incision

The incision starts 2 cm lateral to the outer canthus of the eye, extending 5 mm below and parallel to the lower eyelid lash-line to the inner canthus. The incision turns inferiorly to follow the junction of the cheek and the lateral nose up to the ala. It then follows the alar groove around and into the nostril. The incision then continues to the midline at the junction of the columella and the lip, at which point it turns inferiorly through 90° and continues in the midline of the philtrum to the midline of the upper vermillion border of the lip.

The incision continues in the midline of the lip and through the superior labial frenulum of the buccal surface of the lip to the midline gingiva between the upper central incisors.

Make a paramedian incision on the hard palate extending from the junction of the hard and soft palate posteriorly to the premaxillary mucosa anteriorly, 7 mm from the midline on the side of the swing. Here, the incision then turns toward the midline and to the gingiva between the two upper central incisors.

The line of the posterior end of the hard palate incision is continued laterally through the mucosa of the soft palate to the posterior aspect of the maxillary tuberosity.

#### 46.6.2.4 Procedure

The soft tissue is dissected to expose bone for osteotomies. A straight horizontal osteotomy is marked at the level of the inferior margin of the infraorbital foramen, from the rim of the pyriform aperture medially to the malar aspect of the zygoma laterally. This osteotomy separates the bony orbit superiorly from the remaining maxilla/zygoma inferiorly. At the lateral end of this osteotomy, a second osteotomy is marked at 90° to the posteroinferior border of the zygoma. This osteotomy will complete the division of the zygoma. A third osteotomy is marked vertically in the midline of the anterior maxilla and extends between the medial incisors. This osteotomy divides the maxilla just off the midline so that the septum remains intact and articulates with the contralateral maxilla (Fig. 46.13).

#### 46.6.2.5 Closure

The osteotomies are fixed with mini plates and screws. The mucosa is closed with 3-0 vicryl, and the skin is closed with 6-0 silk.

#### 46.6.2.6 Complications

1. Bleeding: Avoided by meticulous haemostasis
2. Facial scar problems: Avoided by meticulous closure of the skin
3. Palatal fistula: Managed by a rotation palatal flap

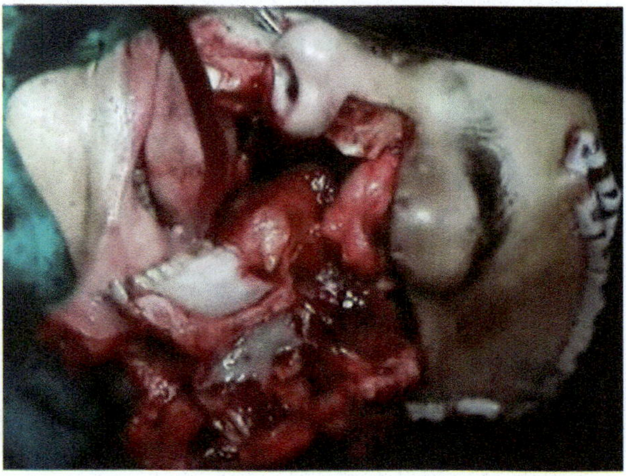

**Fig. 46.13** Maxillotomy

## 46.6.3 Weber Ferguson Approach [16, 17]

### 46.6.3.1 Indications

The Weber Ferguson approach is indicated for access for tumours involving the maxilla extending superiorly to the infraorbital nerve and into or involving the orbit. It provides wide access to all areas of the maxilla and orbital floor. Radical maxillectomy has usually been done by the classical Weber Ferguson incision since age-old times and still is being used widely due to its advantage of excellent exposure and minimal scarring as the incision follows the natural skin crease.

### 46.6.3.2 Contraindications

1. Lymphoreticular tumours that are best treated by nonsurgical means.
2. Extensive tumours that require bilateral maxillectomy.

### 46.6.3.3 Incision

The same as in maxillary swing but the lip-splitting incision is extended in two directions. Another incision turns laterally in front of the incisor and extends along the gingivobuccal sulcus to meet the first incision behind the maxillary tuberosity (Fig. 46.14).

### 46.6.3.4 Procedure

After dissecting the soft tissues, osteotomies start by dividing the zygomatic arch, continuing medially to the lateral part of the infraorbital fissure, extending across the anterior part of the floor of the orbit to include the infraorbital rim until it joins the pyriform aperture. The medial wall of the maxilla and the hard palate are transected. Inserting a curved osteotome between the maxillary tuberosity and the pterygoid plate will mobilize the maxilla completely and any attached soft tissue is divided with scissors (Fig. 46.15).

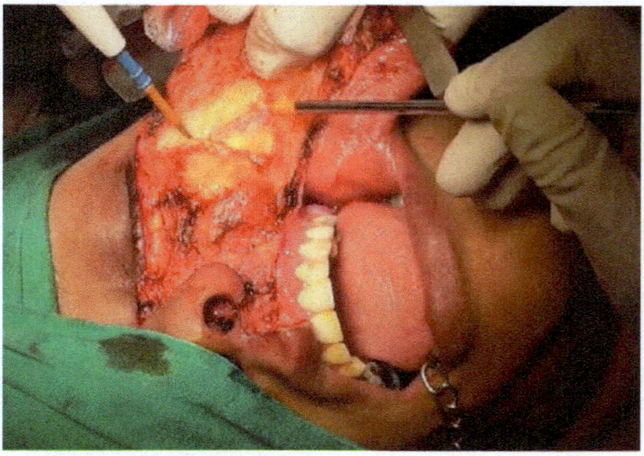

**Fig. 46.14** Elevation of the skin flap

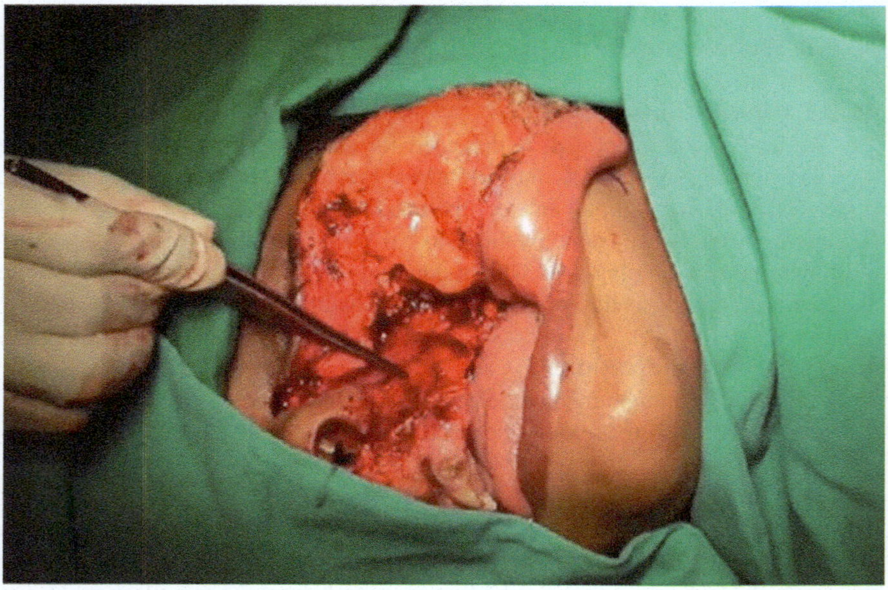

**Fig. 46.15** Excision of maxilla

#### 46.6.3.5 Closure

A split-thickness skin graft is used to cover raw areas and a temporary prosthesis is used to maintain the facial contour. A dental plate is attached to the dentition on the opposite side. The check flap is returned, and the wound is closed in layers.

#### 46.6.3.6 Complications

1. Bleeding: Avoided by the nasal pack and temporary prosthesis
2. Cosmetic problems such as ectropion: Avoided by making the incision not too close to the eyelid

## 46.7 Ethmoid Sinus

### 46.7.1 External Ethmoidectomy [18]

#### 46.7.1.1 Indications

The indications for external ethmoidectomy have been reduced by the advent of the endoscope, which is now mostly used in the management of ethmoid sinus disease.

1. Repair of nasal-orbital-ethmoid fractures
2. Acute ethmoiditis with orbital or periorbital abscess
3. Tumours of the ethmoid sinus
4. Approach to the sphenoid sinus and pituitary
5. Approach to the optic foramen for decompression and biopsy

#### 46.7.1.2 Contraindications

1. Coagulation defects
2. Acute infection in the absence of a complication
3. Low skull base or skull base erosion

#### 46.7.1.3 Incision

A curvilinear incision of 2–3 cm in length through the skin, subcutaneous tissue and periosteum is placed between the nasion and the medial canthus. The incision is positioned such that one-third of the incision extends above the medial canthus and two-thirds extend below the canthus.

#### 46.7.1.4 Procedure

1. The angular vessels are identified and ligated.
2. The lacrimal sac is elevated out of the lacrimal fossa.
3. The ethmoid labyrinth is entered, and the ethmoid mucosa is removed completely to enter the nasal fossa.
4. The anterior two-thirds of the lamina papyracea are removed.
5. The dissection through the ethmoid air cells is continued to reach the anterior wall of the sphenoid sinus.
6. Limits of dissection
   (a) Superiorly: Frontoethmoid sutures and anterior ethmoid artery (landmark of fovea ethmoidalis and base of the skull)
   (b) Posteriorly: Posterior ethmoid artery
   (c) Medially: Middle turbinate
   (d) Laterally: Posterior third of lamina papyraecea to protect the optic nerve
7. The anterior ethmoid artery is usually ligated, while the posterior ethmoid artery should not be ligated.

#### 46.7.1.5 Closure

1. Reapproximate the medial canthus to the periosteum.
2. Subcutaneous layer is closed with vicryl.
3. Skin is closed with subcuticular proline.

#### 46.7.1.6 Complications

1. Diplopia: If the trochlea fails to reattach postoperatively.
2. CSF leak: If there is dissection above the frontoethmoid suture line.
3. Facial scar: If the closure is not meticulous.

### 46.7.2 Transorbital Ethmoidectomy [19]

#### 46.7.2.1 Indications

1. Access to orbital floor in blowout fractures
2. Orbital decompression especially in Graves' disease

#### 46.7.2.2 Contraindications

If the lesion could be managed endoscopically to avoid cosmetic problems.

#### 46.7.2.3 Incision

The incision extends from the inner canthus below the lower lid to the midpoint of the orbital rim. The incision is made down to the bone.

#### 46.7.2.4 Procedure

The periosteum is elevated from the orbital floor and medial orbital wall. In the case of orbital decompression, bone can be removed laterally as far as the infraorbital nerve and superiorly as far as the ethmoidal vessels.

#### 46.7.2.5 Closure

The orbicularis muscle is sutured with vicryl, and the skin is closed with subcuticular proline.

#### 46.7.2.6 Complications

1. Epiphora
2. Diplopia
3. Cosmetic problems

## 46.8 Sphenoid Sinus

### 46.8.1 Sublabial Transseptal Approach [20, 21]

#### 46.8.1.1 Indications

1. Resection of lesions located in the middle of the skull base
2. The procedure of choice for the surgical treatment of pituitary adenomas with a primary sellar extension

#### 46.8.1.2 Contraindications

1. Acute sphenoid sinusitis

2. Intrasellar vascular anomalies
3. Ecstatic midline carotid arteries
4. Significant lateral suprasellar extension of the tumour

#### 46.8.1.3 Incision

Anterior hemitransfixion incision is made of the nasal septum on the left side. Anterior and posterior tunnels are raised and the decussating fibres separating the two tunnels are divided. A gingivobuccal sulcus incision from premolar to premolar is made down to bone.

#### 46.8.1.4 Procedure

All soft tissues are elevated off the bone. The bone of the posterior septum is removed. The anterior face of the sphenoid is exposed. The sphenoid is entered through its ostium or a natural dehiscence. The front wall of the sphenoid is removed maximally by a punch forceps.

#### 46.8.1.5 Closure

Flaps are approximated with each other with vicryl. The gingivobuccal incisions are closed with 3-0 vicryl. Splints and packing are often used.

#### 46.8.1.6 Complications

1. Injury of the carotid artery
2. Injury of the optic nerve
3. CSF leakage

### 46.8.2 External Sphenoethmoidectomy Approach [22]

During external ethmoidectomy, the sphenoid sinus can be opened by removing its anterior wall. Diseased mucosa, polyps or tumours can be removed.

## 46.9 External Ligation of Ethmoidal Arteries [23, 24]

### 46.9.1 Indications

Uncontrolled epistaxis above the middle turbinate.

### 46.9.2 Contraindications

Anatomical deformity or vascular lesions endangering the optic nerve.

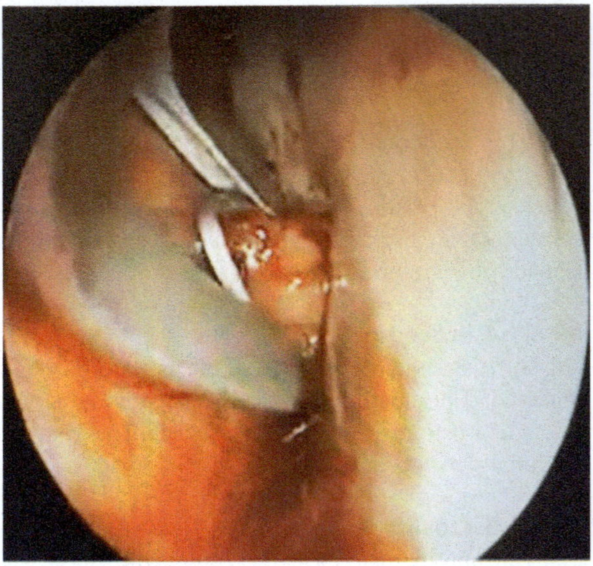

**Fig. 46.16** Clipping of anterior ethmoid artery

### 46.9.3 Incision

A curved incision of about 3 cm in length is made medial to the inner canthus. The periosteum is incised and elevated to expose the fronto-maxillo-lacrimal suture.

### 46.9.4 Procedure

The angular vessels are identified and ligated. The anterior ethmoidal artery is identified by following the frontoethmoid suture line (13-18 mm), two sliver clips are placed and the vessel is transected. About 10-13 mm from the anterior ethmoidal artery, the posterior ethmoid artery is identified, two silver clips are placed and the vessel is transected taking care of the optic nerve which is just 4-7 mm posteriorly (Fig. 46.16).

### 46.9.5 Closure

The wound is closed in layers with a drain.

## 46.10 Ligation of Internal Maxillary Artery [25, 26]

### 46.10.1 Indications

Epistaxis posteriorly after failure of nasal packing.

### 46.10.2 Contraindications

Anatomical deformity or vascular malformations.

### 46.10.3 Incision

A Caldwell-Luc operation with a large opening is done.

### 46.10.4 Procedure

An operating microscope may be used for magnification. The periosteum of the posterior wall of the maxillary sinus is elevated and based laterally. The thin posterior inferior wall of the sinus is removed by a burr. Adipose tissue is dissected to identify the main trunk of the internal maxillary artery. The artery is occluded with clips proximally and distally and may be transected.

### 46.10.5 Closure

The mucoperiosteal flap is replaced, and the Caldwell-Luc incision is closed with 4-0 vicryl.

### 46.10.6 Complications

1. Facial numbness and pain
2. Infection of the pterygomaxillary space

## References

1. Saumik D, Pranabashish B, Anup D, Ramanuj S. Lateral rhinotomy—revisited. Indian J Otolaryngol Head Neck Surg. 2007;59(3):215–20.
2. Hussain A, Hilmi OJ, Murray DP. Lateral rhinotomy through nasal aesthetic subunits. Improved cosmetic outcome. J Laryngol Otol. 2006;116(9):703.
3. Zachariah T, Neelakandan RS. Utility of the midface degloving approach for extended exposure in maxillary pathologies. J Maxillofac Oral Surg. 2020;19(2):217–24.
4. Ferreiraa LM, Nascimento AS, Gomesc EF, Azevedod JF, Araújoe RP, Moraesf RB. Midfacial degloving - access to nasal cavity and paranasal sinuses lesions. Braz J Otorhinolaryngol. 2006;72(2):158–62.
5. David M, Poetker MD, Todd A, Loehrl MD, Robert J, Toohill MD. Frontal sinus trephination for acute sinusitis. Oper Tech Otolaryngol Head Neck Surg. 2010;21(2):130–3.
6. Megía R, Lobo D, Viera J. Indication of frontal sinus trephination procedure. In: Atlas of frontal sinus surgery. Cham: Springer; 2022. p. 201–6.

7. Neel HB, McDonald TJ, Facer GW. Modified Lynch procedure for chronic frontal sinus disease: rationale, technique, and long-term results. Laryngoscope. 1987;97:1274–9.
8. Kennedy DW, Hwang PH, Stammberger HR. Diseases of the nose, sinuses, and skull base: external approaches to the paranasal sinuses. In: External frontoethmoidectomy. Stuttgart: Georg Thieme Verlag KG; 2012.
9. Manuel TR, Pulido R, Alcántara GL. Current indications for the osteoplastic flap. Acta Otorrinolaringol Esp. 2016;67(1):33–9.
10. Pagella F, Maiorano E, Turri-Zanoni M, Ferrari M, Carena P, Zoia C, Czaczkes C, Conti C, Schreiber A, Battaglia P, Emanuelli E, Pelucchi S, Bignami M, Nicolai P, Castelnuovo P. The role of the osteoplastic flap in the endoscopic era: a retrospective multicentre experience on revision surgery. Acta Otorhinolaryngol Ital. 2023;43(Suppl. 1):S34–40.
11. Lawson W, Ho Y. Open frontal sinus surgery: a lost art. Otolaryngol Clin North Am. 2016;49(4):1067–89.
12. Huang YC, Chen WH. CaldwellLuc operation without inferior meatal antrostomy: a retrospective study of 50 cases. J Oral Maxillofac Surg. 2012;70(9):20804.
13. Kim E, Duncavage J. Caldwell-Luc procedure. Oper Tech Otolaryngol Head Neck Surg. 2010;21(3):163–5.
14. Kalra GS, Midya M, Bedi M. Access to the skull base—maxillary swing procedure—long term analysis. Ann Maxillofac Surg. 2018;8(1):86–90.
15. Gonzalez MA, Pieper DR, Cambra JB, Simman R, Jackson IT. Skull base tumors: a comprehensive review of transfacial swing osteotomy approaches. Plast Reconstr Surg. 2005;115:711–20.
16. Rajasekhar G, Vura NG, Sudhir R, Srikanth Dhanala S, Alwala AM. Versatility of Dieffenbach's modification of Weber Fergusson's approach for treatment of maxillary pathologies. J Maxillofac Oral Surg. 2012;11(4):416–9.
17. Amy L, Pittman MD, Chad A, Zender MD. Total maxillectomy. Oper Tech Otolaryngol Head Neck Surg. 2010;21(3):166–70.
18. Neal GD. External ethmoidectomy. Otolaryngol Clin. 1985;18(1):55–8.
19. Desouza C, Menezes CA, D'souza M, Shah A, Morris MS. Pediatric proptosis and transorbital fronto-ethmoidectomy. Orbit. 1990;9(1):19–27.
20. Eisele DW, Flint PW, Janas JD, Kelly WA, Weymuller EA Jr, Cummings CW. The sublabial transseptal transsphenoidal approach to sellar and parasellar lesions. Laryngoscope. 1988;98(12):1301–8.
21. Mark S, Persky MD. The sublabial transseptal approach to the pituitary gland. Oper Tech Otolaryngol Head Neck Surg. 2003;14(3):199–203.
22. Unlu HH, Songu M, Ovali GY, Nese N. (External sphenoethmoidectomy). Inverted papilloma with new bone formation: report of three cases. Am J Rhinol. 2007;21(5):607.
23. Kulvin M. Epistaxis: control by ligation of anterior ethmoidal artery. Arch Otolaryngol. 1955;62(1):84–9.
24. Manjila S, Cox E, Robert T, Geertman T. Extracranial ligation of ethmoidal arteries before resection of giant olfactory groove or planum sphenoidale meningiomas: 3 illustrative cases with a review of the literature on surgical techniques. Neurosurg Focus. 2013;35:E13.
25. Lin G, Bleier B. Surgical management of severe epistaxis. Otolaryngol Clin. 2016;49(3):627–37.
26. Hirsch C. Ligation of the internal maxillary artery in patients with nasal haemorrhage. Arch Otolaryngol. 1936;24(5):589–93.

# 47 Primary Open Rhinoplasty

Wael Khamis Hussien

**Key Points**

- The external nose is a visible component of the face and can be divided topographically into three units: the frontal, lateral, and basal units.
- The lower lateral cartilages are the most important structure for tip projection and support, while the lateral crura are important for tip definition and shape.
- The internal nasal valve (INV) is the narrowest segment of the nasal airway and is typically located approximately 1.3 cm from the nares. The external nasal valve is formed by the caudal septum, the medial crura of the alar cartilage, and the lateral nasal wall. The nasal valves play an important role in regulating the flow and resistance of air entering the nasal cavity during breathing.
- Patient evaluation is a critical component of the rhinoplasty process. It involves a thorough assessment of the patient's medical history, physical characteristics, expectations, and desires for the outcome of the procedure.
- Nasal analysis is an essential part of the evaluation process for rhinoplasty. During nasal analysis, the surgeon evaluates the structure, shape, and size of the nose to determine the underlying anatomy and to identify potential issues that need to be addressed during surgery.
- External rhinoplasty, also known as open rhinoplasty, is a surgical approach used to reshape the nose. It provides better access to the nasal framework.

W. K. Hussien (✉)
Department of Otolaryngology, Alexandria University, Alexandria, Egypt
e-mail: wael.khamis@alexmed.edu.eg


S. Elwany (ed.), *Current Rhinology*,
https://doi.org/10.1007/978-3-031-70077-4_47

Nasal reconstruction may seem like a fairly modern procedure because of its association with celebrities, but, in fact, rhinoplasty has a very rich history. The origins of rhinoplasty can be traced back as far as ancient Egypt, where criminals were sometimes punished by having their noses cut off. Some of the earliest recorded surgical techniques for reconstructing the nose date back to the Roman Empire, as described in Aulus Cornelius Celsus' De Medicina. In India, the physician Sushruta described a plastic surgical operation for reconstructing a nose destroyed by rhinectomy in the sixth century BCE. The history of rhinoplasty continued to evolve and develop over time, with notable advancements and contributions from various cultures and individuals throughout history. Today, rhinoplasty is a common plastic surgery procedure with a range of techniques and approaches available to surgeons [1].

## 47.1 External Nose Anatomy

The external nose is a visible component of the face and can be divided topographically into three units: the frontal, lateral, and basal units. The frontal region includes the bridge of the nose, the root, and the apex. The lateral region includes the sides of the nose and the nasal alae, and the basal region includes the nostrils and the nasal septum which separates the nostrils. The external nose is made up of skin, subcutaneous tissue, muscles, and cartilage, and its shape and size vary greatly among individuals and populations.

### 47.1.1 External Nasal Skin and Soft Tissue

The external skin of the nose is composed of several specific anatomical and histological subunits that determine the aesthetic appearance of the nose. The majority of the nasal skin is made up of sebaceous skin, and whenever possible, scar lines should be placed along relaxed skin in order to minimize their visibility. The skin over the cartilaginous part of the nose is thicker and contains numerous sebaceous glands. Some sebaceous noses cannot be reduced in size because of redundant skin. The external nasal skin is supplied by ophthalmic (V1) and maxillary (V2) branches of the trigeminal (CN V) nerve [2].

### 47.1.2 Nasal Bones and Cartilages

The nose is supported by both bone and cartilage. The nasal skeleton is a combination of bone and cartilage, which forms both what we can see as the external nose and the internal nasal septum. The bone supports the back and bridge of the nose, while the cartilage supports the front of the nose, including the septum, the bilateral alar and lateral cartilages, and the upper lateral cartilages that underlie the nasal bones cephalically and articulate with the nasal septum medially. The nasal septum consists of bone posteriorly and cartilage anteriorly, with the perpendicular plate of the ethmoid bone superiorly and the vomer inferiorly making up the bony part of the septum.

The bony structures of the nasal framework are located caudal to the cartilaginous structures. The two upper lateral cartilages are paired and are attached caudally to the nasal bone. The middle third of the nose's strength is determined by how well the upper lateral cartilages adhere to the nasal bones where they overlap. Stronger overlap between the upper lateral cartilages and longer nasal bones results in stronger middle third strength. When longer nasal bones are present, dorsal reduction of the nose may be more tolerable with less aesthetic and functional deformity of the middle third of the nose. In the scroll region, the lower lateral cartilages roughly correspond to the upper lateral cartilages. The nasal ala is created when the lower lateral cartilages medially oppose one another and curl outward at the nasal tip. The cartilaginous septum, which is made up of the quadrangular cartilage that lies ventrally to the bony nasal septum, provides additional structural support. The nasal septum is attached dorsally to the upper and lower lateral cartilage which provides structural support.

The nasal vault refers to the bony and cartilaginous framework of the nose. It is divided into three main parts: the upper third, which is made up of bone; and the middle and lower thirds, which are made up of cartilage. The upper third is composed of the two nasal bones, which are attached to the frontal bone superiorly and laterally to the maxillary bones. The middle vault represents the middle third of the nose, which consists anatomically of the two upper lateral cartilages and the dorsal part of the septal cartilage. The lower third is composed of the lower lateral cartilages, which form the tip of the nose and the paired sesamoid cartilages at the base of the nasal septum. These cartilages provide structural support and shape to the nose. Surgical manipulation of the nasal vault may be necessary to correct structural defects or to improve aesthetic appearance [3].

### 47.1.3 Nasal Tip

The nasal tip is an important subunit of the nose and can be divided into several structures including the lower lateral cartilages, medial crura, lateral crura, domes, and soft tissue envelope. The lower lateral cartilages are the most important structures for tip projection and support, while the lateral crura are important for tip definition and shape. The medial crura connects the lower lateral cartilages to the nasal septum, and the domes are the most distal part of the lower lateral cartilages, contributing to tip definition and refinement. The soft tissue envelope, including the skin and subcutaneous tissue, also plays an important role in the appearance of the nasal tip (Fig. 47.1).

A thorough understanding of nasal tip anatomy is important for performing rhinoplasty and achieving optimal aesthetic results. Knowledge of the complex three-dimensional relationship between the various nasal tip structures is essential, as is an understanding of the underlying functional anatomy involved in nasal breathing.

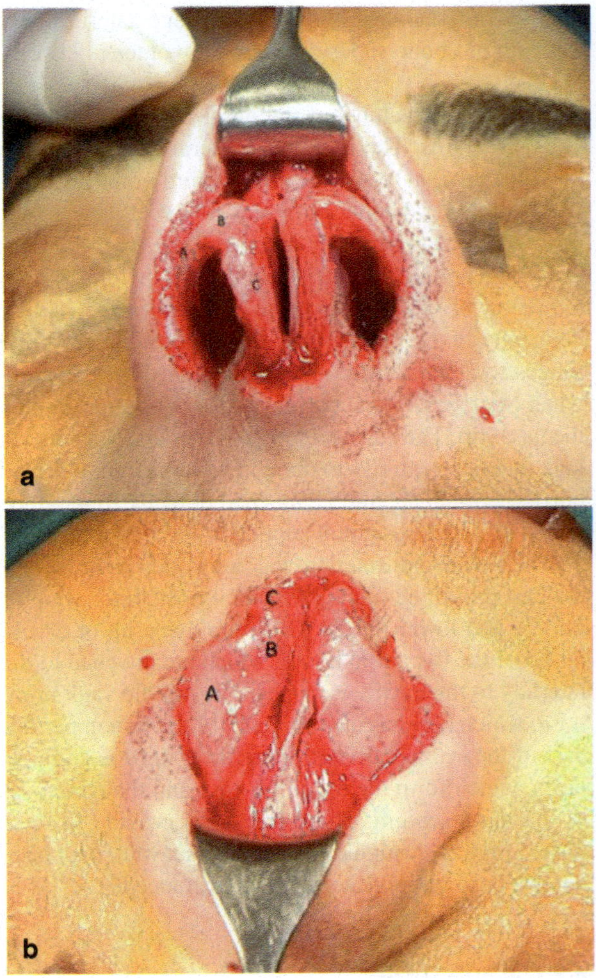

**Fig. 47.1** Overview of the units of the alar cartilage. (**a**) Lateral crus. (**b**) Intermediate or domal crus. (**c**) Lateral crus

Anderson's tripod model is a concept in rhinoplasty (nose job) surgery that describes the structural support of the nasal tip. It was first introduced by Dr. Jack Anderson in 1969 and describes the nasal tip support provided by three key structures: the medial crura, lateral crura, and the caudal septum. These structures form a tripod-like framework that supports and shapes the nasal tip. The tripod model explains that any changes made to one of the structures will affect the position of the others, making it a useful concept for understanding how rhinoplasty procedures can alter the shape and projection of the nasal tip [4].

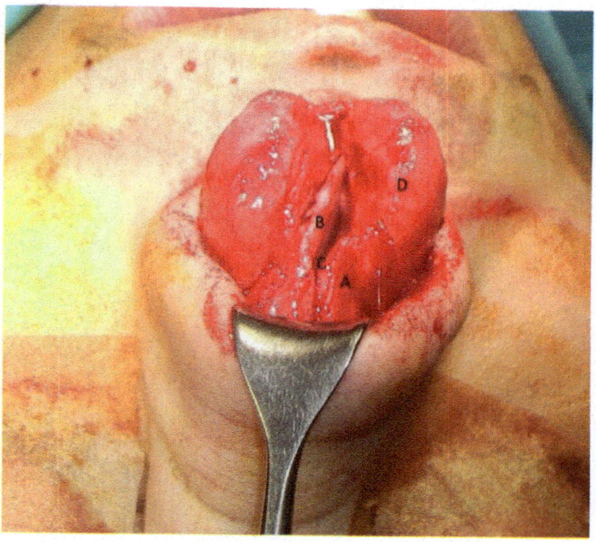


**Fig. 47.2** (**a**) Upper lateral cartilage. (**b**) Caudal cartilaginous septum. (**c**) Internal nasal valve angle. (**d**) Alar cartilage

### 47.1.4 Internal Nasal Valve

The internal nasal valve (INV) is the narrowest segment of the nasal airway and is typically located approximately 1.3 cm from the nares. It is considered to be the most significant point of nasal airway resistance, accounting for a larger part of the nasal resistance. The INV is bounded by the caudal margin of the upper lateral cartilage laterally, the nasal septum medially, and the head of the inferior turbinate inferiorly. The INV is where the nasal walls come closest together, and it is covered by skin with hair and vibrissae [5] (Fig. 47.2).

The upper lateral cartilage defines the caudal margin of the INV, from its caudal border to its attachment at the piriform aperture, and it is also known as the internal nasal valve area. The lower lateral cartilage, located below the upper lateral cartilage, and the septum, located medially, are also important in defining the nasal valve complex.

The INV is subject to collapse, particularly during inspiration, which can result in a decrease in nasal airflow and increased nasal resistance, leading to nasal obstruction. Surgical procedures aimed at increasing the dimensions of the INV are commonly performed to alleviate nasal obstruction. These procedures can include a variety of techniques such as spreader grafts, batten grafts, alar rim grafts, and inferior turbinate reduction.

Overall, understanding the anatomy of the internal nasal valve is important for the management of patients with nasal obstruction and for performing surgical procedures intended to alleviate it.

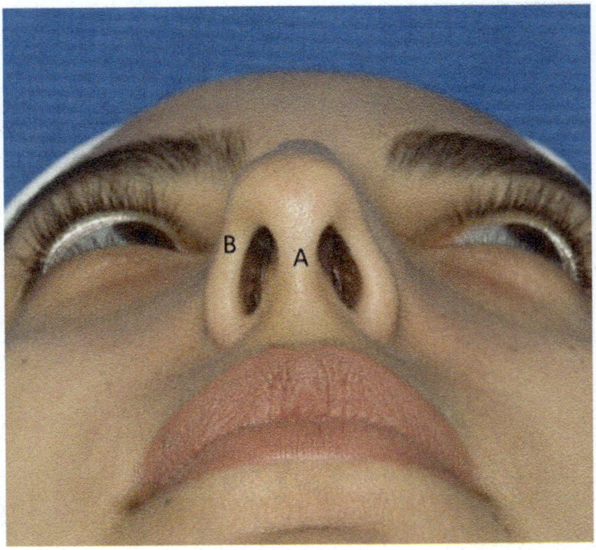


**Fig. 47.3** External nasal valve angle formed by the (**a**) caudal septum, the medial crura of the alar cartilages and (**b**) the lateral nasal wall

### 47.1.5 External Nasal Valve

The external nasal valve is an anatomical structure located in the nasal vestibule. It is formed by the caudal septum, the medial crura of the alar cartilage, and the lateral nasal wall. The external nasal valve plays an important role in regulating the flow and resistance of air entering the nasal cavity during breathing. Dysfunction in the external nasal valve can lead to nasal obstruction, which is a common complaint among patients seeking nasal surgery. Appropriate diagnosis and treatment of external nasal valve dysfunction is important for maintaining adequate nasal function and quality of life [6] (Fig. 47.3).

## 47.2 Patient Evaluation in Rhinoplasty

Patient evaluation is a critical component of the rhinoplasty process. It involves a thorough assessment of the patient's medical history, physical characteristics, expectations, and desires for the outcome of the procedure. A comprehensive evaluation should be conducted to determine if the patient is a good candidate for the surgery and to develop a customized surgical plan that will achieve the desired results.

The following are some key factors that are typically evaluated during the patient evaluation process in rhinoplasty.

1. Medical history: The surgeon will review the patient's medical history to identify any preexisting medical conditions, allergies, and medication use that may affect the surgery.

2. Nasal anatomy: The surgeon will evaluate the patient's nasal anatomy, including the shape, size, and symmetry of the nose, as well as any structural issues such as a deviated septum or nasal obstruction.
3. Skin quality: The surgeon will assess the quality and thickness of the patient's nasal skin, as this can impact the surgical approach and potential outcomes.
4. Goals and expectations: The surgeon will discuss the patient's goals and expectations for the procedure and assess whether they are realistic and achievable through surgery.
5. Psychological assessment: The surgeon may conduct a psychological assessment to determine whether the patient has a healthy mindset and realistic expectations for the surgery.

## 47.3 Nasal Analysis

Nasal analysis is an essential part of the evaluation process for rhinoplasty, which is a surgical procedure performed to reshape the nose. During nasal analysis, the surgeon evaluates the structure, shape, and size of the nose to determine the underlying anatomy and to identify any potential functional or aesthetic issues that need to be addressed during the procedure.

The nasal analysis typically includes a detailed examination of the external and internal structures of the nose, including the nasal bones, cartilage, septum, and nasal passages. The surgeon will also evaluate the patient's facial proportions, skin type, and overall facial symmetry to determine the optimal surgical approach.

Based on the results of the nasal analysis, the surgeon will develop a customized surgical plan that is tailored to the patient's individual needs and goals. This plan may involve reshaping the nasal bones, reducing or augmenting the cartilage, adjusting the position of the septum, or addressing other functional or cosmetic concerns.

Overall, nasal analysis is an important step in the rhinoplasty process, as it allows the surgeon to develop a safe and effective surgical plan that can achieve the desired results while minimizing the risk of complications.

While rhinoplasty surgery is part art, defining the problem areas of the nose can be done in a more structured, reproducible method. A systematic assessment of the nose's anatomy in relation to other facial characteristics is necessary to identify any elements that can cause actual or perceived incongruity or asymmetry [7].

The principle of dividing the face into horizontal thirds and vertical fifths is a useful method of evaluating facial features. The division into these units allows for the definition of symmetry of the face. The Frankfort horizontal is a theoretical line drawn from the superior point of the external auditory canal to the inferior aspect of the infraorbital rim or the border of the lower eyelid–cheek junction. The face can be divided into thirds by horizontal lines drawn parallel to this line at the trichion, glabella, subnasale, and menton. The upper third is from the trichion to the glabella, the middle third from the glabella to the subnasale, and the lower third extends from the subnasale to the menton. For patients with receded hairlines, the middle third is

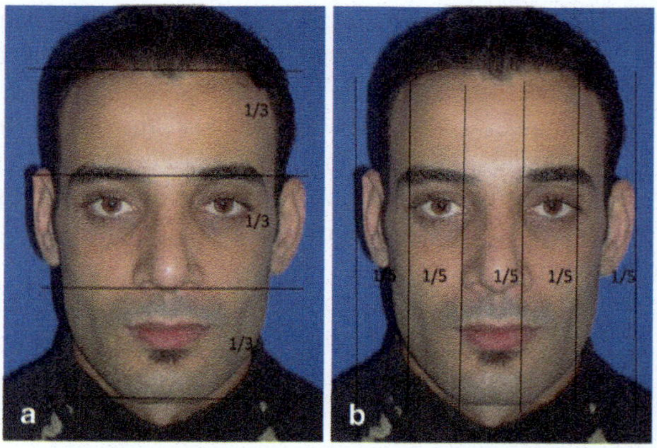


**Fig. 47.4** (**a**, **b**) Face is divided into horizontal thirds and vertical fifths to evaluate the symmetry of the facial features

used as the main unit of reference. Vertical fifths are divided using vertical parallel lines with each fifth equal to the width of an eye. The width of the nose should equal a vertical fifth. These reference units are important to utilize in evaluating the nose in relation to the face and to note any imbalances that may affect the perception of the nose (Fig. 47.4a, b).

### 47.3.1 Frontal View

When assessing the nose from the frontal view, there are several features that are typically evaluated.

1. Nasal symmetry: The nose should appear symmetrical and balanced when viewed from the front. Any asymmetries or deviations may be corrected during rhinoplasty.
2. Nasal width: The width of the nose should be proportional to the width of the face. If the nose is too wide or narrow, it may be adjusted during rhinoplasty.
3. Nasal tip position: The position of the nasal tip should be in line with the upper lip and the center of the face. If the tip is too high or low, it may be adjusted during rhinoplasty.
4. Nasal tip shape: The shape of the nasal tip should be proportional to the rest of the nose and the face. The tip can be rounded, pointed, or a combination of both, depending on the patient's preference.
5. Nostril size and shape: The nostrils should be proportionate to the rest of the nose and the face. If the nostrils are too wide, narrow, or asymmetrical, they may be adjusted during rhinoplasty.

### 47.3.2 Lateral View

When assessing the nose from the lateral (side) view, there are several features that are typically evaluated.

1. Nasal bridge: The height and shape of the nasal bridge should be proportionate to the rest of the face. A hump or depression in the bridge may be adjusted during rhinoplasty.
2. Nasal tip rotation: The angle between the upper lip and the nasal tip should be in the range of 90–105° for women and 90–95° for men. If the angle is too acute or obtuse, it may be adjusted during rhinoplasty. However, the nasolabial angle may be affected by anatomic variables unrelated to the nasal tip such as a prominent anterior nasal spine or maxillary protrusion.
3. Nasal tip projection: The amount that the nasal tip extends from the face should be proportionate to the rest of the nose and the face. If the tip is too prominent or recessed, it may be adjusted during rhinoplasty.
4. Nasal length: The length of the nose should be proportionate to the rest of the face. If the nose is too long or short, it may be adjusted during rhinoplasty.
5. Nasofrontal angle: The angle between the forehead and the nose should be in harmony with the rest of the face. If the angle is too steep or shallow, it may be adjusted during rhinoplasty. This angle converges at the nasion and is typically between 115 and 130°, with a more obtuse angle appealing in female noses and a more acute angle appealing in male noses.

### 47.3.3 Basal View

The nostrils, columella, infratip lobule, and alar base can all be seen in the basal view. A bulbous tip would give the nose a more trapezoidal form. The curvature of the alar rim can be used to assess the symmetry of the lower lateral cartilages. The nostrils should be symmetric and pear-shaped with a 30–45° angle from the midline. This view reveals the width of the alar base, which should be nearly equivalent to the intercanthal distance.

## 47.4 Photography in Rhinoplasty

Photography plays an important role in rhinoplasty, both in the pre-operative planning and post-operative assessment of the results. Here are some ways in which photography is used in rhinoplasty.

1. Preoperative planning: Before performing rhinoplasty, the surgeon will typically take several photographs of the patient's face, including various views of the nose. These photographs can be used to create a digital 3D model of the nose,

which the surgeon can use to plan the surgical approach and communicate the intended changes with the patient.
2. Intraoperative guidance: During the surgery, the surgeon may use photography to guide the placement of incisions and the reshaping of the nose. For example, they may use photographs to ensure that the nasal bridge is straight and that the nostrils are symmetrical.
3. Postoperative assessment: After the surgery, the surgeon will take photographs of the patient's face and nose to assess the results of the procedure. These photographs can be compared with the preoperative photographs to evaluate the success of the surgery and identify any areas that may require further refinement.

Overall, photography is a valuable tool in rhinoplasty, helping surgeons to plan and execute the surgery with greater precision and accuracy, as well as providing a means of objective assessment of the results.

## 47.5 Indications of Rhinoplasty

Rhinoplasty is a cosmetic surgical procedure that is performed to enhance the appearance of the nose. There are some situations in which rhinoplasty is indicated. Here are some indications for rhinoplasty.

1. Cosmetic concerns: Rhinoplasty is often performed to improve the aesthetic appearance of the nose. People may choose to undergo this surgery to address issues such as a large, wide, or asymmetrical nose, a prominent hump on the bridge of the nose, a bulbous or drooping tip, or a deviated septum.
2. Breathing difficulties: Rhinoplasty can also be performed to correct structural abnormalities in the nose that may be causing breathing difficulties. These abnormalities may include a deviated septum, collapsed nasal valves, or enlarged turbinates.
3. Trauma or injury: A broken nose or other injury to the nose can also be a reason for rhinoplasty. This type of surgery can help to repair the damage and restore the natural shape and function of the nose.
4. Congenital defects: Some people are born with congenital defects that affect the appearance or function of the nose. Rhinoplasty can be used to correct these defects and improve the overall appearance and function of the nose.

## 47.6 Contraindications of Rhinoplasty

Rhinoplasty is generally a safe and effective procedure, but it may not be suitable for everyone. Here are some contraindications for rhinoplasty.

1. Age: Most plastic surgeons recommend that patients wait until their nasal bone growth is complete before undergoing rhinoplasty. For most people, this occurs around the age of 16 for girls and 18 for boys.
2. Medical conditions: Certain medical conditions may make rhinoplasty unsafe or increase the risk of complications. These conditions may include bleeding disorders, uncontrolled high blood pressure, diabetes, and some autoimmune diseases.
3. Mental health issues: Patients with certain mental health conditions, such as body dysmorphic disorder, may not be good candidates for rhinoplasty. These patients may have unrealistic expectations or become excessively preoccupied with their appearance.
4. Smoking: Smoking can impair the healing process and increase the risk of complications following surgery. For this reason, plastic surgeons typically advise patients to quit smoking before and after rhinoplasty.
5. Pregnancy: It is generally recommended that women wait until after they have given birth and finished breastfeeding before undergoing rhinoplasty.

It is important to discuss your medical history and any potential risk factors with a qualified plastic surgeon before undergoing rhinoplasty.

## 47.7 Preparations for Rhinoplasty

Preparing for rhinoplasty is an important step in ensuring a successful outcome. Here are some general guidelines to help you prepare for your procedure.

1. Medical evaluation: The surgeon should request a medical evaluation to assess your overall health and any potential risk factors. They may also request blood tests and imaging studies such as X-rays or a CT scan.
2. Medications and supplements: The surgeon will ask you to stop taking certain medications or supplements that could increase the risk of bleeding or interfere with the anesthesia. These may include aspirin, nonsteroidal anti-inflammatory drugs (NSAIDs), and herbal supplements.
3. Quit smoking: Patients should quit smoking for several weeks before and after theisurgery. Smoking can interfere with the healing process and increase the risk of complications.
4. Arrange for help: Patients will likely need someone to drive them home after surgery and help with basic activities during the first few days of recovery.
5. Prepare for recovery: Specific instructions on how to care for the nose and manage any discomfort during the recovery period. This may include taking pain medications, using cold compresses to reduce swelling, and avoiding strenuous activities for several weeks.
6. Anesthesia and operative site preparation: During the open rhinoplasty, general anesthesia or intravenous methods (e.g., propofol) are recommended. Muscle relaxants are a possibility if general anesthesia is used. Preoperative delivery of a single intravenous antibiotic dose covering skin flora is required. A single

intravenous steroid injection (for example, 8 mg of dexamethasone) may aid reduce edema. A single intravenous dosage of tranexamic acid (10 mg/kg) may help to minimize intraoperative bleeding. In order to avoid distorting the look of the nose, local anesthetic is infused throughout the septum, columella, border, soft tissue triangle, sidewalls, and dorsum. Nasal decongestant-soaked pledgets are applied to the bilateral nasal cavity. Vibrissae are clipped to improve visibility and reduce crusting after surgery.

## 47.8 Open (Primary) Rhinoplasty

### 47.8.1 Introduction

External rhinoplasty, also known as open rhinoplasty, is a surgical approach used to reshape the nose. In this approach, the surgeon makes a small incision on the columella. This incision allows the surgeon to lift the skin and soft tissue of the nose, providing better access to the nasal framework.

External rhinoplasty is often preferred for more complex nasal deformities or when significant structural changes are required. This approach allows the surgeon to directly visualize the nasal anatomy and make more precise modifications to the underlying cartilage and bone.

The decision to use an external or internal approach for rhinoplasty depends on the individual's unique nasal anatomy, the extent of the desired modifications, and the surgeon's experience and preference. It is important to consult with a board-certified plastic surgeon who has expertise in both techniques to determine the most appropriate approach for your specific needs.

### 47.8.2 Incision

A useful tool is to mark the skin for the deformities that are diagnosed preoperatively to aid in the reach of the prober shape. Marking of the amount of the hump needed for removal, the medial and lateral osteotomies, the skin incision, and the alar reduction lines are the most common markings needed in rhinoplasty (Fig. 47.5).

A double skin hook is inserted beneath the right nostril to evert the alar margin, while the operator's nondominant index finger everts the ala, exposing the caudal margin of the right lateral crural crus (LLC's) lateral crus. The same incision is repeated on the left side. The soft tissues covering the lateral crura, medial crura, and domes are elevated from the underlying frame using a pair of baby Metzenbaum scissors by spreading and cutting the tissues with the scissors. The dissection is carried out cephalically in order to reveal the anteromedial two-thirds of the lateral crura (Fig. 47.6a, b).

Then an incision is marked in the narrowest portion of the columella. The most common design of the incision is the inverted V design. This is used to ensure by disturbing a straight incision of the columella by an inverted V incision in the

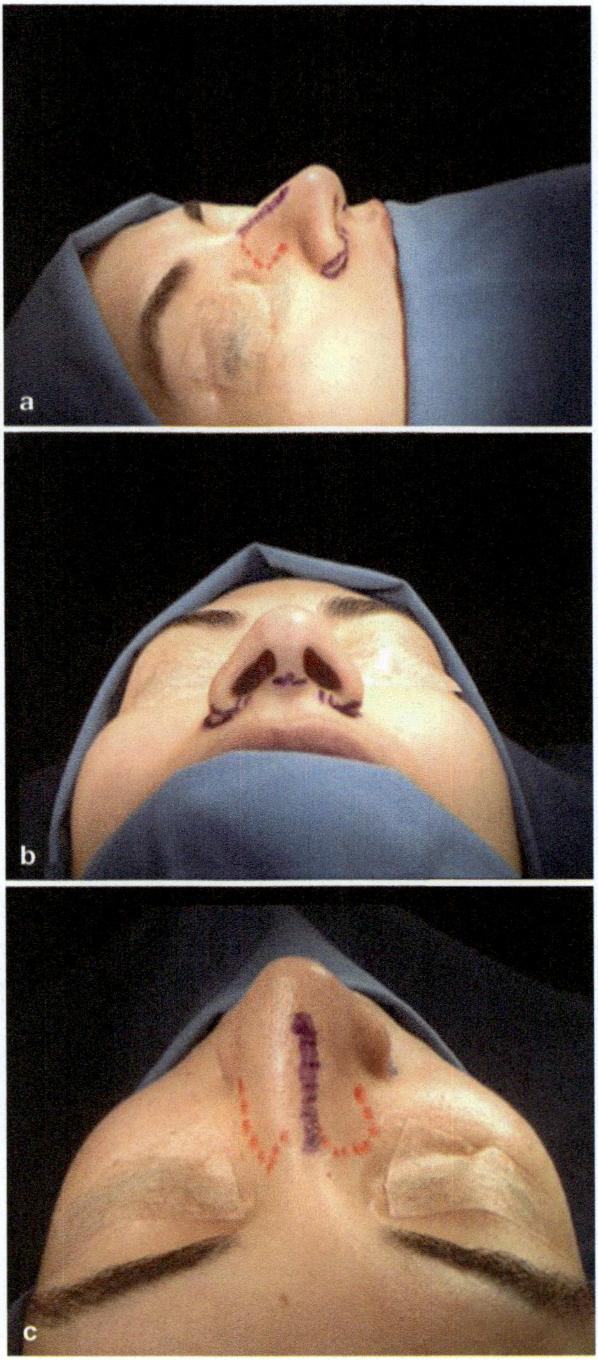

**Fig. 47.5** (a–c) Skin marking prior to incision to i the hump, osteotomy lines, skin incision, and alar reduction

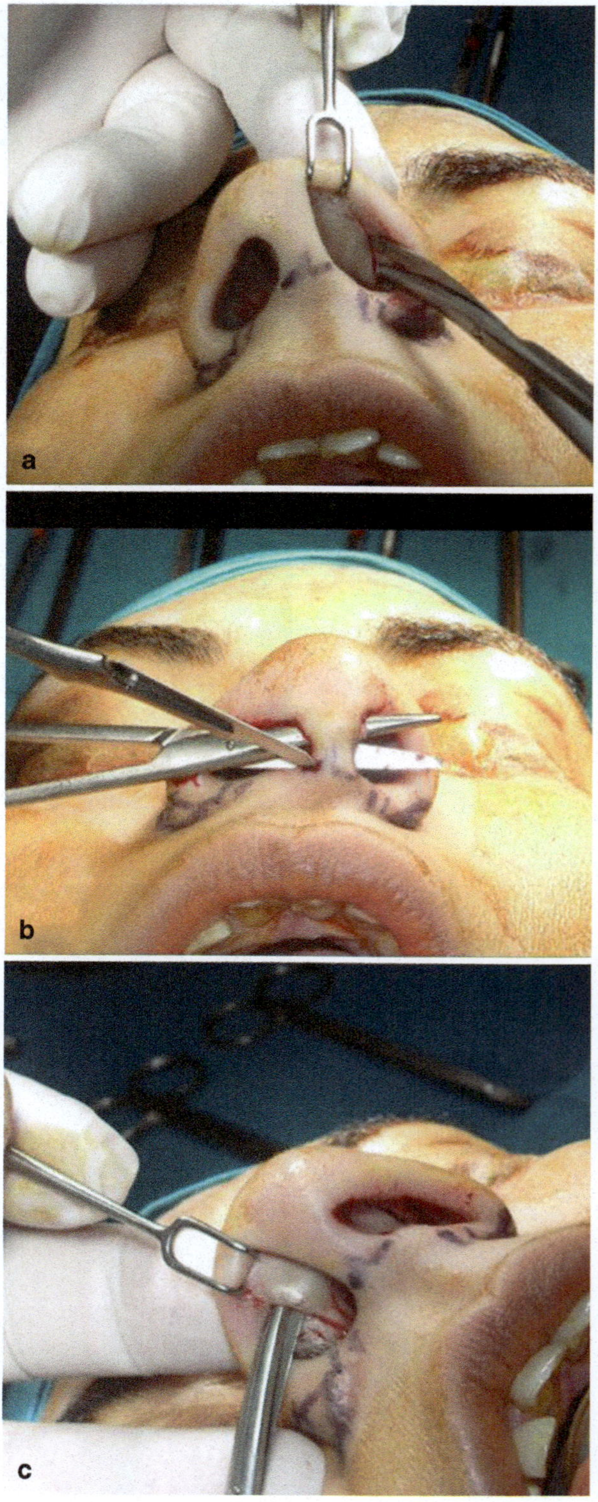

**Fig. 47.6** (**a**, **b**) Left and right infracartilagenous skin incision. (**c**) Columellar incision using an inverted V design and two lateral horizontal incisions

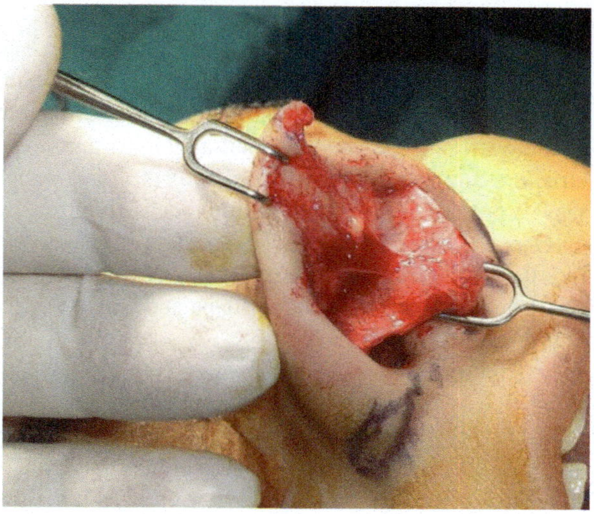

**Fig. 47.7** Exposure and dissection plane over the lower lateral cartilage

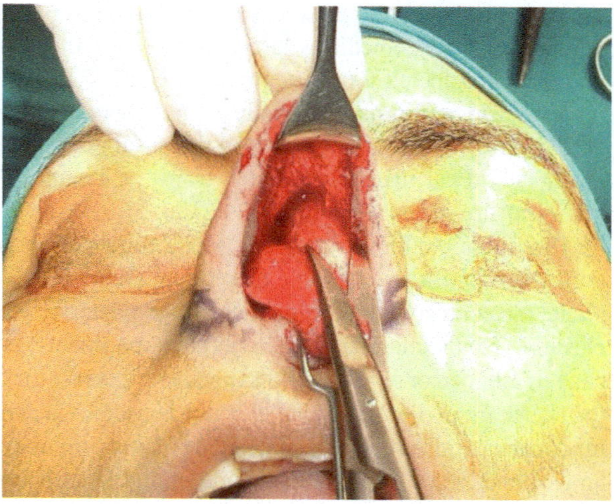

**Fig. 47.8** Dissection is continued using the Joseph scissors back over the dorsum until the nasal bones are reached

middle of the incision. This design will make the scar less straight and hence less visible. A pair of scissors is inserted beneath the skin to ensure that the incision is not too close to the medial crura cartilage (Fig. 47.6c).

The dissection is continued using the Joseph scissors back over the dorsum until the nasal bones are reached. At this phase, a periosteal elevator is utilized to raise the periosteum from the dorsum while attempting to keep the dissection on the sub-periosteal plane. Preservation of the periosteum will help in covering the sculpted nasal bones and aid in preserving the natural appearance of the nose after the surgery. Also, this will lead to less telangiectasis of the skin over the bone that is a common sequela that happens with a supra periosteal plane of flap elevation (Figs. 47.7 and 47.8).

### 47.8.3 Anteroinferior Septal Angle

During rhinoplasty surgery, gaining access to the caudal end of the upper lateral cartilages (ULCs) and the dorsum of the nose often requires the removal of the soft tissue overlying the caudal septal angle. To minimize the disruption of the nasal structure and preserve the integrity of the mucoperichondrium, the surgeon may leave a portion of the tissue intact to act as an intrinsic spreader graft.

Once the tissue is removed, the surgeon will use a pair of Joseph scissors to separate the ULCs from the dorsum. This separation allows the surgeon to modify the cartilage to achieve the desired shape and contour of the nose.

### 47.8.4 Septoplasty

The procedure involves the elevation of the septal mucoperichondrium, which is the lining that covers the cartilage of the nasal septum, through an anterior approach by elevation of a left-sided mucoperichondrial flap or a left-side Killian incision. The mucoperichondrium is dissected off the caudal septum if repositioning is required. Separation of the medial crura can increase the septal exposure if an anterior approach is selected for the septoplasty (Fig. 47.9a, b).

A free elevator is used to create a tunnel between the septum and the upper lateral cartilage cephalically to the level of the nasal bones. Next using Joseph scissors, the upper lateral cartilage is separated from the septum to facilitate further dissection and exposure of the septum (Fig. 47.10a, b).

To initiate the elevation of the septal mucoperichondrium, the periosteal elevator's sharp end is used for the dissection. Once the dissection has entered the right plane, it can be continued cephalically and posteriorly with the dull end of the septal elevator. This technique helps to expose the underlying cartilage and bone, which can be reshaped or repositioned as needed to correct the deviated septum (Fig. 47.11).

The sharp end of the septal elevator is used to incise the septal cartilage after the mucoperichondrium has been lifted to its maximum extent on the left side, leaving an L-shaped strut for the dorsal and columellar support, with at least 15 mm maintained anteriorly and 10 mm caudally. It is a prevalent finding that the maxillary crest of the vomer bone or the entirety of the vomer bone displays a deviation, often accompanied by a spur on one side of the septum. It is imperative to take out the deviated segment of the vomer bone utilizing a rongeur.

In many conditions, the maxillary crest is found to be deviated to one side, and in some conditions, this deviation could be a contribution to airway blockage. For correction, we have to remove the deviated part of the maxillary crest with a rongeur or osteotome. Care must be taken not to injure the neighboring flaps. In some other conditions, the anterior nasal spine is found to be deviated or excessively protruded, and this could be corrected using an osteotome.

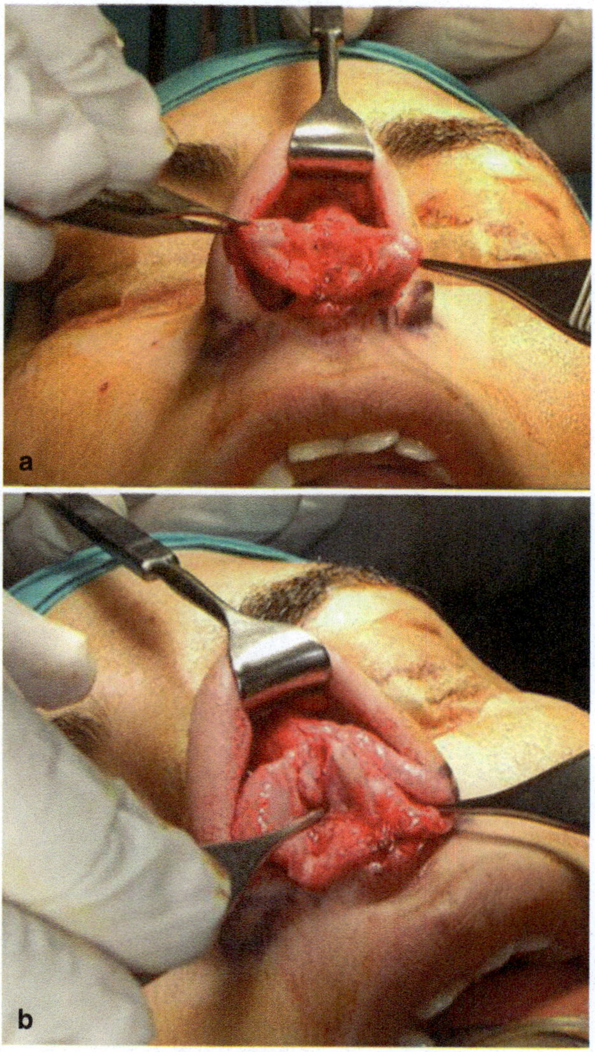

Fig. 47.9 (a) Anterior approach of septoplasty. (b) Exposure of the septal cartilage by lateral retraction of the medial crira

#### 47.8.4.1 Role of Septal Deviation in Crooked Nose

Problems with the nasal function and appearance might result from deviation of the dorsal portion of the septum. The resultant nasal deviation may affect the entire nasal pyramid. On rare occasions, localized deviations with varied degrees of deformity to the upper, middle, or lower section may occur. Rohrich et al. classified internal nasal septal deviations based on three broad categories including caudal septal deviations, concave dorsal deviations, and concave/convex dorsal deviations (S-shaped). Caudal septal deviations and concave dorsal deformities were further divided into subtypes by the authors: straight septal tilt, concave deformity and S-shaped deformity for caudal septal deviation, and C-shaped dorsal deformity and reverse C-shaped dorsal deformity for concave dorsal deformity [8].

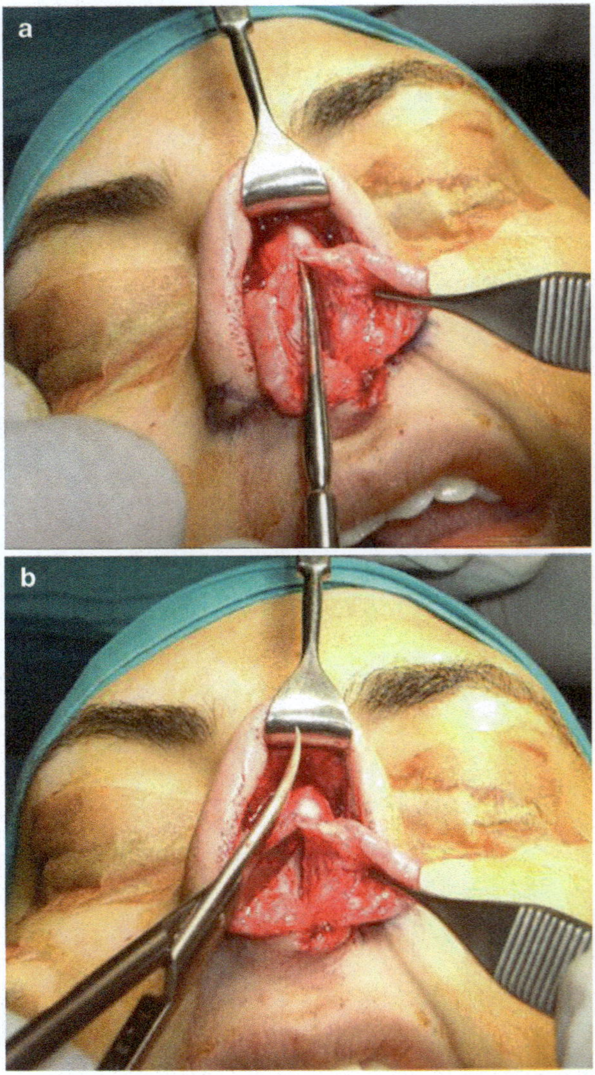


**Fig. 47.10** (**a**) Tunnel dissection between the upper lateral cartilage and the septum using a freer elevator. (**b**) Separation of the septum from the upper lateral cartilage

The primary component of a deviated nose is a deviated nasal septum, which serves as the foundation for the external nasal framework. The combined septal and corrective rhinoplasty should be performed in a single procedure because septum surgery often plays a crucial role in the effective management of the externally deviated nose. Even if there are no functional issues, septal surgery may still be necessary to fix slight septal abnormalities that could interfere with the proper alignment of the external nasal pyramid [9].

In patients with moderate deflections of the dorsal segment of the nasal septum, sutured in-place spreader grafts are placed between the dorsal edge of the cartilaginous septum, and the upper lateral cartilages are straightforward techniques to address this deformity (Fig. 47.12a, b).

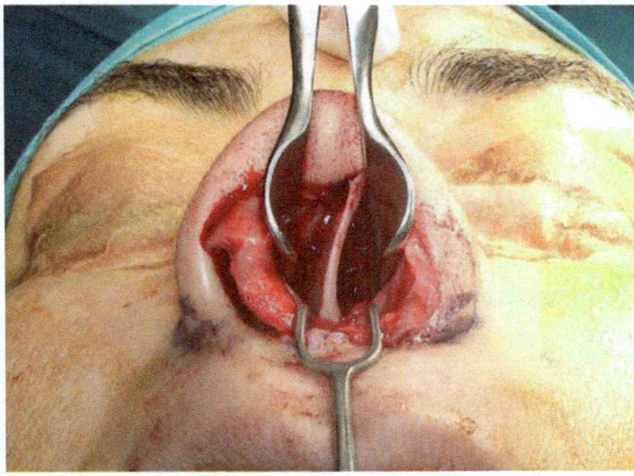

**Fig. 47.11** Exposure of the nasal septum

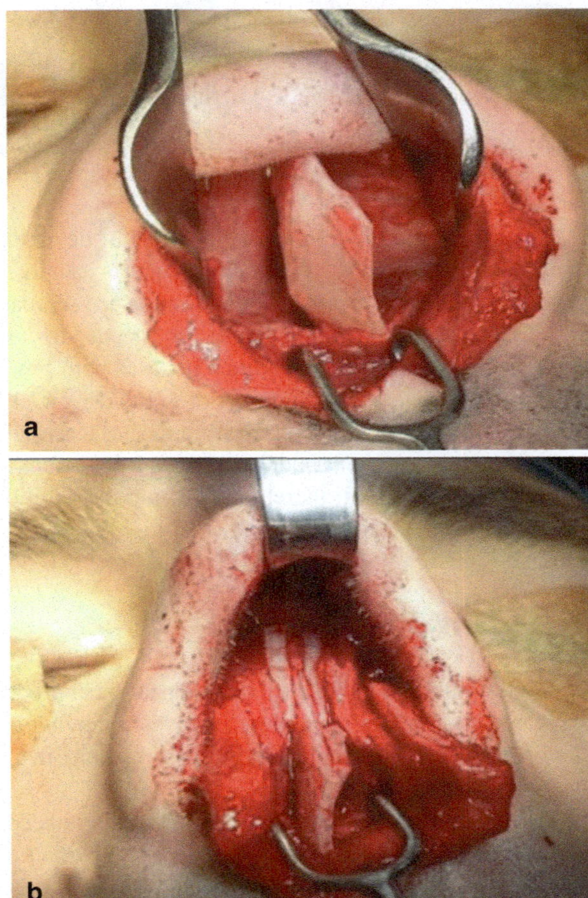


**Fig. 47.12** (**a**) Severely deviated nasal septum with the deviation reaching higher parts of the septum. (**b**) Use of spreader grafts and septal grafts to correct the deviation

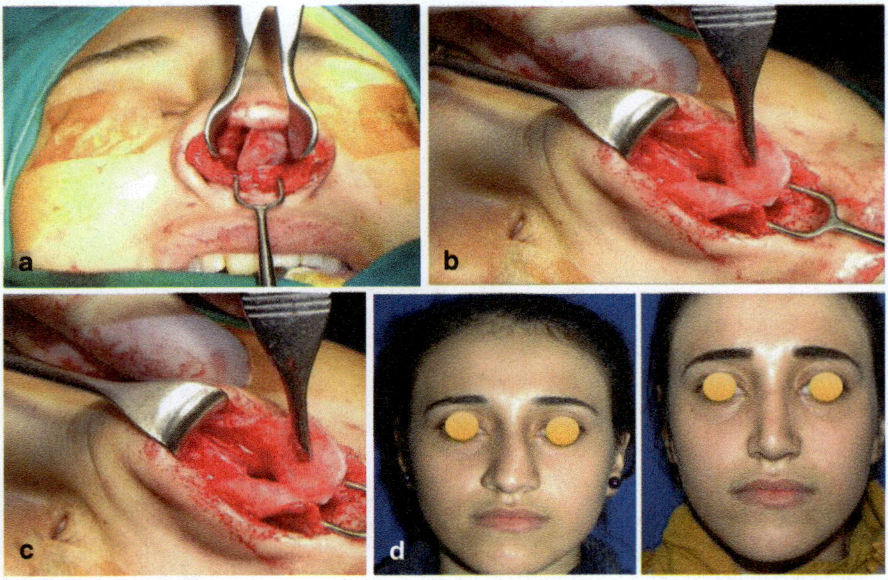


**Fig. 47.13** (**a**, **b**) Showing a severe septal deviation. (**c**) Using multiple grafts for correction of the septal deviation. (**d**) Before and after rhinoseptoplasty using multiple septal grafting techniques

Patients having multiple or high grades of deviation usually require the use of multiple grafts. Application of multiple grafts usually entitles the need for sectioning of the original harvested cartilage and hence decreases the strength of the splints besides increasing the intraoperative time needed to complete the procedure. Still, it is considered an effective technique in cases with few deviations that can be properly corrected with a lesser number of grafts (Fig. 47.13a–d).

A single batten graft harvested from the nasal septum provides an excellent alternative for correction of caudal and dorsal deviations in a single step without the need to divide the graft; thereby preserving the additional support provided by the undivided cartilage graft [10] (Fig. 47.14a–e).

### 47.8.5 Dorsal Hump Removal

Rhinoplasty hump removal is a common surgical procedure used to reduce the size of a dorsal hump. The procedure involves removing or reshaping the excess bone and/or cartilage on the bridge of the nose, resulting in a smoother and more aesthetically pleasing profile.

The dorsal hump is removed once the radix is deepened. The nasion should be deeper than the remainder of the dorsum in a perfect nasal frame to accommodate the heavier soft tissues that cover this area of the nose. The bony hump is subsequently removed using a rasp.

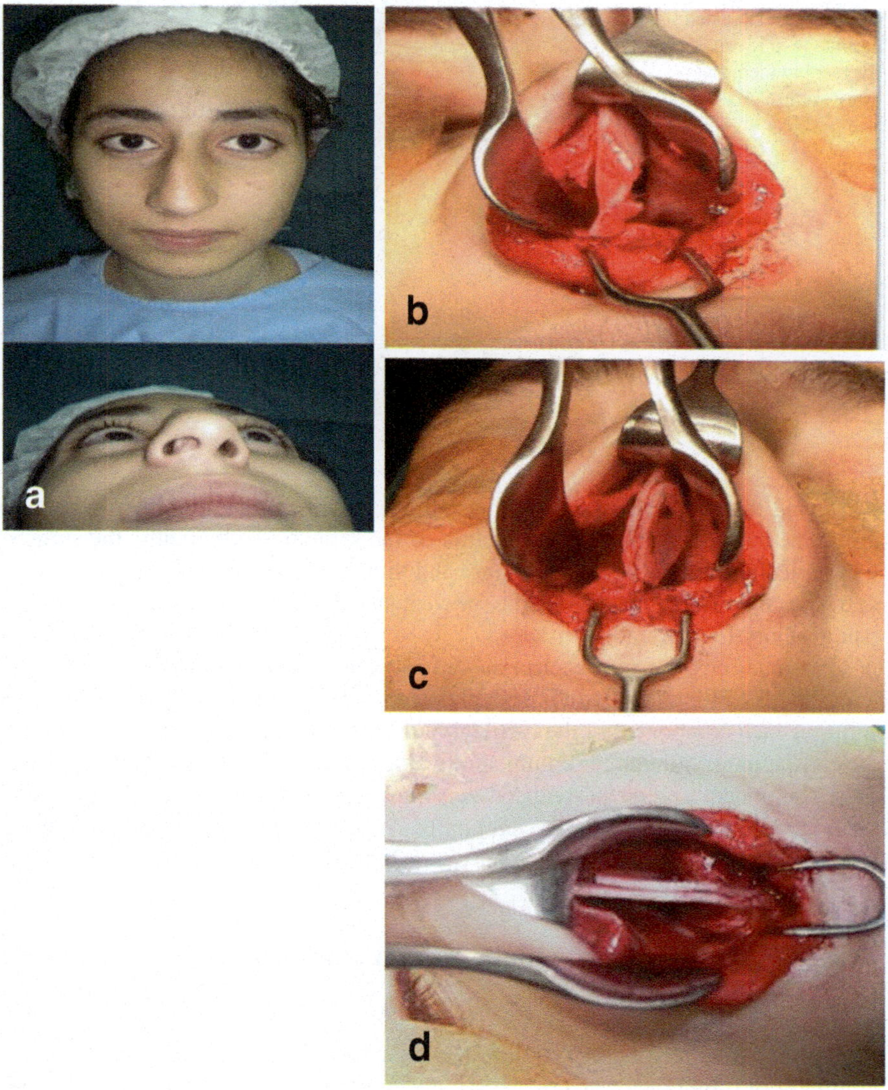


**Fig. 47.14** (**a**) Showing a crooked nasal deviation associated with a severe septal deviation. (**b**) Intraoperative septal deviation after dissection. (**c**, **d**) Correction of the septal deviation using large batten graft septoplasty technique. (**e**) Before and after septorhinoplasty using batten graft septoplasty

The use of a tungsten carbide rasp in a push-and-pull maneuver is a common technique for removing a bony hump during rhinoplasty surgery. The rasp is designed to remove bone in a controlled manner, allowing the surgeon to reshape the nose (Fig. 47.15).

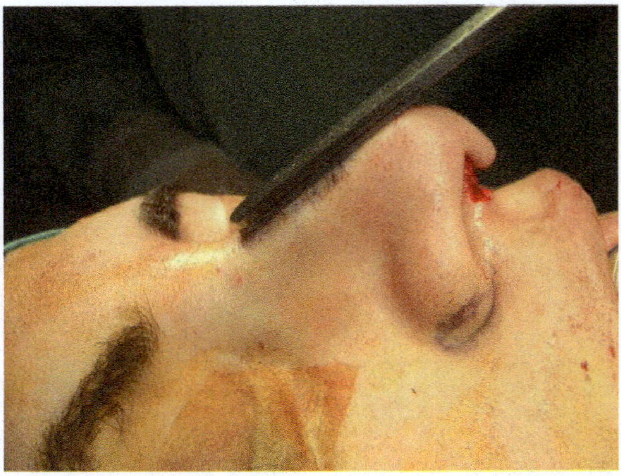

**Fig. 47.15** Tungsten carbide rasp is usually used for rasping the nasal bony hump

During the procedure, the surgeon will use the rasp in an oblique direction to minimize the risk of inadvertent fracture of the septum. Additionally, the surgeon will typically use their left index finger and thumb to provide support and stability to the nasal bones, which can help to prevent slipping of the rasp and minimize the risk of injury to surrounding tissues.

Once the bony dorsum reaches the requested level designed preoperatively, we manage the cartilaginous hump. It is preferred to tackle the cartilaginous hump by splitting each component of the cartilaginous hump. There are three components of the cartilaginous hump: the septum and two upper lateral cartilages. After splitting, each component should be reduced separately starting with the septum using a straight scissor to remove the excess hump. Then, on each side, upper lateral cartilage is reduced using the same scissor to reach the desired level.

### 47.8.6 Removal of the Cephalic Margin of the Lower Lateral Cartilages

The width of the lateral crus is reduced, and the extra cartilage is excised, leaving a minimum of 6 mm of lower lateral cartilage anteriorly and 8 mm or more posteriorly. A number 15 blade is used to make the cartilage incision, and the excess cartilage is then dissected out with a pair of scissors. If feasible, the mucoperichondrium is kept whole. The excised cartilage may be used as an alar rim transplant if it is thick and rigid enough. Since lower lateral cartilages are frequently not symmetrical, to begin with, it is crucial to leave a symmetric amount in place after removal (Fig. 47.16a, b).

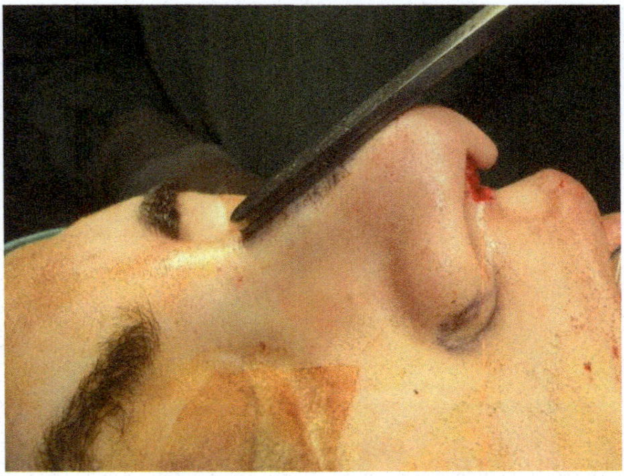

**Fig. 47.16** (a, b) Before and after cephalic trimming of the lateral crus of the lower lateral cartilage

### 47.8.7 Osteotomies

After dorsal hump resection, lateral osteotomy is performed either percutaneously or endonasally in order to close the open roof of the nose, correct the deviation of bony noses, narrow the upper third of the nose, and fix the curved lateral nasal wall. The lateral osteotomies can be performed at any time during the operative sequence although they are usually performed during the final stages. The osteotomies frequently used in primary rhinoplasty are medial and lateral. The medial osteotomy is done through the open approach of rhinoplasty. The lateral osteotomy is performed through either a percutaneous external perforated technique or endonasally. There is debate over whether the internal or external technique is superior although the indications are generally consistent. Although they are typically carried out in the final stages of the operation, lateral osteotomies can be carried out at any point.

Osteotomies are performed after a significant hump reduction to narrow the open roof. To guarantee complete mobilization of the lateral wall, an original paramedial medial osteotomy parallel to the septum was previously described. However, if the true medial osteotomy is extended cephalically, it may cause the fused radix bone to break, creating a "rocker deformity." At the highest point of the open roof, typically 0–3 mm from the septum, a paramedian osteotomy is made. Currently, the majority of surgeons favor a medial oblique osteotomy, which descends toward the medial canthus level at an angle of typically between 15 and 25° from the midline. It is best done with a straight-guarded osteotome to allow palpation and exact level determination.

The goal of lateral osteotomies is to decrease the base bony width of the nose as measured at its widest point. The low-to-high and low-to-low osteotomies, which are the two most used techniques, are different in their direction of movement, bony fracture severity, and motion. The maxillary nasal process's pyriform aperture serves as the starting point of the low-to-high osteotomy, which proceeds tangentially across it to the nasal bone suture line at the level of the medial canthus. In

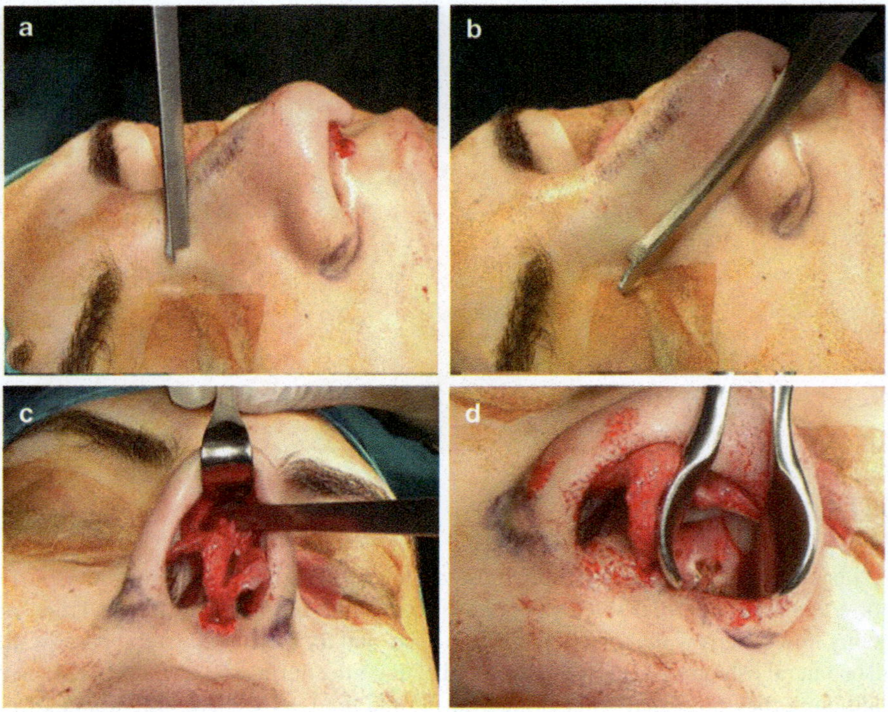


**Fig. 47.17** (**a**) Showing the direction of the medial osteotomy using a straight guarded osteotome. (**b**) Showing the direction of the lateral osteotomy high to low using a curved guarded osteotome. (**c**) Medial osteotomy. (**d**) Transvestibular incision made by electrocautery for the insertion of the lateral osteotomy above the level of the head of the inferior turbinate

contrast, the low-to-low osteotomy is done using a curved osteotome. It begins at the pyriform aperture on the nasal process of the maxilla and passes straight up the lateral wall to end at the level of the medial canthus. A speculum is inserted in the nostril to view the pyriform aperture. A transverse cut is made in the mucosa using above the level of the head of the inferior nasal turbinate by a scalpel or using cautery incision for the lateral osteotomy made perpendicular to the pyriform rim to prevent circumferential scarring. The osteotome is inserted with the guard outward to facilitate palpation. The surgeon holds the curved osteotome in the dominant hand and palpates the guard with the other hand. The lateral osteotomy continues to the level of the medial canthus or the base of the previous medial osteotomy (Fig. 47.17a–d).

The intermediate osteotomy is considered a double-level lateral osteotomy. This technique is used to correct a severe convexity of the lateral nasal bony wall at the suture line of the nasal bone and the frontal process of the maxilla. An osteotome passes from caudal to cephalic along the suture, thus decreasing the convexity of the lateral nasal bones allowing straighter nasal walls. It is done after performing the medial osteotomy and before performing the lateral osteotomy.

Piezoelectric instrumentation (PEI) has recently proven to be more advantageous than conventional hand-held osteotomies. Little harm has been done to the soft tissue surroundings. The surgeon can more precisely diagnose and treat osseocartilaginous vault abnormalities with extensive exposure. Osteotomies are no longer indicated, performed, and evaluated blindly, allowing for far higher precision. It is possible to remove the bony cap surgically, minimizing stress to the cartilaginous vault beneath.

### 47.8.8 Spreader Grafts

Spreader grafts have a significant role in rhinoplasty that should not be understated. They are useful in restoring the aesthetics of the nasal dorsum, supporting the nasal valve, and preserving the straightened position of the deviated cartilaginous dorsum. Sheen popularized spreader grafts in rhinoplasty in the 1980s as a way of repairing the internal nasal valve and recontouring the cosmetic look of the nasal dorsum. Spreader grafts have been routinely used in situations of primary and secondary rhinoplasty since that period. The grafts were designed to function as volumetric expanders, stabilizing and shifting the upper lateral cartilage away from the dorsal septum in order to enhance the internal nasal valve angle [11].

Spreader grafts are typically made from septal cartilage and it might be harvested from conchal cartilages in secondary rhinoplasties. Spreader grafts are fashioned into rectangular bars that are 2–3 cm long, 3–5 mm broad, and 1.5 mm thick. The harvested cartilages are then placed on both sides between the upper lateral cartilage and the upper section of the septal cartilage. It is crucial, however, that the spreader graft extends to encompass the k-area, particularly under the nasal bones. Finally, the cartilages are joined using a 5-0 polydioxanone suture (Fig. 47.18).

### 47.8.9 Tip Surgery

Open tip suture technique is our recommendation to produce an aesthetic tip. It has flexibility and control that are impossible with any other tip-modifying techniques.

#### 47.8.9.1 Columellar Strut

The columellar strut and suture offer three significant advantages: tip stability, tip projection, and columellar reshaping. Suturing the medial crura to the strut results in a more cohesive tip complex and better symmetry. The columellar strut is usually cut 20 mm long, 2–3 mm wide, and 1.5 mm thick. This graft is shaped to the desired dimensions using a #15 blade. A pocket is made between the alar cartilages, and the strut is inserted down. A vertical suture of 5-0 PDS is placed to sandwich the strut between the two middle crura (Fig. 47.19).

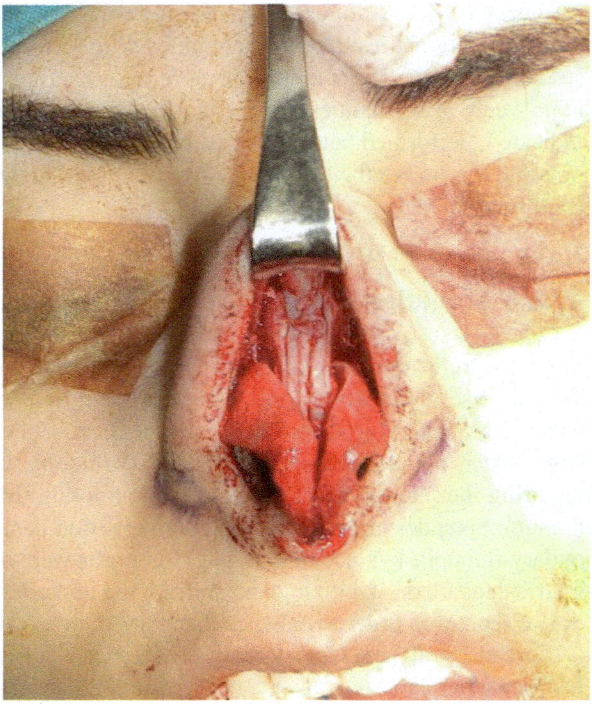

**Fig. 47.18** Bilateral septal spreader grafts

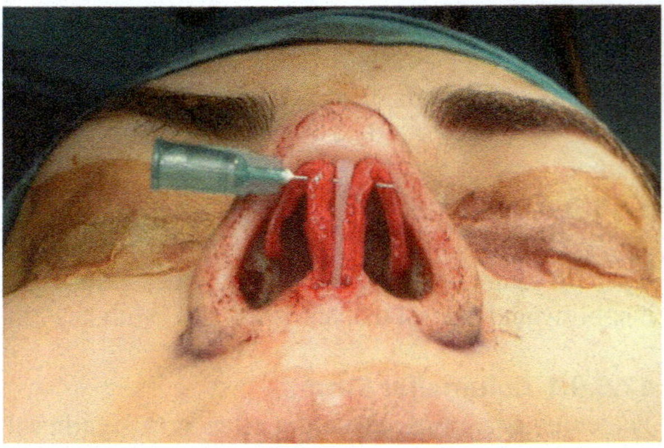

**Fig. 47.19** Placement of the columellar strut

#### 47.8.9.2 Dome Creation Suture

The dome creation suture defines the tip by forming the ideal domal architecture from flat or concave cartilages. To form a convex domal segment, a horizontal mattress suture is inserted across the domal segment at the domal notch and cinched down. Then, from medial to lateral, a horizontal mattress suture is applied with the knot secured medially. Gradually tightening the tension until the correct domal convexity is obtained. Although the domal convexity is the focus, the reality is a progressively increasing domal convexity.

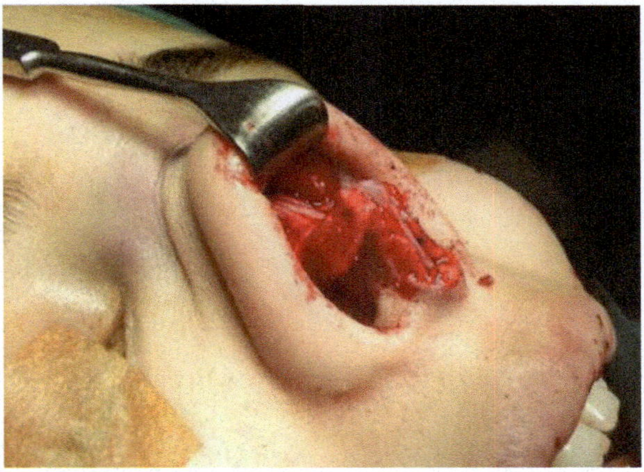

**Fig. 47.20** Dome creation and approximation sutures

#### 47.8.9.3 Dome Approximation Suture

The infralobule and dome widths are both reshaped by the interdomal suture. It is a straightforward vertical suture that enters one crus at the same level as the domal creation suture, leaves above the crural suture, and then enters the opposite crus next to the domal creation suture. Up until the proper width is reached, the knot is tightened. This is done to create a single pointy tip commonly known as the "tip diamond" concept (Fig. 47.20).

### 47.8.10 Alar Base Reduction

Alar base modification is carefully planned preoperatively and performed very conservatively; aggressive excisions can be disastrous and irreparable. There are three surgical techniques: (1) nostril sill excision to reduce nostrils, (2) an alar wedge excision to reduce nostril flare, and (3) a combined sill/wedge excision. The study of the nasal base with the other aspects of the face during preoperative nasal analysis is critical for a favorable outcome. The shape, size, position, and symmetry of the alar base must be evaluated from frontal and basal views. The width of the alar base is best measured from the front. The basal view is critical for assessing the anatomy of the nasal base, alar flare, nostril circumference, and asymmetries (Fig. 47.21).

#### 47.8.10.1 Nostril Sill Excision

Callipers are used to measure and mark the distance from the midcolumellar point to the alar crease, which is typically 10–12 mm from the midcolumellar point. The area that will be excised is marked. The excess nostril sill to be excised is marked by two lines almost parallel to each other. The width of the excised wedge can vary between 1 and 4 mm. A subcutaneous suture using vicryl 4.0 will decrease the tension over the cutaneous sutures. The cutaneous sutures can be established using polypropylene 6.0 sutures.

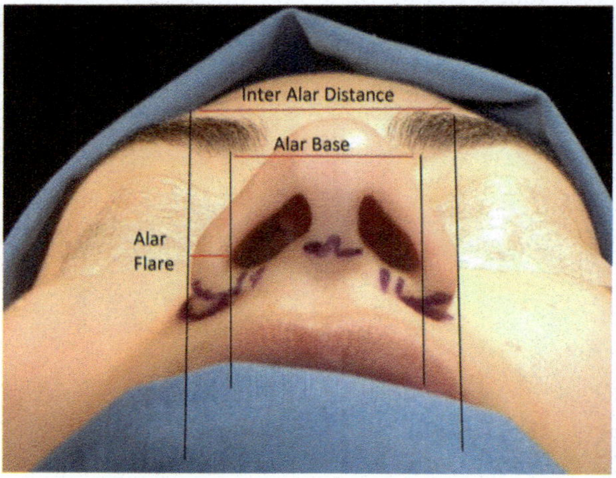


**Fig. 47.21** Showing the interalar distance, alar base, and alar flare dimensions

#### 47.8.10.2 Alar Flare Reduction

The alar wedge excision is an elliptical incision in the alar crease. It is used to minimize the size and vertical length of the alar lobule, as well as to rectify excessive flaring in the frontal view. Before injecting a local anesthetic solution, markings should be done methodically and precisely with callipers. A No. 15 blade is used to make an incision in the alar crease. The removed wedge contains the skin as well as deeper tissue such as alar musculature and fibrofatty tissue. A subcutaneous 4.0 vicryle absorbable stitch is used to approximate edges. Skin is closed meticulously with 6.0 polypropylene sutures.

### 47.8.11 Closure and Postoperative Management

All incisions are sutured. Beginning with the transcolumellar incision: first, the midline suture at the apex of the V for alignment; second, the lateral corner sutures to ensure redraping of the skin; and finally, the columellar pillar sutures all done with polypropylene 5.0 sutures. The nose is then taped with 0.5-in. wide paper tape which compresses the skin envelope and reduces edema. A metal Denver or Brown splint is then placed and secured in place over the nose with paper tape of the same width (0.5 in.). The postop medications are confirmed (analgesics for pain and oral antibiotic for 7 days). The patient is reminded to clean all suture lines free of crusts three times a day with hydrogen peroxide and apply antibiotic ointment. After 7 days, the dressings are removed.

## References

1. Celsus AC, Constantin R, Casaubon I, Almeloveen TJ. Aur. Corn. Celsi De medicina libri octo. Amstelaedami: Apud Joannem Wolters; 1687. p. 48, 574, 26.
2. Sand M, Sand D, Thrandorf C, Paech V, Altmeyer P, Bechara FG. Cutaneous lesions of the nose. Head Face Med. 2010;6:7.

3. Sachs ME. Mastering revision rhinoplasty, vol. xiii. New York: Springer; 2006, 394 p.
4. Hetzler L, Givens V, Sykes J. The tripod concept of the upper nasal third. JAMA Facial Plast Surg. 2019;21(6):498–503.
5. Patel B, Virk JS, Randhawa PS, Andrews PJ. The internal nasal valve: a validated grading system and operative guide. Eur Arch Otorrinolaringol. 2018;275(11):2739–44.
6. Hamilton GS 3rd. The external nasal valve. Facial Plast Surg Clin North Am. 2017;25(2):179–94.
7. Tardy ME. Rhinoplasty : the art and the science. Philadelphia: Saunders; 1997.
8. Rohrich RJ, Gunter JP, Deuber MA, Adams WP Jr. The deviated nose: optimizing results using a simplified classification and algorithmic approach. Plast Reconstr Surg. 2002;110(6):1509–23; discussion 1524–5.
9. Foda HM. The role of septal surgery in management of the deviated nose. Plast Reconstr Surg. 2005;115(2):406–15.
10. Wael Khamis H, Remon B. Batten graft septoplasty: evaluation of a preferred technique. Egypt J Ear Nose Throat Allied Sci. 2015;16(3):223–9.
11. Sheen JH. Spreader graft: a method of reconstructing the roof of the middle nasal vault following rhinoplasty. Plast Reconstr Surg. 1984;73(2):230–9.

# Hybrid Rhinoplasty

# 48

Giuseppe Cottone, Ali Abd Alameer Khazaal, and Enrico Robotti

**Key Points**

- For some surgeons born and raised to the structural approach, integrating preservation principles in their practice would be made easier by a "hybrid" approach. On the other hand, it is also evident that reintegrating some key "open" structural points makes the difference, especially when approaching difficult cases (e.g., severe dorsal asymmetries/crookedness or extremely "dysfunctional" noses).
- Hybrid means to combine different elements, sometimes opposite, to reach the best result: dorsal preservation and tip structure, preservation principles and full open dissection, manual instruments and power-assisted devices, and piezoelectric and power burrs.
- We present our hybrid approach, the "modified dorsal split (MDS) hybrid preservation rhinoplasty": a fully open approach with an initial supraperichondrial dissection then transitioning to a subperichondrial–subperiosteal dissection, dorsal preservation along with a structural tip combining piezo and power tools and eventually finalized by reestablishing nose ligaments and compartments.

**Supplementary Information** The online version contains supplementary material available at https://doi.org/10.1007/978-3-031-70077-4_48.

G. Cottone
Milan, Italy

A. A. A. Khazaal (✉)
Baghdad, Iraq

E. Robotti
Bergamo, Italy


S. Elwany (ed.), *Current Rhinology*,
https://doi.org/10.1007/978-3-031-70077-4_48

## 48.1 Background

The new scenario in which we are living, both scientifically and socially, is undoubtedly dominated by social media and strong competition. As much as surgical techniques are advancing and increasing the level of complexity, the patient's desires and expectations are continuously and similarly growing, too. This is probably, although partially, the result of the new universal trend of sharing surgical results (as well as surgical "spots" and "nuances") on social networks so that the surgeon's material is becoming public and available to everyone.

For these and many other reasons, rhinoplasty surgeons are faced with the need to provide increasingly high-standard results to this increasing plethora of highly demanding (often quite "educated" from the surgical point of view) patients.

The outcome that stems from this new and complex background is quite understandable and characterizes contemporary rhinoplasty: to develop and adopt a multitude of advanced techniques with the aim of achieving "high standard" and "finesse" rhinoplasty results. Much of this can be attributed to the resurgence of preservation rhinoplasty (PR) [1, 2], which has essentially been made possible both by a better understanding of anatomy [3–8], as well as by expanding the toolbox that surgeons use [9–15].

Taking a step back, let us try to quickly resume the last 40 years, which represented a quite short period of big changes in rhinoplasty. It all started with the monumental *Aesthetic Rhinoplasty* by Sheen, published in 1978 [16], which summarized three key concepts [1]: (a) the conceptualization of the rhinoplasty as truly aesthetic and standardized procedure and not just as "functional" surgery, (b) the replacement of the "reduction-only" concept described by Joseph [17–19] with a more balanced and modern concept of reduction/augmentation (often by using a well-standardized set of specific grafts) primary rhinoplasty, and (c) a more focused and conscious "know-how" on revision rhinoplasty, resulted from a growing experience on this kind of surgery. To achieve a good function along with a pleasant and natural look of the nose became the new standard in every rhinoplasty.

While the revolutionary concepts of the "open structural" rhinoplasty were reaching their apogee, the "closed" approach was losing popularity because of a long-lasting period of stalemate without any significant innovations. Thanks to the crucial works of many pioneers such as Goodman [20], Anderson [21], Daniel [22], and Gunter [23], "open structural" rhinoplasty started to receive always more and more consent for number of reasons: extremely better visualization of the surgical field, great potential to reach and easily work on the bony vault, midvault, septum (key for complex septal reconstructions) and tip and, last but not least, shorter learning curve for young surgeons. From that moment on, the rhinoplasty surgery became one of the most requested facial procedures worldwide, and the "open structural" approach was definitely the master.

Despite an evident improvement in both the functional and aesthetic results, it was clear soon that the structural approach, mainly in not expertised hands, resulted in destruction leading to a huge number of complications often asking for surgical revisions.

To address this persisting problem, a group of surgeons started to think of a new way to perform the rhinoplasty, trying to replace resection with preservation, excision with gentle manipulation, full degloving with minimal surgical dissections (often coming back to a pure "closed" approach), and secondary rib reconstruction with minimal revisions [1, 24]: this marked the birth (a kind of resurrection and a return to origins) of the preservation rhinoplasty. Differently from the past, this resurrection was made possible (as well as strongly "scientific") by new accurate anatomical studies [3–8, 25, 26]; an intense brainstorming (characterized by hundreds of publications and congresses/courses) leading to new elegant techniques [27–33] and refinements of old surgical techniques [2, 34, 35]. The new wave of PR represented (and still represents) the great vogue of the last decade; the wagon where a lot of young—and "young at heart"—wanted to get on.

However, history is a circle, and also PR's issues recently started to come to a head: increasing number of complications (often due to excessive septal destabilization with subsequent saddling), the tendency to generate scooping deformity—often due to poor basis of nose "structure" in the youngest surgeons—and tip over projection/over-rotation (which is becoming a kind of demodé in certain countries) along with a correct learning curve which is appearing slower of how it was thought.

It is quite frequent, especially in the scientific world, that new techniques and ideas are initially met with enthusiasm, and subsequently with later caution as challenges emerge and problems arise. Similarly, the "pure" preservation rhinoplasty has recently started to be considered not the exclusive and only "best and contemporary approach" in contrast to the old-fashioned "disruptive" structural rhinoplasty. It is becoming obvious that the pendulum is moving back toward the middle, nowadays. So, "hybrid" approaches, which blend the rationale (considering both advantages and disadvantages) of preservation and structure, recognizing the merits of the former, but without entirely renegading the latter, are gaining more and more popularity. Those "hybrid" techniques can be resumed as essentially employing dorsal preservation methods (for managing the nasal dorsum), while the tip remains "structural" (i.e., managed by a structural approach), however, dissecting on proper anatomical planes and respecting/reconstructing ligaments as far as possible [10, 11, 36–42].

## 48.2 Hybrid Concepts

What the term "hybrid" stands for and what is our hybrid philosophy? The goal of this paragraph (as well as of the entire chapter) is to answer these questions trying to give the readers a detailed description along with a rattled-off version of the preservation-structure hybrid principles that we pursue every day in our daily rhinoplasty practice.

It became evident that, for some surgeons—like the authors of this chapter—born and raised to the structural approach, integrating preservation principles in their practice would be made easier by a "hybrid" approach. On the other hand, after the first "preservationist" big wave, it also became evident that reintegrating some

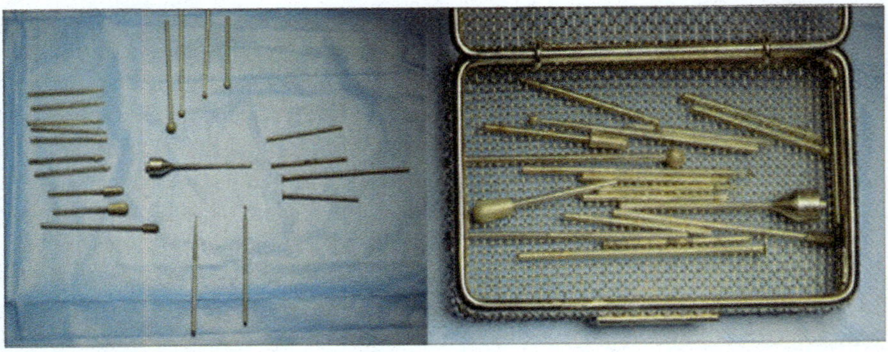

**Fig. 48.1** Burrs menu: different shapes and sizes of burrs used in our rhinoplasty practice

key "open" structural points makes the difference, especially when approaching difficult cases (e.g., severe dorsal asymmetries/crookedness or extremely "dysfunctional" noses) where a full reestablishment along with a full open view makes the surgical workflow easier. For us and others, this essentially means an open dissection rhinoplasty with preservation of the dorsum and structural reediting of the tip while preserving/reconstructing nasal ligaments as far as possible. However, our "hybrid" philosophy is not only limited to the preservation-structure duality but also to the "hybridization" (i.e., the combined, sometimes simultaneous) use of both manual and mechanical instruments and, among these latter, the full logical combination of the piezo technology and power tools (Fig. 48.1) [43, 44].

## 48.3 Open Approach and Planes of Dissection

For us and many others, "to open" a nose does not mean "to sacrify" the original anatomy, but rather to fully view the surgical field with plenty of control of the underlying anatomical structures. This is the main reason why we always adopt an open dissection with a full degloving of the soft tissue envelope (a partial, sometimes limited—but still always "open"—degloving becomes our choice in a minority of cases where a limited or focused midvault/bony vault work is needed while the tip issues represent the main concern) (Fig. 48.2) [25, 36–38].

We used to start by using a mid-columellar inverted-V incision (which represents our only choice except for those extremely rare cases of nonfeasibility or when we decide to use—or to fix—the scar of a previous nose surgery). We approach our dissection over the lower lateral cartilages (LLCs) on a supraperichondrial plane (Fig. 48.3). Although the subperichondrial LLCs dissection, as described by Cakir and Coskun [42], could be seen as an elegant alternative, we found that it is likely to weaken the alar cartilages, especially under a fully open approach and particularly in thick skin patients (where our experience has thought us that LLCs tend to be weaker and, also, where it makes no sense to stay under the perichondium for camouflage-related reasons or if you consider a subsequent soft tissues' debulking

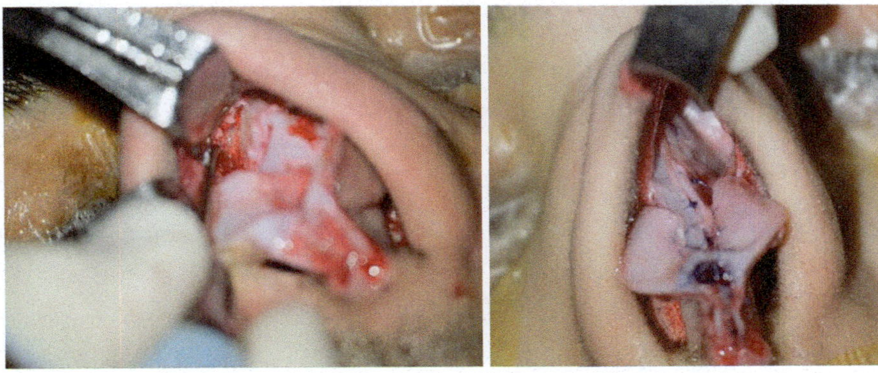

**Fig. 48.2** Wide degloving and clear anatomy

**Fig. 48.3** LLCs supraperichondrial plane of dissection

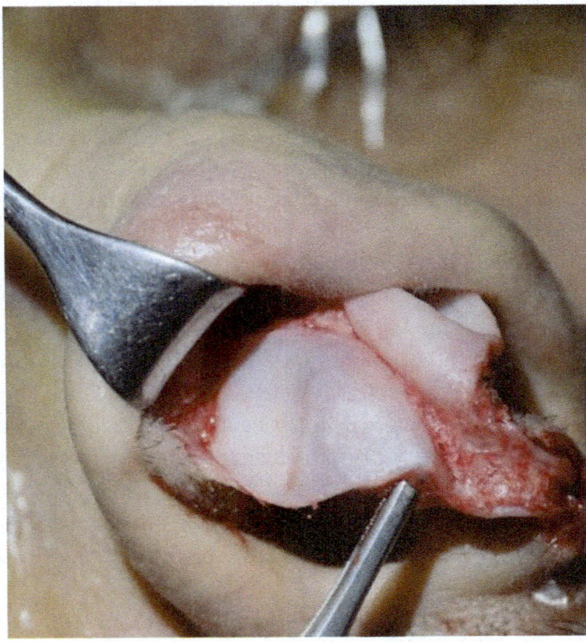

of the tip) [38]. Even if in one of our last published papers, we considered different planes of dissection based on the skin quality and the LLCs' weakness [38], in the last 3 years we definitively switched to a supraperichondrial dissection of the LLCs in 100% of our cases, because we are firmly convinced that this initial approach is easier, quicker, and safer. We invariably transition to a subperichondrial plane at the level of the scroll area (Fig. 48.4) (i.e., where the scroll cartilages are or are supposed to be anatomical, although sometimes they are hypoplastic or even absent). This is the anatomical landmark of the vertical scroll ligament, which joins with the longitudinal scroll ligament between the cranial edge of the LLCs and the caudal

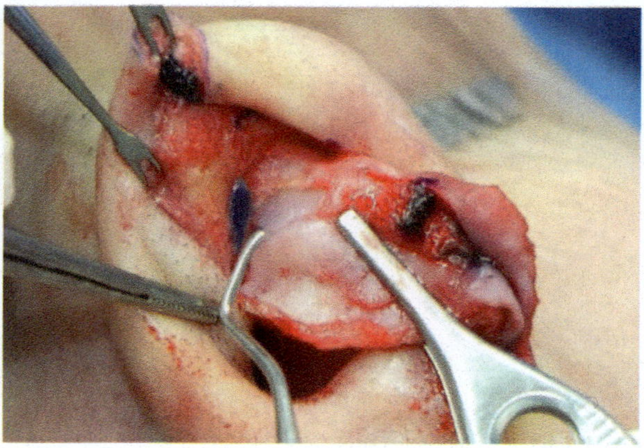

**Fig. 48.4** Transition from supraperichondrial plane to subperichondrial plane: lower lateral cartilages (LLCs) are usually dissected leaving the perichondrium intact (i.e., following a supraperichondrial dissection); the subperichondrial plane is usually entered at the upper edge of the LLCs at the level of the scroll area. The scroll cartilages, when present, are marked with methylene blue

edge of the upper lateral cartilages (ULCs). The dissection will then progress cranially, under the perichondrium, with a full degloving and exposition of the ULCs until reaching the caudal edge of the nasal bones (i.e., the keystone area). From that point onwards, the surgical dissection continues in a subperiosteal plane until a full bony degloving is obtained, too. As we already outlined, this kind of dissection can be more limited laterally in unusual circumstances where no bony work will be necessary to the lateral nasal base. This technique allows us to define three specific points, which become important during the final closure steps: right and left scroll cartilages and supraseptal grooves. This "3 points compartmentalization" technique will let us reduce the dead space and redrape the single plane dissection in an anatomically correct position enhancing nasal contour (Fig. 48.4) (from 3 points article) [38].

In the minority of cases where we choose a fully structural approach (severe dorsal asymmetries/crookedness), the dissection will still be the same.

## 48.4 Dorsal Preservation and Tip Structuring

As we already explained, in these last years, having recognized the clear advantages of the preservation rhinoplasty concepts but always having taken into account the effectiveness—sometimes even the essentiality—of the structural approach, we switched our minds to a hybrid preservation-structure way of performing rhinoplasty. This is true for the majority of our cases except for the ones—although rare—in which we still prefer a classic full structural open approach by means of a component separation and incremental reduction as popularized by Rohrich [45]. This essentially means that, nowadays, we perform dorsal preservation along with a structural re-editing of the tip while preserving/reconstructing the ligaments as far as possible, and after an accurate supraperichondrial (at the level of the LLCs)/ subperichondrial (from the scroll area onwards)/subperiosteal (at the bony vault) open dissection.

We believe that re-editing the dorsum under direct vision is the key, and this is the clear reason why we always "open" our noses. We also believe that preserving the beauty and the function of the natural keystone areas (both the dorsal keystone areas—DKA—and the lateral ones—LKAs) must be considered always mandatory, except for those rare sparse cases where there is nothing to preserve (although preservation approaches are expanding more and more for these latter, too) [46–51]. Dorsal preservation undoubtedly plays a crucial role in avoiding aesthetic drawbacks (such as "open roof" or "inverted V" deformities, as well as minimal surface irregularities to touch) and functional sequelae, by additionally avoiding the reconstruction of the midvault subsequent to the dorsum de-humping.

On the other hand, we continue to think "structural" when addressing the tip: dedicated tip sutures along with strong and durable support (i.e., a tailored septal extension graft), sometimes with further conformational elements (i.e., a tip shield graft and/or a columellar "spacer" strut) for better tip and/or nasolabial angle definition, still represent our way of doing to prevent the postoperative loss of tip projection/support, particularly at long-term follow-up.

## 48.5 Combining Piezo and Power Tools

Our idea of "hybrid" goes beyond what we outlined in the previous paragraph. As a matter of fact, our daily surgical practice is nowadays characterized by the combined—hybrid—use of manual, sometimes tailored or made-to-order and electric instruments. Regarding this last group of electric tools, we invariably combine power instruments (Fig. 48.1) (e.g., power burrs) with the piezoelectric technology.

The introduction of piezoelectric technology into rhinoplasty was widely popularized by Gerbault [9] and then adopted by many as the ideal instrument for bony management while respecting soft tissue and perichondrium [12–14, 52–54]. Many papers have been published over the last years emphasizing such advantages as well as also claiming, sometimes arbitrarily, that piezo technology would reduce edema and favor more rapid healing [55, 56].

The enthusiasm with which piezo has been met in the surgical community, founded on undeniable advantages accompanied by significant marketing, carried the consequence of laying aside, at least partially, the use of power tools, which came to be seen as "old-fashioned" and, essentially, more destructive.

But power tools, differently from piezo, are universally available in most operating rooms and different systems will usually, but not uniformly, fit most of the burrs commercially available.

The value of power tools in rhinoplasty was first described by Toriumi and Becker in 1997 [57], who compared manual and powered tools in dorsal reduction, emphasizing the advantage of using power for sculpting bone. Also, Guyuron in 1989 proposed a guarded burr as an effective and safe way of deepening the nasofrontal angle [58]. Davis and others widely reported the use of power tools for bone reshaping [15, 59–61].

Interestingly, power tools had been described much before piezo in rhinoplasty, but essentially they never enjoyed the same popularity. A possible reason could be that piezo came to be introduced in parallel with those new accurate anatomical concepts that steered rhinoplasty toward the preservation and, substantially, required greater precision in osteotomies. If one, however, steps back and sets aside the urge to swiftly replace older technologies with newer ones, it becomes evident that each specific tool possesses distinct advantages and disadvantages. The next logical step is to combine the use of different tools for specific indications, designating for which indication one instrument works better than the other. This comes together with the undeniable fact that certain instruments may perform better in one surgeon's hands than another's, thus entering the realm of a surgeon's manual dexterity and personal preference.

We feel to summarize our daily, long-lasting, experience with this kind of electric tool by giving a few effective take-home messages [43]: (1) piezo remains the ideal tool for cutting bone, regarding osteotomies and septoplasty (i.e., for cutting the posterior bony part of the septum—the perpendicular plate of the ethmoid—or in the case of vomerine spurs); (2) cylindrical and conical burrs are ideally suited for precise bone reshaping (i.e., osteoplasty). They will not damage soft tissue or cartilage if handled with due care; (3) piezo can equally be used for bone reshaping, however, with limitations as compared to burrs; and (4) thin, discoid, rotating burrs are an alternative to piezo in confined spaces where their design provides an obvious advantage.

## 48.6 Modified Dorsal Split Hybrid Preservation

After the first description of the "hybrid" structure-preservation approach to primary rhinoplasty [36], which actually came quite contemporary with other authors [62, 63], we gradually transitioned to this "new way" which nowadays represents almost 90% of our approach on primaries. The authors preferred technique is the *modified dorsal split (MDS) hybrid preservation rhinoplasty* [36] which is characterized by the following surgical steps and/or variations.

### 48.6.1 Tip and Dorsum Dissection

After a mid-columellar inverted-V incision, dissection over the LLCs is usually done on a supraperichondrial plane (Fig. 48.3), as we mentioned. We invariably transition to a subperichondrial plane at the level of the scroll cartilages. Often visible, but at times, just delineated by a gray transition line, they mark the level of the vertical scroll ligament. The dissection continues cranially fully exposing the ULCs below the perichondrium and continuing to the edge of the nasal bones, becoming eventually subperiosteal. This dissection technique allows us to define three specific points: right and left scroll cartilages and supraseptal grooves. This "3 points compartmentalization" technique is one of the many expedients we adopt to reduce the dead space and redrape the single plane dissection in an anatomically correct position enhancing nasal contour and supraalar definition (Fig. 48.5) [38].

.

### 48.6.2 Bony Vault Reshaping and Sculpturing

The dissection then progresses to a fully open approach, which can be more limited laterally in unusual circumstances where no bony lateral work will be necessary. Then, either a cartilaginous pushdown or a full letdown will follow. While the preferred option has already been selected by clinical examination and viewing the bony cap on sagittal cut Cone Beam Computed Tomography (CBCT) (Fig. 48.6) [64], however, we await a final decision once the dorsum is fully opened. Subsequently, we proceed with initial osteoplasty, which can be sufficient per se for managing the bony dorsum or be preliminary to a full letdown.

(a) In case of a *cartilaginous pushdown*, the relatively small bony cap is efficiently lowered by burrs. Typically, this is done by cylindrical, conical, or reversed conical burrs at low RPM and with ice-cold constant irrigation.
(b) In case of a *full letdown*, initial osteoplasty will often serve to convert an S-shaped bony cap to a V-shaped configuration [8]. It is self-evident that this

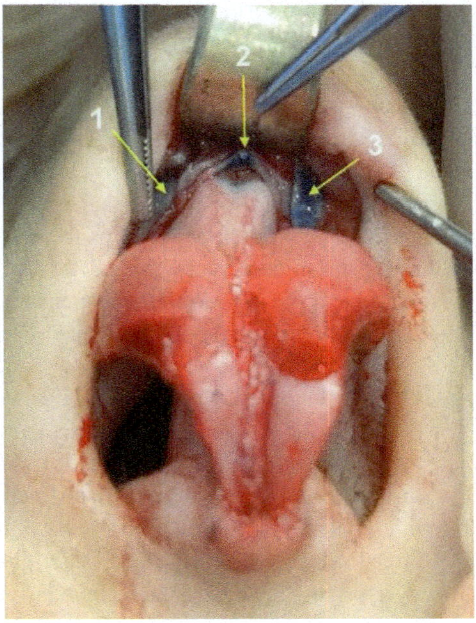


**Fig. 48.5** Concept of the 3 points compartmentalization technique is shown in this figure: all three points are marked (1: right scroll cartilage, 2: supraseptal groove, and 3: left scroll cartilage). They will be resutured, at the end of the surgery and before the final closure, to re-compartmentalize again the nose

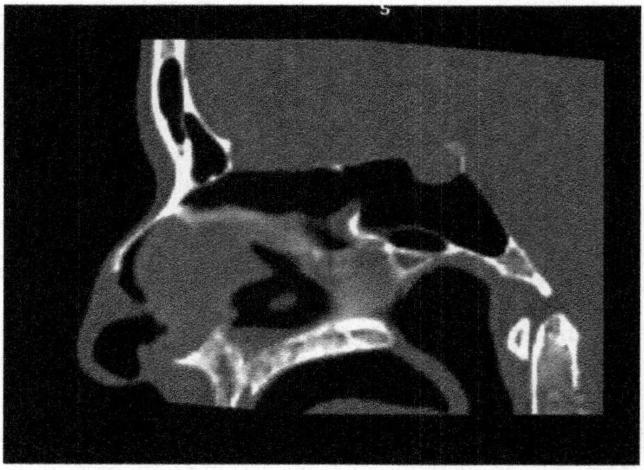

**Fig. 48.6** Bony cap on sagittal section CBCT, preoperative analysis

will be possible only with a fully open approach and will significantly expand the conventional indications of the letdown procedure.

The extent of osteoplasty can be planned preoperatively by assessing the thickness of the bone in CBCT and needs to be performed intraoperatively with care, noting that a color change of the bone from white to pink will signal the limit to sculpture. Of course, specific piezo inserts can be used as an alternative option for osteoplasty, but we believe that cylindrical and conical burrs are faster and allow a better, wider, and uniform contact area for shaping and polishing the bone. One can obviously state that piezo will offer a better guarantee toward injury or even avulsion of the ULCs, but the use of burrs, if handled with care, won't cause any injury to the underlying cartilage; moreover, burrs have the privilege of sculpturing with a smoother surface.

### 48.6.3 Middle Vault Dorsal Split and Osteotomies Where Needed

Splitting the middle vault along the septal "T" follows next, according to the MDS preservation technique, which aims to preserve the DKA, while allowing liberty in reshaping the middle vault as needed [36, 37]. Different osteotomies may now be necessary, and piezo becomes indispensable for this purpose. Its use will be facilitated by the previous osteoplasty done by burrs.

(a) In case of a *cartilaginous push down* with minimal bony component, the whole bony dorsum may solely be addressed by osteoplasty, including the possibility of proper definition of aesthetic dorsal lines. Otherwise, a combination of low-to-low osteotomies together with median oblique, and/or transverse osteotomies will allow a reduction of the bony width without further loss of height after lowering the bony cap. Proper planning of such osteotomies is facilitated by assessing the CBCT, and the underlying key concept is to avoid full fractures, while rather achieving greenstick mobilization [11, 39]. Sometimes, power tools are again called for, by the use of the Luer lock adapter for Transcutaneous Transosseous Cerclage Suture (TTC) suturing as described by Haack and Gubisch [65, 66]. This will allow when needed, effective stabilization of the mobilized nasal bones. If nasal bone asymmetry is an issue, usually the case being greater convexity on one side, this will be addressed by criss-cross or even fishbone piezo osteotomies, as described by Martins and Goksel [12, 40].

(b) In case of a *full letdown*, circumferential osteotomies will be carried out with the appropriate piezo inserts, staying as low as possible in the nasofacial groove and with the help of a suction elevator. This can be done symmetrically or asymmetrically by the removal of differential bony wedges if the bony orientation is different. In fact, it is indeed striking how effective an asymmetric letdown can be in managing bony deviation. Although many authors have different opinions regarding how to perform the transverse bony cut at the radix, the senior author prefers to employ a small disc burr which can be inserted in an inevitably narrow space with a precise cut although not allowing the same superior oblique direction of the osteotomy which could be achieved with a transcutaneous osteotome at the radix. When coupled, however, with a long piezo insert to incrementally and carefully excise small bony wedges from the perPendicular Plate of Ethmoid (PPE) until it meets the transverse osteotomy, this will allow avoiding a drop-down of the radix. Should this drop of the radix instead be desirable, a burr will finally have to be used to smooth off the remaining sharp edges. In both cases above, the high-middle septal strip is suture-fixated under direct vision to the septum, in end-to-end or end-to-side fashion, after vertical scoring to release tension and straighten the dorsum, with the "Vitruvian man" maneuver as described by Neves [41]. Appropriate trimming of the ULC and, if needed, selective spreader grafts are used to finalize the dorsal lines. The middle vault is finally resutured along the borders of the septal "T," without any need for an LKA release. Obviously, the septoplasty (to be illustrated below) will be completed before resuturing the middle vault.

In case of a more significant bony cap, but still not necessitating a full letdown or where the radix is already low, a modification of the cartilaginous pushdown is possible by including a portion of the bony cap within the pushed-down DKA segment. Essentially, the osteochondral junction at the DKA is partially extended to comprise the distal portion of the bony cap, which has already been reduced by burr osteoplasty. This modification, proposed independently by Khazaal [67] and Furtado [68], involves performing small additional medial oblique osteotomies starting at the keystone using piezo. A bony-cartilaginous flap is thus created. Instead of a transverse cut at the radix, a transverse cut is precisely executed at the point of the bony dorsum where the hump initiates (Fig. 48.7) [67]. This can be accomplished with either a disc diamond burr for a superficial partial thickness cut or using a pin diamond burr (1 mm) (Fig. 48.8) for a subdorsal transverse cut, strategically weakening the bone precisely at the hump's starting point, following the subdorsal "green-stick" concept described by Ferreira et al. [69]. An additional step involves

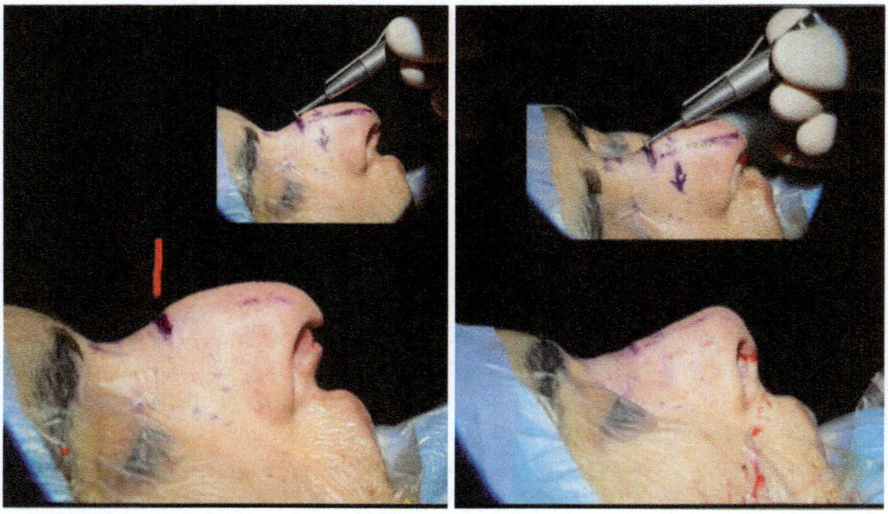

**Fig. 48.7** Weakening the bony hump just where the hump begins, either subdorsal using disk burr as shown in this figure or weakening the bone below the bony cup

**Fig. 48.8** 1 mm burr and 2 mm burr

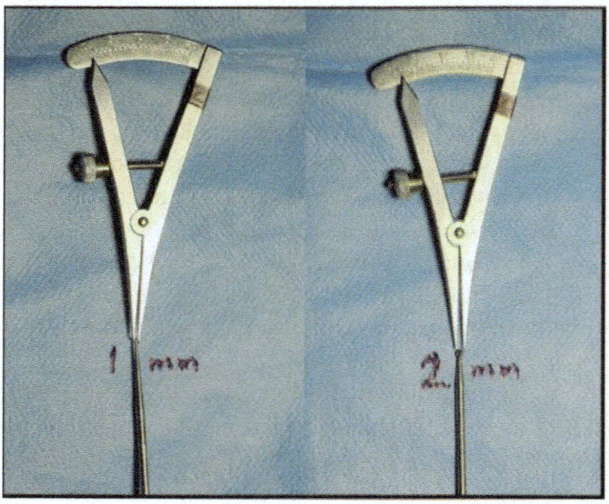


a subdorsal longitudinal cut of the PPE, removing a piece of bone equal to the desired hump reduction. This meticulous process ensures that the bony hump descends with full control in continuity with the split and scored septal "T," preserving the DKA. If needed, piezo can be used to remove small wedges of bone laterally, adjacent to the medial oblique cut, in a similar way to that described by Ferreira in his spare roof type B technique [69]. This additional step provides the necessary space to ease the downward movement of the bony-cartilaginous flap without resistance.

## 48.7 Septoplasty

No matter if we are going to deal with a septal deviation or just harvest a septal graft, the concept and the strategy are almost the same. The MDS preservation technique usually facilitates an L-strut septoplasty together with a high middle strip, although a Cottle technique can be employed in selected cases. Piezo once again comes into play as an indispensable tool for both parallel superior and inferior longitudinal cuts in the bone after a Freer septum knife has been used for the cartilaginous portion. The superior cut will be done in the PPE where it joins with the quadrangular septal cartilage and the latter in the vomer. This will have to follow the high-middle strip removal, and a long piezo insert becomes invaluable here. Piezo will allow a clean cut and, importantly, will safeguard the integrity of the remaining posterior connection of the L-strut and prevent its collapse with the consequent saddling. Once the superior and inferior longitudinal cuts are made, a small and long, thin narrow disc burr is employed vertically to finalize the transection of the remaining connection posteriorly (Fig. 48.9) so that the septal segment to be removed can be taken in its entirety. Although the space is tight, it will be enough for the disc burr with the aid of a Killian thin speculum. This method prevents unwanted piecemeal resection of multiple septal segments and will allow the obvious advantage of obtaining essentially a single and a big bony cartilaginous graft (Fig. 48.10). The harvested graft can then be liberally used as needed, including composite combinations of cartilage and bone, as well as perforated PPE segments for splinting different areas, where perforations are done by a piezo conical tip. Finally, in those instances where spine manipulation is needed, piezo is again used either for creating slots or for drilling holes or bisecting the spine on whichever side, then replacing the septum in the middle with proper suture fixation. Piezo technique here is once again uniquely efficient and also safe regarding the potential of soft tissue and nerve injury. Last but not least, piezo will allow, where a significant spur exists, to bisect the spur and extract it carefully thereafter.

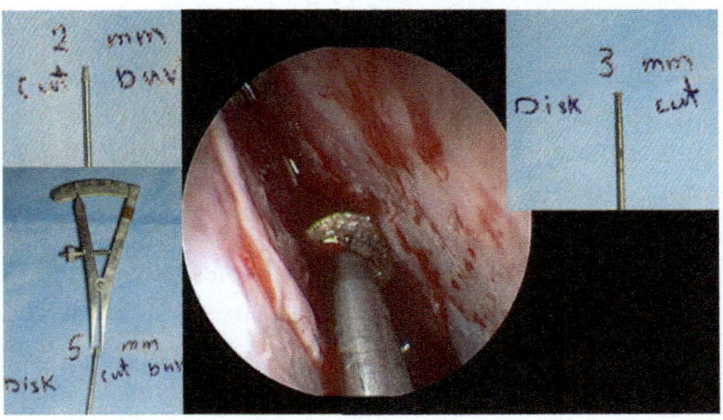


**Fig. 48.9** Disc burr of different sizes used to make clear vertical cut cephalically on the PPE or vomer

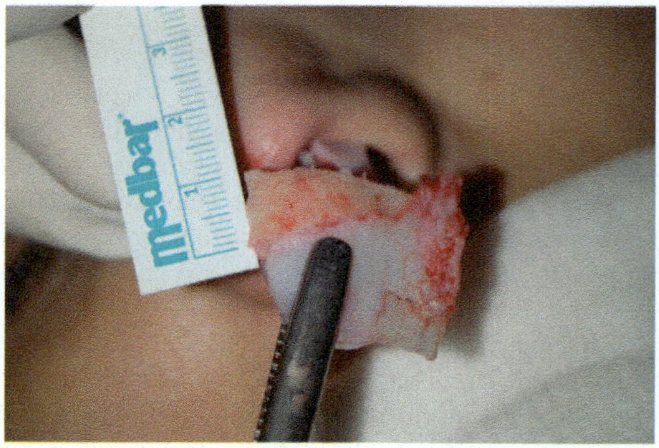


**Fig. 48.10** Big bony cartilaginous piece harvested from the septum using piezo and disc burr

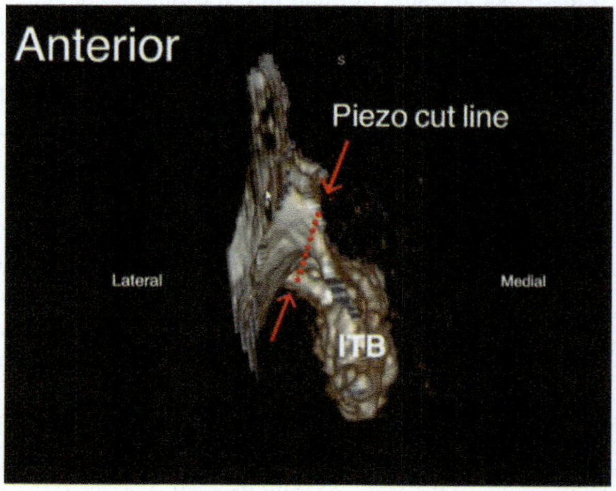


**Fig. 48.11** 3D reconstruction CT from one of our patients showing the hypertrophied bony component of the inferior turbinate which matters more than the soft tissue in such a case

## 48.8 Turbinoplasty [53]

Our novel technique for inferior turbinates (IT) treatment was described years ago and still, although with some refinements, we continue to use it. Piezo is used for turbinoplasty after assessing the volume and relative percentage of bone versus mucosa in CBCT views. The indication will obviously be turbinates with a significant bony component particularly in compensatory inferior turbinate hypertrophy (ITH) (Fig. 48.11). A small full-thickness incision through the anterior–inferior surface of the turbinate is made by a fine-angled microsurgical needle in the cutting mode. Once the Bovie tip touches the bone, a short tunnel is made between the mucosa and the inferior turbinate bone, using a small sharp elevator, with the dissection only extending a few millimeters distal to the bony edge. Next a long, angled, or straight piezo insert is inserted into the tunnel. The same insert used in other portions of the rhinoplasty is essentially reemployed. The insert is moved in a direction from caudal to cephalic, perpendicular to the line of attachment of the

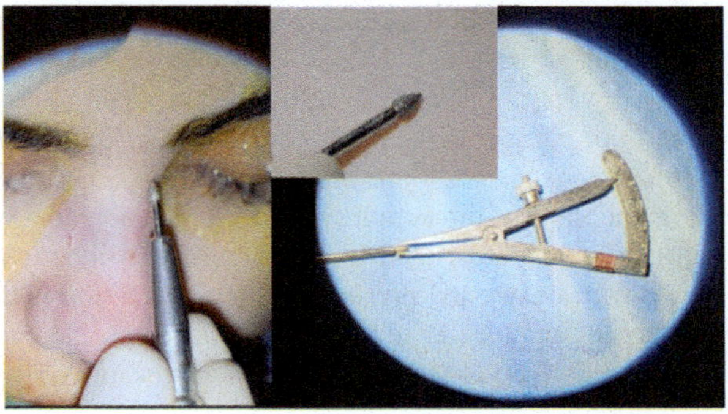

**Fig. 48.12** Small unique burr "Duomo Burr" from Dr. Robotti's burrs menu selected for radix sculpture

turbinate bone to the lateral nasal wall, which is in fact the site of maximum angulation. This is different and distinct from the line of conventional (manual) outfracture, which occurs more laterally, along the weakest point of the bone. It is striking to note that at this point the inferior turbinate easily lateralizes passively, actually almost spontaneously. Next, the same Bovie tip cautery is introduced submucosally along its full length, prevalently in the inferomedial portion of the turbinate. A coagulation current is used while the needle is withdrawn progressively, thus achieving a submucosal intraturbinal microcauterization to reduce the soft tissue volume by fibrosis without the direct damage caused by surface electrocautery. Once the above steps mentioned before are completed, large Mayo scissors are introduced, placed flat on the turbinate, and used to complete lateralization of the turbinate.

## 48.9 Final Osteoplasty: Beveling and Polishing

After completing the tip work, which will be done structurally (identifying, preserving, or reconstructing ligaments and using small septal extension grafts, strut spacer grafts, and appropriate maneuvers to achieve correct sidewall straightening and orientation as needed), a final osteoplasty is usually necessary before closure and re-compartmentalization of the dorsum [38]. This is done both by round diamond burrs when beveling is necessary on the sharp edges of osteotomies as well as by flat-surfaced, conical, and cylindrical burrs for final smoothing of bony contour. Essentially, sharp edges are flattened, and small surface irregularities are polished. Moreover, reassessing and revisiting the radix height and width to finalize by sculpting it accordingly with a unique conical small burr of 3 mm, "Duomo Burr" (Fig. 48.12).

## 48.10 Conclusions

This chapter resumes the "quintessence" of our thinking and approach to primary rhinoplasty. It appears clear how much we believe a "hybrid" approach, which we carefully described to the readers, could really make a difference. It embodies the pros of both structural and preservation techniques by minimizing their pitfalls and weak points. From our "hybrid" perspective, we definitely advocate dorsal preservation by splitting the midvault under an open approach and this is actually the excerpt of our technique of choice: the *modified dorsal split hybrid rhinoplasty for cartilaginous pushdown or full letdown applications*. We also believe that selecting the right plane of dissection (we invariably adopted a supraperichondrial dissection until the scroll area, then transitioning to a subperichondrial/subperiosteal plane) along with ligaments' preservation/reconstruction is the key. Eventually, we think that combining piezo and power tools is a game changer in terms of speed of surgical execution, postoperative recovery, and beauty of the final result.

**Cases**

**Case 1**

**Preoperative** (Fig. 48.13)

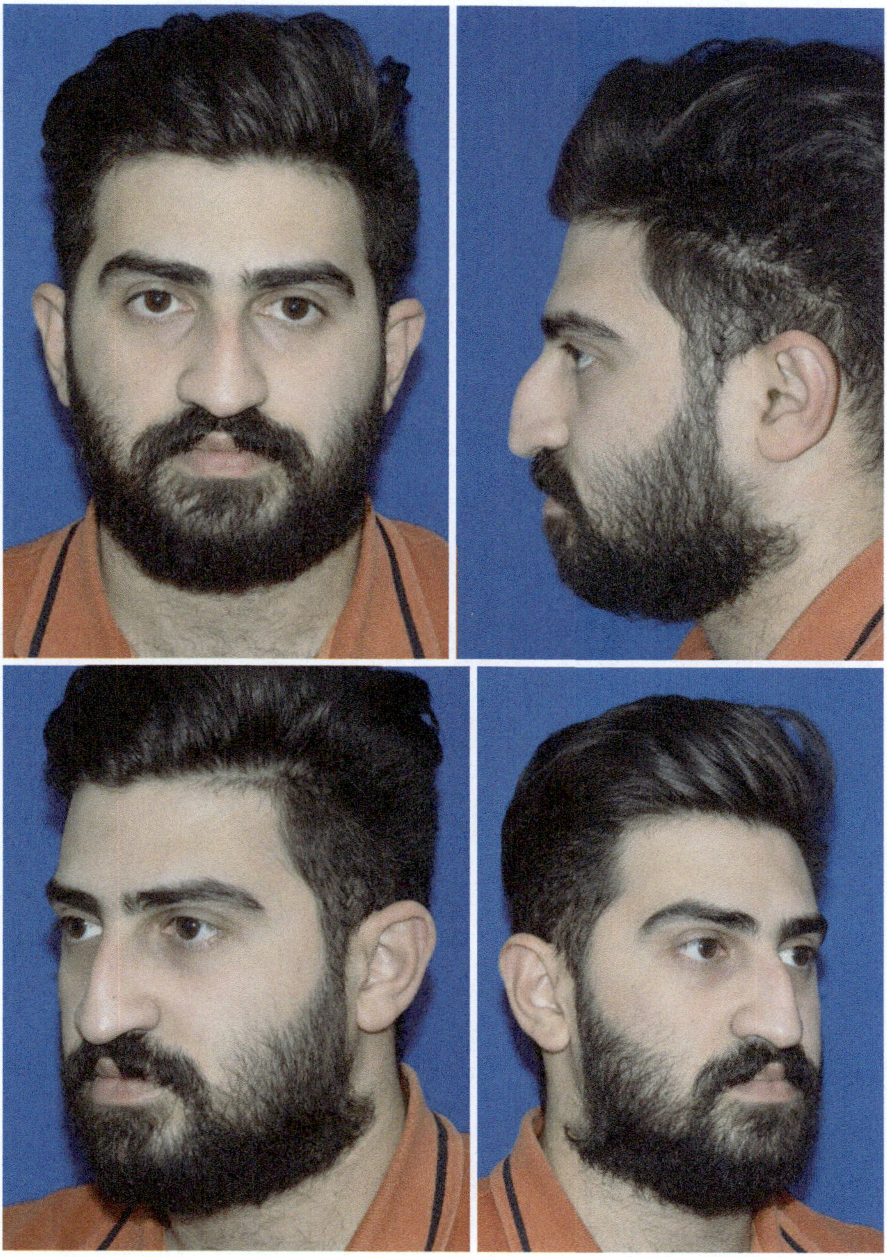

**Fig. 48.13** Preoperative (4 months): frontal, oblique left, profile left, oblique right, profile right, smiling frontal, smiling left, smiling right, and basal view

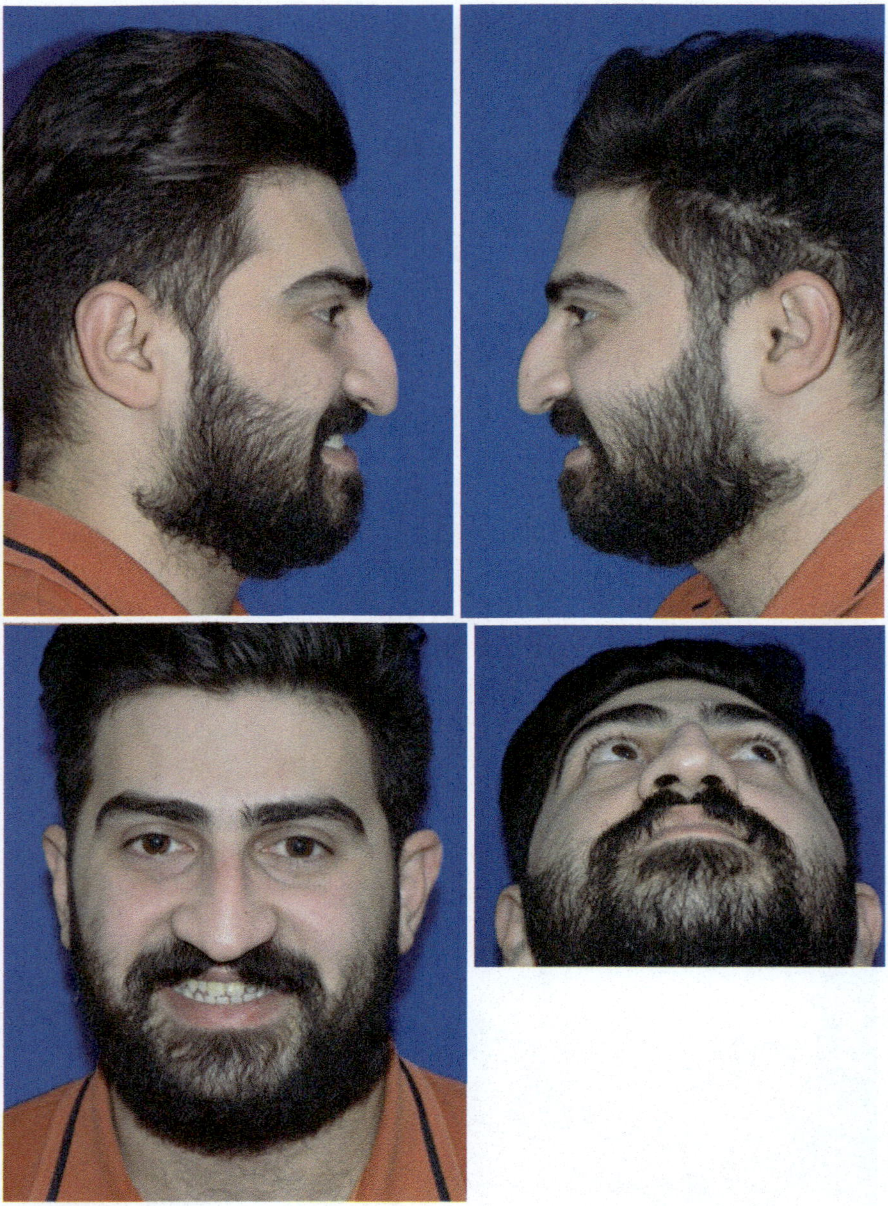

**Fig. 48.13** (continued)

**Postoperative** (Fig. 48.14)

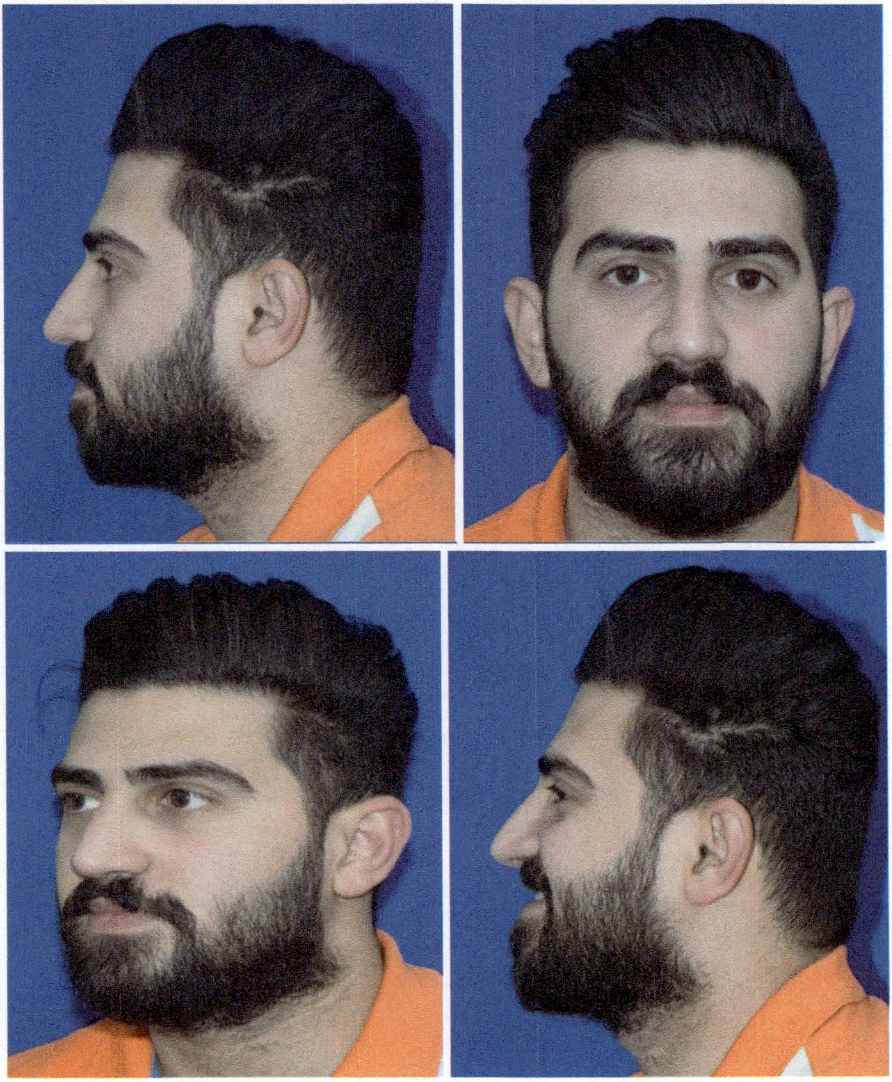

**Fig. 48.14** Postoperative (4 months): frontal, oblique left, profile left, oblique right, profile right, smiling frontal, smiling left, smiling right, and basal view

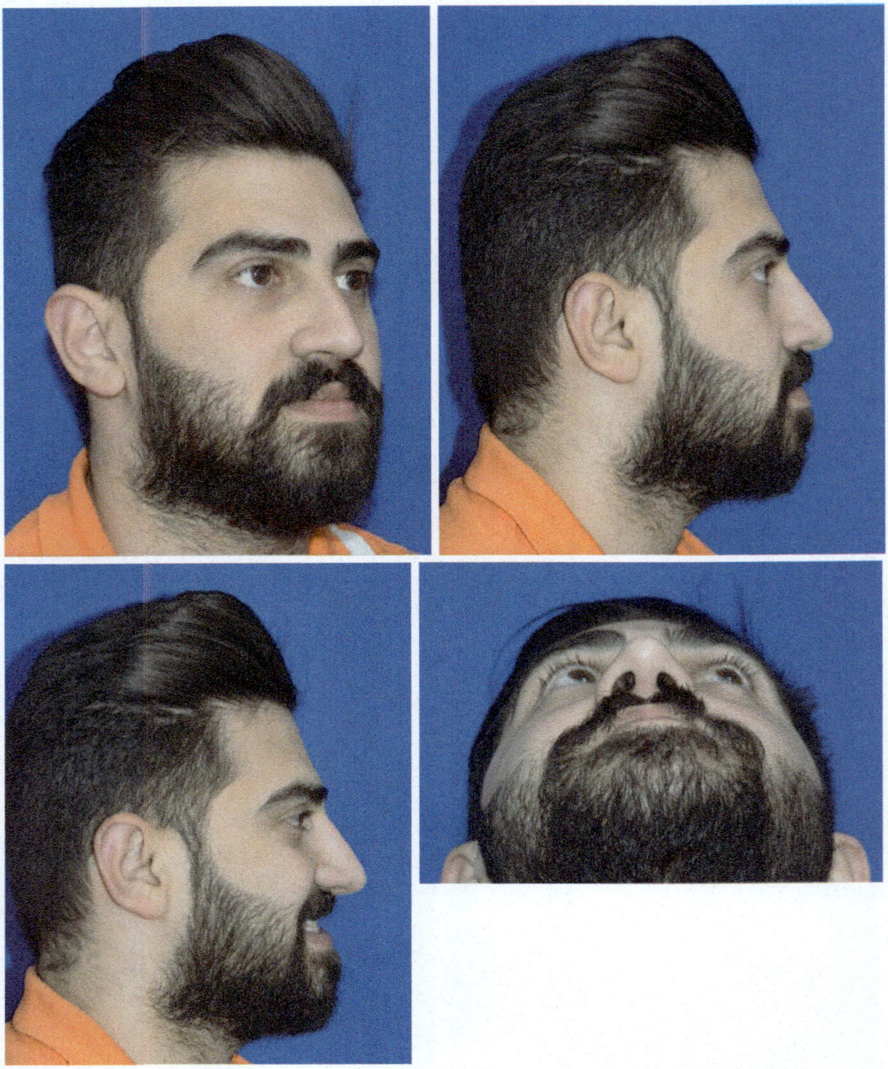

**Fig. 48.14** (continued)

**Case 2** (Figs. 48.15 and 48.16)
**Preoperative**
**Postoperative**

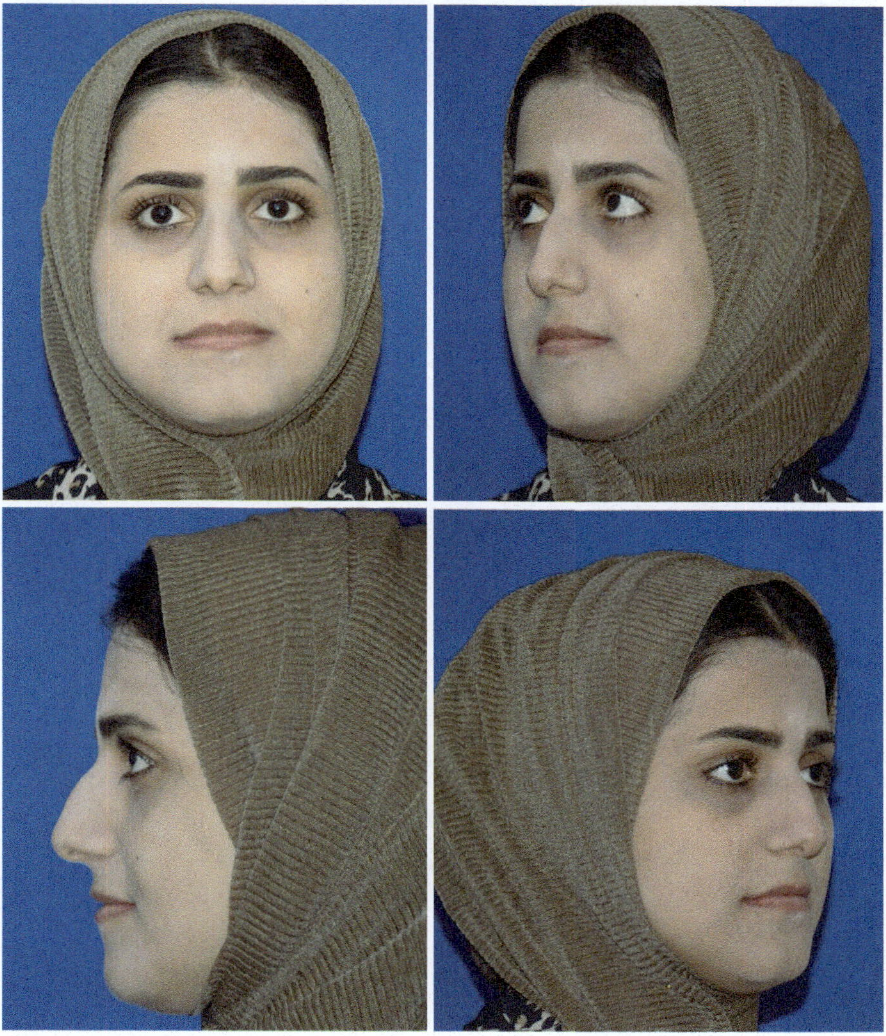

**Fig. 48.15** Preoperative (8 months): frontal, oblique left, profile left, oblique right, profile right, smiling frontal, smiling left, smiling right, and basal view

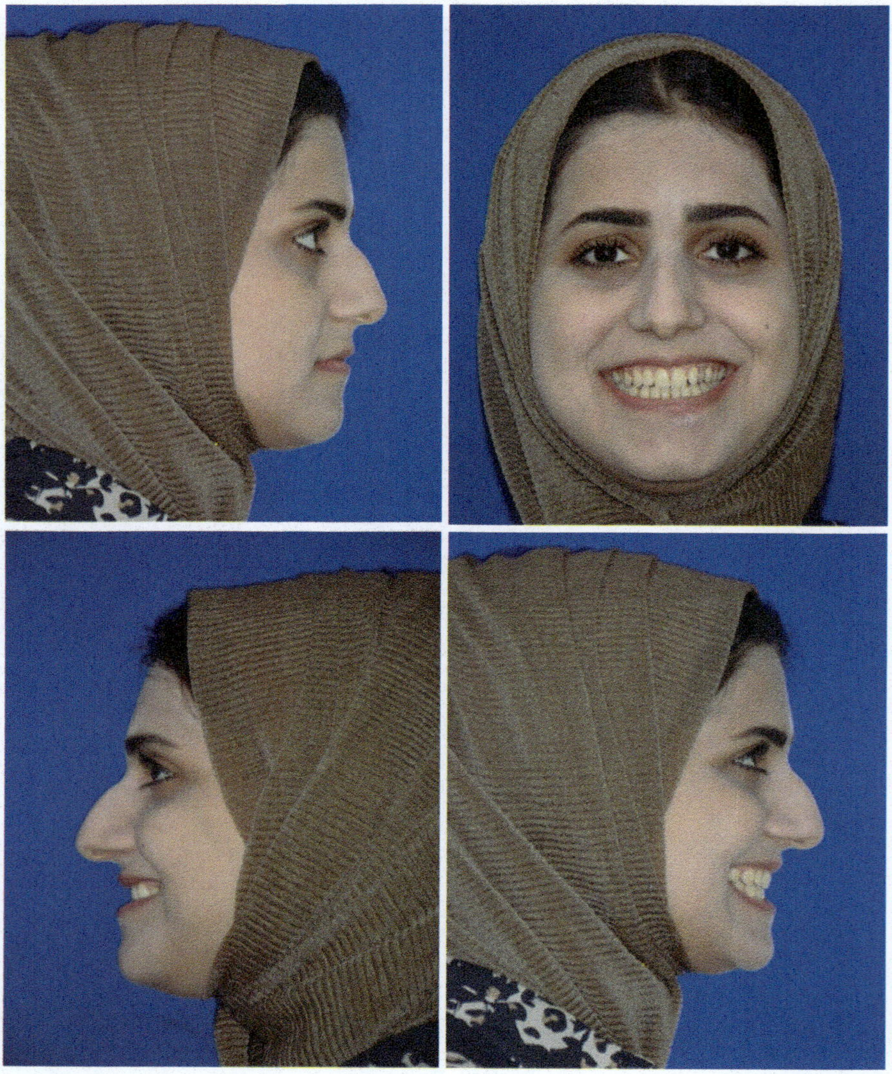

**Fig. 48.15** (continued)

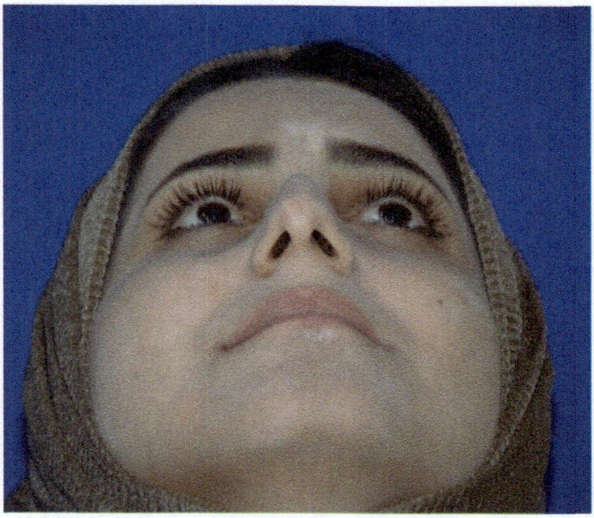

**Fig. 48.15** (continued)

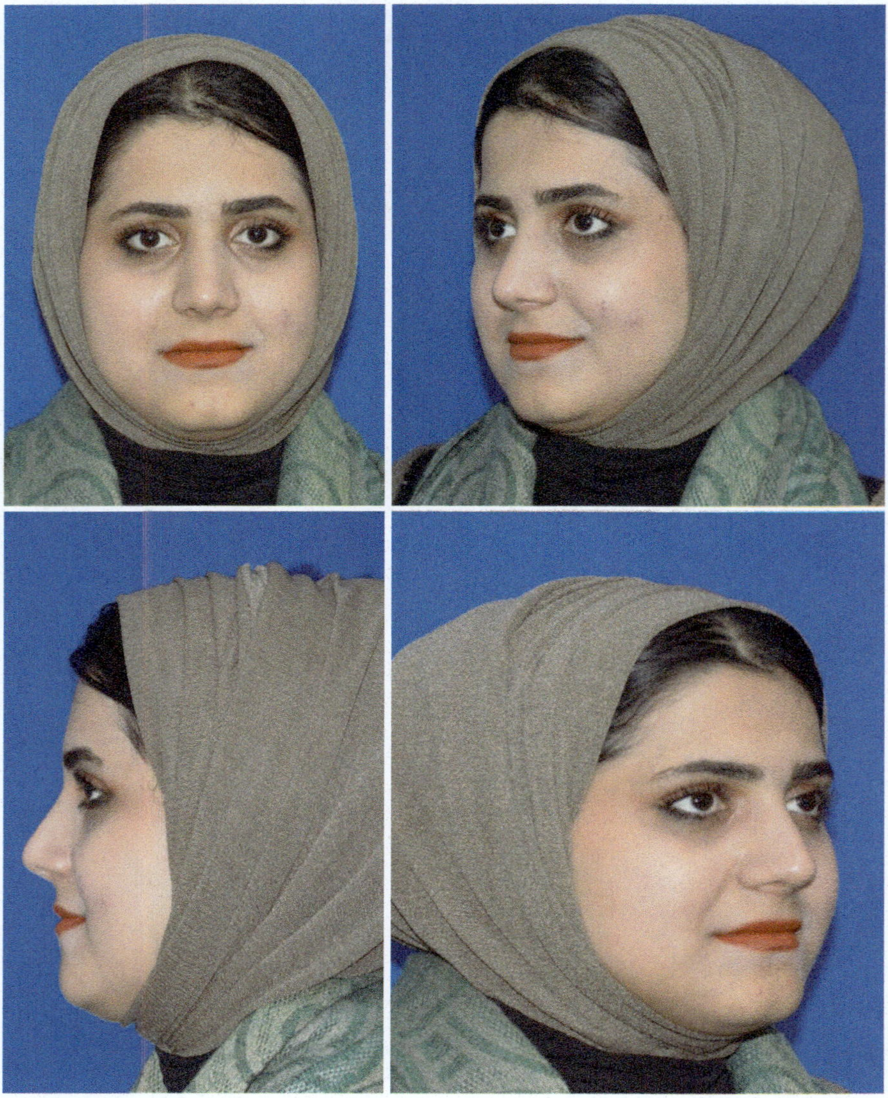

**Fig. 48.16** Postoperative (8 months): frontal, oblique left, profile left, oblique right, profile right, smiling frontal, smiling left, smiling right, and basal view

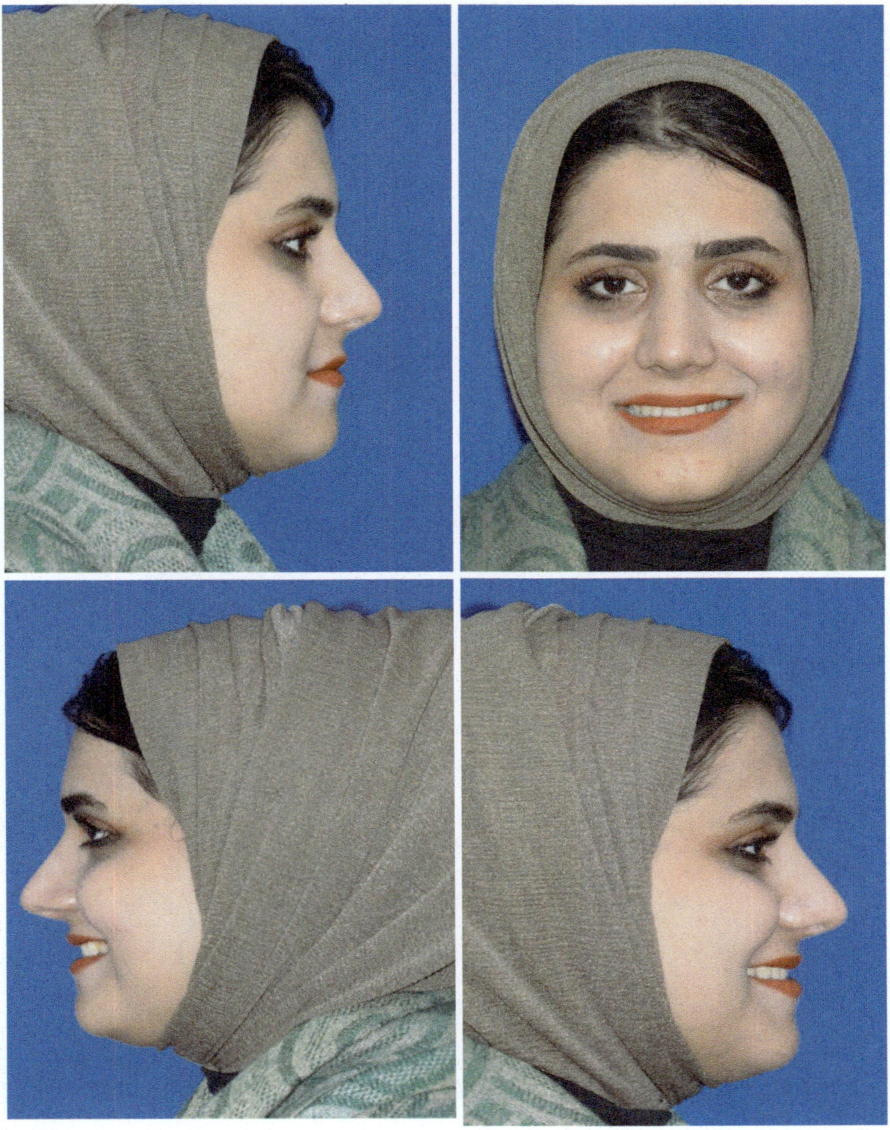

**Fig. 48.16** (continued)

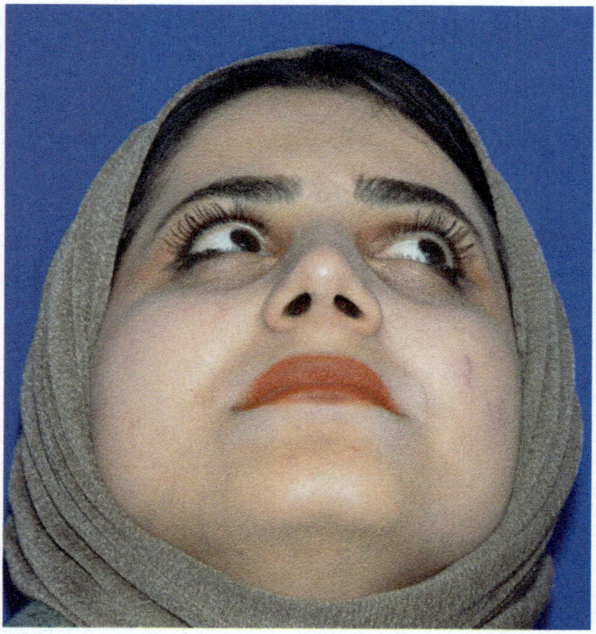

**Fig. 48.16** (continued)

## References


1. Daniel RK. The preservation rhinoplasty: a new rhinoplasty revolution. Aesthet Surg J. 2018;38(2):228–9. https://doi.org/10.1093/asj/sjx258. PMID: 29319790.
2. Saban Y, Daniel RK, Polselli R, Trapasso M, Palhazi P. Dorsal preservation: the push down technique reassessed. Aesthet Surg J. 2018;38(2):117–31. https://doi.org/10.1093/asj/sjx180. PMID: 29319787.
3. Daniel RK, Palhazi P. The nasal ligaments and tip support in rhinoplasty: an anatomical study. Aesthet Surg J. 2018;38(4):357–68. https://doi.org/10.1093/asj/sjx192. PMID: 29365051.
4. Daniel RK, Palhazi PR. An anatomical and clinical atlas. Cham: Springer; 2018.
5. Irmak F, Ertaş A, Kaleci B, Özkan S, Şentürk GE, Kuran I, Karşidağ S. The keystone, scroll complex, and interdomal area of the nose: histologic and anatomical observations. Plast Reconstr Surg. 2020;146(1):75–9. https://doi.org/10.1097/PRS.0000000000006895. PMID: 32590646.
6. Daniel RK, Palhazi P, Saban Y, Cakir B. Chapter 2. In: Preservation rhinoplasty. 3rd ed. Chicago: Septum Publishing; 2020.
7. Alfertshofer MG, Frank K, Ehrl D, Freytag DL, Moellhoff N, Gotkin RH, Mardini S, Beleznay K, Swift A, Cotofana S. The layered anatomy of the nose: an ultrasound-based investigation. Aesthet Surg J. 2022;42(4):349–57. https://doi.org/10.1093/asj/sjab310. PMID: 34363459.
8. Lazovic GD, Daniel RK, Janosevic LB, Kosanovic RM, Colic MM, Kosins AM. Rhinoplasty: the nasal bones—anatomy and analysis. Aesthet Surg J. 2015;35(3):255–63. https://doi.org/10.1093/asj/sju050. PMID: 25805278.
9. Gerbault O, Daniel RK, Kosins AM. The role of piezoelectric instrumentation in rhinoplasty surgery. Aesthet Surg J. 2016;36(1):21–34. https://doi.org/10.1093/asj/sjv167. Epub 2015 Nov 6. PMID: 26545389.

10. Gerbault O, Daniel RK, Palhazi P, Kosins AM. Reassessing surgical management of the bony vault in rhinoplasty. Aesthet Surg J. 2018;38(6):590–602. https://doi.org/10.1093/asj/sjx246. PMID: 29432541.
11. Zholtikov V, Golovatinsky V, Palhazi P, Gerbault O, Daniel RK. Rhinoplasty: a sequential approach to managing the bony vault. Aesthet Surg J. 2020;40(5):479–92. https://doi.org/10.1093/asj/sjz158. PMID: 31157882.
12. Göksel A, Patel PN, Most SP. Piezoelectric osteotomies in dorsal preservation rhinoplasty. Facial Plast Surg Clin North Am. 2021;29(1):77–84. https://doi.org/10.1016/j.fsc.2020.09.004. PMID: 33220846.
13. Goksel A, Tran KN. Open preservation rhinoplasty using the piezo electric instrument. Facial Plast Surg Clin North Am. 2023;31(1):59–71. https://doi.org/10.1016/j.fsc.2022.08.007. PMID: 36396289.
14. Robotti E. Shaping the nasal dorsum. HNO. 2018;66(2):92–102. https://doi.org/10.1007/s00106-017-0425-x. PMID: 29085975. English.
15. Racy E, Fanous A, Benmoussa N. Powered rhinoplasty: a simple step-by-step approach. Plast Reconstr Surg. 2021;147(1):65–7. https://doi.org/10.1097/PRS.0000000000007505. PMID: 33370051.
16. Sheen JH. Aesthetic rhinoplasty. St Louis: Mosby; 1978.
17. Joseph J, Aufricht G. Operative reduction of the size of a nose (rhinomiosis). Plast Reconstr Surg. 1970;46(2):178–83. https://doi.org/10.1097/00006534-197008000-00014. PMID: 5423485.
18. Joseph J. The classic reprint: nasal reductions. Plast Reconstr Surg. 1971;47(1):79–83. https://doi.org/10.1097/00006534-197101000-00015. PMID: 4921911.
19. Aufricht G. Joseph's rhinoplasty with some modifications. Surg Clin North Am. 1971;51(2):299–316. https://doi.org/10.1016/s0039-6109(16)39378-1. PMID: 4930522.
20. Goodman WS. External approach to rhinoplasty. Can J Otolaryngol. 1973;2(3):207–10. PMID: 4791580.
21. Anderson J, Ries W. Rhinoplasty: emphasizing the external approach [book review]. Plastic and reconstructive surgery. 1988;81(1):132–3.
22. Daniel RK. Rhinoplasty: creating an aesthetic tip. A preliminary report. Plast Reconstr Surg. 1987;80(6):775–83. PMID: 3317462.
23. Gunter JP, Rohrich RJ. External approach for secondary rhinoplasty. Plast Reconstr Surg. 1987;80(2):161–74. https://doi.org/10.1097/00006534-198708000-00001. PMID: 3602167.
24. Toriumi DM. Structure rhinoplasty: lessons learned in 30 years. Chicago: DMT Publishers; 2018.
25. Goksel A, Saban Y, Tran KN. Biomechanical nasal anatomy applied to open preservation rhinoplasty. Facial Plast Surg. 2021;37(1):12–21. https://doi.org/10.1055/s-0040-1715622. Epub 2021 Jan 27. PMID: 33506451.
26. Kosins AM, Daniel RK. Decision making in preservation rhinoplasty: a 100 case series with one-year follow-up. Aesthet Surg J. 2020;40(1):34–48. https://doi.org/10.1093/asj/sjz107. PMID: 30958525.
27. Çakır B, Öreroğlu AR, Daniel RK. Surface aesthetics in tip rhinoplasty: a step-by-step guide. Aesthet Surg J. 2014;34(6):941–55. https://doi.org/10.1177/1090820X14537643. Epub 2014 Aug 1. PMID: 24936094.
28. Gonçalves Ferreira M, Toriumi DM. A practical classification system for dorsal preservation rhinoplasty techniques. Facial Plast Surg Aesthet Med. 2021;23(3):153–5. https://doi.org/10.1089/fpsam.2021.0030. Epub 2021 Apr 16. PMID: 33861635.
29. Patel PN, Abdelwahab M, Most SP. A review and modification of dorsal preservation rhinoplasty techniques. Facial Plast Surg Aesthet Med. 2020;22(2):71–9. https://doi.org/10.1089/fpsam.2020.0017. PMID: 32130066; PMCID: PMC7312707.
30. Patel PN, Most SP. Overview of dorsal preservation rhinoplasty. Facial Plast Surg Clin North Am. 2023;31(1):1–11. https://doi.org/10.1016/j.fsc.2022.08.003. PMID: 36396280.
31. Kovacevic M, Veit JA, Toriumi DM. Subdorsal Z-flap: a modification of the Cottle technique in dorsal preservation rhinoplasty. Curr Opin Otolaryngol Head Neck Surg. 2021;29(4):244–51. https://doi.org/10.1097/MOO.0000000000000726. PMID: 34183554.

32. Çakır B, Genç B, Finocchi V, Haack S. My approach to preservation rhinoplasty. Facial Plast Surg Clin North Am. 2023;31(1):25–43. https://doi.org/10.1016/j.fsc.2022.08.014. PMID: 36396287.
33. Finocchi V, Vellone V, Mattioli RG, Daniel RK. A 3-level impaction technique for dorsal reshaping and reduction without dorsal soft tissue envelope dissection. Aesthet Surg J. 2022;42(2):151–65. https://doi.org/10.1093/asj/sjab261. PMID: 34175938.
34. Arancibia-Tagle D, Neves JC, D'Souza A. History of dorsum conservative techniques in rhinoplasty: the evolution of a revived technique. Facial Plast Surg. 2021;37(1):86–91. https://doi.org/10.1055/s-0041-1724031. Epub 2021 Feb 23. PMID: 33621985.
35. Most SP. Preservation rhinoplasty: revitalization of an age-old technique. Facial Plast Surg Clin North Am. 2021;29(1):xiii–xiv. https://doi.org/10.1016/j.fsc.2020.09.011. PMID: 33220849.
36. Robotti E, Chauke-Malinga NY, Leone F. A modified dorsal split preservation technique for nasal humps with minor bony component: a preliminary report. Aesth Plast Surg. 2019;43(5):1257–68.
37. Robotti E, Cottone G, Leone F. Modified dorsal Split preservation hybrid rhinoplasty for cartilaginous pushdown and full letdown applications: a PROM-based review of 100 consecutive cases. Facial Plast Surg. 2023;39(4):441–51.
38. Robotti E, Leone F, Malfussi VA, Cottone G. The "3 points compartmentalization" technique in subperichondrial-subperiosteal dissection in primary rhinoplasty to reduce edema and define contour. Aesth Plast Surg. 2022;46(4):1923–31.
39. Neves JC, Erol O, Arancibia-Tagle D, Ilhan E. Precision segmental preservation rhinoplasty: avoiding widening, defining new dorsal Esthetic lines in dorsal preservation rhinoplasty. Facial Plast Surg Clin North Am. 2023;31(1):155–70.
40. Martins L, Fagundes MSC, Koener HN, Fakih-Gomez N, D'Souza AR. The fish bone technique: an innovative approach for the bony nasal pyramid. Facial Plast Surg. 2024;40:93.
41. Neves JC, Arancibia Tagle D, Dewes W, et al. The split preservation rhinoplasty: "the Vitruvian man split maneuver". Eur J Plast Surg. 2020;43:323–33.
42. Neves JC, Zholtikov V, Cakir B, Coşkun E, Arancibia-Tagle D. Rhinoplasty dissection planes (subcutaneous, Sub-SMAS, supra-perichondral, and sub-perichondral) and soft tissues management. Facial Plast Surg. 2021;37(1):2–11. https://doi.org/10.1055/s-0041-1723825. Epub 2021 Feb 25. PMID: 33634451.
43. Robotti E, Cottone G, Khazaal A, De Bernardis R, Leone F. Combining piezo and power tools for a better outcome in hybrid "structural-preservation" rhinoplasty. To be submitted for publication.
44. Robotti E. Master lecture: "Modern rhinoplasty—where the journey is taking me". In: IMRHIS 2023, third Joint International Meeting of Rhinoplasty Societies, Berlin; 29 June–2 July 2023.
45. Rohrich RJ, Muzaffar AR, Janis JE. Component dorsal hump reduction: the importance of maintaining dorsal aesthetic lines in rhinoplasty. Plast Reconstr Surg. 2004;114(5):1298–308; discussion 1309–12. https://doi.org/10.1097/01.prs.0000135861.45986.cf. PMID: 15457053.
46. East C. Preservation rhinoplasty and the crooked nose. Facial Plast Surg Clin North Am. 2021;29(1):123–30. https://doi.org/10.1016/j.fsc.2020.09.007. PMID: 33220837.
47. Finocchi V, Vellone V, Ramieri V, de Angelis F, Marianetti TM. Pisa tower concept: a new paradigm in crooked nose treatment. Plast Reconstr Surg. 2021;148(1):66–70. https://doi.org/10.1097/PRS.0000000000008064. PMID: 34181604.
48. Rodrigues Dias D, Santos M, Sousa E, Castro S, Almeida E, Sousa C, Gonçalves FM. The spare roof technique as a new approach to the crooked nose. Facial Plast Surg Aesthet Med. 2022;24(3):178–84. https://doi.org/10.1089/fpsam.2021.0368. Epub 2022 Apr 11. PMID: 35404125.
49. Finocchi V, Vellone V. Managing the severe septal deviation using dorsal preservation. Facial Plast Surg Clin North Am. 2023;31(1):107–17. https://doi.org/10.1016/j.fsc.2022.08.009. PMID: 36396281.
50. Yorgun M, Çekiç E, Evlice A. Mobile bony cap (Meysem Yorgun technique): an innovative technique in preservation rhinoplasty for crooked nose deformity. Plast Reconstr Surg

Glob Open. 2023;11(4):e4919. https://doi.org/10.1097/GOX.0000000000004919. PMID: 37063499; PMCID: PMC10101306.
51. Tremp M, Schneider J, Raghu RBN, Goksel A, Saban Y. A systematic analysis of the nasal septum in crooked noses and suggested treatment algorithm according to preservation rhinoplasty (PR) principles. Aesth Plast Surg. 2023;47(4):1499–507. https://doi.org/10.1007/s00266-023-03293-3. Epub 2023 Feb 24. PMID: 36826521; PMCID: PMC10390351.
52. Taglialatela Scafati S, Regalado-Briz A. Piezo-assisted dorsal preservation in rhinoplasty: when and why. Aesth Plast Surg. 2022;46(5):2389–97.
53. Robotti E, Khazaal A, Leone F. Piezo-assisted turbinoplasty: a novel rapid and safe technique. Facial Plast Surg. 2020;36(3):235–41.
54. Verkest V, Pingnet L, Fransen E, Declau F. Piezo-assisted turbinoplasty versus partial turbinectomy in external septorhinoplasty: a prospective comparative study in 100 patients. Aesth Plast Surg. 2022;46(3):1323–31.
55. Wähmann M, Riedel F, Kovacevic M, Hopf A, Albers AE. Vergleich von piezoelektrisch assistierter und konventioneller Osteotomie bei der Rhinoplastik: Ein systematisches Review [Comparison of piezoelectric and conventional osteotomy in rhinoplasty: a systematic review]. HNO. 2019;67(2):98–109. German.
56. Ilhan AE, Cengiz B, Caypinar EB. Double-blind comparison of ultrasonic and conventional osteotomy in terms of early postoperative edema and ecchymosis. Aesthet Surg J. 2016;36(4):390–401.
57. Becker DG, Toriumi DM, Gross CW, Tardy ME Jr. Powered instrumentation for dorsal reduction. Facial Plast Surg. 1997;13(4):291–7.
58. Guyuron B. Guarded burr for deepening of nasofrontal junction. Plast Reconstr Surg. 1989;84(3):513–6.
59. Davis RE, Raval J. Powered instrumentation for nasal bone reduction: advantages and indications. Arch Facial Plast Surg. 2003;5(5):384–91.
60. Ghassemi A, Ayoub A, Modabber A, Bohluli B, Prescher A. Lateral nasal osteotomy: a comparative study between the use of osteotome and a diamond surgical burr—a cadaver study. Head Face Med. 2013;9:41.
61. Avşar Y. Nasal hump reduction with powered micro saw osteotomy. Aesthet Surg J. 2009;29(1):6–11.
62. Cakir B, Goksel A, Gerbault O, et al. Discussion at: advanced aesthetic rhinoplasty course, Saint Petersburg, Russia; 24–27 Oct 2019.
63. Toriumi DM, Kovacevic M, Kosins AM. Structural preservation rhinoplasty: a hybrid approach. Plast Reconstr Surg. 2022;149(5):1105–20.
64. Robotti E, Daniel RK, Leone F. Cone-beam computed tomography: a user-friendly, practical roadmap to the planning and execution of every rhinoplasty-a 5-year review. Plast Reconstr Surg. 2021;147(5):749e–62e. https://doi.org/10.1097/PRS.0000000000007900. PMID: 33835107.
65. Rezaeian F, Gubisch W, Janku D, Haack S. New suturing techniques to reconstruct the keystone area in extracorporeal septoplasty. Plast Reconstr Surg. 2016;138(2):374–82.
66. Haack S, Hacker S, Mann S, Gubisch W. Bony fixation of the nasal framework. Facial Plast Surg. 2019;35(1):23–30.
67. Khazaal A. A modified dorsal split preservation technique for nasal humps with major bony component. Rhino Egypt 29th ed., Cairo; 4–6 March 2021.
68. Furtado S. 7th Bergamo open rhinoplasty course, Bergamo; 24–26 March 2022.
69. Gonçalves Ferreira M, Ishida LC, Ishida LH, Santos M. Ferreira-Ishida technique: spare roof technique B. Step-by-step guide to preserving the bony cap while Dehumping. Plast Reconstr Surg. 2022;149(5):901e–4e.

# Spare Roof Technique: Preservation Rhinoplasty in the Era of Osteo and Chondroplasty

49

Miguel Gonçalves Ferreira and Mariline Santos

**Key Points**

- The chapter explores preservation rhinoplasty techniques, particularly the spare roof technique (SRT), focusing on maintaining nasal structures while addressing dorsal hump deformities.
- The chapter outlines anatomical considerations and expands on indications for dorsal preservation, emphasizing surface modification.
- Additionally, it details the SRT and its variants, such as SRT-B, highlighting meticulous surgical steps for achieving optimal aesthetic outcomes, especially in crooked noses.
- Furthermore, it introduces the reverse spare roof technique (rSRT) for correcting saddle nose deformities, offering insights into its applications in nasal contour restoration and augmentation rhinoplasty.

M. G. Ferreira (✉)
Centro Hospitalar Universitário do Porto, Instituto Ciências Biomédicas Abel Salazar, Porto University, Porto, Portugal

Hospital Luz Arrábida, Vila Nova de Gaia, Portugal

Clínica Nariz e Face, Porto, Portugal

M. Santos
Centro Hospitalar Universitário do Porto, Instituto Ciências Biomédicas Abel Salazar, Porto University, Porto, Portugal


S. Elwany (ed.), *Current Rhinology*,
https://doi.org/10.1007/978-3-031-70077-4_49

## 49.1 Introduction

The majority of Caucasian aesthetic rhinoplasty patients complain about a noticeable hump in profile view [1]. This makes the adequate reduction of a prominent dorsum a significant determinant of success in these patients [1]. However, dorsal hump reduction can create both aesthetic and functional problems if performed incorrectly because the "keystone area" is a natural area of weakness of the middle third [2, 3].

Since the beginning of rhinoplastic procedures, the middle third has been the most challenging segment regarding its stability, functionality, and aesthetic lines [2, 4]. This is a transition segment between the bony pyramid and the tip, comprising only one T-shaped or M-shaped cartilage that, owing to academic and historical purposes, is divided into two upper lateral cartilages (ULCs) and one quadrangular septal cartilage, with different thermo-mechanical characteristics [5].

Based on the integrity of the ULCs, there are two different ways to dehump a nose: the structural techniques (resection/reconstruction) and the preservation techniques [6].

After the first resection procedures described by Jacques Joseph, J. Sheen made the first consistent description of reconstruction with "spreader grafts." [7] This fact can be assumed as the beginning of the "structural" techniques. In 1954, M Cottle published the first consistent description of the "push-down"—the beginning of "preservation" techniques [8].

The structural techniques consist of splitting the ULCs (among them) and the dorsal septum, achieving a complete separation of this M-shaped segment into three parts [2, 9]. In the classical *en bloc* humpectomy, there is always some degree of avulsion of the ULCs, most of the time reconstructed with spreader grafts [4, 7]. "Spreader flaps" had been developed by multiple surgeons and led to the beginning of the component dorsal reduction [10, 11]. In this technique, there is a simple separation between both ULCs and the dorsal aspect of the septum, most of the time with confection of auto spreader flaps [9].

## 49.2 Preservation Rhinoplasty

Preservation rhinoplasty is resurgent worldwide as surgeons see the benefits of preserving critical anatomic nose structures. The descriptive title "preservation rhinoplasty" was coined by Rollin K. Daniel and has become a rather popular movement in recent years [12–14].

Dorsal preservation (DP) was introduced many years ago by Goodale in 1899, Lothrop in 1914, and Cottle in 1946 [12]. There has been a resurgence in recent years, introducing new innovative techniques to manage the dorsal hump. According to Toriumi, DP has experienced a revival because the method preserves the favorable anatomy of the upper two-thirds of the nose and minimizes the need for spreader grafts and spreader flaps [14].

Component reduction of the dorsal hump requires amputating the top of the bony nasal vault and reconstructing the open roof. This potentially introduces rough bony edges, irregularities, depressions, or prominences that may require soft tissue camouflage in the form of temporalis fascia grafts, diced cartilage and fascia grafts, and other soft tissue grafts. Minimizing this risk for irregularities is a significant advantage of DP in managing the dorsal profile [15].

DP is a complex area of rhinoplasty due to the number of new techniques and modifications developed in recent years. The contemporary definition of DP does not require preserving the continuity of the bony-cartilaginous dorsum or treating this unit *en bloc*. It is widely accepted that the real anatomical frontier of dorsal preservation rhinoplasty is the cartilaginous middle vault. Essentially, in all DP cases, the middle vault preservation remains true [15].

Acceptance of the preservation principle in rhinoplasty surgery has increased dramatically, and surgeons worldwide are now performing preservation rhinoplasty, leading to an expanding list of indications and techniques [16–19].

### 49.2.1 Different Techniques for Dorsal Preservation

Conceptually and structurally, two classes of DP techniques have been described: foundation techniques (FTs) and surface techniques (STs) [20].

FTs are based on dorsal impaction, which involves impaction of the nasal pyramid into the face, requiring impaction osteotomies—push-down or let-down—a disruption between the skull and nasal pyramid [20].

STs are based on dorsal modulation; the hump is treated superficially with modulation of the middle vault, without impaction osteotomies—no bony push or let-down [20]. Ishida cartilaginous push-down (1999), septorhinoplasty by disarticulation described by Jankowski (2013), spare roof technique A (2016), spare roof technique B (2022), and cartilage-only push-down described by Kosins (2017) are some examples [15].

### 49.2.2 Indications for Dorsal Preservation

#### 49.2.2.1 Anatomic Considerations

The most recent anatomic concepts in DP are the W-point, E-point, V-shaped, and S-shaped nasal bones, lateral and dorsal keystone areas, and impaction osteotomies' predictability [21–24].

The W-point is the point where the more caudal aspect of the upper lateral cartilage is fused with the septal cartilage [21]. This point is essential due to the preservation of the cartilaginous middle vault and, in the high strip, the preservation of the W-anterior septal angle segment.

The E-point represents where the ethmoid's perpendicular plate meets the nasal bones' undersurface [23]. A recent study in Caucasian patients found that 97% of the nasal humps begin caudally to the E-point [23]. Thus, in most cases, the hump is not supported by the perpendicular plate of the ethmoid (PPE), highlighting that it is a rare need to excise PPE while dehumping.

In the Caucasian hump, there are two main types of nasal bone configuration: S-shaped nasal bones (SSNBs) and V-shaped nasal bones (VSNBs) [24]. The SSNBs have been reported to account for the vast majority (88%), and they have a kyphotic configuration, which means that the caudal aspect of the nasal bones is convex. This means it is virtually impossible to dehump a nose by classical FT. The only efficient way to flatten a significantly kyphotic bony hump is by performing dorsal modulation in which ostectomy is performed—bone must be removed.

All the techniques to dehump, either structured or preserved, have somewhere a triangular ostectomy as one of the most important steps. Due to the geometric proprieties of the nasal pyramid/hump, in structured rhinoplasty or preservation rhinoplasty by ST, the triangular ostectomy is smaller than in FT. This might lead to higher unpredictability in FT [15].

The keystone area was divided into lateral (LKA) and dorsal (DKA)—"bony cap"—by Palhazi et al. [21] This division is very important because it allows a more accurate description of the areas treated by surgeons. Preserving the DKA—called "bonny cap"—can be done by DP. Release of the LKA is one of the most critical structural steps in DP, either in FT or ST. Releasing the LKA allows the split of two structures strongly connected in the middle vault—bone and cartilage. This release allows the flattening of the convex (humped) dorsum [15].

### 49.2.3 Expanding Conventional Indications

One of the big issues related to classical dorsal preservation (push or let-down) was the "indications." Due to many limitations of the technique proposed by Cottle, the item "indications" was a must in preservation meetings.

Things have changed after the appearance of surface techniques: we believe there is no contraindication for DP in primary and secondary rhinoplasties with intact upper lateral cartilages (ULCs)—cartilaginous middle vault. However, if not diagnosed and corrected, some features can contribute to suboptimal results or be considered contraindications for DP such as the S-shaped nasal bones, ULCs shoulders, dorsal irregularities, asymmetries, low radix, low anterior septal angle (ASA) (supratip control), crooked nose, big humps (hump recurrence), and irregular dorsal aesthetic lines [15, 25].

Regarding the S-shaped nasal bones, ULC shoulders, and dorsal irregularities, the ability to perform surface modification of the bony dorsum in the form of bony cap removal and shaving or burring the shoulders of the ULCs has been essential in converting questionable candidates for DP to good candidates for DP [25]. Sculpting the bony cap and dorsum is a big part of this. If the middle vault is asymmetric or deformed, surface adjustments can be performed to make the case a candidate for DP, such as using the piezotome to burr down the bony cap or trim the prominent edges of the ULCs. The release of LKA also allows for improved symmetry of the ULCs due to the ability to sink the excess of ULCs in the LKA.

If there is a low radix, a small tissue radix graft can help camouflage a potential residual hump and aesthetically improve the nasofrontal angle [19].

The supratip control: low supratip is a classical contra-indication for the push or let-down technique. After the tip surgery, which typically increases rotation and projection, the supratip gets even worse if one does not predict and fix that. While performing the classical Cottle low-strip, the advancement/rotation of the septum is excellent for this control. The first author has developed a new flap—the septal advancement flap (SAF)—designed to achieve control/smoothness in this area in the medium long-term follow-up [26].

In cases of crooked nose, the axis deviation of the nose can be challenging to manage with spreader grafts and spreader flaps. DP techniques allow the axis of the nose to be tilted to the midline with great precision. Treatment of the deviated nose is one of the strengths of the DP techniques. One can shift the bony and cartilaginous vault (axis deviations) to the midline with asymmetric bone reduction and overlapping subdorsal segments, which might be considered one of the most significant advantages of the DP techniques [19, 27].

Finally, the lateral keystone release is essential, particularly in more prominent dorsal humps, because this can act as a blocking point [15]. It can help to prevent hump recurrence with more prominent dorsal humps. It is mandatory to perform in all cases of DP once it allows splitting the bony and cartilaginous part of the middle vault—achieving the new anatomical relation while flattening the middle vault.

Dorsal aesthetic lines (DALs) are rhinoplasty's most relevant surface anatomic landmarks. With ST, it is straightforward to preserve or create new DALs—mainly with the spare roof technique B, where the bony cap is preserved exactly with the tailor of the new DALs [28]. With conventional FT in DP, it is still possible to improve DALs with new devices such as piezo or diamond burrs.

## 49.3 Spare Roof Technique

To treat the middle third conservatively, in 2016, Ferreira MG et al. described the spare roof technique (SRT) as a middle-third preservation technique [6]. The SRT is designed to preserve the natural roof of the upper and middle third based on the old Cottle concept—"as the septum goes, so goes the nose." This technique allows the surgeon to isolate the entire cartilaginous roof of the middle third without splitting the upper lateral cartilages among them.

As concerns the bony cap, the SRT has been subdivided into two types: A and B.

### 49.3.1 Spare Roof Technique A

SRT-A includes ostectomy of the bony cap [29]. However, considering the clinical and surgical experience acquired over the years, for patients with VSNB and up to medium SSNB, it would be possible to dehump the nose while preserving the DKA. Thus, based on a rational anatomical basis for acquired experience with

SRT-A described by Ferreira MG and colleagues and cartilaginous push-down with preservation of the bony cap described by Ishida LC and colleagues, both authors designed a new technique named SRT-B or "Ferreira-Ishida technique." This technique, named the spare roof technique B (or the Ferreira-Ishida technique), is specially designed for patients with a dorsal hump and V-shaped nasal bones. It preserves the bony cap and ensures intact brow-tip dorsal aesthetic lines. In SRT-B, the treatment of the bony hump includes paramedian high parallel osteotomies just below the dorsal aesthetic lines followed by inferior osteotomies to obtain a triangular shape of bone on each side of the bony cap [28].

### 49.3.2 Spare Roof Technique B

SRT-B includes six main steps (Figs. 49.1 and 49.2):

*Step 1:* Draw the desired dorsal brow-tip aesthetic lines on the skin's surface, the pyriform aperture, the rhinion, the amount of triangular bone that must be taken out to allow pushing down the bony cap, and the transversal line at the beginning of the nasal hump.

*Step 2:* Dissect both lateral walls through an intercartilaginous incision (with a Colorado needle) [30].

*Optional:* Dissect the dorsum only if there is any bony or cartilaginous defect. The bony defect (S-shape is the most common) should be managed with piezo or diamond burr, and the cartilaginous irregularities (visible shoulders are the most common) should be managed with a "Colorado needle."

Perform the two triangular ostectomies (just out of the DALs) and release the LKA.

*Step 3:* Release the ULCs from the dorsal septum ("high/medium septal strip") or perform the septal advancement flap (SAF), advancing the caudal aspect of the septum in an L-shaped fashion—from the nasal spine till the E-point [26].

*Step 4:* Take out the amount of dorsal septum necessary to dehump.

*Step 5:* Perform partial ultrasonic ostectomy endonasal, below the nasal bones in the midline, to promote the weakening of the transverse fracture line in the sagittal plane just above the E-point—subdorsal ostectomy [31]. Gently push down the rectangular bony cap in a greenstick fashion. The left thumb must apply one force in the caudal direction.

*Step 6:* Perform regular L-shaped septoplasty. Perform lateral osteotomies—low-low-high—based on the Barn doors concept, and three contiguous greenstick fractures are combined [32].

*Step 7:* In medium/big humps with a convex shape of the ULCs, the "lateral division maneuver" must be done. This maneuver allows the flattening of the convex cartilaginous segment, achieving, if necessary, a straight or even a concave shape.

Spongostan nasal packing and Silastic with side tubes are placed and removed after 7 days.

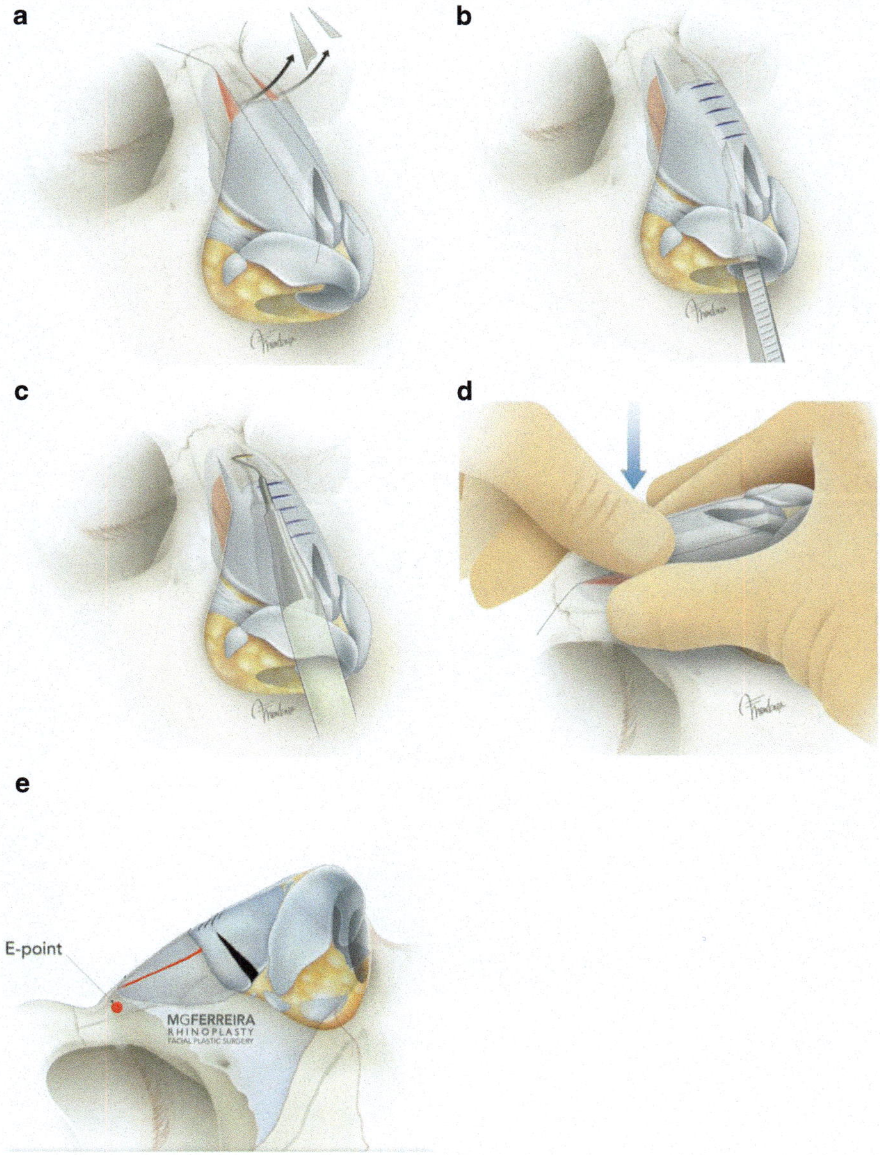


**Fig. 49.1** (**a**) Lateral paramedian triangular ostectomy, following the dorsal aesthetic lines. (**b**) Subdorsal cartilaginous scoring. (**c**) Subdorsal partial radix ostectomy. (**d**) Gentle execution of greenstick dorsal fracture—cranio-caudal direction of thumb movement. (**e**) Lateral division maneuver—is needed—to flatten or turn concave the cartilaginous hump

Postoperative care is the same as in all other rhinoplasty techniques: analgesia (Paracetamol 1000 mg 8/8 h) and Amoxicillin and Acid Clavulanic (875 + 125 mg 12/12 h). Doyle and thermic nasal splints are typically taken out 7–8 days after the surgery.

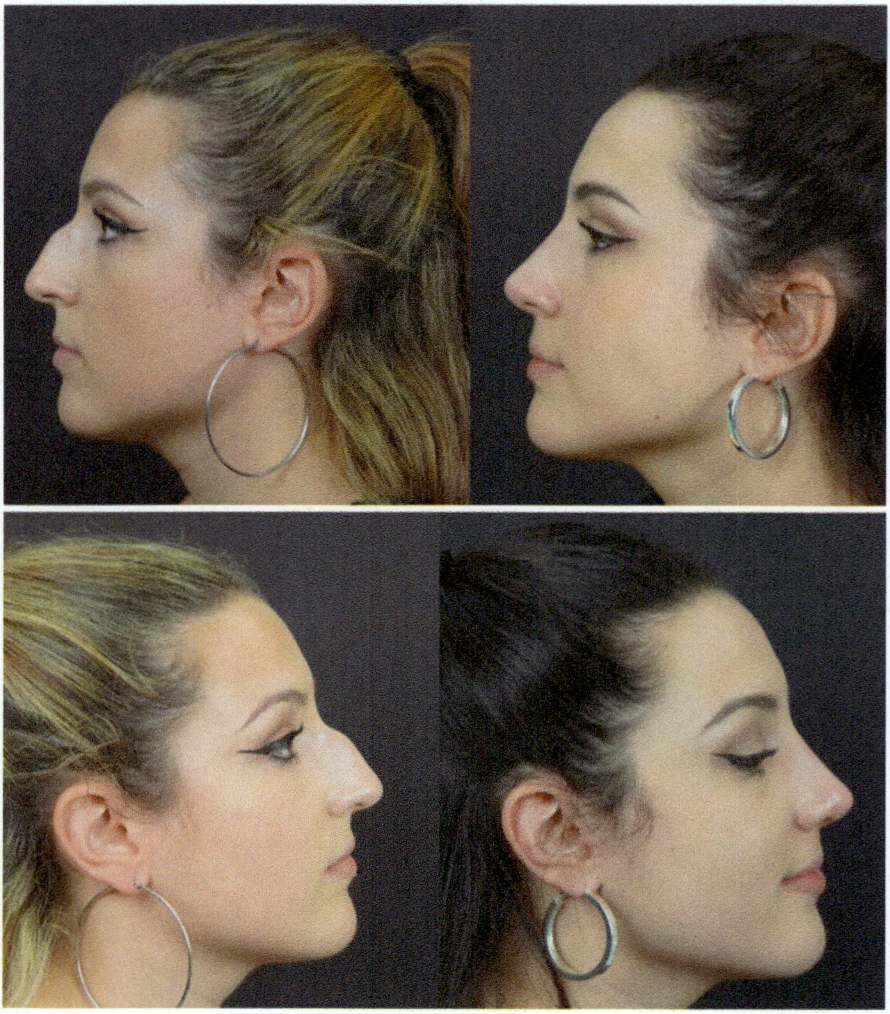

**Fig. 49.2** Clinical case: before and 12 months after SRT-B

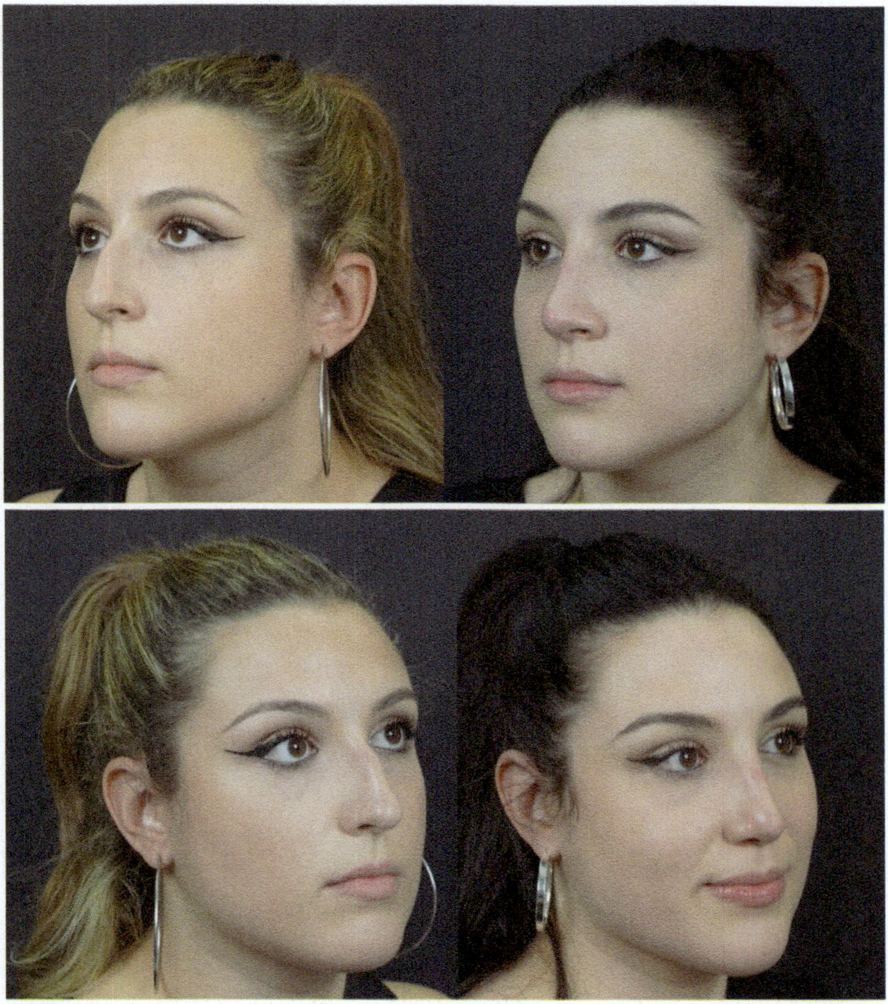

**Fig. 49.2** (continued)

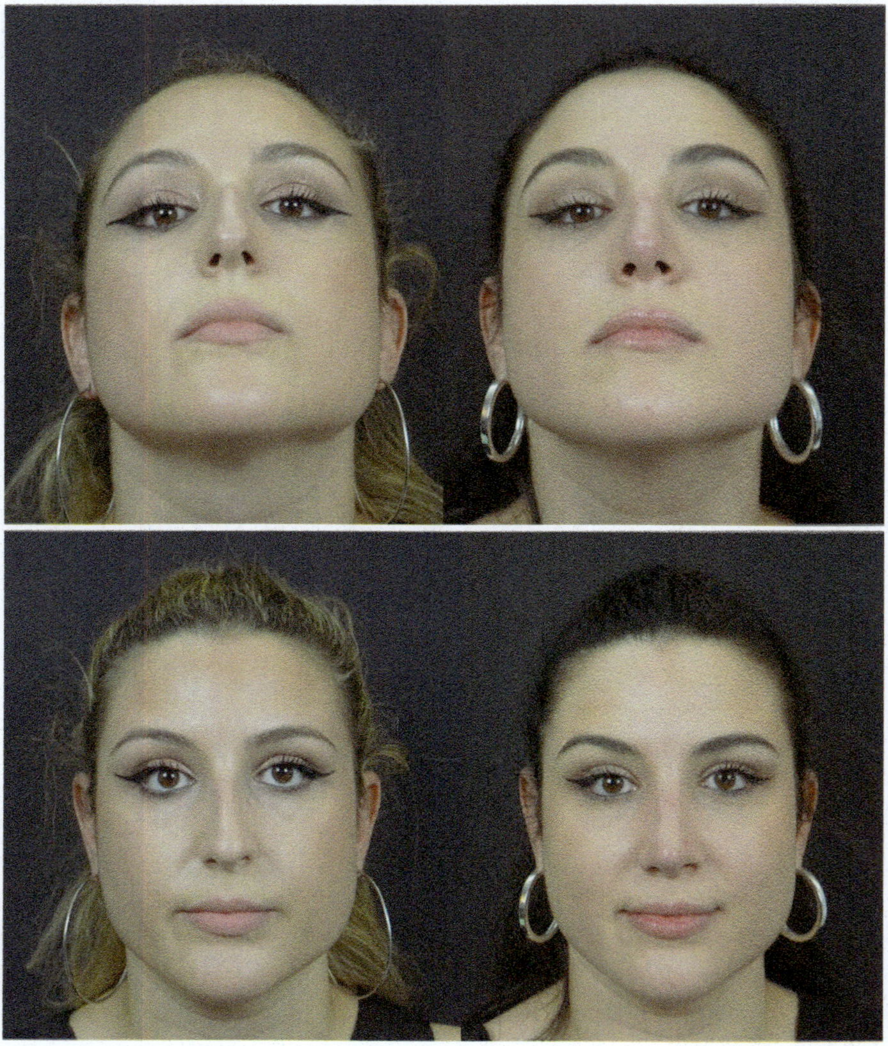

**Fig. 49.2** (continued)

### 49.3.3 Spare Roof Technique in the Crooked Nose

Following the only rhinoplasty dogma, "the nose goes as the septum goes," one should understand that once the high/medium strip is done, the cartilaginous middle vault immediately goes to the midline. At this stage, one has a different nose—pyramid straight and the septum still crooked.

The second stage has to do with the strategy for the septum deviation. A traditional L-shaped septoplasty should be performed if it is a simple septal deviation. If the septal deviation is complex, an extra-corporeal septoplasty must be done.

The SRT significantly improves patient body image perception about the nasal appearance in crooked nose patients, achieving consistent results in the long term [27].

### 49.3.4 Reverse Spare Roof Technique

Saddle nose deformity (SND) is a pathologic entity resulting from loss of dorsal height caused by a substantial decrease in the cartilaginous vault or bony vault, and it can occur following various nasal pathologic conditions. Most saddle nose deformities are secondary to surgery or trauma, but congenital causes exist.

Therefore, repairing the saddle nose represents one of the most challenging problems in nasal surgery, requiring long-term structural support while avoiding sacrificing aesthetics. Various materials have been employed to achieve the desired results for nasal contour restoration. The most used grafts are autologous cartilages. Septal cartilage is ideal for reconstruction but often insufficient except in mild cases. Thus, conchal and costal cartilage grafts are the most used in moderate and severe nasal saddling.

The reverse spare roof technique (rSRT) is only indicated when the cartilaginous middle vault is not violated [33]. The main applications are as follows:

- Closed trauma
- Post-preservation rhinoplasty
- Cocaine noses
- Septal perforations due to septoplasty or other medical conditions
- "Infantiloid" noses
- Primary dorsal augmentation surgery—Asian and Negroid noses

### 49.3.5 Surgical Technique

The rSRT was designed for patients with SND with the integrity of ULCs, and it can be performed using either a closed or open approach. It depends on the surgeon's skills.

Before starting rSRT, the surgeon should expose the quadrangular septum and ULCs by submucosal dissection. Then, the dorsum is accessed by subpericondrium and subperiosteal dissection to achieve complete skeletonization of the cartilaginous middle vault—ULCs.

rSRT for correction of SND consists of four main steps:

*Step 1:* The longitudinal cut of the dorsal septum, from the anterior nasal angle to the perpendicular plate of the ethmoid, 1 mm below the ULCs, separating the dorsal aspect of the septum from the ULCs, preserving the union among the ULCs (which remain preserved).

*Step 2:* It consists of doing the subdorsal osteotomy (a transverse subdorsal osteotomy), two high paramedian osteotomies till the E-point level, and finally, releasing the LKA to allow the osseocartilaginous dorsal vault to be gently elevated [31].

*Step 3:* Subdorsal insertion of the graft below the intact ULCs. This step is more accessible by an open approach. In a closed approach, the Aufricht retractor should be raised as high as possible to achieve the best surgical exposure of the nasal dorsum.

*Step 4:* It consists of suturing the "roof" (ULCs) to the subdorsal graft with absorbable polydioxanone 4-0 to stabilize the roof. Any part of the horizontal part of the L-Strut can be used to "anchor" the sutures to the graft.

Until now, less severe deformities, where supporting structures remain strong, are usually treated with dorsal onlay grafts. However, with rSRT, this technique allows to correct the SND with preservation rhinoplasty concepts and is also used to correct the dorsal hump in a specific group of patients.

Interposing a graft between the remaining septal structure and the cartilaginous middle vault allows for achieving a stable and smooth dorsum with excellent outcomes in the long-term evaluation. Additionally, the rSRT allows any tip technique the surgeon might want.

The ultimate and most promising application of *rSRT* is in augmentation rhinoplasty, regularly done in a large amount of *Asian* and *Negroid* noses/patients.

## References


1. Lohuis PJ, Faraj-Hakim S, Knobbe A, Duivesteijn W, Bran GM. Split hump technique for reduction of the overprojected nasal dorsum: a statistical analysis on subjective body image in relation to nasal appearance and nasal patency in 97 patients undergoing aesthetic rhinoplasty. Arch Facial Plast Surg. 2012;14(5):346–53. https://doi.org/10.1001/archfacial.2012.606.
2. Rohrich RJ, Muzaffar AR, Janis JE. Component dorsal hump reduction: the importance of maintaining dorsal aesthetic lines in rhinoplasty. Plast Reconstr Surg. 2004;114(5):1298–312. https://doi.org/10.1097/01.prs.0000135861.45986.cf.
3. Simon PE, Lam K, Sidle D, Tan BK. The nasal keystone region: an anatomical study. JAMA Facial Plast Surg. 2013;15(3):235–7. https://doi.org/10.1001/jamafacial.2013.777.
4. Daniel RK. Mastering rhinoplasty: a comprehensive atlas of surgical techniques with integrated video clips. Berlin: Springer; 2010.
5. Natvig P, Sether LA, Gingrass RP, Gardner WD. Anatomical details of the osseous-cartilaginous framework of the nose. Plast Reconstr Surg. 1971;48(6):528–32. https://doi.org/10.1097/00006534-197112000-00002.
6. Ferreira MG, Monteiro D, Reis C, Almeida e Sousa, C. Spare roof technique: a middle third new technique. Facial Plast Surg. 2016;32(1):111–6. https://doi.org/10.1055/s-0035-1570503.
7. Sheen JH. Spreader graft: a method of reconstructing the roof of the middle nasal vault following rhinoplasty. Plast Reconstr Surg. 1984;73(2):230–9.
8. Cottle MH. Nasal roof repair and hump removal. AMA Arch Otolaryngol. 1954;60(4):408–14. https://doi.org/10.1001/archotol.1954.00720010420002.
9. Gruber RP, Melkun ET, Woodward JF, Perkins SW. Dorsal reduction and spreader flaps. Aesthet Surg J. 2011;31(4):456–64. https://doi.org/10.1177/1090820X11404401.
10. Oneal RM, Berkowitz RL. Upper lateral cartilage spreader flaps in rhinoplasty. Aesthet Surg J. 1998;18(5):370–1. https://doi.org/10.1016/s1090-820x(98)70095-0.

11. Seyhan A. Method for middle vault reconstruction in primary rhinoplasty: upper lateral cartilage bending. Plast Reconstr Surg. 1997;100(7):1941–3. https://doi.org/10.1097/00006534-199712000-00068.
12. Patel PN, Most SP. Overview of dorsal preservation rhinoplasty. Facial Plast Surg Clin North Am. 2023;31(1):1–11. https://doi.org/10.1016/j.fsc.2022.08.003.
13. Daniel RK. The preservation rhinoplasty: a new rhinoplasty revolution. Aesthet Surg J. 2018;38(2):228–9. https://doi.org/10.1093/asj/sjx258.
14. Toriumi DM. My first twenty rhinoplasties using dorsal preservation techniques. Facial Plast Surg Clin North Am. 2023;31(1):73–106. https://doi.org/10.1016/j.fsc.2022.08.008.
15. Ferreira MG, Santos M. Recent evidence of advanced preservation rhinoplasty. Curr Opin Otolaryngol Head Neck Surg. 2023;31(4):248–53. https://doi.org/10.1097/MOO.0000000000000896.
16. Daniel RK, Kosins AM. Current trends in preservation rhinoplasty. Aesthet Surg J. 2020;2(1):ojaa003. https://doi.org/10.1093/asjof/ojaa003.
17. Kosins AM, Daniel RK. Decision making in preservation rhinoplasty: a 100 case series with one-year follow-up. Aesthet Surg J. 2020;40(1):34–48. https://doi.org/10.1093/asj/sjz107.
18. Patel PN, Kandathil CK, Buba CM, Neves JC, Cobo R, Robotti E, López-Ulloa F, Ferraz M, Saedi B, Pham T, Saleh HA, Most SP. Global practice patterns of dorsal preservation rhinoplasty. Facial Plast Surg Aesthet Med. 2022;24(3):171–7. https://doi.org/10.1089/fpsam.2021.0055.
19. Kosins AM. Expanding indications for dorsal preservation rhinoplasty with cartilage conversion techniques. Aesthet Surg J. 2021;41(2):174–84. https://doi.org/10.1093/asj/sjaa071.
20. Gonçalves Ferreira M, Toriumi DM. A practical classification system for dorsal preservation rhinoplasty techniques. Facial Plast Surg Aesthet Med. 2021;23(3):153–5. https://doi.org/10.1089/fpsam.2021.0030.
21. Palhazi P, Daniel RK, Kosins AM. The osseocartilaginous vault of the nose: anatomy and surgical observations. Aesthet Surg J. 2015;35(3):242–51. https://doi.org/10.1093/asj/sju079.
22. Rolling K, Daniel PP. Osteocartilaginous vault. In: Rhinoplasty: an anatomical and clinical atlas. Cham: Springer; 2018.
23. Ferreira MG, Dias DR, Cardoso L, Santos M, Sousa CA, Dourado N, Santos J, Amarante J. Dorsal hump reduction based on the new ethmoidal point classification: a clinical and radiological study of the keystone area in 138 patients. Aesthet Surg J. 2020;40(9):950–9. https://doi.org/10.1093/asj/sjaa030.
24. Lazovic GD, Daniel RK, Janosevic LB, Kosanovic RM, Colic MM, Kosins AM. Rhinoplasty: the nasal bones—anatomy and analysis. Aesthet Surg J. 2015;35(3):255–63. https://doi.org/10.1093/asj/sju050.
25. Ferreira MG, Toriumi DM, Stubenitsky B, Kosins AM. Advanced preservation rhinoplasty in the era of osteoplasty and chondroplasty: how have we moved beyond the Cottle technique? Aesthet Surg J. 2023;43(12):1441–53. https://doi.org/10.1093/asj/sjad194.
26. Gonçalves FM. Septal advancement flap: preserving, restructuring, and reshaping the nasal tip contour with a novel flap. Facial Plast Surg Aesthet Med. 2023;25(4):279–84. https://doi.org/10.1089/fpsam.2023.0060.
27. Rodrigues Dias D, Santos M, Castro SSE, Sousa CAE, Gonçalves Ferreira M. The spare roof technique as a new approach to the crooked nose. Facial Plast Surg Aesthet Med. 2022;24(3):178–84. https://doi.org/10.1089/fpsam.2021.0368.
28. Gonçalves Ferreira M, Ishida LC, Ishida LH, Santos M. Ferreira-Ishida technique: spare roof technique B. Step-by-step guide to preserving the bony cap while dehumping. Plast Reconstr Surg. 2022;149(5):901e–4e. https://doi.org/10.1097/PRS.0000000000009060.
29. Gonçalves Ferreira M, Santos M, Rosa F, Sousa CA, Santos J, Dourado N, Amarante J. Spare roof technique: a new technique for hump removal-the step-by-step guide. Plast Reconstr Surg. 2020;145(2):403–6. https://doi.org/10.1097/PRS.0000000000006512.
30. Ferreira MG, Santos M. Letter to the editor on incisions in rhinoplasty: the usefulness and safety of Colorado microdissection needle. Aesth Plast Surg. 2023;47(Suppl 1):118–9. https://doi.org/10.1007/s00266-022-03055-7.

31. Ferreira MG, Santos M, Dias D. Subdorsal osteotomy and complete dorsal preservation—a new paradigm in preservation rhinoplasty? Laryngoscope. 2022;132(4):769–71. https://doi.org/10.1002/lary.29832.
32. Ferreira MG, Santos M. The barn doors greenstick fracture-a new 3D geometry for common osteotomies in rhinoplasty: the first 50 patients with 1-year follow-up. Facial Plast Surg. 2023;39(4):434–40. https://doi.org/10.1055/s-0043-1766101.
33. Ferreira MG, Santos M. Preservation rhinoplasty in the saddle nose: the reverse spare roof technique. Facial Plast Surg Aesthet Med. 2022;24(3):168–70. https://doi.org/10.1089/fpsam.2022.0036.

# Reshaping the Medial Nostrils and Columellar Base

# 50

Palmyra J. Geissler and Nicolas Baldini

**Key Points**

- Both nasal aesthetics and nasal function may be compromised when excessive columella width occurs. Reducing columella width requires a working knowledge of nasal cartilage support and a complete understanding of the role of soft tissue in nostril function.
- Equally important is an understanding of the evolution of a more conservative approach when shaping columella width.
- Any tissue resection should be performed cautiously, following a graduated technique.

## 50.1 Background

The nasal base is probably one of the least understood and most complex areas of the nose [1]. The term "nasal base" refers to the bottom third of the nose, as seen in the upward view, when the head is tilted back. It can be divided into an upper cartilaginous portion and a lower soft tissue portion.

One can arbitrarily define the lower nasal base as the soft tissue component of the nasal base incorporating the columellar base, nostril sills, and alar lobules [2].

P. J. Geissler (✉)
Rio de Janeiro, Brazil

Plastic Surgery Department, The University of Texas Southwestern Medical Center, Dallas, TX, USA
e-mail: palmyrageissler@gmail.com

N. Baldini
University of Bordeaux College of Health Sciences, Bordeaux, France

Anatomy Laboratory, University of Bordeaux College of Health Sciences, Bordeaux, France



S. Elwany (ed.), *Current Rhinology*,
https://doi.org/10.1007/978-3-031-70077-4_50

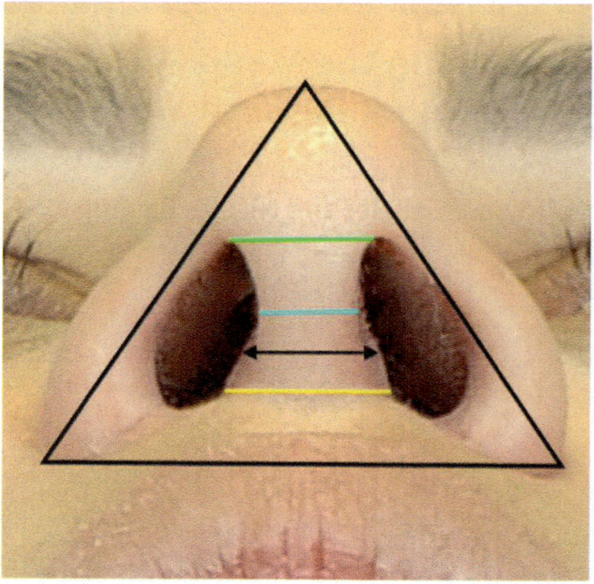

**Fig. 50.1** Columella: a three-dimensional structure: width

The static shape and dynamic function of the lower nasal base are determined by the skin and subcutaneous tissue, including the tela subcutanea cutis and nasal muscles [3]. The columellar base can be arbitrarily defined as extending vertically from the divergence point of the medial crura down to the subnasale. Transversely, the columellar base slopes downward from the footplates to the nostril sills. The transverse width of the columellar base is related to the separation of the footplates and the quantity of intervening soft tissues. Two muscles located in the nasolabial angle, the depressor septi nasi in depth and the orbicularis oris muscle superficially, are separated by a small fat compartment. However, the amount of soft tissue may vary dramatically [2]. The nostril sill is the floor of the nostril aperture. In most cases, it is a distinct segment with a "roll" border. The alar lobule represents the sidewall of the nasal base and is most visible in the lateral view. Essentially, the alar lobule is outlined by the alar groove, beginning at the nostril rim and then running in an almost circular shape down to the alar crease.

Each of these components contributes to the overall shape of the nasal base, and appropriate proportions are paramount. The nasal columella, in particular, plays a pivotal role in determining the shape of the nasal base. Deviations in the columella and variations in its width and height lead to distortion of nostril shape and frequently compromise function.

When seeking to achieve a more aesthetic, shorter, or narrower columella, one must act on the middle segment and the base of the columella. Narrowing and reshaping the medial nostrils and columellar base requires a sequential approach with good anatomical knowledge and aesthetic analysis [4]. As a three-dimensional structure, the columella must be analyzed along three axes: horizontal (thickness or width), vertical (height), and sagittal (nasolabial angle) [1] (Figs. 50.1, 50.2, and 50.3).

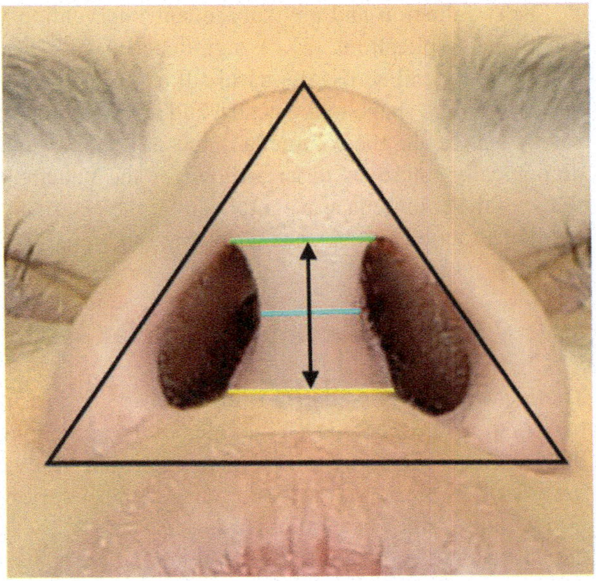

**Fig. 50.2** Columella: a three-dimensional structure: height

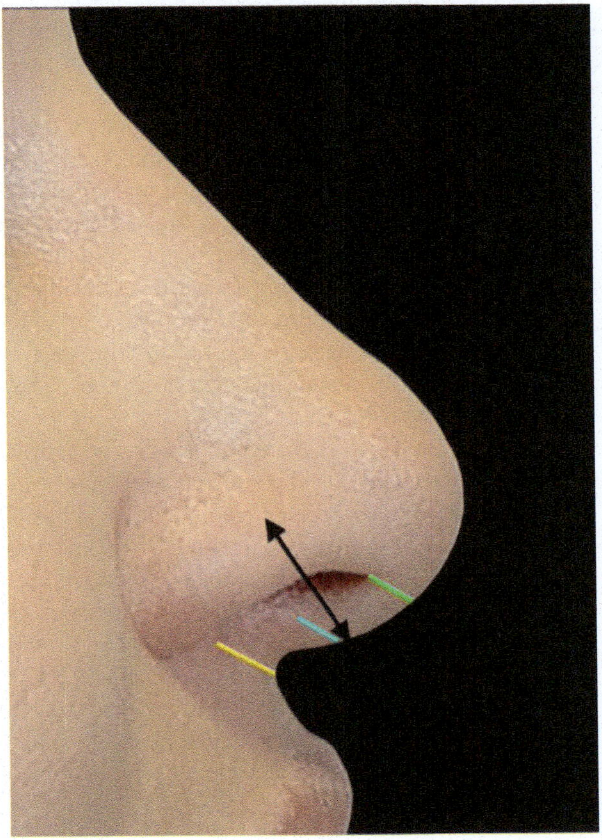

**Fig. 50.3** Columella: a three-dimensional structure: sagittal

Such evaluation and any subsequent intervention will have both aesthetic and functional implications [5]. A significantly wide columella with splayed medial crura may extend across the nasal sill as far as the alar-facial insertion, creating a narrow slit-like shape to the nostril and significantly decreasing airflow to the nasal cavity. Narrowing the columella in these situations increases the nasal aperture and dramatically improves nasal airflow for the patient [6]. Failure to recognize the shape of the columella as a component of the external valve can potentially result in nasal obstruction that persists following functional nasal surgery.

## 50.2 Artistic Anatomy: Columellar Aesthetics

The ideal nostril possesses a teardrop shape with a long axis extending from the base to the apex. There is a slight medial tilt of the long axis toward the midline [7, 8]. The columella serves as the medial border of the nostrils, begins at the apex of the nostril, is inferior to the lobule, and extends inferiorly until it transitions laterally into the nasal sill. The cartilaginous and, to a lesser degree, the bony framework of the columella is composed of paired medial crura, caudal septal cartilage, and the nasal spine. Soft tissue components contribute to the shape of the columella and include the septal membranes, depressor nasi septi muscle, fat pads, and intervening soft tissue between the medial crura. To date, descriptions of the aesthetic columellar ideals are limited, and there is a paucity of literature examining the various configurations of columellar shapes.

First and foremost, one must recognize that the aesthetic columellar shape should not be the focal point of the nasal base; rather, attention should be drawn to achieving symmetry between the nostrils and understanding how the shape of the columella influences this. The ideal columella starts at the apex of the nostril with a width approximately equal to that of the tip-defining points. The columella then tapers symmetrically, reaching its narrowest width approximately at the junction between the middle one-third and lower one-third of the height of the columella. At this point, the columella starts to gradually broaden. At the base of the columella, the width is slightly greater than that at its apex. The transition to the nasal sill is gentle but distinguishable.

The overall ideal aesthetic nasal base has been described as having the shape of an equilateral triangle. Ideal columella width has been described as one-fifth of the total nasal base [7, 8], with the medial crura responsible for the bulk of the volume [9]. The height of the columella should be two-thirds the height of the base and therefore twice the height of the lobule (Fig. 50.4).

Clinically, the shape of the columella varies considerably. A short columella is seen in noses with inadequate tip projection and weak medial crura such as ethnic noses. The columella-to-lobule ratio may approach 1:1. The medial crura may splay at the base of the columella, adding excess width and causing the nostrils to have a rounder appearance rather than a more favorable oblique teardrop configuration. A triangular-shaped columella is seen when an extremely wide columella extends to

**Fig. 50.4** Aesthetics of the nasal base

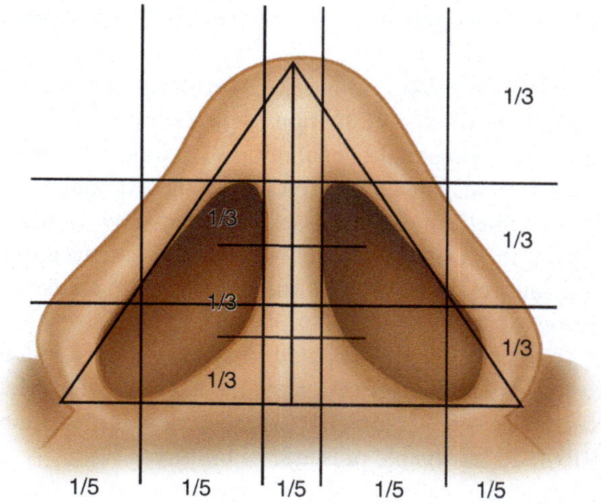


the alar-facial groove, resulting in slit-like nostril shapes. Frequently, this is caused by medial crura that diverge increasingly as they extend inferiorly and approach the corner of the nasal sill [4].

## 50.3 Classification of Medial Nostrils and Columellar Base Deformities

The origin of the columella deformity determines whether it should be classified as primary or secondary. Primary deformities are those that originate from an intrinsic problem, such as medial crura footplates with excess convexity or excessive soft tissue at the columella base. Most commonly, a widened or asymmetric columella is the result of premature or excessive medial crura footplate flaring.

Secondary deformities of the columella result from the influence of adjacent structure(s). Such deformities are often the result of caudal septum cartilage abnormalities (deviation, thickness or width excess). In addition, deformities of the nasal spine, soft tissue pathologies, and iatrogenic causes should be mentioned as possible origins.

(a) Primary Deformities
- Medial Crural Footplate Splay
- Excessive soft tissue between the medial crura and the depressor nasi septi

(b) Secondary Deformities
- Caudal septal deformities (deviation, thickness, and width)
- Nasal spine (deviation, thickness, and width)
- Soft tissue pathologies (tumors)
- Iatrogenic (grafts and scarring)

## 50.4 Recognizing Columellar Disproportion

A complete nasal evaluation is performed and photodocumented. Included in the examination is the evaluation of the external nasal valve from the base view, recognizing the potential contribution of a weak alar rim and wide columella to a narrowed valve. The entire structure of the external nasal valve including the shape of the columella should be assessed both passively and actively with deep nasal inspiration. It is critical that before performing anterior rhinoscopy with the speculum, one must examine the columella and alae to assess whether the external valve may be restricted.

The columella is palpated to assess the position and shape of the medial crura, soft tissue fullness between the medial crura, and relative length and position of the caudal septum. Columellar skin thickness is also appreciated, as thin skin may contribute to the visible presence of bifidity.

In profile view, the alar–columellar relationship is assessed for columellar show or alar retraction. The tip is also palpated to determine the degree of support.

In revision cases, a wide columella may be due to numerous causes, and it is helpful to assess the reason preoperatively. Previously placed columellar struts, tip grafts, and caudal septal extension grafts may all contribute to the shape of the columella. All medical records and operative reports from previous nasal surgeries are evaluated when available.

## 50.5 Addressing Medial Nostrils and Columellar Base Deformities

When the columellar base deformity has a secondary origin, the surgical approach addressing the main cause of the deformity should be performed first.

For example, whenever any tumor resection at the columellar base or correction of a deviated septum is required, these are accomplished before the medial crura footplate approximation.

The medial crura footplate approximation is performed in five surgical steps (Fig. 50.5):

1. The location and extent of the splayed footplates are marked by two symmetrical lines parallel to the columella along the inferior medial portion of the nasal sill.
2. An excision of the minimal mucosa overlying the marked area of the medial crural footplate is performed.
3. A 5-0 polydioxanone horizontal mattress spanning suture is passed across the columella, securing the medial crural footplates.
4. A second 4-0 chromic catgut horizontal mattress suture is used to capture the soft tissue mass at the base of the columella.
5. Mucosal closure is performed with 5-0 chromic catgut.

Alar base resection, when planned, is performed after medial crura footplate approximation. A medial crura footplate approximation suture is placed first to set

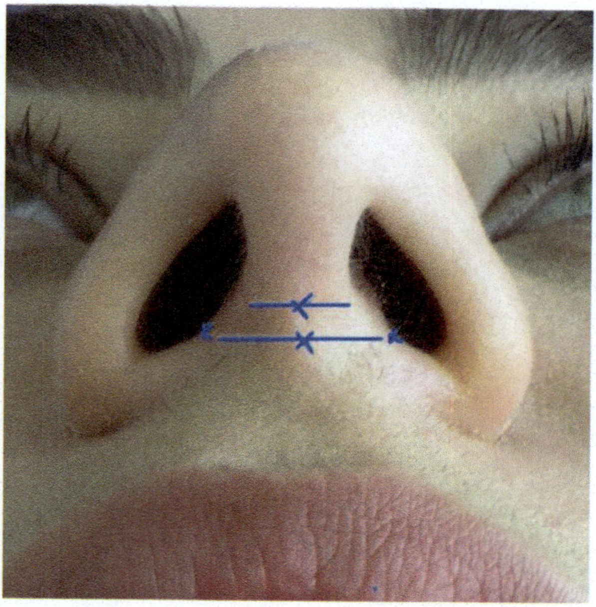

**Fig. 50.5** Diagram illustrating the sutures used for correction of the columellar base deformity. 5.0 PDS matress suture is passed across the columella to secure the medial crura footplates. 4.0 chromic catgut matress suture is used to capture the soft tissue at the columela base. Mucosal incision is closed with 5.0 chromic catgut suture

the medial portion of the nasal sill and more accurately determine the necessary resection.

Soft tissue approximation at the caudal portion of the columella is associated with limited mucosal resection, and cartilage repositioning is sufficient to achieve a pleasant contour in most cases.

However, when an excessive amount of soft tissue is present on the columellar base, it can be necessary to perform resection. Soft tissue between the medial crura footplate and a portion of the depressor nasi septi muscle can be resected when indicated.

In addition, patients with a wide columella may have an excess membranous septum and redundant skin at the columella. In these cases, it is important to excise an amount of membranous septum and excess skin to correct the columella width and achieve an ideal result.

This soft tissue resection should be limited and performed with caution.

Furthermore, in some severe cases, when suture positioning and soft tissue resection cannot address the deformity appropriately, a small trimming of the feet of the medial crura can be necessary.

Three core principles constitute the basis for the medial crura footplate approximation [5]:

1. Limited mucosal resection is used to address the expansion of the nasal lining and soft tissue that results from laterally displaced/excessively flared medial crura.
2. A medial crura fixation suture is used to reposition the cartilage via a cartilage preservation technique, thereby achieving correction of footplate angulation.
3. Soft tissue approximation allows for repositioning and compression of excessive tissue in most patients.

## Case Examples

**Case 1** (Fig. 50.6)

**Case 2** (Fig. 50.7)

**Case 3** (Fig. 50.8)

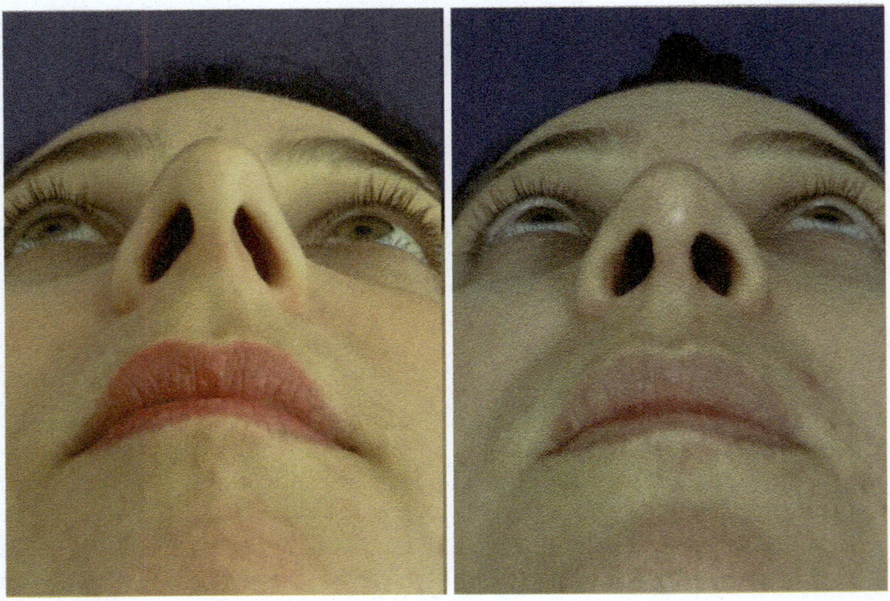

**Fig. 50.6** Patient with medial nostril and columellar base deformity (left) treated with medial crura footplate approximation. Two years postoperative photograph (right)

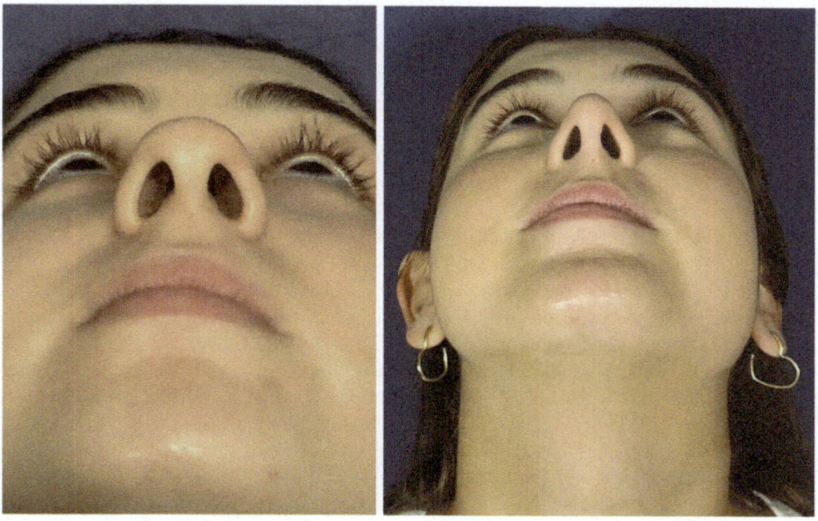

**Fig. 50.7** Patient with medial nostril and columellar base deformity (left) treated with medial crura footplate approximation. One year postoperative photograph (right)

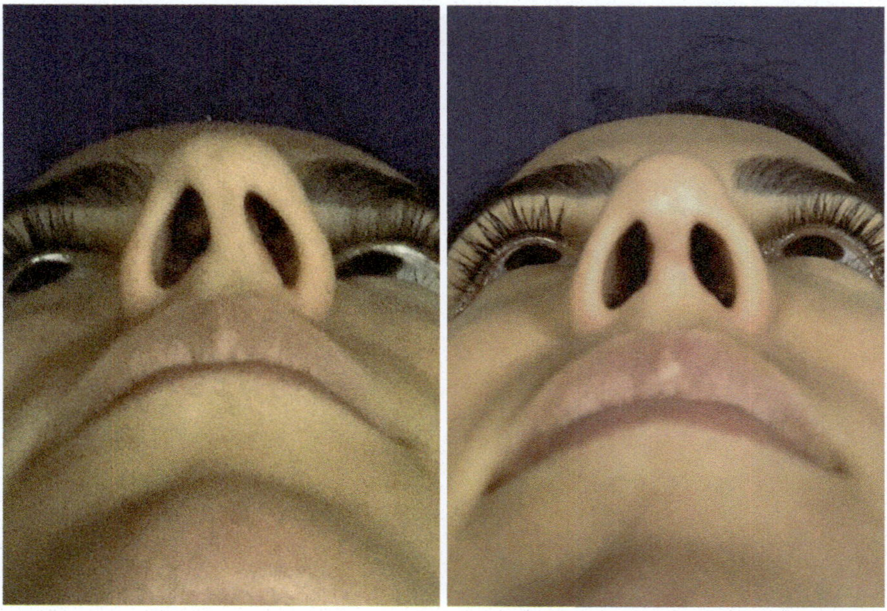

**Fig. 50.8** Patient with medial nostril deformity, columellar base deformity and caudal septum deviation (left) treated with caudal septum repositioning and medial crura footplate approximation. One-year postoperative photograph (right)

## References

1. Baldini N, Alomani M, Fonseca E, Saban Y. A nasal columellar base stabilizing suture technique. Plast Reconstr Surg. 2024;153(2):331e–3e. https://doi.org/10.1097/PRS.0000000000010745.
2. Daniel RK, Glasz T, Molnar G, Palhazi P, Saban Y, Journel B. The lower nasal base: an anatomical study. Aesthet Surg J. 2013;33(2):222–32. https://doi.org/10.1177/1090820X12472695.
3. Daniel RK, Palhazi P. Chapter 5: Nasal base. In: Rhinoplasty an anatomical and clinical atlas. Cham: Springer; 2018. p. 213–58.
4. Kridel RWH, Kwak ES, Watson JB. Columellar aesthetics in open rhinoplasty. Facial Plast Surg. 2016;32(4):333–8. https://doi.org/10.1055/s-0036-1585575.
5. Geissler PJ, Lee MR, Roostaeian J, Unger JG, Rohrich RJ. Reshaping the medial nostril and columellar base: five-step medial crural footplate approximation. Plast Reconstr Surg. 2013;132(3):553–7. https://doi.org/10.1097/PRS.0b013e31829ad2d5.
6. Ghidini A, Dallari S, Marchioni D. Surgery of the nasal columella in external valve collapse. Ann Otol Rhinol Laryngol. 2002;111(8):701–3. https://doi.org/10.1177/000348940211100808.
7. Daniel RK, Farkas LG. Rhinoplasty: image and reality. Clin Plast Surg. 1988;15(1):1–10.
8. Farkas LG, Hreczko TA, Deutsch CK. Objective assessment of standard nostril types—a morphometric study. Ann Plast Surg. 1983;11(5):381–9.
9. Crumley RL. Aesthetics and surgery of the nasal base. Facial Plast Surg. 1988;5(2):135–42. https://doi.org/10.1055/s-2008-1064745.

# Revision Rhinoplasty

# 51

Ali Abd Alameer Khazaal, Giuseppe Cottone, and Enrico Robotti

**Key Points**

- Revision rhinoplasty is a complicated surgery that requires an expert surgeon to be performed.
- Universally rhinoplasty is considered the most demanding procedure in facial plastic surgery. Secondary rhinoplasty is more complex and its crown jewel, and so highly fascinating.
- Preoperative analysis in secondary rhinoplasty is considered a crucial step of this procedure which includes proper history taking, nasal examination, and investigation; Cone beam computed tomography (CBCT), the proper preoperative analysis will raise the success rate and concomitantly the patient and surgeon satisfaction.
- In many secondary rhinoplasty procedures, the rib is an essential tool, and thus some finesse points have to be mastered, and some important concepts should be well understood. This will provide a stable, elegant, and identical reconstruction if applicable.
- New techniques and innovations add more precision and finesse to the results such as the sandwich of perichondrium and fascia SPF, or sandwich of perichondrium, rib lamination and fascia SPLF. Thinking of the SPF–SPLF graft as a hybrid graft that mediates best the gap between the washed-out appearance of diced cartilage in fascia and the sharp edge visibility of solid rib grafts.

**Supplementary Information** The online version contains supplementary material available at https://doi.org/10.1007/978-3-031-70077-4_51.

A. A. A. Khazaal (✉)
Baghdad, Iraq

G. Cottone
Milan, Italy

E. Robotti
Bergamo, Italy


S. Elwany (ed.), *Current Rhinology*,
https://doi.org/10.1007/978-3-031-70077-4_51

## 51.1 Background

Rhinoplasty is considered as one of the most technically challenging aesthetic procedures due to the fact of intricate structural nasal components, which comprise both shape and function, adding to that the critical nose location on the face: central and prominent [1]. Revision is a more complex and demanding procedure, which often represents a final opportunity to correct both functional and aesthetic issues after previous nasal surgeries. The use of rib cartilage in these procedures has become a game-changer, offering unparalleled structural support and versatility. This chapter delves into the finesse required in performing revision rhinoplasty with rib cartilage, exploring its challenges, benefits, and the meticulous skills it demands.

The steady and quick evolution of notion and practice in this procedure in the last decades acknowledges progressively the influence of maintaining the structures in primaries and to rebuild these structures in secondaries. The paradigm is no longer to achieve a thin, small, and pointy nose, but rather a natural, elegant, and well-proportioned nose that breath well [2].

The psychology of the patient is the single most rigorous challenge in revision procedure. Primary rhinoplasty patients are oftentimes optimistic and hopeful; on the contrary, the revision rhinoplasty patient is usually upset, hesitant, and skeptical of what can be achieved after the failure of previous attempts to fulfill their goals. It is quite important to realize the original patients' concerns before they went to their first surgery, in addition to the current concerns and for this reason, it is foremost to listen carefully to the patient's own words and concerns in all the consultations. The most common complications that can be seen after a revision rhinoplasty procedure relates to lateral alar sidewalls and mid-nasal pyramid. These complications can be diminished by taking important steps to lessen the risk. The key in both situations is to guarantee strong structural support, preserving the support after hump reduction and preserving and adding support to the sidewalls [3].

In any event, the challenges for the surgeon are to determine:

1. If the deformity is imagined or real.
2. The ability of the surgeon to correct the deformities.
3. The surgeon's ability to achieve the patient's goal.
4. Realistic expectations of the patients coupled with the likelihood of satisfaction after surgery or not [4–6].

The latter is the most critical part of the decision-making because it can be capricious. It is quite important to make reasonable assumptions during the process of consultation based on the patient's deportment and personality [3]. Doctor–patient relationship and trust must be built laying the foundations for extended counseling to convey a realistic outcome for any revision surgery [7].

In secondary rhinoplasty, constructing a proper dorsum is closely related to reconstructing the tip by retrieving the proper proportions and appropriate length, width, and projection of the nose. Recovering an adequate function is closely linked with tip and dorsum reconstruction [2]. A stable "L-Strut" configuration and a straight midline septum are fundamental to the whole concept of attaining symmetric, aesthetic dorsal lines using strong stable spreaders on both sides. It is evident that one needs a graft that is straight, robust, and long enough to fit the purpose. Thus, a properly shaped rib lamina, if chosen correctly and fashioned well by delicate lamination, will be exemplary for this purpose. The septum is obviously the first-choice grafting material for the tip if it is available. If not, then the rib can be sculptured and fashioned to provide a grafting material that can structure and support the nasal tip and reshape the sidewalls. Eventually, costal cartilage is an abundant material from which to obtain diced cartilage; moreover, the same access supplies fascia and perichondrium to structure an innovative construct for reshaping the dorsal contour (harvested rib menu after lamination with the perichondrium).

If we compare the rib to alternative ear cartilage, the advantages of the rib over the ear cartilage are abundant supply, diversity of straight segments, and versatility. In our experience, all these advantages well compensate for the relative disadvantage of somewhat more intricate harvesting. On the other hand, we find conchal cartilage is brittle and convoluted and lacks the desired rigidity for structural support in most indications (Fig. 51.1) [2]. Another easy-to-find option is the homologous (i.e., human cadaver-derived) irradiated rib, even if considerable data available in the literature showed a higher rate of long-term resorption [8].

Rib cartilage introduction as a grafting material has revolutionized the revision rhinoplasty practice. Whenever the septum is insufficient, we will turn directly to the rib without hesitation. The decision to harvest the rib cartilage is usually delayed after obtaining full exposure if there is a doubt about the septum availability, otherwise, we do it as a first step of the surgery. There is no doubt that the septum is the first choice and is the best possible grafting material, while costal cartilage is the next choice. For this reason, we often use the rib to craft strong spreaders and new robust L-strut, while if the whole or partial septum is still available, it remains the first choice for the tip restructuring, lateral crura as well as septal extension graft (SEG) and strut [2].

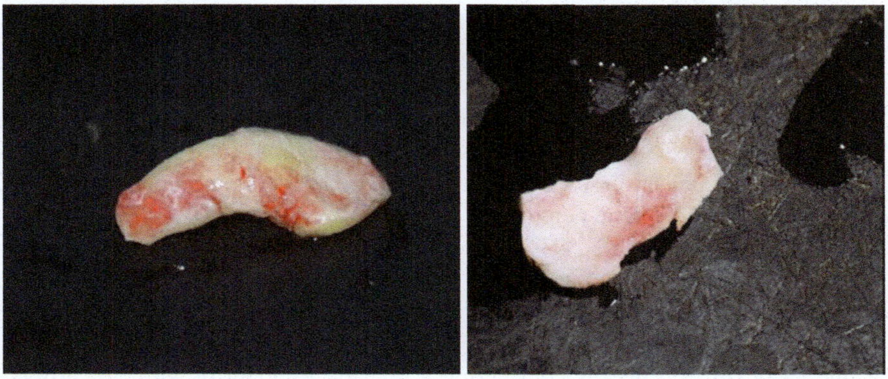

**Fig. 51.1** Brittle convoluted ear cartilage

There is a consensus by most of the authors that revision rhinoplasty surgery should be delayed for at least 1 year after the last rhinoplasty [9, 10]. This time will allow the scar to mature, reducing the risk of deformity due to poor healing of the tissue after the subsequent surgery. Whereas this remains a standard general guideline, early touch-ups of minor deformities may ease the anxieties of patients without compromising the result.

## 51.2 Challenges and Complexities

Revision rhinoplasty with rib cartilage is not free from challenges:

- *Scar tissue management:* overcoming the difficulties posed by scar tissue from previous surgeries
- *Structural and aesthetic balance:* achieving a balance between functional restoration and aesthetic enhancement
- *Harvesting rib cartilage:* addressing the technical and aesthetic considerations in rib cartilage extraction

### 51.2.1 Surgical Finesse and Expertise

The successful execution of this procedure requires a surgeon with exceptional skill and a deep understanding of nasal anatomy. Key aspects include the following:

- *Tailored grafts:* custom shaping of the rib cartilage to suit the individual's nasal structure.
- *Precise placement:* strategic placement of grafts within the nose is paramount to ensure both functional and aesthetic improvements. Surgeons must secure the grafts to provide long-term structural support while avoiding any visible or palpable irregularities.
- *Minimizing complications:* expertise in reducing potential complications associated with rib cartilage harvesting and transplantation.
- *Soft tissue management:* the soft tissues of the nose, such as the skin and mucosa, play a significant role in the final aesthetic outcome. Surgeons must handle these tissues with finesse, ensuring a harmonious result. The senior author described a new technique called *three points compartmentalization* that is applicable in primary and secondary cases, and it has an important rule in reducing edema and better defining the nasal contour [11].

### 51.2.2 Patient Perspective

Rhinoplasty surgeon who is considering a revision rhinoplasty with rib cartilage should pose particular attention to the following:

- *Patient evaluation:* a meticulous preoperative assessment is crucial. Surgeons must understand the patient's goals, assess the current nasal anatomy, and consider previous surgical interventions. Preoperative CT analysis is crucial and obligatory in all our revisions, and we thoroughly described this aspect in a dedicated article published in 2021 [12]. This comprehensive evaluation guides the surgical plan.
- *Expectation management:* understanding the realistic outcomes and limitations of revision surgery.

### 51.2.3 Significance of Rib Cartilage in Revision Rhinoplasty Strength

Rib cartilage grafts have emerged as a preferred material in revision rhinoplasty due to their strength, and they provide a robust framework for reconstructing the nasal structure, particularly in cases where previous surgeries have left little native cartilage.

- *Durability:* rib cartilage grafts offer long-term structural support.
- *Availability:* rib cartilage offers abundant material for reconstruction.
- *Versatility and adaptability:* they can be carved and shaped to address a wide range of nasal deformities.
- *Reduced rejection risk:* as an autologous material (i.e., autograft), rib cartilage has a lower risk of rejection compared to synthetic implants.

## 51.3 Method and Workflow

### 51.3.1 Harvesting a Full-Thickness Segment with Anterior Perichondrium and Rectus Fascia

#### 51.3.1.1 Placing of the Incision

The ideal scar after rib harvest should be the least in visibility on a similar concept as the trans-columellar incision, especially in female patients. For this reason, we changed our paradigm: from the concept of "look for the best rib" we shifted to "look for the lowest possible visibility," adjusting our access to such choice and adjusting our rib harvest to it. Currently, in females, we are always using a 2 to 3.5-cm inframammary incision, specifically in the fold inframammary fold (IMF), no matter which rib is there (usually it is the sixth but sometimes the fifth), and we modify progressively our technique from that described by Gunter in 2008 [13]. The incision length depends on the underlying tissue thickness: 2–2.5 cm in thin patients will be enough (Fig. 51.2).

The precise location of the incision is somewhat more medial in comparison to the one used in breast augmentation: it starts at the cross point between a vertical line drawn 1 cm medial to the areola and the IMF, extending medially. If we start

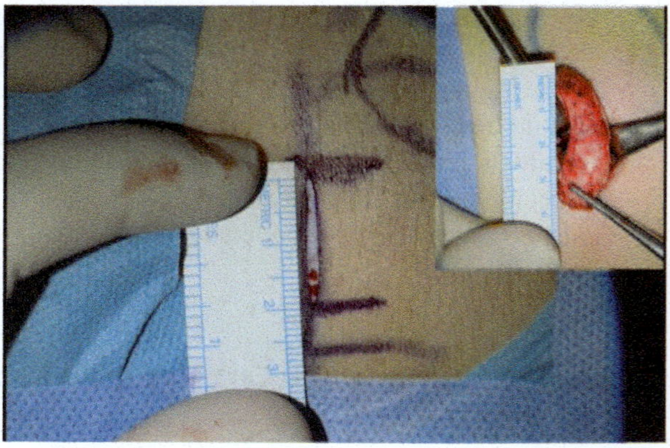

**Fig. 51.2** Small incision 2 cm at the rib donor site, with long harvested rib segment 4 cm

too lateral, then the incision will end up over the bony segment of the rib, rather than the cartilaginous part. If a scar from previous augmentation/reduction/pexy is already present in the fold, the same scar can be used or just lengthened (e.g., in the case of a previous short-scar breast augmentation). The presence of a breast implant is not considered an issue since our dissection for the rib harvesting is going to be performed around the lower edge with no actual exposure of the implant. Palpation and marking of the targeted rib segment follow. There is usually an option to choose between the superior or the inferior rib since there is some leeway in moving the skin. Once completely healed, the scar is usually hardly identifiable (Fig. 51.3).

In male patients with a tendency toward gynecomastia, we still locate the incision in the same place at the fold. Otherwise, we will go for the best-relaxed skin tension line. In these cases, the choice would be the seventh or even the eighth rib, and the scar will be more visible. It is very clear that one can harvest the costal cartilage via a small incision, which can be directly done over a straighter rib segment which is the seventh usually [14], but this, in our experience, may cause more scars spreading, although short, due to stretching and tension with a subsequent distorted healing.

#### 51.3.1.2 Harvesting

After the dermis and the underlying fat are incised, the superficial layer of fascia becomes clear. We prefer to mark this fascia with methylene blue to facilitate the accurate suturing of this layer later. Below the superficial layer of fascia, the fat becomes obvious; and by means of a large elevator and with a sweeping motion, we expose the rectus fascia and clean it of fat lobules (Fig. 51.4). A portion of rectus fascia (usually approximately 3 × 2 cm) is carefully elevated from the rectus muscle using a fine Bovie tip. The fascia is cleansed of all the muscle fibers attached to the underlying surface of it, fixed to a silicone pad with small needles covering it with a wet sponge, and left for later use. The amount of rectus fascia will be more than enough to construct an SPF or SPLF structure, together with the harvested perichondrium as will be delineated later [15].

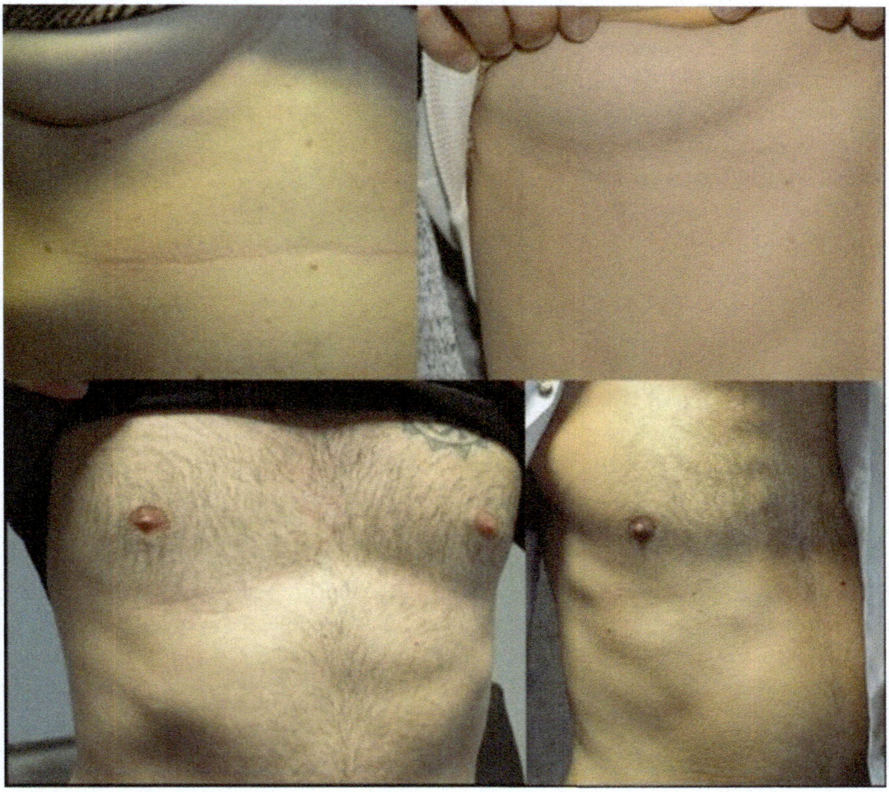

**Fig. 51.3** Invisible healed scar of rib harvest donor site

**Fig. 51.4** Glistening rectus Fascia

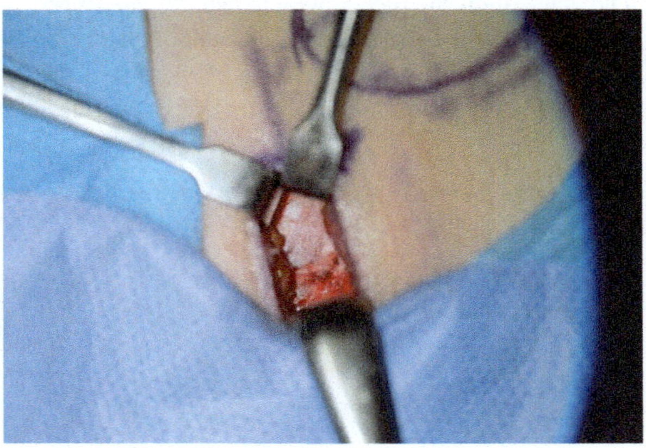

The fibers of the rectus muscle at this point are precauterized by bipolar along their axis and then split and separated as far as possible, avoiding cutting them across, thus with the inframammary incision's original direction. At this point, the

rib is readily visible with its bony cartilaginous junction that is differentiated by its different hue (grayish tinge is distinctive for the bone), and needle palpation is used to confirm that (Fig. 51.5). Then, a full-thickness rib piece of 3–4 cm is harvested circumferentially, keeping the overlying rectangular perichondrium attached to the rib to be harvested together as shown, by dissecting superior and inferior borders, but leaving the perichondrium below the rib intact and stuck to the chest wall to avoid injuring the pleura. Curved small elevators (Robotti rib elevators, Marina Medical Inc., FL, USA), appropriately tailored, facilitate this crucial step. Synchondroses that may exist with the underlying rib should be divided carefully using the sharp-edged large elevator. The remnant cartilaginous sharp edges at the periphery of the donor site are softened by a large curette or a small rongeur.

#### 51.3.1.3 Closure of the Donor Site

Before closing the wound, the donor site is filled with saline, and the anesthesiologist is asked to apply a positive pressure (i.e., a Valsalva maneuver) to check for any pleural injury or leak. Closure starts by resuturing the splayed muscle fibers, superficial fascia, dermis, and skin, in independent layers consecutively. A large bore IV cannula tip is slipped under the muscle repair, and then tapping the catheter to the skin after withdrawing the guiding needle. As a final step of this procedure, 10 mg of ropivacaine (Naropin®) is inoculated through the catheter (we suggest repeating this administration the day after, before removing the catheter and discharging the patient). In our practice, we found this will relieve postoperative pain predictably and efficiently.

### 51.3.2 Fashioning the Rib Segment

The harvested rib piece, which usually measures 3–3.5 cm, is often relatively straight (a curved rib will still allow enough straight long piece). After peeling off the perichondrium by sharp wide elevator, we then start with the rib lamination (Fig. 51.6). A unique solid rib segment is never used. In our practice, the ideal graft

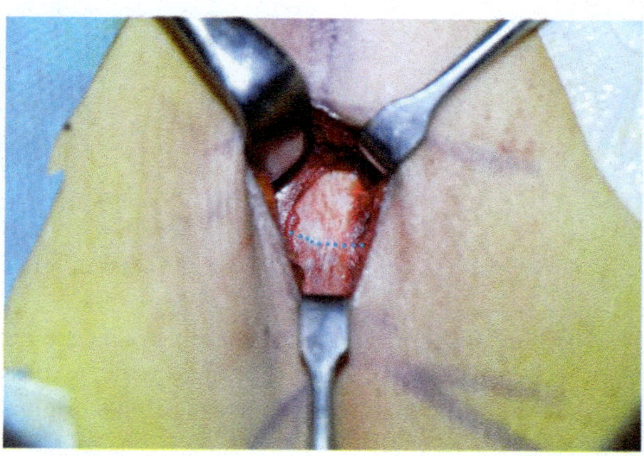

**Fig. 51.5** Rib bony cartilaginous junction that is differentiated by its different hue (greyish tinge is distinctive for the bone)

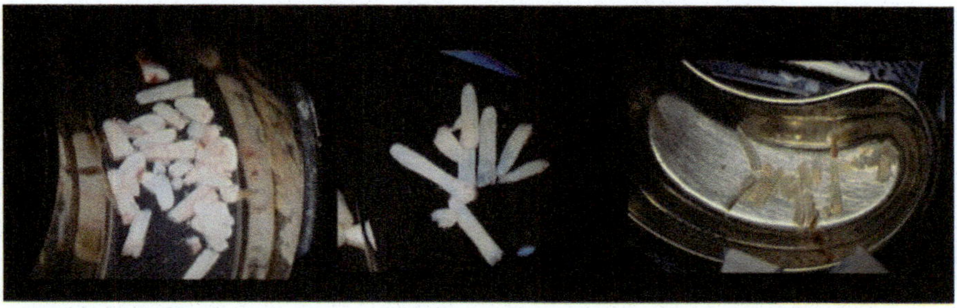

**Fig. 51.6** Different rib segments length from three different patients (short segments, long segments and third patient mixture of different length)

material that one can use to camouflage the tip or as a contour/augmentation graft for the final dorsum management is the perichondrium. Hair transplant blades are used for rib lamination, and these blades can be handled more easily than the taller, more flexible, and wider blades used by pathologists (but, of course, it depends on the rib thickness, and you can choose what you think is the best in your hands). Other devices are described for this purpose, like the one by Foulad et al. [16]. It is well-known clinically that the longer, straighter, and less prone to warping pieces of rib are the longitudinal inner pieces.

Several studies have demonstrated the advantage of balanced cross-sectional carving with harvesting the central cartilage, along with oppositional suturing whenever bending is noticed, and peripheral pieces of the rib are known to be more vulnerable to warping than central pieces [17, 18].

However, experimental studies often do not match everyday practice so, practically, it is clinically difficult to strictly rely on the notion of central carving in all the cases. With progressive experience, what matters and becomes evident is to have an ample choice of rib segments to test their proneness to warp after letting them "swim" into an antibiotic solution for a sufficient time (approximately half an hour), and then rigidly fixating those segments which need to maintain their straightness for a long time. Generally, long, strong straight spreaders are best carved from the rib core, while rib laminas from the peripheral part (often owning some convexity) may be useful for the sidewall reconstruction like the lower lateral crus replacement/reconstruction. Other authors may prefer other carving techniques, like "oblique" carving [19], although clearly oblique segments can be still taken from the rib after the longitudinal core has been laminated, because we still prefer to use the longitudinal lamination.

As the experience of the surgeon grows, one can decide from the beginning of the lamination the kind of segment that will best fit each purpose: struts, spreaders, septal extension grafts, lateral crural struts, interpositional grafts, alar contour grafts, etc. Slicing the segments longitudinally, precisely, forcing the blade, if necessary, when we met calcifications, and following the rib axis is the key here. The "menu" of these multiple laminas, along with the perichondrium, is always put into a kidney dish filled with antibiotic solution as previously shown in Video 51.1. In the literature, it is well-known that rib warping will take place quickly to be easily recognizable, while the surgery goes on in the senior author's experience. To declare itself, the warping tendency will not need more than half an hour, and the segments usually are left much longer in the antibiotic saline. Pieces destined to bend will obviously bend. It is thus clearly advantageous to take and laminate the rib as a first step of the surgery, before starting the rhinoplasty itself, but this is not possible in every case because sometimes the need for a rib can be assessed only after exposing all the nose structures.

According to the senior author's experience (E.R.), computed tomography is not worthwhile to be performed preoperatively to look for rib calcifications. An intraoperative assessment of the rib situation will be enough. It never happens, in daily practice, since there are so many calcifications to decide to renounce harvesting.

The use of piezo, which recently has been introduced for calcified rib harvesting, is irrelevant in our hands. When significant calcification is found, one may harvest another piece of rib from the adjacent rib. Sculpturing segments that contain some calcifications may be eased using a power tool with profuse irrigation. Sometimes, piezo is used just to laminate, on the table, extremely calcified ribs. Practically, the presence of calcification is considered a two-edged sword: apparently, it confirms more rigid and strong grafting configurations, but it restricts the potential of the laminated rib to bend. This characteristic could be helpful when selecting adequate strong and straight segments—without any tendency to bend—as dorsal spreader grafts (Fig. 51.7).

Substantially, the general rule is to have plentiful options to pick up from for the specific needs of the patient. When well dimensioned, well planned, and well executed, using the proper segment for the right indication will deliver a correct, not bulky structure [20].

### 51.3.3 Use of Rib for the Dorsum

The essential concept that matters here is rebuilding the proper dorsal aesthetic lines, with a correct width and a straight nasal axis, and then introducing harmonic proper contour/camouflage above. This is achieved by proper septum

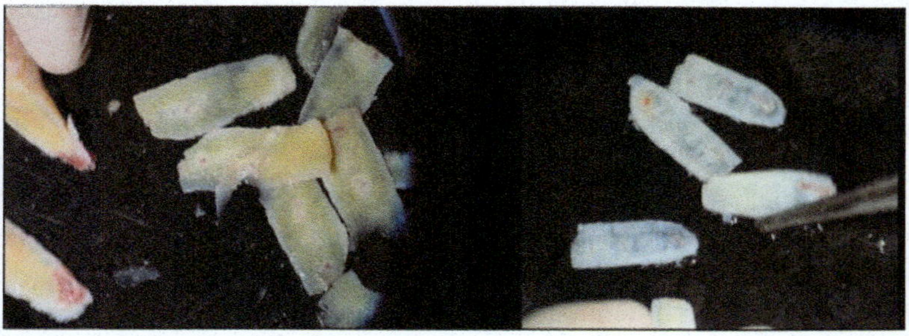

**Fig. 51.7** white and yellow rib segments with central calcifications (from two different patients)

straightening and accomplishing dorsal aesthetic lines by rib spreaders, while eventually finalizing the contour by using perichondrium, fascia, and rib laminas in different configurations. The key to the reconstruction of a symmetrical nasal pyramid (and this is always true both in primary and secondary rhinoplasty) is the proper configuration of the septum, the "L-strut" building/rebuilding, along with pleasant aesthetic dorsal lines (i.e., a straight midline septum in a stable "L-strut" configuration) [21, 22].

The open approach makes the "top–down" exposure of the septum possible, and the residual septum assessment follows, with variable decisions to be made. Those depend on residual deviations and residual septum and thus may lead to straightening the deviated residual septum by using a perforated thin ethmoidal lamina derived from the perpendicular plate of ethmoid (PPE), along with a septal extension graft (SEG) to lengthen it, usually derived from a rib lamina sutured to the nasal spine to deliver a solid vertical segment of L-strut, buttressing it on one or two sides with robust and straight segment, and many other structures (Fig. 51.8).

An ethmoid plate left posteriorly from previous surgery is usually enough to splint the septum or the rib structures, fashioned with a burr to a paper-like thickness and perforated with piezo.

The common scenario we usually find is that the original septum is deficient or unavailable, and in such case, the plan will be to reconstruct a solid L-strut by means of rib segments or to reestablish/strengthen the residual septum with rib segments. Rib spreaders are an essential requisite to confirm the septum to the midline and to give proper dorsal aesthetic lines by establishing the lateral desired width. In this context, you need to pay attention to choosing the best rib pieces which are the straightest among those laminas which have been kept floating in saline after lamination. Such grafts from the rib can be custom-made (including shaping the lateral/cranial/caudal edges) on the base of shape and width to achieve a symmetric dorsal aesthetic contour by asymmetric or symmetric placement [23].

In all situations, it is essential to ensure that the reconstructed septum is positioned centrally. Secure fixation should be positioned distally to the nasal spine and proximally to the upper lateral cartilage. Furthermore, as outlined in more recent

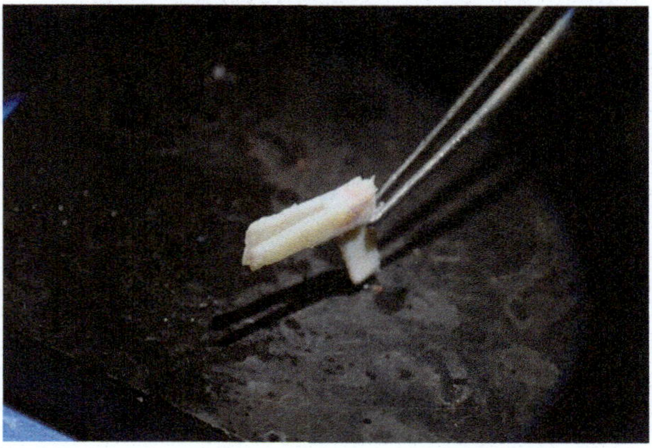

**Fig. 51.8** L strut reconstruct (pistol shape construct

descriptions, attention should be given to achieving a solid fixation with the nasal bones too [24].

This passage delves into the intricate technical details involved in shaping the spine, using tools such as piezo or power devices. It also discusses the optimal arrangement of transosseous sutures linking the proximal septum to the nasal bones, which includes encircling the rib segments employed as spreaders in a cerclage manner [25]. The L-strut's vertical component, viewed either as an SEG or a distal septal replacement graft, must be firmly anchored to the nasal spine to ensure structural integrity, necessitating transosseous sutures. Care must be taken to avoid excessive protrusion of the graft at the spine, as it might cause a transverse skin crease during smiling. This can be managed by reducing the cartilage's thickness over the spine and/or placing a small, soft tissue cushion. While not the main focus of this discussion, it is important to note that correcting residual asymmetrical nasal bones often requires osteoplasty and osteotomy techniques, preferably executed with piezoelectric tools and facilitated by the broad access provided by a full exposure. Similarly, the radix might need to be made deeper using a guarded burr or repeated osteotomies might be necessary either to close an open roof or to reverse a previous over-narrowing of the nasal bones. In some instances, the nasal bones may require to be sculptured in different fashion at the cranial or distal ends due to thickness variability per se, or in other cases, osteotomy might need to be doubled side to side. When using bilateral extended rib spreader grafts, it is crucial to ensure that they don't overly and congest the tip area where they meet the central vertical element of the L-strut. This can be achieved by appropriately shortening one of the spreaders. Additionally, it is vital that they are securely sutured to the remaining septum, highly positioned (proximally), and that each nasal bone at the keystone area has a custom-fitted groove to accommodate the spreader itself (Fig. 51.9).

Using piezo or a cutting burr is effective for accurately creating the groove where the spreaders will be placed. Additionally, adjustments in height can be made concerning the residual septum's remaining height. Specifically, the spreaders can extend beyond it and be fixed slightly higher on each side. This step is crucial for

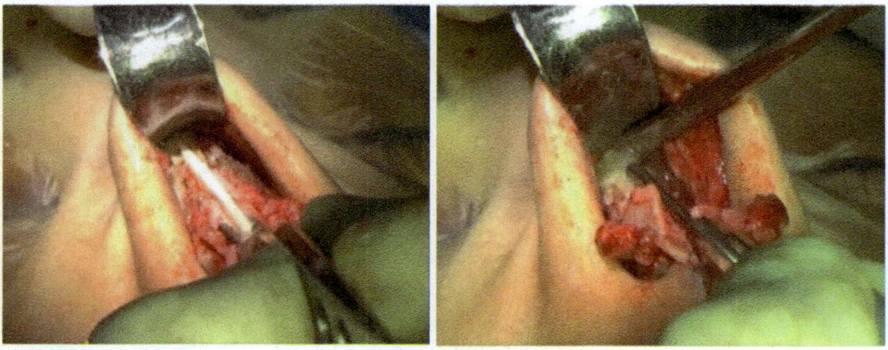

**Fig. 51.9** Bone grooves preprepared with Piezo cutting insert to lunch the spreaders or the cephalic part of the L construct

establishing the structural base upon which the final shape will be crafted. On each side, the upper lateral cartilages, often embedded in scar tissue, must be aligned with the spreaders and firmly sutured. In these situations, the use of rib material is highly valued for its straight form and structural firmness. The key is to use segments that are straight and sturdy, yet not overly thick. In contemporary secondary rhinoplasty, most surgeons typically employ one of these two approaches for reconstructing the dorsal plateau: using a solid segment of rib or employing diced cartilage wrapped in various materials [15]. Solid rib has a long history of use, but it has also faced issues with displacement and warping. To address these problems, a variety of stabilization methods and different carving techniques have been proposed [26–28].

There is a widespread recommendation for using rib segments shaped through cross-sectional balance carving, frequently involving central harvesting. This approach has recently been enhanced by the addition of oppositional suturing techniques [28].

Notable modifications involve scratching the bone "bed" and then attaching a strip of perichondrium to the inner surface of the rib segment to ensure improved adhesion. Additionally, perichondrium grafts sourced from the ear or rib have been demonstrated to possess capabilities for revascularization and secure fixation [14, 29, 30].

Over the last 10 years, diced cartilage fascia has gained popularity due to its straightforwardness and minimal risk of warping. This approach originated from the crucial idea of "composite" reconstruction [4, 31]. This method has developed into an increasingly sophisticated and accurately measured structure, typically incorporating a temporalis fascia wrap and, more recently, using rectus fascia [31–34].

Diced cartilage may be utilized independently or combined with various binding agents [35–38]. In secondary dorsal reconstruction, it typically requires a sheath. While clinical practice usually observes minimal to no resorption, there are contrasting experimental findings reported in the literature [38–40].

#### 51.3.3.1 Challenges for Dorsum Reconstruction with Rib

Both solid rib and diced cartilage fascia techniques come with their own set of drawbacks: solid rib is prone to displacement, warping, and visible edges, even when fixed properly; diced cartilage fascia, while useful, doesn't suffice for structural needs and may lead to contour irregularities and poor definition on the sides, resulting in less aesthetically pleasing dorsal lines. This issue is exacerbated when it is used for augmenting the dorsum rather than being strategically placed for limited fill atop a restructured framework. The ongoing challenge is to create a structure that ensures proper dorsal aesthetic lines (DALs) definition without being overly sharp or appearing flat and uninteresting. This is the reason the senior author (E.R.) has been motivated to seek a more reliable method. Beginning in September 2017, a novel technique: the sandwich of perichondrium and fascia (SPF) and sandwich of perichondrium, rib lamina, and fascia (SPLF)—was developed and from that time on, it was used in more than 500 cases of revision rhinoplasties. This technique will be fully discussed in the next section.

#### 51.3.3.2 SPF–SPLF Technique

This recipe necessitates three key ingredients: perichondrium, rib lamina, and rectus fascia. These components are assembled into either an SPF or SPLF structure. Conveniently, all three elements are sourced from the same donor area. Once a dorsal plateau of the correct height and width is formed using a straight and stable L-strut with various configurations of rib spreaders and the residual septum, exact measurements of the final dorsal graft needed for contouring and slight additional height can be added. These measurements typically are 1 cm in width for male patients and 0.8 cm for female patients, with a length of approximately 3 cm. Following this, the three elements are processed in specific ways: (1) the perichondrium is trimmed to the exact size measured on the dorsum and to be placed facing down as in its natural position in the rib; (2) the rectus fascia is cut about 2 mm wider using a similar template; and (3) a suitable, nonwarped rib lamination of the necessary thickness for the required dorsal augmentation (if needed) is selected. If any remaining laminations show slight warping, one is chosen such that its mild concavity faces the dorsum, to give a gentle and natural dorsal convex "movement." This lamina—as the entire construct—is perfectly tailored, about 2 mm narrower than the measured dorsal width and is rectangular or slightly broader at the junction of its proximal third with the distal two-thirds, especially in male patients to create a subtly fusiform shape at the keystone. Its edges are smoothed out. The selected combination is then assembled into the final construct. The technical nuances of completing the dorsal contour with SPF–SPLF grafts are the following:

- *SPF:* here, the perichondrium acts as a comparably thick base layer with suitable consistency, placed with its inner surface (which was adjacent to the native rib) onto the dorsum. It uniformly covers the newly formed dorsal plateau and a segment of bone at the cephalic end, reshaped using either a piezo or a burr. The fascia is then stitched on top with a continuous 5-0 PDS (Ethicon, Inc., Somerville, N.J.) suture. Two sutures are intentionally left extended at each side of the graft's cephalic end as "guiding" sutures to be passed through the skin at the radix.
- *SPLF:* this method involves adding the rib lamina into its designated slot with a precise, snug fit, and no excess. In both techniques, the caudal end remains open. Insertion and stitching occur after the tip work is complete, with precise stabilization being crucial since forming a tight subperiosteal pocket is often unfeasible. The two extended sutures at the cephalic end are threaded through the skin at the radix and secured with Steri-Strips (3M, Maplewood, Minn.). The soft-tissue margins on each side of the graft (where the fascia and perichondrium meet) are sutured from the caudal to the cephalic end as feasible, to the edges of the right and left upper lateral cartilage. This process effectively finalizes a precise contour matching the width and length of the dorsal plateau. Additionally, to mitigate any lateral movement at the cephalic end, a transosseous cerclage suture is sometimes positioned atop the SPF–SPLF structure without excessive tightening, following the method described by Rezaeian et al. [24].

- The large-bore needle positioned on a specific power drill as described by Haack and Gubisch is very useful for the precise placement of this suture [23].
- *SPLFP (SPLF + Rib Plaster):* In some cases of thin skin patients, when we plan to use the SPLF graft, we may add a rib plaster on top of the rib lamina to soften the edges of this structural graft that may provide a minimal convexity on top of that graft.
- The graft's caudal end is subsequently stitched and sealed [41].
- The surgery then proceeds in a standard manner, concluding with skin closure, the application of Doyle splints, and taping. The SPF–SPLF construct has been implemented in a lot of cases from September 2017 to January 2024. Consistently with the senior author's practice, follow-ups in these rhinoplasty cases occur at 3, 6, and 12 months. A significant number of these cases reached a full 6-year follow-up at the time of this writing. Notably, none of these cases have exhibited any resorption or axis deviation during the follow-up, suggesting the construct's long-term stability when securely fixed (Fig. 51.10).

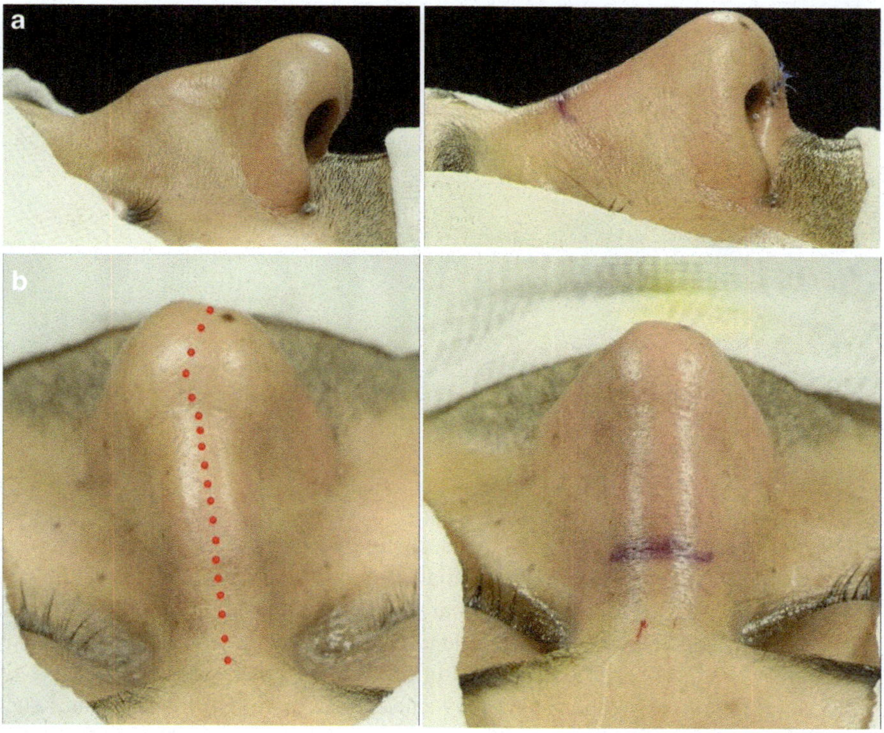


**Fig. 51.10** (**a–d**) This figure demonstrates how a bad septoplasty can lead to destruction of the nose: crooked nose, severe septal deviation after septoplasty, retracted columella due to caudal septal resection with supra-tip depression due to anterior septal angle resection. On table result with costal cartilage, reconstruction of L strut as a foundation, SPLF over the L construct. The beauty of SPLF in reflecting straight aesthetic lines is clear

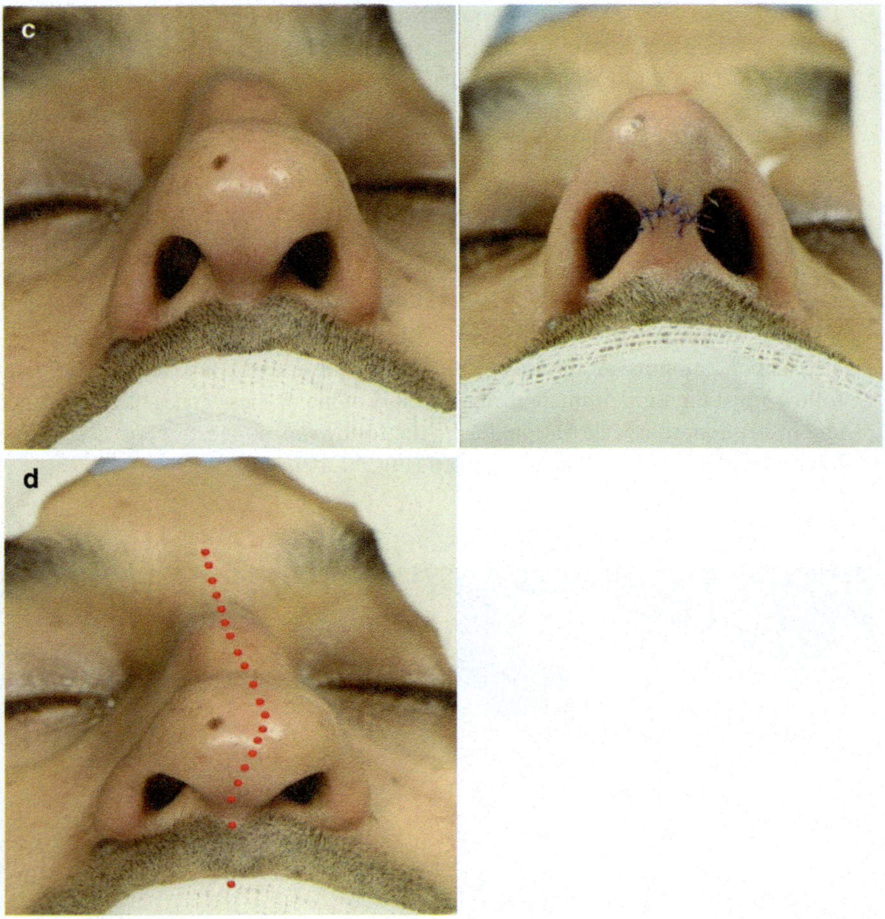


**Fig. 51.10** (continued)

## 51.4 Reconstructing the Tip

The lower lateral cartilages might have been compromised or excessively trimmed, and the support and structure of the medial crura could be disrupted. Since the septum essentially supports the tip, the initial step in tip reconstruction involves restoring a straight septal L-strut with sufficient length and projection, as previously mentioned. Disruption at the distal end of the septum can result in inadequate tip support, while excessive shortening may cause over-rotation of the tip. Issues such as underresection/overresection, dome division, bossae, and asymmetries vary, often affecting nasal proportions. Alar retraction can also occur, particularly if the lateral crura is excessively trimmed cephalically. This issue, combined with unrecognized cephalic malposition (Fig. 51.11), can lead to a "ball tip" configuration,

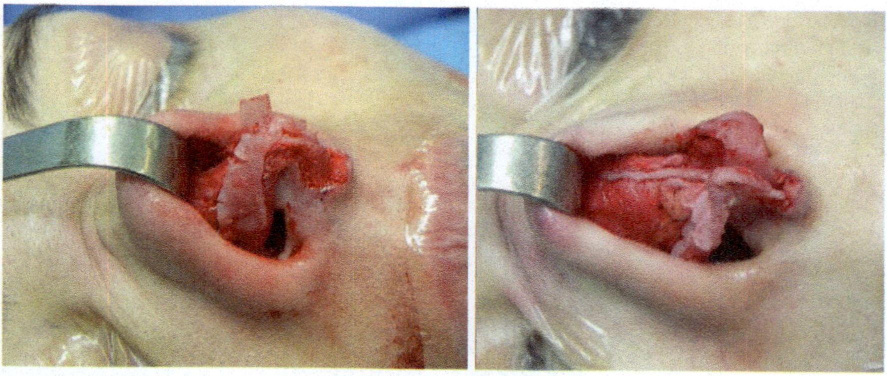

**Fig. 51.11** Bad trimming and different complications from previous surgeries

lacking proper triangulation and sidewall structure. While the potential complications are numerous, the reconstructive strategy generally revolves around reconstructing a straight and stable L-strut, leading to partial or complete reconstruction of the M-arch in almost all cases.

### 51.4.1 Partial M-Arch Reconstruction

The aim of partial reconstruction of the M-arch is to revitalize the tip cartilages on the existing residual elements, thereby re-establishing strong, straight, and elongated lateral crura. This typically involves the reconstruction of the original lateral crura, often using lateral crural strut grafts that are appropriately long, yet thin, and finely beveled (as shown in Fig. 51.12a). The beveling process can be performed with a knife blade or a fine-powered burr with continuous irrigation (Fig. 51.12b). It is an ideal material for these straight segments as they don't need to bend and are less likely to break. As mentioned earlier, a straight and carefully selected rib segment, attached with transosseous sutures to the spine, is often utilized as a distal septum replacement graft or SEG. This helps stabilize the medial crura and reconstruct the vertical portion of the M-arch unless a suitable piece of septum is available for this purpose. In cases, where no sizable or usable lateral crus segment exists lateral to the domes, another common approach is the use of "articulated alar rim grafts (AARGs)," as described by Davis (Fig. 51.12c) [42]. A This sophisticated technique differs fundamentally from the use of alar contour grafts in nonanatomical pockets. It effectively connects the tip to the sidewall in a stable and predictable manner. Additionally, akin to the use of alar contour grafts in primary rhinoplasty, when necessary, small, and slender rim grafts (micro-alar rim grafts) crafted from straight rib elements can be strategically placed in distinct pockets along the alar rim.

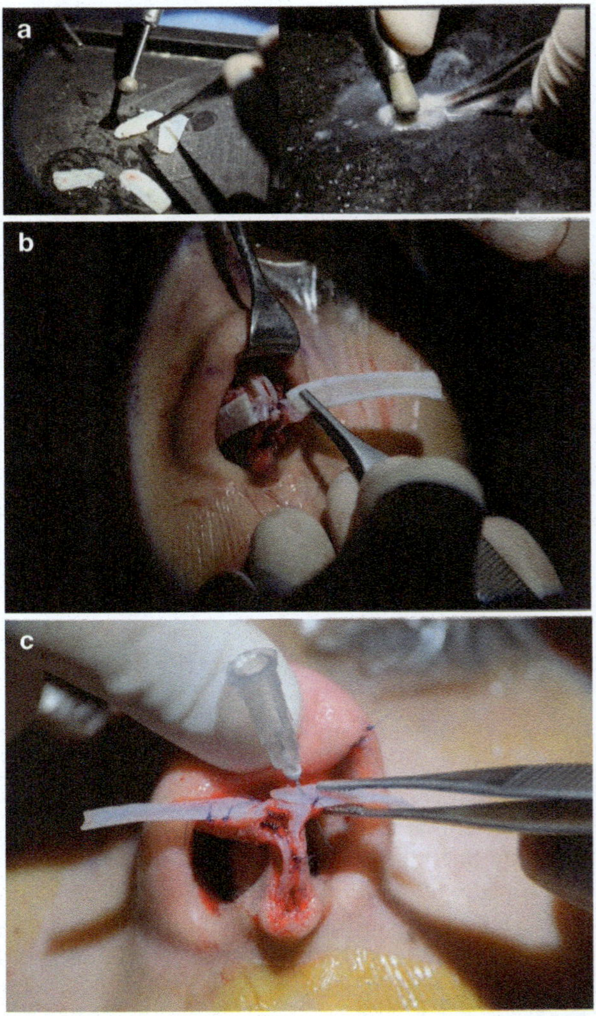

**Fig. 51.12** (**a**) LLC strut. (**b**) Different burr fashioning the lamina. (**c**) Articulated rim graft

## 51.4.2 Total Reconstruction of the M-Arch

Ideally, one would use thin and flexible cartilage for this purpose, with the septum being the optimal choice if it is still available. If not, rib serves as a suitable alternative, preferable to concha due to its useful structural properties. The rib offers straight segments that can be bent variably, barring any mild to severe calcifications. In numerous instances, SEGs or distal septum replacement grafts are also necessary, especially if further projection, lengthening, or rotation of the tip is needed. Such a configuration securely anchors the tip to the dorsum, offering more predictability than traditional floating columellar strut grafts. Often, this needs to be accompanied by meticulous scar release to address mucosal shortages, which are typically due to scarring rather than an actual lack of mucosa. Expanding the width of the lower lateral cartilages through grafting and inserting interpositional laminated grafts (to bridge the gap between the reconstructed lateral crus's upper edge and the upper lateral cartilage's lower edge) when needed will aid in maintaining this lengthening. Clearly, composite grafts also play a role in cases of extreme mucosal shortage [43]. In the author's experience, rib usage in secondary rhinoplasty is primarily for restructuring the dorsum. Frequently, enough septum is available to complete the tip work; however, if this is not the case, the rib is also used here, even though septum is a superior choice. A range of different scenarios can present in the tip during secondary rhinoplasty, and these are best addressed by adhering to the fundamental principle of restructuring rather than merely applying onlay camouflage grafts, which could add unnecessary bulk (Fig. 51.13) [42, 44].

Total M-arch reconstruction in selected—though not uncommon—cases requires the thinner rib laminas available so that they can be bent progressively to reconstruct M-arches bilaterally (Fig. 51.14) [45]. This approach provides a superb anatomical reconstruction of the lower lateral complex, yet it is true that these constructs can sometimes fracture, potentially leading to the loss of the domal angle. In these instances, the ideal solution is the application of AARGs and/or the use of perichondrium to soften the sharp edges.

### 51.4.3 Use of Rib, Perichondrium, and Fascia for Touchups

Adding subtle finishing touches to small dorsal irregularities and the constructed tip with available tissue often enhances the refinement of a revision case, particularly with thin and scarred skin. A small piece of rectus fascia, which can be

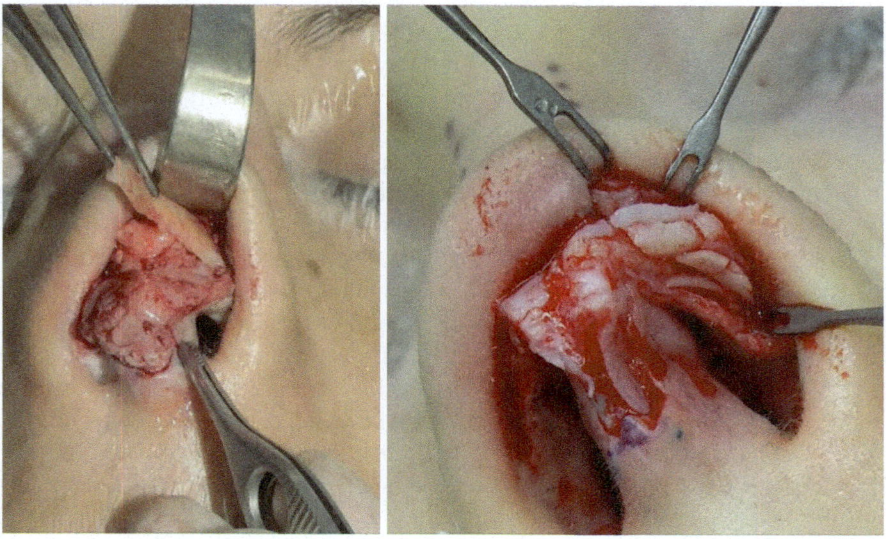

**Fig. 51.13** Bulky massy unwise grafts from bad previous revisions

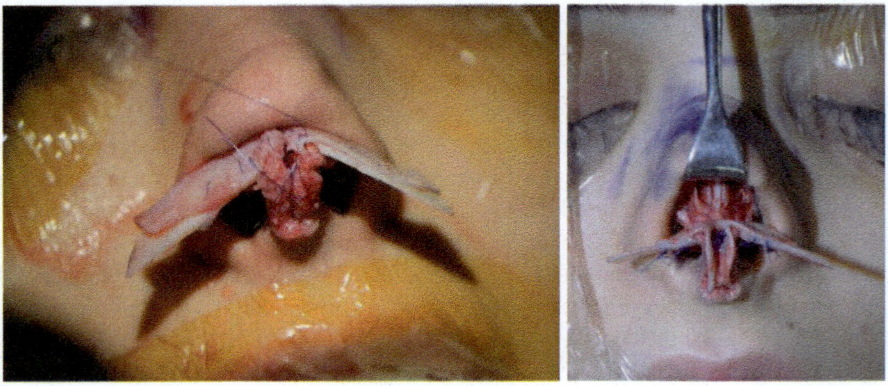

**Fig. 51.14** Total reconstruction of the M arch

**Fig. 51.15** Perichondrium over tip to soften the diamond

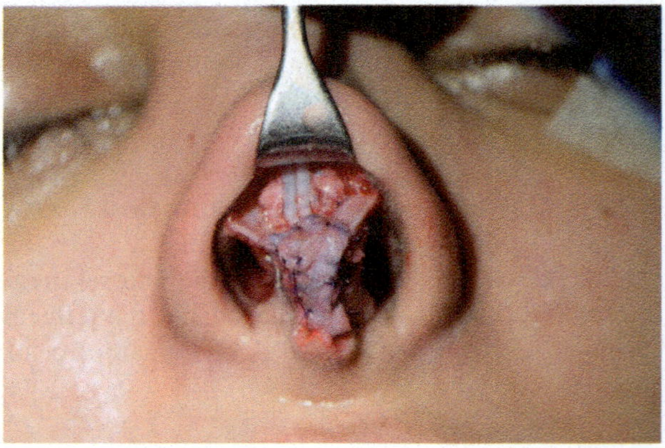

folded, if necessary, serves well as an onlay camouflage. Similarly, perichondrium, known for its ability to soften the tip, works excellently when positioned within the desired "tip diamond" area (Fig. 51.15). In some instances, a small alar contour graft can be meticulously crafted using a #11 blade from the outer edge of a rib lamination. It is important to recognize that this peripheral whitish area differs in color and consistency from the central, broader, and yellow region, which displays a palisade-like structure and is prone to calcification. This outer area more closely resembles the septum and is ideal for creating very thin yet robust segments for placement along the alar rim. Lastly, when a full-thickness rib segment is harvested, there is always ample material left to be minced, placed in a syringe, and used as a "filler" at the end of the procedure for any final adjustments [37]. Unlike septum, rib cartilage, even when finely diced, has a distinct consistency and is prone to obstructing a cannula if it is too narrow. For this reason, the senior author (E.R.) opts for a specially designed trocar for this task.

## 51.5 Long-Term Follow-Up

Regular follow-up is essential to assess the healing process and address any complications early. Long-term follow-up is important in primary rhinoplasties and crucial in secondaries.

## 51.6 Conclusion

Revision rhinoplasty with rib cartilage stands as a testament to the surgical artistry and precision required in modern plastic surgery. It offers a ray of hope to patients seeking correction of complex nasal issues postprimary surgery. It involves a careful evaluation of the patient's goals and anatomy, precise surgical techniques, and thoughtful postoperative care. This procedure demands not only a deep understanding of nasal anatomy and a unique set of skills but also an artistic sensibility and eye, as well as a comprehensive approach toward patient care and expectation management all together to restore both function and beauty to the nose and achieve natural and harmonious results. By combining the surgeon's expertise with the advantages of rib cartilage grafts, revision rhinoplasty can achieve remarkable results, providing both improved aesthetics and function for the patient. As the field advances, the use of rib cartilage in revision rhinoplasty will continue to evolve, further refining the balance between reconstructive necessity and aesthetic desire. Nonetheless, it is imperative for patients to have realistic expectations and trust in the expertise of their surgeons throughout the process.

**Cases**
**Case 1 (Fig. 51.16):**
**Case 2 (Fig. 51.17):**
**Case 3 (Fig. 51.18):**

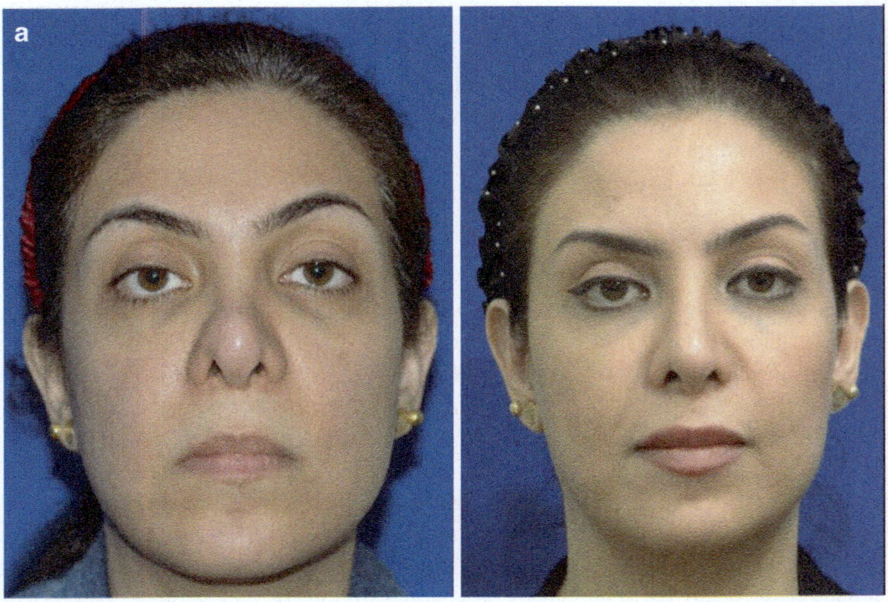


**Fig. 51.16** (**a–h**) Six months post revision septorhinoplasty with costal cartilage, (**i**) demonstrate 3D reconstruction as part of preoperative analysis, (**j**) shows a permanent filler coming out immediately after columellar incision which was injected after her first surgery

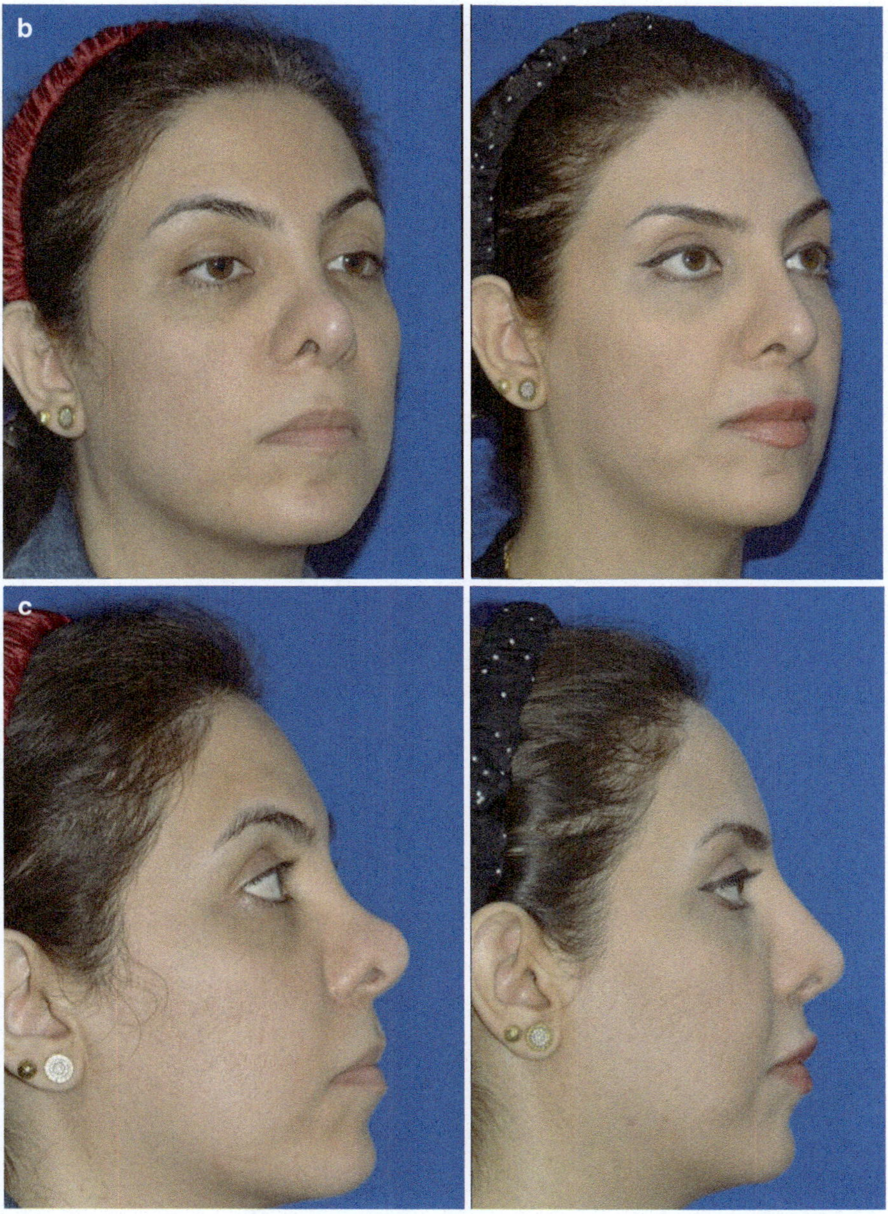


**Fig. 51.16** (continued)

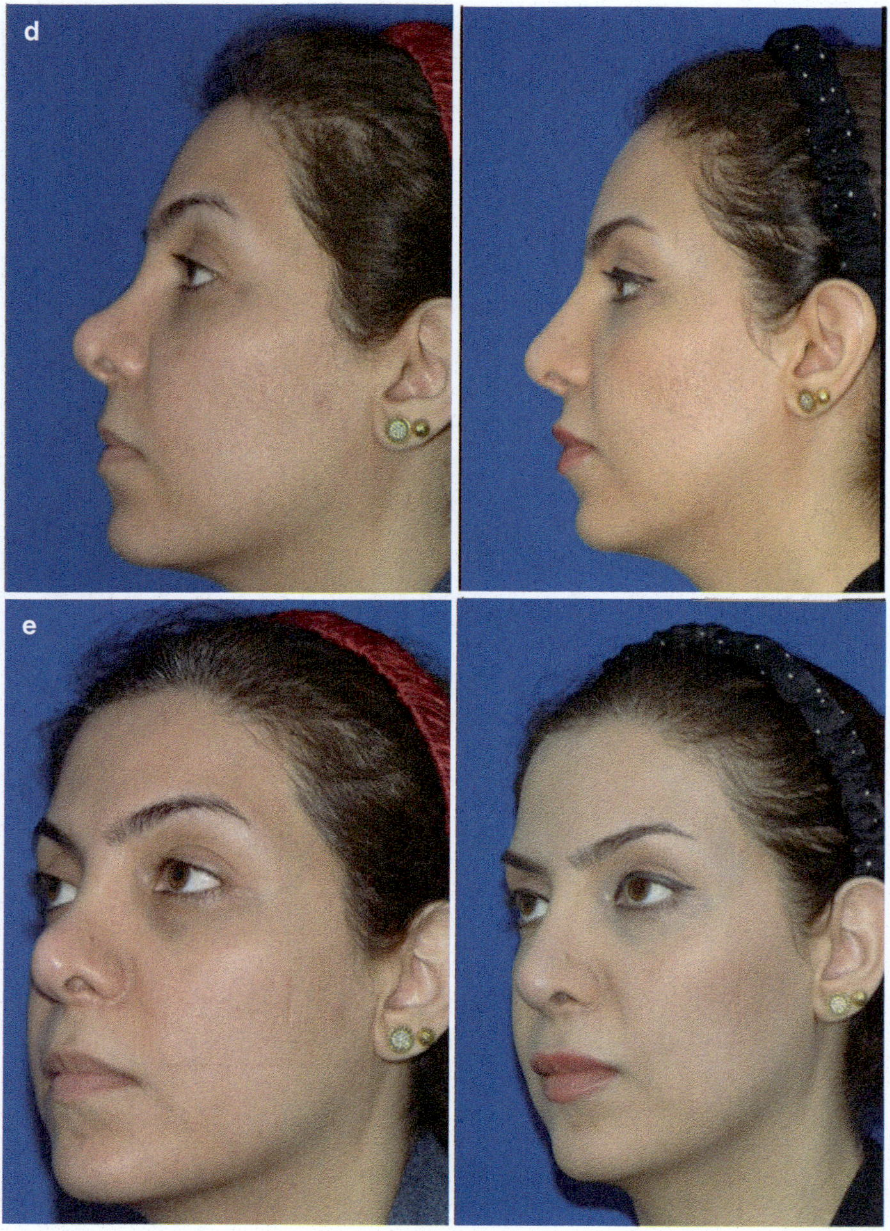


**Fig. 51.16** (continued)

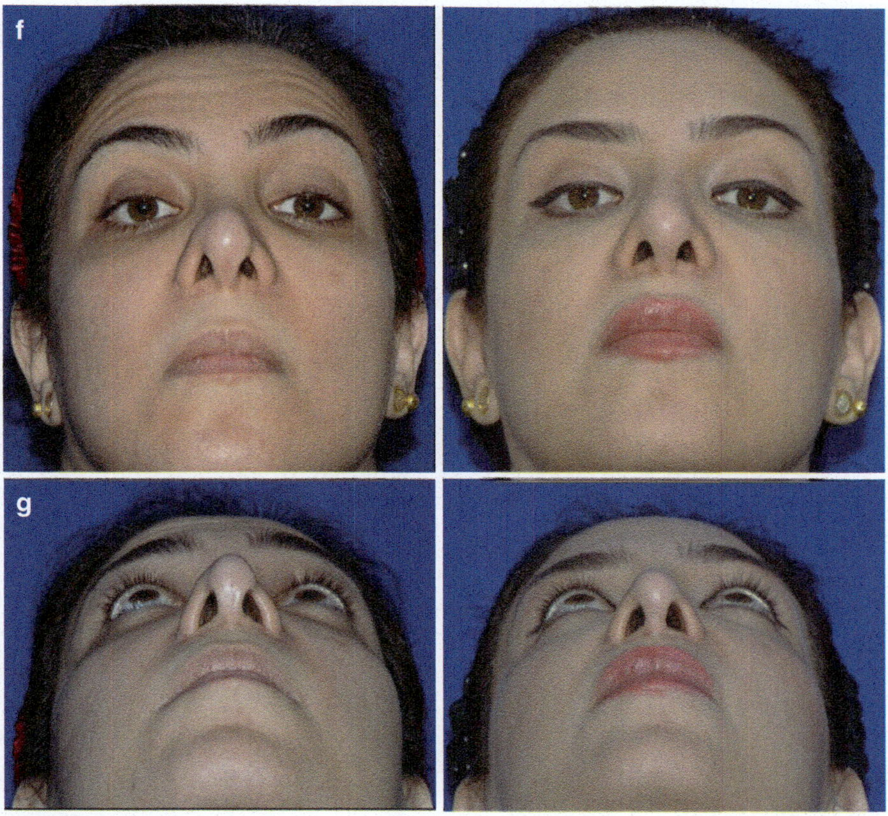


**Fig. 51.16** (continued)

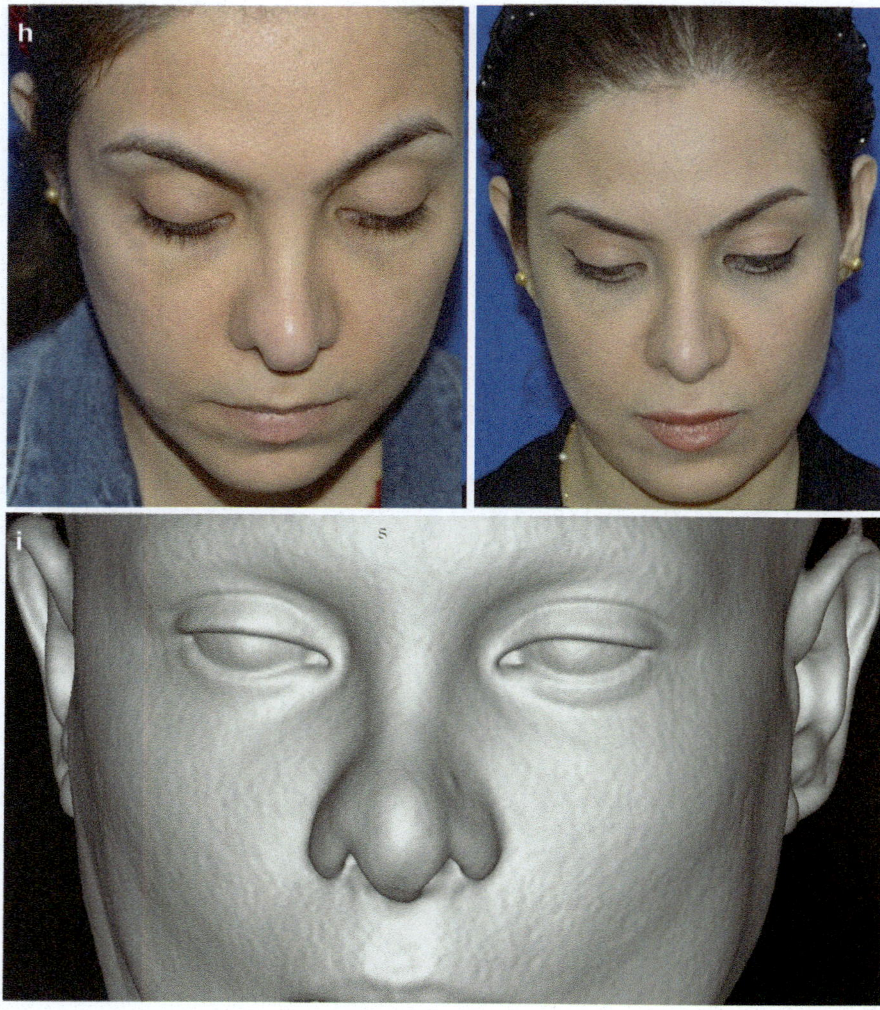


**Fig. 51.16** (continued)

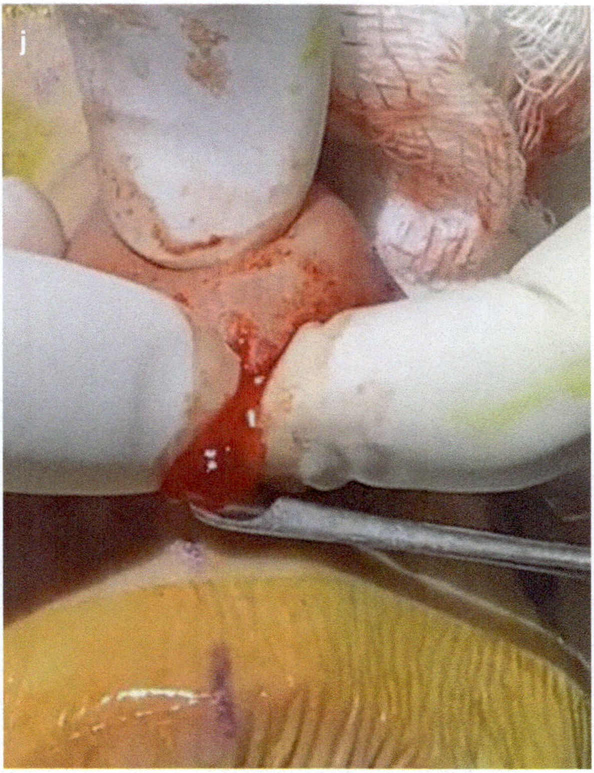


**Fig. 51.16** (continued)

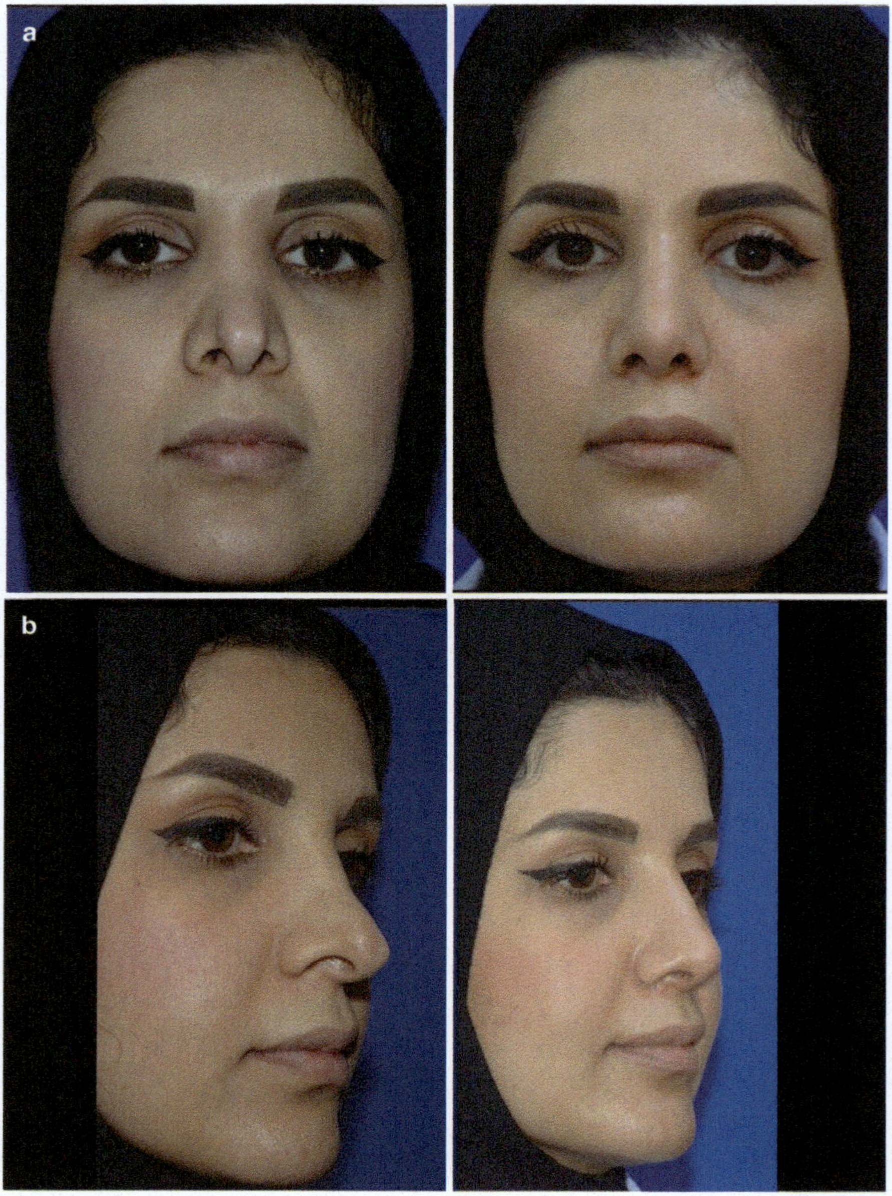


**Fig. 51.17** (**a–f**) Five months post revision septorhinoplasty with costal cartilage, (**g**, **h**) 3D Volume rendering from preoperative patient CT

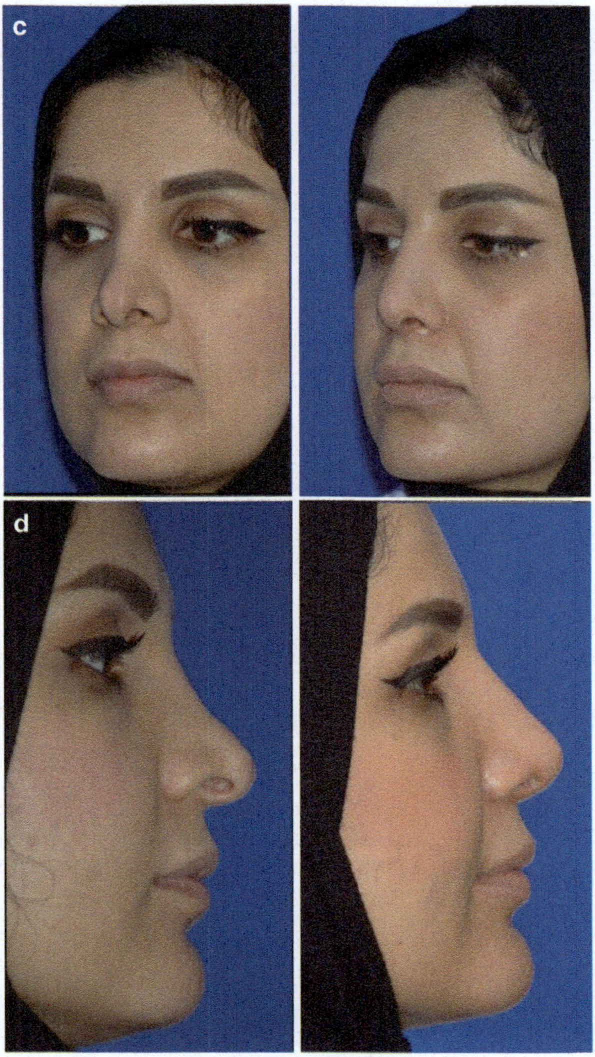


**Fig. 51.17** (continued)

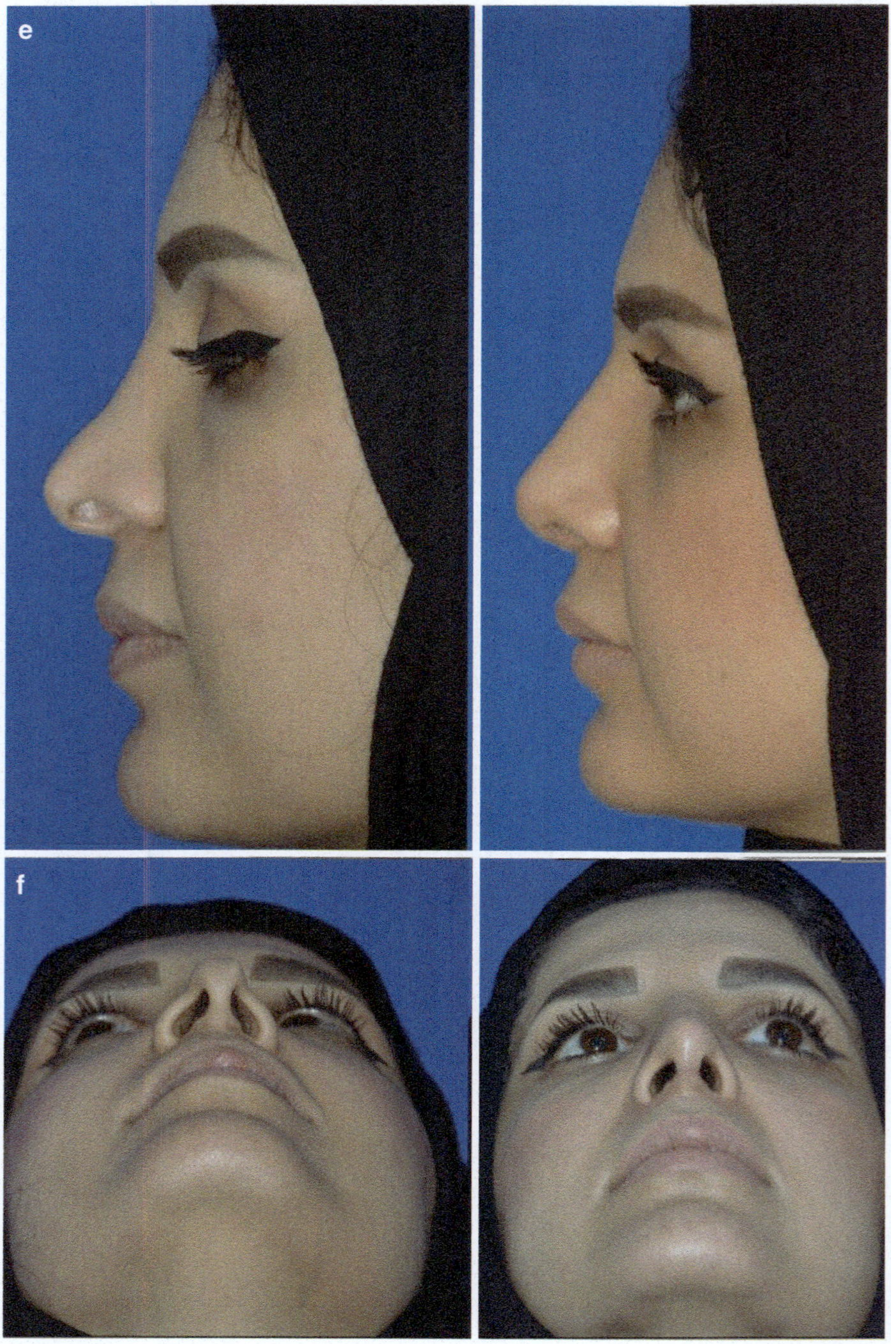


**Fig. 51.17** (continued)

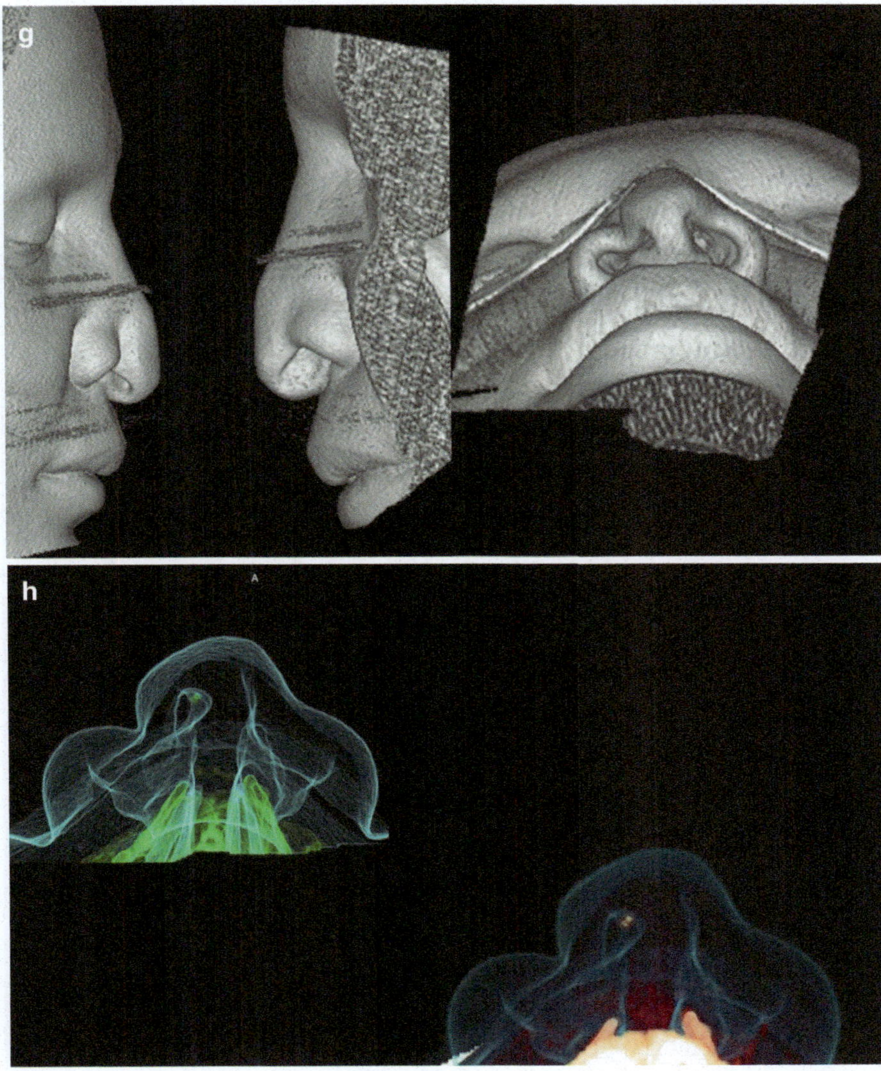


Fig. 51.17 (continued)

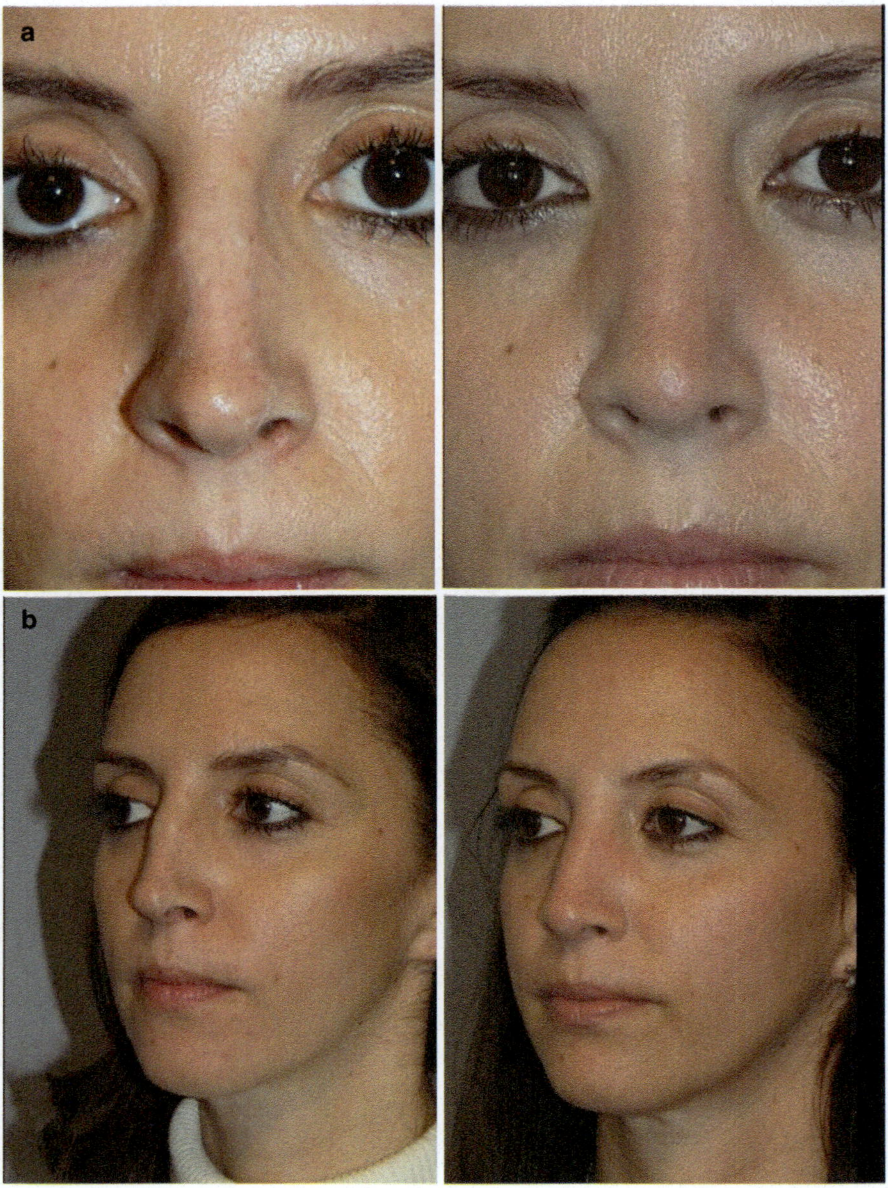


**Fig. 51.18** This 40-year-old patient underwent revision rhinoplasty with rib grafting following her previous rhinoplasty performed 1 year before. Her concerns regarding her function, as well as her nasal appearance. She underwent correction of her still asymmetric nasal bones by osteoplasty and osteotomy (**a–f**), bilateral rib spreaders (**k**) to correct her distal septal deviation together with a perforated ethmoid splint (**j**), septoplasty (**i**), turbinoplasty, as well as extended lateral crura struts (**l**) from rib laminas (**g**) shows a transverse cut of the rib piece; (**h**) shows the rib laminas "menu" for her sidewall and external nasal valve. The result is shown 1 year following her revision-wide

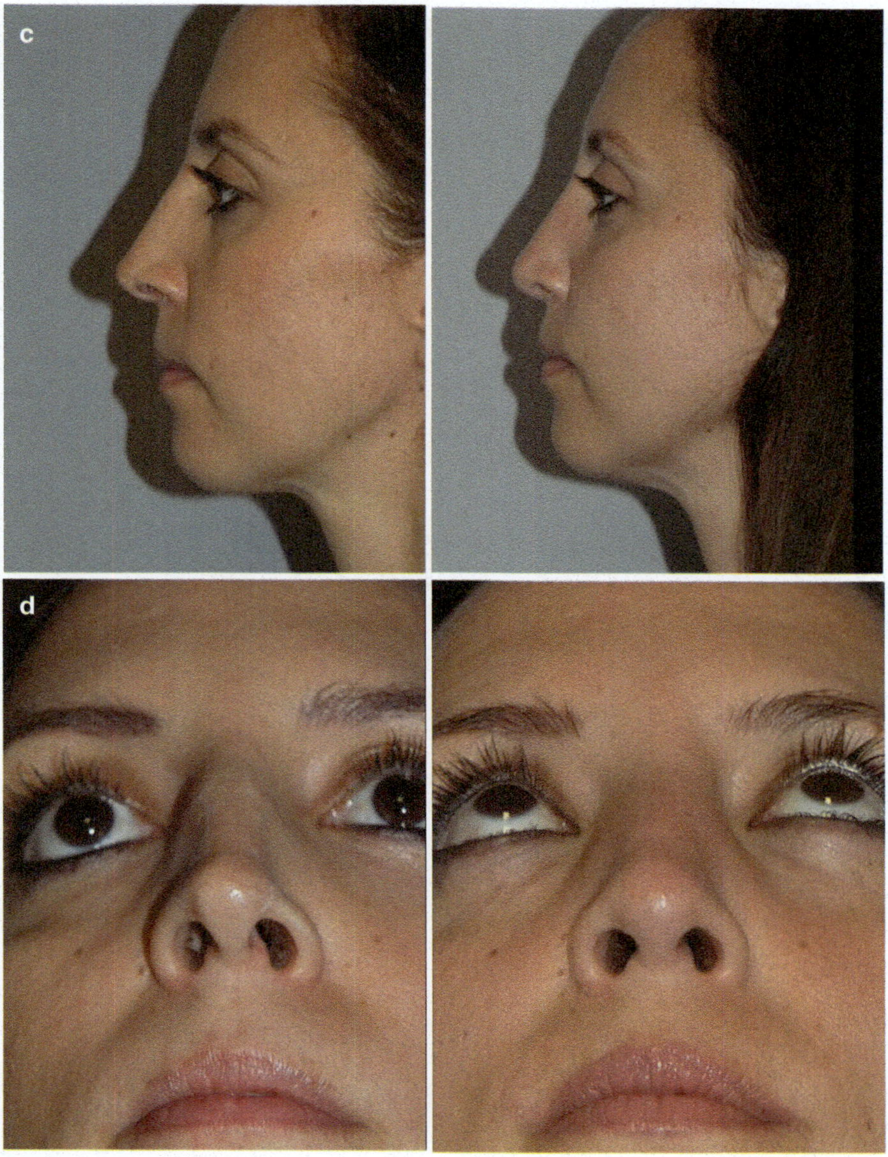


**Fig. 51.18** (continued)

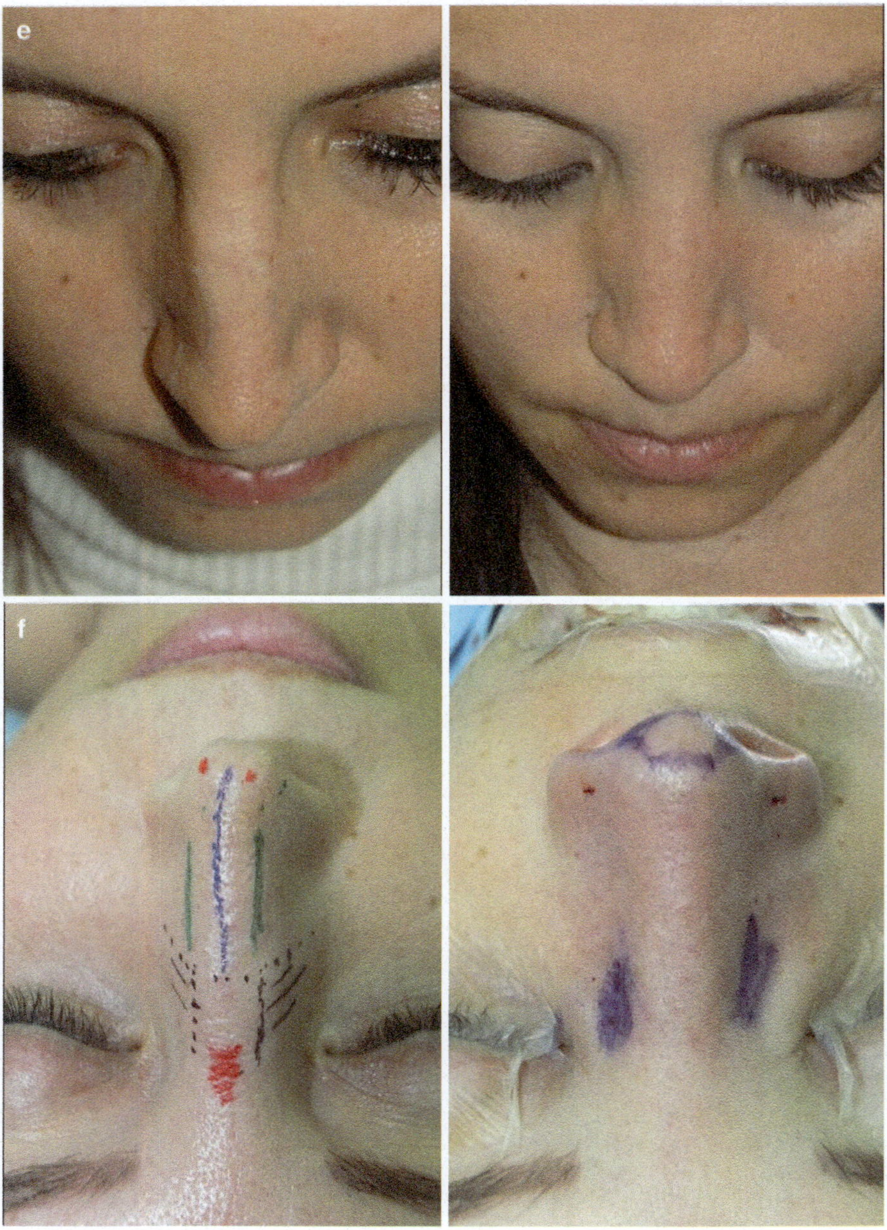


**Fig. 51.18** (continued)

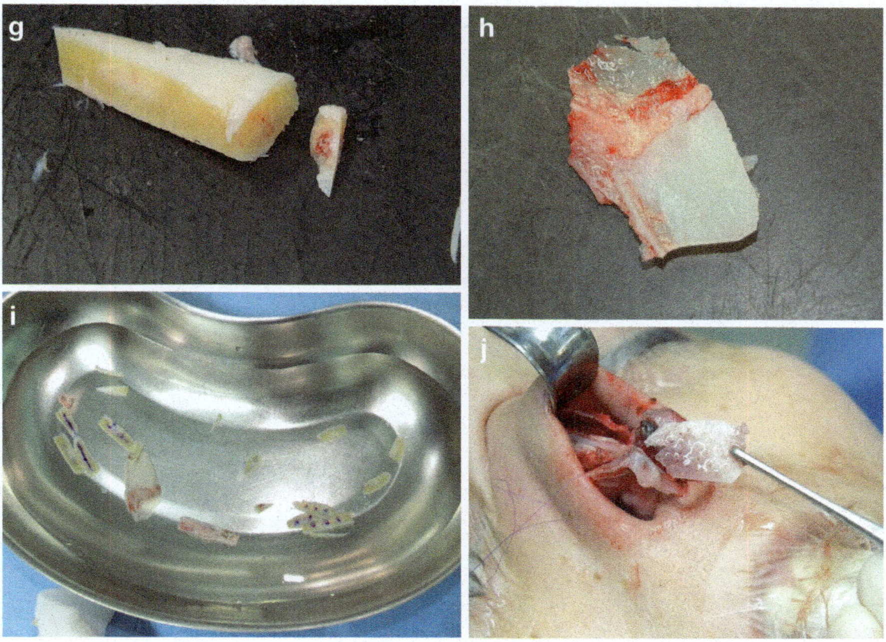


**Fig. 51.18** (continued)

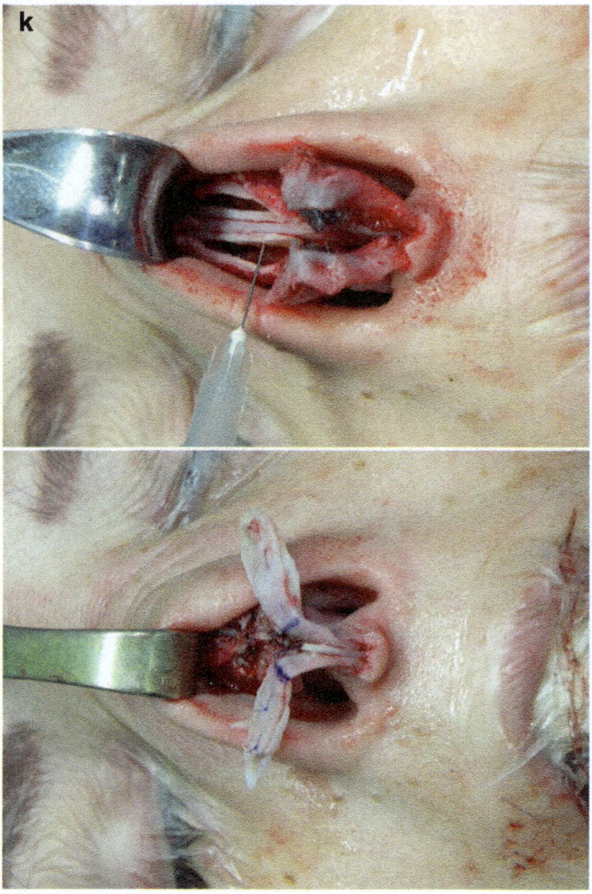


**Fig. 51.18** (continued)

## References


1. Alsarraf R. Outcomes research in facial plastic surgery: a review and new directions. Aesthetic Plast Surg. 2000;24(3):192–7.
2. Robotti E, Penna WB. Current practical concepts for using rib in secondary rhinoplasty. Facial Plast Surg. 2019;35(1):31–46. https://doi.org/10.1055/s-0039-1677801. Epub 2019 Feb 13. PMID: 30759459.
3. Adamson PA, Warner J, Becker D, Romo TJ III, Toriumi DM. Revision rhinoplasty: panel discussion, controversies, and techniques. Facial Plast Surg Clin North Am. 2014;22(1):57–96. https://doi.org/10.1016/j.fsc.2013.09.002. PMID: 24290995.
4. Daniel RK. Diced cartilage grafts in rhinoplasty surgery: current techniques and applications. Plast Reconstr Surg. 2008;122:1883–91.
5. Toriumi DM. Management of the middle nasal vault in rhinoplasty. Oper Tech Plast Reconstr Surg. 1995;2(1):16–30.
6. Losquadro WD, Bared A, Toriumi DM. Correction of the retracted alar base. Facial Plast Surg. 2012;28(2):218–24.

7. Paun SH, Nolst Trenité GJ. Revision rhinoplasty: an overview of deformities and techniques. Facial Plast Surg. 2008;24(3):271–87. https://doi.org/10.1055/s-0028-1083082. Epub 2008 Oct 24. PMID: 18951315.
8. Wee JH, Mun SJ, Na WS, et al. Autologous vs irradiated homologous costal cartilage as graft material in rhinoplasty. JAMA Facial Plast Surg. 2017;19(03):183–8.
9. Adamson PA. The failed rhinoplasty. Curr Ther Otolaryngol Head Neck Surg. 1990;4:137–44.
10. Tardy ME, Watson D, Chand M. Secondary rhinoplasty. In: Papel ID, editor. Facial plastic and reconstructive surgery. 2nd ed. New York: Thieme Medical Publishers; 2002. p. 439–51.
11. Robotti E, Leone F, Malfussi VA, Cottone G. The "3 points compartmentalization" technique in subperichondrial-subperiosteal dissection in primary rhinoplasty to reduce edema and define contour. Aesthetic Plast Surg. 2022;46(4):1923–31. https://doi.org/10.1007/s00266-022-02957-w. Epub 2022 Jun 3. PMID: 35657393.
12. Robotti E, Daniel RK, Leone F. Cone-beam computed tomography: a user-friendly, practical roadmap to the planning and execution of every rhinoplasty-a 5-year review. Plast Reconstr Surg. 2021;147(5):749e–62e. https://doi.org/10.1097/PRS.0000000000007900. PMID: 33835107.
13. Marin VP, Landecker A, Gunter JP. Harvesting rib cartilage grafts for secondary rhinoplasty. Plast Reconstr Surg. 2008;121(04):1442–8.
14. Toriumi DM. Dorsal augmentation using autologous costal cartilage or microfat-infused soft tissue augmentation. Facial Plast Surg. 2017;33(02):162–78.
15. Robotti E, Leone F. The SPF-SPLF graft: building the ideal dorsum in revision rhinoplasty. Plast Reconstr Surg. 2020;145(6):1420–4. https://doi.org/10.1097/PRS.0000000000006865. PMID: 32459772.
16. Foulad A, Hamamoto A, Manuel C, Wong BJ. Precise and rapid costal cartilage graft sectioning using a novel device: clinical application. JAMA Facial Plast Surg. 2014;16(02):107–12.
17. Farkas JP, Lee MR, Lakianhi C, Rohrich RJ. Effects of carving plane, level of harvest, and oppositional suturing techniques on costal cartilage warping. Plast Reconstr Surg. 2013;132(2):319–25.
18. Rosenberger ES, Toriumi DM. Controversies in revision rhinoplasty. Facial Plast Surg Clin North Am. 2016;24(03):337–45.
19. Taştan E, Yücel ÖT, Aydin E, Aydoğan F, Beriat K, Ulusoy MG. The oblique split method: a novel technique for carving costal cartilage grafts. JAMA Facial Plast Surg. 2013;15(03):198–203.
20. Robotti E. The role of preoperative planning in secondary rhinoplasty. In: Rohrich R, Ahmad J, editors. Secondary rhinoplasty by the global masters. Boca Raton: Thieme CRC Press; 2016. p. 1–1816.
21. Toriumi DM. Subtotal septal reconstruction: an update. Facial Plast Surg. 2013;29(6):492–501.
22. Gubisch W. Secondary septoplasty. In: Gubisch W, editor. Mastering advanced rhinoplasty. Cham: Springer; 2017. p. 37–123.
23. Gubisch W. Twenty-five years' experience with extracorporeal septoplasty. Facial Plast Surg. 2006;22(04):230–9.
24. Rezaeian F, Gubisch W, Janku D, Haack S. New suturing techniques to reconstruct the keystone area in extracorporeal septoplasty. Plast Reconstr Surg. 2016;138(02):374–82.
25. Haack S, Hacker S, Mann S, Gubisch W. Bony fixation of the nasal framework. Facial Plast Surg. 2019;35(1):23–30. https://doi.org/10.1055/s-0039-1677767. Epub 2019 Feb 13. PMID: 30759458.
26. Gunter JP, Clark CP, Friedman RM. Internal stabilization of autogenous rib cartilage grafts in rhinoplasty: a barrier to cartilage warping. Plast Reconstr Surg. 1997;100:161–9.
27. Cochran CS, Gunter JP. Secondary rhinoplasty and the use of autogenous rib cartilage grafts. Clin Plast Surg. 2010;37:371–82.
28. Farkas JP, Lee MR, Rohrich RJ. Technical maneuvers to decrease warping of peripheral costal cartilage grafts. Plast Reconstr Surg. 2016;138:228e–32e.
29. Kim JH, Jang YJ. Use of diced conchal cartilage with perichondrial attachment in rhinoplasty. Plast Reconstr Surg. 2015;135:1545–53.

30. Boccieri A, Marianetti TM. Perichondrium graft: harvesting and indications in nasal surgery. J Craniofac Surg. 2010;21:40–4.
31. Calvert J, Kwon E. Techniques for diced cartilage with deep temporalis fascia graft. Facial Plast Surg Clin North Am. 2015;23:73–80.
32. Kelly MH, Bulstrode NW, Waterhouse N. Versatility of diced cartilage-fascia grafts in dorsal nasal augmentation. Plast Reconstr Surg. 2007;120:1654–9; discussion 1654–9.
33. As'adi K, Salehi SH, Shoar S. Rib diced cartilage-fascia grafting in dorsal nasal reconstruction: a randomized clinical trial of wrapping with rectus muscle fascia vs deep temporal fascia. Aesthet Surg J. 2014;34:NP21–31.
34. Cerkes N, Basaran K. Diced cartilage grafts wrapped in rectus abdominis fascia for nasal dorsum augmentation. Plast Reconstr Surg. 2016;137:43–51.
35. Tasman AJ. Advances in nasal dorsal augmentation with diced cartilage. Curr Opin Otolaryngol Head Neck Surg. 2013;21:365–71.
36. Codazzi D, Ortelli L, Robotti E. Diced cartilage combined with warm blood glue for nasal dorsum enhancement. Aesthetic Plast Surg. 2014;38:822–3.
37. Kreutzer C, Hoehne J, Gubisch W, Rezaeian F, Haack S. Free diced cartilage: a new application of diced cartilage grafts in primary and secondary rhinoplasty. Plast Reconstr Surg. 2017;140:461–70.
38. Bullocks JM, Echo A, Guerra G, Stal S, Yuksel E. A novel autologous scaffold for diced-cartilage grafts in dorsal augmentation rhinoplasty. Aesthetic Plast Surg. 2011;35:569–79.
39. Tabbal N, Tepper OM. Diced cartilage versus solid grafts in rhinoplasty. Aesthetic Plast Surg. 2011;35:580–1.
40. Fatemi MJ, Hasani ME, Rahimian S, Bateni H, Pedram M, Mousavi SJ. Survival of block and fascial-wrapped diced cartilage grafts: an experimental study in rabbits. Ann Plast Surg. 2012;69:326–30.
41. Robotti E, Leone F, Malfussi V, Cottone G. RIB plaster: a versatile, moldable derivative from scraping the periphery of the rib. Plast Reconstr Surg. 2023; https://doi.org/10.1097/PRS.0000000000010742. Epub ahead of print. PMID: 37220333.
42. Davis RE. Revision of the overresected nasal tip complex. Facial Plast Surg. 2012;28(04):427–39.
43. Rao N, Toriumi DM. Auricular composite grafting in functional rhinoplasty. Facial Plast Surg. 2017;33(4):405–10. https://doi.org/10.1055/s-0037-1604107. Epub 2017 Jul 28. PMID: 28753714.
44. Cerkes N. Nasal tip deficiency. Clin Plast Surg. 2016;43(01):135–50.
45. Gubisch W. Tip refinements in secondary rhinoplasty. In: Gubisch W, editor. Mastering advanced rhinoplasty. Cham: Springer; 2017. p. 635–805.

# Complications of Rhinoplasty

# 52

Amr Gouda

**Key Points**
- Complications versus iatrogenic sequelae
- Functional and aesthetic complications
- How to avoid and how to manage each complication

## 52.1 Introduction

Rhinoplasty is widely recognized as one of the most difficult and challenging surgeries within plastic surgery. Despite its complexities in obtaining the best functional and aesthetic outcomes, leaving little room for error, rhinoplasty has remained one of the most frequently performed cosmetic operations.

Complications in rhinoplasty refer to unexpected and adverse events that can occur during or after the surgery. These complications can arise due to various reasons, including surgical technique, patient's anatomy, healing process, or other factors. They can range from mild issues such as swelling and bruising to more severe problems such as infection, bleeding, or breathing difficulties. On the one hand, complications, in many cases, are inherent risks associated with any surgical procedure and may not necessarily imply malpractice.

Malpractice, on the other hand, refers to a situation where a healthcare provider, in this case, a rhinoplasty surgeon, fails to meet the standard of care expected in their field, leading to harm or injury to the patient. Malpractice in rhinoplasty could involve negligence, errors in judgment, lack of informed consent, improper surgical technique, or failure to provide adequate postoperative care.

A. Gouda (✉)
Department of Otolaryngology, Ain Shams University, Cairo, Egypt


S. Elwany (ed.), *Current Rhinology*,
https://doi.org/10.1007/978-3-031-70077-4_52

Here is how complications and malpractice in rhinoplasty differ:

Complications are unexpected events or outcomes that can occur despite the surgeon following proper procedures, employing appropriate techniques, and providing adequate care. Not all complications are a result of malpractice; they can sometimes be an inherent risk of the surgery.

Malpractice: it involves a breach of the standard of care expected from a competent and qualified rhinoplasty surgeon. Malpractice occurs when a surgeon fails to perform the surgery with reasonable skill and care, leading to avoidable harm or injury to the patient.

It is important to note that not all complications automatically indicate malpractice. However, certain complications might arise due to the negligence or incompetence of the surgeon, which could be considered malpractice. Establishing whether a complication resulted from malpractice often requires careful evaluation of the circumstances, evidence, and whether the surgeon deviated from the accepted standards of care.

Patients who suspect malpractice or have concerns about their surgery outcomes should consult with another qualified surgeon for a second opinion. Legal recourse might be an option in cases where negligence or malpractice is suspected and has caused significant harm or injury to the patient.

In this chapter, complications associated with rhinoplasty will be discussed along with explanations of their potential causes and recommended management approaches.

## 52.2 Complications

### 52.2.1 Open Roof Deformity (Fig. 52.1a, b) [1, 2]

- Possible etiology:
  - Excessive dorsal reduction without performing proper lateral osteotomies
- How to manage:
  - Revision of proper lateral osteotomies
  - Dorsal onlay graft if needed

### 52.2.2 Bony Step Deformity (Fig. 52.2) [3, 4]

- Possible etiology:
  - Improper lateral osteotomies (can be seen if one of the lateral osteotomies is made medial to the naso-facial groove, with a ridge visibly seen on that side of the nose)
- How to manage:
  - Proper placement of the lateral osteotomies in the ascending process of the maxilla

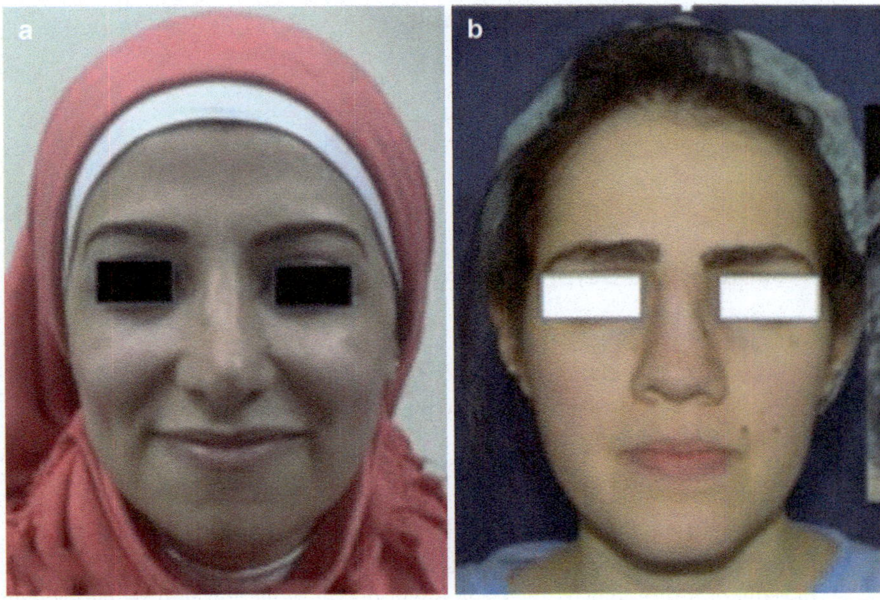


**Fig. 52.1** Open roof deformity

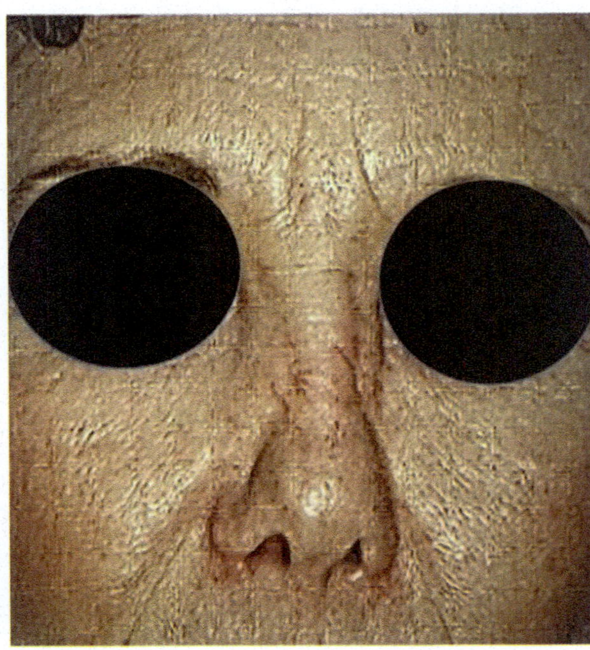

**Fig. 52.2** Bony step deformity

### 52.2.3 Asymmetry of the Bony Vault

- Possible etiology:
  - Asymmetric osteotomies
- How to manage:
  - Proper osteotomies

### 52.2.4 Saddle Nose Deformity (Fig. 52.3) [5, 6]

- Possible etiology:
  - Aggressive dorsal reduction
  - Aggressive septoplasty without leaving proper dorsal strut
  - Inadequate cartilaginous support
- How to avoid:
  - Proper osteotomies.
  - In septoplasty, maintain a 1.5-cm dorsal strut.
  - Dorsal preservation will be better than reduction rhinoplasty.
  - In reduction rhinoplasty, the component dorsal reduction will be better than en-block reduction.
- How to manage:
  - Minor saddle deformity: revision with dorsal onlay camouflage graft
  - Severe cases: sliced rib cartilage graft reconstruction

**Fig. 52.3** Saddle nose deformity

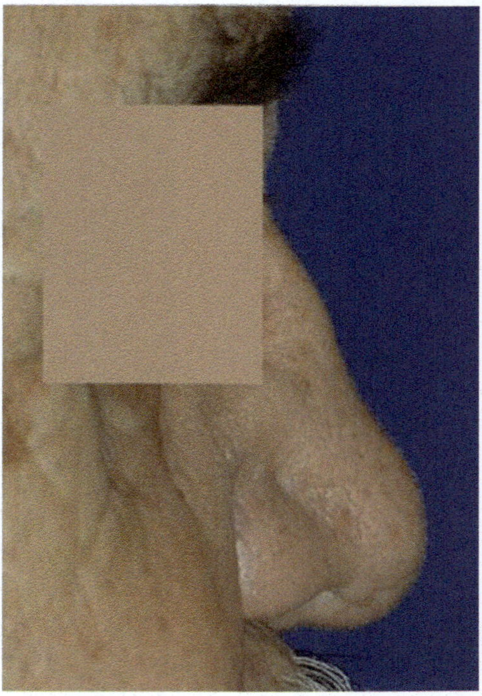

### 52.2.5 Inverted V Deformity (Fig. 52.4) [7–9]

- Possible etiology:
  - Dissection deep to the nasal bones instead of subperiosteal dissection
- How to avoid:
  - Use of spreader grafts or autospreader grafts
- How to manage:
  - Revision with the use of spreader grafts.
  - Onlay crushed or diced cartilage camouflage grafts.
  - Osteotomies to narrow the bony base if this is a contributing factor.

### 52.2.6 Rocker Deformity [7, 10]

- Possible etiology:
  - Carrying osteotomies higher in the thicker part of the frontonasal junction
- How to avoid:
  - Proper planning of the osteotomies
  - In endonasal lateral osteotomy, palpate the guarded portion of the osteotome to ensure proper direction
- How to manage:
  - Transverse percutaneous osteotomies

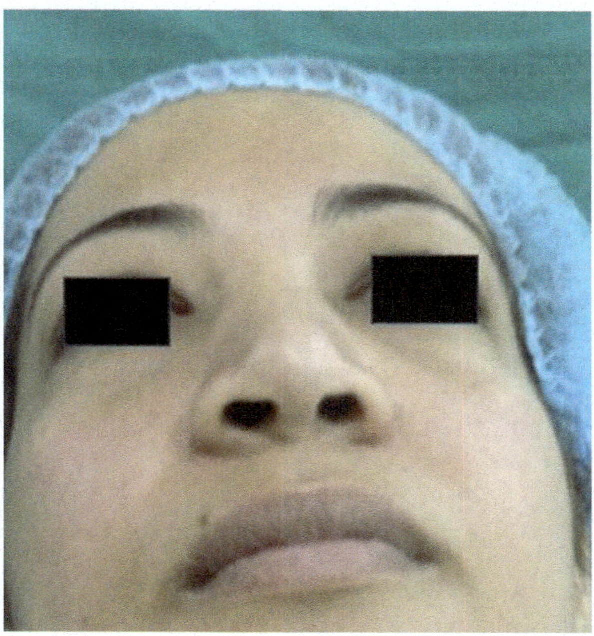

**Fig. 52.4** Inverted V deformity

### 52.2.7 Pollybeak Deformity (Fig. 52.5) [11–13]

The lower third of the dorsum is more projected than the tip.

- Possible etiology:
  - Overresection of nasal bones
  - Underresection of the anterior part of the dorsal septum
  - Loss of tip support with subsequent tip ptosis
  - Postoperative soft tissue edema or fibrosis
- How to avoid:
  - Appropriate planning of dorsal reduction, both bony and cartilaginous dorsum
- How to manage:
  - Proper balance of the nasal dorsum either using dorsal onlay graft, or appropriate cartilaginous dorsal reduction to that of bony dorsal reduction.
  - Postoperative edema may require local steroid injections postoperatively.

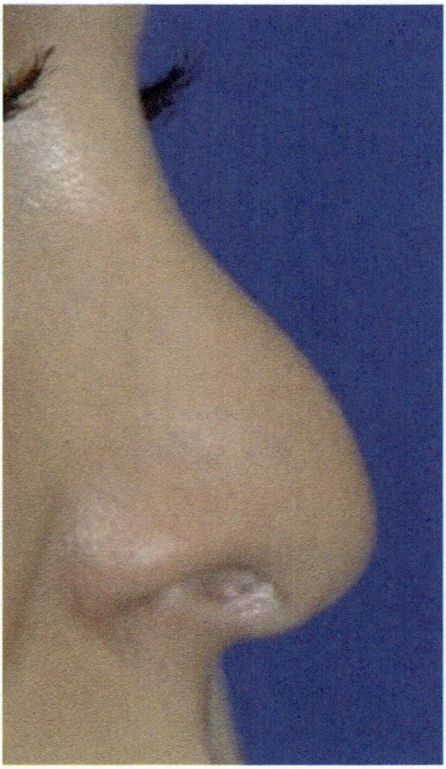

**Fig. 52.5** Pollybeak deformity

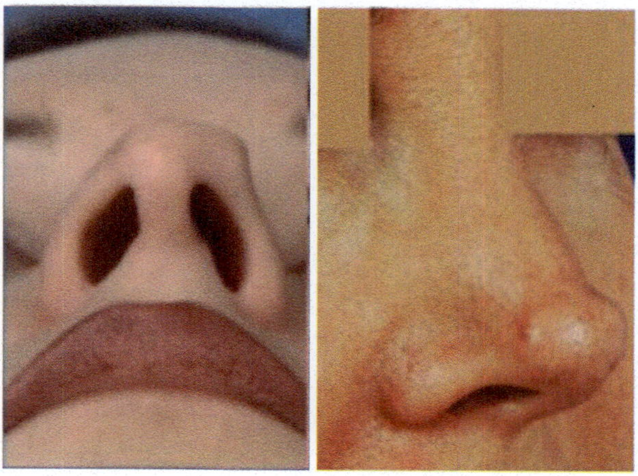

**Fig. 52.6** Bossae

### 52.2.8 Bossae (Fig. 52.6a, b) [14, 15]

- Predisposing factors:
  - Tip bifidity, thin skin, and strong alar cartilages
- Possible etiology:
  - Aggressive cephalic trim of lateral crura
- How to avoid:
  - Maintaining the strength and integrity of the alar cartilage
  - Structural grafting when necessary
  - Symmetric reconstitution of the tip domes with proper tip sutures
- How to manage:
  - Revision with structural grafting of lateral crura (lateral crural strut grafts)
  - Crushed diced cartilage and/or fascia to camouflage any irregularities

### 52.2.9 Alar Retraction (Fig. 52.7) [9, 16]

- Possible etiology:
  - Overresection of lateral crura during cephalic trim
  - Overly tight lateral crural spanning sutures
  - Malpositioning of the lateral crura
  - Overly tight closure of the marginal incision
  - Contracture from wound healing
- How to manage:
  - Minor cases: lateral crural strut grafts and alar rim grafts
  - Severe cases: auricular composite grafts
  - Removal/revision of any offending tip sutures

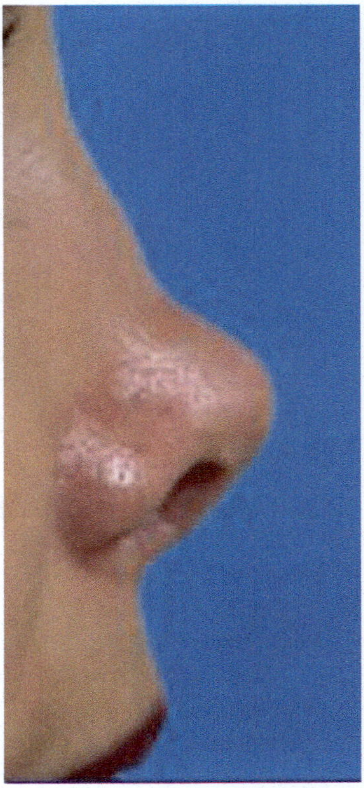

**Fig. 52.7** Alar retraction

### 52.2.10 Pinched Tip (Fig. 52.8) [4, 10]

- Possible etiology:
  - Overresection of lateral crura during cephalic trim
  - Malpositioning of lateral crura
  - Contracture from wound healing
- How to avoid:
  - Spare at least 7–9 mm rim strip
  - Ensure appropriate orientation and positioning of lateral crura
- How to manage:
  - Lateral crural strut grafts
  - Possible crushed cartilage grafts for camouflage
  - Removal/revision of any offending tip sutures

### 52.2.11 Columellar Retraction [4, 9]

- Possible etiology:
  - Overresection of the caudal septum.

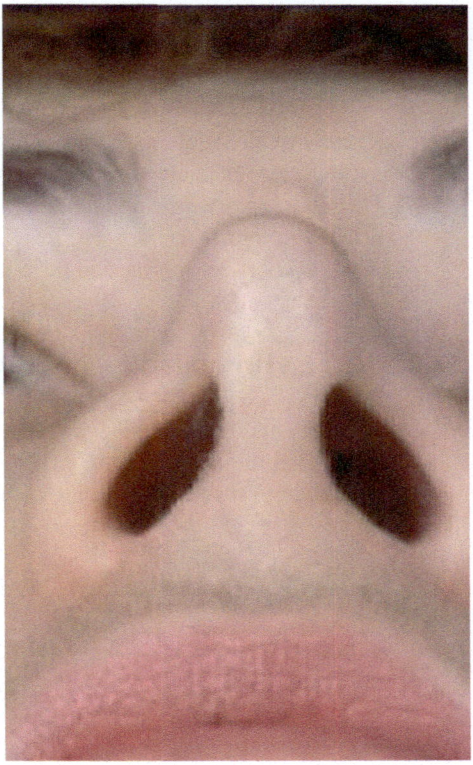

**Fig. 52.8** Pinched tip

- Excessive setback of the medial crura during tongue-in-groove.

- How to avoid:
  - Avoid overresection.
  - Avoid excessive setbacks.
- How to manage:
  - Caudal septal extension graft, columellar strut graft, and columellar plumping graft.
  - Septo-columellar sutures can be used to help prevent contracture during wound healing.

### 52.2.12 Functional Complications: Nasal Obstruction [3, 7]

1. Possible etiology:
   (a) External nasal valve collapse
   - How to avoid:
     - Maintain integrity and appropriate position of lateral crura, and avoid overaggressive narrowing of the alar base.
   - How to manage:
     - Lateral crural strut grafts and possible alar rim grafts.

(b) Internal nasal valve collapse:
- How to avoid:
  - Avoid overaggressive narrowing of the bony base and use spreader grafts or autospreader grafts to maintain patency.
- How to manage:
  - Spreader or autospreader grafts.

(c) Deviated septum or turbinate hypertrophy:
- How to manage:
  - Proper septoplasty and turbinate reduction.

### 52.2.13 Dorsal Irregularities or Visible Graft (Fig. 52.9) [13–15]

- How to avoid and how to manage:
  - Proper osteotomies with proper rasping.
  - Use diced or crushed cartilage to camouflage any irregularities.

### 52.2.14 Surgical Complications [1, 5, 6, 9, 11–13]

1. Bleeding:
   (a) How to avoid:
   - Aspirin should be discontinued 10 days before the procedure.
   - Preoperative injection using local anesthetic mixed with epinephrine into the subcutaneous tissues and topical vasoconstrictive drugs with adequate time given for the onset of these drugs.

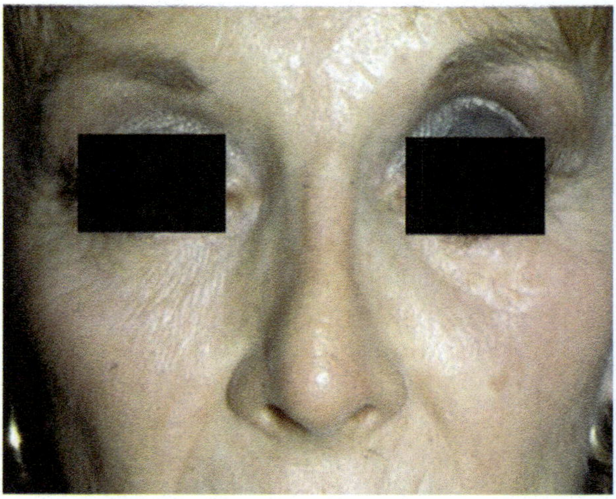

**Fig. 52.9** Dorsal irregularities

- Dissection in the correct tissue planes, by maintaining dissection in the subperichondrial plane (dissection should be deep to the superficial musculoaponeurotic system (SMAS) layer).

(b) How to manage:

- Cauterizing a bleeding site, or suturing an open area in the incision or at the columella-septum junction.

2. Erythema:
   (a) A red flag to the surgeon that rhinoplasty incision and dissection may have jeopardized the nasal soft tissue vascularity causing congestion.
   (b) Postoperative erythema can also signal an allergy to topical adhesives used as dressings. The surgeon is advised to remove the dressings and allow the area to resolve without the dressing.
   (c) Lastly, erythema may be the result of an infectious inflammatory condition.
3. Infection:
   (a) Extremely rare.
   (b) Regional erythema or cellulitis.
   (c) The surgeon must rule out an allergic reaction to tape or ointment. If it is felt that the response represents a true infection, then the patient should be started on oral antibiotics and intranasal antibiotic cream.
   (d) In severe presentations, the patient should be admitted for intravenous antibiotics.
4. Edema and ecchymosis:
   (a) Should be expected after rhinoplasty.
   (b) Patient education is key to minimizing postoperative anxiety for the patient: patients must understand that the "final" result should not be expected for about a year.
   (c) Perioperative steroids were shown to decrease periorbital edema.
5. Skin loss:
   (a) Rare complication
   (b) Predisposing factors: defatting of the tip, an aggressive alar base reduction, and excessive use of cautery or tight postoperative wrapping
   (c) Also, early revision rhinoplasty (better to wait 1 year before revision surgery)
6. Olfactory:

   Anosmia or hyposmia may occur due to the following:
   (a) Iatrogenic cribriform plate fracture.
   (b) Temporary hyposmia subsequent to nose surgery is associated with swelling and direct injury to the neuroepithelium.
   (c) Postoperative neurotrophic viral infection may be another surgery-related factor.
   (d) Psychogenic factors can be accountable as well.
7. Cerebrospinal Fluid rhinorrhea (CSF) rhinorrhea

Rare due to unrecognized injury to the cribriform plate or anterior cranial fossa

8. Septal perforation
9. Septal hematoma
10. Orbital problems.
    (a) Edema may hinder lacrimal drainage.
    (b) Rarely laceration of the lacrimal sac may result in acute purulent dacryocystitis and must be handled by intubating the lacrimal system.

### 52.2.15 Patient Dissatisfaction

- Causes:
  - Inappropriate patient selection.
  - Inappropriate preoperative counseling to set patient expectations appropriately.
- A full discussion of the risks, benefits, and potential complications of rhinoplasty is necessary.
- Thorough discussion and understanding of the possible need for additional procedures to achieve the patient's desired outcome is important.
- Expected changes over the long-term course should be addressed.

## References


1. Rettinger G. Risks and complications in rhinoplasty. GMS Curr Top Otorhinolaryngol Head Neck Surg. 2007;6:Doc08.
2. Khansa I, Khansa L, Pearson GD. Patient satisfaction after rhinoplasty: a social media analysis. Aesthet Surg J. 2016;36(1):NP1–5.
3. Spataro E, Piccirillo JF, Kallogjeri D, Branham GH, Desai SC. Revision rates and risk factors of 175 842 patients undergoing septorhinoplasty. JAMA Facial Plast Surg. 2016;18(3):212–9.
4. Eytan DF, Wang TD. Complications in Rhinoplasty. Clin Plast Surg. 2022;49(1):179–189.
5. Layliev J, Gupta V, Kaoutzanis C, et al. Incidence and preoperative risk factors for major complications in aesthetic rhinoplasty: analysis of 4978 patients. Aesthet Surg J. 2017;37(7):757–67.
6. Uzun L, Ugur MB, Peksoy I, Cabuk M, Cinar F. The effect of lateral osteotomy of septorhinoplasty on nasolacrimal duct functions: a radionuclide imaging study. Am J Rhinol. 2005;19(4):388–94.
7. Romo T, Sonne J, Choe KS, Sclafani AP. Revision rhinoplasty. Facial Plast Surg. 2003;19(4):299–307.
8. Cameron Heilbronn MD, Dalan Cragun BS, Wong BF. Complications in rhinoplasty: a literature review and comparison with a survey of consent forms the radix graft in cosmetic rhinoplasty. Facial Plast Surg Aesthet Med. 2020;22(1):50.
9. Surowitz JB, Most SP. Complications of rhinoplasty. Facial Plast Surg Clin N Am. 2013;21(4):639–51.
10. Neaman KC, Boettcher AK, Do VH, et al. Cosmetic rhinoplasty: revision rates revisited. Aesthet Surg J. 2013;33(1):31–7.

11. Rodman R, Kridel R. A staging system for revision rhinoplasty: a review. JAMA Facial Plast Surg. 2016;18(4):305–11.
12. Kara CO, Kara IG, Yaylali V. Subconjunctival ecchymosis due to rhinoplasty. Rhinology. 2001;39(3):166–8.
13. Gryskiewicz JM. Visible scars from percutaneous osteotomies. Plast Reconstr Surg. 2005;116(6):1771–5.
14. Wee JH, Park MH, Oh S, Jin HR. Complications associated with autologous rib cartilage use in rhinoplasty: a meta-analysis. JAMA Facial Plast Surg. 2015;17(1):49–55.
15. Gryskiewicz JM, Gryskiewicz KM. Nasal osteotomies: a clinical comparison of the perforating methods versus the continuous technique. Plast Reconstr Surg. 2004;113(5):1445–56.
16. Kar M, Cingi C, Thomas R. Complications of rhinoplasty. Cham: Springer; 2020.

SPRINGER NATURE

# GPSR Compliance

*The European Union's (EU) General Product Safety Regulation (GPSR) is a set of rules that requires consumer products to be safe and our obligations to ensure this.*

*If you have any concerns about our products, you can contact us on ProductSafety@springernature.com*

In case Publisher is established outside the EU, the EU authorized representative is:

Springer Nature Customer Service Center GmbH
Europaplatz 3
69115 Heidelberg, Germany

The manufacturer's authorised representative in the EU is Springer Nature Customer Service Centre GmbH, Europaplatz 3, 69115 Heidelberg, Germany. If you have any concerns regarding our products, please contact ProductSafety@springernature.com

Printed and bound by CPI Group (UK) Ltd, Croydon, CR0 4YY
30/09/2026
02225454-0018